Medical Emergencies in Children

Revised Fifth Edition

Medical Emergencies in Children

Revised Fifth Edition

Meharban Singh

MD, FAMS, FIAP, FIMSA, FNNF, Hony. FAAP

Former Professor and Head
Department of Pediatrics and Neonatal Division
WHO Collaborating Center for Training and
Research in Newborn Care
All India Institute of Medical Sciences
New Delhi

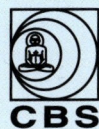

CBS Publishers & Distributors Pvt Ltd

New Delhi • Bengaluru • Chennai • Kochi • Kolkata • Mumbai

Bhopal • Bhubaneswar • Hyderabad • Jharkhand • Nagpur • Patna • Pune • Uttarakhand • Dhaka (Bangladesh) • Kathmandu (Nepal)

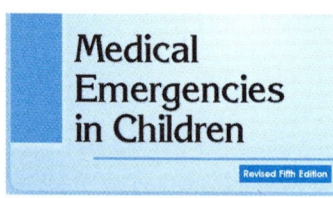

Medical Emergencies in Children

Revised Fifth Edition

ISBN: 978-81-239-2898-2

Revised Fifth Edition: 2016
 Reprint 2017, 2020
First Edition: 1988
Second Edition: 1993
Third Edition: 2000
Fourth Edition: 2006
Fifth Edition: 2012

Published by Satish Kumar Jain and produced by Varun Jain for

CBS Publishers & Distributors Pvt Ltd
4819/XI Prahlad Street, 24 Ansari Road, Daryaganj, New Delhi 110 002, India.
Ph: 23289259, 23266861, 23266867   Fax: 011-23243014   Website: www.cbspd.com
                                                                e-mail: delhi@cbspd.com; cbspubs@airtelmail.in.

Corporate Office: 204 FIE, Industrial Area, Patparganj, Delhi 110 092
Ph: 011-4934 4934   Fax: 011-4934 4935   e-mail: publishing@cbspd.com; publicity@cbspd.com

Branches

- **Bengaluru:** Seema House 2975, 17th Cross, K.R. Road,
  Banasankari 2nd Stage, Bengaluru 560 070, Karnataka
  Ph: +91-80-26771678/79   Fax: +91-80-26771680   e-mail: bangalore@cbspd.com
- **Chennai:** 7, Subbaraya Street, Shenoy Nagar, Chennai 600 030, Tamil Nadu
  Ph: +91-44-26260666, 26208620   Fax: +91-44-42032115   e-mail: chennai@cbspd.com
- **Kochi:** 42/1325, 1326, Power House Road, Opp KSEB Power House, Ernakulam 682 018, Kochi, Kerala
  Ph: +91-484-4059061-65   Fax: +91-484-4059065   e-mail: kochi@cbspd.com
- **Kolkata:** No. 6/B, Ground Floor, Rameswar Shaw Road, Kolkata-700014 (West Bengal), India
  Ph: +91-33-2289-1126, 2289-1127, 2289-1128   e-mail: kolkata@cbspd.com
- **Mumbai:** 83-C, Dr E Moses Road, Worli, Mumbai-400018, Maharashtra
  Ph: +91-22-24902340/41   Fax: +91-22-24902342   e-mail: mumbai@cbspd.com

Representatives

- Bhopal   0-8319310552
- Jharkhand   0-9811541605
- Pune   0-9623451994
- Kathmandu (Nepal)   977-9818742655
- Bhubaneswar   0-9911037372
- Nagpur   0-9421945513
- Uttarakhand   0-9716462459
- Hyderabad   0-9885175004
- Patna   0-9334159340
- Dhaka (Bangladesh)   01912-003485

Printed at: Magic International, Greater Noida, UP

to

my teachers
SS Manchanda; OP Ghai; BNS Walia
who taught me the philosophy of child care
and
critically ill children through whom
I learnt the art of pediatrics

Preface to the Fifth Edition

It is a matter of great satisfaction to me that the fourth edition of *Medical Emergencies in Children* has been accorded such an overwhelming reception and response by a large number of postgraduate medical students and pediatric consultants. The book has served as a useful catalyst to initiate and enthuse young pediatricians to take interest in pediatric emergency medicine and establish pediatric intensive care units. There is a welcome trend for development of a large number of pediatric intensive care units both in the government sector and private hospitals. Of late, an increasing number of specially trained pediatric intensivists is managing these units. The medical knowledge and intensive care technology are expanding so fast that a book dealing with management of critically sick children must be revised and updated periodically to incorporate the latest advances in the field in order to offer the current state-of-the-art information for optimal and rational management of children presenting with life-threatening medical emergencies.

The book has been extensively revised, updated and practically rewritten. The contents have been streamlined and book has been subdivided into six sections. Eight new chapters dealing with medico-legal issues in the emergency department, acute fever without a focus, raised intracranial tension, neonatal jaundice, acute flaccid paralysis, hematologic emergencies, electrocution and lightning, pain relief and sedation have been incorporated. All the chapters have been revised and updated to incorporate latest comprehensive information pertaining to pathophysiology, diagnosis and management of common childhood medical emergencies. Additional illustrations, photo-graphs and algorithms have been incorporated to enhance the clarity of contents. The list of references have been updated to serve as a useful resource for indepth study of specific disorders. The major emphasis of the book is placed on providing immediate first aid followed by comprehensive and detailed management in the pediatric intensive care unit. The book has evolved as a comprehensive textbook of critical care in children which has a uniform format and is characterized by clarity of expression, and a problem-oriented approach with a large number of pragmatic flow charts for ease of comprehension and assistance for making prompt management decisions. The book continues to be a harmonious blend of current pathophysiologic basis of common pediatric emergencies and a simplified approach for their optimal and rational management within the constraints of resources and equipment faced by healthcare professionals in the developing countries.

I am most grateful and appreciative of a large number of distinguished contributors from India and abroad who have most willingly devoted their precious time and energy to write, revise and update their chapters. I greatly honor their gracious gesture of personal friendship in acceding to my request for submitting the revised chapters within the stipulated deadline. I would like to specially thank my enterprising wife Kaushal for her support and encouragement during the gestational period of the book. Shri Chandra Shekhar Pant has done an excellent job in diligently inserting the manuscript in the word processor and composing the book. My special thanks are due to CBS Publishers & Distributors for their enthusiasm and efforts to bring out the revised fifth edition of the book. I am confident that *Medical Emergencies in Children* shall continue to fulfill my hope, concern and aspirations to enthuse pediatricians to establish pediatric intensive care units in the country and improve survival of children with complex life-threatening medical disorders.

Child Care Center
625, Arun Vihar, Sector 37
Noida 201 301
Tel: 0120-4346451, 9818888772
e-mail: drmbsk@gmail.com

Meharban Singh
MD, FAMS, FIAP, FIMSA, FNNF, Hony. FAAP

Preface to the First Edition

Children are delicate, functionally immature and vulnerable to develop a variety of life-threatening emergencies. Like flowers they can readily wither following an acute illness but are endowed with tremendous recuperative capabilities and when tended with care and concern for their physiological handicaps, they bloom back to life with equal ease. The body homeostatic mechanisms are immature and labile in children. They readily develop electrolyte disturbances, acid base imbalance and biochemical alterations following a variety of systemic conditions. The knowledge and understanding of these mechanisms is essential for scientific and rational management of critical disorders in children.

In this comprehensive treatise on medical emergencies in infants and children, the emphasis is laid on physiologic background, etiopathogenesis, clinical spectrum, diagnosis and management of critically sick children. The book has been designed to provide problem-oriented approach to common medical emergencies in children. The main focus of the book is on management which has been discussed in detail. Acute failure of different organs of the body; central nervous system, heart, lungs, liver, kidneys, etc. have been accorded extensive coverage. Life-threatening infections and metabolic disturbances are exceedingly common in children and have been accorded special focus. Accidental poisonings and emergencies due to physical agents like burns, drowning, animal bites and foreign bodies take a heavy toll of life in developing countries and have been covered in-depth. A detailed description of life-saving emergency procedures (including assisted ventilation) and a compendium of emergency drugs have been appended.

It is a common observation that unlike adults, most children are admitted to the hospital with a life-threatening acute disorder. Despite this fact, most pediatric units in the teaching hospitals and nursing homes are ill equipped to manage pediatric emergencies. Recently, interest in the care of high risk newborn babies has resulted in the creation of special care neonatal units in several hospitals but intensive care of critically sick children has received scant attention. There is an urgent need to establish pediatric intensive care units (PICUs) to cater to the special needs of critically sick children and I do hope that the chapter on organization of a pediatric intensive care unit would provide the relevant information and basic guidelines to create such units in the country.

A number of individuals and organisations have inspired me to conceive, plan and produce this volume. I am most grateful to a large number of distinguished contributors from India and abroad who have most willingly devoted their precious time and energy to compile the latest state-of-the-art information and their own personal experience pertaining to emergencies of their special interest. I am most appreciative of their gesture of personal friendship in meeting the deadline for submission of manuscripts. They have been also kind enough to give me the liberty to prune, revise and edit the material to present to you a comprehensive manual of uniform format which is characterized by clarity of expression and problem-oriented approach; and is replete with simple practical tips and pragmatic flow charts for ease of comprehension. The book is a harmonious blend of latest pathophysiologic basis of critical disorders and a current simplified approach for their management within the constraints of resources and equipment faced in the developing countries.

I am indebted to my dear colleagues, Dr Vinod K Paul and Ashok K Deorari for their assistance and support during the preparation of the book. I would like to thank my enterprising wife Kaushal for her patience, understanding and encouragement during the travails of editing process. My special thanks and gratitude is due to my friend and publisher, Shri Narinder K. Sagar who personally supervised every aspect of printing and production to bring out the book in a record time. I am confident that this book would fill a void and fulfill my hope and concern for better care of critically sick children in India and South-East Asia.

All India Institute of Medical Sciences
New Delhi
October 2, 1988

Meharban Singh MD

Contributors

Ramesh Agarwal MD, DM (Neonatology)
Associate Professor
Division of Neonatology
Department of Pediatrics
WHO Collaborating Centre for Training and Research
in Newborn Care
All India Institute of Medical Sciences
New Delhi-110 029
E-mail: ra.aiims@gmail.com

Neonatal emergencies in the delivery room

Sandeep Agarwala MS, MCh
Additional Professor
Department of Pediatric Surgery
All India Institute of Medical Sciences
New Delhi-110 029
E-mail: sandpagr@hotmail.com

Acute abdomen

Pankaj Ailawadhi MS, MCh
Senior Research Fellow
Department of Neurosurgery
All India Institute of Medical Sciences
New Delhi-110 029
E-mail: pankajailawadhi@yahoo.co.in

Head injury

Arvind Bagga MD, DNB, FIAP, FAMS
Professor of Pediatrics
Incharge Nephrology Division
All India Institute of Medical Sciences
New Delhi-110 029
E-mail: arvindbagga@hotmail.com

Acute kidney injury

Anurag Bajpai MD, FRACP (Australia)
Consultant Pediatric and Adolescent Endocrinologist
Regency Hospital Ltd.
A2 Sarvodya Nagar, Kanpur-208 005
E-mail: dr_anuragbajpai@yahoo.com
          dr_anuragbajp1@hotmail.com

Endocrinal emergencies

M Bajpai MS, MCh, FRCS (Glasgow), PhD, FAMS
Professor of Pediatric Surgery
All India Institute of Medical Sciences
New Delhi-110 029
E-mail: bajpai2@hotmail.com

The child with polytrauma

Sameer Bakhshi MD, DABP
(Pediatric Hematology and Oncology)
Professor of Pediatric Oncology
Department of Medical Oncology
Dr. BRA Institute Rotary Cancer Hospital
All India Institute of Medical Sciences
New Delhi-110 029
E-mail: samb@hotmail.com

Oncological emergencies

Shinjini Bhatnagar DNB (Pediatrics), PhD, FNASc
Professor and Head
Pediatric Biology Centre
Translational Health Science and Technology Institute
496 Udyog Vihar, Gurgaon
E-mail: shinjinibhatnagar@rediffmail.com

Acute gastroenteritis

Veeresshwar Bhatnagar MS, MCh, FNASc, FIMSA, FAMS
Professor of Pediatric Surgery
All India Institute of Medical Sciences
New Delhi-110 029
E-mail: veereshwarb@hotmail.com

Foreign bodies in the aero-digestive tract

Mona K Chaturvedi MD
Senior Research Officer
Department of Pediatrics
All India Institute of Medical Sciences
New Delhi-110 029

Acute gastroenteritis

Deepak Chawla MD, DM (Neonatology)
Assistant Professor
Department of Pediatrics
Government Medical College Hospital
Chandigarh

Neonatal sepsis

Krishan Chugh MD, MNAMS
Chairman, Department of Pediatrics
Consultant Pediatric Pulmonologist and Intensivist
Sir Ganga Ram Hospital, New Delhi-110 060
E-mail: chughk2000@yahoo.co.in

Cardio-pulmonary resuscitation

Tanuj Dada MD
Additional Professor
Dr Rajendra Prasad Center
for Ophthalmic Sciences
All India Institute of Medical Sciences
New Delhi-110 029
Email: tanujdada@rediffmail.com

Ophthalmic emergencies

Ashok K Deorari MD, FAMS
Professor of Pediatrics
WHO Collaborating Center for Training and Research
in Newborn Care
All India Institute of Medical Sciences
New Delhi-110 029
E-mail: ashokdeorari_56@hotmail.com

Emergency procedures

Hitesh Dhawan MD
Senior Resident in Pediatrics and Critical Care
Dayanand Medical College and Hospital
Ludhiana-141 001

Electrocution and lightning

TD Dogra MD
Professor and Head
Department of Forensic Medicine and Toxicology
All India Institute of Medical Sciences
New Delhi-110 029
E-mail: tddogra@hotmail.com

Medico-legal issues in the emergency department

Sourabh Dutta MD, PhD, FRCPS (Neonotology)
Additional Professor of Pediatrics
Division of Neonatology
Advanced Pediatric Center
Postgraduate Institute of Medical Education and Research
Chandigarh-160 012
E-mail: sourabhdutta@yahoo.co.in

Hyperpyrexia, heat exhaustion and heat stroke
Neonatal seizures

Subodh Ganu MD
Senior Registrar
Pediatric Emergency and Intensive Care Medicine
Women's and Children Hospital
Adelaid, Australia
E-mail: subodh.ganu@gmail.com

Hyperpyrexia, heat exhaustion and heat stroke

Shaila Garg MD, DM, MRCP
Cardiology Fellow
Cedars Sinai Medical Center
University of California
Los Angeles School of Medicine
Los Angeles, CA
Email: shailagarg@yahoo.com

Congestive heart failure

Sheffali Gulati MD
Associate Professor of Pediatrics
Child Neurology Division
All India Institute of Medical Sciences
New Delhi-110 029
E-mail: sheffalig@yahoo.com

Status epilepticus

Deepak Kumar Gupta MS, MCh
Associate Professor
JPN Apex Trauma Center and
Neurosciences Center
All India Institute of Medical Sciences
New Delhi-110 029
E-mail: drdeepakgupta@gmail.com

Head injury

L K Gupta MD
Assistant Professor
Department of Dermatology, Venereology and Leprosy
RNT Medical College, Udaipur

Dermatological emergencies

Namita Gupta MBBS
Senior Research Officer
All India Institute of Medical Sciences
New Delhi-110 029

Hematologic emergencies

Pankaj Hari MD
Additional Professor of Pediatrics
Division of Nephrology
All India Institute of Medical Sciences
New Delhi-110 029
E-mail: pankajhari@hotmail.com

Drowning

Yogesh Jain MD
Pediatrician and Public Health Physician
Jan Swasthya Sahyog (People's Health Support Group)
Guniyari, Bilaspur
Chhattisgarh-495 001
E-mail: jethuram@gmail.com

Cerebral and other forms of severe malaria

Rajnish Juneja MD, DM (Cardiology)
Professor of Cardiology
Cardiothoracic Center
All India Institute of Medical Sciences
New Delhi-110 029
E-mail: rjuneja2@rediffmail.com

Cardiac emergencies in newborn babies
Cardiac arrhythmias

Madhulika Kabra MD
Professor of Pediatrics
Chief Genetics Unit
All India Institute of Medical Sciences
New Delhi-110 029
E-mail: mkabra_aiims@yahoo.co.in

Emergencies due to inborn errors of metabolism

SK Kabra MD
Professor of Pediatrics
Incharge Pediatric Pulmonology Division
All India Institute of Medical Sciences
New Delhi-110 029
E-mail: skkabra@hotmail.com

Dengue fever and severe dengue infection

Sujatha Kannan MD
Assistant Professor of Pediatrics
Staff Intensivist
Children's Hospital of Michigan
Division of Critical Care Medicine
3901 Beaubien Boulevard
Detroit, Michigan 48201
E-mail: skannan@med.wayne.edu

The child with multiple-organ dysfunction syndrome

Anju Kataria MD
Pediatrician
Jan Swasthya Sahyog (People's Health Support Group)
Guniyari, Bilaspur
Chhattisgarh-495 001

Cerebral and other forms of severe malaria

Utkarsh Kohli MD
Senior Resident
The Carman and Ann Adams
Department of Pediatrics, Children's Hospital of
Michigan, Detroit, MI, USA

Shock

Praveen Kumar MD, DNB, DM (Neonatology)
Professor and Head of Neonatal Unit
Department of Pediatrics
Advanced Pediatric Center
Postgraduate Institute of Medical
Education and Research
Chandigarh-160 012
E-mail: drpkumarpgi@gmail.com

Transport of sick children
Neonatal jaundice

Rashmi Kumar MD
Professor of Pediatrics
King George Medical University
Lucknow
E-mail: rashmik@sancharnet.in

Viral encephalitis and encephalopathies

Sanjeev Lalwani MD
Associate Professor
Department of Forensic Medicine and Toxicology
All India Institute of Medical Sciences
New Delhi-110 029

Medico-legal issues in the emergency department

Rakesh Lodha MD
Associate Professor
Department of Pediatrics
All India Institute of Medical Sciences
New Delhi-110 029
E-mail: rakesh_lodha@hotmail.com

Supportive care of critically sick children
Shock
Dengue fever and severe dengue infection
Poisoning in children
Assisted ventilation

S Mahadevan MD, PhD, MNAMS
Professor of Pediatrics
Jawaharlal Institute of Post-graduate Medical
Education and Research
Puducherry-605 006
E-mail: smaha1232@rediffmail.com

Animal and insect bites

AK Mahapatra MS, MCh, DNB
Professor and Head
Department of Neurosurgery
Neurosciences Center
All India Institute of Medical Sciences
New Delhi-110 029
E-mail: akmahapatra_22000@yahoo.com

Head injury

Ankur Mandelia MS
Senior Resident
Department of Pediatric Surgery
All India Institute of Medical Sciences
New Delhi-110 029

Acute abdomen

Mukta Mantan MD, DNB
Associate Professor of Pediatrics
Maulana Azad Medical College
and Associated Hospitals
New Delhi
E-mail: muktamantan@hotmail.com

Acute kidney injury

P Ramesh Menon MD
Assistant Professor
Department of Pediatrics
Govt. TD Medical College
Vandanam, Allepey
Kerala-688 005
E-mail: rpmpgi@gmail.com

Poisoning in children

Gayatri Munghati MS
Senior Resident
Department of Pediatric Surgery
All India Institute of Medical Sciences
New Delhi-110 029
E-mail: drgayatrism@gmail.com

The child with polytrauma

Srinivas Murki MD, DM (Neonatology)
Consultant Neonatologist
Fernandez Hospital, Bogulkunta
Hyderabad-500 001
E-mail: srinivasmurki2001@yahoo.com

Neonatal jaundice

JPS Narula MD, DM, PhD, FACC, FAHA
Professor of Medicine
Chief Division of Cardiology
Associate Dean
University of California
Irvine School of Medicine, Irvine CA
E-mail: narula@uci.edu

Congestive heart failure

RP Naryan MS, MCh, FICS, FIAS
Former Professor and Head
Department of Burns, Plastic and Maxillo-Facial Surgery
Vardhman Mahavir Medical College and
Safdarjung Hospital, New Delhi
E-mail: rpn@vsnl.com

Burns

Gouri Rao Passi MD, DNB, MNAMS
Consultant Pediatrician
Choithram Hospital and Research Center
Indore
E-mail: gouripassi@hotmail.com

Serious bacterial infections

Vinod K Paul MD, PhD, FIAP, FAMS
Professor and Head
Department of Pediatrics
Incharge WHO Collaborating Center
for Training and Research in Newborn Care
All India Institute of Medical Sciences
New Delhi-110 029
E-mail: vinodkpaul@hotmail.com

Neonatal sepsis
Animal and insect bites

GCM Pradeep DCH, DNB, DM (Neonatology)
Assistant Professor and Consultant Neonatologist
M S Ramaiah Medical College and Hospital
Bangalore
E-mail: pgcm@yahoo.com

Neonatal seizures

Arun K Pramanik MD
Professor of Pediatrics and Chief Neonatology Section
School of Medicine in Shreveport
Louisiana State University Medical Center
1501 Kings Highway, Post Office Box – 33932
Shreveport, LA 71130-3932
E-mail: aprama1998@yahoo.com

Respiratory distress in newborn babies
The bleeding neonate

M Ramam MD
Additional Professor
Department of Dermatology and Venereology
All India Institute of Medical Sciences
New Delhi-110 029
E-mail: mramam@hotmail.com

Dermatological emergencies

RK Sabharwal MD, DM (Neurology)
Senior Consultant
Child Neurology and Epilepsy
Centre for Child Health
Sir Ganga Ram Hospital
New Delhi-110 029
E-mail: mukpran@yahoo.com

Acute flaccid paralysis

Sunil Saharan MD
Senior Resident
Miami Children's Hospital
Miami, Florida (USA)

Supportive care of critically sick children

Naveen Sankhyan MD, DM (Pediatric Neurology)
Assistant Professor
Department of Pediatrics
Advanced Pediatric Center
Postgraduate Institute of Medical Education and Research
Chandigarh-160 012
E-mail: drsankhyan@yahoo.co.in

Raised intracranial pressure

Ashok P Sarnaik MD, FCCM
Professor of Pediatrics
Chief Critical Care Medicine
Wayne State University School of Medicine
Children's Hospital of Michigan
3901 Beaubien Boulevard
Detroit, Michigan 48201
E-mail: asarnaik@med.wayne.edu

The child with multiple-organ dysfunction syndrome

K Sasidaran MD, DM (Pediatric Critical Care)
Senior Resident
Advanced Pediatric Center
Postgraduate Institute of Medical Education and Research,
Chandigarh

Fluids, electrolytes and acid-base disorders

Anita Saxena MD, DM (Cardiology), FACC
Professor of Cardiology
Cardio-Thoracic Center
All India Institute of Medical Sciences
New Delhi-110 029
E-mail: anitasaxena@hotmail.com

Cardiac emergencies in newborn babies
Cardiac arrhythmias

Vineet Sehgal MD
Consultant Pediatric Pulmonologist
Max Hospital, Pitampura and Max Super-speciality
Hospital, Saket, New Delhi
E-mail: vineetdoc@hotmail.com

Acute severe asthma

Rachna Seth DNB, MNAMS
Associate Professor
Division of Pediatric Oncology
Department of Pediatrics
All India Institute of Medical Sciences
New Delhi-110 029
E-mail: drrachnaseth@yahoo.co.in

Hematologic emergencies

GR Sethi MD
Director Professor of Pediatrics
Maulana Azad Medical College and Lok Nayak Hospital
New Delhi
E-mail: yogodan@vsnl.com

Acute severe asthma

Kapil Sikka MS, DNB
Assistant Professor
Department of Otolaryngology and Head Neck Surgery
All India Institute of Medical Sciences
New Delhi-110 029

Otolaryngological emergencies

Daljit Singh MD, FIAP, FNNF, FIMSA
Principal and Professor of Pediatrics
Dayanand Medical College and Hospital
Ludhiana-141 001
E-mail: drdaljit@yahoo.com

Electrocution and lightning

Digvijay Singh MD
Senior Resident
Dr Rajendra Prasad Center for Ophthalmic Sciences
All India Institute of Medical Sciences
New Delhi-110 029

Ophthalmic emergencies

Meharban Singh MD, FAMS, FIAP, FIMSA, FNNF, Hony. FAAP
Former Professor and Head
Department of Pediatrics and Neonatal Division
WHO Collaborating Center for Training and
Research in Newborn Care
All India Institute of Medical Sciences
New Delhi
E-mail: drmbsk@gmail.com

Organization of a pediatric intensive care unit
Ethical issues, dilemmas and legal aspects of
  critically sick children
The crying infant and toddler
Acute fever without a focus
Neonatal emergencies in the delivery room
Neonatal sepsis
Acute gastroenteritis
Cerebral and other forms of severe malaria
Status epilepticus
Oncological emergencies
Pain relief and sedation
Emergency procedures
Compendium of emergency drugs
Appendices

Surjit Singh MD, DCH (London)
Professor of Pediatrics
Incharge Pediatric Allergy and Immunology Unit
Advanced Pediatric Center
Postgraduate Institute of Medical
Education and Research,
Chandigarh-160 012
E-mail: surjitsinghpgi@rediffmail.com

Anaphylaxis
Acute fever with a skin rash

Tanu Singhal MD, MSc (Tropical and Infectious Diseases)
Kokilaben Dhirubhai Ambani Hospital and
Medical Research Institute,
Mumbai
E-mail: tanu.singhal@relianceada.com

Dengue fever and severe dengue infection ARDS in children

Pratibha D Singhi MD, FIAP
Professor of Pediatrics
Chief, Pediatric Neurology and Neurodevelopment
Advanced Pediatric Center
Postgraduate Institute of Medical
Education and Research
Chandigarh-160 012
E-mail: medinst@pgi.chd.nic.in

The comatose child

Sunit Singhi MD, FIAP
Professor and Head
Department of Pediatrics
Advanced Pediatric Center
Postgraduate Institute of Medical
Education and Research
Chandigarh-160 012
E-mail: drsinghi@glide.net.in

Fluids, electrolytes and acid base disorders
Acute respiratory distress and respiratory failure
The comatose child

Sindhu Sivanandan MD
Fellow Neonatal–Perinatal Medicine
Foothills Medical Centre
Division of Neonatology
University of Calgary
Alberta, Canada
E-mail: drsindhusivanandan@gmail.com

Assisted ventilation

M Srinivas MS, MCh
Additional Professor
Department of Pediatric Surgery
All India Institute of Medical Sciences
New Delhi-110 029

Foreign bodies in the aero-digestive tract

Anshu Srivastava MD, DM (Gastroenterology)
Associate Professor
Department of Pediatric Gastroenterology
Sanjay Gandhi Postgraduate Institute of Medical
Sciences
Lucknow-226 014
E-mail: avanianshu@yahoo.com

Acute gastro-intestinal bleeding

R Tandon MD, FAMS, FICC, FISC
Professor Emeritus
Cardiothoracic Center
Department of Cardiology
All India Institute of Medical Sciences
New Delhi-110 029

Congestive cardiac failure

Alok Thakar MS, FRCS
Additional Professor
Department of Otolaryngology and Head
Neck Surgery
All India Institute of Medical Sciences
New Delhi-110 029
E-mail: drthakar@gmail.com

Otolaryngological emergencies

Anu Thukral MD, DM (Neonatology), DNB, MNAMS
Senior Research Associate
Department of Pediatrics
All India Institute of Medical Sciences
New Delhi-110 029
E-mail: dranuthukral@yahoo.com

Emergency procedures

Soonu Udani MD, DABP, DABPNM
Chief Pediatric Intensivist
PD Hinduja National Hospital and Medical Research
Centre,
Mumbai
E-mail: drsudani@gmail.com

ARDS in children

Anju Virmani MD, DNB (Endocrinology)
Consultant Pediatric Endocrinologist
Indraprastha Apollo Hospital and Max Hospital,
New Delhi
E-mail: virmani.anju@gmail.com

Diabetic ketoacidosis

Pankaj Vohra MD, DABP
(Pediatric Gastroenterology)
Consultant Pediatric Gastroenterology and Hepatology
Pushpawati Singhania Research Institute for Liver,
Renal and Digestive Diseases and
Max Healthcare, Saket, New Delhi
E-mail: pankajvohramd@yahoo.com

Acute liver failure

Surender Kumar Yachha MD, DM
(Gastroenterology), FIAP
Professor and Head
Department of Gastroenterology
Sanjay Gandhi Postgraduate Institute of
Medical Sciences
Lucknow-226 014
E-mail: skyachha@sushrut.sgpgi.ac.in

Acute gastro-intestinal bleeding

Acknowledgements

I would like to express may appreciation and gratitude to my erstwhile students and faculty colleagues of the Department of Pediatrics, All India Institute of Medical Sciences, New Delhi, who provided suggestions, guidance and material to bring out the revised edition. My special thanks are due to the post-graduate and post doctoral students in pediatrics and its sub-specialities who reviewed the fourth edition and made outstanding contributions and suggestions to bring out the revised and updated fifth edition.

Meharban Singh

Contents

1

Organization, Resuscitation and Stabilization

Organization of a Pediatric Intensive Care Unit

Meharban Singh

As opposed to ambulatory services, the emergency services are poorly organized in most developing countries. During the past decade or so, a number of teaching institutions and private corporate hospitals have established intermediate level intensive care facilities for newborn babies. The pediatric intensive care services have now engaged the serious attention of Indian pediatricians[1]. In order to provide optimal medical care to children with life-threatening disorders, there is a need to establish pediatric intensive care units (PICU) in major pediatric centers in the country. Knowledge of pathophysiology of life-threatening conditions and technological advances to monitor and treat children with critical life-threatening disorders have progressed dramatically during the past 3 decades. The major constraints of delivery of intensive care to children in a developing country are lack of satisfactory infrastructure, high costs of electronic equipment and emergency drugs and lack of specially trained medical and nursing manpower.

Children have specialized physiologic, pharmacologic and psychologic needs, and it is appropriate to provide them critical care by pediatric intensivists in a specialized units of excellence[2-4]. The old fashioned concept of treatment rooms for providing emergency care must be replaced by PICUs. Children with multisystem diseases and serious dysfunction of one or more vital organs demand a concerted team approach for their proper evaluation, monitoring and management. Children are vulnerable and delicate due to several biological handicaps. Because of instability of the homeostatic mechanisms and functional immaturity of vital organs, children are susceptible to develop life-threatening dehydration, hyperthermia, shock, intractable seizures, accidents, poisonings, etc., which demand urgent attention to prevent irreversible biophysiological alterations. Most pediatric emergencies present with organ dysfunction of an acute onset and there is a very good chance for complete recovery when life support is provided during the crucial early stages of the disease process. The potentiality for complete recovery is remarkable in children as long as life is sustained during the acute phase of illness. As compared to adults, chances of survival and functional recovery are much more favorable in children receiving intensive care. The special needs of the critically ill children demand a high level of expertise provided by a team of physicians, nurses and ancillary staff with the help of sophisticated equipment. PICU should look after the physical, psychosocial, emotional and spiritual needs of children with life-threatening conditions and their families[5].

PHYSICAL DESIGN AND FACILITIES

The Indian Academy of Pediatrics (IAP) intensive care chapter and Indian Society for Critical Care Medicine (ISCCM) pediatric section have jointly developed guidelines for establishment of Pediatric Intensive Care Unit (PICU)[6].

Location and Size

PICU should be located adjacent to children ward and should have an easy access to a ramp, elevators, emergency department, operation theater, radiology department and laboratory. The optional number of PICU beds (intermediate and critical patients) are estimated to vary between 10 and 15 percent of the total children beds. There is higher demand for PICU beds in a referral or tertiary care hospital. Additional beds are required if unit is expected to cater to post surgical patients. A unit of less than 6 beds is not justified due to considerable cost involved for infrastructure, equipment and maintenance[7-10]. It is, therefore, desirable to regionalize intensive care facilities for children for cost-effective utilization of meagre resources.

Unit Design

The unit should be provided with generous space keeping in mind the need for a large number of ancillary facilities. Apart from open bay area (intermediate care), there should be single bed (assisted ventilation or intensive care) and two bed rooms (critical care), and isolation room. The isolation room should be located at the far end of the unit and provided with ante-room with hand-washing and gowning facilities. The open ward type facility with movable partitions should be allocated with 150-200 sq feet area per patient. The open bay is used for care of convalescing patients who need close monitoring but are not on life support system. It is advisable to provide at least 250 sq feet area for the single bedroom and 200 sq feet area for each bed in the two bedroom facility. The rooms should have glass partitions to facilitate constant observation of patients. The design should be flexible keeping in mind the needs of a wide spectrum of patients. Wash basins and hand sanitizing facilities should be available for every 2–3 beds. The area around the bed should have enough space for housing monitoring equipment and for performing routine ICU procedures such as cardio-pulmonary resuscitation (CPR), placement of central lines and chest tube. The unit should provide easy access for portable X-ray machine, portable ultra-sound, echocardiograph and electro-encephalograph machines. The total floor area needed is about 3 times of the space required for the beds to accommodate ancillary facilities.

The unit should be provided with glazed tiles, PVC antistatic flooring and equipped with high sound absorption capabilities. The unit should be double-walled, dust and sound proof and preferably air conditioned (Figure 1.1). Facilities for centralized suction, oxygen, compressed medical air and running water around-the-clock should be available. Hanging pendants for centralized gas line supply and suction facilities and wall-mounted shelves for placing electronic monitoring equipment provide unencumbered space in the unit.

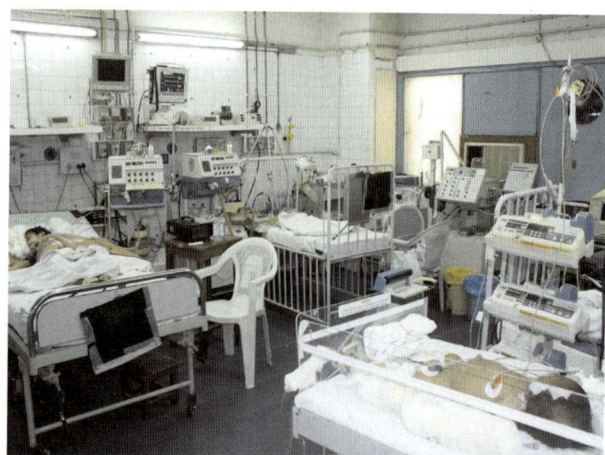

Figure 1.1 Pediatric intensive care unit of AIIMS

Beds

The ratio of adult sized to pediatric beds should be 4:1. There should be easy and rapid access to the head end of all beds for prompt CPR when required. There should be easy maneuverability of head and foot ends of beds. All beds should be provided with a railing to prevent accidental fall of the child. At least two air/water matteresses should be available to prevent bed sores in children with coma. Each bed should be provided with two outlets each for oxygen, compressed air and suction and at least ten electrical outlets which should be located at least 4 feet above the floor level[11]. One multi-channel vital sign monitor should be available for each bed. Facilities should be available for providing extra light and warmth by overhead radiant warmer to each patient as and when needed.

Back-up emergency power and reserve gas supply (oxygen and compressed air) should be available to meet any oxigencies of the failure of the centralized facilities. Each bed should have emergency alarm button and intercom facility. A cart should be available at the bedside to hold personal belongings and disposables. The room should have windows to prevent a sense of isolation. Adequate lighting, child-friendly wall papering, paintings or cartoons of bright colors provide vibrant look to the unit.

Power Supply and Temperature Control

The unit should preferably be centrally air conditioned (with cooling and watering facilities) and ambient temperature should be maintained between 25° and 26°C. The unit should be provided with uninterrupted power supply with back-up power sources such as automode invertors and generators of sufficient wattage in accordance with the load of various equipment. Effective air ventilation of PICU is essential to reduce noso-comial infections. The most satisfactory ventilation is achieved with laminar flow system but it is rather expensive. When centralized air-conditioning is used, minimum of 12 changes of room air per hour are recommended. The air-conditioning ducts should be provided with millipore filters of 0.5 μ size to restrict the entry of microbes. A constant positive air pressure should be maintained in the PICU so that the contaminated air from the carridors does not gain access into the unit.

Central Station

A well equipped central station from where all the patients can be easily observed through their glass partitions is mandatory in a modern PICU[11].

The chief nurse can constantly watch all the patients and working staff from the central station. The central station also serves the important function of exchange of information and communication with parents through alarm bells, intercom, mobiles and direct-line external phone. At least two telephone lines and one mobile facility should be available. One landline telephone number should be dedicated to incoming calls for ease of communication with parents and for prompt implementation of transport requests. In advanced centers, a central electronic patient monitoring facility is installed but it does not substitute the bed side observations. A computer or microprocessor with a printer is useful for the resident staff for creating patient documents and having computerized link to the laboratory for collection of laboratory reports. The central station should have enough space for resident doctors and secretarial staff for documentation.

Ante-room for Handwashing

Handwashing facilities should be available at the enterance. It should be provided with liberal space with self-closing doors. The sink should be large and deep (24″ wide × 16″ front-back and 10″ deep) and made of porcelain or stainless steel and without any counter slab or shelf. Street shoes are changed by PICU slippers, followed by thorough handwashing and gowning. The use of mask is controversial and usually recommended to personnel suffering from acute respiratory infection. Hand-free elbow or foot-operated water tap and liquid soap dispenser are recommended. Pictorial handwashing instructions should be affixed on the wall next to the sink. Hands should be dried with a single use or disposable napkins. The walls adjacent to the sink should be made of non-porous or non-absorbant material to prevent growth of moulds. The unit should be provided with 24-hour un-interrupted water supply.

Store Room

A store room should be located within or closely adjacent to PICU to store equipment, drugs and disposables. A refrigerator is a must to store life saving perishable drugs. Portable X-ray machine should be housed next to patient care area. Next to PICU, an area should be earmarked for stacking stretchers, trolleys and wheel chairs.

Clean and Dirty Utility Rooms

The clean utility room is used for storage of clean linen, procedure sets and disposables. Dirty utility room should be located preferably near the exit and away from the clean utility area. Covered bins with plastic hampers should be available in the patient care area. The soiled linen and waste material should be shifted to dirty utility hold without any delay. The dirty utility room should have an area for emptying and cleaning bed pans and urine bottles, and stocking brooms, detergents and cleaning material.

Waste Disposal

The disposal of contaminated waste (garbage, contaminated and infected medical waste), syringes, needles and sharp objects should be in accordance with standard pollution control guidelines. Covered bins with plastic hampers should be provided along each bed for disposal of soiled linen and contaminated waste materials.

Stat Laboratory

A mini laboratory with facilities for arterial blood gases, blood sugar, electrolytes, urine examination, cytology for body fluids from serosal cavities, CSF, urine with Gram staining facilities should be available in the PICU. In addition to mini stat laboratory in the PICU, the main centralized laboratory should provide round-the-clock facilities for urgent biochemical tests with turn around time (reporting time) of less than one hour.

Room for Preparation of Intravenous Fluids and Special Feeds

A separate room should be earmarked and provided with laminar flow for preparation of intravenous fluids, parenteral nutritional formulations, entral feeds and medications. Boiling and autoclaving facilities should be available adjacent to this room.

Staff Rooms

Space should be provided adjacent to PICU to meet the personal, professional and administrative needs of the resident staff on duty. A comfortable room with intercom, telephone, computer terminal and WC facilities is mandatory. A change room for nurses is required for changing the formal street clothes to a smart shirt and trouser dress as stipulated by the PICU.

Conference Room

A room for holding academic meetings, discussion of difficult cases, deaths and administrative meetings for improvement of quality of care etc. should be available. The room should be equipped with audio-visual facilities and have a small library with ready access to the important books on emergency and intensive care, journals and policy manuals. The conference room can be used for discussion and counseling of parents and attendants of patients admitted in the PICU.

X-ray Viewing Area

In the PICU, an area should be earmarked for keeping the illuminated viewing panels to examine a series of X-ray films during the rounds.

Crash Cart

A crash cart with emergency drugs and portable monitor/defibrillator should be available in the PICU.

Receptionist Desk

A receptionist should control the entry of visitors in the PICU. The area should be monitored by security personnel.

Waiting and Rest Rooms for Attendants

Waiting area for parents and attendants should be earmarked in the close vicinity of PICU. It should be provided with comfortable chairs, drinking water, television and WC facilities. Separate toilets and wash room facilities should be available for patients and their parents and attendants.

PERSONNEL

Medical Staff

A dedicated, disciplined and adequately trained medical and supportive staff should be available round-the-clock. There should be an equal distribution of staff during three shifts of working. The staff should receive constant in-service and on-going training in the art and science of cardio-respiratory resuscitation (PALS certified) and management of pediatric emergencies. The floating staff should be kept to the barest minimum to ensure continuity of service and maintenance of routines and rituals of the unit. A full-time pediatric intensivist should be incharge of the unit along with one senior resident or registrar for eight beds. There is a need to start DM programs for pediatric intensive care because of acute shortage of pediatric intensivists in our country. One junior resident (preferably 3rd year resident) should be available for four patients round-the-clock. There is evidence to suggest that availability of a fully trained and qualified pediatrician round-the-clock improves the survival of patients admitted in the PICU[12]. Other pediatric specialists like anesthesiologist, surgeon, cardiologist, neurologist, neurosurgeon, orthopedic surgeon, ENT specialist, psychiatrist or psychologist, etc. should be available on call.

Nursing Staff

The availability of adequately trained nurses in the art of intensive care is most crucial for the success of PICU. The nursing director should have specialized training in pediatric intensive care management and life support and should be responsible for coordination of in-service education and nursing administration. It should constitute an independent nursing unit and one nurse should be available for one or two patients throughout 24 hours. A ventilated or unstable patient (shock, apnea, hypoxemia) should preferably be looked after by one trained nurse round-the-clock. For example, for 8-bedded PICU 15 staff nurses are required in order to post at least four nurses in each 8-hour shift. During morning hours, one dynamic senior staff nurse should function as a nursing chief to coordinate efficient functioning of the unit. The staff nurses in the unit should be trained in pediatric resuscitation procedures, respiratory care, correct handling of various electronic monitoring devices and should be able to recognize the psychological needs of children and their families. Essential skills should also include the ability to recognize, interpret and record the waxing and waning symptoms and vital signs of critically ill patients. They should be trained to administer life saving drugs and perform specialised nursing procedures.

Ancillary Staff

There is a need to have at least one biomedical technical assistant and respiratory therapist to supervise ventilatory therapy, provide physiotherapy and look after the maintenance of the equipment. They can also be trained for drawing blood samples and establishing an intravenous line by serving as perfusionists. A biochemistry technician should be available round-the-clock to undertake urgent biochemical laboratory tests. A part-time specially trained pharmacist and nutritionist should be available[13]. A social worker can provide much needed emotional and financial support and liaison with parents and relatives so that physicians and nurses can expend their valuable time more usefully in the care of serious patients[14]. At least one nursing aide and a janitor should be available round-the-clock. They should be specially trained, efficient and sensitive to the urgent patient care needs.

The PICU staff must demonstrate exemplary dedication, highest level of technical skill, compassion, confidence and courtesy. The parents must be constantly kept informed about the condition of their wards and repeatedly assured that whatever is humanly possibly is being done to save the life of their child. This type of a rapport with the parents is essential because in the unfortunate event of death of a patient, it becomes easier to provide emotional cushion to the family and obtain necessary permission for autopsy.

EQUIPMENT

Equipment required to provide cardiopulmonary resuscitation, airway management, oxygen delivery, mechanical ventilation, vital sign monitoring with continuous ECG tracing, CVP monitoring, nutritional support, precise therapeutic interventions with infusion pumps and adequate transport facilities. The organization of a PICU demands considerable financial inputs for purchase of a variety of diagnostic, monitoring and therapeutic equipment (Table 1.1).

Table 1.1 Equipment for 8-bedded PICU	
List of equipment	**Qty.**
■ *Cardio-respiratory resuscitation trays:* Ambu bags with masks of different sizes, laryngoscopes with straight blades, ET tubes, laryngeal mask airways, plastic oral airways, oral suction traps, suction catheters etc.	4 sets
❑ Multichannel automated vital sign monitors with alarms	4
❑ Non-invasive blood pressure monitors and sphygmomanometers	4
❑ Volume-controlled pressure-limited ventilators	4
❑ High frequency ventilators	2
❑ Portable transport ventilators	2
❑ Double-probe electronic thermometers	4
❑ Volumetric micro infusion pumps	15
❑ Oxygen head boxes	15
❑ Pulse oximeters	8
❑ Mistogen and heavy duty nebulizers	2
❑ Radiant warmers with servo control system	4
❑ Portable ECG, EEG and Doppler ultrasonography and echocardiography machines	One each
❑ Facilities to monitor central venous pressure, pulmonary arterial pressure and intracranial pressure	2 each
❑ Surgical procedure trays: Vascular cut-down, tracheostomy, cricothyroidotomy, thoracostomy, pericardiocentensis, paracentesis	2
❑ Phototherapy units	2
❑ Overhead warmers	2
❑ Exchange transfusion sets and blood warmers	2
❑ Peritoneal dialysis kits	2
❑ Facilities for fiberoptic flexible endoscopes to visualize upper air passages, proximal and distal GI tract	
❑ Emergency ("code" or "crash") cart: Defibrillator with pediatric and adult paddles (4.5 cm, 8.0 cm), cardioverter and pace makers	2
❑ Ophthalmoscope and otoscope sets	2
❑ Procedure lamps	2
❑ Weighing scales for infants and children with stadiometer	2 each
❑ Refrigerator for storing life saving drugs, sera and blood products	2
❑ *Miscellaneous small items:* Disposable gamma-irradiated small-vein infusion sets, intraosseous needles, burette sets, medicaths or catheter-over-needle devices, central catheters, feeding tubes, suction catheters, endotracheal tubes, laryngeal mask airways, nasopharyngeal and oropharyngeal airways, nasal prongs, T-tubes, thoracostomy tubes, tracheostomy tubes, disposable syringes and needles, lumbar puncture and biopsy needles, urine collection bags, sterile gloves, Sengstaken tubes, rectal tubes, tape measures, torches, pediatric restraining devices, extremity splints, etc.	

Level 3 or tertiary care PICUs provide high-end intensive care facilities to patients with complete failure of one or multiple body organs with state-of-the-art facilities for super speciality surgical disciplines and organ transplant facilities. They are equipped with specialized monitoring, diagnostic and therapeutic equipment like flexible laryngoscope, flexible bronchoscope, non-invasive ventilators (High frequency, jet ventilation), nitric oxide or heliox ventilation, end-tidal CO_2 monitor, intracranial pressure monitor, and ECMO facilities.

Mere acquisition of newer equipment does not necessarily ensure better services and outcome. The physicians and nurses must be conversant with the working and limitations of various equipment. It is an unfortunate fact that equipment worth millions of foreign exchange are lying useless in several hospitals in developing countries due to non-availability of spares and lack of expertise to commission them. The equipment should be purchased only after thorough scrutiny and one should avoid the trap of buying outmoded models from foreign companies. Apart from cost, the other major considerations that should be taken into account before ordering new equipment include evaluation of equipment by demonstration, reliability of the firm, information regarding frequency of break-downs from other users, built-in alarm systems, maintenance services and other facilities offered by the company[15-17]. It is desirable to buy most of the equipment from one or two local suppliers who have established their credibility for prompt after sales preventive and breakdown maintenance services.

Enough essential accessories must be purchased at the time of buying the equipment. The size of equipment should conform to the needs of all the children who vary in size from birth to adolescence. It is desirable to train technical assistants for proper preventive maintenance of vital equipment. Availability of a biomedical engineer in the PICU team would go a long way for optimal utilization of our meagre resources spent on the purchase of expensive equipment[17].

Laboratory facilities should be available round-the-clock for prompt evaluation of several biochemical parameters which are crucial for the management of critically sick children (Table 1.2). A specially trained technician should be available round-the-clock to manage PICU laboratory. It is unwise to expect a resident doctor to expend his valuable time in the laboratory.

ORGANIZATION AND ADMINISTRATION

A network of strategically located PICUs together with an efficient referral and transport system can go a long way in providing regionalized intensive care facilities and improving child survival. It is desirable to adopt a two-tier approach for creating PICUs in the country. Basic PICUs should be developed at the district level and in small to medium private hospitals to provide facilities for effective monitoring and therapy of critically sick children with involvment of single body system. These units should have transfer arrangements with

Table 1.2 Laboratory facilities for PICU
❑ Facilities for complete hemogram, microscopic examination of peripheral blood, cytology and Gram's staining of cerebrospinal fluid, urine and stools, biochemical examination of urine and stools with reagent strips
❑ Portable 3 phase-generator 100 mA X-ray facilities with automatic developer
❑ Blood gas and acid-base analyzer
❑ Microchemistry* facilities for estimation of blood glucose (glucometer), urea, creatinine, electrolytes, calcium, lactate, ammonia, and clotting studies
❑ Drug screening and toxicology screen*
❑ Culture facilities
❑ 12-lead portable ECG machine
❑ Doppler ultrasonography and echocardiography machine
❑ Portable EEG machine
❑ Osmometer and refractometer
*Centralized laboratory facility is more cost-effective and is satisfactory if reports are available within one hour

an advanced PICU with the help of a well equipped transport team. Advanced level state-of-the-art PICUs should be established on a regional basis at tertiary care centers and major teaching hospitals[18, 19]. However, the benefits of intensive care can be achieved only if patients are referred and transferred at the earliest before they deteriorate to multi-organ failure or decompensated state. The advanced PICU should have optimal facilities to manage children having life-threatening complex medical emergencies with multi-organ failure. Some beds in the PICU should be earmarked for intermediate care to look after patients who are weaned off the ventilator or recovering from syndrome of multi-organ dysfunction.

A fully trained pediatric intensivist should be the leader and incharge of PICU. The medical director of the unit should be a pediatric intensivist who is specially trained and experienced in critical care of children. He is charged with following responsibilities: (i) Smooth functioning of PICU with implementation of policies and management protocols including admission and discharge criteria, (ii) Quality assurance of clinical care, (iii) Communica-tion and interface with parents and attendants, (iv) Purchase and maintenance of equipment, (v) Establishing teaching and training program for medical, nursing and ancillary staff, (vi) Implementing policies for infection control in the PICU, (vii) Maintaining statistics for spectrum of morbidity and mortality in the unit, (viii) Organizing and implementing transport facilities to pick critically sick children from the referring hospital and (ix) Maintaining liaison with other team members of PICU like nursing director, pediatric subspecialities including surgical colleagues, hospital administrator, laboratory, imaging department and blood bank representatives. The ethical and medico-legal issues including value-judgement regarding benefits to the child, family and society should be jointly taken in close consultation with the parents or surrogates.

There should be a close collaboration between the pediatrician, surgeon and anesthetist for management of critically sick patients. There should be a cadre of nurses specially trained in the art of intensive care and they should not be posted to cold areas. There should be an on-going commitment for education and training of medical, nursing and supportive staff working in the PICU. All the staff members and professionals working in the PICU should attend regular continuing education programs, regional and national meetings in pediatric critical care medicine and advanced life support[20]. Because of nursing constraints and our unique socio-cultural matrix, at least one of the parents should be allowed in the PICU with their critically sick child. They serve as valuable observers and can be trained effectively to discharge simple nursing chores. The familiar face and voice of parent is reassuring to the child and accelerates the process of healing and recovery. The incidence of nosocomial infections is higher in PICU because cell-mediated immunity is depressed in a critically ill patient, nutrition is suboptimal and invasive procedures are performed with haste[21]. Unnecessary traffic into the critical care unit should be restricted to reduce the risk of hospital-acquired infections (HAIs).

Facilities should be available for effective hand washing before entering the PICU and in-between the patients. Over-shoes or slippers should be worn before entering the unit. The use of gown and mask has not shown any reduction in the spread of noso-comial infections or vascular catheter colonization rates in a PICU[22]. *All health workers in the PICU must rigorously follow universal precautions as a safeguard against contracting HIV and HBV infections while sampling, doing procedures and handling specimens.* It is essential to have a procedure manual for residents so that there is uniformity in the routines and policies being followed in the PICU. The manual should provide detailed instructions for indications for admission of patients to the intensive care unit (Table 1.3).

Table 1.3 Indications for admission to the PICU

General

Cardio-respiratory arrest, central cyanosis, shock, hyperpyrexia, acute poisoning, acute hemorrhage, severe anemia, severe dehydration and dyselectrolytemia, severe acid-base disorders, severe protein-energy malnutrition, diabetic ketoacidosis, near-drowning, polytrauma, postoperative patients.

Central nervous system

Coma, intractable seizures, tetanus, acute intracranial infection, paralysis of respiratory muscles (Polio/LGB), head injury.

Cardiovascular system

Cardiac arrest, arrhythmias, pulmonary edema, intractable heart failure, hypertensive emergencies.

Respiratory system

Acute respiratory distress and respiratory failure due to any cause, gasping breathing with apneic attacks, obstructed breathing, croup, status asthmaticus, foreign body.

Abdomen

Upper and lower gastrointestinal bleeding, hepatocellular failure, acute renal failure.

In view of limited resources and scarcity of available PICU beds, there is a need to prioritize admissions[23]. The patients with reasonable chance of intact survival should get priority over terminal patients with untreatable underlying conditions. Priority should also be given to acutely ill patients needing short term care in the PICU. The guidelines for admission and discharge should be clearly written down to avoid any misunderstanding with colleagues and patients. The policies for admission and plan for monitoring and management should be periodically reviewed so that facilities of PICU are most cost-effectively and optimally used.

If resources permit, an ambulance equipped with life support facilities can be commissioned for transport of emergencies from peripheral hospitals and nursing homes[24]. The criteria for transfer of a patient from PICU to an intermediate or a minimal care facility should be clearly defined. The policies regarding record of vital signs, body weight, routine investigation, etc. should be clearly stated. The responsibilities of all the staff members working in the PICU should be clearly identified. The residents and nurses should be conversant with all the equipment being used in the PICU. *Management protocols and algorithms should be developed to ensure rational and prompt management of common pediatric emergencies*[25]. It is desirable to have clearly written down policies and protocols for management of common medical emergencies, procedures, administration of life-saving medications, nursing care. Detailed monitoring charts for nurses and resident doctors should be available to record vital signs, level of consciousness, fluid intake and output, hydration status, functional status of major body organs, progress notes, etc. When facilities are available, PICU should be linked with National Poison Control Center to seek prompt information regarding specific management of a child with accidental poisoning. A list of emergency drugs available in PICU along with their dosages should be displayed (Table 1.4)[26, 27].

The resident doctors should be instructed to write problem-oriented case records and maintain flow charts for evaluation and treatment. Computerized data collection is desirable for on-going evaluation and quality control. Strict record of daily input and output should be maintained for all patients. The evaluation and monitoring must assess the efficacy of services in terms of patient outcome, resource utilization and cost effectiveness. Uniform criteria should be used to assess the severity of condition and risk of mortality for internal quality control and for comparing data with other PICUs[28–30].

A log book for all the available equipment in the PICU should be maintained incorporating address and telephone numbers of the supplier, date of purchase, cost, break downs, list of accessories in stock, etc.[17] The decision regarding withdrawal of life support or declaration of death should be based on specified guidelines and left to the discretion of a senior resident or consultant. In case of death, the family should be prepared by sympathetic handling for autopsy both in the interest of the advancement of medical knowledge and safeguarding health of other siblings. If autopsy is refused, tissue biopsies should be obtained from the

---

Table 1.4 List of emergency drugs

1. **Infusates**

   Fluids, plasma expanders and electrolyte solutions like Ringer's lactate, physiological saline, saline 3%, dextrose 5%, 10% and 50%, salt-poor albumin 5%, 10% and 20%, fresh frozen plasma, hemeccel, mannitol 20%, lomodex, protein hydrolysate or amino acid mixture, intralipid, fluids for peritoneal dialysis, sodium bicarbonate 7.5%, potassium chloride 15% and clacium gluconate 10%.

2. **Circulatory support**

   Epinephrine 1:1000 and 1:10,000 solution, atropine sulfate, adenosine, hydrocortisone, dexamethasone or betamethasone, cortisone acetate, methyl prednisolone, dopamine, dobutamine, norepinephrine, metarminol and nikethamide.

3. **Sedatives and anticonvulsants**

   Phenobarbital, phenytoin, diazepam, lorazepam, midazolam, thiopental, etomidate, propofol, paraldehyde, morphine, fentanyl, pethidine (meperidine), ketamine, droperidol, chlorpromazine, magnesium sulfate, oral chloral hydrate, phenergan, and triclofos sodium.

4. **Cardiotonics and antihypertensives**

   Hydralazine, nifedipine, diazoxide, verapamil, amiodarone, captopril, propranolol, methyl dopa, reserpine, sodium nitroprusside, digoxin, furosemide, aminophylline, isoproterenol, quinidine, bretylium tosylate, procainamide hydrochloride, lidocaine, tolazoline, and adenosine.

5. **Antibiotics and chemotherapeutic agents**

   Benzyl penicillin, ampicillin or amoxycillin, amoxycillin with sulbactum or clavulanate, cefuroxime axetil, aztreonam, co-trimoxazole, chloramphenicol, gentamicin, amikacin, carbenicillin, cloxacillin, vancomycin, teicoplanin, tigecycline, cefotaxime, ceftriaxone, cefixime, cefpodoxime proxetil, cefepime, cefoperazone, piperacillin, ceftazidime, imipenem with cilastatin, meropenem, linezolid, flouroquinolones, quinine dihydrochloride, artemether, artesunate, acyclovir, amphotericin B, fluconazole, flucytosine, and metronidazole.

6. **Specific antidotes**

   Calcium-ETDA, nalorphine, naloxone hydrochloride, cyanide kit, flumazenil, diphenhydramine hydrochloride, neostigmine, N-acetyl cystein, pralidoxime chloride, penicillamine, desferoxamine, methylene blue, diphenhydramine, protamine sulfate, sodium nitrite, sodium thiosulfate, polyvalent snake antivenin, scorpion antivenin, antitetanic and antidiphtheritic sera.

7. **Miscellaneous drugs**

   WHO-ORS, ipecac syrup, apomorphine, succinylcholine, pancuronium, vercuronium, edrophonium chloride, ranitidine, sucralfate, glucagon, heparin, crystalline insulin, paracetamol, ibuprofen, domperidone, ondansetron hydrochloride, dicyclomine hydrochloride, vasopressin, tetanus toxoid, pyridoxine, kayaxelate, vitamin K, beclate, salbutamol, terbutaline, ipratropium bromide, metered dose inhalers, nebulizer solutions, etc.

For dosages of drugs, refer to Singh M, Deorari AK. Drug Dosages in Children, 9th edition, CBS Publishers & Distributors, New Delhi, 2015.

suspected diseased organs. There should be a constant interaction and discussions among various personnel working in the PICU to update, revise and improve existing policies for its effective implementation in order to provide optimal intensive care facilities. It is mandatory to review all deaths to identify the underlying conditions, cause and mode of death and whether outcome could have been improved by more aggressive or alternative therapy. A critical care unit committee should be formed to approve the policies and procedures pertaining to control of nosocomial infections, safety measures, traffic control, parent visitation, admissions and discharges including use of a triage system. Above all, the atmosphere in a PICU must be positive, pleasant and full of optimism and hope to adequately cushion the anxiety and concern of the parents.

PREVENTION OF NOSOCOMIAL INFECTIONS

The hospital-acquired infection (HAI) is defined as an infection which occurs in a patient admitted in the hospital or health care facility, in whom the infection was not present or incubating at the time of admission. Intensive care units are notorious for spread of nosocomial infections by multi-drug resistant hospital-acquired pathogens because critically sick children are immuno-compromised. There is a potential risk of transmission of life-threatening viral infections like HIV and HBV to personnel working in the PICU unless due precautions are taken. There is an increasing scare of emergence of a new genre of multi-drug resistant deadly super bugs which have been designated as NDM1 (New Delhi metallo-beta-lactamase 1). They can be warded off by effective preventive measures but cannot be treated at present by currently available antibiotics. A detailed guidelines for prevention of hospital-acquired infections are provided by World Health Organization.[31] The following guidelines should be followed to ensure asepsis which would go a long way to improve the survival of patients admitted in the PICU.

Entry to the PICU

1. Remove street shoes and wear PICU sleepers before entering.

2. Effective and thorough hand washing before entering the PICU and after touching each patient is the most important measure for prevention of nasocomial infection. The nails should be kept short and trimmed. Scrub thoroughly both hands and forearms upto elbows with a soapy solution and water for at

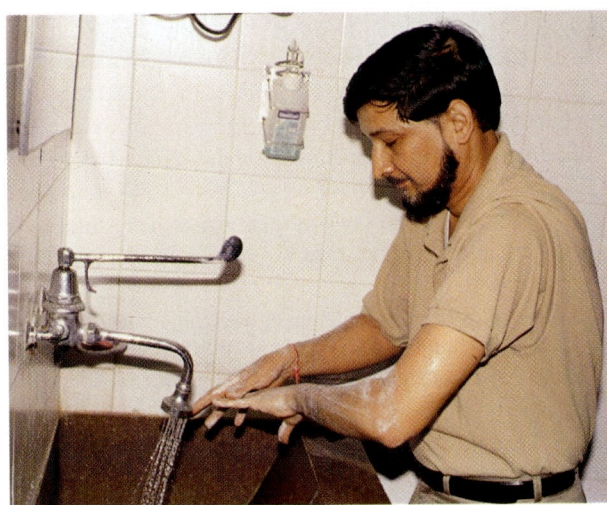

Figure 1.2 The correct technique of thorough hand washing upto elbows before entering PICU

least 2 minutes after removing the watch, rings, bangles, etc. (Figure 1.2). Dry with single use sterile napkin and rinse the hands with sterilium. Thereafter, before touching any child, rinse the hands with sterilium in-between patients. If sterilium is not available, rewash the hands with soap and water for at least 30 seconds.

3. Mask should be worn if the person working in the PICU is suffering from an acute respiratory tract infection.

House-keeping Rituals[32]

1. Universal precautions for prevention of HIV (and HBV) should be followed at all times (Table 1.5).

2. The floor and wash basins must be mopped with 3% phenol or 5% lysol once in each duty shift.

3. Use gloves for handling blood, blood products and all discharges and secretions. Wash hands immediately if they are accidentally contaminated with blood products or patients' body fluids.

4. Soiled and infected linen must be removed from PICU immediately.

5. Walls, windows, furniture and shelves must be cleaned with phenol solution once a week.

6. The plastic waste buckets (with polythene hampers) provided at each bed side must be emptied during each shift.

7. Holes and crevices in the floor and wall should be plugged and anticockroach measures deployed once in every 3 months.

8. The cold sterilization solutions must be freshly prepared daily.

Table 1.5   Universal precautions
❑   Treat every specimen of blood or body fluid as potentially infectious.
❑   Wear gloves for handling all bodily fluids and while performing phlebotomy.
❑   For all procedures where splashing of body fluids or droplets may occur, wear waterproof gown, mask and goggles.
❑   Avoid re-capping, bending or breaking of needles, but when recapping is unavoidable it should be done with a single hand to avoid accidental needle stick injury to the finger.
❑   Wear gloves for patient care, if exudative or weeping dermatitis is present.
❑   Handwashing is a must in-between examination of patients, after any procedure and on removal of gloves.
❑   Promptly clean any blood spills or bodily fluids by pouring 1% bleach solution or 0.5% sodium hypo-chlorite over the spill and leave it soaked for at least 10 minutes.
❑   Disinfect or sterilize re-usable devices as recommended.
❑   Safe disposal of needles and other sharps into puncture resistant containers. Dispose puncture resistant disposable container for decontamination or incineration when three-quarters full.
❑   Wear heavy-duty rubber gloves for cleaning instruments, handling soiled linen or dealing with spills of blood and body fluids.

Disinfection of Equipment

1. Cheatle forceps and thermometers should be kept in dry sterile cotton or 5% savlon freshly prepared every day. Inscribe the date of preparation on the bottle.

2. Oxygen tubings and humidifier chamber should be changed and filled with sterile water daily and in-between patients. Oxygen hood should be cleaned with soap and water or cidex after each use.

3. Suction bottle and tubings should be changed daily and in-between patients. Fill the suction bottle with 5% savlon daily. Switch on the suction machine and suck in formaline solution to sterilize inner lining of the suction tubes daily.

4. The inspiratory and expiratory ports of Ambu bag should be opened and cleaned with cidex or korsolex after each use. Silicon bags and masks can withstand autoclaving. Laryngoscope blade should be cleaned with 70% surgical alcohol or sterillium after each use.

5. The ventilator circuit tubing should be changed every day. It is preferable to use disposable single-use ventilator circuit tubing.

6. Open care systems, incubators, monitors, etc. should be cleaned daily with a detergent followed by 2% bacillocid solution. After drying they should be wiped with a cloth soaked in cidex. Alcohol should not be used for cleaning plastic or acrylic canopies as it will cause opacification.

Asepsis during Procedures

Strict aseptic precautions should be followed while performing any procedure in the PICU. Wash hands with sterilium and wear sterile gloves. *All the disposable items must be discarded after a single use.*

Establishing IV line

Clean the skin site with spirit-betadine (30 seconds)- spirit. If more than 3 attempts are futile, use another brand new venflon. Avoid using heparinized stock solution for rinsing, instead use normal saline ampoules for flushing IV cannula. Use betadine or neosporin ointment at puncture site and affix it with two strips of micropore followed by support with sticking plaster. Change the IV infusion set daily and the IV line should be routinely changed after every 2–3 days. If thrombophlebitis develops, remove the venflon and send its tip for culture. Apply betadine ointment and bandage with ichthyol glycerin dressing. *Never try to reinsert the needle into its plastic cover, instead it must be discarded unsheathed in the waste bucket and destroyed.*

For administration of medicines, do not disconnect the cannula from the drip set. Instead use an IV line connection with a latex side channel. Swab the latex side channel with spirit-betadine-spirit before inserting the needle.

Central venous line

Tunnel the tip of the central line catheter at least 2 cm through the subcutaneous tissue before entering the vein. Keep the infusion running through the central line all the time to maintain its patency. After reading the CVP, remember to restart the intravenous drip to prevent clotting of the line. Keep the venipuncture site sterile by application of betadine or neosporin ointment and a light dressing. Do not maintain the central line for more than 72 hours and when central catheter is removed, its tip should be sent for culture.

Endotracheal intubation

Sedation and use of atropine is desirable in an elective intubation. The endotracheal tube should be changed after every 48 hours and its tip must be sent for culture. The tracheal aspirate should be sent for culture and Giemsa stain to look for polymorphs and pathogens after every 48 hours.

Suction of endotracheal tube

Nurse and assistant must wear gloves to undertake this procedure. Bag and mask the patient with 100% oxygen for 2–3 minutes before undertaking the suction. Suck the ET tube intermittently while withdrawing the suction catheter. If the secretions are thick and viscid, instil a mixture of 0.7 ml normal saline and 0.3 ml sodium bicarbonate through the endotracheal tube before suction. The suction catheter should be discarded if it accidentally touches any object.

Bladder catheterisation

Continuous bladder catheterisation with the help of an indwelling catheter is advocated in children with shock and acute renal failure. Change the urinary catheter after 48 hours. For most clinical situations, intermittent catheterisation is preferable to the use of indwelling catheter. The catheter should never be disconnected from urobag tubing. Urine may be drained from the side port of the urobag once in every shift for measuring the urine output. Do not open the urobag more frequently because of the potential risk of ascending infection.

Peritoneal dialysis

Use strict aseptic precautions as in a surgical procedure by wearing gown, mask and gloves. Do not allow the dialysis procedure to go on for more than 48 hours. In a case of messy dialysis, start appropriate antibiotics which can also be instilled into the peritoneal cavity. After the procedure, send peritoneal fluid for cytology and culture. The tip of dialysis catheter should also be sent for culture.

Chest tube drainage

Ensure strict aseptic precautions. Do not disconnect the drainage set or its tubings at any point and do not try to flush the tubings. Change the sealed bottle of water daily and affix the label at the upper level of the fluid in the drainage bottle.

Abdominal paracentesis

Take strict aseptic precautions. Apply betadine or neosporin ointment at the puncture site and affix properly to the skin. Connect the draining IV set to a closed urobag instead of leaving the tip open in a bottle.

The infection control officer should coordinate the surveillance activities and ensure compliance of strict housekeeping rituals to maintain asepsis. The cultures should be sent from various high-risk areas and equipment of PICU once every month. The nature of bacterial isolates and their antibacterial sensitivity pattern should be recorded in a software or log book. The Infection Control Committee must hold regular meetings to identify the incidence of nosocomial infections and various predisposing conditions and situations contributing to their occurrence.

REFERENCES

1. Vidyasagar D, Singh M, Bhakoo ON, *et al*. Evolution of neonatal and pediatric critical care in India. *Crit Care Clinics* 1997; 13:331-346.

2. Singhi S. Pediatric intensive care: concept and issues (Editorial). *Indian Pediatr* 1995; 32:147-157.

3. Vidyasagar D, Holbrook P. The scope of pediatric critical care. *Crit Care Med* 1980; 8:535.

4. Rosenberg DI, Moss MM, and the American College of Critical Care Medicine of the Society of Critical Care Medicine. Guidelines and levels of care for pediatric intensive care units. *Crit Care Med* 2004; 32:2117-2127.

5. Consensus Guidelines for Pediatric Intensive Care Units in India. Indian Society of Critical Care Medicine (Pediatric section) and Indian Academy of Pediatrics (Intensive Care Chapter). *Indian Pediatr* 2002, 39: 43-50.

6. Consensus guidlines for pediatric intensive care units in India. Indian society of Critical Care Medicine (Pediatric Section) and Indian Academy of Pediatrics (Intensive care chapter). *Indian Pediatr* 2002, 39:43-50.

7. American Academy of Pediatric Committee on Pediatric Emergency Medicine. Guidelines for pediatric emergency care facilities. *Pediatrics* 1995; 96:526-537.

8. Boutros AR. Pediatric intensive care in general hospital. *Pediatric Clin N Amer* 1980; 27:493.

9. Guidelines for pediatric intensive care units. *Pediatrics* 1983; 72:364-72.

10. Driscoll S, Flemming M, Khilnani P. Establishing a new Pediatric Intensive Care Unit. *Indian J Pediatr* 1993, 60(3): 331-339.

11. Committee on Hospital Care and Pediatric Section of the Society of Critical Care Medicine. Guidelines for Pediatric intensive care units. *Crit Care Med* 1993, 21: 1077-1086.

12. Tenner PA, Dibrell H, Taylor RP. Improved survival with hospitalization in a pediatric intensive care unit. *Crit Care Med* 2003; 31:847-852.

13. Mann HJ. Pharmacy technology of the ICU: Today and tomorrow. *Crit Care Clin* 2000; 16:641-658.

14. Rothstein P. Psychological stress in families of children in a pediatric intensive care unit. *Pediatr Clin N Amer* 1980; 27:613.

15. American College of Emergency Physicians: Pediatric equipment guidelines (Policy statement) *Ann Emerg Med* 1995; 25:307-309.

16. Guidelines for pediatric equipment and supplies for emergency departments. Committee on pediatric equipment and supplies for emergency departments, National Emergency Medical Services for Children Resource Alliance. *Pediatr Emerg Care* 1998; 14:62-64.

17. Deorari AK, Paul VK (Eds.). Neonatal Equipment: Everything you wanted to know. *Sagar Publications, New Delhi,* Fourth edition 2010.

18. American Academy of Pediatric Committee on Hospital Care and Society of Critical Care Medicine, Pediatric Section: Guidelines and levels of care for pediatric intensive care units. *Pediatrics* 1993; 92:166-175.

19. Yeh TS. Regionalization of pediatric critical care. *Crit Care Clin* 1992; 8:23-25.

20. Pollock MM, Patel KM, Ruttiman E. Pediatric critical care training programs have a positive effect on pediatric intensive care mortality. *Crit Care Med* 1997; 25: 1637-1642.

21. Clendenen WW, Ryan ME. Infections in the pediatric intensive care unit. How to minimize the risk? *Postgrad Med* 1985; 77:139.

22. Donowitz LG. Failure of the overgown to prevent nosocomial infection in a pediatric intensive care unit. *Pediatrics* 1986; 77:35.

23. Task force on Guidelines. Society of Critical Care Medicine. Recommendations for intensive care unit admission and discharge criteria. *Crit Care Med* 1988, 16: 807-808.

24. Dobrin RS, Block B, Gilman J, *et al.* The development of emergency transport system. *Pediatr Clin N Amer* 1980; 27:633.

25. Kabra SK, Lodha R. Pediatric Intensive Care Protocols of AIIMS. *The Indian Journal of Pediatrics,* New Delhi, 2011.

26. Baren JM, Seidel JS. Emergency drugs. *Pediatr Rev* 1994; 15:224-238.

27. Singh M, Deorari AK. Drug Dosages in Children, *CBS Publishers & Distributors Pvt Ltd, New Delhi,* 9th edition, 2015.

28. Pollack MM, Ruttimann UE, Glass NL, *et al.* Monitoring patients in pediatric intensive care unit. *Pediatrics* 1985; 76:719.

29. Pollack MM, Ruttiman UE, Getson PR. Pediatric risk of mortality (PRISM) score. *Crit Care Med* 1988; 16:1110-1116.

30. Thukral A, Lodha R, Irshad M, Arora NK. Performance of pediatric risk mortality (PRIMS), Pediatric index mortality (PIM) and PIM2 in a pediatric intensive care unit in a developing country. *Pediatric Crit Care Med* 2006, 7: 356-361.

31. Ducel G, Fabry J, Nicolle L. Prevention of hospital-acquired infections: A practical guide. World Health Organization, second edition, 2002.

32. Singh M. House keeping routines. *In:* Care of the Newborn. *CBS Publishers & Distributors Pvt Ltd, New Delhi,* 8th edition 2015 pp 66-73.

Ethical Issues, Dilemmas and Legal Aspects of Critically Sick Children

Meharban Singh

> *"No other gift is greater than the gift of life! The patient may doubt his relatives, his sons and even his parents, but he has full faith in his physician. He gives himself up in the doctor's hands and has no misgivings about him. Therefore, it is the physician's duty to look after him as his own".*
>
> **—Charaka (300 BC)**

The term ethics refers to moral principles, or a set of moral values which determine the code of conduct as stipulated by the medical profession. The ethical decisions are based upon a system of moral values that serve the best interests of society in a humane and caring way. The moral values are governed by the society and they extoll what is correct, righteous, virtuous, noble, desirable and acceptable.

There is a tremendous age old faith, trust and respect towards physicians in Indian culture. The doctor is often viewed as a demi-god (some even behave like that!) and his advice is usually considered as a gospel truth without any doubt and misgivings thus imposing an onerous responsibility on him to be ethical, up-to-date and honest in his approach and dealings with his patients. The physicians must realize that they are both morally and legally accountable to the society.

Due to rapid strides in medical technology over the years, the care of critically ill children with life-threatening disorders in the Pediatric Intensive Care Unit (PICU) has unfolded complex medical, social, ethical, philosophical, moral and legal issues[1-3]. It is a sad reality that physicians are allowing technology to de-humanize medicine. The focus has gradually shifted from the whole patient to his systems, organs, tissues, cells and even DNA! Several physicians have fallen into the trap of treating laboratory reports rather than viewing the patient in the wider context of his disease and social milieu.

Apart form tremendous financial cost of pediatric intensive care to the parents and society, there is incalculable cost in terms of pain, suffering, grief, anxiety, inadequacy, frustration and guilt not only to parents but also for the treating medical and nursing team of PICU.

Principles Governing Ethical Decisions

Ethical decisions are based on the five *prima facie* principles of beneficence, non-maleficence, parental autonomy, correct medical facts and justice[4-7]. Beneficence refers to the mandate that we should be the best advocates of our patients and safeguard their "best interests" in accordance with the age old Hippocratic tradition. It stipulates that physicians should be concerned with saving life and they should avoid doing any wilful harm to their patients, i.e., they should be non-maleficence in their diagnostic and therapeutic actions. Hippocrates said that the first dictum of patient care is *"Primum non nocere"* i.e. above all, do no harm. Almost 1000 years ago, according to Manu's code for the physicians, it was ordained that *"Dedicate yourself entirely for helping the sick, even though this may be at the cost of your own life. Never harm the sick, not even in your thoughts or dreams. May the gods help you if you follow this rule. Otherwise may the gods be against you".*

The autonomy and wishes of parents or guardians as surrogate decision makers should be honored and they should be taken into confidence while making a decision regarding the medical care of their children through a process of informed consent. The principle of justice demands that we seek the morally correct distribution of resources, ensure cost-effectiveness of therapeutic interventions by balancing medical benefits and burdens to the family and society. Distributive justice demands that no one is denied access to a reasonable level of essential care regardless of their socio-economic status.

A large number of other factors and considerations are taken into account while making a decision for various complex issues prevailing in the PICU[8, 9]. Is there a reasonable chance of survival of the child with the available technology or are the efforts likely to be futile? In what clinical situations, medical intervention is considered as futile at present? Would the quality of life be worthwhile if the child survives with aggressive management? How to assess the burdens and benefits of a therapy? Can the family afford expensive management? Should we be concerned with the "best interests" of the patient alone or global interests of the family, society and state? In what clinical situations intensive life support therapy should be withheld? Should HIV-infected child be admitted to the PICU? Should an unsalvageable child be hooked off the ventilator when a relatively better risk child who needs assisted ventilation is admitted to the PICU? There are several other confounding variables and dilemmas like cultural considerations, fertility of the parents, inter-parental harmony, gender of the child, the concept of destiny or will of God, the doctor-knows-the-best attitude, education and economic status of parents, available social support system and national priorities. However, whatever final decision is taken jointly by the medical team of experts and parents, it should be without any ambiguity and recorded in the case file with full justifications.

The Consumer Protection Act

> *"....what is not negotiable that our profession exists to serve the patient, whose interests come first. None but a saint could follow this principle all the time, but so many doctors have followed it so much of the time that the profession has been generally held in high regard."*
>
> **—Sir Theadore Fox**

Physicians are expected to provide efficient and effective medical services to the best of their abilities in a humane and compassionate manner. They are liable for penal action under the existing criminal law for acts of negligence. But, the legal procedure is time-consuming, expensive and tedious. The Medical Council of India and State Medical Councils do have the power to penalize doctors indulging in professional misconduct and malpractice. Unfortunately they have failed in their responsibility to impose deterrent punishment to medical practitioners indulging in unfair and negligent medical practices. To rectify this anomaly and ensure speedy compensation to aggrieved

persons, the apex court has decreed that the medical practitioners shall be liable under the Consumer Protection Act (CPA) 1986. Individuals and institutions who provide medical services by charging the professional fees come under the purview of CPA. When a physician or hospital provides services free of charge to all patients, the CPA cannot be invoked for claiming any damages.

The medical fraternity believes that CPA is unjustified because medical service is neither a commodity nor a contract. It is imposible to predict and judge the outcome of any treatment due to numerous variables and dynamic nature of the human body. Moreover, the CPA may further enhance the cost of medical care because doctors would indulge in "defensive" medicine (with unnecessary laboratory tests) and recover the cost of their indemnity insurance from patients. Doctors may also refuse to treat critically ill patients to avoid litigation. Above all, it has been argued that CPA may further erode the doctor-patient relationship of trust and faith, so crucial for promoting the process of natural healing.

It is true that most patients do not suspect the competence and technical expertise of doctors. They, however, do want a doctor who would listen to them, analyze their medico-psychosocial problems and they should have the option to see the same doctor as and when required. Patients want a competent, caring and concerned doctor rather than a highly trained technocrat. Despite the gradual erosion of doctor-patient relationship, a recent survey in Britain showed that 80 percent patients still trust their physicians while only 5 percent of people trust politicians. Even in the highly litigious society of the USA, it has been found that most patients sue their doctors because of lack of communication rather than due to lack of expertise and medical knowledge. In a study conducted by Association of Consumer Action Safety and Health (ACASH) it has been found that lack of proper communication is indeed the commonest reason for taking recourse to CPA (Table 2.1).

Legal Issues and Concerns

The pediatrician on duty in the emergency department may be sued either for civil or criminal offence. The civil suit is usually lodged with the consumer court to seek compensation for suboptimal care leading to avoidable complications and disability on follow-up. The parents may lodge an FIR with police leveling criminal charges against the physician for gross negligence leading to the death or disability of the patient. If found guilty by

Table 2.1 Common reasons for taking recourse against doctors under CPA*
• Lack of proper communication.
• Instigation by jealous professional "friends".
• Rude, inconsiderate, unsympathetic and casual behavior of members of health care team.
• Unsatisfactory and unfriendly hospital ethos and facilities.
• Unsatisfactory medical record keeping.
• Substandard, defective and malfunctioning medical equipment.
• Indiscriminate use of hi-tech expensive investigations.
• Lack of clear, unambiguous expert opinion.
• Lack of knowledge and expertise.
* Based on a study conducted by Association of Consumer Action Safety and Health (ACASH)

the court, the pediatricians may have to serve a term in jail and/or asked to pay compensation to the aggrieved party. The onus of providing the neglect by the physician (defendant) solely rests with the plaintiff suing the physician by providing evidence that the physician did not provide the "standard care" and negligence on his part was responsible for the death or disability of the patient. It is an unfortunate fact that the information and evidence of neglect may be provided to the parents by "professional friends" of the physician. This is in contrast with the basic tenet or principle extolled by Sir William Osler; *"Never let your tongue say a slighting word against your colleague".*

In a recent judgement, Supreme Court of India has opined that doctors cannot be charged as criminals for the death or disability of the patients under their care unless there is an evidence for gross and glaring professional neglect and incompetence. In order to reduce the menace of criminal proceedings against doctors on frivolous grounds and provide healing touch to the deteriorating doctor-patient relationship, The Supreme Court of India has made an historic judgement on February 10th, 2010 which states "......*It is the bounden duty of the civil society to ensure that the medical professionals are not unnecessarily harassed by the complainants who use the criminal process as a tool for pressurizing the medical professionals and hospitals for extracting uncalled for compensation. It would not be conducive to the efficiency of the medical profession, if a doctor is to administer medicine with a halter (nooze) around his neck."*

In order to reduce the risk of litigation, the following guidelines are useful as a safeguard against civil or criminal cases of neglect and should be followed by health care professionals.

1. The parents and patients should be treated as clients with due respect, care, concern and compassion. The interaction with parents and attendants should be pleasant and our behavior should not be abrasive, rude or crude. Most parental complaints are made when there is lack of cordial parent-physician relationship.

2. Emergency care should not be denied or delayed to any patient. Cardiopulmonary resuscitation (CPR) and stabilization care should be provided to every patient before he is referred to a higher level of care[10]. Every emergency room should have adequate quota of supplies of disposables and functional equipment to provide effective CPR.

3. Pediatric intensive care unit (PICU) should be run in a business-like manner with adequate supplies and well trained residents, nurses and support staff. The family must be made to perceive that whatever was humanely possible was done for the care of their child. Whenever consultation is required from another expert, it should be sought without any delay.

4. At the time of admission of the child to the hospital and before conducting any diagnostic or life saving therapeutic procedure, proper informed consent must be taken after explaining the likely risks and complications of the procedure[11]. The consent can be given/ signed by any one of the parents and in their absence by anyone who has brought the patient to the emergency department like a relative, neighbour, teacher, care taker, etc. In a case of life saving procedure like CPR, when consent cannot be taken, the procedure should not be delayed. However, indications and details of procedure should be recorded in the case file.

5. Maintain an uptodate medical record of the patient because in a case of legal dispute it is likely to be reviewed by an expert appointed by the court. The record should have patient's name and age, father's name, address and hospital number on each page. The entries should be dated and timed and written in detail clearly and legibly. No attempt should ever be made to "modify" the entries at a later date by deletions, alterations or additions. When there are several alterations or over writings in the medical record, the lawyer or judge is likely to assume that the record is "doctored" or tampered.

6. When a patient is suffering from a complex medical problem and the treating hospital does not have the necessary expertise and technology to manage it, the patient should be referred to a higher level of care after explaining all the pros and cons to the family. The reasons for referral should be recorded in the case file.

7. When a sick child is taken home by the parents against the advice of the treating doctor, it should be recorded in the case file as "left against medical advice" and duly counter signed by the parent.

8. It is desirable that every physician who deals with medical emergencies should obtain indemnity insurance as a safeguard against any litigation. Many hospitals pay for the malpractice insurance of their employees.

The Need and Quality of Pediatric Intensive Care Facilities

Society must make sincere efforts to provide basic or essential medical care facilities to all children irrespective of their habitat, caste, religion or social class to honor the principle of distributive justice[12]. In view of our economic constraints we should follow the philosophy of utilitarian ethics based on the concept of "value for money" and focus our resources and efforts for care of salvage-able babies.

Nevertheless, it is not only justified but highly desirable to establish PICUs in all district and state level hospitals both in the private and government sector in a phased manner throughout the country. It is mandatory to ensure equitable development of health care services for children at all levels. In order to ensure effectivity and credibility of the referral system, it is desirable to establish highly specialized medical care facilities for children suffering from life-threatening critical disorders. If cardiac intensive care units and cancer critical care units for adults is an accepted norm by the society, establishment of PICUs should be more readily acceptable because they are more cost-effective. Saving the life of an adult with stroke or cancer provides a lease of longevity for 2 to 5 years but saving the life of a child is associated with a productive life of several decades. Moreover, it is easier to salvage the life of a critically sick child due to their better recuperative capabilities and lack of degenerative changes and functional derangements in the body organs.

The modern PICU should be equipped with the state-of-the-art technology and run with business-like efficiency. It should be staffed with skillful, dedicated and trained paramedics, nurses and resident doctors. But above all, they should be enthused and equipped with qualities of human warmth, compassion and consideration. The general atmosphere of PICU should exude overall optimism rather than the gloom of hopelessness despite all the odds. It is desirable to maintain a balanced approach in various management protocols in order to avoid both under and over treatment. The PICU procedure manual should outline details of admission policies and indications for do-not-resuscitate (DNR) and for withholding/withdrawing life support systems[13,14].

In view of the shortage of nurses and local cultural considerations, at least one of the parents should be allowed to remain with the critically sick child and perform certain dedicated tasks and provide a routine conventional parenting role. They should be provided with an accurate information regarding the condition of the child on a regular and continuous basis in an easily understandable language without any medical jargon. There should be one identifiable physician for regular interaction with the family in a relaxed manner in a rest room located adjacent to the PICU. The parents greatly honor the availability of a caring, credible, considerate and compassionate health team. They need the assurance and transparency that every possible effort is being made to save the life of their sick child.

Should every Dying Child be Admitted to the PICU?

In view of limited availability of PICU beds and financial constraints, a policy of prioritization should be followed for admitting patients to the PICU. To serve the utilitarian concept of value-for-money, the priority should be accorded to critically sick children having potentially salvageable medical disorders. It is futile to admit children having irreversible terminal conditions with no chances of recovery (massive brain hemorrhage, severe hypoxic-ischemic brain damage, metastatic cancer, advanced multi-organ failure, etc.) or children with persistent vegetative state with hardly any chances of meaningful existence. Due to tremendous gap between the "haves" and "have-nots" in our society and lack of health insurance facilities, it is an unfortunate reality that intensive care is available mostly to those who can afford it and is being denied to the poor and needy segment of society. It is true but unfortunate that in a developing country, economic and social realities may outweigh ethical considerations. This situation is against the basic tenets of our constitution in which individual's right to life is enshrined in Article 21. It is, therefore, mandatory to ensure equitable development of health care services for children at all levels. In the meantime clearcut guidelines should be formulated (refer to Chapter 1) for admission and discharge of patients to the PICU to avoid any confusion and misunderstanding among the colleagues, patients and their attendants.

Importance of Communication to strengthen Doctor-patient Relationship

> *"Thou shall behave and act without arrogance and with undistracted mind, humility, and constant reflection. Thou shall pray for the welfare of all creatures...."*
> —*Charak Samhita*

Most parental complaints in the PICU originate due to lack of communication or because of abrasive, insensitive and callous attitude of the members of the health team rather than due to lack of skills or faulty technical management of the patient. We must be polite, courteous, transparent and competent in our dealings with parents and attendants. Even if the questions of parents are irrelevant, repetitive, and irritating; we must answer them with grace, equanimity and calmness without any hurry, anger or arrogance. *It is an amazing fact that most parents are grateful even when we are unable to save the life of their child especially if one showed concern, care and compassion and they were made to perceive that whatever was humanely possible was done for the care of their child.* It is important to communicate "with" parents by literally coming down to their level and by maintaining an eye-to-eye contact. It is crucial to listen and talk to the parents at least twice a day in a relaxed unhurried manner[15–18].

Humility, concern, empathy and compassion are crucial to generate faith and provide emotional support to the family at this critical juncture. The pediatrician should be careful and tactful not only in deciding "what to tell" to the parents but also "how to tell it". The parents should be told about the condition of the child in a simple, easily understandable language. We should be pragmatic and honest but always try to keep the hope alive which has tremendous healing capabilities. Avoid creating confusion in the minds of parents due to conflicting messages given by different physicians.

In a critically sick child, always give a guarded prognosis which can be tempered with hope and godly benevolence. *The health team should not only try to do their best, but the family must be made to perceive and appreciate that whatever was humanely possible in the circumstances was actually done for their child.* The parents should be encouraged to touch and talk with their critically sick child, whether he is an infant or a child in coma, because it transmits healing messages. The religious faith of the family should be honored and if the parents wish they may be allowed to use any *mantras* or amulets to enhance the process of healing through faith. By and large, efforts should be made to honor all the wishes of the parents of critically sick child if they are not obviously harmful or contrary to the recommended therapies in a specific situation.

The Concept of Medical Futility

Despite tremendous advances in medical knowledge and technology in the recent past, medicine cannot achieve immortality. Based on known medical facts, when an intended therapy is likely to fail in 100 percent cases, it is considered as futile to continue with aggressive management[13,19]. The medical therapy that merely prolongs life of a patient with permanent unconsciousness in a persistent vegetative state (PVS) or when survival is likely to be associated with virtual or total lack of cognition without any meaningful existence, the therapy becomes meaningless or a futile effort. However, in actual clinical practice these decisions are rather dificult as rightly said by Sir William Osler, *"medicine is a science of uncertainty and an art of probability"*.

Persistent Vegetative State (PVS)

Ethics and Humanities Subcommittee of the American Academy of Neurology has provided clear clinical guidelines for the diagnosis of PVS[20,21]. The common etiologic syndromes of PVS in children include near-drowning, hypoxic-ischemic encephalopathy, meningitis, encephalitis/ encephalo-pathies and degenerative CNS disorders. It is characterized by protracted coma with open eyes. There is no voluntary action or behavior of any kind though they do have periods of wakefulness and physiological sleep. They are unable to experience any suffering, pain and pleasure. They lack coordinated chewing and swallowing and thus require oro-gastric feeding. They are likely to have prolonged survival if provided with fluids and nutrition. In view of their meaningless existence without any purpose, the American Academy of Neurology has sanctioned the withdrawal of nutrition and fluids in patients with PVS if agreed by their care providers and parents through the process of informed consent. However, this approach is controversial on basic humanitarian grounds because feeding hungry people is considered as a great act of compassion while starving a dependent person is viewed with utmost aborrhence and disbelief. Therefore, they may be denied aggressive medical care but must be provided with basic needs of warmth, fluids and food with tender love and compassion.

Financial Considerations

The PICU care is highly cost-intensive and daily cost of care may be more than the monthly salary of the family. Apart from out of pocket expenses for PICU care in private sector, there are additional financial implications to the family due to lost wages, travel expenses, expenses on drugs, special diets, disposables, etc. Lack of medicare insurance coverage and profound economic disparities and unequitable social justice in developing countries further complicate the complex economic realities. The patients are often completely drained off monetarily by private corporate hospitals and then referred to the government hospitals when they are at the brink of bankruptcy and near the threshold of death. The overall gloomy prognosis and outcome both in terms of immediate survival and quality of life after survival, often makes economic drainage unbearable leading to several adverse consequences to the family dynamics for several months and years.

The Decision Making Process

Ethical decisions are based upon a system of values that serve the best interests of the society in a humane and caring way. They are based on clear understanding of a large number of complex issues. The underlying medical facts pertaining to the patient should be properly analyzed in the light of available information and technology. Sound ethical decisions can only be based on correct medical facts[22, 23]. It should be known with fair degree of confidence whether the intended therapy in a particular patient is likely to be rewarding or futile. We should carefully evaluate the burdens (suffering, death, disability) and benefits of the proposed intervention to the child, family and society (value conflicts). A team approach should be followed by taking into confidence all the medical and nursing experts for identification of various options and for

making a reasonable and right opinion The issue should be discussed with the parents to seek their opinion through a process of informed consent. The various confounding conflicts should be resolved to arrive at a mutually acceptable option through a process of consensus. The final decision should be recorded in the case file with full justifications and endorsement by the parent/s.

Withholding/Withdrawal of Life Support Therapies

There is no significant medical and moral distinction between withholding and withdrawing the life-sustaining treatment. When it is futile to treat because the condition is either irreversible and terminal or patient is in PVS or brain dead, it is undesirable and unrealistic to continue with overzealous aggressive medical therapy. The core consideration in making such a decision is evaluation of burdens and benefits of a therapy to the child, family and society ("best interest standards"). Instead of continuation of life prolonging therapy, it is desirable to provide palliative care to relieve pain and suffering. Humanistic teachings in general and philosophies of all the major religions of the world recognize that there comes a time in the care of every patient when it is appropriate for the doctor to stop further attempts to prolong unnecessarily the process of dying. A policy of passive euthanasia or "mercy killing" may be practiced by withholding CPR, life saving surgery, assisted ventilation, dialysis, vasopressors, blood and blood products and expensive antibiotics[2].

The provision of fluids and nutrition is also a form of medical therapy but its denial is controversial and often considered inhuman and cruel. Although switching off a ventilator is an "act of commission" but active euthanasia (say by intravenous administration of potassium chloride) is considered as morally, ethically and legally unjust. There is a risk of error, possibility of an abuse and likelihood of erosion of trust in the doctor-patient relationship[22]. The sanctity and dignity of life should not be sacrificed at any cost. However, unintended but foreseen consequences of over dosage of conventional drugs in the management of terminally sick patient, e.g., overdose of analgesic-sedative to a patient with cancer is practised at times without raising any eye brows. It is mandatory and desirable that all patients must be treated with love and compassion and provided adequate analgesia and sedation to relieve their pain and suffering[24].

Cardiopulmonary resuscitation is withheld if a patient is terminally sick or it is believed that the available therapies are likely to be futile and in the event of survival there will be virtual or total loss of cognition for any meaningful existence (Table 2.2). The decision should be taken after due deliberations among various experts and by taking family into confidence through the process of informed consent. The decision should be recorded in the case file along with full medical justifications and should be duly signed by the parent/surrogate. This approach is duly approved by the leading professional and academic bodies of the world. The policy is rational and logical and is aimed at reducing the suffering and misery of both the dying patient and his close relatives but it lacks legal sanction and protection[24]. Recently, The Supreme Court of India has made the historical judgement, that passive enthanasia may be practiced in selected cases after recording full medical justifications by a panel of experts and by taking the informed consent of the parents/guardian.

Table 2.2 Indications for do-not-resuscitate (DNR) orders
1. Advanced metastatic malignancy
2. Multisystem end-stage organ failure
3. Severe irreversible CNS disorder: Trauma, bleeding, and tumor
4. Severe underlying neuromotor disability
5. Persistent vegetative state
6. Brain dead*
* Usually it is an indication for withdrawal of life support

The Criteria for Diagnosis of Death

Availability of advanced life support systems has posed practical difficulties in making the diagnosis of death. There are three main reasons for declaring a patient as brain dead; (i) to save the agonizing bed-side vigil of the relatives, (ii) to reduce the financial burden to the family and make available the PICU bed to a more salvageable patient and (iii) to harness the possibility of cadaveric transplantation of certain organs such as liver, heart and kidneys. When there is irreversible cessation of circulatory and respiratory functions and CPR efforts diligently performed over a period of 30 minutes have failed, death can be certified. In patients maintained on assisted ventilation, criteria of brain death are used for declaring the patient as dead (Table 2.3)[25]. However, it must be remembered that spinal segmental responses and deep tendon jerks may persist even in the presence of brain death. After brain death and cessation of spontaneous breathing, the heart may continue to beat if mechanical ventilation maintains adequate oxygenation of blood.

Table 2.3 Clinical criteria for brain death in children
• Irreversible coma
• Absence of motor responses to pain
• Absence of pupillary responses to light and pupils are fixed at midposition (4–6 mm)
• Absence of corneal reflexes
• Absence of caloric responses (vestibulo-ocular reflex)
• Absence of gag reflex or coughing in response to tracheal suctioning
• Absence of sucking and rooting reflexes
• Absence of respiratory drive at a $paCO_2$ of 60 mmHg or 20 mmHg above the normal baseline values
• *Observation period between two evaluations on the basis of child's age. The second neurologic assessment should be done by a different attending physician but second apnea testing should be done by the same physician*
(i) Term baby up to 30 days: 24 hours
(ii) >30 days to <18 year: 12 hours
(iii) >18 years: Interval is optional
• *Confirmatory tests* (EEG and radionuclide cerebral blood flow)
(i) When clinical examination and apnea testing cannot be completed safely due to the underlying medical condition.
(ii) When there is uncertainty about the result of neurological examination.
(iii) If medication effect is present.
(iv) To reduce the inter-examination observation period.
Adapted from Nakagawa TA, Ashwal S, Mathur M, Mysore MR et al. Guidelines for the determination of brain death in infants and children. An update of the 1987 Task Force Recommendations. *Crit Care Med* 2011, 39:2139–2155.

The clinical diagnosis of brain death is based on absence of brain stem responses[26]. There are no reliable clinical criteria of brain death in preterm babies and term babies below the age of 7 days. In infants between the age of 7 days to 2 months, the brain stem responses should be absent during an observation period of 48 hr, between 2 months to 1 year for 24 hr and children older than 1 year for 12 hr before death is declared. Due to increased possibility of recovery, the observation period is prolonged in children with narcotic poisoning, exposure to severe cold, near-drowning, hypoxia, carbon monoxide exposure, electrocution, head injury, neuromuscular blockade, etc. In view of the increasing importance of early diagnosis of brain death due to the emerging possibilities of cadaveric organ donation for transplant programs, a large number of sophisticated laboratory procedures are available, but the lack of their universal availability, portability and affordability undermines their practical utility (Table 2.4).

Table 2.4 Confirmatory tests for diagnosis of brain death

- **Electroencephalography**

  Recordings are obtained for least 30 minutes with a 16- or 18-channel instrument.

  Interelectrode impedance should be between 100 and 10,000 Ω.

  The integrity of the entire recording system should be tested.

  The distance between electrodes should be at least 10 cm.

  The sensitivity should be increased to at least 2 µV for 30 minutes with inclusion of appropriate calibrations. The high-frequency filter setting should not be set below 30 Hz, and the low-frequency setting should not be above 1 Hz.

  Electroencephalography should demonstrate a lack of reactivity to intense somatosensory or audiovisual stimuli.

- **Cerebral angiography**

  The contrast medium should be injected under high pressure in both anterior and posterior circulations. No intracerebral filling should be detected at the level of entry of the carotid or vertebral artery to the skull. The external carotid circulation should be patent. The filling of the superior longitudinal sinus may be delayed.

- **Transcranial Doppler ultrasonography (TCD)**

  There should be bilateral insonation. The probe should be placed at the temporal bone above the zygomatic arch or the vertebrobasilar arteries through the suboccipital transcranial window. The abnormalities should include a lack of diastolic or reverberating flow and documentation of small systolic peaks in early systole. A finding of a complete absence of flow may not be reliable owing to inadequate transtemporal windows for insonation.

- **Cerebral scintigraphy or radionuclide brain scan (technetium Tc 99m hexametazime)**

  The isotope should be injected within 30 minutes after its reconstitution. A static image of 500,000 counts should be obtained at several time points, i.e. immediately, between 30 and 60 minutes later, and at 2 hours.

  A correct intravenous injection may be confirmed with additional images of the liver demonstrating uptake (optional).

  Brain death is confirmed if there is no radionuclide localization in the middle cerebral, anterior cerebral and basilar artery territories of the cerebral hemispheres (Hollow skull phenomenon). No tracer is seen in the superior sagittal sinus although minimal tracer may come from the scalp.

The Child with an Incurable Disease

Pediatricians often face several situations in clinical practice wherein a child is diagnosed to have a potentially fatal disease (AIDS, malignancy, genetic disorder) or develops an acute life-threatening disorder. The news of an incurable or difficult-to-manage intractable disease should be given to both the parents in a relaxed manner with due consideration and compassion. Parents must be given opportunity to ask questions and ventilate their feelings and we must listen attentively and provide appropriate answers to relieve their anxiety, concerns and worries. It is controversial as to how much information should be given to the child and whether he should be taken into confidence and told about the nature of the disease or it should be kept as a guarded secret. By and large, it depends upon the age, inquisitiveness, sensitivity and emotional maturity of the child whether he should be told about the nature of disease or not but you must seek the advice of parents in this matter. The news about the "bad" disease should never be conveyed bluntly like a bolt from the blue. We should be honest and pragmatic in our approach and the news of "gloomy prognosis" must be tempered with due optimism and godly benevolence to keep the hope alive in order to augment the process of healing. We do know that time, patience, hope, prayer, positive thinking and will power have tremendous healing capabilities and they should be effectively harnessed in our day-to-day clinical practice.

How to Communicate Death of the Child?

"Death is certain for the born and rebirth is inevitable for the dead. You should not, therefore, grieve over the inevitable".

—*Bhagvad Gita*

Although we are all destined to die and death is the greatest truth, it is always unacceptable especially so when life is cut short in the bud without fullfilment of purpose of existence or when it is due to an unnatural cause. *Despite all the technological advances, medicine cannot achieve immortality.* It is easier to face death when it is anticipated and family is adequately prepared for the eventuality. The family should be prepared emotionally and spiritually before declaration of death[27]. The news of death should be conveyed with compassion and utmost care but in no unmistakable terms that the child has died despite our best intentions and efforts. Acceptance of death becomes difficult when a child dies in the emergency department due to an acute life-threatening disease or road accident. A large number of emotions like anger, hostility, shock, grief, guilt, denial, depression, etc. need to be handled with poise, sympathy, utmost care and compassion so that reality is accepted with grace as a will of God or nature's ordain. While CPR is provided (if DNR is not applicable), the relative/attendant should be escorted to the rest room and allowed to ventilate his/her feelings. Family's wishes for religious support and ceremonies (use of amulets, *mantras*, holy water, etc.) or their desire that death should occur in the familiar atmosphere of home rather than hospital, should be honored as far as possible[28,29]. When a child is conscious and dying, the family should be at his bed side and talk with him to allay his fears and assist him to express his concerns, desires and emotions. Silent listening and support at this stage is valued more than unnecessary talking.

During their formative years some resident doctors and nurses may feel extremely frustrated and angry due to their inadequacy and inability to save life despite maximal efforts. They also need emotional support, guidance and advice to avoid unnecessary identification and attachment with the family. They should be assisted to learn the art of detachment, imperturbability and poise at all odds. After taking relevant postmortem biopsies, family should be approached with caution and tact to seek permission for autopsy. Do not give the impression that autopsy is needed for making a diagnosis but for helping the medical science and family regarding the prevention of disease among contacts and siblings and for possible genetic counseling. After completing urgent formalities, a detailed death certificate should be prepared. Provide courtesy, compassion and conveyance to the family for a dignified journey of the dead child to the mortuary or home. The coping of the death of a child in PICU is a painful and challenging experience but one that can also provide profound respect for humanity and life. Death deflates our ego and teaches us humility and provides strength to face and accept the greatest reality and truth of life, with equanimity and grace.

Ethics of Organ Transplantation

The enaction of Human Organ Transplant Act by the Indian Parliament in 1994 has opened opportunities for cadaveric transplant of heart, lungs, liver, kidneys, pancreas etc. which should be fully exploited. The possibility of positive contribution through their tragedy that their child may be able to see the world or live through somebody's else's eyes and organs, may be accepted with enthusiasm. The issue of organ donation should not broached if there are well recognized contraindications for donation of organs like primary immunodeficiency disorder, genetic defect, HIV, HBsAg-positivity, viremia and septicemia[30]. However, it is estimated that merely 1.0 percent of all perinatal deaths are due to brain death[31]. In Europe, physicians have removed organs from anencephalic infants without waiting for their death on the ground that these infants are "brain absent". This approach is not generally favored and is considered illegal in most countries.

When death occurs due to cardiorespiratory failure, it compromises the perfusion and viability of organs required for transplantation. The transplantation of cadaveric organs demands; (i) early and reliable diagnosis of brain death, (ii) the donor organs are free from transmissible viral diseases, (iii) the family is willing to donate the organs of their dead child, (iv) the organs are properly preserved and (v) the recipient/s can be readily called on a short notice. These logistic difficulties are indeed insurmountable in Indian setting thus denying the potential benefits of transplant of cadaveric organs. Children with anencephaly and persistent vegetative state are not brain dead and should not be "killed" or exploited for organ transplantation. It is unethical, illegal and immoral to trade body organs for transplantation for peculiar or financial considerations. Xenotransplantation (animal-to-human transplant) of cells, tissues and organs with or without genetic engineering is fraught with serious hazards of transmission of animal viruses, rejection, social injustice, moral and religious considerations.

Conclusions and Recommendations

Every society has the obligation to ensure that no child dies due to lack of minimal essential care regardless of the socio-economic status of their parents. The continuing process of erosion of doctor-patient relationship and trust due to insensitive and commercialized attitude of upcoming physicians (especially due to exorbitant cost of medical education in private sector) and overdemanding attitude of educated and well informed computer-savvy parents need to be checked against further disintegration. In view of the fact that services of doctors have been included in the purview of Consumer Protection Act for redressal of grievances and grant of compensation by the consumer courts, it is essential for the doctors to be more cautious, considerate and ethical in their dealings with their patients to avoid any unnecessary legal actions. It is desirable that all medical colleges in the country should initiate regular education programs in the field of behavioral sciences and medical ethics for graduate and postgraduate medical students[32]. Ethics committees should be established in all hospitals and they should serve as a watch dog to monitor and maintain the sanctity of all ethical decisions[33].

The physicians should be enthused and imbued with the qualities of sensitivity, compassion and genuine concern towards their patients through a process of role modeling by the teachers. We must learn the art of treating our patients not only with our head but also with our heart. It is nice to be a well informed doctor but it is much nicer to be a good human being in order to provide holistic care rather than mere cure to one's patients. Mother Teresa has rightly extolled that *"Medicine is a mission. It is not a profession and it is not a business"*. The physicians should make concerted efforts to resurrect medical ethics, master the sublime art of medicine and acquire the divine gift of healing.

REFERENCES

1. American Academy of Pediatrics. Committee on Bioethics. Ethics and care of critically ill infants and children. *Pediatrics* 1996; 98:149-152.

2. American Academy of Pediatrics. Committee on Bioethics. Guidelines on foregoing life-sustaining treatment. *Pediatrics* 1994; 93:532-536.

3. Singh M. Ethical and legal issues in clinical practice. In: Pediatric Clinical Methods, *CBS Publishers & Distributors Pvt Ltd,* New Delhi 5th edition, 2015, p309-319.

4. Beauchamp TL, Childress JF (eds.). Principles of Biomedical Ethics. *New York, Oxford University Press, 2001.*

5. Pellegrino AD. The metamorphosis of medical ethics. *JAMA* 1993; 269: 1158-1162.

6. Singh M. Ethical issues in perinatal medicine: Indian perspective. *Indian Pediatr* 1995; 32:953-958.

7. Singh M, Kumar S, Mittal S, *et al.* Ethical issues in perinatology: A panel discussion. *Natl Med J India* 1996; 9: 32-37.

8. Burns JP, Truog RD. Ethical controversies in pediatric critical care. *New Horiz* 1997; 5:72-84.

9. Jeena PM, Mc Nally LM, Stobie M, *et al.* Challenges in the provision of ICU services to HIV infected children in resource poor settings: a South African case study. *J Med Ethics* 2005, 31: 226-230.

10. Macro CA. Ethical issues of resuscitation. *Emerg Med Clin N Amer* 1999, 17: 527-538.

11. Lidz CW, Applelbaum DS, Meisel A. Two models of implementing informal consent *Arch Int Med* 1988, 148: 1385-1387.

12. Sarnaik AP, Daphtary K, Sarnaik AA. Ethical issues in pediatric intensive care in developing countries: combining western technology and Eastern wisdom. *Indian J Pediatr* 2005; 72 (4) :339-342.

13. The Ethics Committee of the Society of Critical Care Medicine. Consensus statement of the Society of Critical Care Medicine's Ethics Committee regarding futile and other possibly inadvisable treatments. *Crit Care Med* 1997; 25: 887-891.

14. Tomlinson T, Brody H. Ethics and communication in do-not-resuscitate orders. *N Engl J Med* 1988; 318: 43-46.

15. Barody BA. Ethical and legal issues in pediatric oncology. In: Clinical Pediatric Oncology, Fernbach DJ, Vietti TJ (Eds.), *St. Louis, Mosby Year Book Inc,* 4th edn. 1991; pp 295-303.

16. Singh M. Ethical considerations in pediatric intensive care unit: Indian perspective. *Indian Pediatr* 1996; 33:271-278.

17. Singh M. Art of Communication. In: A Manual of Essential Pediatrics. *Thieme Medical and Scientific Publishers Pvt Ltd,* New Delhi 2nd edition 2013, p6.

18. Singh M. Communication as a bridge to build a sound doctor-patient/parent relationship. *Indian J Pediatr.* 2015, doi 10.1007/s 12098-015-1853-9.

19. Schneiderman L, Jecker L, Jonsen A. Medical futility: Its meaning and ethical implications. *Ann Intern Med* 1990; 112:949-954.

20. Munsat TL, Stuart WH, Cranfort RE. Guidelines on the vegetative state: Comments on the American Academy of Neurology Statement. *Neurology* 1989; 39:123-124.

21. Position of the American Academy of Neurology on certain aspects of the care and management of the persistent vegetative state patient. *Neurology* 1989; 39:125-126.

22. Glover JJ, Holbrok PR. Ethical considerations. In: Textbook of Pediatric Critical Care. Holbrook PR (Ed.). *Philadelphia, W.B. Saunders Company,* 1993; pp 1124-1130.

23. Rustiton CH, Glover JJ. Involving parents in decisions to forego life-sustaining treatment for critically ill infants and children. *Critical Care Nursing* 1990; 1:206-210.

24. Blendon RJ, Szalay US, Knox RA. Should physicians aid their patients in dying? The public perspective. *JAMA* 1992; 267:2658-62.

25. Nakagawa TA, Ashwal S, Mathur M, et al. Guidelines for the determination of brain death in infants and children. An update of the 1987 Task Force Recommendations. *Crit Care Med* 2011, 39:2139-2155.

26. Report of Special Task Force: Guidelines for determination of brain death in children. *Pediatrics* 1987; 80:298-300.

27. Howell DA, Martinson IM. Management of the dying child. In: Principles and Practice of Pediatric Oncology. Pizza PA, Poplack DG (Eds.). *Philadelphia, J. B. Lippincott Co,* 1993; pp 1115-1124.

28. Kohler JA, Radford M. Terminal care of children dying of cancer: Quantity and quality of life. *Br Med J* 1985; 291:115-116.

29. Lauer ME, Camitta BM. Home care for dying children: A nursing model. *J Pediatr* 1980, 97:1032-1035.

30. Henderson DP. Death of a child. In: Pediatric Emergency Medicine. Barkin RM (Ed.). *St Louis, Mosby Year Book,* 1992; pp 60-65.

31. Singh M. Ethical issues and dilemmas in the care of newborn babies in the developing world. *Semin Neonatal* 1999; 4:151-157.

32. Singh M. Behavioral sciences and medical ethics for undergraduate students. *Indian J Med Educ* 1994; 33:30-34.

33. Singh M. Ethical and social issues in the care of newborn babies. *Indian J Pediatr* 2003; 70:417-420.

Cardiopulmonary Resuscitation

Krishan Chugh

Death of a child is a major catastrophe for a family and a challenge for health care professionals. Medical science has advanced to a stage wherein impending death can be recognized and many a times the child can be 'revived' even after all the discernible signs of life have ceased. The series of coordinated interventions designed to restore adequate ventilation and circulation in a child whose vital functions have ceased is called cardiopulmonary resuscitation (CPR). Two separate levels of skills and medical care have been defined in the context of CPR: *Basic Life Support (BLS) and Advanced Life Support (ALS)*.

Pediatric Basic Life Support (PBLS) consists of sequential assessments and motor skills designed to support or restore effective ventilation and circulation in a child in respiratory or cardiorespiratory arrest (CPA). Ideally, PBLS should begin within seconds after it is recognised that a need for it exists, because the only tools required are rescuer's mouth, hands and a sincere will on his/her part to save a life. However, if adjuncts such as bag and mask are readily available they should be used if the rescuer ('Provider') is trained in their use. Thus, PBLS is mainly for out-of-hospital CPA. PBLS training should ideally be made available to all the responsible citizens. However, teachers, day care boarding professionals, sports supervisors, life guards and parents of children suffering from chronic illnesses should be the special targets for training.

When CPA has occurred or is impending, prompt access to pediatric advanced life support (PALS) would also be required. It may be provided at the out-of-hospital location or within the health care facility. PALS consists of PBLS plus advanced airway management, quick vascular access, use of drugs and defibrillator to stabilize the victim. PALS can be provided by medical personnel or paramedics under the supervision of a physician. PALS training should be mandatory for all prehospital and hospital personnel who are involved in the medical care of the infants and children. Further, the CPR training

(PALS course) should be revised at regular intervals.

This chapter will focus on the pre-resuscitation, resuscitation and post resuscitation aspects of cardiopulmonary arrest (Table 3.1) and emphasise the assessment, action and reassessment cycle (Figure 3.1).

Table 3.1 The components of CPR
◆ Emphasising age-related differences
◆ Recognition of CPR situation
◆ Providing pathophysiological background
◆ Describing methods and skills of CPR
● PBLS
● PALS
◆ Emphasising steps of post CPR stabilization

OUTCOME OF CPR

Unlike adults, CPA due to primary cardiac events is less likely in children. Infact, ventricular fibrillation has been reported in less than 10 to 15 percent of children less than 10 years age who experience pulseless arrest outside the hospital[1,2]. Respiratory conditions are by far the most common cause of cardiac arrest. Many a times the child has isolated respiratory arrest when life support measures are started. However, if there is a delay, respiratory arrest leads to hypoxemia and acidosis which culminate in bradycardia or asystole. It has been seen that of all the arrhythmias associated with cardiac arrest, asystole accounts for 78 percent, bradyarrhythmias account for 12 percent and ventricular arrhythmias remaining 10 percent[3].

Rapid and effective bystander CPR is associated with successful return of spontaneous circulation (ROSC) and neurologically intact survival in children following out-of-hospital cardiac arrest.[4,5] Bystander resuscitation may have the greatest impact for out-of-hospital respiratory arrest,[6] because survival rates >70% have been reported with good neurologic outcome.[7] Bystander resuscitation may also have substantial impact on

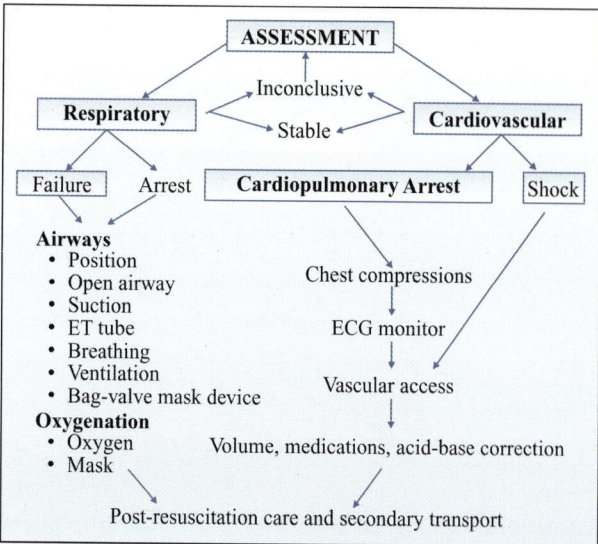

Figure 3.1 The resuscitation process

survival from primary ventricular fibrillation (VF), because survival rates of 20% to 30% have been documented in children with sudden out-of-hospital witnessed ventricular fibrillations (VF)[8].

Overall only about 6% of children who suffer an out-of-hospital cardiac arrest and 8% of those who receive prehospital emergency response resuscitation survive, but many suffer serious permanent brain injury as a result of their arrest.[8-11] Out-of-hospital survival rates and neurological outcome can be improved with prompt bystander CPR,[7,12] but only about one third to one half of infants and children who suffer cardiac arrest receive bystander CPR.[10,13] Infants are less likely to survive out-of-hospital cardiac arrest (4%) than children (10%) or adolescents (13%), presumably because many infants included in the arrest figure are found dead after a substantial period of time, due to sudden infant death syndrome (SIDS).[9] As in adults, survival is greater in pediatric patients with an initial rhythm of VF or pulseless ventricular tachycardia (VT) than in those with asystole or pulseless electric activity.[8,9]

Results of in-hospital resuscitation are better with an overall survival of 27%.[14,15] The 2008 pediatric data from the National Registry of Cardio-Pulmonary Resuscitation (NRCPR) recorded an overall survival of 33% for pulseless arrests among the 758 cases of in-hospital pediatric arrests that occurred in the participating hospitals. Pediatric patients with VF/pulseless VT had a 34% survival to discharge, while patients with pulseless electric activity had a 38% survival. The worst outcome was in patients with asystole, only 24% of whom survived to hospital discharge. Infants and children with a pulse, but poor perfusion and bradycardia

who required CPR, had the best survival (64%) to discharge. Children are more likely to survive in-hospital arrests than adults,[14] and infants have a higher survival rate than children.

Once the respiratory arrest is prolonged, tissue hypoxia leads to multiple organ failure. When heart and breathing stop, the likelihood of recovery without brain damage is best if effective CPR is started within first 4 minutes. As time elapses, the chances of brain damage increase greatly[16,17]. Hypoxia and ischemia cause permanent cellular injury leading to an immediate or delayed death. In the former, CPR is unable to reestablish spontaneous circulation. In the latter, perfusion is temporarily restored but critical organ dysfunction continues. It may manifest as recurrent cardiac arrests, hypoxic encephalopathy with severe brain damage or complete brain death, acute pulmonary injury, disseminated intravascular coagulation, acute tubular necrosis, hepatic failure, sepsis and multiple organ failure.

Primary goal of CPR is to restore spontaneous circulation before the point of irreversibility is reached. Secondary attention is then shifted to treating the underlying cause and enhancing the degree of neurologic recovery. However, efforts at cerebral resuscitation have been disappointing[18,19]. These low percentages of survival and even lower chances of survival with intact brain functions is indeed depressing but one must draw motivation from those survivors who are useful to the society. After all, the only alternative to CPR is a certain death.

CAUSES AND CORRELATES OF CARDIOPULMONARY ARRESTS

In majority of children, CPA is the culmination of a cascade of pathophysiological changes that have been going on for a period of time before the CPA actually occurs. In other words, CPA can be anticipated most of the times. The conditions which lead to CPA vary according to age and the type of population studied (Table 3.2).

Table 3.2 Common causes of cardiopulmonary arrest
• Anaphylaxis
• Respiratory diseases e.g. Aspiration, pneumonia, ARDS
• Sepsis and meningitis
• Gastroenteritis
• Airway obstruction (including foreign body aspiration)
• Seizures
• Accidents: Trauma, burns and drowning

Children in PICU are always at a higher risk for CPA because of the nature of their underlying illness and unstable hemodynamic status. Several interventions, which can precipitate CPA in such children, are listed in Table 3.3.

Children with certain specific conditions are more vulnerable to develop CPA and should be closely watched for development of complications which can culminate in CPA (Table 3.4).

PATHOPHYSIOLOGY OF CARDIOPULMONARY ARREST

Final common pathway leading to cardio-pulmoanry arrest is the same regardless of the underlying disease and its complication and is shown in Figure 3.2.

Respiratory failure is defined as a clinical state characterised by inability to deliver adequate oxygen to meet the demands of the tissues. As long as the child is able to meet these demands by increasing work of breathing he is in potential respiratory failure (respiratory distress).

Shock is defined as a clinical state charactersied by inability of circulation to meet the oxygen and metabolic demands of tissues. As long as the blood pressure is normal it is known as compensated shock and when the blood pressure falls the patient has gone into decompensated stage of shock. Inadequate delivery of substrate and oxygen to the tissues leads to anerobic metabolism (accumulation of lactic acid and fall in pH), organ dysfunction and finally organ death. Hypotension is defined as a systolic blood pressure

Table 3.4 Special conditions predisposing to cardiopulmonary arrest	
Conditions	**Complications**
Trauma	• CNS injury • CNS depression • Cervical spinal injury • Hemorrhagic shock • Upper airway obstruction • Pneumothorax • Flail chest
Burns	• Hypovolemic shock • Inhalation injury • Airway obstruction • Carbon monoxide poisoning
Gastroenteritis	• Hypovolemic shock, dyselectrolytemia
Seizures	• Upper airway obstruction • Respiratory depression • Drugs leading to apnea
Coma	• Aspiration, blocked airways
Critically ill child	• Raised intracranial tension • Natural history of life threatening disease • Complications of treatment • Premature withdrawal of life support • Unintentional withdrawal of life support
Immediate post-CPR	• Life support stopped too soon • Precipitating event recurs • Hypoxic ischemic vital-organ damage
During IPPV	• Endotracheal tube displacement • Pneumothorax • Endotracheal tube obstruction • Equipment failure
Tracheostomy	• Obstruction • Dislodgement

Table 3.3 High risk procedures that may lead to CPA	
Intervention	**Cardiopulmonary outcome**
• Sedation	Respiratory depression
• Suctioning • Passage of nasogastric tube • Intubation • Manipulation of airways	Bradycardia due to vagal stimulation
• Rectal temperature measurement • Lumbar puncture • Patient restraint • Painful procedures	Bradycardia due to Valsalva's maneuver
• Decreasing oxygen support • Decreasing ventilator support • Extubation	Respiratory distress/failure
• Oral feeding	Aspiration
• Chest physiotherapy	Airway obstruction by mobilizing secretions

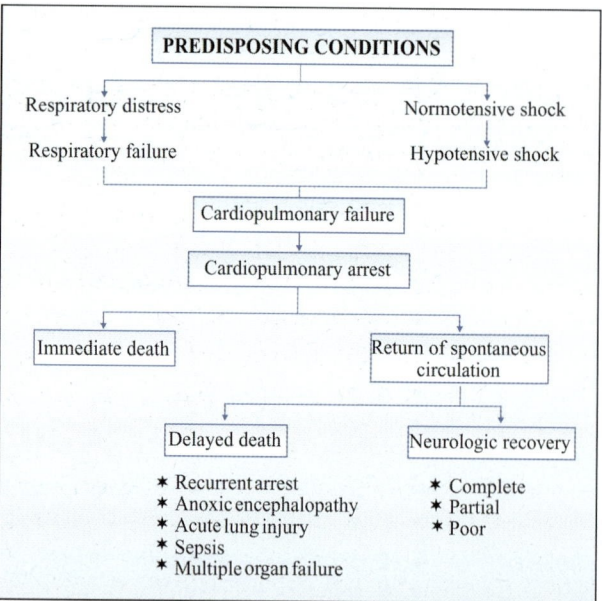

Figure 3.2 Pathophysiology of pediatric cardiopulmonary arrest

less than the 5th percentile of normal for age[20], as given below:

- <60 mm Hg in term neonates (0 to 28 days)
- <70 mm Hg in infants (1 month to 12 months)
- <70 mm Hg + (2 x age in years) in children 1 to 10 years
- <90 mm Hg in children ≥ 10 years of age

RAPID CARDIOPULMONARY ASSESSMENT

To provide optimum therapy to a critically ill child who develops cardiopulmonary failure or arrest, an accurate but rapid assessment is necessary. The three components of this assessment are A, B, and C i.e. **A**irway, **B**reathing and **C**irculation (Table 3.5).

The airway may be (a) clear or patent, (b) maintainable by non-invasive methods like head positioning or suctioning or (c) not maintainable without invasive methods like endotracheal intubation, needle cricothyrotomy, and foreign body removal maneuvers, etc.

Increased rate of breathing is an early sign of respiratory failure while slow, irregular or gasping breaths are ominously late signs. The breathing should be assessed by minute ventilation (tidal volume × respiratory rate). The clinical correlates of these parameters can be assessed on the bed side by observing the chest rise and auscultating the breath sounds (tidal volume) and counting the respiratory rate. The work of breathing is assessed clinically by the degree of respiratory distress.

Table 3.5 Rapid cardiopulmonary assessment	
Respiratory assessment	**Cardiovascular assessment**
A. Airway patency ◆ Able to maintain independently ◆ Requires adjuncts/assistance **B. Breathing** ◆ Rate ◆ Mechanics • Retractions • Grunting • Accessory muscles use • Nasal flaring ◆ Air entry • Chest expansion • Breath sounds • Stridor • Wheezing • Paradoxical chest movements ◆ Color • Pink • Blue • Pale • Mottled	**C. Circulation** ◆ Heart rate ◆ Blood pressure ◆ Volume/strength of central pulses ◆ Peripheral pulses • volume/strength • Present/absent ◆ Skin perfusion ◆ Capillary refill time ◆ Difference in the core and toe temperature ◆ Pink, blue, pale or mottled skin **CNS perfusion** ◆ Responsivenss (AVPU) • **A**wake • Responds to **v**oice • Responds to **p**ain • **U**nresponsive ◆ Recognizes parents ◆ Muscle tone ◆ Pupil size ◆ Posturing

Circulation is dependent on the cardiac output and the peripheral vascular resistance. Cardiac output is a product of stroke volume and heart rate. Stroke volume in turn depends on the preload, myocardial contractility and afterload. It is essential to remember these principles of pathophysiology because an assessment of each one of these components is possible clinically. Further, therapeutic interventions are available to manipulate and regulate them.

Early recognition of poor circulation (shock) is dependent on assessment of perfusion of various organs like skin, brain, kidneys, etc. as fall in blood pressure is a late sign (decompensated shock). Skin perfusion can be assessed on the bed side and is an early sign of shock. Prolonged capillary refill time (> 2 sec) is abnormal if the ambient temperature is not very low. Cold extremities occur late in the course of shock. Pink color of the skin usually indicates normal tissue perfusion while pallor indicates ischemia, cyanosis indicates hypoxemia and mottling of skin indicates either or both. CNS perfusion is best reflected in the level of responsiveness. For rapid assessment, Glasgow coma scale is not recommended, instead 4 levels as listed in Table 3.5 are easy to assess.

Urine output is a very important parameter for assessment of perfusion of kidneys, and indirectly other vital organs. However, it can be assessed only over a period of time. Hence, it has a limited value for rapid assessment of perfusion in a child with CPA.

PRIORITIES IN MANAGEMENT

The purpose of rapid cardiorespiratory assessment is to quickly decide the priorities of the medical team. An experienced physician should be able to complete the rapid assessment in 30 seconds and categorise the child in the clinical states listed in Table 3.6. The priorities in management can then be decided.

Although a large number of variables can be monitored there are only a few which are helpful in improving the outcome, others are merely distracting. The child should be assessed at frequent intervals, at least every 3-5 minutes regarding the parameters listed in Table 3.7. It is very important to constantly monitor the technique of CPR and the ability of the rescuers to carry out the tasks assigned to them. Similarly, it is not uncommon for the equipment failure to go unnoticed in the supercharged atmosphere of CPR.

The most important electronic monitor is the electocardiographic monitor because different interventions are required for different types of cardiac electrical activity. Continuous $EtCO_2$ measurement is useful to assess the effectiveness of CPR. A rising $EtCO_2$ value generally indicates return of spontaneous circulation[17,21]. A low $EtCO_2$ value may indicate poor pulmonary blood flow or an esophageal intubation[3, 22].

Diagnosis of barotrauma (leading to pneumothorax) is also made clinically during CPR and empirical treatment is recommended without awaiting for confirmation by a chest radiograph. Measurement of blood pressure by an indwelling arterial catheter provides invaluable information. Aortic diastolic pressure relates directly to the adequacy of coronary perfusion during CPR[23]. Myocardial blood flow is a major determinant of return of spontaneous circulation following CPR[24]. Coronary perfusion pressure has prognostic value. $EtCO_2$ has also been correlated with the coronary perfusion pressure[25].

PEDIATRIC BASIC LIFE SUPPORT

The purpose of performing CPR is to provide oxygen to the vital organs, the heart and brain, until

Table 3.6 Categorization of children with CPA	
Categories	**General actions**
1. Stable	Observe, reassess
2. Potential respiratory failure or shock	Sequential assessment and laboratory studies. Prompt, gentle actions like position of comfort, supplemental oxygen, normal ambient temperature and withholding feeding
3. Definite respiratory failure or shock	A. **A**irway: Maintain patency B. **B**reathing: Maximize oxygenation C. **C**irculation: Vascular access D. **D**rugs
4. Cardiopulmonary failure	All the steps listed above (A, B, C, D). Priority actions are ventilation and oxygenation

Table 3.7 Monitoring during CPR
The Patient
• Chest expansion with each assisted breath on both sides
• Any spontaneous breathing
• Color
• Breath sounds in axillae
• Heart rate
• Central pulses, peripheral pulses
• Pupillary reflexes
• Abdominal distension
• Level of consciousness
The Rescuer
• Position of rescuer's hands
• Depth, and quality of chest compressions
• Rescuer's exhaustion
The Monitors
• ECG
• Pulse oximeter
• Non-invasive blood pressure monitor
• Arterial pressure (when line obtained)
• CVP (when line obtained)
• Capnometer (EtCO$_2$)
• Temperature
The Laboratory Tests
No laboratory test is generally recommended during CPR
The Equipment
• Oxygen turned on or not, flow rate
• Oxygen tubing connected to bag + reservoir assembly
• Vascular access site
• Suction pressure adequate or not
The Drugs
Leader of the team keeps a mental/written record of drugs being administered and decides on the need for repeating/stepping up the doses.
The Time
• For timing of repeated doses of drugs
• For timing of recovery
• For deciding when to abandon CPR

normal circulation is restored. A systematic approach has been designed to standardize the technique so as maximum benefit may be provided to the critically ill child without causing any harm.

The sequence of starting CPR in BLS in children has now been modified from "ABC" to "CAB"[26], i.e chest compressions, airway and then breathing on the basis of adult studies in whom VF cardiac arrest is more common and for whom chest compressions are more important for return of spontaneous circulation.[27,28]

Asphyxial cardiac arrest is more common than VF cardiac arrest in infants and children, and ventilations are extremely important in pediatric resuscitation. Animal studies[29] and a recent large pediatric study[30] show that resuscitation results for asphyxial arrest are better with a combination of ventilations and chest compressions. It is, however, unknown whether it makes a difference if the sequence begins with ventilations (ABC) or with chest compressions (CAB). Starting CPR with 30 compressions followed by 2 ventilations should theoretically delay ventilations by only about 18 seconds for the lone rescuer and by an even shorter interval for 2 rescuers. The CAB sequence for infants and children is recommended in order to simplify training with the hope that more victims of sudden cardiac arrest will receive bystander CPR. It offers the advantage of consistency in teaching rescuers, whether their patients are infants, children, or adults.[26]

Healthcare providers are more likely to work in teams and less likely to be lone rescuers. Activities described as a series of individual sequences are often performed simultaneously (e.g. chest compressions and preparing for rescue breathing) so there is less significance regarding what is performed first. It is reasonable for healthcare providers to tailor the sequence of rescue actions to the most likely cause of arrest.[26] Figure 3.3 summarizes international pediatric basic life support algorithm.

BEGINNING CPR

The guidelines delineate a series of skills as a *sequence* of distinct steps depicted in the Pediatric BLS Algorithm, but they should be performed *simultaneously* (e.g. starting CPR and activating the emergency response system) when there is more than one rescuer.

Safety of the Rescuer and Victim

Always make sure that the area is safe for you and the victim. Care should be taken to move the child gently, especially if trauma to the neck or spine is suspected. However, it is mandatory to move the victim if he is found in a dangerous location (e.g. a room full of smoke) or if CPR cannot be performed where he is found. When the child is moved the head and body must be held and moved as a unit and head and neck firmly supported so that head does not roll, wobble, twist or tilt.

Assess Need for CPR

To assess the need for CPR, the lay rescuer should assume that the cardiac arrest is present if the victim is unresponsive and not breathing or only gasping.

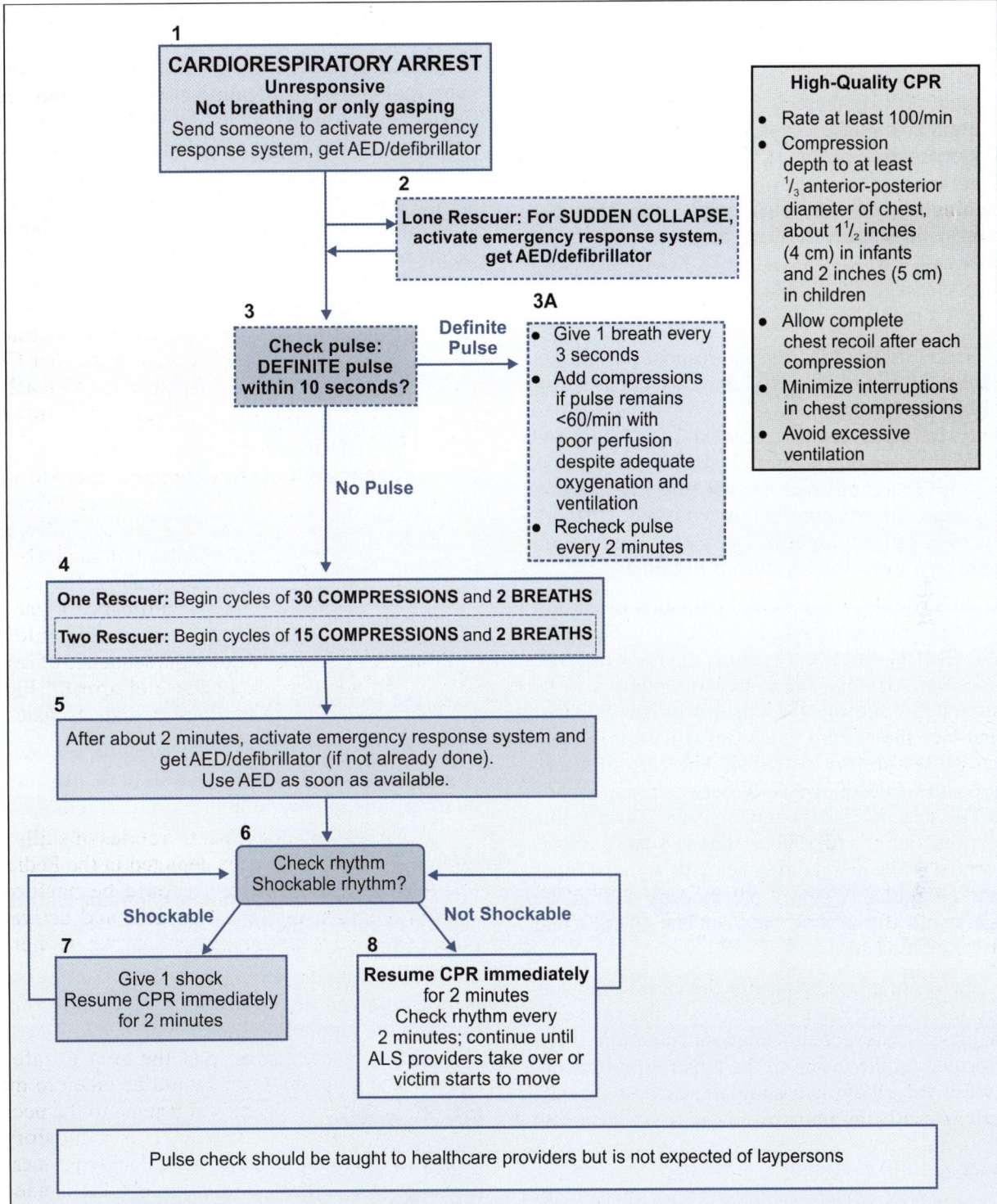

1

CARDIORESPIRATORY ARREST
Unresponsive
Not breathing or only gasping
Send someone to activate emergency
response system, get AED/defibrillator

2

Lone Rescuer: For SUDDEN COLLAPSE,
activate emergency response system,
get AED/defibrillator

High-Quality CPR

- Rate at least 100/min
- Compression
  depth to at least
  $1/3$ anterior-posterior
  diameter of chest,
  about $1^1/_2$ inches
  (4 cm) in infants
  and 2 inches (5 cm)
  in children
- Allow complete
  chest recoil after each
  compression
- Minimize interruptions
  in chest compressions
- Avoid excessive
  ventilation

3

Check pulse:
DEFINITE pulse
within 10 seconds?

Definite
Pulse

3A

- Give 1 breath every
  3 seconds
- Add compressions
  if pulse remains
  <60/min with
  poor perfusion
  despite adequate
  oxygenation and
  ventilation
- Recheck pulse
  every 2 minutes

No Pulse

4

One Rescuer: Begin cycles of **30 COMPRESSIONS** and **2 BREATHS**

Two Rescuer: Begin cycles of **15 COMPRESSIONS** and **2 BREATHS**

5

After about 2 minutes, activate emergency response system and
get AED/defibrillator (if not already done).
Use AED as soon as available.

6

Check rhythm
Shockable rhythm?

Shockable   **Not Shockable**

7

Give 1 shock
Resume CPR immediately
for 2 minutes

8

Resume CPR immediately
for 2 minutes
Check rhythm every
2 minutes; continue until
ALS providers take over or
victim starts to move

Pulse check should be taught to healthcare providers but is not expected of laypersons

Figure 3.3 Algorithm for basic life support

Check for Response

Gently tap the victim and ask loudly, "Are you okay?" Call the child's name if you know it. If the child is responsive, he or she will answer, move, or moan. Quickly check to see if the child has any injuries or needs medical assistance. If you are alone and the child is breathing, leave the child to phone the emergency response system, but return quickly and recheck the child's condition frequently. Children with respiratory distress often assume a position that maintains airway patency and optimizes ventilation. Allow the child with respiratory distress to remain in a position that is most comfortable. If the child is unresponsive, shout for help.

Check for Breathing

If you see regular breathing, the victim does not need CPR. If there is no evidence of trauma, turn the child onto the side (recovery position), which helps maintain a patent airway and decreases risk of aspiration. If the victim is unresponsive and not breathing (or only gasping), begin CPR. Treat the victim with gasps as though there is no breathing and begin CPR.

Pulse Check

If the infant or child is unresponsive and not breathing (gasps do not count as breathing), healthcare providers may take up to 10 seconds to attempt to feel for a pulse (brachial in an infant and carotid or femoral in a child). If, within 10 seconds, you don't feel a pulse or are not sure if you feel a pulse, begin chest compressions. It can be difficult to feel a pulse, especially in the heat of an emergency, even for healthcare providers.

In an adult or older child palpation of carotid pulse is recommended because of ready accessibility to the rescuer performing the ventilation. Usually, there are no clothings to be removed for feeling the carotid pulse. Further, sometimes the carotid pulse can still be felt when other pulses are not palpable. The carotid artery lies on the side of the neck between the trachea and the sternocleidomastoid muscle. To feel this artery the victim's thyroid cartilage (Adam's apple) is located while maintaining head tilt with the other hand. The pulse is gently palpated by sliding the fingers into the groove between the trachea and sternocleidomastoid.

In an infant, palpation of the carotid pulse is more difficult because of the short and fat neck. Brachial pulse is recommended for palpation. It can be located on the inside of the upper arm, midway between the elbow and shoulder, as it is pressed gently towards the humerus.

Chest Compressions

During cardiac arrest, high-quality chest compressions generate blood flow to vital organs and increase the likelihood of ROSC. If the infant or child is unresponsive and not breathing, give 30 chest compressions.

Chest compressions are serial, rhythmic compressions of the chest that result in circulation of oxygen containing blood to the vital organs (heart, lungs and brain) until advanced life support can be provided. To perform chest compressions, the victim must be placed supine on a hard surface, like a board, ground or floor. For an infant this hard surface can also be the rescuer's hand with the palm supporting the infant's back. The victim's head should not be higher than the chest otherwise gravity will impede flow of blood to the brain.

In case of infants the area of compressions is the lower half of the sternum. Index finger is kept just below the infant's nipples on the sternum. The middle finger is placed adjacent to the index finger. Sternal compressions are performed approximately one finger below the level of the nipples using two or three fingers (Figure 3.4). Alternatively the chest of the infant may be encircled by both the hands supporting the back and the thumbs placed on the lower sternum to deliver the compressions (Figure 3.5). The sternum is compressed approximately one-third the depth of the chest.

At the end of each compression the sternum should be allowed to return back briefly to its normal position. However, during pressure release the fingers should not be lifted off the chest. A smooth compression-relaxation rhythm should be developed at least at a rate of 100 per minute. The 2 thumb encircling hands chest compression technique is the preferred technique for 2 rescuer infant CPR. The 2 finger technique is recommended for 1 rescuer infant CPR to facilitate rapid transition between compression and ventilation and to minimize interruptions in chest compressions. It remains an acceptable alternative method of chest compressions for 2 rescuers.

To perform chest compressions in children, using two fingers the lower margin of the rib cage is traced towards the midline into the notch where the sternum and the ribs meet. The heel of this hand is placed over the lower half of the sternum; between the nipple line and the notch, avoiding the

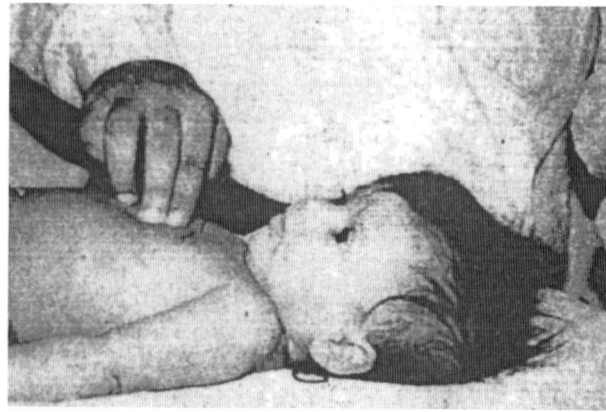

Figure 3.4 External cardiac massage in an infant. Two fingers are placed over the lower sternum 2 cm below the internipple line to compress heart. The infant should lie on a hard surface

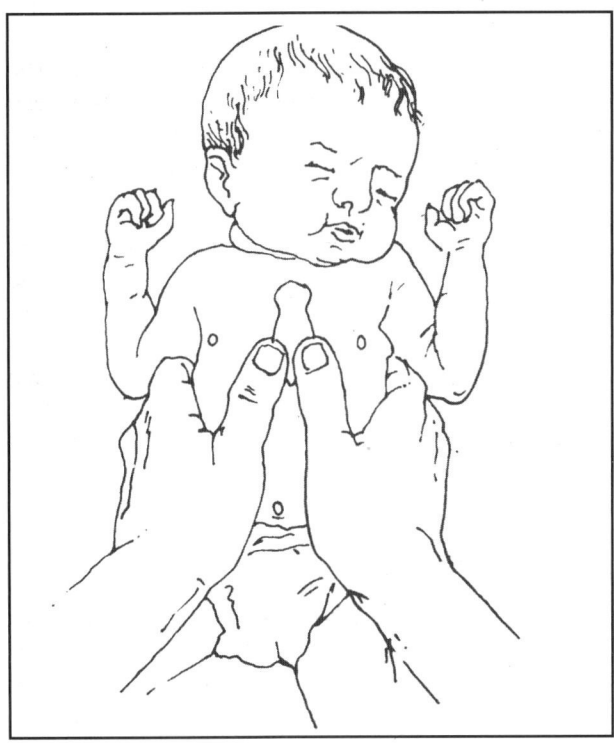

Figure 3.5 External cardiac massage by using thumbs of both hands

xiphoid process. The long axis of the heel is over the long axis of the sternum. The chest is compressed to approximately one-half to one-third of its total depth. The compression rate is kept at 100 per minute. Both the 1 and 2 hand techniques for chest compressions in children are acceptable provided that the rescuers compress the lower part of the sternum to a depth of approximately one-third of the anterior-posterior diameter of the chest.

The following are characteristics of high-quality or effective CPR:

(i) Chest compressions of appropriate rate and depth. "Push fast": push at a rate of at least 100 compressions per minute. "Push hard": push with sufficient force to depress at least one third the anterior-posterior (AP) diameter of the chest or approximately $1^{1}/_{2}$ inches (4 cm) in infants and 2 inches (5 cm) in children. Inadequate compression depth is common even by health care providers[31].

(ii) Allow complete chest recoil after each compression to assist the heart to refill with blood.

(iii) Minimize interruptions of chest compressions.

(iv) Avoid excessive ventilation.

Chest compressions are preferably delivered on a firm surface for better results.[32] For an *infant,* rescuers should compress at least one third the depth of the chest, or about 4 cm (1.5 inches). Do not press on the xiphoid or the ribs. For a *child,* compress the lower half of the sternum *at least* one third of the AP dimension of the chest or approximately 5 cm (2 inches) with the heel of one or both hands. Do not press on the xiphoid or the ribs. Because children and rescuers come in all sizes, rescuers may use either 1 or 2 hands to compress the child's chest.

After each compression, allow the chest to recoil completely because complete chest reexpansion improves the flow of blood returning to the heart and thereby blood flow to the body during CPR[33]. During pediatric CPR incomplete chest wall recoil is common, particularly when rescuers become fatigued[31]. Incomplete recoil during CPR is associated with higher intrathoracic pressures and significantly decreased venous return, coronary perfusion, blood flow, and cerebral perfusion. Rescuer fatigue can lead to inadequate compression rate, depth, and recoil.[31] Rescuers should, therefore, rotate the compressor role approximately every 2 minutes to prevent compressor fatigue and deterioration in quality and rate of chest compressions. The switch should be accomplished as quickly as possible (ideally in less than 5 seconds) to minimize interruptions in chest compressions.

Resuscitation outcomes in infants and children are best if chest compressions are combined with ventilations, but if a rescuer is not trained in providing ventilations, or is unable to do so, he should continue with chest compressions ("Hands-Only" or compression-only CPR) until help arrives.

Open the Airway and give Ventilations

For the lone rescuer a compression-to-ventilation ratio of 30:2 is recommended. After the initial set of 30 compressions, open the airway and give 2 breaths. In an unresponsive infant or child, the tongue may obstruct the airway and interfere with ventilations.[34]

Head tilt-chin lift. If there is enough tone in the muscles of the jaw, tilting the head back will cause the mandible to move forward and open the airway. In the absence of sufficient muscle tone, as is often the case in an unconscious child, a head tilt alone will be inadequate to open the airway[23]. When this is the case, the mandible may need active support by lifting the chin. To perform this technique one hand is placed on the child's forehead and the head is tilted backwards into a neutral position. The neck is slightly extended. The fingers (without the thumb) of the other hand are placed under the bony

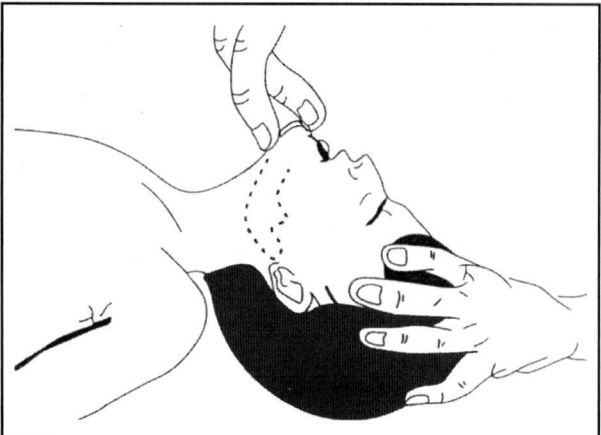

Figure 3.6 Opening the airway by head tilt-chin lift maneuver

part of the lower jaw at the chin and the mandible is lifted forwards and upwards (Figure 3.6). Care is taken not to close the mouth or push on soft tissues under the chin, because this may obstruct rather than open the airway.

Jaw thrust. In a victim of suspected neck injury extension of the neck can be dangerous. Hence, jaw thrust is the safer method compared to the head tilt-chin lift. Two or three fingers are placed under each side of the lower jaw at its angle and the jaw is lifted upwards and outwards (Figure 3.7). If this method is unsuccessful, the head may be extended very slightly and another attempt made to ventilate.

To give breaths to an infant, use a mouth-to-mouth-and-nose technique (Figure 3.8); to give breaths to a child, use a mouth-to-mouth technique (Figure 3.9).[35] Make sure the breaths are effective (i.e. the chest rises). Each breath should take about one second. Pause between breaths to breathe. If the chest does not rise, reposition the head, make a better seal, and try again.[35] It may be necessary to move the child's head through a range of positions to provide optimal airway patency and effective rescue breathing.

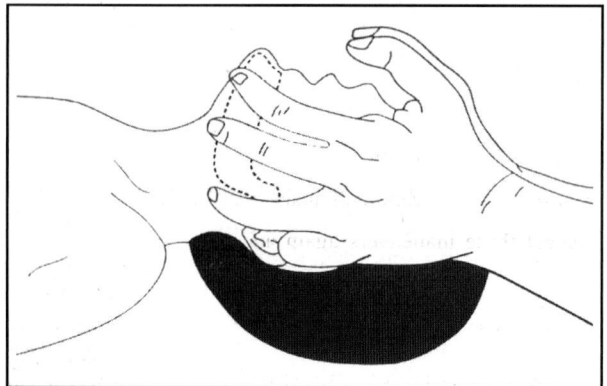

Figure 3.7 Opening the airway with the jaw thrust maneuver

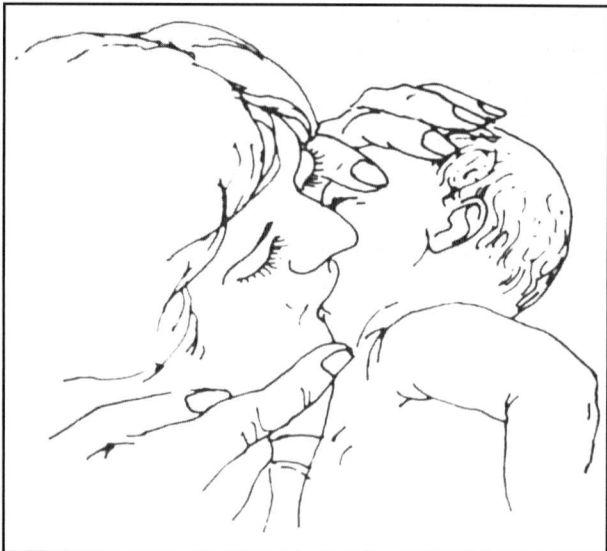

Figure 3.8 Mouth-to-mouth resuscitation with nose seal in an infant. Oral air (rather then exhaled breath) should be blown into baby's mouth and nose

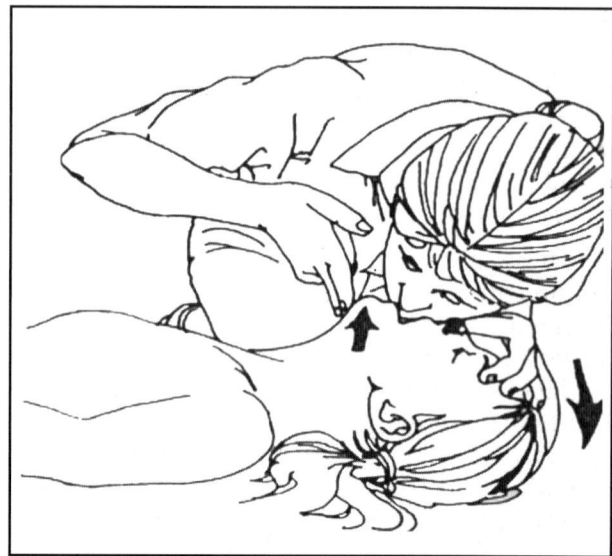

Figure 3.9 Mouth-to-mouth breathing in a child. In older children mouth-to-mouth seal is made during artificial breathing while pinching the nose of the victim

In an infant, if you have difficulty making an effective seal over the mouth and nose, try either mouth-to-mouth or mouth-to-nose. If you use the mouth-to-mouth technique, pinch the nose closed. If you use the mouth-to-nose technique, close the mouth. In either case make sure the chest rises when you give a breath. If you are the only rescuer, provide 2 effective ventilations using as short a pause as possible after each set of 30 chest compressions.

To minimize the pressure required for ventilation and to prevent the development of gastric distension, breaths should be delivered slowly[36]. An appropriate tidal volume is that which causes the chest to rise. Patency of the airway should be checked if air does not enter freely. An obstruction should be suspected if the chest wall does not rise. Other possible causes may be less volume or delivery of air under low pressure.

Mouth-to-barrier device ventilation is preferred by some, in view of the possibility of transmission of infections, including HIV. Masks and face shields have been designed for this purpose and may be used if readily available. However, care should be taken not to waste any time in procuring such a device. Further, the correct size of the mask is mandatory as otherwise the seal may not be airtight.

Coordinate Chest Compressions and Breathing

After giving 2 breaths, immediately give 30 chest compressions. The lone rescuer should continue this cycle of 30 chest compressions and 2 breaths for approximately 2 minutes (about 5 cycles) before leaving the victim to activate the emergency response system, if one exists, and provide an automated external defibrillator (AED) if one is nearby.

If an advanced airway is in place, cycles of compressions and ventilations are no longer delivered. Instead the compressing rescuer should deliver at least 100 compressions per minute continuously without pauses for ventilation. The ventilation rescuer delivers 8 to 10 breaths per minute (a breath every 6 to 8 seconds), being careful to avoid excessive ventilation in the stressful environment of a pediatric arrest.

Activate Emergency Response System

If there are 2 rescuers, one should start CPR immediately and the other should activate the emergency response system (if one exists) and obtain an AED, if one is available. Most infants and children with cardiac arrest have an asphyxial rather than a VF arrest; therefore 2 minutes of CPR are recommended before the lone rescuer activates the emergency response system and gets an AED if one is nearby. The lone rescuer should then return to the victim as soon as possible and use the AED (if available) or resume CPR, starting with chest compressions. Continue with cycles of 30 compressions to 2 ventilations until emergency response rescuers arrive or the victim starts breathing spontaneously.

OTHER CONDITIONS

Foreign Body Airway Obstruction

Foreign body aspiration into the airway causing complete obstruction followed by cardiopulmonary arrest is a common cause of airway obstruction, especially in infants and toddlers. However, differentiation from infective or other causes is important. If infection is the cause, maneuvers to dislodge the foreign body are dangerous and may result in inappropriate delay in transporting or treating the patient. Infection may be suspected if the patient has fever or evidences of cough and cold.

A foreign body may cause partial or complete obstruction. If the patient is acyanotic, conscious and has an adequate air exchange he should be encouraged to cough forcefully and breathe sponta-neously.

Relief of airway obstruction should be attempted only if signs of complete airway obstruction are observed. These signs include ineffective cough (loss of sound), increased respiratory difficulty accompanied by stridor, development of cyanosis and loss of consciousness. If there is no chest rise during CPR rescue breaths in an unconscious patient, despite the correct position of the head and jaw, should raise strong suspicion of a foreign body in the airway.

Maneuvers to relieve airway obstruction caused by a foreign body depend on age of the victim (Table 3.8). Heimlich's maneuver (subdiaphragmatic abdominal thrusts) increases the intrathoracic pressure, creating an artificial cough that forces air and may force the foreign body out of the airway. In an infant abdominal thrusts are not recommended because of potential risk of injury to the unprotected upper abdominal organs leading to laceration of liver, rupture of stomach, diaphragm and jejunum.

Table 3.8 Methods to relieve airway obstruction due to foreign body	
Infant	Back blows (5 times) Chest thrusts (5 times)
Child	Heimlich maneuver (5 times)
Adult	Heimlich maneuver (5 times)
Repeat these maneuvers again and again till the victim expels the foreign body or becomes unresponsive.	

Finger Sweeps

Blind finger sweeps should not be performed in infants and children because the foreign body may be pushed back into the airway causing further obstruction or injury to the supraglottic structures. In the unconscious adult patient, the finger sweep is performed by opening the mouth by grasping the tongue between the thumb and fingers and lifting the mandible. This maneuver alone may relieve the obstruction. Otherwise, the finger of the free hand may be inserted along the inside of the cheek and deeply into the throat down to the base of the tongue. A hooking action should be used to dislodge the foreign body.

The Infant

When the infant is conscious he is straddled over the arm of the rescuer with face down and head lower than the trunk. The infant's head is supported with the rescuer's hand around the chest and the jaw. When support is adequate 4-5 back blows are rapidly delivered with the heel of the hand between the infant's shoulder blades (Figure 3.10). Now, the free hand is placed over the infant's back, holding the infant's head. The infant is effectively sandwiched between the two arms and hands of the rescuer. The infant is turned and held supine on the rescuer's thigh. The infant's head remains lower than the trunk all this while. Up to five quick downward chest thrusts are given in the same location and manner as external chest compressions for cardiac arrest.

The airway may now be opened by using the head tilt-chin lift, and if spontaneous breathing is absent and the chest does not rise on rescue breathing, the maneuvers may be repeated till either the foreign body is expelled or the infant becomes unconscious.

If the infant becomes unconscious, the airway is opened using the tongue-jaw lift and if a foreign body is seen it is removed with a finger sweep. Rescue breathing is now attempted. If chest does not rise adequately the back blows and chest thrusts described above are repeated until the ventilation is established.

The Child

In children and adults, the Heimlich maneuver is recommended to dislodge a foreign body. To perform the maneuver the rescuer stands behind the conscious victim and wraps his hands around the patient's waist. He grasps one fist with the other hand and places the thumb side of his fist against the patient's abdomen in the midline slightly above the naval and well below the tip of the xiphoid process. The rescuer then presses his fist 5 times into the patient's abdomen with a quick inward and upward thrust, each thrust being separate and a

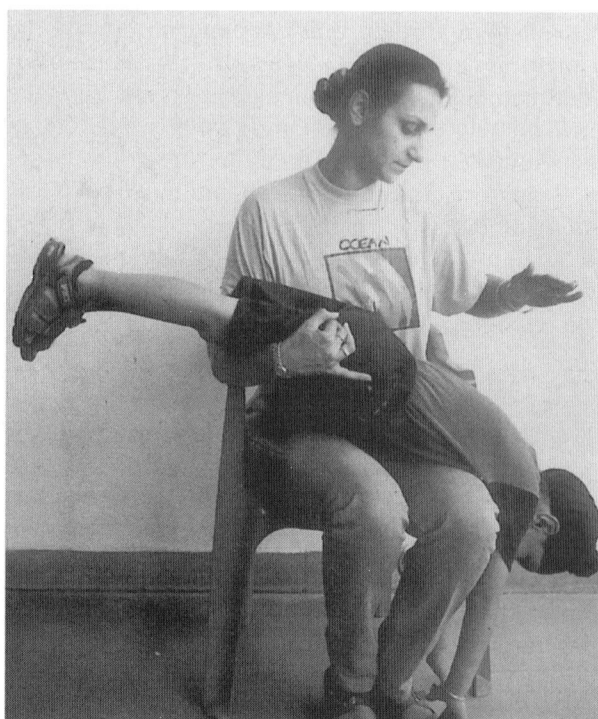

Figure 3.10 Procedure for dislodging foreign body in a child. The toddler is suspended upside down on the arm or legs and thumped firmly on the back between the shoulder blades

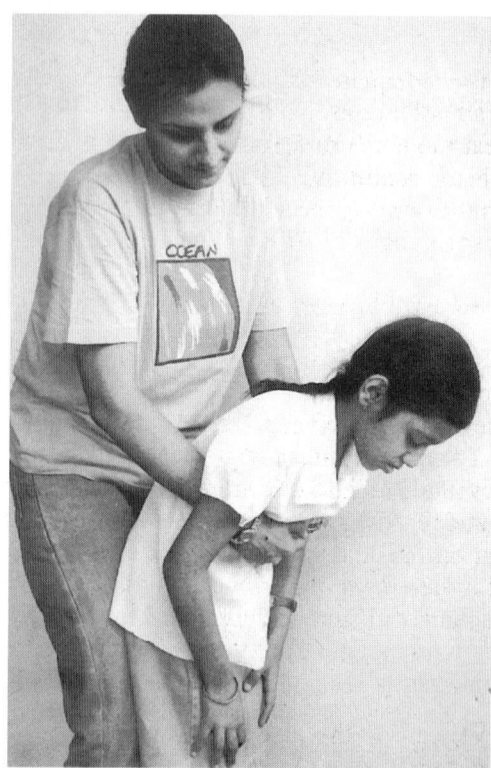

Figure 3.11 Heimlich's maneuver. The child is firmly held from behind by interlocking your hands over the center of the abdomen just below the rib cage. The locked hands are sharply pulled upwards with thrusting movements to raise the pressure inside the abdomen and chest

distinct movement. These thrusts are repeated till the child expels the foreign body or loses consciousness (Figure 3.11).

If the child loses consciousness finger sweep may be performed carefully as described earlier. To perform this maneuver on an unconscious child he should be placed supine. The rescuer should kneel beside the victim or straddle his hips. The rescuer places his one hand in the midline slightly above the naval and well below the xiphoid process. The other hand is placed on top of the first. Both hands are pressed into the abdomen with a quick upward thrust. A series of 5 such thrusts are performed. At the end of five thrusts the airway is opened with tongue-jaw lift and finger sweep performed if foreign body is seen. Rescue breathing is attempted again. If unsuccessful, Heimlich's maneuver is repeated.

Abdominal and chest thrusts have been noted to cause rupture or laceration of abdominal or thoracic viscera. Regurgitation of abdominal contents and aspiration may also occur as a result of abdominal thrusts. During Heimlich maneuver upto one liter of air is expelled by a thrust with an average pressure of 31 mmHg[37].

Inadequate Breathing with Pulse

If there is a palpable pulse >60 per minute but there is inadequate breathing, give rescue breaths at a rate of about 12 to 20 breaths per minute (1 breath every 3 to 5 seconds) until spontaneous breathing resumes. Reassess the pulse every 2 minutes but spend no more than 10 seconds doing so.

Bradycardia with Poor Perfusion

If the pulse is < 60 per minute and there are signs of poor perfusion (ie, pallor, mottling, cyanosis) despite support of oxygenation and ventilation, begin chest compressions. Because cardiac output in infancy and childhood largely depends on heart rate, profound bradycardia with poor perfusion is an indication for chest compressions because cardiac arrest is imminent and beginning CPR prior to full cardiac arrest results in improved survival.[38]

Defibrillation

VF can be the cause of sudden collapse[39] or may develop during resuscitation attempts.[40] Children with sudden witnessed collapse (eg, a child collapsing during an athletic event) are likely to have VF or pulseless VT and need immediate CPR and rapid defibrillation. VF and pulseless VT are referred to as "shockable rhythms" because they respond to electric shocks (defibrillation). Many AEDs have high specificity in recognizing pediatric shockable rhythms, and some are equipped to decrease (or attenuate) the delivered energy to make them suitable for infants and children < 8 years of age.[41] For infants a manual defibrillator is preferred when a shockable rhythm is identified by a trained healthcare provider. The recommended first energy dose for defibrillation is 2 J/kg. If a second dose is required, it should be doubled to 4 J/kg. If a manual defibrillator is not available, an AED equipped with a pediatric attenuator is preferred for infants. An AED with a pediatric attenuator is also preferred for children < 8 year of age. If neither is available, an AED without a dose attenuator may be used. AEDs that deliver relatively high energy doses have been successfully used in infants with minimal myocardial damage and good neurological outcomes.[42] Rescuers should coordinate chest compressions and shock delivery to minimize the time between compressions and shock delivery and to resume CPR, beginning with compressions, immediately after shock delivery. The AED will prompt the rescuer to re-analyze the rhythm every 2 minutes. Shock delivery should ideally occur as soon as possible after compressions.

Defibrillation Sequence Using an AED

Turn the AED on.

(i)   Follow the AED prompts.
(ii) End CPR cycle (for analysis and shock) with compressions, if possible
(iii) Resume chest compressions immediately after the shock.

Minimize interruptions in chest compressions.

The BLS maneuvers have been summarized in Table 3.9. In general, the recent recommendations have emphased that the quality of CPR should be increased by the recommendations: *"Push hard, push fast, minimize interruptions; allow full chest recoil, and do not hyperventilate"*.

ADVANCED LIFE SUPPORT (ALS)

Vascular Access

Rapid vascular access is one of the key aspects of successful CPR because drugs and fluids are critical for effective management of CPA. It is often difficult to establish a "life line" in children, more so in infants. Crucial time is sometimes wasted in trying to secure an intravenous access. Peripheral veins are usually collapsed and

Maneuver	Infant (< 1yr)	Child (1to 8 yr)	Child and adult (> 8 yr)
o **Airway**	Head tilt-chin lift*	Head tilt-chin lift*	Head tilt-chin lift*
o **Breathing**			
• Initial	Two breaths at 1 to 1½ sec/breath	Two breaths at 1 to 1½ sec/breath	Two breaths at 1 to 1½ sec/breath
• Subsequent	20 breaths/min	20 breaths/min	20 breaths/min
o **Circulation**			
• Pulse check	Brachial/femoral	Carotid	Carotid
• Compression area	Lower half of sternum	Lower half of sternum	Lower half of sternum
• Compression width	2 or 3 fingers	Heel of one hand	Two hands stacked together
• Depth	Approximately one-third the depth of the chest or 1.5 inches	Approximately one-third the depth of the chest or 2 inches	1.5-2 inches
• Rate	At least 100/min	100/min	80-100/min
• Compressions- ventilation ratio			
Two rescuers	15:2	15:2	15:2
Single rescuer	30:2	30:2	30:2
o **Maneuver for removal of foreign body**	Back blows/chest thrust	Heimlich maneuver	Heimlich maneuver

Table 3.9 Summary of BLS maneuvers

* If trauma is present, use only jaw thrust

unidentifiable in a patient in CPA. In two studies[43,44] with a combined experience of almost 100 children in arrest, one-fourth had no intravenous access even after 10 minutes. Venous cutdowns are no better[45]. Limiting the time spent attempting to establish peripheral venous access in a critically ill or injured child is of paramount importance[46]. There are many possible routes of access. They have been classified as direct and indirect (Table 3.10).

Table 3.10 Vascular access during CPR

Direct vascular access
* Intravenous
   Central
   Peripheral
* Intraosseous
* Intraarterial
* Intracardiac

Indirect vascular access
* Endotracheal
* Sublingual

Priorities of Access

During CPR or decompensated shock, prompt availability of vascular access is more important than the site of access. The best site of access depends on provider's expertise and clinical circumstances[20].

A plan best suiting the environment, skills, and resources of the resuscitation team should be prospectively devised. Such a protocol saves time and increases the chances of success. In children upto 6 years of age a brief attempt is made to start peripheral intravenous line. If no access is achieved promptly, then an intraosseous needle should be placed (Table 3.11).

Table 3.11 Vascular access on the basis of age of the child

Infants and children (younger than 6 years)
* Attempt a peripheral line (including antecubital vein)
* If IV access in not rapidly achieved try intraosseous access
* Later, central line placement (femoral, subclavian, external or internal jugular veins; femoral is preferred)

Children (older than 6 years) and adults
* First attempt: Peripheral line
* Second attempt: Intraosseous access or central line placement

In the older child peripheral venous access is generally easier than in younger patient. If peripheral intravenous placement fails, then an intraosseus access or femoral vein or another central vein cannulation may be attempted. Efforts should be made to ensure sterility of the procedure without compromising on time.

Peripheral Venous Access

This is the safest method of intravenous access. Generally, a large vein such as the antecubital vein is chosen because of ease of cannulation, its relatively fixed anatomical position (and hence chance of success even in 'blind' placement when it is not visible due to vascular collapse) and no interference with ventilation and chest compressions that are likely to be performed simultaneously by other members of CPR team. Although it has been shown that supradiaphragmatic and central veins are better[47], the peripheral vein is acceptable. To avoid delay in drugs reaching the heart, it is essential to follow each medication by a saline flush. Half to one ml/kg of saline is usually sufficient for peripheral and intraosseous line[48] with a minimum of 5 ml. The needle cannulas (angiocaths) have now more or less replaced the butterfly needles for establishing peripheral venous access.

Central Venous Access

The central venous lines are the gold standard against which other routes of resuscitative drug delivery are compared[48, 49]. The central venous drug administration produces more rapid onset of drug action and higher peak drug levels than peripheral venous drug administration in adults. However, this advantage does not appear to be present in pediatric animal models or clinical studies[50,51]. Because peripheral routes compare favorably when properly flushed and because of the risks involved, attempts at subclavian or internal jugular catheterisation are best avoided in an infant or a small child during CPR. Further, these attempts are likely to interfere with ventilation and chest compressions. Femoral venous access is much safer. Over the needle catheter (Seldinger technique) or through the needle catheters, both have been used in pediatric age group. Seldinger technique is usually preferred. Placement of a central venous catheter requires training and experience, and the procedure can be time consuming. Therefore central venous access is not recommended as the initial route of vascular access in an emergency[52].

Intraosseous Access

The major merits of intraosseous (IO) technique are its rapidity, high success and low complication rates. Intraosseous access can be reliably achieved in 30 to 60 seconds in most cases,

even by healthcare providers with minimal experience[53,54]. This route delivers the drugs or fluids into the noncollapsible marrow venous plexus from where emissary veins carry them to the general circulation. It being a large vascular bed, rapid infusions required for volume resuscitation in cases of shock can also be administered by this route. Blood transfusions, irritant infusions, catecholamine infusions and even viscous drugs have been successfully administered through this route[55]. In addition to infusion, the procedure allows bone marrow aspiration which can be analysed for pH, pCO_2, blood culture and blood typing and cross matching[56].

The technique of IO line placement is simple. A bone marrow needle with stylet or the specially designed intraosseous needles are recommended. However, in a desperate situation any wide bore strong needle, especially if it has a stylet can be used. The needle is inserted into the medial surface of tibia 1-3 cm below the tibial tuberosity. This point is generally one finger width below and just medial to the tibial tuberosity. The needle is directed slightly inferiorly to avoid damage to the epiphyseal plate. The needle should be kept approximately perpendicular to the surface of the bone. The advancing force over the needle head is released as soon as a sudden decrease in resistance to forward motion of the needle is felt. A test injection of 10 ml normal saline can be used to ascertain the position of the needle. Insertion is successful and the needle is clearly in the marrow cavity if the following conditions are fulfilled: (i) a sudden decrease in resistance occurs as the needle passes through the bony cortex into the marrow, (ii) the needle can remain upright without support, (iii) marrow can be aspirated and (iv) fluid flows in freely through the needle without evidence of subcutaneous infiltration. If there is an evidence of infiltration or if test injection fails, a second attempt at intraosseous cannulation should be performed on the contralateral tibia.

Distal femur, medial malleolus and anterior superior iliac spine are the alternative recommended sites for children. IO access can be used in all age groups, including preterms. In older children and adults, distal tibia, anterior superior iliac spine, distal radius or distal ulna can be used. Sternal IO cannula for adults are now available[20].

The complication rates with IO technique are usually less than 1 percent[57,58]. Reported complications include osteomyelitis, tibial fracture, compartment syndrome and skin necrosis.

Intra-arterial access

The arterial catheterisation during CPR should only be used in selected cases and that too only by specially experienced CPR team members who have expertise in performing the procedure and interpreting the data.

Endotracheal access

During CPR attempts to established intra-venous access may fail sometimes, especially in infants. In such situations endotracheal route can be used for administration of some of the drugs (Table 3.12). It can serve as a temporary route till direct intravascular route is established. Ionized medications such as sodium bicarbonate or calcium chloride cannot be given by the endotracheal route.

Table 3.12 Endotracheal route for administration of drugs

Drugs that can be given
- Epinephrine
- Lidocaine
- Atropine
- Naloxone

Dosages
- Epinephrine 10 times of IV dose
- Others 2 to 3 times of IV dose

Methods of drug administration
- Dilute in 3-5 ml normal saline, instill directly, give IPPR
- Instill via catheter, flush with 3-5 ml normal saline, give IPPR

The drugs reach the pulmonary tree which has a large surface area and rich vascularity. In some studies rate of absorption and physiological effects of epinephrine and atropine administered by the endotracheal route compared favorably with intravenous route[23]. However recent animal studies suggest that the concentration of drugs in blood after ET administration is low. Lower concentration of epinephrine can cause hypotension, lower coronary artery perfusion pressure and flow, and reduced potential for return of spontaneous circulation[59]. Another risk associated with the endotracheal route of administration is the formation of an intra-pulmonary depot of the drug, which may prolong the drug's effect. This could result in postresuscita-tion hypertension or the recurrence of fibrillation after normal circulation is restored[23]. Thus, intra-osseous or IV are the preferred routes of drug delivery.

Sublingual access

The deep sublingual region has a large venous plexus, which facilitates rapid drug absorption. During CPR epinephrine is probably the only drug worthy of this extraordinary route of administration.

ADJUNCTS FOR AIRWAYS AND VENTILATION

Oxygen Therapy

During CPA there is profound hypoxemia of the tissues. Hence, maximum or high concentration of oxygen should be delivered to the lungs. Oxygen toxicity is not a hazard during short period of cardiopulmonary resuscitation and no patient during CPR should be denied 100 percent oxygen.

However, once the child has been 'revived' and stabilized, oxygen delivery to the lungs may be reduced under close clinical and pulse oximeter monitoring to a safer level. It is only at this stage,

Table 3.13 Oxygen delivery devices		
Device	**Flow rate**	**Oxygen (%)**
Low flow systems		
1. Nasal cannula	1-6 L/min	Maximum 45%
2. Nasal catheter	-do-	-do-
3. Face mask	5-10 L/min	35-60%
4. Venturi type masks	5-10 L/min	25-60%
High flow systems		
1. Oxygen hood	10-15 L/min	upto 80-90%
2. Partial rebreathing mask	10-12 L/min	50-60%
3. Non-rebreathing mask	10-12 L/min	upto 90%
4. Anesthesia bag with non-rebreathing mask	10-12 L/min	upto 95%
During CPR only 90– 100 percent oxygen delivery devices are advised. Other delivery systems are recommended only after stabilization.		

(when spontaneous respiration is effective) that other oxygen delivery devices may be used. Oxygen delivery systems may be high flow or low flow systems (Table 3.13).

Low flow systems are those in which room air is entrained because the gas flow is insufficient to completely meet the inspiratory flow requirements Low flow systems generally provide 23-60 percent oxygen and they are not very reliable. High flow systems, because of higher flow rates and the addition of reservoirs provide adequate gas flow to meet the total inspired flow requirements of the patient, so entrainment of room air does not occur. High flow systems can reliably deliver either low or high oxygen inspired concentrations. Hence, they are preferred in the emergency settings.

Patient size and minute ventilation has a profound effect on oxygen delivery[60]. Thus, a low flow device like the nasal cannula delivering just 1 L/min oxygen to a 2 kg newborn acts almost as efficiently as a high flow device with 10-12 L/min oxygen for an older child of say 20 kg.

Suction

To maintain a clear airway one may have to suck out secretions, blood, vomitus or meconium from the oropharynx, nasopharynx or trachea. Both, portable and installed suction equipment should be available for CPR. An installed suction unit should be capable of generating a vacuum of 300 mm Hg when the tube is clamped. A suction force of 80-120 mm Hg is generally necessary to suck the airway of an infant or child.

Appropriate sized flexible plastic suction catheters for the endotracheal tube or tracheostomy, a nonbreakable collection bottle, and a supply of sterile water for clearing tubes and catheters should be available. Thicker, wide bore, more rigid suction catheters are advisable for removing thick secretions and particulate matter from the pharynx. All possible sterile precautions should be taken and endotracheal suctioning time should not exceed 5 seconds each time. Further, each attempt should be preceded and followed by a short period of ventilation with 100 percent oxygen to minimise hypoxemia.

Oropharyngeal Airways

Appropriate sized airway when inserted into an unconscious patient is a great help as it prevents falling back of the tongue. However, when introduced into a conscious or stuporous patient, laryngospasm or vomiting may be induced besides excessive secretions and agitation. Improper placement of the oropharyngeal airway usually results in backward displacement of the tongue into the pharynx and worsening of airway obstruction.

Airway sizes of 4 to 10 cm in length are used for infants and children. Appropriate size for the child may be estimated by placing the orpharyngeal airway next to the face and measuring the length from the corner of the mouth to angle of the jaw. If the oropharyngeal airway is too large it may obstruct or traumatize the laryngeal structures.

Masks

During CPR in hospital and more frequently in pre-hospital setting ventilation is performed via a mask with a bag–valve–mask system. Currently, disposable, soft–plastic, transparent face masks are available in various sizes. A proper sized mask should allow an airtight seal. A mask should reach from the midportion of the bridge of the nose to the protuberance of the chin without extending over the end of the chin. Thus, it must enclose both the nose and mouth but avoid compression of eyes.

Bag and Mask Ventilation

Self inflating bags with valves and attached reservoir are used for resuscitation for providing ventilation during CPR by most providers. However, trained personnel can use the anesthesia bag as an alternative. A correct size bag is chosen. Generally, 450-500 ml bag is recommended for full term newborn infants, infants and younger children. For, older children and adults 750 ml or a larger sized bag is recommended for resuscitation.

Technique of ventilation requires some training and skill. The provider should be able to deliver effective oxygenation and ventilation keeping the airways open and assessing the effectiveness of ventilation. The rescuer should use only the force and tidal volume necessary for the chest to rise visibly. Excessive ventilation volumes and pressures may compromise cardiac output, overdistend the alveoli, increase the chances of aspiration and pneumothorax.

Currently, the E-C clamp technique is recommended for holding the mask over the face. The thumb and forefinger form a "C" shape to tightly seal the mask onto the face while the remaining fingers of the same hand form an "E" shape to lift the jaw, pulling the face toward the mask[61]. If the airway resistance is high or lung compliance is not good, two rescuers may be required to provide sufficient ventilation. One rescuer uses both hands to open the airway and maintain a tight E-C clamp mask-to-face seal while the other rescuer compresses the ventilation bag.

Endotracheal Tubes

After a brief period of bag–valve–mask breathing with 100% oxygen a translaryngeal endotracheal tube should be placed. The ET tube should be sterile, disposable, transparent, appropriate sized and not too pliant. Either cuffed or uncuffed endotracheal tubes can be used for intubation in both infants and children.[52] Moreover, under certain circumstances (e.g. poor lung compliance, high airway resistance and large glottic air leak), cuffed tracheal tubes may be preferable.

The size of ET tube is chosen according to the size and age of the child. A popular formula to calculate the diameter of the ET tube is given below:

$$\text{ET tube size (inner diameter in mm)} = \frac{\text{Age (yr)}}{4} + 4$$

In addition to the calculated ET tube size, a 0.5 mm size smaller and a 0.5 mm size larger tubes are kept ready. By looking at the laryngeal opening through the laryngoscope the experienced rescuer decides which of the above 3 chosen sizes would be most appropriate for a particular child. When cuffed ET tube is being used the size chosen is 0.5 mm less than the one calculated by the above formula.

Length-based resuscitation tapes are helpful and more accurate than age-based formula estimates of endotracheal tube size for children up to approximately 35 kg,[62] even for children with short stature.[63] Length of the tube to be inserted (from the gum margin to the midtrachea) is estimated by the formula:

$$\text{Length (cm)} = \frac{\text{Age (yr)}}{2} + 12$$

Another popular formula for estimating the length of ET tube is:

Depth of insertion = inner diameter x 3.

Table 3.14 gives the average size of endotracheal tubes and suction catheters required in infants and children.

Once the tube has been inserted, its position is checked to ensure correct placement by following features:

(i) Auscultation of breath sounds in both axillae. They should be equal on two sides.

(ii) Absence of breath sounds over the stomach area.

(iii) Symmetrical chest expansion with positive pressure breaths.

(iv) Improvement in color, heart rate and perfusion.

(v) Direct visualization of the vocal cords and "glottic marker" on the ET tube through laryngoscope.

(vi) Improvement in oxygenation as measured by pulse oximeter and increasing end–tidal CO_2 strip.

(vii) After stabilization, the precise location of ET tube may be checked by radiography. Flexion and extension of the neck can produce relatively large movements of the tip of the ET tube resulting in extubation (during extension) or bronchial intubation (during flexion). Hence, due care should be taken to maintain neutral position, especially during nursing procedures and transportation.

Although all the above steps are useful, it is recommended that in all settings (i.e. pre-hospital, emergency departments, intensive care units, operating rooms), confirmation of tracheal tube placement should be achieved using detection of exhaled CO_2 in intubated infants and children with a perfusing cardiac rhythm. This may be accomplished using a colorimetric detector (CO_2 strip) or capnometry[64]. During cardiac arrest, if exhaled CO_2 is not detected, tube position should be confirmed using direct laryngoscopy[52].

The ET tube should be properly fixed using adhesive tape that ensures stability without damaging the skin (especially during removal).

A properly secured ET tube serves the following purposes:

- Provides a secure, and stable airway for oxygenation and ventilation
- Protects the airway against gross aspiration
- Allows removal of secretions
- Reduces dead space
- Helps avoid gastric distension
- Provides route for drug delivery
- Allows hyperventilation in patients with raised intracranial pressure.

If ET tube is confirmed to be correctly placed but bagging is not producing adequate chest expansion (and there is no improvement in SaO_2, $EtCO_2$ and arterial blood gas analysis) one of the following conditions should be ruled out:

(i) ET tube is too small. The airleak can be minimized by putting a larger size tube

(ii) Air is leaking at one of the joints / connections. The air leak should be detected and corrected.

(iii) Inadequate size or poor compression of the resuscitation bag is giving inadequate tidal volume.

(iv) Pop-off valve of the bag is not occluded so that the air-oxygen mixture escapes into atmosphere.

(v) Poor compliance of lungs or airway obstruction may require higher pressures to be applied.

(vi) ET tube is blocked

(vii) Lungs are being compressed from outside eg air or fluid in the pleural cavity or profound abdominal distension.

When a patient with ET tube shows sudden deterioration, one of the following conditions should be looked for which can be remembered by the acronym DOPE.

Displaced tube:

- ET tube too far down into one of the main bronchus – withdraw the tube
- ET tube 'out'–reinsert the tube
- ET tube in the esophagus – reinsert the tube

Obstructed tube: Do suction, if it is completely or severely obstructed, replace the tube

Pneumothorax: Urgent decompression .

Equipment failure: Identify the 'failed' equipment and replace it.

Sellick maneuver. During emergency endotracheal intubation an assistant applies pressure over the cricoid by palpating the cricoid cartilage between the thumb and second finger and exerting downward pressure. During this the esophagus is occluded between the trachea and the cervical vertebrae, thereby preventing aspiration. Further, this maneuver helps in better visualization of the glottis. Once the position of the ET tube has been confirmed to be correct, the cricoid pressure can be released. There is insufficient evidence to recommend routine cricoid pressure application to prevent aspiration during endotracheal intubation in children. Do not continue cricoid pressure if it interferes with ventilation or the speed or ease of intubation[52].

Laryngeal Mask Airway (LMA)

LMA has been used in the operation theater by anesthetists for short anesthesia with satisfactory

Table 3.14 Guidelines for endotracheal tube and suction catheter sizes		
Age	Distance from teeth/ gums to mid trachea (cm)	Suction catheter (Fr)
Premature baby	8	5-6
Term infant	9-10	6-8
6 months	10	8
1 year	11	8
2 years	12	8
4 years	14	10
6 years	15	10
8 years	16	10
10 years	17	12
12 years	18	12
Adolescent	20	12

control of airways during the past few years. The LMA may be an acceptable initial alternative airway adjunct for experienced providers during pediatric cardiac arrest when tracheal intubation is difficult to achieve.[65,66] However, its use is associated with a higher incidence of complications in young children.[67,68] If an advanced airway is in place during CPR (e.g. endotracheal tube, LMA), ventilate at a rate of 8 to 10 times per minute without pausing for chest compressions. In the victim with a perfusing rhythm but absent or inadequate respiratory effort, give 12 to 20 breaths per minute. One way to achieve this rate with a ventilating bag is to say "squeeze-release-squeeze" at a normal speaking rate[20].

Cricothyrotomy

In rare situations when the intensivist fails to intubate the trachea of a child, cricothyroid membrane can provide a temporary access to the airway. A 14 or 16 gauge intravenous cannula is passed in the midline through the cricothyroid membrane located between the inferior edge of the thyroid cartilage and the upper edge of cricoid cartilage. Once the attached syringe is able to suck the air easily, the entry into trachea is confirmed and now the plastic catheter is advanced into the trachea. Normally, the connector from 3.0 mm endotracheal tube fits snugly onto the intravenous cannula. Though this procedure is purely temporary and not free of complications, the intensivist should not delay the decision to try this route to avoid irreversible brain damage because of prolonged hypoxia which is bound to occur if other means to access the airway have failed.

Tension Pneumothorax

Once air starts leaking into the pleural cavity, its pressure is likely to progressively increase with every positive pressure breath. This can cause profound shift of the mediastinum and compression of not only ipsilateral but even the contralateral lung thereby making adequate ventilation impossible. Further, mediastinal shift and high intrathoracic pressure would also impede venous return and reduce the cardiac output. Results would be disastrous unless immediate steps are taken.

Immediate needle decompression must be attempted even without radiological confirmation. An 18 size intravenous cannula attached to a 10 or 20 ml syringe should be inserted in the second intercostal space in the midclavicular line and plunger withdrawn to suck out air. In younger infants, a scalp vein needle can be inserted keeping the open end of the attached tubing under water or saline in a bowl. Gush of air confirms the diagnosis. Subsequently, more definitive treatment in the form of chest tube insertion can be undertaken.

FLUID THERAPY

Hypovolemia and resulting shock are important factors leading to cardiopulmonary arrest. Hence, aggressive fluid therapy to achieve rapid correction of hypovolemia is a logical step in the treatment of shock. However, the situation is not so clear once cardiopulmonary arrest has actually set in. Venous volume loading during CPR increases cardiac output initially[69,70]. However, the resultant increase in right atrial pressure diminishes coronary blood flow and myocardial activity. This is obviously harmful. Experimentally it has been shown that arterial volume loading improves myocardial and cerebral perfusion but it is not technically feasible in most CPR situations. Thus, the present consensus is to treat hypovolemic shock with volume loading while normovolemic cardiac arrest is managed mainly with vasopressors.

In cases of shock, 20 ml per kg of saline or Ringer's lactate should be infused rapidly. Usual intravenous drip sets and tubings are unable to allow the administration of such large amounts of fluids. The best way to ensure rapid infusion of fluids is to manually push large size syringe fulls of the fluid into a large bore intravenous cannula or intraosseous needle. The bolus is repeated if no improvement is observed. Volume expansion must continue until signs of shock are no longer observed. Recently, the importance of infusing large volumes of fluids in the initial few minutes of resuscitation has been emphasized[71]. A child in hypovolemic shock may require 40–60 ml/kg of fluid during the first 15 minutes of resuscitation[72].

Although it is well known that crystalloids stay within the intravascular compartment for much shorter period of time than colloids (e.g. blood, fresh frozen plasma, 5 percent albumin, haemaccel, starch preparations) but crystalloids are the preferred fluids during initial resuscitation. In later phases of fluid resuscitation in patients with shock colloids may be useful.

Blood and blood products are reserved for specific situations of blood loss or correction of coagulopathies. In situations of blood loss (e.g. trauma) blood should be administered as soon as it is available when despite two boluses (i.e. 40 ml/kg) of fluids child has not shown adequate improvement.

During resuscitation for cardiac arrest, volume loading is indicated only in following situations:

1. Prehospital cardiac arrest, cause not known; child not responding to oxygenation, ventilation, chest compressions, and epinephrine. At this juncture correction of 'probable' hypovolemia may be tried.

2. Known or strongly suspected hypovolemia e.g. internal hemorrhage due to trauma or shock due to gastroenteritis.

Hyperglycemia during resuscitation is associated with poor neurological outcome. Hence, glucose containing solutions in resuscitation fluids are indicated only when hypoglycemia has been documented. Thus, for boluses only Ringer's lactate (and not dextrose Ringer lactate) and normal saline (0.9 percent NaCl) are recommended. When hypoglycemia is documented, glucose should be administered as a separate bolus.

PHARMACOTHERAPY

Drugs are life-saving in many situations but they have a limited role for the management of CPA. Of the many drugs recommended or tried during pediatric CPR, only epinephrine is of some proven value. Atropine and sodium bicarbonate are of limited utility and their use is optional, provided they do not distract from proven therapy.

Epinephrine

Many workers have demonstrated that epinephrine is useful in pediatric CPR[73,74]. Epinephrine elevates perfusion pressure generated during chest compressions, stimulates spontaneous contraction during asystole, improves the myocardial contractility state and makes the cardiac conduction system more responsive to the effect of electrical defibrillation in ventricular fibrillation states[73].

These beneficial effects are obtained mainly through alpha-adrenergic effects and not the beta adrenergic effects of epinephrine. The alpha and beta adrenergic effects of ephinephrine in relation to CPR are summarized in (Table 3.15).

Table 3.15 Alpha-adrenergic and beta-adrenergic agonist effects of epinephrine
Alpha adrenergic effects   • Constriction of peripheral vessels   • Maintain aortic diastolic pressure   • Improve coronary blood flow   • Improve cerebral blood flow   • There are no metabolic stimulatory effects   **Beta adrenergic effects**   • Vasodilation of peripheral vessels   • Decrease in aortic diastolic pressure   • Increase in cellular metabolic rate   • Increase in heart rate and/or arrhythmias following resuscitation

Indications. Epinephrine is indicated in all forms of pediatric cardiac arrest. Epinephrine stimulates the electrical and mechanical activity of the heart in asystole or bradyarrhythmia. Even in ventricular fibrillation it may be useful as it makes the fibrillation more responsive to electrical defibrillation.

Dose. The standard dose of ephinephrine is 0.01 mg/kg (0.01 ml/kg of 1:1000 solution), given by intravenous or intraosseous route. Although, in a pediatric CPR study the use of higher dose of epinephrine (0.2 mg/kg) has been shown to be safe and more effective[75], a deleterious effect with a ten fold increase in second and subsequent doses has been observed in other studies. Hence, unless intra-arterial monitoring indicates otherwise, usual second and subsequent recommended dose currently is 10 mcg/kg[18]. The dose of epinephrine may be repeated after every 3 to 5 minutes.

Epinephrine is absorbed from the mucosa of the airways and can be administered through the endotracheal tube if intravenous or intraosseous access are not available. The starting endotracheal dose is 0.1 mg/kg which should be diluted in 3 to 5 ml of saline and instilled into the ET tube. The administration of epinephrine should be followed immediately by several positive pressure breaths.

In a CPR scene of urgency and stress one has often noticed that the nurse fills up the full ampoule of epinephrine into the syringe and the physician injects the whole amount into the vein without checking the amount handed over. This should be avoided. Epinephrine should not be added to a bicarbonate infusion since catecholamines are inactivated by alkaline solution.

Vasopressin

There is a lot of interest in the use of vasopressin after epinephrine during CPR. However, presently there is insufficient evidence to recommend the routine use of vasopressin during cardiac arrest in children[52]. Pediatric and adult case series/reports suggest that vasopressin or its long-acting analogue, terlipressin, may be effective in refractory cardiac arrest when standard therapy fails[76, 77]. A large pediatric NRCPR case series, however, suggested that vasopressin is associated with lower ROSC, and a trend toward lower 24-hour and discharge survival.[78] A majority of controlled trials in adults do not demonstrate a benefit[79, 80].

Sodium bicarbonate

Routine administration of sodium bicarbonate is not recommended in cardiac arrest .[52,81] Sodium bicarbonate may be administered for treatment of some toxidromes or special resuscitation situations such as hyperkalemic cardiac arrest. During cardiac arrest or severe shock, arterial blood gas analysis may not accurately reflect tissue and venous acidosis.[82] Excessive sodium bicarbonate may impair tissue oxygen delivery; cause hypokalemia, hypocalcemia, hypernatremia, and hyperosmolality; decrease the VF threshold; and impair cardiac function[83].

Calcium

Calcium ions are useful for all muscular activity and are essential for myocardial excitation-contraction coupling. It also enhances ventricular automaticity during asystole and increases myocardial contractility. Based on these physiologic effects and the evidence that severe ionized hypocalcemia was present in adult patients suffering from out-of-hospital cardiac arrest[84], calcium therapy during CPR was favoured till recently, especially in settings of asystole and electromechanical dissociation (EMD). However, no significant beneficial effects of calcium therapy have been demonstrated in these settings[85].

Indications. When hypocalcemia is known to be present it should be considered as the cause of arrest and treated aggressively. Similarly, when a child develops cardiorespiratory arrest and has an underlying disease which is associated with hypocalcemia (e.g. Long term use of loop diuretics, hypoparathyroidisim, renal failure) calcium may be given. Other indications for administration of calcium are hyperkalemia, hypomagnesemia and an overdose of calcium channel blockers.

Dose. Calcium chloride is the preferred salt and the recommended dose is 0.20 to 0.25 ml per kg of 10 percent solution. This delivers 5 to 7 mg/kg of elemental calcium. Since, calcium gluconate 10 percent solution contains only one-third the amount of elemental calcium (9 mg/ml compared to 27.2 mg/ml in 10 percent calcium chloride) the dose of calcium gluconate should be three times higher.

Precautions. Calcium salts can sclerose the vein and cause severe chemical burns if extravasation occurs. Rapid administration of calcium causes bradycardia and even cardiac asystole. Calcium salts form insoluble precipitates in the presence of sodium bicarbonate.

Atropine

Atropine is a parasympatholytic agent that increases the heart rate and shortens the AV node conduction time. It has no significant effect on systemic vascular resistance, myocardial perfusion pressure or myocardial contractility.

Indications. In young children cardiac output is heart-rate dependent, and symptomatic brady-cardia (heart rate of less than 60 per minute is associated with poor perfusion) must be treated even if blood pressure is normal. Since bradycardia usually results from hypoxemia, efforts should be focussed on improving ventilation and oxygenation. The potential indications for administration of atropine include severe bradycardia, heart block (second and third degree), slow idioventricular rhythm, asystole and electromechanical dissocia-tion. However, it must be emphasised that it is uncertain whether atropine is useful in the treatment of asystole. Laboratory animal and clinical studies have failed to demonstrate any efficacy of atropine in cardiac arrest[86].

Dose. The recommended dose of atropine is 0.02 mg/kg with a minimum dose of 0.1 mg and a maximum single dose of 0.5 mg for a child and 1.0 mg for an adolescent. This dose may be repeated every five minutes for a maximum total dose of 1.0 mg for a child and 2.0 mg for an adolescent. When intratracheal route is adopted because of the non–availability of an intravenous or intraosseous route, the dose should be increased 2 to 3 times.

Precautions. Tachycardia is a recognized side effect of atropine. On the other hand, low doses of atropine may be accompanied by a paradoxical bradycardia in infants. Thus, a minimum dose of 0.1 mg should be administered in children. Atropine produces pupillary dilatation but does not affect the pupillary constrictive response to light.

Glucose

Glucose is the major metabolic substrate for the brain and neonatal myocardium. Stores of glucose in sick newborn babies and infants are limited. Hypoglycemia is known to depress the myocardial and brain functions. Hence, it is prudent to prevent hypoglycemia and treat it if it is present. Thus, if bedside glucose testing is not available, empiric treatment with glucose should be considered, especially when the infant is at risk for hypoglycemia or standard treatment is not showing the desired effect.

However, hyperglycemia must be avoided. There are several studies, both experimental and clinical which show harmful effects of hyperglycemia on the mature brain during CPR[87,88]. During ischemia, under normoglycemic conditions, brain lactate concentration reaches a plateau while in hyperglycemic milieu, brain lactate concentration continues to rise for the duration of the ischemic period[89]. Lactic acidosis appears to exacerbate the ischemic brain injury.

Dose. The recommended dose of glucose is 0.5 to 1.0 g/kg intravenously i.e. 2-4 ml/kg of 25% glucose solution. When the child also needs volume expansion a bolus of 10 to 20 ml/kg of dextrose–normal saline (5 percent glucose with 0.9 percent sodium chloride) or dextrose Ringer's lactate may be used. This will provide 0.5 to 1.0 g/kg of glucose. However, glucose containing solutions are not routinely recommended for bolus therapy.

Precautions. 25% glucose solution being hypersmolar, sclerosis of peripheral veins can occur. Repeated doses of glucose may cause hyperglycemia and lead to poor neurological outcome.

Naloxone

When narcotic overdose or poisoning is suspected an intravenous or endotracheal dose of naloxone is recommended to reverse the respiratory and circulatory depression. The currently recommended dose of naloxone is 0.1 mg/kg. Even at higher doses, naloxone is safe. Hence, it may be repeated frequently till the desired effects are produced.

Lidocaine

Lidocaine is an antiarrhythmic agent that causes a decrease in automaticity and in spontaneous depolarization of pacemaker tissue. Lidocaine abolishes re-entry ventricular arrhythmias and prevents or terminates ventricular arrhythmias due to accelerated ectopic foci. Lidocaine is thus useful to raise the threshold for ventricular fibrillation and to suppress postcardioversion ventricular ectopy, especially with recurrent ventricular fibrillation or tachycardia. Ideally, it should be administered before cardioversion if vascular access and the drug are readily available.

Dose. To achieve and maintain therapeutic levels of the drug, a bolus dose of lidocaine should be immediately followed by a constant infusion. Without an initial bolus, approximately 5 half-lives (half life 108 min) are required to achieve plateau concentration[90]. A loading bolus of 1 mg/kg is administered, followed by an infusion of 20 to 50 mcg/kg per minute. If the arrhythmia recurs, a second intravenous bolus at the same dose can be given.

Precautions. In higher doses lidocaine produces CNS as well as myocardial and circulatory disturbances. The CNS side effects include seizures, psychosis, drowsiness, paresthesias, disorientation, muscle twitchings, agitation and respiratory arrest. Conversion of second degree heart block to complete heart block and further slowing of sinus bradycardia have been described. These potential side effects do not prohibit careful use of lidocaine.

Electrical Therapy

Three modes of electrical therapy may be used in children in the CPR situation; defibrillation, cardioversion and cardiac pacing. Defibrillation is the untimed, asynchronous depolarization of a critical mass of myocardial cells to allow spontaneous organised myocardial depolarization to resume. Ventricular fibrillation (VF) and pulseless ventricular tachycardia (VT) are the definitive indications for defibrillation.

Synchronised cardioversion also results in depolarization of myocardium, but is timed to be synchronous with patient's intrinsic electrical activity. It can convert atrial flutter, atrial fibrillation and supraventricular tachycardia and ventricular tachycardia into normal sinus rhythm when current is synchronised with the R waves. In children, cardioversion is reserved for above rhythms refractory to drug therapy and overdrive pacing or in cardiovascular collapse.

Emergency transcutaneous ventricular pacing is rarely resorted to in children, although with modern technology it is easy to apply and has been used for postoperative cardiac patients. There is anecdotal success in patients with symptomatic bradycardia[88].

Ventricular fibrillation is uncommon in children compared to adults and accounts for only 5-15% of all pediatric victims of out-of-hospital cardiac arrest and is reported in up to 20% of pediatric in-hospital arrests at some point during the resuscitation. The incidence increases with age. Treatment consists of continuing with oxygenation, ventilation and chest compressions until defibrillation can be arranged. A starting dose of 2–4 joules/ kg is recommended[52]. Unfortunately, during defibrillation CPR maneuvers have to be interrupted and precious time is wasted if normal rhythm is not achieved soon. Hence, search for reliable parameters which would predict the success of defibrillation procedure continues[91].

Generally, 'infant paddles' are suitable for children weighing less than 10 kg (up to one year) and 'adult paddles' for older and bigger children. Electrode cream must be applied over two separate areas in such a way that heart is between them e.g. one electrode below the right clavicle and the second to the left of left nipple, in midaxillary line. If only 'adult' paddles are available, one paddle is placed on anterior chest and the other on the back. Defibrillation is a potentially dangerous procedure since electrical current is being passed through the body. Thus, the operator, all helpers and all bystanders should be 'clear' off the electrical fields when the discharge buttons are pushed.

For the past few years Automated External Defibrillators (AEDs) have become available. With further advances in technology many AEDs can accurately detect VF in children of all ages and differentiate shockable from unshockable rhythms with a high degree of sensitivity and specificity even in children.

For automated defibrillation, ILCOR pediatric task force recommends an initial pediatric attenuated dose for children 1 to 8 years of age and up to about 25 kg (55 pounds) and 127 cm (50 inches) in length. There is insufficient information to recommend for or against the use of an AED in infants <1 year of age. A variable dose manual defibrillator is preferred for defibrillation in an infant. If this is not available, an AED able to recognize pediatric shockable rhythms and equipped with dose attenuation is preferred. If such a defibrillator is not available, a standard AED with standard electrode pads may be used. A standard AED (without a dose attenuator) should be used for children ≥ 25 kg (about 8 years of age), adolescents and adult victims[20].

Dosages of drugs and electrical defibrillation therapy for a 10 kg child are shown in the Table 3.16 and the algorithms to be followed[20] in patients of bradycardia and asystole and pulseless arrest are shown in Figures 3.12 to 3.14.

POSTARREST STABILIZATION AND TRANSPORT

Once the patient has been resuscitated successfully the second phase of management begins for the resuscitation team. The CPR team has to stabilize the child and transport him to the PICU which, at times may be several kilometers away. The objectives of post resuscitation stabilization are to prevent secondary organ injury and to deliver the patient in optimal condition to a tertiary care center. These objectives are best accomplished by reassessing the ABCs and evaluating the other important organ systems repeatedly on an ongoing basis. At this stage a quick attempt is also made to evaluate the patient for underlying cause of the arrest and planning for any specific measures that may be required immediately.

Table 3.16 Drugs and their doses for a 10 kg patient during CPR			
Drug and concentration	**Dosage**	**Calculated dose and volume (10 kg infant)**	
Adenosine (3 mg/ml)	0.1mg/kg (max 6 mg) Repeat 0.2 mg/kg (max 12 mg)	1 mg 2 mg	0.33 ml 0.66 ml
Amiodarone (50 mg/ml)	5mg/kg IV/IO Repeat upto 15 mg/kg (max 300 mg)	50 mg	1 ml
Atropine sulfate (0.1 mg/ml)	0.02 mg / kg IV or ET; may repeat in 5 min	0.2 mg	2.0 ml
Calcium choride 10% (100 mg/ml)	20 mg/ kg IV; may repeat in 10 min	200.0 mg	2.0 ml
Dextrose, 25% (0.25 g/ml)	0.5 g/kg IV, 2 ml/ kg (D25 W)	5.0 g	20.0 ml
Epinephrine 1:10,000 (0.1 mg / ml syringe prepared by diluting 1:1000 solution ten times)	0.01 mg / kg IV; repeat q 5 min	0.1 mg	1.0 ml
Epinephrine, 1:1000 (1 mg/ ml)	0.1 mg / kg ET or 2nd dose IV in pulseless arrest (May use up to 0.2 mg / kg IV)	1.0 mg	1.0 ml
Lidocaine, 2% cardiac (20 mg / ml)	1 mg / kg IV or ET, then 0.5 mg / kg q 20 min	10.0 mg 5.0 mg	0.5 ml 0.25ml
Cardioversion	0.5–1.0 J/Kg	5 to 10 joules	
Defibrillation	2-4 J/kg	20 to 40 joules	

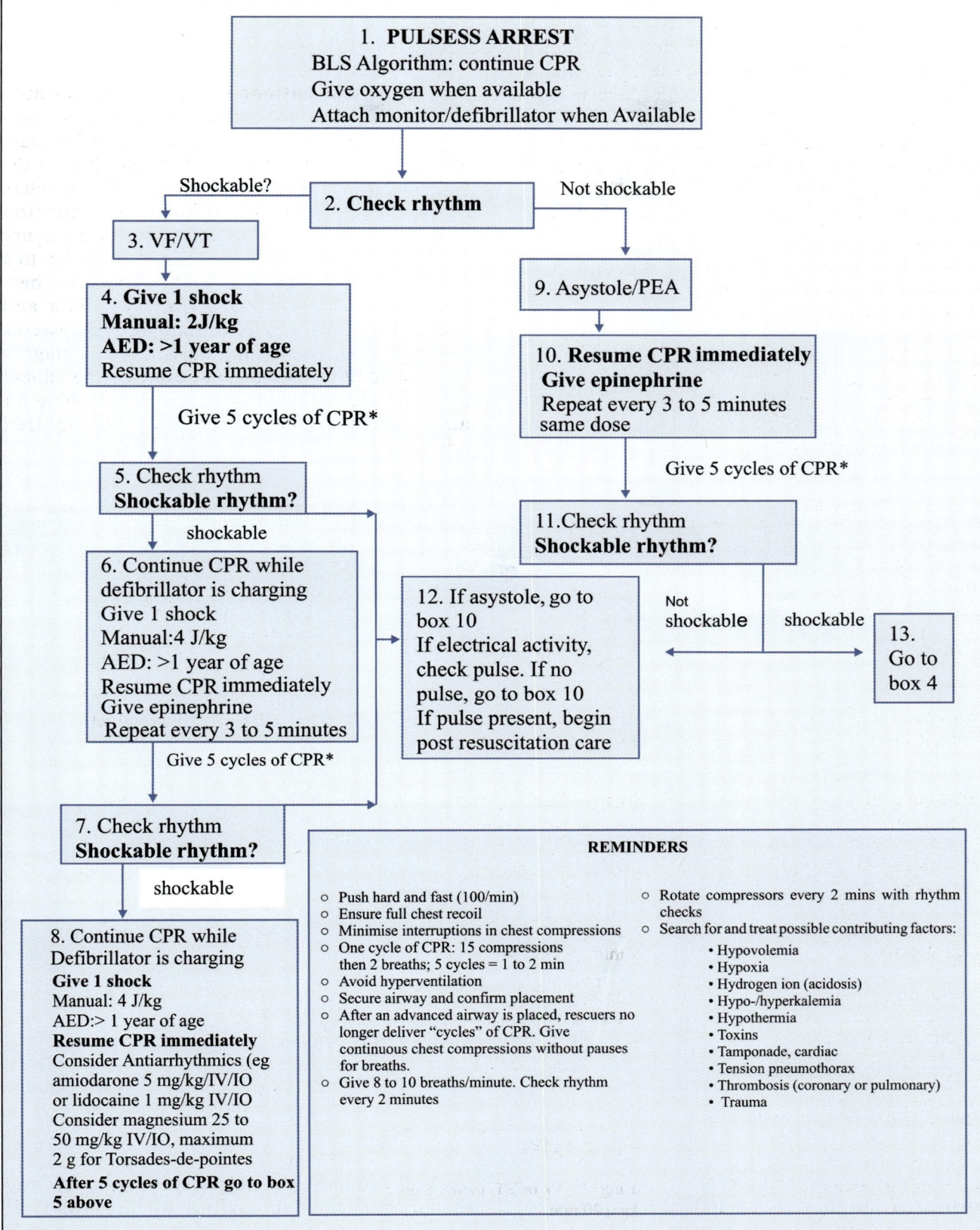

Figure 3.12 Algorithm for pulseless cardiac arrest

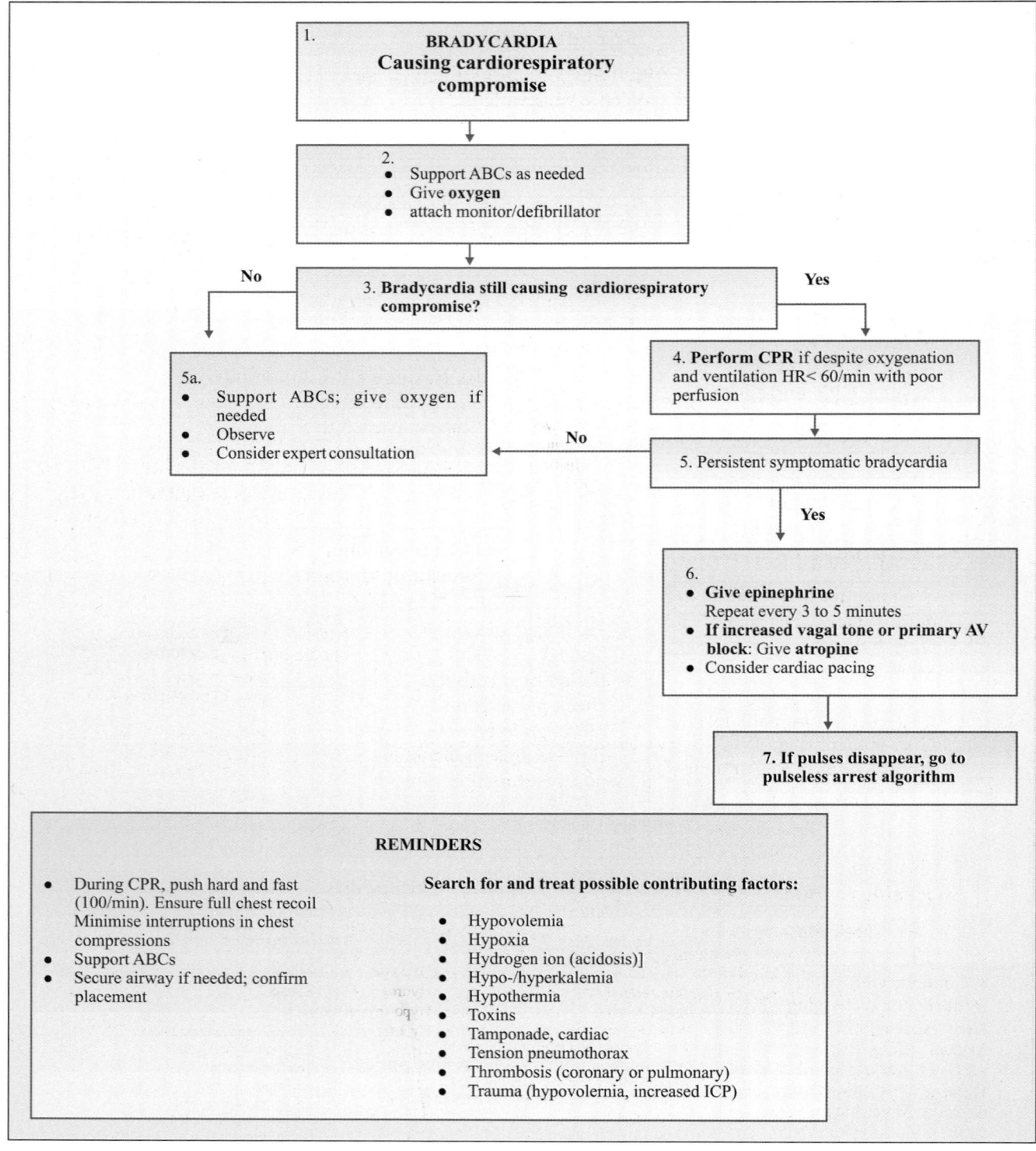

Figure 3.13 Algorithm for bradycardia

Airway is assessed repeatedly by chest rise, use of accessory muscles, nasal flaring, patient color and auscultation of breath sounds on both sides. Non intubated patient is at a greater risk for loss of control of airway during transport. Hence, such a child should be reassessed for the need for endo-tracheal intubation at this stage. A chest X-ray should be obtained for confirming the position of the ET tube and possibility of pneumothorax (this complication can also occur in patients resuscitated by bag–valve–mask without ET tube). A nasogastric tube should be inserted for deflating the stomach.

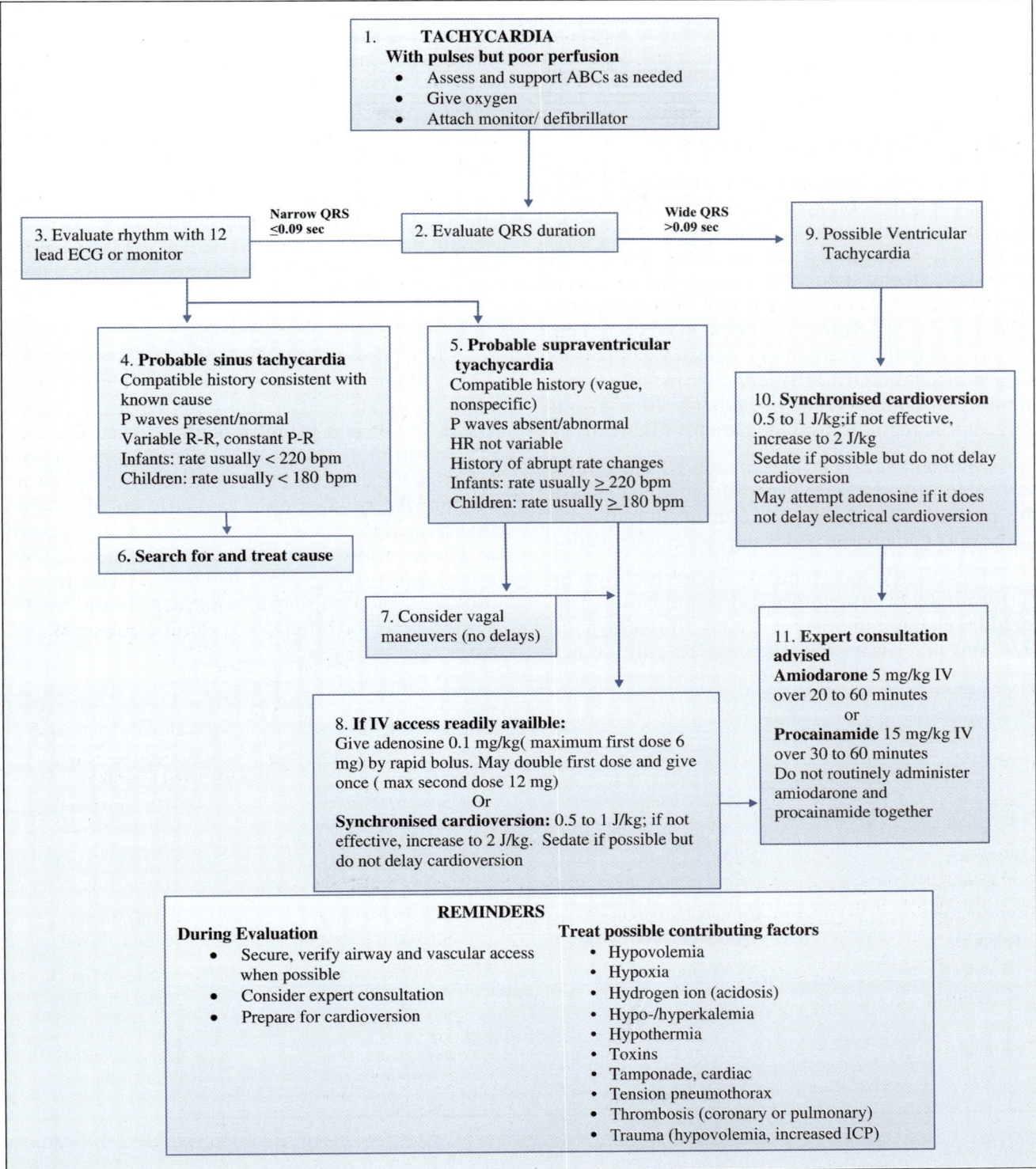

Figure 3.14 Algorithm for tachycardia

The child should be assessed for any need for sedation and use of muscle relaxant. An agitated child is unlikely to allow proper maintenance of airway during transport. Diazepam or morphine in a dose of 0.1 to 0.2 mg / kg by slow intravenous injection may be used. Adequacy of breathing is assessed by clinical examination and use of pulse oximeter and $EtCO_2$ monitor and blood gas measurement whenever possible. Clinical parameters like adequate bilateral chest expansion, equal bilateral breath sounds, absence of cyanosis, absence of nasal flaring or use of accessory muscles of respiration and absence of agitation should be looked for.

In a study comparing mechanical and manual ventilation during transport it was shown that respiratory parameters were more stable on mechanical than on manual ventilation[92].

Circulation is evaluated on an ongoing basis by assessing the color, capillary refill, pulse rate, rhythm and quality and blood pressure. Electronic monitors, though useful are not absolutely necessary. Mental status and urine output are useful indicators of end organ perfusion. When required repeat bolus of fluid for shock may be given. Majority of children are likely to need vasopressors after resuscitation. Usually, epinephrine infusion is the drug of choice. However, other pressor agents may also be required in some patients (Table 3.17).

Maintenance fluids must be started and volume and composition adjusted according to the needs of the patient. Measurement of urine output by a indwelling catheter provides important information

Disability assessment is carried out by performing a brief neurological examination. This includes evaluation of level of consciousness, pupil size and reactivity and response to pain. When increased intracranial pressure is suspected, hyperventilation is generally recommended as an emergency measure to reduce the intracranial pressure. Post-ischemic seizures should be treated aggressively. Adequate cerebral perfusion requires support of optimal cardiac output and systemic oxygen delivery (Table 3.18).

Blood glucose should be checked before and during transport. Hypoglycemia when present should be treated and child reassessed for need for more glucose. While hyperglycemia carries a poor outcome its treatment by insulin is not recommended at this stage.

Induction of hypothermia (32°C to 34°C) for 12 to 24 hours should be considered in children who remain comatose after resuscitation from cardiac arrest.[52,93] It is a useful modality for adolescents resuscitated from sudden, witnessed, out-of-hospital VF cardiac arrest. Although there are no randomized studies in the pediatric population on the effect of therapeutic hypothermia, it is of benefit in adults[94] following witnessed out-of-hospital VF arrest and in asphyxiated newborns[95]. Health care providers should prevent hyperthermia and treat it aggressively in infants and children resuscitated from cardiac arrest.

Table 3.17 Medications for a 10 kg patient during post CPR stabilisation			
Drug and Concentration	**Dosage**	**Concentration**	**Calculated dose**
Dobutamine (12.5 mg/ml)	5-15 ug/kg/min	6 mg/kg/100 ml at 1ml/hr=1ug/kg/min	60.0 mg/100 ml (4.8 ml/100ml)
Dopamine (40 mg/ml)	2-20 ug/kg/min	6 mg/kg/100 ml at 1ml/hr=1ug/kg/min	60.0 mg/100 ml (1.5 ml/100ml)
Epinephrine (1mg/ml)	0.1 ug/kg/min (upto 20 ug/kg/min in pulseless arrest)	0.6mg/kg/100 ml at 1ml/hr=0.1ug/kg/min	6.0 mg/100ml (6.0ml/100 ml)
Lidocaine (20mg/ml)	20-50 ug/kg/min	120 mg/100 ml at 1ml/kg/hr (10.0ml/hr) =20 ug/kg/min	120 mg/100ml (6ml /100ml)
Amrinone	0.75-1mg/kg over 5 mins loading; 5-10 ug/kg/min infusion	6 mg/kg/100ml at 1 ml/ hr = 1ug/kg/min	60 mg/100ml 12ml/100ml

Table 3.18 Important parameters for ongoing assessment		
Respiratory	**Cardiovascular**	**Neurologic**
• Chest rise • Breath sounds • Cyanosis • Agitation • Pulse oximetry • End–tidal CO_2	• Heart rate/rhythm • Pulse quality • Capillary refill • Blood pressure • Urine output	• Level of consciousness • Pupillary response to light

Whenever laboratory backup is available complete blood counts, blood glucose, electrolytes, blood urea nitrogen and creatinine along with an ABG should be obtained. Results of these parameters, if not available by the time of transport may be communicated to the tertiary care center as soon as possible. A toxicology screen may be taken whenever indicated.

Transporting the post resuscitation child to a pediatric tertiary care center is a difficult and challenging task. Advance preparation, clear policies and administrative protocols are necessary. If the tertiary care center is given advance information adequate preparations can be made at that end. Mode of transport will depend to a large extent on the availability of facilities. However, a fully equipped ambulance is likely to give best results. The transport team can be from the referring hospital. The team should ideally consist of a pediatric intensive care trained pediatrician, trained nurses and technicians. Adequate facilities and skills for monitoring the child for any deterioration and remedial actions should be available. In most situations it is better to spend that extra time necessary for stabilizing the child at the referring hospital rather than quickly rushing an unstable child to the tertiary care center. Thus, 'stay and play 'is a better policy than 'scoop and run'.

Communication between the CPR team and the tertiary care facility form an important part of CPR management for the continuing care of the patient as well as for medicolegal purposes. A brief history, all the details of treatment and assessment at various stages of CPR, the current clinical status and any skiagrams etc. must be provided. To ensure that no communication gaps occur, the physician and nurse from one center should speak directly to the physician and the nurse of the other center.

COMPLICATIONS OF CPR

CPR is a procedure which is performed in an atmosphere full of tension. At times the paramedics and medics may not be fully trained to conduct the CPR. The maneuvers like chest compressions, endotracheal intubation, and bag and mask ventilation etc. have some complications even when performed by fully trained personnel. Further, CPR is often performed without ideal monitoring facilities in majority of cases. All these factors contribute towards high complication rates. Complications may develop in as many as 43% of all cases receiving CPR[96]. Common complications to the victim and to the rescuer are listed in Tables 3.19 and 3.20.

Table 3.19 Complications of CPR

Thoracopulmonary
- Rib fractures
- Sternal fractures
- Upper airway injury
- Anterior mediastinal hemorrhage
- Pulmonary edema
- Cardiac contusion, laceration or rupture
- Aspiration pneumonia
- Barotrauma

Neck
- Trauma to hyoid bone, thyroid cartilage

Abdominal
- Abdominal visceral injury
- Abdominal distension

Metabolic
- Electrolyte disturbances : hypokalemia, hyperkalemia, acidosis, alkalosis
- Hyperglycemia, hypoglycemia

Related to vascular access
- Trauma to bone
- Infection at the site

Table 3.20 Dangers of CPR to the rescuers

- **Exhaustion**
- **Transmission of diseases from victim to the rescuer**
  - Hepatitis B and C
  - HIV
  - Respiratory infections
  - Tuberculosis
- **Medicolegal liability in case of injury or death of the victim**

PROGNOSTIC FACTORS

Clinical variables associated with survival include length of CPR, number of doses of epinephrine, age of the victim, witnessed versus unwitnessed cardiac arrest, and the first and subsequent rhythm.[97-99] None of these associations, however, predict outcome. Witnessed collapse, bystander CPR, and a short interval from collapse to arrival of professionals improve the chances of a successful resuscitation. Intact survival has been documented after unusually prolonged in-hospital resuscitation.[100]

Overall it has been observed that survival is better if the patient had isolated respiratory (and not cardiorespiratory) arrest, had bradycardia and not asystole, required only PBLS and not PALS, and the pulse returned in the field itself. The outcome is more favourable for CPR conducted in the hospital rather than out-of-hospital setting (Table 3.21).

Table 3.21 Prognostic correlates of pediatric CPR	
Favorable	**Unfavorable**
• CPR conducted in the hospital • Isolated respiratory arrest • Bradycardia • Witnessed arrest • Hypothermia • Only BLS required • Pulses return in field • No cardiotonic drugs required • Prompt PALS given • Ventricular fibrillation on arrival to the hospital • Traumatic etiology	• Out-of-hospital CPR • Cardiorespiratory arrest • Asystole • Unwitnessed arrest • Normothermia • PALS required • Pulseless at arrival in the hospital • More than two doses of epinephrine are required • No underlying disease • Chronic illness

TERMINATION OF CPR

The paramedics, must continue CPR and the decision to stop CPR should not to be made by them because termination of CPR amounts to virtually declaring death, and this job can be performed only by the physicians. Hence, paramedics can terminate CPR only when they are physically exhausted and cannot carry on any further or when the victim has been handed over to a more qualified team.

The decision to terminate CPR is far more difficult for the physician. Rigid criteria cannot be laid down. Underlying disease, type of cardiac rhythm, duration of CPR and response of the child to various interventions help the physician to make the decision. Poor neurologic function or brain death during CPR are totally unreliable. Hence, these criteria cannot be used to terminate CPR. Most authorities believe that except for cases of profound hypothermia (temperature less than 30°C) and occurrence of recurrent rather than persistent cardiac arrest, prolonged efforts at resuscitation are not indicated in pediatric patients after an out-of-hospital cardiopulmonary arrest. If after an optimal CPR efforts for 20-30 minutes, there are neither spontaneous breaths nor cardiac pulsations, resuscitation efforts can be abandoned and child declared dead[11].

NEWER AND EXPERIMENTAL TREATMENT MODALITIES

Use of cardiopulmonary bypass, ECMO and inhaled nitric oxide followed by ECMO[101] are the examples of application of newer modalities in the management of cardiorespiratory arrest. Consideration should be given to early activation of extra-corporeal life support (ECLS) for a cardiac arrest that occurs in a highly supervised environment, such as an ICU, with the clinical protocols in place and the expertise and equipment available to initiate it rapidly. ECLS should be considered only for children in cardiac arrest refractory to standard resuscitation attempts, with a potentially reversible cause of arrest.[52] When ECLS is employed during cardiac arrest, outcome for children with underlying cardiac disease is better than the outcome for children with noncardiac disease. With underlying cardiac disease, long-term survival when ECLS is initiated in a critical-care setting has been reported even after 50 minutes of standard CPR.[102-104]

The newer vasopressors which need to be studied in cardiac arrest are endothelin-1 and vasopressin. These vasopressors have been shown to improve organ perfusion in subjects with prolonged cardiac arrest in experimental animals. Perhaps optimal vasopressor therapy in the future will include vasopressin with or without other vasopressors. Though some adult human studies are now available for use of vasopressin, data for pediatric population needs to be generated before firm recommendations can be made[52].

There has been a recent interest in the use of sodium nitroprusside (SNP) instead of epinephrine during CPR. Though this may seem paradoxical, the rationale proposed is that SNP causes vasodilation which may increase forward blood flow during each chest compression. This has been studied in a porcine model and better resuscitation rates, improved hemodynamics and 24-hr survival rates with good neurological function as compared to standard CPR were found.[105] Though there is a need for further investigations on the safety of SNP during CPR and on its mechanisms of action, this SNP-CPR, by targeting small resistance vessels, has the potential to become an important adjunct to ameliorate organ perfusion during CPR and ultimately improve outcome of CPR.[106]

Summary of recent changes in pediatric BLS and ALS guidelines

The American Heart Association has been updating the guidelines for pediatric basic and advanced life support at regular intervals. The latest update was published in 2010[26,52]. The major changes with regard the previous recommendations are as follows:

1. Initiation of CPR with chest compressions rather than rescue breaths (C-A-B rather than A-B-C); leads to a shorter delay to first compression. This will possibly decrease bystander hesitancy and increase the absolute number of children receiving CPR.

2. Modification of recommendations regarding adequate depth of chest compressions to one-third of the AP diameter of the chest (earlier 1/3rd to ½); this corresponds to approximately 1 ½ inches (4 cm) in most infants and about 2 inches (5 cm) in most children.

3. Removal of "look, listen and feel for breathing" from the sequence; CPR is initiated with chest compressions if the child is unresponsive and not breathing (or gasping)

4. De-emphasis of the pulse check for healthcare providers: Healthcare providers may not reliably detect presence of a pulse; in an unresponsive child who is not breathing, if a pulse is not detected within 10 seconds, begin CPR.

5. Automated external defibrillator (AED) in infants: In infants, a manual defibrillator is preferred to an AED with a pediatric dose attenuator. If neither is available, AED without a pediatric dose attenuator may be used. (Earlier there was no recommendation for or against using an AED in infants)

6. New information is provided on resuscitation of infants and children with selected congenital heart defects and pulmonary hypertension, including possible early consideration for extracorporeal life support (ECLS).

7. After CPR, titrate inspired oxygen, once spontaneous circulation has been restored to maintain SpO_2 >= 94% but < 100% to avoid the risk of hyperoxemia induced free radical injury.

8. Calcium administration is not recommended in CPR except in very specific circumstances.

9. The definition of wide-complex tachycardia has been changed from QRS duration of >0.08 second to >0.09 second.

10. Indications for postresuscitation therapeutic hypothermia have been clarified.

REFERENCES

1. Lewis JK, Minter MG, Eshelman SJ, Witte ML. Outcome of pediatric resuscitation. *Ann Emerg Med* 1983; 12:297–299.

2. O' Rourke PP. Outcome of children who are apneic and pulseless in the emergency room. *Crit Care Med* 1986; 14:466 – 468.

3. Williams PG, Primm PA. Cardiopulmonary arrest and resuscitation. In: Essentials of Pediatric Intensive Care (volume - II) Levin DL, Morriss FC (Eds) *New York. Churchill Livingstone* 1997; p 1287–1302.

4. Kyriacou DN, Arcinue EL, Peek C, Kraus JF. Effect of immediate resuscitation on children with submersion injury. *Pediatrics* 1994; 94 (pt 1):137–142.

5. Hickey RW, Cohen DM, Strausbaugh S, Dietrich AM. Pediatric patients requiring CPR in the pre-hospital setting. *Ann Emerg Med* 1995; 25: 495–501.

6. Kuisma M, Alaspaa A. Out-of-hospital cardiac arrests of non-cardiac origin: epidemiology and outcome. *Eur Heart J* 1997;18:1122–1128.

7. Lopez-Herce J, Garcia C, Rodriguez-Nunez A, *et al.* Long-term outcome of paediatric cardiorespiratory arrest in Spain. *Resuscitation* 2005;64:79–85.

8. Mogayzel C, Quan L, Graves JR, *et al.* Out-of-hospital ventricular fibrillation in children and adolescents: causes and outcomes. *Ann Emerg Med* 1995; 25: 484–491.

9. Atkins DL, Everson-Stewart S, Sears GK, *et al.* Epidemiology and outcomes from out-of-hospital cardiac arrest in children: The Resuscitation Outcomes Consortium Epistry-Cardiac Arrest. *Circulation* 2009; 119:1484 –1491.

10. Sirbaugh PE, Pepe PE, Shook JE, *et al.* A prospective, population-based study of the demographics, epidemiology, management, and outcome of out-of-hospital pediatric cardiopulmonary arrest. *Ann Emerg Med* 1999; 33: 174 –184.

11. Schindler MB, Bohn D, Cox PN, *et al.* Outcome of out-of-hospital cardiac or respiratory arrest in children. *N Engl J Med* 1996; 335:1473–1479.

12. Lopez-Herce J, Garcia C, Dominguez P, *et al.* Characteristics and outcome of cardiorespiratory arrest in children. *Resuscitation* 2004; 63:311–320.

13. Pell JP, Sirel JM, Marsden AK, *et al.* Presentation, management, and outcome of out-of-hospital cardiopulmonary arrest: comparison by underlying aetiology. *Heart* 2003; 89: 839–842.

14. Nadkarni VM, Larkin GL, Peberdy MA, *et al.* First documented rhythm and clinical outcome from in-hospital cardiac arrest among children and adults. *JAMA* 2006; 295:50 –57.

15. Tibballs J, Kinney S. A prospective study of outcome of in-patient paediatric cardiopulmonary arrest. *Resuscitation* 2006;71:310–318.

16. Schindler MB, Bohn D, Cox PN, *et al.* Outcome of out–of–hospital cardiac or respiratory arrest in children. *New Eng J Med* 1996; 335:1473 –1479.

17. Suominen P, Rasanen J, Kivioja A. Efficacy of cardiopulmonary resuscitation in pulseless paediatric trauma patients. *Resuscitation* 1998; 36: 9-13.

18. Abramson NS, Safar P, Detre K, *et al.* Brain Resuscitation Clinical Trial (BRCT) I Study Group: Randomized clinical study of thiopental loading in comatose survivors of cardiac arrest. *N Engl J Med* 1986; 314:397– 403.

19. Abramson NS, Sutton–Tyrell K, Safar P, *et al.* A randomized clinical study of a calcium–entry blocker (lidoflazine) in the treatment of comatose survivors of cardiac arrest. Brain Resuscitation Clinical Trial II Study Group. *N Engl J Med* 1991; 324:1225-1231.

20. American Heart Association. Pediatric Advanced Life Support. *Circulation* 2005; 112:167-187.

21. Falk JL, Rackow EC, Weil MH. End–tidal carbon dioxide concentration during cardiopulmonary resuscitation. *N Engl J Med* 1988; 318:607-611.

22. Idris AH, Staples Ed, O' Brien DJ, *et al.* End–tidal carbon dioxide during extremely low cardiac output. *Ann Emerg Med* 1994; 23:568.

23. Schleien CL, Kuluz JW, Hal saffner D, Roger MC. Cardiopulmonary resuscitation. In: Textbook of Pediatric Intensive Care. Roger MC (Ed). *Williams & Wilkins, Baltimore,* 1992; pp 3-51.

24. Niemann JT. Differences in cerebral and myocardial perfusion during closed–chest resuscitation. *Ann Emerg Med* 1984; 13:849-853.

25. Sanders AB, Ewy GA, Bragg S, *et al.* Expired pCO_2 as a prognostic indicator of successful resuscitation from cardiac arrest. *Ann Emerg Med* 1985; 14:948-952.

26. Berg MD, Schexnayder SM, Chameides L, *et al.* Part 13: pediatric basic life support: 2010 American Heart Association Guidelines for Cardiopulmonary Resuscitation and Emergency Cardiovascular Care. *Circulation* 2010;122 (suppl 3): S862–S875.

27. Rea TD, Cook AJ, Stiell IG, *et al.* Predicting survival after out-of-hospital cardiac arrest: role of the Utstein data elements. *Ann Emerg Med* 2010; 55:249 –257.

28. Assar D, Chamberlain D, Colquhoun M, *et al.* Randomised controlled trials of staged teaching for basic life support, 1: skill acquisition at bronze stage. *Resuscitation* 2000; 45:7–15.

29. Berg RA, Hilwig RW, Kern KB, *et al.* Simulated mouth-to- mouth ventilation and chest compressions (bystander cardiopulmonary resuscitation) improves outcome in a swine model of prehospital pediatric asphyxial cardiac arrest. *Crit Care Med* 1999; 27:1893–1899.

30. Kitamura T, Iwami T, Kawamura T, *et al.* Conventional and chest-compression-only cardiopulmonary resuscitation by bystanders for children who have out-of-hospital cardiac arrests: a prospective, nationwide, population-based cohort study. *Lancet* 2010; 375 (9723):1347–1354.

31. Sutton RM, Niles D, Nysaether J, *et al.* Quantitative analysis of CPR quality during in-hospital resuscitation of older children and adolescents. *Pediatrics* 2009;124: 494–499.

32. Nishisaki A, Nysaether J, Sutton R, *et al.* Effect of mattress deflection on CPR quality assessment for older children and adolescents. *Resuscitation* 2009; 80:540 –545.

33. Aufderheide TP, Pirrallo RG, Yannopoulos D, *et al.* Incomplete chest wall decompression: a clinical evaluation of CPR performance by EMS personnel and assessment of alternative manual chest compression-decompression techniques. *Resuscitation* 2005; 64: 353–362.

34. Ruben HM, Elam JO, *et al.* Investigations of pharyngeal X-rays and perfomance by laymen. *Anesthesiology* 1961; 22:271–279.

35. Zideman DA. Paediatric and neonatal life support. *Br J Anaesth* 1997; 79:178 –187.

36. Melker R, Cavallaro D, Krischer J. One rescuer CPR- a reappraisal of present recommendations of ventilation. *Crit Care Med* 1981; 9:423.

37. Heimlich HJ, Hoffmann KA, Canestri FR. Food choking and drowning deaths prevented by external subdiaphragmatic compression: Physiological basis. *Ann Thorac Surg* 1975; 20:188-195.

38. Donoghue A, Berg RA, Hazinski MF, *et al.* Cardiopulmonary resuscitation for bradycardia with poor perfusion versus pulseless cardiac arrest. *Pediatrics* 2009; 124: 1541–1548.

39. Atkins DL, Jorgenson DB. Attenuated pediatric electrode pads for automated external defibrillator use in children. *Resuscitation* 2005; 66: 31–37.

40. Samson RA, Nadkarni VM, Meaney PA, *et al.* Outcomes of in-hospital ventricular fibrillation in children. *N Engl J Med* 2006; 354:2328 –2339.

41. Atkinson E, Mikysa B, Conway JA, *et al.* Specificity and sensitivity of automated external defibrillator rhythm analysis in infants and children. *Ann Emerg Med* 2003;42: 185–196.

42. Bar-Cohen Y, Walsh EP, Love BA, Cecchin F. First appropriate use of automated external defibrillator in an infant. *Resuscitation* 2005; 67: 135–137.

43. Brunette DD, Fischer R. Intravascular access in pediatric cardiac arrest. *Am J Emerg Med* 1998; 6:577.

44. Rossetti VA, Thompson BM, Aprahamian C, *et al.* Difficulty and delay in intravascular access in pediatric arrests. *Ann Emerg Med* 1984; 13:40.

45. Iserson KV, Criss EA. Pediatric venous cutdowns: Utility in emergency situations. *Pediatr Emerg Care* 1986; 2:231-234.

46. Kanter RK, Zimmerman JJ, Strauss RH, Stoeckel KA. Pediatric emergency intravenous access. Evaluation of a protocol. *Am J Dis Child* 1986;140:132–134.

47. Doan LA. Peripheral versus central venous delivery of medications during CPR. *Ann Emerg Med* 1984; 13: 784-786.

48. Andropoulos DB, Soifer SJ, Schreiber MD. Plasma epinephrine concentrations after intraosseous and central venous injection during cardiopulmonary resuscitation in the lamb. *J Pediatr* 1990; 116:312-315.

49. Spivey WH, Lathers CM, Malone DR, *et al.* Comparison of intraosseous, central, and peripheral routes of sodium bicarbonate administration during CPR in pigs. *Ann Emerg Med* 1985; 14:1135-1140.

50. Fleisher G, Caputo G, Baskin JM. Comparison of external jugular and peripheral venous administration of sodium bicarbonate in puppies. *Crit Care Med* 1989; 17:251–254.

51. Orlowski JP, Porembka DT, Gallagher JM, *et al.* Comparison of intraosseous, central intravenous and peripheral intravenous infusions of emergency drugs. *Am J Dis Child* 1990; 144:112 -117.

52. Kleinman ME, Chameides L, Schexnayder SM, *et al.* Part 14: Pediatric advanced life support: 2010 American Heart Association Guidelines for Cardiopulmonary Resuscitation and Emergency Cardiovascular Care. *Circulation* 2010;122(suppl 3):S876 –S908.

53. Fuchs S, LaCovey D, Paris P. A prehospital model of intraosseous infusion. *Ann Emerg Med* 1991; 20: 371-374.

54. Glaeser PW, Losek JD, Nelson DB, *et al.* Pediatric intraosseous infusions: impact on vascular access time. *Am J Emerg Med* 1988; 6:330–332.

55. Camercon Jl, Pontanarosa PB, Passalaqua AM. A comparative study of peripheral to central circulation delivery times between intraosseous and intravenous injection using a radionuclide technique in normovolemic and hypovolemic canines. *J Emerg Med* 1999; 7: 123-127.

56. Kissoon N, Peterson R, Murphy S, *et al.* Comparison of pH and carbon dioxide tension values of central venous and intraosseous blood during changes in cardiac output. *Crit Care Med* 1994; 22:1010 –1015.

57. Christensen DW, Vernon DD, Banner W Jr, Dean JM. Skin necrosis complicating intraosseous infusion. *Pediatr Emerg Care* 1991; 7:289-290.

58. Galpin RD, Kronick JB, Willis RB, Frewen TC. Bilateral lower extremity compartment syndromes secondary to intraosseous fluid resuscitation. *J Pediatr Orthop* 1991; 11:773-776.

59. Vaknin Z, Manisterski Y, Ben-Abraham R, *et al.* Is endotracheal adrenaline deleterious because of beta adrenergic effect? *Anesth Analg* 2001; 92:1408-1412.

60. Hazinski MF, Zaritsky AL, Nadkarni VM, *et al. PALS Provider Manual.* American Heart Association (pub) 2002: p 88-89

61. Hazinski MF, Zaritsky AL, Nadkarni VM, *et al. PALS Provider Manual.* American Heart association (pub) 2002:p 92-98

62. Hofer CK, Ganter M, Tucci M, *et al.* How reliable is length-based determination of body weight and tracheal tube size in the paediatric age group? The Broselow tape reconsidered. *Br J Anaesth* 2002; 88:283–285.

63. Daugherty RJ, Nadkarni V, Brenn BR. Endotracheal tube size estimation for children with pathological short stature. *Pediatr Emerg Care* 2006; 22:710 –717.

64. Bhende MS, Thompson AE, Cook DR, Saville AL. Validity of a disposable end-tidal CO_2 detector in verifying endotracheal tube placement in infants and children. *Ann Emerg Med* 1992; 21:142-145.

65. Carenzi B, Corso RM, Stellino V, *et al.* Airway management in an infant with congenital centrofacial dysgenesia. *Br J Anaesth* 2002;88:726 –728.

66. Fraser J, Hill C, McDonald D, Jones C, Petros A. The use of the laryngeal mask airway for inter-hospital transport of infants with type 3 laryngotracheo-oesophageal clefts. *Intensive Care Med* 1999;25: 714–716.

67. Lopez-Gil M, Brimacombe J, Alvarez M. Safety and efficacy of the laryngeal mask airway. A prospective survey of 1400 children. *Anaesthesia* 1996;51:969–972.

68. Lopez-Gil M, Brimacombe J, Cebrian J, Arranz J. Laryngeal mask airway in pediatric practice: a prospective study of skill acquisition by anesthesia residents. *Anesthesiology* 1996; 84:807– 811.

69. Ditchey RV, Lindenfeld J. Potential adverse effects of volume loading on perfusion of vital organs during closed-chest resuscitation. *Circulation* 1984; 69: 181–189.

70. Voorhees WS, Ralston SH, Kougias C, Schmitx PM. Fluid loading with whole blood or Ringer's lactate solution during CPR in dogs. *Resuscitation* 1987; 15:113–123.

71. Carcillo JA, Fields AI. Clinical practice parameters for hemodynamic support of pediatric and neonatal patients in septic shock. *Crit Care Med* 2002; 30: 1365-1378.

72. Dellinger RP, Carlet JM, Masur H, *et al.* Surviving sepsis campaign guidelines for management of severe sepsis and septic shock. *Crit Care Med* 2004; 32:858-872.

73. Michael JR, Cuerci AD, Koehler RC, *et al.* Mechanisms by which epinephrine augments cerebral and myocardial perfusion during cardiopulmonary resuscitation in dogs. *Circulation* 1984; 69:822–835.

74. Pearson JW, Redding JS. Influence of peripheral vascular tone on resuscitation. *Anesth Analg* 1965; 44:746.

75. Goetting MG. Mastering pediatric cardiopulmonary resuscitation. *Ped Clin N Am* 1994; 41:1147–1182.

76. Mann K, Berg RA, Nadkarni V. Beneficial effects of vasopressin in prolonged pediatric cardiac arrest: a case series. *Resuscitation* 2002; 52: 149–156.

77. Lindner KH, Prengel AW, Brinkmann A, *et al*. Vasopressin administration in refractory cardiac arrest. *Ann Intern Med* 1996;124:1061–1064.

78. Duncan JM, Meaney P, Simpson P, *et al*. Vasopressin for in-hospital pediatric cardiac arrest: results from the American Heart Association National Registry of Cardiopulmonary Resuscitation. *Pediatr Crit Care Med* 2009;10:191–195.

79. Callaway CW, Hostler D, Doshi AA, *et al*. Usefulness of vasopressin administered with epinephrine during out-of-hospital cardiac arrest. *Am J Cardiol* 2006; 98:1316 –1321.

80. Gueugniaud PY, David JS, Chanzy E, *et al*. Vasopressin and epinephrine vs. epinephrine alone in cardiopulmonary resuscitation. *N Engl J Med* 2008; 359:21–30.

81. Meert KL, Donaldson A, Nadkarni V, *et al*. Multicenter cohort study of in-hospital pediatric cardiac arrest. *Pediatr Crit Care Med* 2009;10:544 –553.

82. Weil MH, Rackow EC, Trevino R, *et al*. Difference in acid-base state between venous and arterial blood during cardiopulmonary resuscitation. *N Engl J Med* 1986; 315:153–156.

83. Aufderheide TP, Martin DR, Olson DW, *et al*. Prehospital bicarbonate use in cardiac arrest: a 3-year experience. *Am J Emerg Med* 1992; 10:4 –7.

84. Urban P, Scheidegger D, Buchmann B, Barth D. Cardiac arrest and blood ionized calcium levels. *Ann Intern Med* 1988; 109:110-113.

85. Dembo DH. Calcium in advanced life support. *Crit Care Med* 1981; 9:358–359.

86. Coon GA, Clinton JE, Ruiz E. Use of atropine for brady– asystolic prehospital cardiac arrest. *Ann Emerg Med* 1981; 10:462-467.

87. Ashwal S, Schenider S, Tomasi L, Thompson J. Prognostic implications of hyperglycemia and reduced cerebral blood flow in childhood near–drowning. *Neurology* 1990; 40:820–823.

88. Longstreth WT, Inui TS. High blood glucose level on hospital admission and poor neurological recovery after cardiac arrest. *Ann Neurol* 1984; 15:59-63.

89. Sesjo, BK. Cerebral circulation and metabolism. *Neurosurgery* 1984; 60:883.

90. Collinsworth KA, Kalman SM, Harrison DS. The clinical pharmacology of lidocaine as an antiarrhythmic drug. *Circulation* 1974; 50:1217–1230.

91. Noc M, Weil MH, Tang W, *et al*. Electrocardiographic prediction of success of cardiac resuscitation. *Crit Care Med* 1999; 27:708-714.

92. Dockey WK, Futterman C, Keller SR, *et al*. A comparison of manual and mechanical ventilation during pediatric transport. *Crit Care Med* 1999; 27: 802–806.

93. Doherty DR, Parshuram CS, Gaboury I, *et al*. Hypothermia therapy after pediatric cardiac arrest. *Circulation* 2009;119:1492–1500.

94. Hypothermia After Cardiac Arrest Study Group. Mild therapeutic hypothermia to improve the neurologic outcome after cardiac arrest. *N Engl J Med* 2002; 346: 549 –556.

95. Gluckman PD, Wyatt JS, Azzopardi D, *et al*. Selective head cooling with mild systemic hypothermia after neonatal encephalopathy: multicentre randomised trial. *Lancet* 2005; 365:663–670.

96. Krischer JP, Fine EG, Davis J, Nagel El. Complications of cardiac resuscitation. *Chest* 1987; 92:287–291.

97. Atkins DL, Everson-Stewart S, Sears GK, *et al*. Epidemiology and outcomes from out-of-hospital cardiac arrest in children: The Resuscitation Outcomes Consortium Epistry-Cardiac Arrest. *Circulation* 2009;119:1484 –1491.

98. Zaritsky A, Nadkarni V, Getson P, Kuehl K. CPR in children. *Ann Emerg Med* 1987;16:1107–1111.

99. Gillis J, Dickson D, Rieder M, *et al*. Results of inpatient pediatric resuscitation. *Crit Care Med* 1986;14:469–471.

100. Parra DA, Totapally BR, Zahn E, *et al*. Outcome of cardiopulmonary resuscitation in a pediatric cardiac intensive care unit. *Crit Care Med* 2000; 28: 3296 –3300.

101. Duncan BW, Ibrahim AE, Hraska V, *et al*. Use of rapid-deployment extracorporeal membrane oxygenation for the resuscitation of pediatric patients with heart disease after cardiac arrest. *J Thorac Cardiovasc Surg* 1998;116:305–311.

102. Morris MC, Wernovsky G, Nadkarni VM. Survival outcomes after extracorporeal cardiopulmonary resuscitation instituted during active chest compressions following refractory in-hospital pediatric cardiac arrest. *Pediatr Crit Care Med* 2004; 5:440–446.

103. Alsoufi B, Al-Radi OO, Nazer RI, *et al*. Survival outcomes after rescue extracorporeal cardiopulmonary resuscitation in pediatric patients with refractory cardiac arrest. *J Thorac Cardiovasc Surg* 2007; 134: 952–959.

104. Lequier L, Joffe AR, Robertson CM, *et al*. Two-year survival, mental, and motor outcomes after cardiac extracorporeal life support at less than five years of age. *J Thorac Cardiovasc Surg* 2008;136:976–983.

105. Yannopoulos D, Matsuura T, Schultz J, *et al*. Sodium nitroprusside enhanced cardiopulmonary resuscitation improves survival with good neurological function in a porcine model of prolonged cardiac arrest. *Crit Care Med* 2011; 39:1269-1274.

106. Fumagalli F, Ristagno G. The patient is in cardiac arrest! Let's be snappy: Prepare a bolus of sodium nitroprusside, while I compress the chest. It's not a joke! *Crit Care Med* 2011; 39:1548-1549.

Anaphylaxis

4

Surjit Singh

The term 'anaphylaxis' or an 'anaphylactic reaction' refers to an acute onset IgE-mediated life-threatening clinical syndrome which occurs when large quantities of inflammatory mediators are rapidly released from mast cells and basophils within a few minutes of exposure to an allergen to which the individual has previously been sensitized[1-3]. The term 'anaphylactoid reaction,' on the other hand, refers to a phenomenon in which the clinical and pathological features may mimic anaphylaxis but there is no discernible allergen-IgE antibody reaction[1,3]. Moreoover, anaphylactoid reactions can occur even at the time of first exposure i.e. prior sensitization is not an essential prerequisite for such reactions. Anaphylactoid reactions are mediated by anaphylatoxins like C3a and C5a[4,5].

Both anaphylactic and anaphylactoid reactions can be life-threatening and can affect any organ system. Death most commonly results from asphyxia (due to either upper airway involvement resulting in laryngeal edema or lower airway involvement resulting in severe bronchospasm) or cardiovascular collapse (i.e. anaphylactic shock) resulting from third space losses as a result of transudation of fluid from the intravascular space.[3-5].

Anaphylactic reactions occur at a frequency of 0.4 cases per million per year in the general population, but are seen much more frequently in hospitalized patients. It is believed that anaphylaxis affects 1-2% of the general population at some time during life[4-6].

ETIOLOGICAL AGENTS

Clinical history is of paramount importance in determining the cause of anaphylaxis. The most common inciting agents are drugs, foods and insect venoms though in a recent study in children Dibs and Baker[4] found latex induced anaphylaxis to be very common.

While most anaphylactic reactions follow parenteral administration of drugs/chemicals, oral intake or mucocutaneous contact can also, at times, result in severe anaphylaxis. The rapidity of development of anaphylaxis is directly related to its severity.

Contrary to common belief, atopic individuals do not have an increased risk of developing anaphylaxis as compared to the general population[4]. Food induced anaphylaxis (eg. after ingestion of peanuts/shellfish) is being increasingly reported from the west but appears to be rather uncommon in our experience[1,4,6-8]. The reason for this is not clear. In western countries food allergens account for 30% of fatal cases of anaphylaxis. Table 4.1 lists the commonly incriminated agents in anaphylaxis.[1,3,9,10]

Table 4.1 Common causes of anaphylaxis and anaphylactoid reactions
Anaphylaxis
Drugs
• Pencillins, cephalosporins, amphotericin B, streptomycin, phenytoin, thiamine, lignocaine and other anesthetic agents, N-acetylcysteine
Biological products
• Blood products, vaccines, antisera, intravenous immunoglobulins, L-asparaginase, allergenic extracts used for desensitization therapy
Foods
• Milk, peanuts, egg-white, sea-foods, treenuts, soya
Insect venoms
• Insects of the order Hymenoptera (wasp, hornet, honey bee, yellow-jacket)
Miscellaneous agents
• Iron-dextran, latex, tick-bite
Idiopathic
• No cause is found in some children
Anaphylactoid reactions
• Nonsteroidal anti-inflammatory drugs (especially aspirin), contrast agents used in diagnostic radiology and IVIG.

PATHOPHYSIOLOGY

An anaphylactic reaction can only occur if an individual with specific IgE antibodies gets exposed to an allergen to which he has previously been sensitized[3,9,10]. These IgE antibodies are fixed on the high-affinity cell surface receptors (FcERI) of mast cells and basophils. On exposure to the incriminated allergen, there is cross-linking of numerous IgE antibody molecules occupying the FcERI receptors. This cross-linking leads to activation of mast cells and results in increased intracellular free calcium levels. Following these signalling events the cytoplasmic granules fuse with one another causing release of mediators of inflammation like histamine, leukotrienes and proteases amongst many others. It must be appreciated that this cascade of events can be initiated by extremely small amounts of allergen. The released mediators have both local and systemic effects, the most notable amongst these being increased vascular permeability, smooth muscle contraction, vasodilation and mucous gland secretion[2,3,11].

The initiating mechanism is somewhat different in anaphylactoid reactions as these are not IgE mediated. Here the incriminated agent may activate the alternative complement pathway by binding to certain serum proteins or by activation of proteolytic enzymes. This activation of the alternative complement pathway results in generation of anaphylatoxins C3a and C5a which bind to specific receptors on the surface of mast cells and basophils, thereby resulting in their degranulation and subsequent release of histamine and other inflammatory mediators. C3a and C5a can by themselves also directly cause smooth muscle contraction and increased mucous gland secretion. It is apparent, therefore, that even though the end inflammatory changes in anaphylactic and anaphylactoid reactions are almost similar, IgE-mediated hypersensitivity is not demonstrable in the latter while it is a *sine quo non* of the former. Most of the hypersensitivity reactions seen with iodinated radiographic contrast media are believed to be anaphylactoid in type[2,4,5].

PATHOLOGY

In fatal cases there is edema and vascular congestion in the mucosa of upper airways. In the lungs there is mucosal and submucosal edema, peribronchial vascular congestion and eosinophilia. Features of shock are also prominent; these include congested liver and spleen and in addition there may be evidences of myocardial ischemia and/or infarction[3,8]. Elevated levels of specific IgE can be demonstrated in the heart blood of patients dying of anaphylaxis by radio-allergo-sorbent-test (RAST) or by SDS-PAGE immunoblotting[3].

CLINICAL FEATURES

It cannot be over-emphasized that both anaphylactic and anaphylactoid reactions occur with extreme rapidity[1-3]. Prompt diagnosis and immediate treatment are the cornerstones of management of such cases. The symptoms usually start within seconds or minutes after exposure to the allergen and sometimes cardiovascular collapse can progress so rapidly that there may be no discernible warning symptoms and signs. Fatal anaphylaxis, occuring suddenly, following ingestion of peanuts is well documented in sensitized individuals[3,4,8].

A tingling sensation, feeling of intense fright or sense of impending doom may herald the onset of reaction. Some patients may complain of feeling 'odd' or have 'sinking/fainting' sensation. These initial symptoms are soon followed by overt involvement of one or more of several organ systems especially respiratory, cardiovascular, skin and gastrointestinal. Involvement of the respiratory tract may present with features of upper airway obstruction (i.e. 'lump' in the throat, hoarseness of voice or stridor) or lower airway involvement (i.e. dyspnea or wheezing). There may be peripheral or central cardiovascular involvement; the former is characterized by generalized arteriolar dilatation and increased vascular permeability, while the latter may result in cardiac arrhythmias. In addition there may be myocardial ischemia and/or infarction due to the shock-like state resulting from rapid fluid shifts from the intravascular to the extravascular spaces. There may be tell-tale evidence in the skin in the form of intense pruritus and a localized or generalized urticarial eruption (which is due to involvement of superficial layers of dermis) or angioedema (which is due to involvement of deeper layers of dermis and subcutaneous tissues). The latter may especially involve tissues of the upper airways, eyelids, lips or tongue. Gastrointestinal involvement results from mucosal edema and contraction of intestinal smooth muscle and may present with crampy abdominal pain and diarrhea[7,8]. At times the patient may suddenly start talking irrelevantly or behaving abnormally. Seizures can also occur.

Patients with severe manifestations may develop multi-organ failure if the shock is not corrected. Hemostatic abnormalities can also be seen because of activation of the intrinsic coagulation pathway resulting in disseminated intravascular coagulation and depletion of clotting factors. Some children can have a biphasic or multiphasic response i.e. recurrence(s) of anaphylaxis after apparent clinical resolution of the initial episode[12-14]. This occurs specially in those children who require higher or multiple doses of adrenaline to control their initial symptoms. Such recurrences of anaphylaxis are usually mild and respond promptly to standard treatment[12-15].

CLINICAL CONDITIONS MIMICKING ANAPHYLAXIS

1. *Hereditary angio-neurotic edema.* This is a rare complement disorder which results from a deficiency of the C_1 esterase inhibitor.[2,3] It is inherited as an autosomal dominant disorder. Children can present with recurrent attacks of angioedema, which persists for periods varying from a few hours to few days. Pruritus is conspicuously absent. It does not respond to adrenaline.

2. *Anaphylactoid reactions* from iodinated radiographic contrast media may be mild or severe and even prove fatal in 1:100,000 cases. Such reactions can occur on first exposure and need not always occur on subsequent exposures. Attempts to demonstrate specific IgE antibodies to such compounds have been unrewarding. These hypersensitivity reactions are, therefore, considered to be anaphylactoid rather than anaphylactic in nature[1-3].

3. *Non-IgE 'anaphylaxis'.* IgA deficient individuals may develop anti-IgA antibodies which are believed to be IgG4 in nature[3]. If such sensitized individuals are given non-IgA depleted blood products, anaphylaxis can result from complement activation and anaphylatoxin generation due to circulating immune complexes of IgA and IgG4-anti-IgA. These anaphylatoxins can result in mast cell activation and release of inflammatory mediators.

4. *Exercise-induced 'anaphylaxis'.* This was first described by Sheffer and Austen in 1980. It is believed to result from mast cell activation secondary to endorphin release during exercise. It is considered an anaphylactoid reaction because IgE involvement has never been demonstrated. Affected individuals need not develop 'anaphylaxis' after each episode of exercise[16].

5. *Aggregate 'anaphylaxis'.* This may result from infusion of intravenous immunoglobulin (IVIG) preparations containing high molecular weight aggregates of gamma-globulins. Such reactions are rare with the highly refined preparations of IVIG that are currently available. These aggregates generate anaphylatoxins (C3a and C5a) which are capable of activating mast cells for mediator release. This is an anaphylactoid reaction[3].

6. *Miscellaneous conditions.* Other conditions which can mimic the symptoms and signs of anaphylaxis include cardiac arrhythmias, severe asthma, vasovagal syncope and anxiety reactions.

LABORATORY INVESTIGATIONS

It cannot be overemphasized that anaphylaxis is a clinical diagnosis and usually no investigations are required to confirm it. The hemogram may show an elevated hematocrit and leucocytosis. Arterial blood gases may reveal variable changes depending on the severity of the episode; severe hypoxia and hypercapnia may be present along with acidosis. Electrocardiography may show nonspecific ST-T wave changes and arrhythmias, especially heart blocks. Serum tryptase levels are elevated and may be used to confirm the diagnosis[5]. Laboratory tests can be helpful to confirm the diagnosis of anaphylaxis or rule out other causes. Proper timing of such tests (e.g. serum tryptase) is essential.

TREATMENT

Treatment of both anaphylaxis and anaphylactoid reactions is similar[1,2] and must be started early to improve the outcome. Treatment should be aimed at managemnt of shock, upper airway swelling and bronchial obstruction – these being the three most important determinants of mortality[6]. Death can occur within minutes after the initial symptoms[5,6,8]. Even if there is any doubt about the diagnosis, it is prudent to administer adrenaline and oxygen, which are the cornerstones of management of anaphylaxis. Delay in initiation of treatment can be fatal, especially in severe reactions.

The mainstay of therapy is intramuscular adrenaline, administration of oxygen and adequate volume replacement. Adrenaline has both alpha and beta agonist activity and results in vascoconstriction, bronchial smooth muscle relaxation and attenuation of increased vascular permeability. The dose is 0.01 ml/kg (1:1000 solution) and can be repeated at 15-30 minute intervals. The intramuscular route (vastus lateralis rather than deltoid) is preferred to the subcutaneous route as recent studies have shown that there may be delayed absorption when the drug is given by the latter route[6,17,18].

In children with severe symptoms or shock, a dependable intravenous line should be established. Adrenaline is given intravenously (0.01-0.05 ml/kg of 1:10,000 solution) along with volume expanders (saline, plasma or albumin). An effective airway must be secured (either by endotracheal intubation or tracheostomy) and adequate ventilation established. Fluids should be infused liberally (20 ml/kg bolus followed by 10 ml/kg/ hour) and if hypotension is still persisting, dopamine should be used as a vasopressor (10–15 µg/kg/min). Replacement of third space losses may require infusion of large amounts of fluids. If there is significant wheezing, nebulized salbutamol (0.15 mg/kg) may be given. The child must be kept recumbent with legs elevated. Arterial oxygen saturation must be checked at frequent intervals[3,5,16-18].

It must be emphasized that corticosteroids have no significant role in the management of anaphylaxis because the onset of their therapeutic effect requires several hours and they do not alleviate any of the life-threatening manifestations of anaphylactic reactions. However, they may prevent and alleviate later recurrence of bronchospasm, hypotension or uticaria[2,3,5]. One should use either methylprednisolone (1-2 mg/kg) or hydrocortisone (5-10 mg/kg) IM or IV every 6 hours. For patients with intractable reactions, glucagon has been found a potentially life-saving supplemental therapy.

Gastrointestinal and skin manifestations (urticaria, angioedema) are usually not life-threatening and respond to antihistaminics (eg.diphenhydramine 1–2 mg/kg IM or IV)[5,7]. Intravenous antihistaminics should always be infused slowly so that there is no hypotension. Oral antihistaminics may suffice for treatment of mild manifestations.

Treatment of anaphylaxis developing during transfusion of blood (or blood products) requires immediate stoppage of the transfusion, maintenance of adequate vascular access and administration of adrenaline/steroids.

If the reaction has been caused by an injected drug, adrenaline should be infiltrated locally (0.1-0.2 ml of 1: 1000 solution) along with application of ice-packs to retard absorption of antigen. If the injected site is over a limb, a tourniquet should be applied proximal to the site of injection, briefly releasing it every few minutes.

For anaphylactic reactions due to Hymenoptera stings (e.g.wasp, hornet, honey bee, yellow jacket) the principles of treatment remain the same. Cold compresses may help to reduce the pain and swelling. In addition, in case of honey-bee stings the venom sac and stinger usually remain in the skin and should be swiftly removed (but ensuring that no compression is done) so as to retard further absorption of venom[3,5].

If the child develops a cardiac arrest during anaphylaxis cardiopulmonary resuscitation and advanced cardiac life support measures should be initiated. High-dose intravenous adrenaline (0.01 mg/kg i.e. 0.1 ml/kg of a 1:10,000 solution up to 10 mg/min rate of infusion), repeated every 3 to 5 min is recommended. Higher dosages (0.1-0.2 mg/kg or 0.1 ml/kg of a 1:1,000 solution) may be required for asystole. Prolonged resuscitation should be continued as many children ultimately recover completely.

Children with mild reactions may be discharged after a few hours of observation. However, those who have had severe reactions, and specially if they required multiple doses of adrenaline for resuscitation, must be hospitalized and kept under observation for 24-48 hours as biphasic and multiphasic anaphylactic reactions can occur under such circumstances[12,13]. Some recent studies suggest that delayed administration of adrenaline can be associated with an increased incidence of biphasic reactions.

Newer therapeutic agents like leukotriene modifiers, tranexamic acid and nitric oxide synthesis inhibitors have been considered for treatment of anaphylaxis but their use is considered only in special circumstances.

PREVENTION

All medical personnel who give intramuscular injections must be prepared to manage an anaphylactic reaction. Ideally all children must be observed for 15-20 minutes after any intramuscular injection. Children with Hymenoptera venom anaphylaxis should reduce their outdoor activities to a bare minimum and must avoid using perfumes and wearing bright clothes (especially orange/yellow) which attract insects. They must be advised to ensure ready availability of adrenaline at all times and, if possible, have a preloaded adrenaline syringe (EpiPen, Ana-Kit)[17]. Adrenaline aerosol spray (Medihaler) is also a useful adjunct for treatment of laryngeal edema and threatened airway obstruction but is not a substitute for intramuscular adrenaline. Venom desensitization procedures are very effective and are recommended for individuals who have experienced systemic anaphylaxis after a sting and who have a significant positive skin test to one or more venoms[19-21]. There is high grade cross-reactivity between yellow-jacket and wasp venom but only low grade cross-reactivity between honey-bee and yellow jacket venoms. Immunotherapy is started with very dilute strengths of the venom (1:10,000 - 1:50,000) which are gradually increased to 1:50. Injections are initially given weekly for a few months and then maintenance therapy is continued at 4-6 weekly intervals. Immunotherapy results in development of "blocking" antibodies of the IgG4 subclass. Treatment can usually be discontinued after approximately 5 years or so, but in some cases life-long maintenance therapy may be necessary.

Children who have had anaphylactoid reactions to iodinated radiographic contrast media should be pretreated with antihistamines and steroids if the contrast needs to be administered again. Many such children would be able to tolerate repeat administration of the contrast without significant reactions[3,4]. Children who have had anaphylactic reactions after exposure to a particular drug should be advised to avoid exposure to related drugs in future. However, the first episode of anaphylaxis cannot be usually predicted. Routine skin testing for antimicrobials (pencillins included) is, strictly speaking, not warranted; such procedures should only be carried out in those individuals who give a history of having had immediate hypersensitivity reactions in the past. Moreover, scratch testing must always precede intradermal skin testing because it is not always realized that some patients may develop anaphylaxis during the latter test procedure itself. In the case of penicillin any meaningful skin testing procedure must include both major and minor antigenic determinants[1,2]. As these determinants are not easily available commercially, routine testing for penicillin hypersensitivity, using benzyl penicillin as is done commonly, does not preclude the occurrence of anaphylaxis even in those individuals who test negative. It should also be noted that anaphylactic reactions to penicillin develop only due to sensitization to the minor antigenic determinants while the major antigenic determinants are responsible for allergic reactions other than anaphylaxis. All patients who have had serious anaphylactic reactions in the past should wear an information bracelet giving details of their allergic predisposition.

PROGNOSIS

Anaphylaxis can be fatal if treatment is delayed. In true anaphylactic reactions, each succeeding exposure to the offending allergen would generally be expected to result in a more severe reaction. However, there may be some loss of sensitivity over a period of time, but this is extremely unpredictable. Exercise induced and idiopathic anaphylaxis can be recurrent in nature.

REFERENCES

1. Sampson HA, Leung DYM. Anaphylaxis. In: Nelson Textbook of Pediatrics, 18th. Kliegman RM, Behrman RE, Jenson HB, Stanton BF. (Eds.) *Saunders Elsevier, Philadelphia,* 2008, pp. 983-985.

2. Lieberman P, Nicklas RA, Oppenheimer J, Kemp SF, Lang DM. The diagnosis and management of anaphylaxis practice parameter: 2010 Update. *J Allergy Clin Immunol* 2010; 126:477-480.

3. Simons FER. Anaphylaxis: Recent advances in assessment and treatment. *J Allergy Clin Immunol* 2009; 124:625-636.

4. Dibs SD, Baker MD. Anaphylaxis in children: a 5-year experience. *Pediatrics* 1997, 99(1): E7.

5. Simons FER. Anaphylaxis. *J Allergy Clin Immunol* 2010; 125:S161-S181.

6. Sampson HA. Anaphylaxis and emergency treatment. *Pediatrics* 2003; 111: 1601-1608.

7. Simons FER, Clark S, Camargo Jr. CA. Anaphylaxis in the community: Learning from the survivors. *J Allergy Clin Immunol* 2009; 124:301-306.

8. Sampsom HA, Mendelson L, Rosen JP. Fatal and near-fatal anaphylactic reactions to food in children and adolescents. *N Engl J Med* 1992; 327: 380-384.

9. Ditto AM, Krasnick J, Greenberger PA, Kelly KJ, McGrath K, Patterson R. Pediatric idiopathic anaphylaxis. *J Allergy Clin Immunol* 1997, 100(3): 320-326.

10. Simons FER. Anaphylaxis: Recent advances in assessment and treatment. *J Allergy Clin Immunol* 2009; 124:625-636.

11. Krasnick J, Patterson R, Harris KE. Idiopathic anaphylaxis: long-term follow-up, cost and outlook. *Allergy* 1996, 51 (10): 724-731.

12. Stevens WJ, Ebo DG, De Clerck LS, Bridts CH, De Gendt CM, Mertens AV. Evolution of lymphocyte transformation to wasp venom antigen during immunotherapy for wasp venom anaphylaxis. *Clin Experiment Allergy* 1998, 28 (2): 249-252.

13. Brazil E, MacNamara AF. "Not so immediate" hypersensitivity- the danger of biphasic anaphylactic reactions. *J Accident and Emerg Med* 1998, 15: 252-253.

14. Brady WJ Jr., Luber S, Carter CT, Guertler A, Lindbeck G. Multiphasic anaphylaxis: an uncommon event in the emergency department. *Acad Emerg Med* 1997, 4 (3); 193-197.

15. Lee JM, Greenes DS. Biphasic anaphylactic reactions in pediatrics. *Pediatrics* 2000; 106: 762-766.

16. Volcheck GW, Li JT. Exercise-induced urticaria and anaphylaxis. *Mayo Clinic Proceedings* 1997, 72 (2): 140-147.

17. Simons FE, Roberts JR, Gu X, Simons KJ. Epinephrine absorption in children with a history of anaphylaxis. *J Allergy Clin Immunol* 1998, 101 : 33-37.

18. Gold MS, Sainsbury R. First aid anaphylaxis management in children who were prescribed an epinephrine autoinjector device. *J Allergy Clin Immunol* 2000; 106: 171-176.

19. Simons FER, Gu X, Simons KJ. Epinephrine absorption in adults: intramuscular versus subcutaneous injection. *J Allergy Clin Immunol* 2001; 108: 871-873.

20. Diez Gomez ML, Quirce Gancedo S, Juliade Paramo B. Venom immunotherapy: Tolerance to a 3-day protocol of rush-immunotherapy. *Allergologia et Immunopathologia* 1995, 23 (6); 277-284.

21. Sturm G, Kranks B, Rudolf C, *et al.* Rush Hymenoptera venom immunotherapy: a safe and practical protocol for high risk patients. *J Allergy Clin Immunol* 2002; 110: 928-933.

Section 1

Fluids, Electrolytes and Acid-Base Disorders

5

Sunit Singhi and K Sasidaran

The integrity of an organism depends on a stable internal environment, which is constituted in a large measure by water and electrolytes, which are maintained within normal limits by a delicate balance. In several disease states, the disturbance in this balance may not be the primary disorder but its correction is mandatory for the complete recovery. The goal of fluid and electrolyte therapy is to maintain normal volume and tonicity of body fluids necessary for supply of nutrition at the cellular level.

PHYSIOLOGIC CONSIDERATIONS

Next to oxygen, water is the most essential element for life. The largest component of body is water. From birth onwards, the relative proportions of bone, fat, muscle, viscera, and water change because of dynamic changes in body size.

Body Water and its Distribution

Total body water (TBW) is higher at birth which gradually declines to 65 percent of body weight by one year of age[1,2]. Almost all the reduction in TBW is contributed by loss of extracellular water (ECW) over time. Table 5.1 provides the percentage of TBW in different age groups.

Total body water is divided into two principle compartments; the intracellular (ICW) and the extracellular water (ECW). After infancy the ICW to ECW ratio reaches 2:1 and remain constant during subsequent years. The ECW compartment is further divided into the interstitial and intravascular spaces, which are separated in a 3:1 ratio. Thus, the intravascular space constitutes 1/12 of the total body water.

When there is an increase in the total body water, this is clinically manifested by an increase in the ECW space, because the ICW compartment is not accessible to direct assessment[1]. Fat is low in water content, therefore, total body water represents a lower percentage of body weight in an obese or chubby infant[3].

Table 5.1 Total body water in different age groups

Age group	Total body water in %	TBW distribution factor (TBWD)
Fetus	90%	0.9
Premature babies	80%	0.8
Term infants	70%	0.7
Young children	65%	0.65
Adolescent	60%	0.6
Adult male	60%	0.6
Adult female	50%	0.5

Electrolyte Composition of Body Fluids

Concentration of electrolytes in body fluids is shown in Table 5.2. Sodium and chloride are the principal electrolytes in the extracellular fluid (ECF) while potassium and phosphates are the principal electrolytes in the intracellular fluid (ICF)[2,3]. Chloride and bicarbonate are major extracellular anions, whereas proteins and phosphate comprise the major intracellular cations.

In the ECF, electrolyte concentration of plasma is somewhat different from that of interstitial fluid. In plasma the protein concentration is higher and the sodium and chloride concentrations are lower than that of interstitial fluid[3].

Volume of distribution for individual solutes[4,5]

Differences in cell permeability and binding characters of specific ions are reflected in the coefficients that are used to determine the volume of distribution for individual solutes. The volume of distribution for sodium is equal to total body water (Table 5.1) but for bicarbonate it is 0.3 times the total body water. Understanding this concept is important to formulate therapeutic regimens to treat disorders of sodium and water balance.

Table 5.2 Electrolyte composition of body fluids

Electrolytes	ICF	ECF	Interstitial fluid
Cations (mEq/L)			
Na$^+$	9.0	140	147
K$^+$	158	4.5	4.0
Ca^{++}	3.0	5.0	2.5
Mg^{++}	30	2.0	1.0
Anions (mEq/L)			
Cl$^-$	4.0	103	114
HCO3$^-$	10.0	25	30
Proteins	65	15	0
Phosphates	95	2.0	2.0
Organic acids	4.0	6.0	7.5
Sulfates	22	-	1.0

Osmolality and Regulation of Body Water

The plasma osmolality (Posm) is equal to the sum of the individual osmolalities of each solute present in the vascular space. This is defined as the number of milliosmoles of solute present per kilogram of water. Since sodium, glucose and urea are the principal intravascular solutes, the osmolality of the plasma can be estimated by the following formula:

$$\text{Plasma osmolality} = 2 \times \text{serum Na}^+ \text{ in mEq/L} + \frac{\text{Glucose (mg/dl)}}{18} + \frac{\text{BUN (mg/dl)}}{2.8}$$

Although there are significant differences in the ionic composition of different body fluid compartments, under equilibrium conditions, the sum of all osmotically active particles is equal in all compartments. Normal plasma osmolality is 285-295 mOsm/kg and this is in equilibrium with interstitial and intracellular fluid.

Effective osmolality or tonicity is calculated by the following formula as glucose and/or BUN become effective osmoles only in diseased states like diabetic ketoacidosis and acute kidney injury

Effective plasma osmolality = 2 × (Serum Na$^+$ in mEq/L)

A change in effective osmolality is the major determinant of movement of water between plasma and interstitial fluid, and interstitial fluid and intracellular fluid. Water will flow from a region of low to high osmolality.[5]

The calculated serum osmolality is normally within 1-2% of value obtained by direct osmometry. Significant "osmolar gap" (measured osmolality – calculated osmolality) indicates accumulation of unmeasured osmoles.

Mechanisms for Maintenance of TBW and Plasma Osmolality

Thirst is activated when ECF water deficit is about 2.0 percent. The center for thirst is situated in the hypothalamus. Thirst remains the major early defense mechanism against hypertonicity and dehydration[5].

Renal mechanisms. Kidneys regulate water balance and the osmolality of body fluids by controlling excretion of solutes and free water under the influence of ADH and natriuretic peptides[4]. ADH secretion from supraoptic-hypophyseal system is regulated by intracellular and plasma osmolality (through osmoreceptors) and by volume of ECF (Volume receptors). *Hypovolemia is a more potent stimulus for ADH secretion than hyperosmolality.* Fall in plasma volume and resultant reduction in renal perfusion triggers the release of aldosterone from adrenal cortex. This hormone causes active transport of sodium at the distal tubular level so that sodium and water is retained in the extracellular space. *Natriuretic peptides are body's defense against plasma volume expansion[4].*

Physiological Requirements of Water and Electrolytes

Physiological requirements of fluids and electrolytes consist of the amount of water and electrolytes necessary to replace obligatory urinary and insensible water losses, and the water required for metabolic activity[6, 7]. These may be computed on the basis of body weight, surface area or metabolic rate (Table 5.3). For every 100 kcals metabolized, a child requires approximately 110 - 115 ml of water, 3 mEq of sodium and 2.5 mEq of potassium. About 10-15 ml of water is produced in the body during oxidation of endogenous and exogenous carbohydrates, proteins and fats. Thus for all practical purposes 100 ml of fluid is sufficient to metabolize 100 kcals[6, 7].

Infants are always at danger of developing fluid imbalance because of several reasons; (i) their body surface area to body weight or lean body mass is 2.7 times more than older children and adults. Hence, their insensible water losses are much more;

Source	Losses per 100 kcals metabolized energy		
	Water (ml)	**Na$^+$ (mEq)**	**K$^+$ (mEq)**
Insensible losses			
Lungs	-15	0	0
Skin	-30	0.1	0.2
Stool losses	-10	0.1	0.2
Urinary losses	-55	3.0	2.0
Water for oxidation	+15		
Total for maintenance	**100 ml**	**3.2 mEq**	**2.4 mEq**

Table 5.3 Physiological losses of fluids and electrolytes[6,7, 15]

(ii) they require more urine volume to excrete solutes, because their maximal renal concentrating capacity is lower than older children and adults; (iii) infants have greater caloric requirement per kg than adults and, therefore, need more water for metabolism; (iv) there is a rapid turnover of water in infants, daily maintenance water requirements being approximately 15 percent of total body water (as opposed to 5% in an adult); (v) they are prone to frequent episodes of diarrhea and (vi) above all,

they are at the mercy of adults to satisfy their fluid requirements.

Fluid requirement increases with patient's age and correlates well with body surface area, caloric requirement and body weight. Table 5.4 shows maintenance requirements of fluids and electrolytes on the basis of body weight and surface area. Clinical conditions that affect water loss from body or the total caloric expenditure require modification of normal maintenance requirement (Table 5.5).

Table 5.4 Daily maintenance requirements of fluids and electrolytes

Requirements	By body weight	By surface area
Water		
Upto 10 kg	100 ml/kg	1500 ml/m^2
11-20 kg	1000 ml + 50 ml/kg for extra weight above 10 kg	(range 1200-1800 ml)
> 20 kg	1500 ml + 20 ml/kg for extra weight above 20 kg	
Sodium	3-4 mEq/kg/day	40-60 mEq/m^2
Potassium	2-3 mEq/kg/day	30-40 mEq/m^2
Chloride	3-4 mEq/kg/day	-

Table 5.5 Factors increasing insensible water loss (ISWL)[15]

Conditions increasing ISWL	Percent change	Volume change in ml	Modified maintenance fluid volume to be started based on BSA
Prematurity	100-300	500-1500/m^2	1500 ml/m^2 + 500 ml/ m^2
Radiant warmer	50-100	250-500/ m^2	1500 ml/m^2 + 250 ml/ m^2
Phototherapy	25-50	125-250/ m^2	1500 ml/m^2 + 125 ml/ m^2
Hyperventilation	20-30	100-150/ m^2	1500 ml/m^2 + 100 ml/ m^2
Increased activity	5-25	25-125/ m^2	1500 ml/m^2 + 25 ml/ m^2
Hyperthermia	12/°C	60/°C	1500 ml/m^2 + 60 ml/°C

In recent years, there has been an ongoing controversy about the appropriate maintenance fluid in hospitalized children. Even though the standard recommendation based on original work by Holliday et al[7] suggest the use of hypotonic saline (0.33 – 0.5% saline), a group of people relate this practice to the increased occurrence of hyponatremia and neurological complications. *It is reasonable to use N/2 saline as maintenance fluid in all acutely ill hospitalized children*[8].

A modification in the volume of maintenance fluid is necessary with altered body temperature, altered ambient temperature and humidity, renal diseases, respiratory, cardiovascular problems and during neonatal period. This happens due to alteration in total amount of insensible water loss from normal (500 ml/m^2) leading to disturbed state of equilibrium.

There are limitations to any protocolized fluid charting approach because (a) ISWL changes due to any factor have a wide range; (b) many factors tilting ISWL on either side may co-exist in an individual patient; and (c) few factors may influence more than other factors

The fluid recommendations given in Tables 5.5 and 5.6 can *only serve as a rough guideline to initiate modified volume of maintenance intravenous fluids in specific conditions* but subsequent titration need to be done based on ongoing volume status assessment, urine output measurement, fluid balance (positive or negative), and myocardial function of an individual patient.

Neonatal Period

Approximately 70 percent of usual maintenance requirements are given during the first 2 days. It is gradually increased to 100 percent by day 4-5. Low birth weight infants require relatively more water because of relatively greater insensible water losses. Table 5.7 provides guidelines for fluid requirements in the neonates.

Above mentioned recommendations are the general guidelines. Ideally, advances in fluids should to be made based on assessment of fluid status. Average maintenance fluid requirements in neonates may require modification because of many factors, which include use of radiant heaters, phototherapy, high ambient humidity, gestational age, fever and hypermetabolic state.

Sodium supplementation is started when cumulative weight loss from birth reaches ≥ 6% of birth weight, after ensuring initial diuresis (urine output ≥ 1 ml/kg/hour) unless serum sodium falls to ≤ 130 mEq/L. We usually start at 2 mEq/kg/day but preterm babies may require incremental dose after 1st week of life.

Potassium supplementation is usually not required till day 3 of life, and should be started based on serum potassium level.

Elemental calcium in a dose of 36-72 mg/kg/day (4-8 ml/kg/day of 10% calcium gluconate) should be initiated in all sick babies and babies < 1500 g from day 1 of life.

Table 5.6 Factors reducing insensible water loss (ISWL)[15]			
Conditions reducing ISWL	Percent change	Volume change in ml	Modified maintenance fluid volume to be started based on BSA
Enclosed incubator	25-50	125-250/m^2	1500 ml/m^2 - 125 ml/ m^2
Humidified air	15-30	75-150/ m^2	1500 ml/m^2 - 75 ml/ m^2
Sedation	5-25	25-125/ m^2	1500 ml/m^2 - 25 ml/ m^2
Decreased activity	5-25	25-125/ m^2	1500 ml/m^2 - 25 ml/ m^2
Hypothermia	5-15	25-75/ m^2	1500 ml/m^2 - 25 ml/ m^2

Table 5.7 Neonatal fluid requirements (ml/kg/day)					
Birth weight	Day 1	Day 2	Day 3	Day 4	Day 5
< 1000 g	80-100	Increase fluids as per hydration status			
1000 – 1500 g	80	100	120	140	150
> 1500 g	60	80	100	120	140

DEHYDRATION

Dehydration is net loss of body water. It is the commonest imbalance of body water in infants and children. The most common cause of dehydration in children is diarrhea and vomiting. It may also occur due to excessive urinary losses because of diabetes insipidus, osmotic diuresis (hyperglycemia), cerebral salt wasting and diuretic use.

Dehydration may be hypotonic, isotonic or hypertonic. The commonest type of dehydration is isotonic. In this form, there is a proportionate loss of water and solutes from ECF. The latter thus remains isotonic. There is no redistribution of fluid as there is no osmotic gradient between ECF and ICF. The intracellular volume remains intact.

In hypotonic dehydration, the depletion of solutes in ECF is much more than the water losses. This leads to movement of water from ECF to ICF, causing a further contraction of ECF and shock. In hypertonic dehydration, there is an excessive loss of water proportionate to the solutes. This leads to movement of water from cells into the ECF causing intracellular dehydration.

The steps in the successful management of dehydration in infants and children include the following:

1. Assessment of degree of dehydration
2. Rapid restoration of intravascular volume
3. Correction of total fluid deficit (rehydration therapy)
4. Replacement of ongoing loses and nutritional support
5. Provision of maintenance fluids and electrolytes
6. Monitoring to prevent resurfacing of fluid deficit and dyselectrolytemia

1. Assessment of Dehydration and Estimation of Volume Deficit

If child's pre-illness weight is known, dehydration can be assessed accurately from the weight loss suffered by the child. But often the previous weight of the child is not known. Clinical history and examination, therefore, remains the mainstay of assessment of dehydration (Table 5.8) though their reliability has been questioned[9].

An attempt should be made to estimate volume of urine output, vomitus and diarrheal losses on the basis of history. Pulse rate, blood pressure and respiratory rate must be interpreted in relation to the child's age. Capillary refilling and skin turgor time of greater than 1.5 sec have been shown to be a reliable marker of dehydration[10].

Clinical signs of tachycardia, decreased skin turgor, sunken eyes and fontanel, lethargic or impaired mental status, and oliguria predict a more than 10% weight loss[9, 10]. A capillary refill time of 2–3 sec corresponds to 50–100 ml/kg loss, 3–4 sec

Table 5.8 Assessment of severity of dehydration			
Characteristics			
Infants	**Mild 1-5%**	**Moderate 6-9%**	**Severe ≥ 10% (> 15% shock)**
Children	**Mild 1-3%**	**Moderate 4-6%**	**Severe ≥ 7% (> 9% shock)**
Pulse	Normal	Tachycardia	Tachycardia, weak pulse
Systolic BP	Normal	Normal-low	Orthostatic hypotension to shock
Urine output	Decreased	Decreased	Oliguria-anuria
Buccal mucosa	Slightly dry	Dry	Parched
Anterior fontanel	Normal	Sunken	Markedly sunken
Eyes	Normal	Sunken	Markedly sunken
Skin turgor/ capillary refill	Normal	Decreased	Markedly decreased
Skin (< 12 months age)	Normal	Cool	Cool, mottling, acrocyanosis

Note: In a malnourished child, subcutaneous tissue is markedly reduced. Reliance on sunken eyeball, fontanel and loss of skin turgor in these children may lead to overestimation of dehydration. On the other hand, in chubby children dehydration may be underestimated. Thirst, dry mucosa, urine flow, metabolic acidosis, and circulatory status, therefore, are more reliable indicators of dehydration in these children.

corresponds to 100–150 ml/kg, and more than 4 sec corresponds to 150 ml/kg[9, 10, 11]. *Signs and symptoms of shock are early and more conspicuous in hypotonic dehydration, while in hypertonic dehydration CNS signs are more prominent.*

Laboratory investigations[12] may help in further assessment of fluid and electrolyte deficits and to guide the fluid therapy in severely dehydrated patients. However, there is no linear relationship between laboratory data and severity of dehydration[12]. These are not essential for starting the therapy. The most helpful investigations are listed below:

(i) **Blood urea and serum creatinine** may be elevated due to hemoconcentration and renal hypoperfusion caused by dehydration, and should alert to the possibility of pre-renal failure. A serum creatinine of more than 2 mg/dl in a dehydrated child suggests a coexisting renal disease rather than pre-renal failure.

(ii) **Serum electrolytes.** Sodium level helps in determining the type of dehydration. Based on serum sodium values, dehydration can be categorized as isotonic (serum sodium within normal range), hypotonic (serum sodium <130 mEq/L) and hypertonic (serum sodium >145 mEq/L). Hypotonic dehydration usually results from replacing losses with low solute fluids such as dilute fruit juice, cola drinks, tea etc. Lethargy and irritability are common and vascular collapse occurs early. Hypokalemia is common in dehydration following diarrhea especially in malnourished children.

(iii) **Plasma osmolality** gives direct indication as to whether a patient has isotonic, hypo or hypertonic dehydration.

(iv) **Acid base status.** Moderate to severe dehydration is associated with metabolic acidosis.

(v) **Urine specific gravity.** During dehydration body attempts to conserve urinary water loss and the urine is concentrated; the specific gravity is more than 1020. In a dehydrated patient if urine specific gravity is less than 1015, it may indicate urinary water loss.

(vi) **Hemoconcentration** as determined by hemoglobin and hematocrit may not be very helpful in assessment of dehydration as many children have pre existing anemia but serial determination may be helpful in monitoring the adequacy of fluid replacement.

2. Rapid Restoration of Intravascular Volume

Patients who have moderate or severe hypovolemia will have compromised effective circulating volume, and rapid expansion of intravascular volume is required to restore perfusion and avoid tissue damage. Rapid restoration of ECF volume can be achieved by infusing 20–40 ml/kg 0.9% saline or Ringer's solution over a one hour period, followed by an additional 20–40 ml/kg if the circulation is not fully restored

Assessment of the patient's perfusion during and at completion of the intravenous bolus would guide us to determine if additional bolus therapy is warranted. Isotonic crystalloid fluid is the only solution recommended for volume repletion; use of hypotonic or hypertonic crystalloid solutions are not recommended. However, patients with decreased oncotic pressure due to illnesses such as nephrotic syndrome may benefit from a colloid solution if they present with hypovolemia. In these patients, initial bolus therapy with 5% albumin may be beneficial.

3. Correction of Total Fluid Deficit

Intravenous Rehydration Therapy

In severe dehydration and hypovolemia, after rapid volume restoration, intravenous rehydration therapy is initiated. If child can drink, he can be started on complete oral rehydration therapy (ORS) about 5 ml/kg/hour after ensuring that child is passing urine and dehydration is isotonic.

The guidelines for intravenous fluid therapy in diarrheal dehydration are given Table 5.9 In severe dehydration caused by diarrheal dehydration. The goal of early intravenous rehydration therapy is to achieve normal urine output, correct K+ deficit and acidosis and enable patient to return to oral rehydration at the earliest. In non-isotonic dehydration, intravenous rehydration therapy may be required for longer duration ($\geq$ 24 hours).

Indications for intravenous rehydration in the emergency room

(i) Severe dehydration
(ii) Persistent vomiting
(iii) Paralytic ileus
(iv) Child is unconscious
(v) Child is too sick to drink ORS

When IV line cannot be established, intraosseous route is suitable for administration of fluids in severely dehydrated children[19]. The total

Table 5.9 Recommended fluid therapy for intravenous rehydration	
Type of fluid therapy	Solution
Maintenance	5% dextrose in 0.45% saline with 20 mEq/L KCl over 24 hr
Isotonic dehydration	5% glucose in 0.45% saline with 20 mEq/L KCl given over 24 hr
Hypotonic dehydration	5% glucose in 0.9% saline with 20 mEq/L KCl given over 12 hr followed by 5% dextrose water in 0.45% saline with 20 mEq/L KCl given over the next 24 hr
Hypertonic dehydration	5% dextrose water in 0.2% saline containing 20 mEq/L KCl to be given over the number of days necessary to lower the Na+ concentration by 10 mEq/day

Table 5.10 Guidelines for intravenous rehydration therapy in severe dehydration			
Time	Type of fluid	Amount of fluid (ml/kg)	
		Infant (< 1 year)	Older children
0-1 hour	Ringer's lactate or 0.9% saline	30	40
1-3 hours	Ringer's lactate or 0.9% saline	40	60
4-6 hours	ORS or N/2 saline in 5% dextrose (+ 1 ml KCL/ 100 ml fluid if urine output is established)	50	50

Note: If child can drink give ORS (about 5 ml/kg/hour) with IV fluids after first 3 hours. If the patient has passed urine he may be placed fully on ORS. If unable to accept orally then deficit is corrected with N/2 saline in 5% dextrose + 1 ml potassium chloride (15% solution)/100 ml fluid

Table 5.11 Intravenous fluid requirement calculation for 10 kg child with moderate dehydration		
Requirement	Type of fluid	Volume
Deficit	N/2 saline in 5% dextrose	7% x 10 kg =700 ml
+ Maintenance	N/5 saline in 5% dextrose	100 ml/kg =1000 ml
+ Concurrent losses*	N/2 saline	3 stools = 300 ml loss
Total		2000 ml

* For each large stool, give 200 ml for older child, 100 ml for infant > 6 months, 50 ml for infant < 6 months. Add potassium chloride (15%) 1 ml to every 100 ml of fluid as soon as urine flow is established.

Table 5.12 Scheme for step-wise intravenous rehydration of a 10 kg infant with moderate dehydration (7%)		
Time line	Volume of fluid	Type of fluid
0-1 hour	20 ml/kg	200 ml normal saline or Ringer's lactate
1-9 hours	1/2 deficit + 1/3 maintenance	400 ml N/2 in D5W 350 ml N/5 in D5W + 8 ml KCL (15%)*
9-24 hours	1/2 deficit + 2/3 maintenance + ongoing losses (say 3 stools)	400 ml N/2 in D5W + 650 ml N/5 in D5W + 150-300 ml N/2 in D5W

* Add potassium once the child has passed urine

fluid deficit can be replaced as half normal saline (0.45%) in 5% dextrose. Conventionally, this is given over a period of 24 hours along with estimated concurrent losses and maintenance requirements. Half of the total calculated volume is given in first 8 hours, and the remaining over the next 16 hours. Rapid intravenous rehydration in emergency room over a period of 3-4 hours has also been found to be safe and equally effective in children who cannot tolerate oral fluids[20].

Hypotonic dehydration

Hypotonic dehydration (Na+ $\leq$ 130 mEq/L) is associated with excessive depletion of ECF solute viz. sodium and chloride, and movement of water from ECF to ICF. Thus all manifestations of dehydration including shock appear early. Rehydration fluid should contain more sodium chloride and the rehydration should be achieved rapidly. A scheme for intravenous rehydration of hypotonic (hyponatremic) dehydration is shown in Table 5.13.

Hypertonic dehydration

Hypertonic dehydration (Na+ > 145 mEq/L) is associated with a deficit of free water. It is best reflected as elevated serum sodium levels, and is thus called as hypernatremic dehydration. Mild grades of hypernatremia (serum sodium 146-150 mEq/L) associated with diarrheal dehydration can be easily and safely treated with oral rehydration therapy.

If serum sodium is more than150 mEq/L, intravenous correction of hypernatremia may be needed[19]. Serum sodium should not be allowed to drop by more than 10 mEq/L/day. Rapid correction often leads to water intoxication, cerebral edema and convulsions. The intravenous rehydration schedule described earlier must be modified so that the sodium deficit is corrected slowly over 48 hours (Table 5.14).

There is a controversy regarding the nature of fluid to be used to correct deficit. N/2 saline (0.45%) in 5% dextrose has the advantage of avoiding rapid change of tonicity; others recommend N/5 saline (0.18%) in 5% dextrose. The volume of free water needed to lower serum sodium by one mEq/L is approximately 4 ml/kg evenly distributed over 48 hours. The fluid should also contain potassium chloride (1 ml of 15% solution per 100 ml) and calcium gluconate (1.0 2.0 ml/kg/day of 10% solution).

Tables 5.13 and 5.14 mention the guidelines to initiate initial fluid therapy in children with hyponatremic and hypernatremic dehydration. Monitoring serum sodium every 4-6 hourly would guide the further fluid titration based on target sodium and achieved sodium levels.

Table 5.13 Scheme for intravenous rehydration of 10 kg infant with hyponatremic dehydration			
Step I	0-1 hour	20 ml/kg	200 ml NS/RL
Step II	1-9 hours	1/2 deficit + 1/3 maintenance	500 ml NS 350 ml N/5 in D5W
Step III	9-24 hours	1/2 deficit + 2/3 maintenance + ongoing losses	500 ml NS 650 ml N/5 in D5W

NS : Normal saline, RL: Ringer's lactate, D5W = Dextrose 5%. Add potassium chloride (15%) 1.5 ml/100 ml i.e. 3 mEq/100 ml after child has passed urine

Table 5.14 Guidelines for treatment of hypernatremic dehydration		
Step 1	Child in shock	20 ml/kg Ringer's lactate or normal saline in first hour followed by 10 ml/kg/hour of N/2 saline in 5% dextrose till child passes urine or dehydration is corrected
Step 2	Slow rehydration (over 48 hours)	60-75 ml/kg/day N/5 saline in 5% dextrose + 3/4th maintenance* requirement as N/5 saline in 5% dextrose + ongoing losses

*Maintenance requirement is reduced by 25% in hypernatremia because of SIADH. Add potassium chloride once child has passed urine.

Oral Rehydration Therapy[21, 22, 23]

Total correction of fluid and electrolyte deficit can be achieved safely and rapidly through oral rehydration therapy (ORT) in most cases with dehydration[13, 14]. Also in patients with severe dehydration, once the intravascular volume deficit has been corrected and urine flow is established, rest of the deficit can be corrected by ORT.

Various types of ORS have been tried in last two decades. These include ORS with maltodextrins like rice based ORS, ORS with amino acids, starch based ORS, liquid or tablet forms of ORS, low osmolar ORS and micronutrients enriched ORS with low osmolarity like ReSoMal[16, 17]. ORS enriched with amino acids like glycine, alanine, glutamate etc. have been tried without any added benefits. Cereals like rice, maize, sorghum and millet have been used in place of glucose in ORS as they contain maltodextrins[16]. Rice-based ORS usually contains 50-80 gm/l of pre-cooked rice.

The World Health Organization (WHO) and the United Nations Children's Fund (UNICEF) have endorsed the use of a low osmolar rehydrating solution that includes: Na 90 mmol/l, Cl 80 mmol/l, K 20 mmol/l, base 30 mmol/l, and glucose 111 mmol/l. The WHO solution has proved useful in many clinical trials conducted for rehydrating children and has also been shown to reduce the morbidity and mortality associated with diarrheal illness regardless of its etiology[13, 14, 15].

The changes in the initial WHO formulation arose from concerns that using an oral rehydrating solution with a sodium content > 60 mmol/l would prove problematic in developed countries where most gastroenteritis is viral in nature and has a lower sodium content than the secretory diarrheas seen in less developed areas. There exists a theoretical concern that hypernatremia might ensue if minimally dehydrated children losing small amounts

Table 5.15 Oral rehydration therapy guidelines[13,14]

Grade of dehydration	Rehydration volume	Rehydration duration
Mild	30-50 ml/kg ORT	3-4 hour
Moderate	50-100 ml/kg ORT	3-4 hour
Severe	100-150 ml/kg ORT	3- 4 hour
If hypernatremia is present	As per grade of dehydration	Atleast 12 hours for ORT. Monitor fall in serum Na^+

- If child wants more ORS, give without any restriction
- Continue breast feeding in breastfed infants
- To infants under 6 months, who are not breast fed, give 100-200 ml clean drinking water along with ORS
- Replace ongoing losses
- Reassess the child after 4 hr, and manage according to the degree of dehydration. If the child's condition worsens, or child continues to vomit, intravenous rehydration should be started.

of sodium in their stools were treated exclusively with WHO solution without provision of extra free water. In cases of mild dehydration, stemming from causes other than secretory diarrhea, solutions with lower sodium contents may be equally useful[18]. In fact, solutions with sodium content ranging from 30 to 90 mmol/l have proved quite effective in this situation[22, 23, 24]. A guide to oral rehydration therapy using WHO ORS according to grade of dehydration assessment is shown in Table 5.15.

A variety of ORS formulations[16, 17] (WHO formula, as well as others) are commercially available in sachets to prepare 200, 250, 500 and 1000 ml of ORS. Composition of these formulations is shown in Table 5.16. The water used for preparing ORS should preferably be boiled and cooled, but clean drinking water can be used.

Table 5.16 New ORS formulations

Product	Concentration in mmol/l					
	Na	K	Cl	Sugar	Base	Osmolality
WHO ORS	90	20	80	111	30	311
Ceralyte 90	90	20	80	220	30	275
Low Na^+ ORS	75	20	65	75	30	245
Rehydralyte	75	20	65	140	30	300
Ceralyte 70	70	20	60	220	30	230
Enfalyte	50	25	45	170	34	167
Pedialyte	45	20	35	140	30	254

4. Replacement of Ongoing Losses and Nutritional Support

If diarrhea continues after rehydration has been achieved, the amount of water and salt lost in diarrheal stools should be replaced by ORS. The child may be given ORS *ad libitum* depending upon the thirst. Alternatively, fluid may be replaced according to the stool frequency. For a *large watery stool in small infants (<6 months) 50 ml/stool, larger infants (>6 months) 100 ml/stool and in older children 200 ml/stool should be replaced with close monitoring of the child*[13, 14] (Table 5.17).

Mother should be advised to continue to breast feed the infant between the drinks of ORS solution or continue whatever formula feeds were being given to the child. For the dietary intake of children with acute gastroenteritis refer to Chapter 26.

ELECTROLYTE DISTURBANCES

Common electrolyte disorders in sick children include hyponatremia, hypernatremia, hypokalemia, hyperkalemia, hypocalcemia, and hypomagnesemia.

Disorders of Sodium Homeostasis

Few basic physiological concepts of sodium and water homeostasis, and mechanisms of intracellular volume and cell integrity maintenance should be understood to devise effective approach and management strategies for dysnatremias. Any solute that cannot cross fluid compartments will dictate water movement into its compartment, creating an osmotic pressure. Such a solute is referred as an *effective osmole*. In contrast, solutes that freely cross fluid compartments, and are therefore not restricted to any one fluid compartment, are considered to be ineffective osmoles because, they do not generate an osmotic pressure. Each body compartment contains a predominant solute that acts as an effective osmole. As discussed in a previous section, sodium and glucose regulate *effective plasma osmolality*.

Two types of solutes are used by cells to adapt to changes in cell volume. These are ionic solutes

Table 5.17 A guide to correction of ongoing loses using ORT		
Type of Dehydration	**Replacement of ongoing loses**	**Nutrition**
Mild	60-120 ml per each diarrheal stool or episode of emesis*	Continue breast milk or age appropriate usual diet
Moderate	60-120 ml per each diarrheal stool or episode of emesis.	Continue breast milk or age appropriate usual diet
Severe	60-120 ml per each diarrheal stool or episode of emesis. Nasogastric tube is used if needed	Continue breast milk or age appropriate usual diet
Accompanying hypernatremia	60-120 ml per each diarrheal stool or episode of emesis. IV fluid therapy, if no reduction in hypernatremia by 12 hours of ORT	Continue breast milk or age appropriate usual diet

* For each large stool, give 200 ml for older child, 100 ml for infant >6 months, 50 ml for infant < 6 months

Steps for oral rehydration therapy

1. Calculate the amount of oral rehydration solution required by the child to correct dehydration; 50-80 ml/kg for some dehydration

2. Advise the mother to give the calculated amount in next 4-6 hours in small quantities at a time, either with a spoon or in small sips. Approximate usual rate of administration should be about 2 ml/kg every 15 min for mild, and 4 ml/kg every 15 min for moderate dehydration (Never give large amounts with a feeding bottle or cup. This may be vomited out, or may stimulate gastro-colic reflex and result in a large watery stool).

3. If the child vomits, wait for 10-15 minutes, and restart the therapy.

4. Replenish ongoing losses by advising the mother to give 50-100 ml ORS to a child < 2 years and 100-200 ml in children between 2-10 years after passage of each diarrheal stool.

5. Reassess the hydration status at the end of 6 hours of therapy. If there are no signs of dehydration; start maintenance therapy. If the child is still dehydrated but somewhat improved, calculate the deficit and restart the therapy as above.

or *electrolytes* and non-ionic organic molecules (*osmolytes*). Initially and overall during states of osmolar stress, intracellular electrolytes (*potassium and chloride*) mainly contribute to cell volume regulation. The osmolytes (previously known as *idiogenic osmoles*) are a group of osmotically active solutes, typically low in molecular weight and uncharged (betaine, taurine, and glutamine) that can change their cell concentration without altering protein structure or function.

In case of dysnatremias, as a response to the creation of a new osmotic gradient, cellular adaptive mechanisms in the brain begin with a change in the cytoplasmic electrolyte content. This begins within 12 hours after the extracellular fluid osmolality has changed. Cerebral cell osmolyte content only begins to change after extracellular fluid osmolar changes have lasted for more than 24 hours. Thus, with acute changes in the plasma sodium concentration, there is no change in the levels of organic osmolytes in brain cells. This forms the basis of rapid correction of dysnatremias.

Hyponatremia

Hyponatremia is defined as serum sodium concentration of less than 135 mEq/L. It can occur due to water retention, sodium loss or redistribution of sodium and water. Hyponatremia can be true or pseudohyponatremia. Serum sodium levels are relatively low due to the expansion of plasma volume in hyperglycemia and hyperlipidemia. Serum sodium concentration is decreased by 1.6 mEq/L for every 100 mg/dl rise of glucose concentration above 100 mg/dl.

Hyponatremia is a common occurrence in hospitalized sick children[25, 27]. The common causes in our experience are acute diarrhea, acute infectious diseases namely pneumonia, meningitis and sepsis, heart failure, renal diseases, and hepatic failure[27-30]. Presence of hyponatremia generally indicates a serious illness and poor outcome in sick children attending emergency service[27].

Hyponatremia with dehydration. This can occur due to excessive salt and water loss from gastrointestinal tract consequent to diarrhea and/ or vomiting, or renal losses due to diuretic therapy, in salt losing nephritis, losses through gastrostomy or ileostomy, and less commonly but often dramatically in congenital adrenal hyperplasia, adrenal insufficiency and cerebral salt wasting syndrome[27, 28]. In hyponatremia due to renal losses, urinary sodium is usually more than 20 mEq/L. Because there is marked ECF depletion,

signs of dehydration and circulatory collapse are more pronounced as compared to actual fluid loss. Child is usually drowsy. *Convulsions and deep coma occurs when serum sodium is less than 115 mEq/L[25, 27].*

Dilutional hyponatremia. Hyponatremia can occur in patients with congestive cardiac failure, nephrotic syndrome, or hepatic failure due to greater increase in the body water as compared to sodium content. The total body sodium in these patients is high and urinary sodium is often less than 5 mEq/L[24, 25]. The primary defense against developing hyponatremia is the ability to dilute urine and excrete free water. Development of dilutional hyponatremia typically requires a relative excess of free water in conjunction with an underlying condition that impairs the ability to excrete free water.

Clinical Features

Hyponatremia is often associated with state of extracellular hypo-osmolality and a tendency for water to move into the cells. This movement of water in the brain, which is encased in a rigid cranium, is responsible for the most clinical manifestations of hyponatremia. The clinical features include nausea, difficulty in concentrating, confusion, lethargy, agitation, headache, seizures, and in extreme cases brain stem herniation, and death due to cerebral edema. In addition to the above symptoms, patients will often have signs of hypovolemia or hypervolemia, which can aid in assessing the cause of the hyponatremia. Hyponatremia can be classified as acute or chronic.

Chronic hyponatremia occurs when serum sodium falls slowly over a period of 48 hours. In this case, the brain will compensate by extruding the solutes into the ECF compartment. Hence a patient with chronic hyponatremia will be less symptomatic than an acutely hyponatremic patient with the same serum sodium level.

Acute hyponatremia occurs when serum sodium fails rapidly, in less than 48 hours. The brain does not have the opportunity to adjust to the change, and brain stem herniation may occur.

Treatment

It is generally agreed that symptomatic hypo-natremia (with seizures/ impaired consciousness) should be treated with IV infusion of 3% saline, 10 ml/kg at a rate of 1 ml/minute, to correct the sodium deficit by about 5 mEq/L[36, 37, 38]. Rest of the correction should be achieved slowly by administration of saline (0.9% or 0.45%). The deficit may be calculated as follows[48-51]:

Sodium deficit = 0.6 × body weight (kg) × (135-observed serum Na$^+$)

Further correction should then proceed at a rate no greater than 0.5 mEq/L/hr or 12 mEq/L/day. Correction is done slowly so that the brain can readjust to the added solutes[35]. Rapid correction may result in demyelination syndrome and cerebral pontine myelinolysis [52].

In asymptomatic hyponatremia, sodium deficit is calculated as above but the correction is achieved over a period of 24-48 hours. The rate of correction should not exceed 10 mEq/L in 24 hours[37]. Chronic hyponatremia should be corrected at a rate of 0.5 mEq/L/hr or 10-12 mEq/L/day[39].

In addition to above, furosemide may be used in patients with dilutional hyponatremia to remove excess water while giving hypertonic saline. Newer agents, termed "aquaretics", that are antagonists of AVP V2 receptors in kidney are the future treatment options to treat hyponatremia[39]. These agents are more effective compared to diuretics in inducing free water diuresis.

Hyponatremia due to SIADH requires fluid restriction to about two-thirds of the normal requirement. Fludrocortisone (0.1 mg) is useful in cerebral salt wasting syndrome and congenital adrenal hyperplasia in reducing urinary sodium wastage.

Syndrome of inappropriate secretion of antidiuretic hormone is the most important cause of euvolemic hyponatremia. This implies excessive secretion of ADH in the presence of low sodium levels and normal or low plasma osmolality[30]. Vasopressin release varies appropriately with serum sodium concentration but begun at lower threshold of serum osmolality in a set of patients implying a "resetting of osmostat".

Criteria for the diagnosis of syndrome of inappropriate secretion of antidiuretic hormone (SIADH)

Essential criteria

(i) Hyponatremia (serum Na < 135 mEq/L)
(ii) Decreased extracellular fluid effective osmolality (plasma osmolality < 270 mOsm/kg H_2O).
(iii) Inappropriate urine concentration (urine osmolality > 500 mOsm/kg H_2O).
(iv) Clinical euvolemia.

(v) Elevated urinary Na (>20 mEq/L) concentration under conditions of normal salt and water intake.
(vi) Absence of adrenal, thyroid, pituitary or renal insufficiency or diuretic use.

Supplemental criteria

(i) Plasma vasopressin level inappropriately elevated relative to plasma osmolality (Any detectable AVP level when serum osmolality is < 270 mOsm/kg H_2O denotes inappropriate elevation).
(ii) Abnormal water load test i.e. inability to excrete atleast 90% of a 20 ml/kg water load in 4 hours and/or failure to dilute urine osmolality to < 100 mOsm/kg H_2O.
(iii) No significant correction of serum sodium with volume expansion but improvement after fluid restriction.

Causes

(i) CNS disorders like infection, malignancy (primary or secondary), trauma, hypoxic ischemic encephalopathy, Guillain-Barre syndrome, cerebral malformations, intracranial hemorrhage.
(ii) Miscellaneous conditions like acute intermittent porphyria, leukemia, and lymphoma
(iii) Pulmonary disorders including infections, malignancy, cystic fibrosis, positive

pressure ventilation
(iv) Post surgical disorders like anesthetic or premedication induced, abdominal, cardiothoracic and neurosurgery procedures, and severe pain can precipitate SIADH

Management

Initial aim is to correct the underlying cause and restrict the fluid intake. If serum sodium is below 120 mEq/L or is associated with CNS symptoms, 3% saline should be given along with furosemide (1 2 mg/kg IV). Isotonic saline or N/2 saline should never be given. Since blood volume is already expanded, fluid administration may lead to pulmonary edema and heart failure.

Cerebral salt wasting syndrome (CSWS). This may share the similar causes and laboratory criteria with patients having Syndrome of Inappropriate Antidiuresis (SIADH) hence the differentiation is important in critical care setting. Table 5.18 shows differences between SIADH and CSWS.

Table 5.18 Differences between syndrome of inappropriate antidiuresis (SIADH) and cerebral salt wasting syndrome (CSWS)

Parameter	SIADH	CSWS
Sodium	Low	Low
Body water	Increased	Decreased
Serum osmolality	< 280 mOsm/l	Decreased
Urine osmolality	>500 mOsm/l	Increased
Urine to serum osmolality ratio	>1	>1
Urine output	Low	High
Urine Na+ concentration	Increased	Increased

CSWS has volume contraction or hypovolemia and hyponatremia in the setting of polyuria and increased urine sodium losses. Treatment is directed towards vigorous extracellular fluid and sodium replacement. Administration of high doses of fludrocortisones (0.2-0.4 mg/day) has proven to be beneficial in some patients.

Hypernatremia

Hypernatremia is defined as serum sodium concentration of more than 145 mEq/L[48]. It represents a deficit of water with respect to body's sodium stores and can result from a net water loss (diarrhea, vomiting, diuresis and burns) or excessive sodium intake[40]. It can, therefore, be associated with any state of hydration i.e. dehydration, over hydration or normal hydration.

Hypernatremia with dehydration is common with acute diarrheal disease when water loss is more than the electrolyte losses and occasionally in patients with diabetes insipidus in whom there is a pure deficit of water[40]. Hyperventilation, fever, excessive sweating, high solute load or inadequate water intake are other factors contributory to hypernatremia. Sometimes it may be iatrogenic due to excessive replacement of sodium in oral or IV fluids, faulty reconstitution of ORS, use of ORS as maintenance fluid, feeding with high solute milk and injudicious use of sodium bicarbonate.

Clinical features. Signs of dehydration are minimal in hypernatremia as ECF is relatively preserved. Hyperosmolality of the ECF results in withdrawing of fluid from the cells causing intracellular dehydration. Severe hyperosmolality may cause cerebral damage with widespread cerebral hemorrhages, thromboses or subdural effusion especially when hypernatremic dehydration is corrected too fast by excessively hypotonic solution.

Skin turgor is maintained and it may feel rather doughy. Atleast 10-15 percent of body weight must be lost before child shows signs of hypovolemia (hypotension, oliguria). CNS symptoms are very prominent. Child is hyperirritable and has a high pitched shrill cry. Seizures may also occur. Subsequently CNS depression may set in leading to lethargy or even coma. There is usually pronounced metabolic acidosis and child manifests deep rapid breathing. The overall mortality due to hypernatremia is around 10 percent. About 15 percent of survivors may develop permanent neuromotor sequelae.

Treatment. If the child is in shock or severely dehydrated, he should receive a rapid intravenous infusion of Ringer's lactate or saline (0.9%) to correct hypovolemia[35]. The next step is to address the underlying cause. It may require controlling GI fluid losses, pyrexia, withholding diuretics, treatment of hypokalemia/hypercalcemia, or correcting faulty ORS. In diarrheal dehydration, ORT with standard WHO oral rehydration solution and water may be used successfully[40].

In patients with hypernatremia that has developed over a period of hours, rapid correction (1 mEq/L/hour) is safe and improves prognosis[40, 41]. Slow correction is advisable in patients with hypernatremia of longer duration, because full dissipation of accumulated brain solutes may take several days[38]. The targeted fall of serum sodium should be 0.5 mEq/L per hour and 10 mEq/L per day[26]. The goal is to bring serum sodium to 145 mEq/L. The preferred route for fluid administration is oral or by a feeding tube if the child is not in shock. Total correction of hypernatremia by IV route should proceed in a step wise manner. Peritoneal dialysis is indicated if serum sodium is 180 mEq/L or more.

If child develops convulsions during correction of hypernatremic dehydration, it is usually due to water intoxication. In such cases 3-5 ml/kg of 3% saline or 20% mannitol IV should be used to reduce cerebral edema. Hypocalcemia usually occurs during treatment and should be taken care of by adding calcium gluconate in the infusate. Maintenance fluid requirements in hypernatremia are reduced by 25 percent as there is SIADH.

Disorders of Potassium Homeostasis

Serum potassium level does not reflect the total body potassium because 98% of total body potassium is intracellular. Clinical importance comes chiefly from the fact that the ratio of intracellular to the extracellular potassium is the primary determinant of the resting membrane potential (E_m). Increased extracellular potassium decreases the ratio and reduces the resting membrane potential; decreased extracellular potassium increases the ratio and hyperpolarizes the membrane. Alterations in E_m disrupt the depolarizing tissues i.e., neural, cardiac and muscular tissues.

The homeostasis goal of adults is to remain in zero potassium balance whereas in infants and children, aim is to maintain a state of positive potassium balance. The net potassium accretion rate correlates with linear growth of children.

Normal serum potassium values

Preterm upto 48 hours	:	3.0-6.0 mEq/L
Term newborn	:	3.7-5.9 mEq/L
Infant	:	4.1-5.3 mEq/L
Child	:	3.4-4.7 mEq/L
Adult	:	3.5-4.5 mEq/L

Average potassium concentration in body fluids

Sweat has 4.5 mEq/L; stool water 85-95 mEq/L; potassium concentration falls with increasing stool volume. In severe cholera, stool potassium is <10 mEq/l; stomach aspirate 10 mEq/L; biliary drainage, duodenal and ileal secretions 5 mEq/L of potassium.

Hypokalemia

Hypokalemia is defined as a serum *potassium level below 4.0 mEq/L.* It occurs due to GI losses (vomiting, diarrhea, and gastric aspiration), urinary losses (prolonged use of diuretics, renal tubular acidosis, hyperaldosteronism, steroid therapy) hypomagnesemia, intracellular K^+ shift (alkalosis, therapy with β-agonists, insulin[42], diabetic ketoacidosis[43]), protein-energy malnutrition, familial hypokalemic periodic paralysis, and therapy with carbenicillin (impermeant anions). In our experience acute gastroenteritis, septicemia, diuretic therapy and hepatic failure are the commonest causes, especially if the child is malnourished[45-47].

Clinical picture. Potassium has an important role in regulating biologic electricity. Hypokalemia mainly affects bioelectric processes, including muscle contraction, nerve conduction and myocardial pacing. It can cause muscular weakness, hypotonia, diminished reflexes and paralytic ileus. Cardiac effects include various arrhythmias and ECG changes. Long standing hypokalemia decreases the concentrating capacity of kidneys (Hypokalemic nephropathy). Various ECG changes are observed when serum potassium falls below 2.5 mEq/L or total body potassium is reduced. These include prominent U-wave, prolongation of QTc (>0.425 sec) which is actually a long QU interval, T wave inversion and flattening or depression of ST segment. With further lowering there is prolonged PR interval, sinoatrial block, and ventricular extra systole. ECG changes may not correlate with serum potassium level; they are helpful if present but are not reassuring if absent.

Life-threatening consequences such as cardiac arrhythmia and arrest especially in children with pre-existing heart disease, respiratory paralysis and paralytic ileus may occur with severe hypokalemia. In our experience mortality in hypokalemic patients was 3.5 times higher than normokalemic patients and correlated with the severity of hypokalemia[47].

Treatment

1. Identify and treat the underlying cause.

2. Dietary supplementation with foods having high potassium content like coconut water, banana, citrus fruits, and potatoes.

3. Oral potassium supplementation may be required in some cases. Table 5.19 shows commercially available potassium formulations.

4. Rapid IV correction is done if serum potassium is less than 2.5 mEq/L, child is symptomatic or there are ECG changes.

   100 ml of stock solution is made by adding 90 ml NS with 10 ml KCL. Infusing the stock solution @ 1.5 ml/kg/hour will deliver 0.33 mEq/kg/hour of potassium. Maximum 0.5 – 1 mEq/kg/hr of KCl can be given (10% KCl, 1ml = 2mEq) under cardiac monitoring. In severe life-threatening hypokalemia, the infusion is given with an infusion pump at a rate of 0.30-0.35 mEq/kg/hour till the ECG changes revert back to normal[46, 47, 48].

   The concentration of K^+ in the maintenance IV fluids should not exceed 60 mEq/L while giving through peripheral line, 80 mEq/L via central line and this should not be mixed with *dextrose solution.*

5. Magnesium repletion is done if Mg deficiency is present.

6. K^+ sparing diuretics can be used.

Table 5.19 Commercially available potassium formulations

Available preparations	Trade name	Composition
Potassium chloride	Syrup potklor	15 ml = 20 mEq
Potassium citrate	Polycitra	K=1 mEq/ml; HCO_3 2 mEq/ml
	Polycitra K	K= 2 mEq/ml; HCO_3 2 mEq/ml
	Potrate	K= 1 mEq/ml
Potassium gluconate	not available	--

7. Acidosis should be corrected slowly when hypokalemia is present.

8. Potassium should be administered only when urinary flow is established.

Hyperkalemia

Hyperkalemia is defined as a serum potassium level of more than 5.5 mEq/L. It usually occurs due to impaired renal excretion (oliguria, acute renal failure, adrenal insufficiency, and chronic renal failure), shift or release of K^+ into ECF as seen in metabolic acidosis, sepsis, acute hemolysis, acute rhabdomyolysis, and tumor lysis syndrome and tissue necrosis.

Clinical picture. Mild hyperkalemia is often asymptomatic. When severe, the effects are mainly seen on the cardiac and skeletal muscles. Muscular weakness and paresthesias, shock, bradycardia or cardiac arrhythmias may occur. Early ECG changes include prolonged PR, tall T waves, shortened QT interval and wide QRS complexes of decreased amplitude. In severe cases absent P waves, first-degree heart block, sine wave (bizarre QRS complexes), ventricular fibrillation and cardiac arrest may occur.

Management[53]

Hyperkalemia with ECG abnormality is an emergency. The treatment modalities are shown in Table 5.20.

1. Stop oral/IV potassium supplementation.
2. Check the list of drugs and stop those that can cause hyperkalemia.
3. Treat the underlying cause.
4. Use the measures outlined in Table 5.20 for acute reduction in serum potassium.
5. *Dialysis is* recommended if above measures are unsuccessful. *CVVH, hemodialysis, peritoneal dialysis are the various options available in the order of their efficacy.*

Hypocalcemia

Normal range of serum total calcium concentration is 8.5 to 10.2 mg/dl (2.1 to 2.5 mmol/

Table 5.20 Treatment options for acute reduction in serum potassium

Drug	Dose	Onset of action	Duration of action
Inj. Calcium gluconate 10%	100 mg/kg/dose (1ml/kg/dose) IV over 5 – 10 min	1 -3 min	30 min
Inj. $NaHCO_3$	1 -2 mEq/kg/dose IV over 5 -10 min	10 -30 min	2 hrs
Glucose + insulin	0.5 gm/kg (2 ml/kg of 25% dextrose) 0.1 u/kg regular insulin IV over 15-30 min	30 min	2 -4 hrs
Nebulized salbutamol	2.5 mg < 25 kg, 5 mg for > 25 kg over 10 min	30 min	120 min 120 min
Sodium polysterene resins*	0.5 -1 gm/kg orally/ rectally	60- 120 min	4-6 hrs
Furosemide (Restricted usage)	1-2 mg /kgIV/IM	15 – 30 min	4-6 hrs

* Sodium polysterene sulfonate (SPS) resin: Mix each gram in 3-4 ml of water and mix with 10% dextrose and give as retention enema which is retained for 15-30 min

l) and ionized calcium is 4.8 to 7.2 mg/dl (1.1 to 1.8 mmol/l). Calcium in the ionized form is essential for myocardial contractility. It is also involved in control of vascular tone, mediation of action of several drugs and hormones, and function of skeletal muscles. It is difficult to predict ionized calcium levels from total serum calcium, even after making corrections for proteins, albumin or pH. Although hypocalcemia is known to cause several signs and symptoms (Table 5.21), it is often a laboratory diagnosis because the clinical manifestations are minimal or absent.

Table 5.21 Signs and symptoms of hypocalcemia

Nervous system : Paresthesias, fasciculations, muscle spasms; Chvostek's and Trousseau's signs; tetany; irritability; movement disorders; seizures; organic brain syndrome; psychosis.

Pulmonary: Bronchospasm

Cardiovascular: Arrhythmias, hypertension or hypotension, congestive heart failure.

Gastrointestinal: Dysphagia, abdominal pain, biliary colic

Sepsis is often associated with hypocalcemia, it may also occur when calcium is chelated *e.g.* after blood transfusion. Changes in acid-base status may also alter total and ionized calcium values. Hypocalcemia is seen in 35% of patients admitted to our PICU. The incidence of ionized hypocalcemia in our patients was 32.2 episodes/100 patient days[50]. Mild degree of hypocalcemia (ionized calcium > 0.8 mmol/l or 3.2 mg/dl) are usually asymptomatic. *Symptomatic ionized hypocalcemia presents with neurological and cardiovascular features.* All signs and symptoms may not be evident in a given clinical setting. One should treat hypocalcemia if symptomatic or if the ionized calcium concentration is <0.8 mmol/l. The dose is 0.5-1.0 ml/kg of calcium-gluconate over 5-10 minutes followed by a continuous infusion 0.1-0.2 ml/kg hour (equal to 0.5 to 2 mg/kg/hr). Bolus doses of calcium increases the serum ionized calcium concentration for a short period of time (1 to 2 hr). With follow-up infusion the concentration usually normalizes over 2 to 4 hours. Thereafter, rate of infusion of elemental calcium should be maintained at a rate of 0.3 to 0.5 mg/kg/hr. Calcium chloride 10% solution, contains 1.36 mEq/ml or 27 mg/ml and calcium gluconate 10% solution has 0.45 mEq/ml or 9 mg/ml of Ca^{++}.

Magnesium Disorders

Magnesium is essential for maintenance of several cellular functions through its role in activation of adenosine triphosphate (ATP). Normal serum Mg^{++} concentration ranges between 1.5–1.9 mEq/L. Magnesium deficiency is common in critically ill children[51]. It frequently develops in a wide variety of clinical conditions such as protein energy malnutrition, malabsorption, hypo-albuminemia, sepsis, following prolonged gastrointestinal suctioning, diarrhea, blood transfusion, aminoglycoside therapy, osmotic diuresis, and use of diuretics etc.

Hypomagnesemia is associated with prolonged PR interval, widened QRS-complex, ST segment depression and low amplitude T-wave on ECG. It may potentiate dysrrhythmia due to hypocalcemia and digitalis toxicity. *Hyper-magnesemia* produces tall peaked T-waves and narrow QRS complexes. Singhi *et al*[56] found that PICU stay was significantly longer in patients with hyper-and hypomagnesemia as compared to those with normal magnesium level[56].

Refractory hypokalemia is a prominent feature of hypomagnesemia[45]. Intractable arrhythmias, muscle weakness, including respiratory muscle weakness, neuromuscular excitability, seizures, and ECG changes such as prolonged QT interval on ECG are other features. Most patients with symptomatic magnesium depletion and normal renal function have an estimated deficit of 1 to 2 mEq/kg. About twice the estimated magnesium deficit is replaced at a rate of 1 mEq/kg for the first 24 hours and 0.5 mEq/kg/day for the next 3 to 5 days. Magnesium sulfate, 50% solution provides 4 mEq/ml of elemental magnesium.

FLUID THERAPY IN SPECIAL SITUATIONS

Parentral fluid therapy may be required in a wide variety of clinical situations to provide normal or adjusted maintenance fluid needs or to replace abnormal deficits as shown in Table 5.22. Modification of maintenance water requirement may be required in certain clinical conditions because of changes in metabolic rate or water losses (Table 5.5). Some of these conditions are briefly discussed below.

GI Losses

Losses through nasogastric tube, ileostomy, and pancreatic fistula needs to be replaced volume for volume with a solution containing appropriate electrolytes (Table 5.23)

> **Table 5.22 Clinical situations requiring parenteral fluid therapy**
>
> - *Maintenance fluids*
>   - o In a comatose or sick child who is unable to take orally.
>
> - *Adjusted maintenance fluids*
>   - o Oliguria/anuria
>   - o Severe community acquired pneumonia[31]
>   - o Syndrome of inappropriate secretion of ADH (SIADH)
>   - o Raised intracranial pressure
>   - o Postoperative patient
>   - o Cardiac failure
>   - o Edema
>
> - *Maintenance plus deficit replacement and replenishment of concurrent losses of fluids*
>   - o Continuing gastro-intestinal fluid losses (vomiting, diarrhea, nasogastric tube drainage and colostomy etc.)
>   - o Burns
>   - o Diabetic ketoacidosis
>   - o Salicylate intoxication
>   - o Pyloric stenosis

Burns

The aim of fluid therapy is to correct hypovolemia and maintain intravascular volume. The electrolytes, proteins and acid base parameters should be monitored and maintained. The fluid deficit requirement in burns is calculated by Parkland formula: 4 ml/kg/percent of the burn area in 24 hours. One half should be given in 8 hours and the remainder in next 16 hours. The fluid should contain 120 mEq/L of sodium and 20 mEq/L of bicarbonate and made isotonic with chloride and dextrose. Ringer's lactate is most suitable for first 24 hours. No potassium should be added in first 24 hours. Successful fluid resuscitation is evidenced by urine output of 1-2 ml/kg/hour, normal sensorium and satisfactory central venous pressure (CVP). Recently, there is a concern about fluid creep which says fluid supplementation according to Parkland formula may be higher than required in a subset of patients. Parkland formula may be used as a guide to initiate fluid therapy but the subsequent titration should be based on hemodynamic parameters and urine output status.

Colloids are usually started after 24 hours. Earlier infusion of colloids (plasma, albumin) is not useful because it may leak out of the damaged capillaries. Mannitol (0.5 g/kg) may be given to promote diuresis and prevent hemoglobinuria after 4-6 hours. Fluid requirement from second day onwards is three fourth of the first day requirement. Repeated clinical assessment is necessary to prevent overhydration and pulmonary edema. For further details regarding fluid and electrolyte resuscitation in children with burns refer to Chapter 50.

Increased Intracranial Pressure (ICP)

An increase in ICP can occur as a result of meningitis, encephalitis, and cerebral edema secondary to hypoxia etc. It is believed that most of these patients have associated SIDAH, and increased body water. Overhydration should, therefore, be avoided. It is controversial whether these patients should receive restricted i.e. 65-75 percent of usual maintenance fluids. In acute meningitis, fluid restriction as had been advocated in the past may be harmful[32, 33]. Close monitoring is required especially when osmotic diuretic such as mannitol is used. Refer to Chapter 18 for details.

Diabetic Ketoacidosis

It is a hyperosmolar state and for all practical purposes most children would have severe dehydration with an estimated fluid deficit between 10%-12%. These patients have moderately low sodium, normal potassium and total body depletion of phosphate. Hypokalemia is frequent occurrence once insulin therapy is started[44].

If in shock, patient needs fluids not insulin[44]. Give one or two 20 ml/kg normal saline or Ringer's lactate boluses in an hour till pulse volume returns to normal. Then give half of estimated deficit + insensible losses + ongoing losses as N/2 saline + 20 mEq/L KCl + 15 mmol/l potassium hypophosphate are given in the first 8

GI fluids	H+	Na+	K+	Cl−	HCO$_3$
Gastric	80	40	20	150	0
Small bowel	0	130	20	120	30
Pancreatic	0	135	15	100	50

Table 5.23 Average electrolyte contents of various GI fluids (mmol/l)

hours. It is followed up with half of estimated deficit + insensible losses as N/2 saline + 20 mEq/L of KCl for next 16 hours. Glucose is added when blood sugar drops down to 250-300 mg/dl. Accurate and frequent monitoring is essential. For further details regarding management of diabetic ketoacidosis refer to Chapter 41.

Oliguria and Anuria

Fluid therapy whether oral or IV should be limited to 300 to 400 ml/m² (15-20 ml/kg or 30-40 ml/100 kcal) per day. Urinary water loss can be added to it every 4-6 hour. Non urinary fluid losses are replaced by an electrolyte free, high caloric fluid (10% glucose solution). Electrolytes are given only if these are being lost. Hyperkalemia or hypokalemia can occur and should be treated as discussed above. Patients with acute volume overload may require renal supportive therapy (peritoneal dialysis or continuous renal replacement therapy). A fall in body weight of 0.5-1.0 percent per day in the absence of circulatory complications is indicative of adequate fluid management. For further details concerning maintenance fluid and electrolyte therapy in children with acute renal failure refer to Chapter 34.

Drowning

Patients with clinical evidences of poor peripheral perfusion should receive volume expanders (saline, Ringer's lactate) at a rapid rate. Monitoring of the central venous pressure and acid base values are mandatory to guide the initial therapy. Subsequent fluid and electrolyte therapy depends upon the status of serum electrolytes and complications such as cerebral edema and "secondary drowning". For further details refer to Chapter 49.

ACID-BASE PHYSIOLOGY

ABG findings correlate with ventilation, oxygenation and metabolic disturbances. Acid base balance is an essential part of fluid and electrolyte management. Acid is a substance that tends to dissociate or give a hydrogen ion (proton donor) whereas base is a substance that tends to bind or associate a hydrogen ion (proton acceptor).

The acidity of body fluids is expressed in term of hydrogen ion concentration (H⁺) as measured in blood. The pH expresses negative algorithm of (H⁺) and is used to denote acidity or alkalinity. The higher H⁺ ion concentration is associated with acidity and low pH. Conversely reduced H⁺ ion concentration

leads to alkalinity and raised pH. The pH of the fluids is expressed by Henderson-Hasselbalch's equation:

$$pH = pK + \log \frac{HCO_3}{H_2CO_3}$$

The value of pK for bicarbonate carbonic acid buffer is 6.1. Thus, in simple terms pH is a function of ratio of plasma bicarbonate and carbonic acid concentration, the latter is determined by $paCO_2$. Usually the HCO_3^- and carbonic acid concentration in plasma is in a ratio of 20:1, the bicarbonate concentration is 25-27 mEq/1 and carbonic acid concentration 1.35 mEq/1 ($paCO_2$ in mm Hg x 0.03). Normal pH of blood is 7.40 (range 7.35 7.45). *As a rule of thumb, 1 mm Hg increase in $paCO_2$ decreases pH by 0.01 and 1mEq/1 decrease in HCO_3 decreases pH by 0.02.*

Regulation of Body pH

Body pH is maintained within normal limits mainly by three mechanisms.

Chemical buffers of the body. A buffer is a substance that can absorb or donate H⁺ ion and thereby mitigate changes in pH. The four important chemical buffer systems in the body include bicarbonate carbonic acid buffer, phosphate buffer, hemoglobin buffer, and protein buffer. Out of these, the bicarbonate-carbonic acid buffer is the most important system that converts strong acids to a weak carbonic acid.

Respiratory regulatory mechanisms. These mediate via the central and peripheral chemoreceptors. Respiratory mechanism by virtue of rapid breathing eliminates CO_2 and regulates concentration of carbonic acid. The buffering is fast and occurs within minutes. Maximal respiratory compensation to acidosis occurs within 12 to 24 hours.

Renal mechanisms help in the elimination of excess acids and bases by reabsorption of bicarbonate in the proximal tubules and excretion of H⁺ ions as phosphate buffer salts and ammonium ions. The buffering occurs over a period of hours or days.

Disturbances in acid base balance can occur due to primary respiratory or metabolic events, with resultant increase or decrease in body acid or base. In general, if acid-base imbalance is predominantly metabolic in nature, changes in pH, HCO_3^- and $paCO_2$ occur in the same direction (all are reduced or increased and the main alteration is in HCO_3^-). In contrast if the disturbance is predominantly respiratory in origin, changes in HCO_3^- and arterial $paCO_2$ are opposite to changes in pH and main alteration is in $paCO_2$ (Table 5.24). The most serious acid base disorders are of mixed type when both respiratory and metabolic disturbances result in pH changes in the same direction.

Arterial blood sampling for ABG analysis

Blood should be collected in a low friction syringe designed to fill under arterial pressure. Excessive heparin and air bubbles should be expressed from the syringe. If analysis is likely to be delayed for more than few minutes, sample should be refrigerated

Radial arteries are the preferred site for arterial blood sampling. Posterior tibial, dorsalis pedis arteries can also be used. With the change of ventilatory parameters or FiO_2, atleast five minutes (30 minutes in case of obstructive airway disease) should be allowed to attain a steady state to reflect in arterial blood sampling.

Processing of ABG sample

Ideally, blood gas machine and co-oximeter both should be available to get all required parameters for complete systematic blood gas analysis. Blood gas machine measures pH, $paCO_2$, paO_2 and calculate the bicarbonate value. The Co-oximeter can measure the hemoglobin content (in gm/dl) and values related to hemoglobin binding: SaO_2, %COHb (carboxy-hemoglobin), %MetHb (methemoglobin). From this information the arterial oxygen content (CaO_2) can be calculated.

Basic facts in ABG interpretation

(i)   Primary acid base disorder: A primary change is in either HCO_3 (metabolic) or in $paCO_2$ (respiratory).

(ii) Compensation: It depends on how much time has elapsed since the disturbance developed.

(iii) Primary and compensatory changes always occur in the same direction. e.g. rise in HCO_3 follows rise in $PaCO_2$. If changes are discordant (i.e. changes are in opposite direction), suspect a mixed acid-base disorder.

(iv) pH and primary parameter change in the same direction suggests metabolic problem.

(v)   pH and primary parameter change in the opposite direction suggests a respiratory problem.

(vi) Careful history and good physical examination is a must. Information gained from ABG is interpreted in context of clinical findings.

(vii) Serum electrolytes are to be measured along with blood gases to help in further defining an acid-base imbalance.

Steps in evaluation of systemic acid base disorder[61, 62]

Step 1: Complete history and clinical examination[60]

- Information about patient's immediate environment i.e. FiO_2 and barometric pressure

- Additional lab data like previous ABG reports, electrolytes, blood sugar, BUN, hemoglobin content or hematocrit, chest X-ray, pulmonary function tests (if available) etc.

- Clinical information, including the history and physical examination with emphasis on patient's respiratory rate and vital signs, degree of respiratory effort, mental status and state of tissue perfusion.

Table 5.24 Identification of the primary disturbance				
Primary disorder	**pH**	**HCO₃**	**PaCO₂**	**Compensation**
Metabolic acidosis	Low	Low	N/low	Fall in $paCO_2$. Acidic urine
Metabolic alkalosis	High	High	N/ high	Rise in $paCO_2$. Alkaline urine
Respiratory acidosis	Low	N/low	High	Acidic urine
Respiratory alkalosis	High	N /high	High	Alkaline urine

Examples
1 : pH 7.3, HCO_3 14 = Primary metabolic acidosis
2 : pH 7.57, HCO_3 42, $paCO_2$ 47 = Primary metabolic alkalosis
3 : pH 7.57, HCO_3 18, $paCO_2$ 18 = Primary respiratory alkalosis
4 : pH 7.2, HCO_3 28, $paCO_2$ 58 = Primary respiratory acidosis

Table 5.25 Compensatory changes in $PaCO_2$ and HCO_3 in response to acidosis and alkalosis

Primary disorder	Compensatory change	Expected compensation
Metabolic acidosis. Fall in HCO_3	Fall in $paCO_2$	$\Delta paCO_2 = 1.2 \times \Delta HCO_3^-$
Metabolic alkalosis. Rise in HCO_3	Rise in $paCO_2$	$\Delta paCO_2 = 0.7 \times \Delta HCO_3^-$
Respiratory acidosis. Rise in $paCO_2$	Rise in HCO_3^-	Acute : $\Delta HCO_3^- = 0.1 \times \Delta paCO_2$ Chronic : $\Delta HCO_3^- = 0.3 \times \Delta paCO_2$
Respiratory alkalosis. Fall in $paCO_2$	Fall in HCO_3^-	Acute : $\Delta HCO_3^- = 0.2 \times \Delta paCO_2$ Chronic: $\Delta HCO_3^- = 0.5 \times \Delta paCO_2$

Step 2: Identify the primary disturbance

1. Assess pH: high / low

    - Low pH i.e. pH < 7.38 - acidemia
    - High pH i.e. pH > 7.42 - alkalemia

2. Is the primary disturbance respiratory or metabolic (Table 5.24)?

Step 3: Calculate the degree of compensation (Table 5.25).

- The respiratory system responds quickly to a metabolic disturbance and most predictably to metabolic acidosis.

- The magnitude of respiratory response to metabolic alkalosis is not easily predictable. $PaCO_2$ will rise above 40 but not > 50-55 mm Hg, to compensate for metabolic alkalosis.

- If changes occur beyond the predicted values of expected compensation, a mixed disorder should be looked for.

- The base deficit/excess is the amount of deviation of the standard bicarbonate from normal.

Step 4: Calculate the anion gap[57], delta anion gap and ΔHCO_3

(i)   Anion gap = $Na^+ - [Cl^- + HCO_3^-]$

Normal anion gap ranges from 8-16 mEq/L (12 ± 4) but it is variable in different labs. In normal anion gap there is no laboratory evidence of anion gap acidosis. This result does not always rule out an anion gap acidosis but certainly makes the diagnosis unlikely. Low or negative anion gap is seen in hypoproteinemia and certain rare conditions like lithium intake and bromism.

Elevated anion gap is more common and may be associated with metabolic acidosis; higher the gap above the normal, the more likely this will be the cause.

(ii) Δ Anion gap = Anion gap – 12

(iii) $\Delta HCO_3^- = 24 - HCO_3^-$

The coexistence of two metabolic acid-base disorders may be apparent by calculating the delta gap. For every unit rise in anion gap, the bicarbonate should be lowered by one (by buffering). Thus, if the delta gap is added to the measured bicarbonate, the result should be in the normal range for bicarbonate i.e., 22-26 mmol/l. Elevations greater than 26 indicates the additional presence of metabolic alkalosis and reduction of less than 22 indicates the co-existence of non AG metabolic acidosis.

Delta AG + HCO_3^- = 22-26 mmol/l (Pre-existing bicarbonate)

'Pre-existing bicarbonate' = Δ Anion gap + measured bicarbonate

It denotes the bicarbonate level that would have existed if the high anion gap metabolic acidosis were absent.

Δ Anion gap = ΔHCO_3^- = Pure high anion gap metabolic acidosis

Δ Anion gap > ΔHCO_3^- = High anion gap metabolic acidosis + metabolic alkalosis

Δ Anion gap < ΔHCO_3^- = High anion gap metabolic acidosis + hyperchloremic metabolic acidosis

Metabolic Acidosis

Metabolic acidosis is a clinical disturbance characterized by decrease in plasma bicarbonate concentration and compensatory hyperventilation resulting in low $paCO_2$. It is due to loss of bicarbonate from the body, impaired ability to excrete acid by the kidneys accumulation of acid (exogenous/endogenous) in the body. The term acidemia is used when blood pH is < 7.35 and acidosis refers to a pathologic process that leads to increase in H^+ ion concentration.

Causes of metabolic acidosis

Normal anion gap acidosis. Diarrhea, renal tubular acidosis, ureterosigmoidostomy and early stage of acute renal failure.

Increased anion gap acidosis. Diabetic ketoacidosis, lactic acidosis, inborn errors of metabolism, salicylate poisoning, methanol poisoning, uremia and starvation.

Clinical Features

(i) There are symptoms and signs related to underlying disorder.

(ii) Manifestations of acidosis are related to degree of acidosis.

(iii) pH < 7.2 is associated with increased risk of cardiac arrhythmias[58,59].

(iv) Increased work of breathing (Kussmaul's breathing) may predispose to superimposed respiratory acidosis.

(v) Exacerbation of hypotension.

(vi) Lethargy, stupor, coma.

(vii) In infants non specific symptoms like vomiting, anorexia, listlessness and failure to thrive.

(viii) Chronic acidemia results in osteopenia, muscle wasting, growth retardation.

Management

1. Avoid further production of H^+ by ensuring a proper airway, adequate peripheral perfusion, and oxygen delivery.

2. Treat the underlying disorder whenever feasible e.g. fluid therapy in diarrhea and appropriate antibiotics in sepsis to prevent worsening of shock and insulin in DKA.

3. *Bicarbonate therapy*

- Intravenous bicarbonate should be used judiciously if the pH is < 7.2 and / or HCO_3 $\leq$ 5 mEq/L with the aim to raise pH to 7.2.

- $NaHCO_3$ should to be diluted by 1:1 concentration for intravenous infusion.

- Amount of bicarbonate to be given = 0.5 x body weight x base deficit.

- Prerequisite for $NaHCO_3$ therapy is adequate ventilation since $PaCO_2$ is expected to rise after $NaHCO_3$ administration.

- Disadvantages of $NaHCO_3$ therapy are hyperosmolality, hypernatremia, hypokalemia, decrease in ionized calcium, intracerebral acidosis, shift of oxygen dissociation curve resulting in worsening of tissue hypoxia and worsening of intra cellular acidosis.

- Oral bicarbonate therapy is given to children with chronic acidosis in the form of sodium bicarbonate tablets, citrate solutions in the form of sodium citrate or potassium citrate mix.

4. *Hemodialysis or peritoneal dialysis* can be done to treat severe metabolic acidosis or if it is associated with renal failure (uremic acidosis), or it is due to poisonings.

Metabolic Alkalosis

Alkalemia is diagnosed when blood pH is >7.45. Alkalosis refers to the pathologic process that causes a decrease in H^+ ion concentration. Metabolic acidosis is characterized by elevation of HCO_3^- > 28-30 mEq/L with a rise in pH > 7.45 and $paCO_2$.

Clinical features

(i) There are symptoms due to hypokalemia and decreased ionized calcium levels.

(ii) Mild metabolic alkalosis (HCO_3^- < 36 mEq/L) is well tolerated and child remains asymptomatic.

(iii) Moderate metabolic alkalosis: (HCO_3^- 36 to 42 mEq/L) Paresthesias, weakness, orthostatic hypotension, fatigue, muscle cramps, lethargy, hyporeflexia and muscular irritability.

(iv) Severe metabolic alkalosis: (HCO_3^- > 45 to 50 mEq/L) Arrhythmias, tetany, seizures, delirium and stupor may occur. The child may develop hypoventilation which could result in hypoxemia, difficulty in weaning from ventilator, increased digoxin toxicity, worsening of hepatic encephalopathy.

Management

A. Chloride responsive

- Treat the underlying cause.

- Correct the hydration status with intravenous 0.9% saline infusion at 10 ml/kg over 10 to 30 minutes. May repeat the bolus, if indicated. *Do not use Ringer lactate.*

- Associated hypokalemia should be corrected with oral or intravenous KCl supplementation including diet rich in potassium.

- Decrease frequency of NG drainage if possible, stop anti-emetics and drugs that inhibit gastric acid secretion.

- In diuretic-induced metabolic alkalosis stop or decrease the dose of diuretics, use K$^+$ sparing diuretics and provide KCl supplementation.

B.   Chloride resistant metabolic alkalosis

- Treat the underlying cause.
- Adrenal adenoma should be surgically resected.
- Primary hyperaldosteronism is treated by restriction of sodium chloride, KCl supplementation and administration spironolactone.
- Bartter's syndrome is treated with K$^+$ supplementation, use of K-sparing diuretics and indomethacin.
- Gitelman's syndrome: K supplementation, K-sparing diuretics, Mg replacement.
- Liddle's syndrome: Salt restriction, K supplementation, K-sparing diuretics (triamterine, amiloride). *Saline infusion is of no use; it will worsen hypertension*

C.   Treatment of difficult metabolic alkalosis

- Life-threatening metabolic alkalosis (HCO3$^-$ > 50 mEq/L) with problems in mechanical ventilation warrants the following therapeutic options:

  Renal replacement therapy; hemodialysis or peritoneal dialysis. Fluid intake should be reduced and replaced by normal saline. CVVH may be preferred because it is effective within 24 hours.

Respiratory Acidosis

In respiratory acidosis there is decreased elimination of carbon dioxide from the body due to poor ventilation, which leads to accumulation of carbon dioxide in the body and generation of carbonic acid. Acute respiratory acidosis is characterized by a primary rise in paCO$_2$ above 45 mm Hg that remains at this high value upto 6 to 12 hours. Sustained elevation of paCO$_2$ beyond 12 hours is defined as chronic respiratory acidosis. During acute respiratory acidosis the rise in HCO$_3$ concentration rarely exceeds 4 mEq/L and renal compensation does not occur. However, chronic respiratory acidosis is accompanied by renal excretion of H$^+$ ions as NH$_4$Cl, and increased bicarbonate production. Hypochloremia is a common feature of chronic respiratory acidosis because of renal chloride excretion.

Acute respiratory acidosis

The common causes include airway obstruction (severe bronchospasm, birth asphyxia, foreign body inhalation or laryngeal edema), hyaline membrane disease, extensive pneumonia, pneumothorax, pulmonary embolism and pulmonary edema, hypoventilation because of neuromuscular disease (poliomyelitis, Guillain-Barre syndrome) and overdose of opium and sedatives.

Chronic respiratory acidosis

It is associated with chronic lung disease (interstitial fibrosis, bronchiectasis, chronic cor pulmonale), kyphoscoliosis, asphyxiating thoracic dystrophy, paralysis or weakness of respiratory muscles.

Clinical features

Signs and symptoms are related to the degree of hypercapnia. Child develops headache with either irritability or depression due to increase in ICP. There is impairment of consciousness varying from drowsiness to deep coma. Muscular tremors

paCO$_2$ (mm Hg)	HCO$_3$ (mEq/l)		
	< 21	21-26	> 26
> 45	Combined metabolic acidosis plus respiratory acidosis	Respiratory acidosis	Mixed *metabolic plus respiratory acidosis
35-45	Metabolic acidosis	Normal	Metabolic alkalosis
< 35	Mixed* metabolic acidosis plus respiratory alkalsois	Respiratory alkalosis	Combined respiratory alkalosis plus metabolic alkalosis

Table 5.26 Recognition of type of disturbance in acid-base balance

* pH reflects which disorder is primary and which is secondary because compensation is never complete.

can occur. Tachycardia, flushing of skin or perspiration may be present. Blood pressure may be low with signs of shock. Ventricular fibrillations may occur.

Management

The immediate dangers of respiratory acidosis are carbon dioxide narcosis and anoxic damage. Treatment is directed at the underlying cause and improvement of alveolar gas exchange by assisted ventilation. Oxygen administration with high flow rates may help to wash out carbon dioxide. However, in breathing in a tight fitting mask or head box may cause a dangerous elevation of $paCO_2$.

If hyperkalemia or ventricular fibrillation develops in a child with acute respiratory acidosis, sodium bicarbonate may be life saving. It should be administered after establishing ventilation. Metabolic alkalosis may develop because of previous chloride losses and will need replacement.

Respiratory Alkalosis

In this condition there is a fall in arterial $paCO_2$. It usually occurs due to hyperventilation (assisted ventilation), psychogenic or neurogenic hyperventilation. It may be one of the earliest signs of sepsis. Acute respiratory alkalosis lasts no longer than 6 to 12 hours. The compensatory response to this condition involves consumption of HCO_3 by body buffers without any renal involvement. In the chronic phase renal suppression of H^+ ion excretion and chloride retention occurs to offset the falling HCO_3. Hyperchloremia is a common feature in chronic phase.

Clinical picture. Usually there is hyperventilation with features of tetany as alkalosis decreases blood levels of ionized calcium.

Treatment. Breathing in a closed circuit would cause accumulation of carbon dioxide. The underlying condition should be treated. Sodium bicarbonate therapy is not indicated.

Table 5.27 Monitoring of clinical and laboratory data during parenteral fluid therapy				
Parameter	Frequency	Normal value	Fluid deficit signs	Fluid overload signs
Bed side*				
1. Clinical	8 hrly	–	Loss of skin turgor, dry mucosa, tachycardia	Puffiness of eyes, sudden increase in liver size, basal rales
2. Weight	Daily		Weight loss	Sudden weight gain
3. Urine volume	6-8 hrly	1-3 ml /kg/hr	<1 ml/kg/hr	>3 ml/kg/hr
4. Urine specific gravity	6-8 hrly	1008-1015	> 1015	< 1004
Laboratory				
1. Urine osmolality** (mOsm/kg)	12 hr	100-300	> 450	< 100
2. Plasma osmolality (mOsm/kg)	Daily	285	> 300	< 270
3. Serum sodium (mEq/l)	24-48 hr	135-145	-	-
4. Serum potassium (mEq/l)	24-48 hr	4 – 5	-	-
5. Blood urea (mg/dl)	24-48 hr	20-40	> 40	-
6. Serum creatinine (mg/dl)	24-48 hr	0.6-1.2	> 1.4	-

*Meticulous clinical monitoring may be sufficient to detect early fluid imbalance, when laboratory facilities are not available.
**A higher urine osmolality may be due to SIADH which needs water restriction; plasma osmolality and serum sodium values are below normal in SIADH.

Mixed Acid-base Disorders

Mixed acid base disturbances are conditions where more than one primary acid disturbance occurs. The four commonly encountered mixed acid base disorders are: respiratory acidosis + metabolic acidosis, respiratory acidosis + metabolic alkalosis, respiratory alkalosis + metabolic acidosis and respiratory alkalosis + metabolic alkalosis (Table 5.26). The most serious acid-base disorders are of mixed type when respiratory and metabolic disturbances result in a pH change in the same direction.

MONITORING OF FLUID AND ELECTROLYTE THERAPY

While fluids and electrolytes are administered according to the guidelines discussed above, it is necessary to closely follow changes in the clinical and biochemical indicators of water and electrolyte status so as to make timely adjustments to maintain homeostasis in an individual child. During intravenous infusion in early resuscitation phase (0 2 hours) pulse rate, blood pressure, capillary refill time and sensorium should be monitored continuously and urine output every one hourly. Subsequently recording of intake and output, body weight and detection of renal compensatory mechanisms or consequences due to fluid excess or deficit are the most important concerns. A chart should be maintained to record the relevant parameters at regular intervals.

Table 5.27 summarizes the clinical and laboratory data that need to be monitored. Clinical parameters should be reviewed at least 8 hourly and laboratory tests daily to adjust intake of water and electrolytes accordingly. The young infant can concentrate the urine to about 800 mOsm/L. During parenteral administration of fluids, it is best not to tax the kidneys to concentrate maximally but provide enough fluids to achieve urine osmolality between 300-400 mOsm/L.

REFERENCES

1. Joseph G. Verbalis. Disorders of body water homeostasis. *Best Practice & Res Clinical Endocrino & Metab* 2003; 17(4): 471–503.

2. Singhi SC, Ganguly NK, Bhakoo ON, *et al.* Body water distribution in newborn infants appropriate-for-gestational age. *Indian J Med Res* 1995; 101:193-200.

3. Leighton L. Body composition, normal electrolyte concentrations and the maintenance of normal volume, tonicity and acid base metabolism. *Pediatr Clin North Amer* 1990; 37:241-256.

4. Levin ER, Gardner DG, Samson WK, Natriureteric peptides. *New Eng J Med* 1998; 339:321-328.

5. Suzanne MA, Joseph GV, Disorders of body water homeostasis in critical illness. *Endocrinol Metab Clin N Amer* 35 2006: 873–894.

6. Boincan GF, Lewy JE. Estimation of parenteral fluid requirements. *Pediatr Clin North Amer* 1990; 37:257-265.

7. Holiday MA, Segar WE. The maintenance need for water in parenteral fluid therapy. *Pediatrics* 1957; 19: 823-832.

8. Singhi S, Jayashree M. Free water excess is not the main cause for hyponatremia in critically ill children receiving conventional maintenance fluids. *Indian Pediatr* 2009 Jul; 46(7):577-583.

9. Mackenzie A, Barnes G, Shann F. Clinical signs of dehydration in children. *Lancet* 1989; 2:605-607.

10. Saavedra JM, Harns GL, Li S, Fineberg L. Capillary refilling (skin turgor) in assessment of dehydration. *Amer J Dis Child* 1991; 145:296 298.

11. Michael LM, Juan CL. Intravenous fluid management for the acutely ill child. *Current Opin in Pediatr* 2011; 23:186–193.

12. Teach SJ, Yates EW, Feld LG. Laboratory predictors of fluid deficit in acutely dehydrated children. *Clin Paediatr* 1997; 395-400.

13. Bhan MK. Current concepts in management of acute diarrhea. *Indian Pediatr* 2003; 40:463-476.

14. Kaleb KK, Roger G. Management of acute gastroenteritis among children. *MMWR (CDC) Recommendations and report* 2003; 21: 52 (RR16): 1-16.

15. Michael JGS. Fluid and electrolyte therapy in children. In: Avners' Textbook of Pediatric Nephrology. *Springer Publication,* 2010; 325-353.

16. Molla AM, Molla A, Nash SK, Khatua M. Food based oral rehydration salt solution for acute childhood diarrhea. *Lancet* 1989; 2:429 431.

17. Alam NH, Hamadani JD, Dewan N, Fuchs GJ. Efficacy and safety of a modified oral rehydration solution (ReSoMaL) in treatment of severely malnourished children with watery diarrhea. *J Pediatr* 2003; 143: 614-619.

18. Whang R, Flink EB, Dyckner T, Wester PO, Aikawa JK, Ryan MP. Magnesium depletion as a cause of refractory potassium depletion. *Arch Intern Med* 1985; 145:1686-1689.

19. Nalin DR, Hirschhorn N, Greenough W, Fuchs GJ, Cash RA. Clinical concerns about reduced osmolarity oral rehydration solutions. *JAMA* 2004; 291:2632-2635.

20. Bannerjee S, Singhi SC, Singh S, Singh M. The intraosseous route is a suitable alternative to intravenous route for fluid resuscitation in severely dehydrated children. *Indian Pediatr* 1994; 31:1511-1520.

21. Snyder JD. Use and misuse of oral therapy for diarrhea: comparisons of US practices with American Academy of Pediatrics recommendations. *Pediatrics* 1991; 87: 28–33.

22. Santosham M, Daum RS, Dillman L, *et al.* Oral rehydration therapy of infantile diarrhea: a controlled study of well nourished children hospitalized in the United States and Panama. *N Engl J Med* 1986; 306:1070–1076.

23. Leung AKC, Taylor PG, Geoffrey L, Darling P. Efficacy and safety of two oral solutions as maintenance therapy for acute diarrhea. *Clin Pediatr* 1988; 27:359–364.

24. Rahman O, Bennish ML, Alam AN, *et al*. Rapid intravenous rehydration by means of a single polyelectrolyte solution with or without dextrose. *J Pediatr* 1988; 113:654 660.

25. Arieff AI, DeFronzo RA. In: Fluids, Electrolytes and Acid-base Disorders. *Churchill Livingstone, New York, 1994 second edition, 1995.*

26. Adrogne HJ, Madias NE. Hypernatremia. *New Eng J Med* 2000; 342:1493-1499.

27. Prasad SVSS, Singhi S, Chugh KS. Hyponatremia in sick children seeking emergency care. *Indian Pediatr* 1994; 31:287-294.

28. Brimioulle S, Vincent J, Dufaye P, Berre J, Degaute J. Kahn RJ. Hydrochloric acid infusion for treatment of metabolic alkalosis: effect on acid base balance and oxygenation. *Crit Care Med* 1985; 13:738-742.

29. Poddar U, Singhi S, Ganguly NK, Sialy R. Water electrolyte homeostasis in acute bronchiolitis. *Indian Pediatr* 1995; 32:59-65.

30. Dhawan A, Narang A, Singhi S. Hyponatremia and the inappropriate ADH syndrome in pneumonia. *Ann Trop Paediatr* 1992;12(4):455-62.

31. Singhi S, Sharma A, Majumdar S. Body water and plasma volume in severe community acquired pneumonia: implications for fluid therapy. *Ann Trop Paediatr* 2005 Dec; 25(4):243-252.

32. Singhi SC, Singhi PD, Srinivas B, Narakesri HP, Ganguli NK, Sialy R, Walia BNS. Fluid restriction does not improve the outcome of acute meningitis. *Pediatr Infect Dis J* 1995 Jun; 14(6):495-503.

33. Kumar V, Singhi P, Singhi S. Changes in body water compartments in children with acute meningitis. *Pediatr Infect Dis J* 1994 Apr; 13(4):299-305.

34. Singhi S, Dhawan A. Frequency and significance of electrolyte abnormalities in pneumonia. *Indian Pediatr* 1992; 29:735-740.

35. Singhi S, Prasad SVSS, Chugh KS. Hyponatremia in sick children: a marker of serious illness. *Indian Pediatr* 1994; 31:19-25.

36. Dass R, Nagaraj R, Murlidharan J and Singhi S. Hyponatremia and hypovolemic shock with tuberculous meningitis. *Indian J Pediatr* 2003; 70:995-997.

37. Decaux G, Soupart A. Treatment of symptomatic hyponatremia. *Amer J Med Sci* 2003; 326:25- 30.

38. Sarnaik AP, Meert K, Hackbarth R, Fleischmann L. Management of hyponatremic seizures in children with hypertonic saline: a safe and effective strategy. *Crit Care Med* 1991; 758-762.

39. Singhi S. Hyponatremia in critically ill children: Current concepts. *Indian J Pediatr* 2004; 21:803-807.

40. Janicic N, Verbalis JG. Evaluation and management of hypo-osmolality in hospitalized patients. *Endocrinol Metab Clin North Amer* 2003; 32:459-481.

41. Palevsky PM. Hypernatremia. In: Primer on Kidney Disease. Greenbergh A. (ed.) 2nd edition, *San Diego, California, Academic Press,* 1998;64-71.

42. Guzman C, Pizzaro D, Castillo B, Posada G. Hyper-natremic diarrheal dehydration treated with oral glucose electrolyte solution containing 90 or 75 mEq/L of sodium. *J Pediatr Gastroenterol Nutr* 1988; 7: 694-698.

43. Singhi S, Jayshree M, Sarkar B. Hypokalemia following nebulized salbutamol in children with acute attack of bronchial asthma. *J Paediatr Child Hlth* 1996; 32: 495-497.

44. Jayashree M, Singhi S. Diabetic ketoacidosis: Predictors of outcome in a pediatric intensive care unit of a developing country. *Pediatr Crit Care Med* 2004; 5: 427-433.

45. Singhi S, Gulati S, Prasad SVSS. Frequency and significance of potassium disturbance in sick children. *Indian Pediatr* 1994; 31:460-463.

46. Singhi S, Marudkar A. Hypokalemia in a pediatric intensive care unit. *Indian Pediatr* 1996; 33:9-13.

47. Kruse JA, Carlson RW. Rapid correction of hypokalemia using concentrated intravenous potassium chloride infusions. *Arch Intern Med* 1990; 150: 613-617.

48. Singhi S, Gautham KS. Safety and efficacy of a concentrated potassium chloride solution infusion for rapid correction of hypokalemia. *Indian Pediatr* 1993; 31(5):565-569.

49. Ammar W, Stephen LA. Serum sodium disorders: Safe management. *Clinical Medicine* 2010; 10(1): 79–82.

50. Hala MA, Arif S, Fatima B. Severe hypernatremia correction rate and mortality in hospitalized patients *Amer J Med Sci.* 2011; 10(15): 1-5.

51. Ira K, Minhtri K, Nguyen A. Simple quantitative approach to analyze the generation of the dysnatremias. *Clin Exp Nephrol* 2003; 7:138–143.

52. Ce´line O, Dang KN, Michel P. Central pontine and extrapontine myelinolysis: from epileptic and other manifestations to cognitive prognosis. *J Neurol* 2010; 257:1176–1180.

53. Annachiara C, Renzo M, Lamberto P Hypernatremia-induced limbic system damage. *Anesthesiology* 2011; 114(5): 175-178.

54. Greenberg A. Hyperkalemia: treatment options. *Semin Nephrol* 1998; 18:46-57.

55. Singhi S, Singh J, Prasad R. Hypocalcemia in a pediatric intensive care unit. *J Trop Pediatr* 2003; 49:298-302.

56. Singhi S, Singh J, Prasad R. Hypo-and hypermagnesemia in an Indian pediatric intensive care unit. *J Trop Pediatr* 2003; 49:99-103.

57. Brenner BE. Clinical significance of high anion gap. *Amer J Med* 1985; 79:289-296.

58. Orchard CH, Kentish JC. Effects of changes of pH on the contractile function of cardiac muscle. *Amer J Physiol* 1990; 258(6, Part 1):967–981.

59. Orchard CH, Cingolani HE. Acidosis and arrhythmias in cardiac muscle. *Cardiovasc Res* 1994; 28(9):1312–1319.

60. Williams AJ. ABC of oxygen: assessing and interpreting arterial blood gases and acid–base balance. *BMJ* 1998;317(7167):1213–1216.

61. Khadra EA. Disorders of the acid base status. In: Pediatric Nephrology in ICU. *Springer Publications,* 2009; pp. 19-31.

62. Emmett M. Anion gap interpretation: The old and the new. *Nat Clin Pract Nephrol* 2006; 2:4–5.

Shock

Utkarsh Kohli and Rakesh Lodha

Shock is a clinical state of acute disruption of circulatory function, resulting in an insufficiency of tissue perfusion, oxygen utilization and cellular energy production. This leads to deranged homeostasis and cellular injury, resulting in organ dysfunction, which may become irreversible unless corrected rapidly. Shock essentially remains a clinical diagnosis, being defined by a constellation of clinical signs that may arise from several etiologies. The circulatory function depends on cardiac function, vascular tone and blood volume. Shock syndromes may result from abnormalities in one or more of these factors or from cellular dysfunction due to inability to utilize substrates delivered by the circulatory system.

CLASSIFICATION

The absence of universally accepted system for classification of shock is because of the complex pathophysiology and its tremendous variability. Also, for any given shock state, these characteristics vary widely over time. Hence it is important to know both the etiology of shock in a patient and the time course of the syndrome. In a given patient, there may be overlaps. Shock can be classified into the following four major categories (Table 6.1).

1. Hypovolemic (reduced intravascular volume)
2. Cardiogenic (failure of the cardiac pump)
3. Distributive or vasogenic (alteration in vascular tone, either primary or secondary to neurologic or neurohormonal changes)
4. Septic shock (this has features of all the above mentioned types).

In addition to the above classification, it is useful to consider the following three stages of shock (Table 6.2).

1. **Compensated.** The homeostatic mechanisms maintain perfusion of the essential organs; hence blood pressure, cardiac function and urine output may appear to be normal.

Table 6.1 Classification of shock

I. **HYPOVOLEMIC**
   1. *Fluid and electrolyte losses*
      (a) Acute gastroenteritis
      (b) Excessive sweating
      (c) Renal diseases
   2. *Plasma loss*
      (a) Burns
      (b) Third space losses
   3. *Hemorrhage*
      (a) External : Trauma, bleeding disorder, gastrointestinal bleeding
      (b) Internal : Visceral injury, vascular injury, fractures
   4. *Endocrinal disorders*
      (a) Adrenal insufficiency
      (b) Diabetes mellitus
      (c) Diabetes insipidus

II. **CARDIOGENIC**
   1. *Cardiac insufficiency*
      (a) Myocarditis
      (b) Cardiomyopathy
      (c) Dysrrhythmias
      (d) Metabolic: Hypoxia, hypoglycemia, acidosis, hypothermia, uremia
      (e) Drug intoxication : Anthracyclines, β-blockers, tricyclic antidepressants
      (f) Congenital heart disease
      (g) Cardiac surgery
   2. *Obstructive lesions*
      (a) Pericardial tamponade, pneumopericardium
      (b) Pulmonary embolism
      (c) Congenital heart disease: Aortic stenosis, coarctation of aorta, critical pulmonary stenosis, interrupted aortic arch
      (d) Tension pneumothorax

III. **DISTRIBUTIVE**
      (a) Anap,ogenic
      (c) Drug toxicity

IV. **SEPTIC SHOCK**

Clinical parameter	Stage I (Pre-shock/ compensated)	Stage II (Organ hypoperfusion/ decompensated)	Stage III (End organ failure/ irreversible)
Mental state	Clear but distressed	Confused or restless	Apathetic or comatose
Skin	Pale, cold	Cool, clammy	Cold, cyanotic and mottled
Peripheral vasoconstriction	Mild	Marked	Intensive
Blood pressure	Normal/slightly elevated	Low	Unrecordable
Urine output	Normal/low	Oliguria	Anuria
Heart rate	Increased	Increased	Increased
Respiratory rate	Increased	Repiratory failure	Respiratory failure
Metabolic change	Respiratory alkalosis	Lactic acidosis	Severe metabolic acidosis
Basis for staging	Activation of compensatory mechanisms	Compensatory mechanisms beginning to fail	Multiple organ failure

Table 6.2 Clinical parameters and staging of shock

2. *Decompensated.* The circulatory compensation fails because of a wide variety of reasons, leading to manifestations of abnormalities in all organ systems.

3. *Irreversible.* Death is inevitable because of significant, irreparable functional damage to the essential organs.

In the developing world, hypovolemic shock resulting from acute gastroenteritis is the leading cause of shock in children[1,2]. Septic shock is also an important cause given the high incidence of various infections in developing countries.

PATHOGENESIS

1. Hypovolemic Shock

Hypovolemic shock is a clinical state characterized by reduced venous return to the heart (preload), resulting in decreased oxygen and other substrate delivery insufficient to meet tissue demands. Physiologic compensatory mechanisms allow children (otherwise healthy) to tolerate acute volume loss of upto 15 percent. This is achieved at the expense of alterations in intracardiac and systemic venous pressures and changes in regional blood flow to skin, mesentery, kidneys and muscles.

The compensatory mechanisms aim to increase the intravascular volume and blood pressure. Increased adrenergic activity, resulting from both increased sympathetic discharge and adrenal release of catecholamines (feedback from baroreceptors and volume receptors) leads to arterial vasoconstriction, venoconstriction with increased venous return and tachycardia. Reduction in cerebral blood flow is a more potent stimulus for sympathetic discharge than that provided by peripheral baroreceptors (Figure 6.1). Also, reduction in hydrostatic pressure in the capillaries along with precapillary arterial constriction, leads to transudation of fluid from extracellular space into the vessels.

Volume reduction also leads to significant increase in vasopressin secretion, which is mediated through baroreceptors and atrial volume receptors. Renin-angiotensin system is perhaps the most potent hormonal compensatory mechanism. These alterations lead to enhanced water and sodium retention.

Compensated phase of hypovolemic shock is characterized by decrease in stroke volume, central venous pressure (CVP) and urine output, with increase in heart rate, systemic vascular resistance and cardiac contractility. The systemic blood pressure is usually normal; but orthostatic changes in arterial blood pressure and heart rate may be present. If appropriate resuscitative measures are instituted, compensated hypovolemic shock has excellent prognosis.

When intravascular fluid losses surpass the body's compensatory mechanisms, decompensated phase appears with profound systemic vasoconstriction, ischemia and hypoxia. Children are frequently hypotensive, lethargic or comatose, oliguric and acidotic. Stroke volume and cardiac

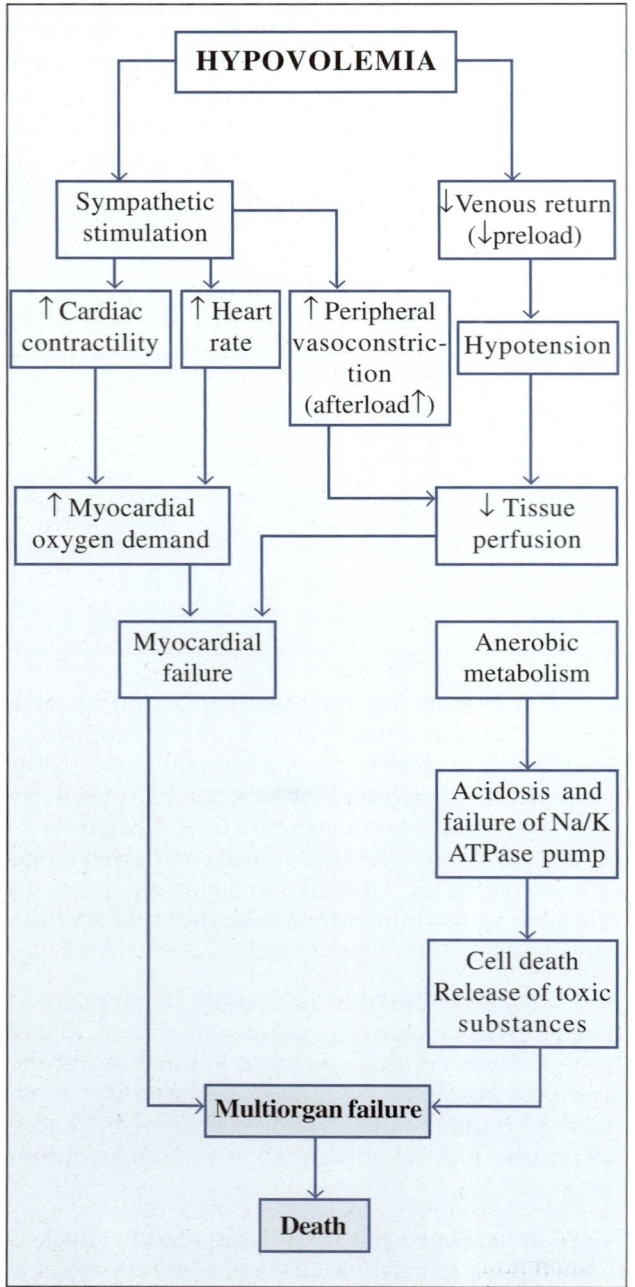

Figure 6.1 Pathophysiology of hypovolemic shock

output are further reduced. Excessive vaso-constriction may reduce the blood flow to the point where cellular damage ensues. Damage to the capillary endothelium leads to loss of proteins and fluid from circulation into third space with further worsening of the hypovolemia. In addition, production and secretion of proinflammatory agents during reperfusion, prolonged severe hypovolemic shock and translocation of toxins from injured gut lead to end organ damage, multiple organ system failure and death[3-5].

2.   Cardiogenic Shock

Cardiogenic shock results from abnormalities of cardiac rhythm or function (pump failure). Commonly, this is caused by impairment in myocardial contractility. Cardiogenic shock can also be caused by mechanical abnormalities. The compensatory mechanisms (as mentioned in section on hypovolemic shock) are activated as the perfusion declines. In the failing heart, the compensatory mechanisms may ultimately become dysfunctional as mentioned below.

1.   The increase in the systemic vascular resistance caused by vasoconstriction, results in increased myocardial afterload. This, along with increased heart rate and contractility raises the myocardial oxygen demand and worsen the ischemia.

2.   The diastolic filling is impaired because of tachycardia leading to decrease in myocardial perfusion.

3.   Fluid retention may increase the intravascular volume significantly to cause increase in preload, pulmonary congestion and hypoxemia.

4.   The ischemia compromises ventricular diastolic compliance, further elevating the left atrial pressure and worsening the pulmonary congestion.

5.   The increased myocardial demand of oxygen and other substrates in the setting of decreased perfusion, leads to worsening of ischemia and a vicious cycle.

6.   The obstructive causes such as pericardial tamponade may cause shock by interfering with the diastolic filling which stimulates the above mentioned compensatory responses. Failure of compensation leads to shock.

3.   Distributive Shock

In this condition, decreased tissue perfusion results from abnormal shunting of normal or increased cardiac output. The important causes are anaphylaxis, drug overdosage and neurogenic shock.

Anaphylactic shock results in a previously sensitized host when an antigen reacts with fixed IgE antibody; triggering a series of reactions involving circulating mast cells, eosinophils, and perivascular connective tissue mast cells, complement activation and vasoactive mediators (histamine, leukotrienes C_4 and D_4, bradykinin and various prostanoid compounds). Widespread vasodilatation, intravascular pooling and decreased venous return are followed by microvascular endothelial injury and intravascular volume depletion via the capillary leak. These lead to decrease in the cardiac output. In addition, airway and pulmonary manifestations of anaphylaxis may be life threatening[6].

Neurogenic shock may occur after high spinal transection, severe brainstem and intracranial injuries. The CNS perfusion is severely affected because of hypotension.

4.   Septic Shock

Septic shock results when infectious agents or infection-induced mediators in the blood stream lead to circulatory decompensation. Various factors contribute to development of shock in sepsis. These include decreased intravascular volume, maldistribution of intravascular volume, impaired myocardial function, and cellular derangements wherein cells and tissues are unable to utilize the substrates delivered to them[7, 8]. The contribution of any of these factors may vary with time. *In contrast to other types of shock, there is early occurrence of impairment of the cellular metabolism in septic shock.*

The infectious agent also triggers a wide variety of beneficial host response mechanisms (endogenous inflammatory mediators). But these may ultimately lead to widely impaired endothelial and cellular functions leading to metabolic dysfunction and circulatory collapse (Figure 6.2).

Toxic effects could result from the microorganisms themselves e.g. from elaboration of exotoxins, and from components of bacterial cell wall known as endotoxins (the lipopolysaccharides in the outer membrane of the Gram-negative bacteria and lipoteichoic acid-peptidoglycan complex of the Gram-positive bacteria[9]. Gram-negative bacteremia leads to greater inflammatory response than Gram-positive bacteremia. Therefore, Gram-negative bacteremia may be associated with higher risk of progression to more severe clinical manifestations such as septic shock rather than Gram-positive sepsis or severe sepsis[10].

Endotoxins are a potent trigger for a wide variety of biologic reactions. They induce an inflammatory response which may protect the host but can result in multiorgan failure and death if released in excessive amounts[11]. The various cell types stimulated would lead to a host of biologic responses including release of several cytokines and

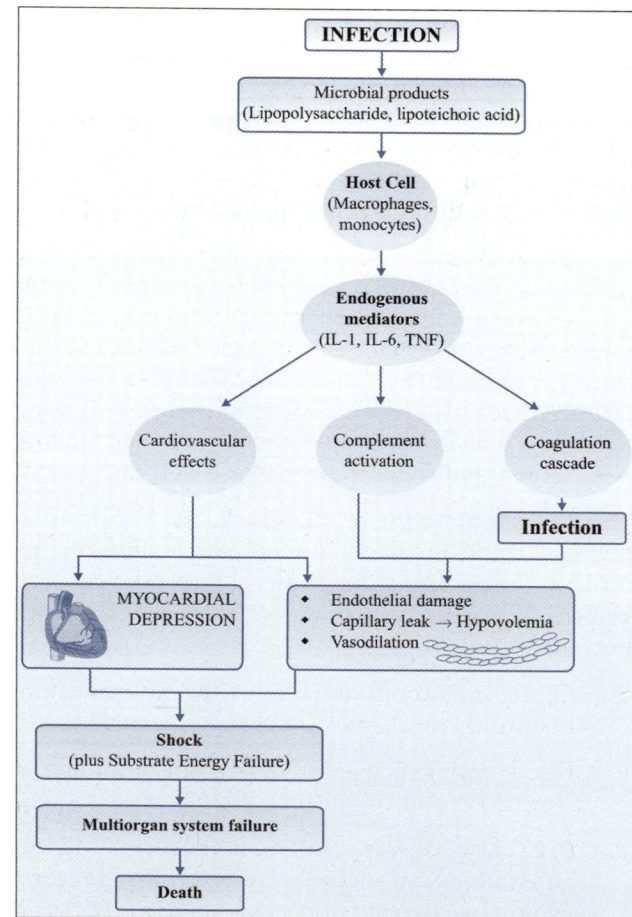

Figure 6.2 Pathophysiology of septic shock

humoral mediators. Cytokines are intercellular signaling peptides which regulate the inflammatory response On exposure to endotoxins, monocytes release TNF and IL-1[12, 13]. These cytokines are critical for regulation of host defences. In addition to their pro-inflammatory effects they also mediate protective anti-inflammatory responses. The anti-inflammatory effects include increased expression of superoxide dismutase, release of acute phase reactants, induction of anti-inflammatory cytokines i.e. IL-4, IL-6, IL-10 and down regulation of TNF and IL-1 receptors[14]. Other humoral mediators include histamine, kinins, endorphins, eicosanoids, platelet-activating factor, collagenases, nitric oxide and complement[11, 13-15].

Both exogenous and endogenous mediators cause peripheral vasodilatation in sepsis. Nitric oxide (NO) is a low-molecular weight, membrane permeable gas which is an important mediator of vasodilatation. NO also functions as a neuro-transmitter, inhibits platelet aggregation and leucocyte adhesion. Endotoxin, TNF and interleukins stimulate calcium independent form of nitric oxide synthase in macrophages and vascular smooth muscle cells. Though NO may be largely responsible for hypotension in septic shock it may also have a role in maintaining microvascular blood flow and countering the vasoconstricting effects of some mediators i.e. thromboxane and endothelin-1[11].

Endotoxemia leads to reduced response of the peripheral vasculature to catecholamines[16]. This may explain the failure of normal adrenergic compensatory mechanisms in septic shock. Other possible explanations for vasodilatation include direct blocking of neurotransmitter release, endotoxin interference with smooth muscle calcium metabolism and membrane ATPase activity.

In patients with septic shock, the ventricular ejection fractions are reduced, even though the cardiac output may be high[17]. The myocardial function may be depressed due to a variety of mechanisms:

(i)   Global metabolic defects of the myocardium resulting from shock.

(ii)   Decreased response to sympathetic stimulation (impaired end organ response).

(iii) Presence of circulating cardioinhibitory substances, myocardial depressant factors (specific myocardial depressant factors [MDFs], histamine, endorphins, complement, interleukins and prostaglandins).

(iv)   Myocardial ischemia resulting from increased workload and reduced supply of energy and oxygen.

(v)   Endocardial endothelial injury (endocardial endothelium has significant influence on myocardial contractility).

(vi)   Nitric oxide production by myocardium/ endocardium.

(vii) Defective myocardial calcium metabolism.

It is important to note that myocardial dysfunction appears to occur not only preterminally but also in the early stages of septic shock[17]. While peripheral vascular paralysis seems to be the major cause of hypotension in early septic shock, myocardial depression does occur, and as the shock progresses, this depression becomes progressively more severe.

Endotoxins also activate the intrinsic coagulation cascade along with fibrinolytic system leading to deposition of fibrin microaggregates in the vasculature and obstructing flow and exacerbating tissue hypoxia[18]. In addition, leukoactivation, complement, oxygen radicals, eicosanoids and platelet activating factor mediate several of pathophysiologic mechanisms occuring in septic shock[19-22].

DIAGNOSIS

It is not difficult to diagnose a full blown case of shock with hypotension, lethargy, poor peripheral perfusion and cold extermities. However, in such cases the likelihood of successful intervention would be limited. *It is important to recognise shock and initiate therapy before it causes irreversible damage to the vital organs.* The early diagnosis of shock requires high index of suspicion. A useful clinical triad to recognize septic shock, before onset of hypotension, includes hyperthermia or hypothermia , altered mental status and peripheral vasodilation (warm shock) or cold extremities (cold shock)[23].

A practical approach is to make a rapid clinical assessment with brief history and physical examination and initiate specific diagnostic modalities to identify the cause and determine the severity of shock. The early diagnosis, recognition and close monitoring of children who are predisposed to shock are crucial to improve survival. Assessment of child's activity, oral intake, responsiveness, mental status, and urine output are valuable in indicating the severity and duration of the abnormality. There may be history of excessive fluid loss because of diarrhea/vomiting or blood loss because of trauma. It is important to elicit details of environmental exposure, previous medical problems, allergies and potential drug ingestion. Septic shock is suspected in a child with history of fever, features suggestive of infection and circulatory collapse. Previous history of disorders such as congenital heart disease, endocrinal or renal disorder offer clues to the etiology.

It is possible to identify signs suggestive of the underlying pathophysiologic process[24]. It must be emphasized that *"hypotension is not the sine quo non of shock"*. It is common to record normal blood pressure in children with early shock. Alteration in mean arterial pressure is a late manifestation of hypovolemic shock in children. A rough estimate of minimal acceptable systolic blood pressure in children is: Systolic blood pressure (mm Hg) = 70 + (age in years × 2)

Hypotension, if present, strongly supports the diagnosis of shock. Initially, the pulse pressure is decreased, often because of some decrease in systolic pressure and an increase in diastolic pressure; later both systolic and diastolic pressures fall, indicating a major hemodynamic compromise. Apart from the blood pressure, pulse characteristics should be carefully noted, as it may give clue to the etiology as well as severity of shock.

Impaired capillary refill is a more sensitive indicator of poor peripheral tissue perfusion. The refill is determined by blanching an area of skin over the face, forehead or sternum by firm compression with finger tip for 5 seconds and then noting the time for the blanching to disappear. Capillary refill which takes longer than 3 seconds is a very sensitive but nonspecific indicator of tissue hypoperfusion[25]. Being a physiological response to intravascular volume depletion, peripheral hypoperfusion in itself does not indicate shock, but it clearly heralds it.

Physical findings of dehydration may be present; these can indicate the severity of hypovolemia. However, these are not sensitive criteria[26]. The measurement of the difference between core and peripheral temperature (e.g. rectal and toe temperature) may be helpful in diagnosis. The difference often exceeds 2.5°C in children with shock[27]. The physical manifestations of metabolic acidosis are primarily respiratory which are characterized by tachypnea and hyperventilation. Initially, there may be respiratory alkalosis. Hypoperfusion of vital organs may manifest as oliguria (renal hypoperfusion) or altered sensorium (CNS hypoperfusion). The physical findings may vary both with the etiology and severity of shock. A wide range of findings are seen especially with septic shock (Table 6.3).

The assessment of the etiology and the severity of shock is greatly assisted by several laboratory investigations like complete blood counts, serum protein/albumin, blood urea/creatinine and serum calcium, preferably ionized calcium. Liver function tests, arterial blood gas analysis, arterial blood lactate and coagulation profile should be checked. X-ray chest and appropriate microbiological studies should be undertaken.

Arterial blood gas analysis is a valuable aid in the management of shock. It helps in determining the adequacy of ventilatory functions. Determination of pH and base deficit aids in the quantification of tissue hypoperfusion, as the degree of metabolic acidosis correlates with the severity of tissue hypoperfusion. A simultaneous mixed venous oxygen tension can help quantifying the oxygen consumption[28].

Table 6.3 Stages of septic shock		
Parameters	**Early (warm)**	**Late (cold)**
Bedside observations		
• Heat rate	Increased	Increased
• Respiratory rate	Increased	Decreased
• Core temperature	Increased	Decreased
• Extremities	Warm and flushed	Cold and pale
• Pulse volume	Bounding	Decreased
• Capillary refilling	Normal	Prolonged
• Blood pressure	Normal or elevated	Decreased
• Pulse pressure	Normal or elevated	Decreased
• Cardiac index	Elevated	Decreased
• Urine output	Adequate or polyuria	Oliguria
• CNS status	Mild mental confusion, irritable, anxious	Lethargy or coma
Laboratory measurements		
• paO_2	Decreased	Decreased
• pH	Respiratory alkalosis (metabolic acidosis is not always present in early phase)	Respiratory/metabolic acidosis
• Arterio-venous oxygen saturation difference	Narrow	Wide
• Blood sugar	Increased	Decreased
• Coagulation abnormalities	Mild	Marked
• Blood lactate	Normal or mildly elevated	Markedly elevated

MONITORING OF A CHILD WITH SHOCK

The aim of monitoring children who are in shock or at risk of developing shock is to detect early alterations in the physiologic status and assess the outcome of the interventions. All children with shock are best managed in a pediatric intensive care unit (PICU). The important components of monitoring include physical parameters, urine output, biochemical parameters, central venous pressure (CVP) and if available pulmonary artery pressure and cardiac index[23]. It is important to emphasize the importance of repeated and careful examination of child's physical status, as this is probably the most sensitive and reliable physiologic monitoring. A monitoring chart should be maintained to document vitals (i.e. temperature, heart rate, respiratory rate, blood pressure), sensorium, fluid input and urine output. Biochemical parameters such as blood glucose levels, calcium, arterial blood gases and serum lactate levels provide useful information to guide the management[23]. In addition continuous electrocardiography, pulse oximetry, and invasive blood pressure monitoring are useful in critically sick children.

Central venous pressure (CVP) monitoring is frequently helpful in the management of a child with shock. CVP catheters can be placed via the external or internal jugular, femoral, basilic or subclavian vein. Before using CVP measurement, it is essential to confirm the position of the tip of the catheter in the right atrium. The central venous pressures are considered to reflect the intravascular volume accurately. However, more than the intravascular volume, right ventricular contractility, right ventricular afterload (pulmonary vascular resistance) and the compliance significantly affect the CVP. The normal CVP, although described as less than 10 mmHg, is usually around 1 to 3 mm Hg, and intravascular volume expansion by as much 30 percent does not significantly alter right atrial pressure[29]. Use of mechanical positive pressure ventilation increases the CVP. This fact should be borne in mind when monitoring CVP. In pure hypovolemic shock without myocardial compromise, it is unlikely that CVP measurement may add anything significant to careful evaluations of peripheral perfusion, blood pressure, urine output and acid base analysis. However, when there is suspicion of myocardial dysfunction or when renal impairment has occured, CVP measurements are useful to avoid excessive fluid infusion. CVP should not be taken as an indicator of left venticular function. There is poor correlation between the CVP and pulmonary artery occlusion pressures, especially in patients with cardiac disease[30].

Hemodynamic variables such as perfusion pressure are helpful to monitor and guide the therapy of shock. The blood flow in the body can be represented as follows:

$$\text{Flow} = \frac{\text{Pressure head}}{\text{Resistance}} = \frac{\text{MAP-CVP}}{\text{TPR}} \text{ where}$$

MAP = mean arterial pressure, CVP = central venous pressure and TPR = total peripheral resistance

This equation illustrates that to achieve good perfusion adequate MAP has to be maintained using fluids and inotropes. It is also clear that if CVP is high then the pressure head for the circulation shall decrease. Vasodilators help as they increase the pressure head by lowering the high CVP due to myocardial dysfunction. High intra-abdominal pressure increases CVP resulting in decreased perfusion. Therapeutic taps in children with refractory septic shock and significant ascites may therefore be helpful in reversing shock (besides improving respiratory embarrassment due to tense ascites).

The *arterial blood gases* should be frequently monitored as these give information about the adequacy of ventilation and tissue perfusion. *Pulmonary artery catheterization* (if available) helps in assessment of pulmonary arterial pressures, cardiac output measurement and evaluation of superior vena cava oxygen saturation. These measurements have been found to increase survival in early goal directed therapy for septic shock[31].

MANAGEMENT

The aim of therapy in children with shock is initially to optimize the perfusion of the vital organs (brain, heart and kidneys), prevent/correct metabolic abnormalities arising from tissue hypoperfusion, and finally to prevent or reverse the defects in cellular substrate delivery and metabolism.

In any form of shock, determining the etiology and treating the underlying cause is mandatory. For suspected sepsis, broad spectrum antibiotics should be administered at the earliest (Table 6.4). However, certain therapies are common to all the forms of shock:

1. Hypoxemia should be prevented and corrected. All children with circulatory

Age	Common organisms	Antibiotics
<2wks	Coliforms, Listeria, Group B streptococci	Ampicillin + gentamicin or cefotaxime
2 wks-2 months	*Streptococcous pneumoniae*, Coliforms, Listeria, *Group B Streptococci.*	Ampicillin + ceftriaxone or cefotaxime
>3 months	*Hemophilus influenzae, Neisseria meningitidis, Streptococcus pneumoniae,* coliforms	Ampicillin + chloramph- enicol or ceftriaxone or cefotaxime
Any age	*Bacteroides fragilis* Meningococcus	Add clindamycin or metronidazole Crystalline penicillin
Immuno-compromised children	*Staphylococcus aureus* and *Pseudomonas aeruginosa*	Ceftazidime + vancomycin

Table 6.4 Rationale for use of antibiotics in septic shock

compromise should receive supplemental oxygen.

2. Assessment of airways and breathing followed by endotracheal intubation and mechanical ventilation is recommended in all cases of shock which are not readily reversible. There may be insufficient oxygen delivery because of decreased respiratory muscle function (due to reduced perfusion, acidosis, hypoxia and metabolic abnormalities), pulmonary edema and noncardiac pulmonary edema (ARDS). In children with cardiogenic shock and pulmonary edema, mechanical ventilation may significantly improve myocardial function by relieving deleterious cardiorespiratory interactions. Intubation and synchronization of ventilation may improve myocardial function by decreasing the afterload effect of excessively negative intrapleural pressures. In addition, the right ventricular function improves as the pulmonary compliance increases and the intrapulmonary shunting decreases.

3. Vascular access should be established rapidly in accordance with Pediatric Advanced Life Support guidelines[32].

4. Optimization and stabilization of the cardiac output and systolic arterial blood pressure by manipulating the preload, heart rate, myocardial contractility, and the after-load.

5. Careful monitoring (*vide supra*).

Early goal-directed therapy for septic shock

Early goal-directed therapy is the latest concept in the treatment of septic shock and this approach has proved useful in decreasing the mortality in adults[31,33]. The same should be applicable to children. In order to optimize resuscitation, the desirable end points should be predifined. In adults the current surviving sepsis campaign guidelines are that during the first 6 hours of resuscitation the goals of therapy should be to achieve CVP of 8-12 mm Hg, MAP >65 mmHg, urine output >0.5 ml/kg/hr and mixed venous O_2 saturation $\geq 70\%$ [31]. In children, early therapeutic end points after one hour of resuscitation are listed below:

- Capillary refill time <2 seconds
- Warm extremities
- No differential between peripheral and central pulses
- Urine output >1 ml/kg/hr
- Normal mental status
- No hypotension
- Normalization of heart rate

Beyond the first hour of therapy in children with septic shock, in addition to the above parameters, the aim is to maintain cardiac index (CI) between 3.3-6.0 L/min/m², decrease lactate and improve base deficit, and achieve mixed venous saturation >70%[23, 31].

Fluid therapy. In a child presenting with shock (except in cardiogenic shock) intravascular volume expansion is frequently adequate to restore the blood pressure and peripheral perfusion. Rapid infusion of 20 ml/kg as a bolus over 5 to 10 minutes can be given safely and repeated if necessary. Aggressive fluid management is the key to success in the management of septic shock. Upto 150-200 ml/kg may be required in the first hour of shock[34,35]. *According to the current recommendations for pediatric septic shock, 20 ml/kg boluses of isotonic crystalloids or isooncotic colloids are given every 5 minutes if required, so that upto 60 ml/kg fluid is infused in first 15 minutes*[23]. At this time a CVP line and invasive hemodynamic monitoring is advisable to guide further therapy in those patients who fail to respond to initial resuscitative efforts. The losses, if any, should be replaced. Simultaneously, maintenance fluid requirements should be given. The response to fluid replacement should be determined by careful monitoring of blood pressure, peripheral perfusion and urine output.

Preload augmentation with fluid infusion in patients with septic shock and myocardial impairment should be monitored by measuring CVP. The CVP line protects against volume overload. In the presence of low CVP, volume overload is highly unlikely, whereas, a CVP that is rising or greater than 10 mm Hg, indicates either fluid overload, myocardial dysfunction or increased right ventricular afterload. In this setting if more fluids are infused, then because of increased venous pressure, perfusion pressure in several critical vascular beds is decreased and vascular leak is increased leading to tissue edema (especially pulmonary edema). Patients with raised intracranial pressure also require careful fluid management. In these patients inotropic support may be started early, even before preload is fully augmented. In patients with severe malnutrition and septic shock, the fluid therapy is given with due caution. Though there are no clear guidelines for this group of patients, the initial fluid boluses generally should not exceed 10 ml/kg over 20 minutes with intensive monitoring for fluid overload and myocardial dysfunction. CVP monitoring is most useful in these patients.

The use of colloid versus crystalloid replacement for shock has been a controversial issue. A large study comparing 4% albumin with normal saline reported similar outcomes in either group[36]. In addition, no difference in outcomes was found between children with dengue shock syndrome treated with colloids or crystalloids in three randomized controlled trials[31,37-39]. Crystalloids such as normal saline and ringer lactate are cheap; convenient to use and free of side effects. But the main disadvantage is that they are rapidly distributed across the intravascular and interstitial spaces so that volume expansion is transient and large volumes of infusion are required. Colloids (i.e. gelatins, starches, dextrans, albumin) result in greater and more sustained increase in plasma volume with associated improvements in cardiovascular function and oxygen delivery. In case of isolated dehydration, the estimated fluid and electrolyte losses should be replaced with crystalloids. For sepsis and trauma, a judicious mixture of crystalloids and blood products should be given to maintain hemoglobin and clotting factors, and colloids (albumin, hemaccel) to maintain colloid oncotic pressure. Colloids may be infused after the child has received 60 ml/kg of crystalloids.

During rapid fluid infusion, the child should be monitored for decrease in tachycardia, improvement in pulse volume, decrease in capillary refilling time, elevation of blood pressure (if initially low) and improvement in sensorium and urine output. Whenever more than 60 to 100 ml/kg needs to be infused over first 1 or 2 hours, more invasive monitoring and diagnostic investigations should be considered. Severe losses of fluids can occur because of capillary leak, but occult hemorrhage should not be missed.

Majority of the patients with hypovolemic shock and about a quarter of patients with septic shock will show improvement with fluid therapy alone. Further fluid therapy would depend on response to initial therapy and etiology of shock. In hypovolemic shock, most commonly seen with diarrhea, the remaining estimated deficit should be infused over next 3-4 hours. The fluid used can be Ringer's lactate or normal saline. In addition, the maintenance fluid needs should be calculated and administered. If the child continues to have diarrhea, ongoing losses should be replaced with half normal (0.45%) saline in 5 percent dextrose with 20 mEq/L of potassium added to the fluid. In septic shock there are no clear guidelines about further fluid therapy. In view of ongoing pathology and capillary leak, the child should be given extra fluids while monitoring for fluid overload. A judicious combination of crystalloids and colloids is suggested.

Vasopressor agents are indicated if the cardiac output and systemic arterial pressures remain low despite adequate fluid infusion; or pulmonary edema develops; or the child has cardiogenic shock. Vasopressor agents are indicated early in the course of septic shock, where the myocardial dysfunction is an early phenomenon. These drugs have their maximum effect only if fluids are infused in adequate quantities. For children, specific inotropic agents with rapid onset of action, and short half lives are prefered. The commonly used inotropic drugs with their doses and adverse effects are listed in Table 6.5[40, 41].

Dopamine is the most commonly used vasopressor agent in shock. As per international

	Table 6.5 Commonly used drugs for management of shock			
	Drug	**Mechanism of action**	**Dose (IV)**	**Comments**
1.	Dobutamine	$\beta_1>\beta_2>\alpha$	1-20 µg/kg/min	Increases cardiac output, vasodilation
2.	Dopamine	$D_1/D_2>\beta>\alpha$ Low dose: D_1, D_2 Moderate dose: β High Dose: $\beta+\alpha$	0.5-4.0 µg/kg/min 4-10 µg/kg/min 10-20 µg/kg/min	Increases mesenteric and renal blood flow Increases cardiac output Systemic vasoconstriction
3.	Epinephrine	$\beta_1=\beta_2>\alpha$	0.05-0.5 µg/ kg/ min 0.1 ml/kg/dose (1:10,000) IV or endotracheal	Positive inotropic and chronotropic effect Asystole and anaphylactic shock
4.	Isoproterenol (isoprenaline)	β_1, β_2	0.05-0.5 µg/kg/min	Positive inotropic and chronotropic effect, peripheral vasodilatation, reduces preload.
5.	Norepinephrine	$\beta_1>\alpha>\beta_2$	0.05-1.0 µg/kg/min	Intense alpha vasoconstrictor
6.	Amrinone	Phosphodiesterase inhibitor	1-3 mg/kg loading dose, followed by infusion @ 5-20 µg/kg/min	Direct acting inotrope
7.	Milrinone	Phosphodiesterase inhibitor	0.3-0.7 µg/kg/min	Inotrope, can cause severe hypotension
8.	Nitroprusside	Vasodilator (Arteries > veins)	0.3-7.0 µg/kg/min	Afterload reduction, can cause cyanide toxicity, and hypotension
9.	Nitroglycerine	Vasodilator (Veins > arteries)	0.5-5.0 µg/kg/min	Preload and afterload reduction, can cause hypotension, and methemoglobinemia

guidelines for management of severe sepsis and septic shock, *if a child fails to respond to aggressive fluid therapy (60 ml/kg in first 15 minutes) then dopamine infusion is started @10µg/kg/min*[31]. It stimulates α-, β- and dopaminergic sympathetic receptors. Dopamine is used to augment cardiac contractility as well as the systemic vascular resistance (especially in septic shock and shock in patients with raised intracranial pressure). *If at the end of one hour the child fails to show adequate improvement despite the fluid resuscitation and dopamine infusion@10µg/kg/min then the shock is regarded as fluid refractory and dopamine resistant. Such patients are then started on catecholamines i.e. epinephrine for cold shock and norepinephrine for warm shock (see Figure 6.3)*[31].

Dobutamine is at present closest to being pure inotropic agent and is the drug of choice for patients with low cardiac index (<2.5 L/min/m²) and elevated systemic vascular resistance despite fluid resuscitation[42]. In addition to improved myocardial contractility, dobutamine can cause peripheral and pulmonary vasodilatation and attenuate pulmonary vascular hypoxic vasoconstriction. Therefore, use of dobutamine may cause significant vasodilatation and increased intrapulmonary shunting, leading to decreased cardiac output and oxygen delivery despite enhanced myocardial contractility. Also, if fall in blood pressure and increase in myocardial oxygen demand occur concurrently, myocardial ischemia is a serious threat. Therefore, a vasopressor such as norepinephrine can be titrated with an inotrope such as dobutamine to simultaneously maintain both MAP and cardiac output.

Epinephrine is recommended for fluid refractory dopamine resistant cold shock[31]. It acts on α- and $\beta_{1,2}$ receptors, leading to a response that mimics generalized autonomic stimulation

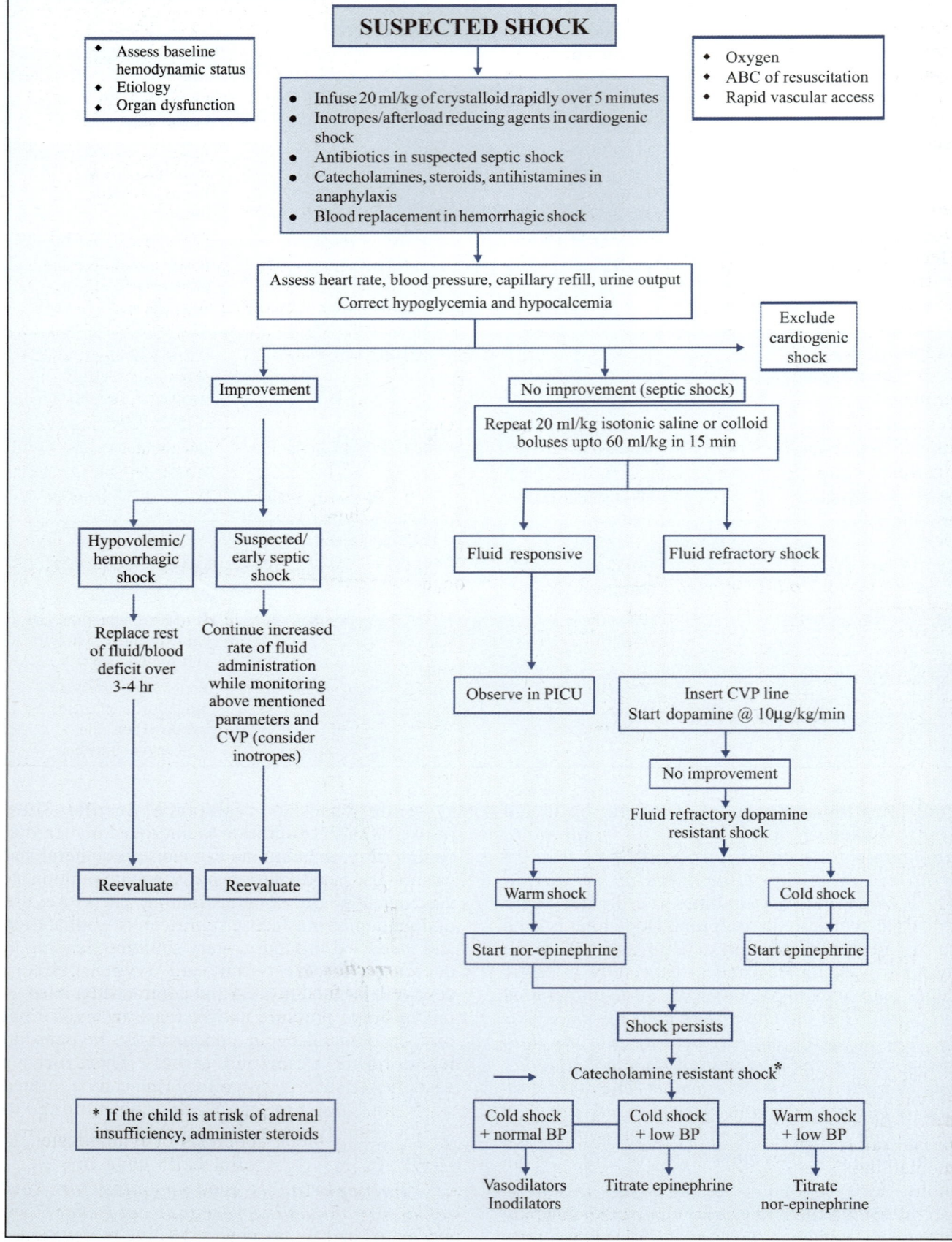

Figure 6.3 Algorithm for the management of septic shock

resulting in increased cardiac output, heart rate and blood pressure, hypermetabolic state and increased myocardial oxygen consumption. There is increase in pulmonary and systemic vascular resistance and renal ischemia is a potential complication. Ventricular tachyarrhythmias are also likely to occur.

Norepinephrine is the drug of choice for fluid refractory, dopamine resistant warm shock[31]. The potent peripheral vasoconstrictor effect of norepinephrine overshadow the positive inotropic effects. When peripheral vascular resistance is low, as in anaphylaxis and in septic shock, enhancing the peripheral vascular tone with norepinephrine may be beneficial. The combination of enhanced contractility and an increase in peripheral vascular resistance rapidly restores blood pressure and perfusion to multiple organs. The clinical use of *isoproterenol* is best reserved for situations requiring potent inotropic stimulation, especially in conjunction with pulmonary vasodilatation.

Inodilators. Amrinone and milrinone belong to the group of *inodilators (inotropes + dilators) that act by* decreasing the myocardial intracellular cAMP degradation by inhibiting phosphodiesterase type III, thus augmenting the myocardial contractility. Since their mechanism of action differs from catecholamines, they can be used in combination with the latter to achieve increase in cardiac output and a decrease in afterload. As these drugs can cause hypotension due to enhanced b_2 action they often require simultaneous institution of fluid boluses or shift from the use of epinephrine to nor-epinephrine[43, 44]. Their use has been recommended in children with normotensive low cardiac output and high vascular resistance despite epinephrine and vasodilator therapy[43-45].

Vasodilators. Reduction of afterload is useful in improving the myocardial function in cardiogenic shock after surgery, myocarditis, in later stages of septic shock with myocardial failure, and in children who require epinephrine/norepinephrine as an inotrope to reduce the α-adrenergic effect of increased vascular resistance. Therefore, vasodilators are recommended for a child with persistent low cardiac output with high systemic vascular resistance despite fluid resuscitation and ionotropic support[46]. Nitroprusside is more potent than nitroglycerine as an afterload reducing agent. Nitroglycerine is a more potent venodilator and pulmonary vasodilator than nitroprusside while nitroprusside has more potent arterial vasodilating effect[47].

Other supportive therapy. In addition to the above measures, the management of multisystem dysfunction is also very important. Renal, CNS, gastrointestinal, hepatic and hematologic abnormalities should be looked for and treated early. Antibiotics should be started within one hour of diagnosing septic shock after obtaining relevant cultures[31].

Renal support is essential to avoid renal failure in hypoperfusion states. Early volume resuscitation and use of low-dose dopamine (0.5-4.0 μg/kg/min) improve the renal blood flow and are beneficial in preventing acute renal failure[48]. Acute renal failure may require treatment with either peritoneal dialysis or hemodialysis. In addition, continuous veno-venous hemofilteration (CVVH) has shown promise in critically ill children with oliguria or anuria and fluid overload. Less fluid overload prior to institution of CVVH has been associated with improved survival in these children; therefore, CVVH should be instituted in critically sick children with anuria or severe oliguria before significant fluid overload occurs[31,49].

Support for hepatic dysfunction includes glucose infusion and replacement of coagulation factors.

Respiratory support is provided by assisted ventilation and has been discussed earlier.

Coagulation profile (including platelet count, PT, PTT) should be monitored. Use of vitamin K, fresh frozen plasma and platelet transfusion corrects most coagulopathies.

Gastrointestinal blood loss from acute gastritis or peptic ulceration can be prevented by using antacids, and H_2-receptor blockers such as ranitidine.

Correction of acid base disturbances allows better cellular function and myocardial performance by reducing systemic and pulmonary vascular resistance. A base deficit of greater than 6-10 mEq/L should be corrected in acute shock states.

Hyperglycemia, hypoglycemia, and variability in blood glucose is associated with adverse outcomes in pediatric patients with septic shock. Therefore, insulin therapy to maintain normoglycemia in pediatric patients should be considered. However, unlike adults, where a blood glucose concentration of <150 mg/dl has been recommended, optimal target blood glucose concentration in pediatric patients is not known. It is important to monitor glucose frequently during continuous insulin administration to prevent hypoglycemia[31,50].

Deep vein thrombosis prophylaxis is recommended in post-pubertal children with severe sepsis. Central venous catheter associated deep vein thrombosis occurs in approximately 25% of children with femoral central venous catheter. Therefore, heparin bonded catheters have been recommended for use in children with severe sepsis[51,52].

Other Modalities for Treatment of Septic Shock

Steroids. Current guidelines recommend that hydrocortisone therapy be reserved for use in children with catecholamine resistance and suspected or proven adrenal insufficiency[31]. Children with severe septic shock and purpura, children who have previously received steroids for chronic illness, and children with pituitary or adrenal illness are at risk for adrenal insufficiency and should be treated with stress dose steroids (hydrocortisone 50 mg/m^2/d).[31] Absolute adrenal insufficiency in the case of catecholamine-resistant septic shock is assumed at a random total cortisol concentration of <18 µg/dL; relative adrenal insufficiency is defined by a post 30- or 60- min ACTH stimulation test increase in cortisol of $\leq$ 9 µg/dL.[31] A retrospective study showed increased mortality in patients with septic shock who were administered steroids.[53] Therefore, steroids are not recommended for use in pediatric patients who do not meet minimal criteria for adrenal insufficiency.

Hormonal therapy. Thyroid hormone deficiency may be present especially in cardiac patients and cause refractory shock. Oral levothyronine or intravenous liothyronine are used if thyroid deficiency is identified[23].

Vasopressin has been found to be a useful adjunct in children with catecholamine refractory septic shock and low peripheral vascular resistance. However, there are no clinical trials to recommend its use in children with sepsis[54,55].

Recombinant human activated protein C (rhAPC). It is recommended that adult patients with sepsis-induced organ dysfunction associated with a clinical assessment of high risk of death as determined by Acute Physiology and Chronic Health Evaluation [APACHE] II $\geq$ 25 or multi-organ dysfunction receive rhAPC. However, in pediatric patients, due to lack of proof of benefit, rhAPC is currently not recommended[31].

Immunotherapy. The use of inhibiting toxic mediators such as antibodies against endotoxin, TNF and IL-1, and specific immunoglobulins has not been documented to be beneficial[56,57]. Intravenous immunoglobulin may be helpful in specific circumstances such as immunodeficiency states. In addition, polyclonal intravenous immunoglobulin has been shown to reduce sepsis and septic shock related mortality in neonates[58]. Granulocyte macrophage colony stimulating factors or white cell transfusions have been found to be useful in children with septic shock with accompanying neutropenia secondary to chemotherapy and in primary white blood cell related immunodeficiencies. Granulocyte macrophage colony stimulating factor given for a period of 7 days was found to be beneficial in a randomized controlled trial in neonates with absolute neutrophil count of < 1500/µl[59].

Nitric oxide synthase inhibitors have not been found to be useful. Some researchers have suggested specific therapeutic goals in children with septic shock[23, 60, 61]. It is important to recognize shock and initiate therapy early in the course of illness. An aggressive multimodal approach consisting of a combination of therapies should be practiced.

Extracorporeal membrane oxygenation (ECMO) is recommended in refractory pediatric septic shock and/or respiratory failure that does not respond to conventional therapies[31]. On long term follow-up, children with sepsis on ECMO have outcomes comparable to children without sepsis[62, 63].

Guiding principles for therapy of cardiogenic shock

Cardiogenic shock is characterized by low perfusion due to myocardial pump failure in the presence of adequate preload. The goal of therapy of cardiogenic shock is to improve tissue perfusion and ensure adequate delivery of oxygen to the tissues. Vasodilators such as nitroglycerine, nitroprusside or nesiritide are beneficial in children with cardiogenic shock and high pulmonary capillary wedge pressure, low cardiac index, and adequate mean arterial pressure whereas children with cardiogenic shock and high pulmonary capillary wedge pressure, low cardiac index, and low mean arterial pressure derive benefit from ionotropic drugs[64].

PROGNOSIS

Aggressive management of shock especially hypovolemic, can be quite rewarding. However, septic shock still has a case fatality rate of more than 50 percent. Adverse outcome is anticipated in following situations:

(i) Multiple organ failure

(ii) Major myocardial damage

(iii) Coagulopathy and DIC

(iv) Renal failure

(v) Repiratory failure

(vi) Uncontrolled sepsis

(vii) Ongoing blood loss.

REFERENCES

1. Perkin RM, Levin DL. Shock in the pediatric patient. Part I. *J Pediatr* 1982; 101:163-169.

2. Witte MK, Hill JH, Blumer JL. Shock in the pediatric patient. *Adv Pediatr* 1987; 34:139-173.

3. Balk RA, Bone RC. The septic syndrome. Definition and clinical implications. *Crit Care Clin* 1989; 5:1-8.

4. Deitch EA, Bridges W, Baker J, *et al*. Hemorrhagic shock-induced bacterial translocation is reduced by xanthine oxidase inhibition or inactivation. *Surgery* 1988; 104:191-198.

5. Deitch EA, Taylor M, Grisham M, Ma L, Bridges W, Berg R. Endotoxin induces bacterial translocation and increases xanthine oxidase activity. *J Trauma* 1989; 29:1679-1683.

6. Haupt MT. Anaphylaxis and anaphylactic shock. In: Current Therapy in Critical Care Medicine. Parrillo JE (Ed.) 2nd ed. *Philadelphia: BC Decker*; 1991.

7. Carcillo JA, Cunnion RE. Septic shock. *Crit Care Clin* 1997; 13:553-574.

8. Parrillo JE. Pathogenetic mechanisms of septic shock. *N Engl J Med* 1993; 328:1471-1477.

9. Westphal O, Jann K, Himmelspach K. Chemistry and immunochemistry of bacterial lipopolysaccharides as cell wall antigens and endotoxins. *Prog Allergy* 1983; 33:9-39.

10. Abe R, Oda S, Sadahiro T, *et al*. Gram-negative bacteremia induces greater magnitude of inflammatory response than Gram-positive bacteremia. *Crit Care* 2010; 14:R27.

11. Natanson C, Hoffman WD, Suffredini AF, Eichacker PQ, Danner RL. Selected treatment strategies for septic shock based on proposed mechanisms of pathogenesis. *Ann Intern Med* 1994; 120:771-783.

12. Cannon JG, Tompkins RG, Gelfand JA, *et al*. Circulating interleukin-1 and tumor necrosis factor in septic shock and experimental endotoxin fever. *J Infect Dis* 1990; 161:79-84.

13. Hesse DG, Tracey KJ, Fong Y, *et al*. Cytokine appearance in human endotoxemia and primate bacteremia. *Surg Gynecol Obstet* 1988; 166:147-153.

14. Dinarello CA. The proinflammatory cytokines interleukin-1 and tumor necrosis factor and treatment of the septic shock syndrome. *J Infect Dis* 1991; 163:1177-1184.

15. Sorensen J, Kald B, Tagesson C, Lindahl M. Platelet-activating factor and phospholipase A2 in patients with septic shock and trauma. *Intensive Care Med* 1994; 20:555-561.

16. Bond RF. Peripheral vascular adrenergic depression during hypotension induced by *E coli* endotoxin. *Adv Shock Res* 1983; 9:157-169.

17. Parker JL, Adams HR. Development of myocardial dysfunction in endotoxin shock. *Am J Physiol 1985*; 248:H818-H826.

18. Beller FK. Sepsis and coagulation. *Clin Obstet Gynecol* 1985; 28:46-52.

19. Fearon DT, Ruddy S, Schur PH, McCabe WR. Activation of the properdin pathway of complement in patients with Gram-negative bacteremia. *N Engl J Med* 1975; 292:937-940.

20. Feuerstein G, Siren AL. Platelet-activating factor and shock. *Prog Biochem Pharmacol* 1988; 22:181-190.

21. Fletcher JR, Ramwell PW. Prostaglandins in shock: to give or to block? *Adv Shock Res* 1980; 3:57-66.

22. Weiss SJ. Tissue destruction by neutrophils. *N Engl J Med* 1989; 320:365-376.

23. Carcillo JA, Fields AI. Clinical practice parameters for hemodynamic support of pediatric and neonatal patients in septic shock. *Crit Care Med* 2002; 30:1365-1378.

24. Wetzel RC, Rogers MC. Pediatric monitoring. In: Textbook of Critical Care. Shoemaker WC, Ayers S, Greuvik A, Holbrook PR, Thompson WL (Eds). *Philadelphia: WB Saunders*; 2011.

25. Saavedra JM, Harris GD, Li S, Finberg L. Capillary refilling (skin turgor) in the assessment of dehydration. *Am J Dis Child* 1991; 145:296-298.

26. Vega RM, Avner JR. A prospective study of the usefulness of clinical and laboratory parameters for predicting percentage of dehydration in children. *Pediatr Emerg Care* 1997; 13:179-182.

27. Aynsley-Green A, Pickering D. Proceedings: Use of central and peripheral temperature measurements in care of critically ill children. *Arch Dis Child* 1974; 49: 242-250.

28. Bergman KS, Harris BH. Arteriovenous pH difference: a new index of perfusion. *J Pediatr Surg* 1988; 23:1190-1192.

29. Sibbald WJ, Calvin J, Driedjer AA. Right and Left ventricular preload and diastolic ventricular compliance: Implications for therapy in critically ill patients. In: Critical Care: Sate of the Art. Shoemaker WC, Thompson WL (Eds). *Fulleston, California: Society of Critical Care Medicine*; 3rd edition, 1982.

30. Civetta JM, Gabel JC, Laver MB. Disparate ventricular function in surgical patients. *Surg Forum* 1971; 22: 136-139.

31. Dellinger RP, Levy MM, Carlet JM, *et al.* Surviving sepsis campaign: international guidelines for management of severe sepsis and septic shock. *Crit Care Med* 2008; 36:296-327.

32. Textbook of Pediatric Advanced Life Support. *American Heart Association;* 2007.

33. Rivers E, Nguyen B, Havstad S, *et al.* Early goal-directed therapy in the treatment of severe sepsis and septic shock. *N Engl J Med* 2001; 345:1368-1377.

34. Carcillo JA, Davis AL, Zaritsky A. Role of early fluid resuscitation in pediatric septic shock. *JAMA* 1991; 266:1242-1245.

35. Tobias JD. Shock in children: the first 60 minutes. *Pediatr Ann* 1996; 25:330-338.

36. Finfer S, Bellomo R, Boyce N, French J, Myburgh J, Norton R. A comparison of albumin and saline for fluid resuscitation in the intensive care unit. *N Engl J Med* 2004; 350:2247-2256.

37. Ngo NT, Cao XT, Kneen R, *et al.* Acute management of dengue shock syndrome: a randomized double-blind comparison of 4 intravenous fluid regimens in the first hour. *Clin Infect Dis* 2001; 32:204-213.

38. Wills BA, Nguyen MD, Ha TL, *et al.* Comparison of three fluid solutions for resuscitation in dengue shock syndrome. *N Engl J Med* 2005; 353:877-889.

39. Dung NM, Day NP, Tam DT, *et al.* Fluid replacement in dengue shock syndrome: a randomized, double-blind comparison of four intravenous-fluid regimens. *Clin Infect Dis* 1999; 29:787-794.

40. Driscoll DJ, Gillette PC, McNamara DG. The use of dopamine in children. *J Pediatr* 1978; 92:309-314.

41. Perkin RM, Levin DL, Webb R, Aquino A, Reedy J. Dobutamine: a hemodynamic evaluation in children with shock. *J Pediatr* 1982; 100:977-983.

42. Jewitt D, Birkhead J, Mitchell A, Dollery C. Clinical cardiovascular pharmacology of dobutamine. A selective inotropic catecholamine. *Lancet* 1974; 2:363-367.

43. Irazuzta JE, Pretzlaff RK, Rowin ME. Amrinone in pediatric refractory septic shock: An open-label pharmacodynamic study. *Pediatr Crit Care Med* 2001; 2:24-28.

44. Lindsay CA, Barton P, Lawless S, *et al.* Pharmacokinetics and pharmacodynamics of milrinone lactate in pediatric patients with septic shock. *J Pediatr* 1998; 132:329-334.

45. Barton P, Garcia J, Kouatli A, *et al.* Hemodynamic effects of intravenous milrinone lactate in pediatric patients with septic shock. A prospective, double-blinded, randomized, placebo-controlled, interventional study. *Chest* 1996; 109:1302-1312.

46. Keeley SR, Bohn DJ. The use of inotropic and afterload-reducing agents in neonates. *Clin Perinatol* 1988; 15: 467-489.

47. Ceneviva G, Paschall JA, Maffei F, Carcillo JA. Hemodynamic support in fluid-refractory pediatric septic shock. *Pediatrics* 1998; 102:e19.

48. Parker S, Carlon GC, Isaacs M, Howland WS, Kahn RC. Dopamine administration in oliguria and oliguric renal failure. *Crit Care Med* 1981; 9:630-632.

49. Foland JA, Fortenberry JD, Warshaw BL, *et al.* Fluid overload before continuous hemofiltration and survival in critically ill children: a retrospective analysis. *Crit Care Med* 2004; 32:1771-1776.

50. Faustino EV, Apkon M. Persistent hyperglycemia in critically ill children. *J Pediatr* 2005; 146:30-34.

51. Pierce CM, Wade A, Mok Q. Heparin-bonded central venous lines reduce thrombotic and infective complications in critically ill children. *Intensive Care Med* 2000; 26:967-972.

52. Krafte-Jacobs B, Sivit CJ, Mejia R, Pollack MM. Catheter-related thrombosis in critically ill children: comparison of catheters with and without heparin bonding. *J Pediatr* 1995; 126:50-54.

53. Markovitz BP, Goodman DM, Watson RS, Bertoch D, Zimmerman J. A retrospective cohort study of prognostic factors associated with outcome in pediatric severe sepsis: what is the role of steroids? *Pediatr Crit Care Med* 2005; 6:270-274.

54. Powell KR, Sugarman LI, Eskenazi AE, *et al.* Normalization of plasma arginine vasopressin concentrations when children with meningitis are given maintenance plus replacement fluid therapy. *J Pediatr* 1990; 117:515-522.

55. Masutani S, Senzaki H, Ishido H, *et al.* Vasopressin in the treatment of vasodilatory shock in children. *Pediatr Int* 2005; 47:132-136.

56. Bone RC, Balk RA, Fein AM, *et al.* A second large controlled clinical study of E5, a monoclonal antibody to endotoxin: results of a prospective, multicenter, randomized, controlled trial. The E5 Sepsis Study Group. *Crit Care Med* 1995; 23:994-1006.

57. Cohen J, Carlet J. INTERSEPT: an international, multicenter, placebo-controlled trial of monoclonal antibody to human tumor necrosis factor-alpha in patients with sepsis. International Sepsis Trial Study Group. *Crit Care Med* 1996; 24:1431-1440.

58. El-Nawawy A, El-Kinany H, Hamdy El-Sayed M, Boshra N. Intravenous polyclonal immunoglobulin administration to sepsis syndrome patients: a prospective study in a pediatric intensive care unit. *J Trop Pediatr* 2005; 51:271-278.

59. Bilgin K, Yaramis A, Haspolat K, Tas MA, Gunbey S, Derman O. A randomized trial of granulocyte-macrophage colony-stimulating factor in neonates with sepsis and neutropenia. *Pediatrics* 2001; 107:36-41.

60. Pollack MM, Fields AI, Ruttimann UE. Sequential cardiopulmonary variables of infants and children in septic shock. *Crit Care Med* 1984; 12:554-559.

61. Pollack MM, Fields AI, Ruttimann UE. Distributions of cardiopulmonary variables in pediatric survivors and nonsurvivors of septic shock. *Crit Care Med* 1985; 13:454-459.

62. Goldman AP, Kerr SJ, Butt W, *et al*. Extracorporeal support for intractable cardiorespiratory failure due to meningococcal disease. *Lancet* 1997; 349:466-469.

63. Meyer DM, Jessen ME. Results of extracorporeal membrane oxygenation in children with sepsis. The Extracorporeal Life Support Organization. *Ann Thorac Surg* 1997; 63:756-761.

64. den Uil CA, Lagrand WK, Valk SD, Spronk PE, Simoons ML. Management of cardiogenic shock: focus on tissue perfusion. *Curr Probl Cardiol* 2009; 34: 330-349.

The Child with Multiple Organ Dysfunction Syndrome

Sujatha Kannan and Ashok P Sarnaik

Inflammation is an essential biologic phenomenon which is necessary for survival. However, an uncontrolled systemic inflammatory response can potentially result in severe pathophysiologic derangements in organs far removed from the initial site of injury. Although bacterial sepsis is the most common predisposing illness, other infectious agents, mechanical and thermal trauma, pancreatitis, organ dysfunction or rejection following solid organ transplantation, and tissue hypoxia are also capable of producing such a widespread systemic inflammatory response. Multiple organ dysfunction syndrome (MODS) is a manifestation of the host's evolving endogenously activated immunoinflammatory cytotoxic response. MODS is characterized by acute but potentially reversible physiologic dysfunction of at least two separate organ systems.

The term MODS is used to emphasize that the syndrome is a continuum of physiologic dysfunction and it represents a process that has common, underlying pathophysiologic mechanisms. For consistent application of terminology associated with MODS, standard definitions for sepsis and organ failure have been developed with international consensus[1,2]. Criteria for sepsis, systemic inflammatory response syndrome (SIRS) and MODS have been adapted to children at the international pediatric sepsis consensus conference in 2002[1,3]. Figure 7.1 summarizes the mechanism of systemic inflammatory response syndrome (SIRS) and pathogenesis of dysfunction of various body organs following severe infection.

PATHOGENESIS

Although diverse in etiology, illnesses leading to multiple organ failure have a common thread i.e. the activation of the inflammatory response. Over the past few years there has been an increasing understanding of the molecular signaling events leading to development of sepsis and MODS. The normal host response to infection is a series of complex immunologic processes which can be broadly classified into following stages mediated by the innate immune system: (a) recognition of pathogen, (b) activation of the inflammatory cascade, and (c) maintaining a balance between pro- and anti-inflammatory mediators. Dysregulation of the orderly immune response is the basis of development of MODS[4].

Recognition of pathogen. Neutrophils, macrophages and natural killer cells recognize foreign molecules such as peptidoglycans in the bacterial cell wall, the protein flagellin in the flagella of bacteria and specific motifs in the chromatin of bacterial DNA. These pathogen-associated molecular patterns are recognized by highly conserved pattern recognition receptors such as CD14 and transmembrane toll like receptors (TLRs) on the host cells. CD14 is a membrane bound receptor expressed by monocytes and neutrophils. One of the materials recognized by CD14 is lipopolysaccharide (LPS) from Gram-negative bacteria. A lipid shuttle molecule termed LPS binding protein (LBP) binds LPS and delivers it to CD14. LPS bound to CD14 forms a quaternary complex after further binding to an extracellular protein (MD2) and TLR4. The LPS-CD14-MD2-TLR4 complex is required to activate host cells exposed to LPS. In the absence of any of these elements, activation of inflammation is ineffective. The transmembrane TLRs are responsible for intracellular transmission of the signal. There are 10 recognized TLRs in the human genome that act as specific receptors for various microbial ligands. The Gram-positive bacterial components peptidoglycans and lipopeptides are recognized by TLR2, TLR6 and TLR1. Gram-negative bacterial LPS are specifically recognized by TLR4. Various TLRs also have specific functions. TLR5 binds directly with flagellin, TLR9 binds with specific chromatin motifs in bacterial DNA, TLR2 binds with mycobacterial cell wall components, TLR6 binds with fungal constituents, and TLR3 binds with

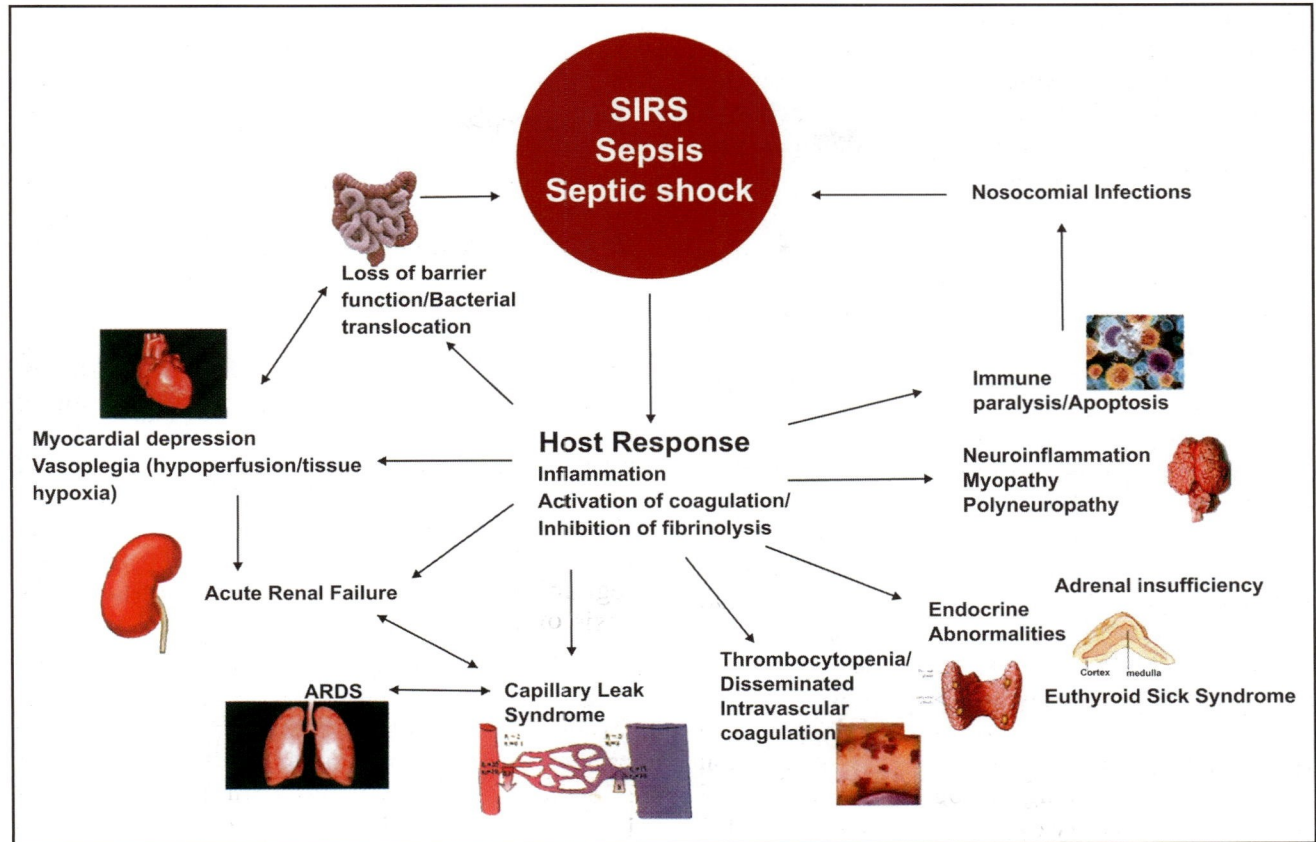

Figure 7.1 Mechanism of systemic inflammatory response syndrome (SIRS) and pathogenesis of dysfunction of various organs following severe infection

double stranded viral RNA. Once the ligand binds the TLR, a series of intracellular signaling events involving tyrosine kinases and mitogen activated protein kinases occur, which leads to activation of transcriptional activators such as NF-kB and activator protein-1 causing the production of pro- and anti-inflammatory cytokines[4, 5]. Several TLR4 and CD14 polymorphisms have been described that increase susceptibility to sepsis and MODS. Genetics thus has significant basis for explanation of the considerable variation in individual response to infection. Although TLRs have been shown to be crucial for an appropriate host defense during infection, studies have shown that deficiency or blockade of TLRs is associated with an enhanced survival rate in sepsis[6, 7]. However, further studies in the clinical setting will be required to develop appropriate therapeutic interventions based on these observations.

Activation of inflammatory cascade. After the initial interaction with the pathogen, the host cells propagate the inflammatory response. PMNs, macrophages, capillary endothelium and epithelial cells release cytokines, chemokines and lipid mediators that attract additional leukocytes. These host leukocytes produce reactive oxygen intermediates, proteolytic enzymes and cationic peptides, which destroy the invading pathogen. One of the cationic peptides, is the bacterial permeability increasing protein (BPI), is a potent antiendotoxin protein with a high affinity to bind Gram-negative bacteria and can also neutralize the biological activity of LPS[4, 5]. Recombinant BPI is currently being evaluated in clinical trials.

Balance between pro-inflammatory and anti-inflammatory responses. The pro-inflammatory mediators include TNF-α, interleukin (IL) 1β, IL-6, IL-8 and eicosanoids. TNF-α and IL-1β have specific receptors on macrophages. They induce vascular monocytes and endothelial cells to express tissue factor that initiates the coagulation cascade. TNF-α causes down-regulation of thrombomodulin and impairs the activation of Protein C resulting in a pro-thrombotic state. TNF-α and IL-1β lead to up regulation of endothelial adhesion molecules E-selectin and P-selectin that help attach activated neutrophils to the endothelial cells. These activated neutrophils release proteases and other pro-inflammatory products mediating vascular injury. IL-8 recruits activated neutrophils to the site of injury. This vascular injury along with the formation of microthrombi leads to tissue ischemia, impaired tissue oxygenation and eventually MODS. Capillary endothelium plays a key role, both as a target and a perpetrator, in sepsis-related acute organ dysfunction.

The anti-inflammatory mediators reduce or terminate the production of pro-inflammatory mediators or protect against their harmful effects. These include disease specific anti-inflammatory mediators such as keratinocyte growth factor in acute lung injury, and nonspecific cytokines such as IL-4, IL-10, IL-6, interferons, heat shock protein, and anticoagulants such as protein C and antithrombin III. The primary role of IL-10 is to counterbalance TNFα and IL-1. IL-10 also inhibits nuclear factor NF-kB which is a promoter of inflammation[5, 8, 9]. Recently, IL-33 has been shown to have beneficial effects on a mouse model of sepsis by decreasing the systemic but not the local pro-inflammatory response[10].

Septic shock and development of MODS. Imbalance between pro-inflammatory and counter-inflammatory response is the basis for circulatory dysfunction and organ damage. Excessive increase in capillary permeability, sludging of platelets, intravascular coagulation, and abnormal vasoregulation are hallmarks of MODS. Dysregulation of the immune system results in extensive inflammatory damage to the capillary endothelium (e.g. intravascular coagulation), epithelial cells (e.g. lungs, kidneys, gut), and parenchymal cells (e.g. cardiac myocytes, hepatocytes) leading to multi organ dysfunction.

Perpetuation of MODS is characterized by 3 major developments; shift from an inflammatory to anti-inflammatory state, a state of anergy, and death of immune cells. Each of these have a profound influence on outcome from MODS. Excessive activity of Th-2 (anti-inflammatory) lymphocytes and their cytokines (IL-4 and IL-10) are associated with increased mortality whereas reversal to Th-1 activation is associated with survival. A state of anergy developing because of apoptotic cell death of large number of lymphocytes is also associated with mortality. Apoptosis induced loss of CD4 T cells, B cells and dendritic cells results in immune suppression and increased vulnerability to fungal and bacterial infections characteristic of MODS lasting for several days to weeks. Genetic factors such as polymorphisms in TNF receptors, IL-1 receptors, Fcg receptors, TLRs and cytokines genes are associated with increased susceptibility to infections and death[11, 12].

The microcirculation and ischemia/reperfusion hypothesis proposes that organ injury is secondary to ischemia and/or endothelial injury. It is suggested that organ failure is the result of a primary injury followed by a subsequent event of ischemia or ischemia/reperfusion, also called the "two hit model"[13]. Excessive inflammation and leukocyte activation leads to formation of microthrombi, microvascular occlusion, ischemia, and organ failure. Reperfusion is associated with the generation of oxygen radicals by either the xanthine oxidase pathway or by activated neutrophils. Oxygen radicals can cause tissue injury resulting in MODS. In addition, ischemia may lead to stress gene expressions, which are programmed cellular responses to environmental stress. Timing of the second insult in relation to the stress response is extremely important.

In the gut-origin hypothesis, the gut is described as the "motor of multiple organ failure"[13]. Loss of gut barrier function and bacterial migration across the epithelium have been shown in animal models and patients with insults such as shock, burns, trauma, and malnutrition. This phenomenon of bacterial translocation may predispose the patient to MODS. Disruption of commensal gut flora with decrease in fewer total obligate anerobes and beneficial bacteria has been noted in patients with severe SIRS and are associated with increased mortality and complications in sepsis[14]. However, it is difficult to separate the effect of bacterial translocation and the response of the gut to the initial insult which results in impaired microcirculation. In both cases, the gut will respond by inflammatory mediator production.

Mitochondrial dysfunction in sepsis and MODS. A central paradigm in multi-organ dysfunction in sepsis appears to be the concept of tissue hypoxia which is related to impaired oxygen utilization at the cellular level. Ultrastructural damage to mitochondria and inhibition of mitochondrial respiration with impaired oxidative phosphorylation and depletion of ATP have been observed in animal models and in the clinical setting, and is associated with poor outcomes in patients with sepsis and MODS[15-17]. Mitochondrial dysfunction may represent a key early cellular event in the development of organ failure. This dysfunction involves (i) impairment of the electron transport system and (ii) marked increase in the production of reactive oxygen species (ROS) with decrease in mitochondrial anti-oxidant capability leading to intracellular oxidative injury. Mitochondrial dysfunction is evident as damage to the inner mitochondrial membrane and organelle swelling which is associated with collapse of the mitochondrial membrane potential resulting in a state called mitochondrial permeability transition (MPT). Opening of specific high conductance channels within the inner mitochondrial membrane is felt to be the key event mediating MPT and is characterized by matrix swelling, uncoupling of oxidative phosphorylation, Ca^{2+} efflux and cytochrome release, triggering apoptotic cell death pathways[18]. This may partly explain the significant discordance noted between histologic findings and extent of organ dysfunction in sepsis. Histologic findings in patients with sepsis and renal failure shows only focal injury with preservation of normal glomeruli and renal tubules and patients who survive often sepsis regain normal baseline renal function[19]. This may suggest that much of the organ dysfunction in sepsis may be explained by "cell hibernating" or "cell stunning". This may be due to decreased oxygen consumption secondary to the depletion of NAD by the enzyme ADP-ribose polymerase that gets activated by oxidants produced during sepsis[11, 19]. These findings are also consistent with the potential for complete functional recovery of organs in patients surviving MODS.

CLINICAL ASPECTS

MODS develops over a period of time after an initial illness resulting in an uncontrolled systemic inflammatory response. The multisystem involvement represents sequential target organ injury resulting from the host's systemic inflammatory response. The clinical manifestations and management are, therefore, to be considered as this process evolves over time.

Circulatory failure

The most common characteristic of the initial illness which incites the inflammatory response resulting in multiorgan dysfunction, is an inadequate blood flow to the tissues to meet their metabolic requirements. This state of shock often has multiple components. Hypovolemia from inadequate fluid intake and increased losses, excessive capillary permeability, metabolic derangements, and poor myocardial contractility often coexist at the time of initial illness. In a previously healthy child, acute overwhelming bacterial or viral infection, trauma and pulmonary aspiration are the commonest precursors of MODS in children. Previously immunocompromised children from chronic debilitating illnesses and malnutrition are especially vulnerable to development of MODS. The incidence of MODS was found to be two-fold greater among children with a co-morbid condition and independently increased the risk of death by 60%[20]. Moreover, the risk of MODS is greater in neonates as compared to older children with higher mortality in this group[21, 22].

The child who is predisposed to MODS often presents with signs and symptoms of decreased cardiac output during the initial phase. Myocardial dysfunction is common in patients with septic shock. TNF-α and IL-1 have been shown to cause decreased cardiac contractility. Also, abnormalities of microcirculation can result in myocardial ischemia. It has been noted that in children with meningococcal septic shock, serum levels of cardiac troponin I inversely correlated with left ventricular ejection fraction. There is also a significant down-regulation of β_1 receptors, uncoupling of the receptors from adenylate cyclase, and decreased generation of cAMP. Typically in adults, vasodilation leading to "warm shock" and hypotension is more common. Myocardial depression is compensated by an increase in heart rate and decrease in SVR, thus maintaining or even increasing the cardiac output. However, in children compensation by increasing SVR resulting in vasoconstriction and "cold shock" is more common. This further worsens cardiac output leading to circulatory failure much sooner in children. Tachycardia, tachypnea, abnormalities of thermoregulation and poor capillary refill are commonly encountered. It is important to recognize that early in the course, the blood pressure may be relatively well maintained by vasoconstriction. Thus, a normal blood pressure does not exclude significantly compromised cardiac output. Cool, vasoconstricted peripheries with prolonged capillary refill time and tachycardia should alert the physician to shock regardless of the blood pressure values. Hypotension is often a late sign in the pediatric age group. Right ventricular decompensation because of increased afterload from pulmonary hypertension is also an important factor in neonates and children[23].

Although hypovolemia is an extremely important component of the clinical state, and aggressive fluid resuscitation initially is crucial, that alone is often insufficient to improve tissue perfusion in a sustained fashion. This is because of excessive capillary permeability resulting in continued loss of fluid into the interstitial space and decreased myocardial contractility. Most patients improve rapidly after appropriate antimicrobial therapy and supportive care. In patients who develop MODS, after a brief period of stabilization lasting from 1-6 hours, sequential organ involvement of varying degrees starts to manifest. The criteria for the diagnosis of dysfunction of various organs are summarized in Table 7.1.

Table 7.1 Criteria for the diagnosis of dysfunction of various organs
Cardiovascular Dysfunction
Despite administration of isotonic IV fluid bolus >40 ml/kg in 1 hour:
Decrease in BP <5th percentile for age or systolic BP < 2SD below normal for age OR
Need for vasoactive drugs to maintain BP in the normal range OR
Two of the following criteria: Unexplained metabolic acidosis; increased arterial lactate, oliguria, prolonged capillary refill; core to peripheral temperature gap > 3°C
Respiratory Dysfunction
PaO_2/FiO_2 <300 in the absence of cyanotic heart disease or preexisting lung disease OR
$PaCO_2$ >65 mmHg or 20 mmHg over baseline OR
>50% FiO_2 to maintain SpO_2 ≥92% OR
Need for mechanical ventilation
Neurologic Dysfunction
Glasgow coma scale ≤11 OR
Acute change in mental status with decrease in GCS ≥3 points from abnormal baseline
Hematologic Dysfunction
Platelet count <80,000/mm³ or 50% decrease in platelet count from baseline OR
International normalized ratio >2
Renal Dysfunction
Serum creatinine > 2 times upper limit of normal for age or 2 fold increase over baseline
Hepatic Dysfunction
Total bilirubin >4mg/dl OR ALT >2 times upper limit of normal for age

Acute respiratory distress syndrome (ARDS)

The lung is one of the most common and the earliest organ involved in the development of multiorgan dysfunction as a result of uncontrolled systemic inflammatory response. In fact, as the management of ARDS has improved in the last two decades to keep the patient alive longer, serious dysfunction of other organ systems has been increasingly encountered. The vulnerability of the lung to edema formation in response to a variety of local and systemic injuries has been known for over a century. Ashbaugh et al[24] described respiratory distress and hypoxemia occurring 1 to 96 hours after the original illness of such diversity as trauma, pancreatitis, drug ingestion, viral pneumonia and aspiration. Regardless of the presenting illness, the clinical pattern of respiratory involvement was remarkably stereotypical in their patients. Severe tachypnea, marked PiO_2-PaO_2 gradient and arterial oxygen desaturation were consistently observed. Postmortem pulmonary findings were also stereotypical. There was hepatization, hyperemia, diffuse atelectasis, and formation of hyaline membranes. Ashbaugh et al stressed the similarities between their patients and neonatal respiratory distress syndrome (hyaline membrane disease)[24]. The term adult respiratory distress syndrome was thus coined to describe patients with diffuse alveolar-capillary damage occurring in a diverse group of disorders. Since such an illness can occur at any age, the word "acute" has replaced "adult".

Subtle clinical changes often precede the development of florid manifestations of ARDS. In the early stage, the chest auscultation and radiographic findings may be normal. Tachypnea is the earliest sign of ARDS, and it is soon followed by chest wall retractions and grunting. Pulse oximetry monitoring or blood gas analysis show evidence of arterial desaturation and increasing alveolar-arterial oxygen gradient. A normal or elevated pH with hypocarbia is typically observed at this time. Subtle changes on chest radiographs include decreased lung volume which may represent microatelectasis or the appearance of streaky infiltrates indicating an increase in lung extravascular water content. In patients with advancing ARDS, hypoxemia is persistent in spite of increase in FiO_2, endotracheal intubation and assisted ventilation. Frothy serosanguinous fluid pouring through the nose, mouth or the endotracheal tube signifies severely increased pulmonary capillary permeability and non-cardiogenic pulmonary edema. Central venous pressure is either low or normal. Chest radiographs at this time show diffuse, bilateral alveolar and interstitial infiltrates with a normal cardiac silhouette. Hypoxemia worsens and hypercapnia develops, both of which may be unresponsive to increasing ventilatory support. Metabolic acidosis with elevated serum lactate may be encountered at any stage of illness signifying decreased oxygen delivery and impaired oxygen utilization.

Hematologic and coagulation abnormalities

The coagulation system and the inflammatory response are highly integrated and work together as a defense mechanism to limit the local inflammation and promote host tissue repair. The coagulation system in sepsis is driven by the tissue factor pathway. Infectious agents and inflammatory cytokines such as TNF-α and IL-1β activate the release of tissue factor from monocytes and endothelium leading to the formation of thrombin and a fibrin clot (Figure 7.2). Inflammatory cytokines and thrombin stimulate the release of plasminogen activator inhibitor (PAI-1) which inhibits tissue plasminogen activator (tPA) preventing endogenous fibrinolysis. Thrombin also activates thrombin activatable fibrinolysis inhibitor

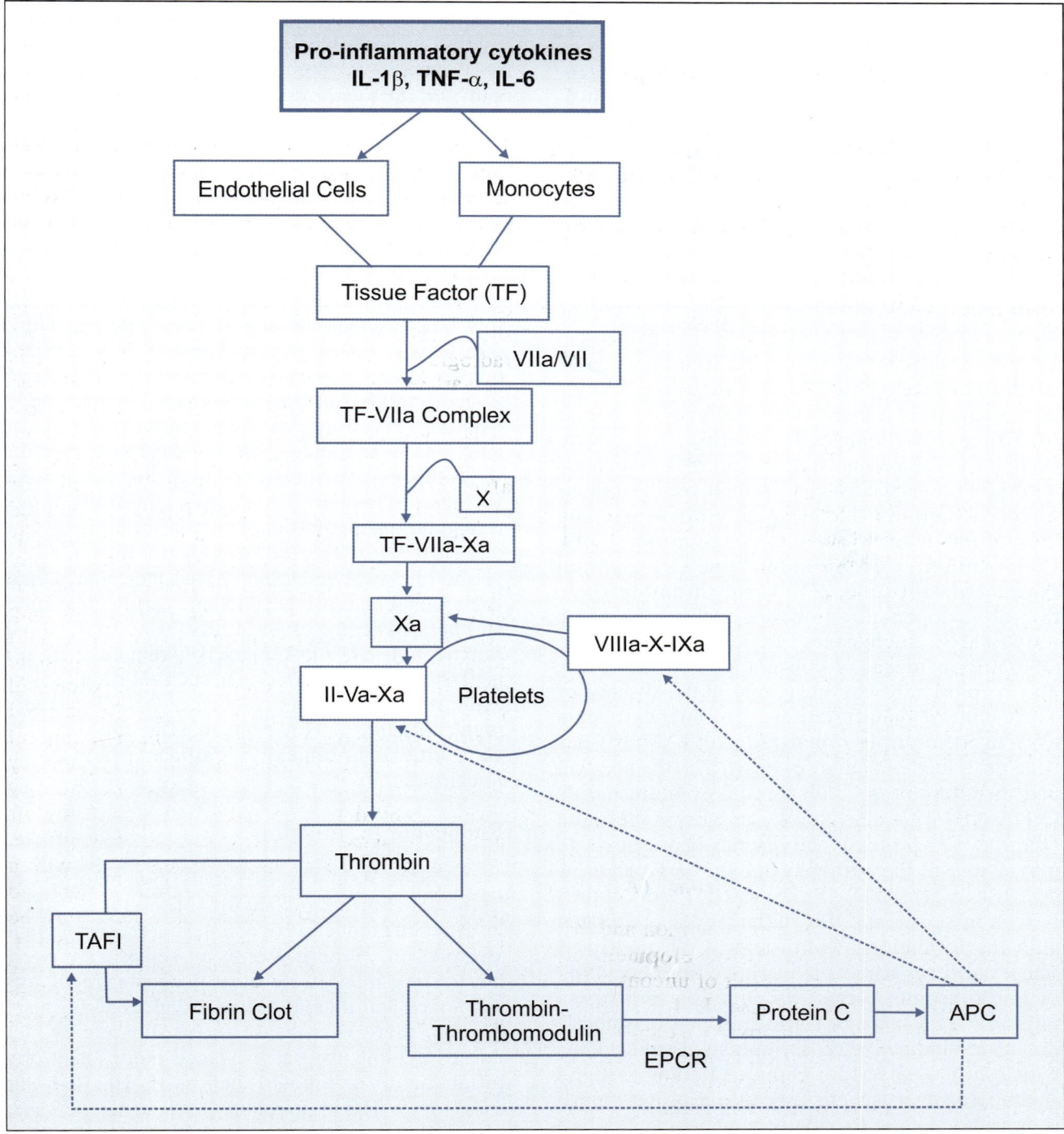

Figure 7.2 The pro-inflammatory cytokines stimulate the release of tissue factor from endothelial cells and monocytes. Tissue factor activates Factor VII to form the TF-VIIa-Xa complex. The activated factor X combines with Va on activated platelets and converts prothrombin to thrombin. Thrombin by a positive feedback loop activates VIII which binds IXa leading to more generation of Xa and further thrombin formation. Thrombin also binds thrombomodulin on the surface of endothelial cells. The thrombin-thrombomodulin complex and endothelial protein C receptor are required for conversion of protein C to activated protein C (APC) that exerts its anti-coagulant effect by degradation of Va and VIIIa and by inhibition of thrombin activatable fibrinolysis inhibitor (TAFI).

(TAFI) that further inhibits endogenous fibrinolysis. Inflammatory cytokines downregulate thrombomodulin and the endothelial Protein C receptor leading to decreased production of activated Protein C (APC). This leads to diffuse endovascular injury, microvascular thrombosis, organ ischemia and MODS[11, 12, 25]. APC can counter these effects by its anti-inflammatory, anti-thrombotic and fibrinolytic actions. The anti-inflammatory effects of APC are due to inhibition of TNF-α production by monocytes, and downregulation of the endothelial expression of E-selectin causing vascular injury. APC accelerates degradation of factors VIIIa and Va limiting the production of thrombin, preventing the activation of TAFI and thus exerting an anti-thrombotic effect. APC also inhibits plasminogen-activator inhibitor type 1 and helps restore normal fibrinolysis[26, 27].

A significant number of children who are destined to develop MODS often show hematologic and coagulation abnormalities early in the course of illness. Widespread petechiae, purpura, ecchymoses and hemorrhagic diatheses associated with poor tissue perfusion are telltale manifestations of overwhelming bacterial or viral sepsis and disseminated intravascular coagulation (DIC). Prolongation of prothrombin time (PT), partial thromboplastin time (PTT) and thrombin time, thrombocytopenia and decreased fibrinogen are universal in such cases. In less severe cases, laboratory evidence of consumptive coagulopathy may be present to varying extent in the absence of overt clinical manifestations. Thrombocytopenia associated multiple organ failure (TAMOF) has been described in pediatric sepsis. The disintergrin and metalloprotease with thrombospondin motifs (ADAMTS-13), also known as von Willebrand factor (vWF) protease activity has been shown to play a role in the pathophysiology of TAMOF. A decrease in ADAMTS-13 activity (<57% of control) is seen in sepsis and this deficiency is associated with the formation of ultra-large vWF multimer. These multimer attract platelets and fibrin resulting in microthrombi, organ dysfunction and organ failure[28, 29]. Presence of fibrin split products and D dimers are indicative of fibrinolysis. Leukocytosis with a shift to the left is a common finding in septic shock. However, severe leukopenia (<3000/mm^3) is considered as a criterion of bone marrow failure and is associated with severity of illness.

Renal dysfunction

Experimental data suggest that during the early stages of sepsis there is renal vasoconstriction with intact tubular function[30]. During early sepsis,

there is induction of nitric oxide synthase by endotoxin leading to NO mediated arterial vasodilation. This leads to arterial underfilling which is sensed by the baroreceptors resulting in an increase in the sympathetic outflow with activation of the renin-angiotensin-aldosterone axis and release of arginine vasopressin from the central nervous system. This causes vasoconstriction with sodium and water retention. TNF-α can cause release of endothelin which is a potent vasoconstrictor and can also cause renal vasoconstriction[19, 31]. Endothelin can also cause capillary leak leading to a decrease in the intravascular volume. At the presentation of the initial illness predisposing to MODS, most patients present with oliguria which at this stage is representative of pre-renal factors resulting from low intravascular volume and low cardiac output due to myocardial depression. If this persists, tubular dysfunction can occur ultimately progressing to acute tubular necrosis. Increased generation of reactive oxygen species and peroxynitrites can also lead to tubular damage. DIC can lead to glomerular microthrombi further worsening the acute renal failure. Despite adequate hemodynamic resuscitation, a significant number of patients who develop MODS also develop evidences of glomerular and tubular injury. In such patients there is a gradual increase in BUN and serum creatinine, and persistence of oliguria. Provision of adequate nutrition is also compromised because of the necessity of fluid restriction in such children. Severe acute renal failure in presence of ARDS carries a high mortality[31]. However, most of the survivors show little or no clinically significant residual renal impairment.

Endocrine dysfunction

Endocrinopathy in sepsis can manifest as hyperglycemia and insulin resistance or as insufficient production of adrenal corticosteroids and vasopressin. Hyperglycemia in sepsis may occur due to stress induced elevation in counter-regulatory hormones and increased hepatic gluconeogenesis. Though there is increase in insulin release, the tissues exhibit insulin resistance induced by pro-inflammatory cytokines such as IL-1β, IL-6 and TNF-α[32, 33]. Hyperglycemia can lead to increased susceptibility to infection, impaired wound healing, increased oxidative stress, hypercoagulability, sympathetic hyperactivity and dyslipidemia. Although tight glycemic control in adult ICUs has been shown to decrease morbidity and mortality, other studies have shown no benefit or potential harm because of increased incidence of hypoglycemia[34-36]. Guidelines for pediatrics are even less defined. Hence use of insulin infusion for glucose control in pediatric sepsis and MODS remains controversial and when used, should be for treatment of sustained hyperglycemia, while taking care to prevent hypoglycemic episodes[37].

Patients with sepsis may have a relative adrenal insufficiency[38, 39]. Some studies have shown that physiologic doses of corticosteroids may improve survival in patients who have persistent shock requiring vasopressors[40]. Patients in septic shock have been shown to have low levels of vasopressin[41, 42]. This may be due to depletion of hypophyseal stores, increased vasopressinase activity, inhibitory effects of nor-epinephrine on vasopressin release and NO mediated inhibition of vasopressin production[42]. The hypothalamic-pituitary-thyroid axis can be affected during sepsis and may lead to acquired transient central hypothyroidism[43]. It has also been proposed that there is decreased peripheral T4 to T3 conversion and there are abnormalities in thyroid binding protein[32]. But there is currently no evidence to show that administration of thyroid hormone is beneficial in sepsis.

Hepatic dysfunction

Liver parenchymal cells are stimulated by TNF alpha, IL-1 and IL-6 to produce acute phase proteins such as C-reactive protein, LBP, haptoglobin, complement C3 and C9, α-macroglobulin, etc. Elevations of transaminases are almost universal in most patients with systemic inflammatory response syndrome. Mild elevation in total and direct bilirubin, prolongation of PT and hypoalbuminemia are also commonly encountered during the subsequent clinical course. However, unlike adults and immunocompromised children, severe liver dysfunction and hepatic encephalopathy are uncommon in previously healthy children with acute illness predisposing to MODS.

Elevated serum lactate is a common finding in sepsis and MODS. This may be due to tissue hypoxia and cytokine mediated increased cellular uptake of glucose leading to increased production of lactate. During sepsis the clearance of lactate by the liver may also be impaired. Other studies have shown that in acute lung injury, the lung may be responsible for lactate production and this increases with severity of the lung injury[44].

Neurologic dysfunction

Changes in sensorium such as disorientation, agitation, confusion, lethargy and obtundation are frequently observed in patients with sepsis. However, although commonly included in the criteria for MODS, significant encephalopathy (Glasgow Coma Score < 5) as a manifestation of systemic inflammatory response syndrome is unusual. Peripheral neuropathy and muscle weakness have been reported in patients with MODS especially those who had received neuromuscular blocking agents for prolonged periods during mechanical ventilation[45]. Animal studies have shown that systemic inflammation induces apoptosis and microglial cell activation in the brain with the hippocampus being the most vulnerable in sepsis[46]. Neonates with early onset sepsis, necrotizing enterocolitis and elevated IL-6, IL-8 and TNF-α levels are at greater risk for developing white matter injury[47].

Gastrointestinal tract

The gastrointestinal tract is an important organ involved in MODS both as the victim as well as the perpetrator of the ongoing inflammatory response. During the acute ischemic/hypoxic phase, blood is diverted away from the splanchnic circulation to preserve the functions of vital organs. After resuscitation, various manifestations of gut injury become apparent. Occult or frank gastrointestinal hemorrhage, indicative of mucosal ulcerations, is frequently encountered. Digestive and absorptive functions can be severely impaired. Intolerance to enteral feeding, abdominal distension, ileus, and diarrhea are commonly encountered. The use of sedatives and paralytics further contribute to gastrointestinal dysmotility. Mucosal ulcerations, overgrowth of Gram-negative bacilli and *Candida*, and loss of gut-barrier function have been implicated in bacterial translocation, perpetuation of the septic state and pathogenesis of MODS[13].

Metabolic abnormalities

Elevation of serum lipase, amylase, and triglycerides are commonly observed. LPS and pro-inflammatory cytokines affect a wide range of enzymes and receptors involved in lipid metabolism leading to an increase in the level of very low density lipoproteins (VLDL). Negative nitrogen balance, poor wound healing and increased susceptibility to nosocomial infection contribute to morbidity and mortality in later stages of MODS.

MANAGEMENT

The management of a child with MODS is based on the following principles:

1. Aggressive treatment of the predisposing illness.
2. Maintenance of adequate tissue oxygenation and cardiovascular support.
3. Attempts to reverse the pathophysiologic processes.
4. Provision of adequate nutritional and metabolic support.
5. Monitoring and assessment of organ function and response to therapy.

Treatment of the initial illness

The most common initial illnesses which subsequently result in MODS are severe systemic viral and bacterial infections, trauma and pulmonary aspiration. Prompt administration of appropriate antibiotics is essential. Shock is a frequent denominator in patients who are prone to develop MODS. Early indicators of decreased perfusion such as tachycardia, decreased toe temperature and prolonged capillary refill time should be vigilantly monitored, rather than relying solely on blood pressure measurements. Intravascular volume depletion, myocardial dysfunction, tissue hypoxia and metabolic derangements often coexist and must be monitored and managed expeditiously. Hypovolemia should be treated aggressively with isotonic fluid expansion. The type of resuscitation fluid remains a matter of controversy. Various factors should be taken into account when choosing fluid for intravascular expansion. These include the type of fluid lost, the amount of volume expansion, availability and cost. Patients with severe diarrhea and vomiting have an overall extracellular fluid (ECF) depletion. Rapid volume expansion with 20 ml/kg isotonic saline or Ringer's lactate is appropriate. Patients with sepsis and trauma have predominantly intravascular depletion with normal or increased interstitial space. A study comparing crystalloids versus colloids for initial fluid resuscitation showed no difference between the two[48]. Patients with septic shock may require rapid administration of large amount of fluids (60-100 ml/kg) to achieve hemodynamic stability. Adequacy of fluid resuscitation during the first hour of presentation has been shown to correlate with survival in septic shock[49]. Hemorrhagic shock should be treated with appropriate amount of blood transfusion. Prolonged tissue ischemia is an important pathogenic factor in the development of subsequent MODS. The need for continued fluid resuscitation should be based on frequent clinical assessments.

Fluid resuscitation alone is insufficient to improve tissue perfusion in a majority of patients with septic shock. Myocardial dysfunction is an important factor compromising tissue perfusion in these patients. If administration of >40-60 ml/kg of crystalloids over 1 hour fails to restore satisfactory hemodynamic status, myocardial insufficiency should be assumed and inotropic support should be initiated. Dopamine and dobutamine at 5 mg/kg/min, either alone or in combination are most widely used inotropic agents in this setting. The dose can be titrated upwards according to clinical assessment. Dopamine in doses > 10-15 µg/kg/min is associated with significant vasoconstriction. Vasopressin infusion should be considered in patients with refractory hypotension despite adequate volume expansion and inotropic agents. Continuous infusion of vasopressin is used at 0.0003 to 0.002 units per kg per min with a maximum of 0.04 units per min[50]. After establishment of adequate blood pressure, reducing the afterload by vasodilators such as milrinone can further enhance tissue perfusion. Continuous arterial blood pressure monitoring is necessary for safe and effective vasodilator therapy. Milrinone is a phosphodiesterase inhibitor, which offers the advantage of combining inotropic effect and afterload reduction without the arrhythmogenic potential of β agonists. Milrinone is given in a loading dose of 50 µg/kg followed by a continuous infusion of 0.5 µg/kg/min. It is important to monitor and promptly treat acidosis, hypoglycemia and hypocalcemia all of which can further impair myocardial contractility. Monitoring the central venous pressure, mixed venous O_2 saturation, arterial-venous oxygenation difference and serum lactate measurement are helpful in assessing cardiac function and oxygen delivery in response to therapy.

Early goal-directed sepsis therapy initiated within the first hour of presentation has been shown to result in a decrease in the incidence of cardiovascular collapse, reduced need for mechanical ventilation and use of vasopressor agents with decrease in the overall morbidity and mortality. The goal-directed therapy involves aggressive volume resuscitation, use of vasoactive and inotropic agents, and blood transfusion, to maintain the goals of mean arterial pressure between 65-90 mmHg, CVP greater than 8 mmHg and mixed venous O_2 saturation > 70%[51].

Management of Sequential Organ Dysfunction

Acute respiratory distress syndrome (ARDS)

ARDS A comprehensive discussion of management of ARDS is given in Chapter 31. The major objectives of managing pulmonary dysfunction in ARDS are (i) continuous assessment of deficiencies in oxygen delivery (DO_2) by invasive and noninvasive monitoring and, (ii) providing adequate DO_2 to meet oxygen requirements while minimizing the complications of therapeutic interventions. Hypoxemia with increased A-aO_2 gradient is a hallmark of ARDS. Important factors which contribute to decreased DO_2 include: decreased FRC, V/Q mismatch and intrapulmonary right-to-left shunting, diffusion barrier and increased right ventricular afterload from pulmonary hypertension resulting in decreased cardiac output[52]. A young child is especially vulnerable to respiratory compromise. Increased chest wall compliance results in greater decrease in FRC compared to adults. Infantile respiratory muscles are not equipped to sustain large elastic load making them susceptible to early fatigue. It is important to identify pulmonary compromise and institute appropriate support early in the course. Patients with marked tachypnea, grunting, significant retractions, SpO_2 < 95% despite supplemental oxygen, and clinical evidences of fatigue are best intubated electively under controlled environment and mechanically ventilated.

Oxygen and PEEP. Providing supplemental oxygen to treat or prevent hypoxemia is the first step in management. The major determinants of arterial oxygen content are the level of hemoglobin and the extent to which it is saturated with oxygen. Maintenance of an adequate hemoglobin level is therefore important. In an acute situation, oxygen should be administered in as high a concentration as possible, the risk of toxicity notwithstanding. When monitoring is available, oxygen$_2$ therapy should be directed to attain PaO_2 at a sufficient level to ensure an oxygen saturation above 95%. Oxygen therapy should be combined with PEEP in intubated patients. Application of PEEP allows for reduction in FiO_2 to maintain satisfactory PaO_2 thus minimizing toxicity associated with prolonged use of oxygen. Although PEEP does not reverse lung injury, it improves oxygenation by several mechanisms. The increased transpulmonary distending pressure results in alveolar stability, recruitment of alveoli, and increased FRC. PEEP also displaces intra-alveolar water into the interstitial and peri-lymphatic spaces with a resultant decrease in venous admixture and improves pulmonary compliance and V/Q matching. An excessively high level of PEEP, however, is associated with decreased venous return and cardiac output. Other detrimental effects of PEEP are overdistension of alveoli, an increase in dead space, and predisposition to barotrauma. The benefit of improved PaO_2 from

PEEP must be weighed against the risk of decreasing cardiac output and barotrauma. The definition of "best PEEP" is debatable. In clinical practice, a gradual increase in PEEP up to 8 to 10 cm H_2O is considered reasonable if each stepwise increase in PEEP is associated with an increase in PaO_2.

Conventional mechanical ventilation. The most efficient mechanical ventilatory support is the one that ensures adequate O_2 delivery and CO_2 removal with lowest possible risk of ventilator-associated injury from oxytrauma, barotrauma, volutrauma and ineffective tracheobronchial toilet. Strategies for improving gas exchange must take into account the pathophysiologic alterations in an individual patient.

Pulmonary mechanics of ARDS are characterized by decreased FRC, low compliance, short time constant and high critical opening pressure. It has been recognized that large changes in tidal volume are more injurious than the levels of mean airway pressure the lungs are exposed to. A study conducted by the NIH ARDS Clinical Trials Network compared the effects of low (6 ml/kg) vs high (12 ml/kg) tidal volume while maintaining plateau pressures less that 30 cm H_2O in adults. There was a 10% reduction in mortality in the group that was treated with low tidal volume[53]. The mechanical ventilation strategy in ARDS is that of recruiting lung volume by appropriate level of PEEP and ventilating at relatively low tidal volumes. Modest elevations in $PaCO_2$ (permissive hypercapnia) are well tolerated. The decreased time constant makes it possible to ventilate at a relatively rapid rate since the time required for lung inflation and deflation is short. Prolongation of inspiration within a given respiratory cycle can improve oxygenation by exposing greater amount of pulmonary capillary blood to a higher PO_2 during inspiration compared to a lower PaO_2 during expiration. Excessively increased inspiratory to expiratory (I:E) ratios, however, can result in auto-PEEP, alveolar overdistension and decreased cardiac output. Most patients with severe ARDS are best managed in pressure controlled, time-cycled ventilatory mode, and require adequate sedation and pharmacologic paralysis to avoid ventilator asynchrony.

High-frequency ventilation. Mechanical ventilation at supraphysiologic rates and low tidal volumes has been shown to improve gas exchange in a selected group of patients with ARDS who do not respond to conventional mechanical ventilation. The major advantage of high-frequency ventilation

(HFV) is the ability to use reduced airway pressure for effective ventilation. The most commonly employed techniques of HFV is that of high-frequency oscillation (HFO) which employs a vibratory diaphragm to generate to-and-fro air movement. Additional air is entrained through a parallel circuit by venturi effect. During expiration air is actively sucked out. The independent controls are respiratory rate, I/E ratio, mean airway pressure (MAP), and change in proximal airway pressure (amplitude). MAP and FiO_2 are main determinants of oxygenation whereas amplitude pressure determines $PaCO_2$. HFV has been an important therapeutic advance added to the physician's armamentarium in the management of ARDS when conventional ventilation is ineffective. Improvement in oxygenation is often dramatic, immediate and sustained. Rapid improvement in oxygenation within 6 hours of institution of HFV predicts a high likelihood of survival[54].

Extracorporeal life support. The use of extracorporeal life support (ELS) has been proposed with the rationale of bypassing the lungs and sparing them from deleterious effects of barotrauma and oxygen toxicity while spontaneous recovery occurs. Selected patients who fail to improve with conventional and high-frequency ventilation, may benefit from ELS. For ELS to be beneficial, it should be instituted before the occurrence of severe irreversible pulmonary injury. However, reasonable entry criteria have not been established for children with ARDS. ELS is invasive, labor intensive, and expensive therapeutic modality.

Surfactant therapy. In ARDS, there is both decreased production and increased destruction of pulmonary surfactant. Exogenous surfactant therapy has been proposed to treat secondary surfactant deficiency, increase FRC and improve compliance. A recent study showed that instillation of natural lung surfactant (calfactant) improved the oxygenation and decreased mortality in infants and children when administered early in the course of ARDS[55]. The optimal timing of such therapy still remains to be established.

Other therapies. Inhaled nitric oxide (iNO), and prone positioning represent unproven forms of respiratory support. NO delivered through the ventilator circuit is proposed to act locally, resulting in selective pulmonary vasodilatation in ventilated areas with improvement in ventilation perfusion mismatch and reduction of intrapulmonary shunt. Although an immediate modest improvement in oxygenation is consistently observed, no long-term benefit on either the oxygenation or the survival has been demonstrated. Small doses (5 to 10 ppm) appear to be as effective as larger doses with less adverse effects such as methemoglobinemia and platelet dysfunction.

It has been shown that pulmonary perfusion is more homogenous resulting in less V/Q mismatch in prone position compared to the traditional supine position of the patient. An improved oxygenation has been observed when patient's position is changed from supine to prone. However, sustained benefit and influence on the final outcome have not been documented.

Hematologic failure

Disseminated intravascular coagulation (DIC) during the initial illness plays an important role in subsequent development of MODS especially in patients with sepsis. While widespread hemorrhagic diatheses is the most clinically obvious consequence of consumptive coagulopathy, it is the microvascular thrombosis, compromising blood flow to the tissues, which is more important in causing end-organ damage and MODS. Treatment of DIC consists of (a) treatment of primary disease, (b) replacement of clotting factors and, (c) inhibition of intravascular coagulation. In early stages, hemorrhagic manifestations of DIC can be effectively treated with 20 ml/kg fresh frozen plasma (FFP). In severe cases, however, the bleeding diatheses and abnormalities of PT and PTT persist despite administration of FFP as clotting factors continue to get consumed. Additionally, there is a concern of "adding fuel to fire" with the administered factors further aggravating intravascular coagulation and worsening tissue ischemia. When coagulopathy persists after FFP, we have found that a two volume exchange transfusion followed by administration of FFP and platelets is effective in managing hemorrhagic manifestations of DIC while improving hemodynamic stability[56].

Theoretical advantages of exchange transfusion include removal of endotoxins, inflammatory cytokines and fibrin degradation products. Plasma exchange has also been shown to replenish ADAMTS-13 activity and remove vWF multimers improving organ function recovery in sepsis and MODS[57, 58]. Antithrombin (AT) III is a physiologic anticoagulant which inhibits intrinsic, extrinsic and the common coagulation pathway. Levels of AT III are decreased in patients with septic shock and the degree of AT III deficiency correlates with outcome. However, it has not been shown to be beneficial in decreasing mortality in clinical trials[59]. In the large double-blinded PROWESS (Human Activated **P**rotein C **W**orldwide **E**valuation in **S**evere **S**epsis) study for treatment of sepsis in adults, a 6.1% absolute reduction in 28 day mortality rate and 20% reduction in the relative risk of death in the treated group was noted. The treatment was found to be effective regardless of the severity of illness, number of dysfunctional organs, site and type of infection[26]. Hence administration of activated Protein C (APC) is recommended in adults with severe sepsis and MOF. However, in children an increase in Protein C activity over time was noted in the ENHANCE trial. Moreover, as per the RESOLVE (Researching Severe Sepsis and Organ Dysfunction on children- a global perspective, F1K-MC-EVBP) trial, there was no difference in mortality or improvement in organ failure upon treatment with APC when compared to placebo, but an increase in incidence of CNS bleeding was noted with APC treatment. Hence APC is not recommended for use in children[60, 37].

Renal, hepatic and gastrointestinal failure

Maintenance of adequate fluid balance, metabolic environment and nutritional intake are critically important in managing a child with MODS. Management of oliguric renal failure requires maintaining the patient in a state of optimum hydration and intravascular volume. Patients with fluid overload should be treated with fluid restriction and diuretics. Prolonged fluid restriction compromises nutritional intake. Early institution of renal replacement therapy with continuous veno-venous hemofiltration (CVVH) should be considered to treat fluid overload and to allow for adequate fluid administration to meet the caloric needs[61]. A meta-analysis of hemodialysis versus continuous renal replacement has not shown an advantage of one method over another for treatment of acute renal failure[62].

Nutritional support

Malnutrition is an important complication of MODS. Whenever possible, enteral feeding with easily absorbed elemental formula, is the preferred method of providing nutrition. Even a small amount of enteral feeding is considered important in maintaining gastrointestinal mucosal integrity and preventing bacterial translocation to the mesenteric lymph nodes. Those patients who cannot tolerate adequate enteral feeding should be treated with parenteral nutrition. While it is important to provide sufficient calories, overfeeding is also deleterious. Children with MODS are often in a severe catabolic state. Positive nitrogen balance may not be achieved even with a relatively large amount of protein intake. A reasonable approach is to provide 1.5 to 2.5 g/kg protein with a calorie to nitrogen ratio of 150 to 250. Carbohydrates should account for 50 to 60% and fats should provide 25 to 30% of total calories. Serum triglycerides and glucose levels should be monitored daily. Carbohydrate and fat intolerance may limit the amount of calories from individual sources. Appropriate amounts of vitamins and trace elements must also be provided in the parenteral nutrition solution. Insulin therapy for treatment of sustained hyperglycemia may be judiciously instituted[37].

Corticosteroids. A study by Annane[40] in 2002 where low dose hydrocortisone (physiologic dose- 50 mg IV every 6 hours) along with fludrocortisone (50 ug per day) were administered for seven days to patients in septic shock showed improved survival when compared to controls. However, results of the CORTICUS study group showed that treatment with hydrocortisone did not show any improvement in survival or reversal of shock in patients with septic shock, even in those who did not have a response to corticotrophin. A recent retrospective analysis of the RESOLVE database showed no difference in improvement in outcome with adjunctive steroid therapy in children with sepsis[63, 64, 37]. Based on these studies, routine use of steroids in sepsis should be avoided, but intravenous administration of physiological doses of hydrocortisone (50 mg/m²/day) in 4 divided doses may be a reasonable approach for children with sepsis who remain hypotensive despite fluid expansion and vasopressor therapy.

Immune modulating therapies. Various therapies directed at modulating cytokine mediated immune response have shown benefits in animal models have not shown similar effects in clinical trials. These include anti-TNF monoclonal antibody, exogenous free radical scavengers, and inhibitors of NO synthase. NFkB inhibitors may be helpful in decreasing the inflammatory response and are being tested experimentally[65]. Antibodies against complement activation product C5a and other strategies that block apoptosis of lymphocytes or gastrointestinal epithelial cells have improved survival in experimental models of sepsis[66]. Future therapies will be directed at manipulating the patient's immune responses to pathogens based on genetic polymorphisms.

PROGNOSIS

The clinical disorder predisposing to development of MODS has a strong influence in determining survival. Patients with preexisting organ dysfunction, underlying malignancy and immunosuppression have a high mortality. Though multiple scoring systems including the Sequential Organ Failure Assessment (SOFA) score, Multiple Organ Dysfunction (MOD) score have been used to predict the mortality from organ dysfunction but they have not been found to be consistently reliable in predicting outcomes[67]. In general, the degree of organ dysfunction at the time of ICU admission predicts mortality[68]. Proulx et al[69] observed that the number of organ systems failure, age < 12 months and the Pediatric Risk of Mortality (PRISM) score were independent risk factors for death in children with MODS[69]. Despite the high mortality, the survivors, without previous organ dysfunction, have few if any sequelae.

REFERENCES

1. Goldstein B, Giroir B, Randolph A, International pediatric sepsis consensus conference: definitions for sepsis and organ dysfunction in pediatrics. *Pediatr Crit Care Med* 2005. 6(1): 2-8.

2. Levy MM, Fink MP, Marshall JC, 2001 SCCM/ESICM/ACCP/ATS/SIS International sepsis definitions conference. *Intensive Care Med* 2003. 29: 530-538.

3. Carcillo JA, Fields A., Task Force Committee Members, Clinical practice parameters for hemodynamic support of pediatric and neonatal patients in septic shock. *Crit Care Med* 2002. 30: 1365-1378.

4. Opal, S. Signaling: How do cells respond to insult? In: 2002 *SCCM/ESICM Summer Conference.* 2002: SCCM.

5. Van Amersfoot ES, Van Berkel T., Kuiper J Receptors, mediators and mechanisms involved in bacterial sepsis and septic shock. *Clinical Microbiol Rev* 2003. 16(3): 379-414.

6. Plitas G, *et al.,* Toll-like receptor 9 inhibition reduces mortality in polymicrobial sepsis. *J Exp Med* 2008, 205:1277–1283.

7. Alves-Filho JC, Freitas A, Souto FO, *et al.,* Regulation of chemokine receptor by Toll-like receptor 2 is critical to neutrophil migration and resistance to polymicrobial sepsis. *PNAS* 2009, 106: 4018-4023.

8. Gerlach, H. Proinflammatory mediators. in 2002 *SCCM/ESICM Summer Conference.* 2002: SCCM.

9. Ward, N. Anti-inflammatory mediators. In: 2002 *SCCM/ESICM Summer Conference.* 2002: SCCM.

10. Alves-Filho JC, Sônego F, Souto FO, *et al,* Interleukin-33 attenuates sepsis by enhancing neutrophil influx to the site of infection. *Nat Med* 2010, 16(6): 708-712.

11. Hotchkiss RS, Karl I, The pathophysiology and treatment of sepsis. *N Engl J Med* 2003. 348: 138-150.

12. Riewald M, Wolfram R, Science review: Role of coagulation protease cascades in sepsis. *Critical Care* 2003. 7: 123-129.

13. Livingston DH, Mosenthal A, Deitch EA, Sepsis and multiple organ dysfunction syndrome: A clinical-mechanistic overview. *New Horiz* 1995, 3: 257-266.

14. Shimizu K, Ogura H, Hamasaki T, *et al,* Altered gut flora are associated with septic complications and death in critically ill patients with SIRS. *Dig Dis Sci* 2011, 56:1171-1177.

15. Mela L, Bacalzo LV, Miller LD, Defective oxidative metabolism of rat liver mitochondria in hemorrhagic and endotoxin shock. *Am J Physiol* 1971 Feb; 220(2):571-577.

16. Brealey D, Karyampudi S, Jacques TS, *et al,* Mitochondrial dysfunction in a long-term rodent model of sepsis and organ failure. *Am J Physiol Regul Integr Comp Physiol* 2004 Mar; 286(3): R491-7. Epub 2003.

17. Brealey D, Brand M, Hargreaves I, *et al,* Association between mitochondrial dysfunction and severity and outcome of septic shock. *Lancet* 2002 Jul 20; 360 (9328):219-223.

18. Anna J. Dare, Anthony R.J. Phillips, Anthony J.R. Hickey, *et al,* A systematic review of experimental treatments for mitochondrial dysfunction in sepsis and multiple organ dysfunction syndrome: Review article. *Radical Biology and Medicine,* 2009, 47 (11), 1517-1525.

19. Schrier RW, Wang W, Acute renal failure and sepsis. *N Engl J Med* 2004. 351: 159-169.

20. Typpo K, Petersen N, Hallman D, *et al,* Impact of premorbid conditions on multiple organ dysfunction syndrome in the PICU. *Pediatr Res* 2007.

21. Leteurtre S, Martinot A, Duhamel A, *et al,* Validation of the paediatric logistic organ dysfunction score: Prospective, observational, multicentre study. *Lancet* 2003; 362: 192–197.

22. Shah P, Riphagen S, Beyene J, *et al.* Multidysfunction in infants with post-asphyxial hypoxic-ischaemic encephalopathy. *Arch Dis Child Fetal Neonatal Ed* 2004; 89:F152–F155.

23. Tabbutt, S., *He*art failure in pediatric septic shock: Utilizing inotropic support. *Crit Care Med* 2001. 29(10): S231-S236.

24. Ashbaugh DG, Bigelow D., Petty TL, *et al,* Acute respiratory distress in adults *Lancet* 1967. 2: 319-323.

25. Cate, H, Pathophysiology of disseminated intravascular coagulation in sepsis. *Crit Care Med* 2000. 28(9): S9-S11.

26. Bernard GR, Vincent J, Laterre PR, *et al.* Efficacy and safety of recombinant human activated protein C for severe sepsis. *N Engl J Med* 2001. 344: 699-709.

27. Matthay, M., Severe sepsis-A new treatment with both anticoagulant and antiinflammatory properties. *N Engl J Med* 2001. 344(10): 759-762.

28. Nguyen TC, Carcillo JA. Bench-to-bedside review: thrombocytopenia-associated multiple organ failure – a newly appreciated syndrome in the critically ill. *Crit Care* 2006;10(6):235.

29. Nguyen TC, Han YY, Kiss JE, *et al.* Intensive plasma exchange increases a disintegrin and metalloprotease with thrombospondin motifs-13 activity and reverses organ dysfunction in children with thrombocytopenia-associated multiple organ failure. *Crit Care Med* 2008, 36 (10):2878-2887.

30. Kikeri D, Pennell J., Hwang KH, *et al.* Endotoxemic acute renal failure in awake rats. *Am J Physiol* 1986, 250: F1098-F1106.

31. Karnik AM, Bashir R., Khan F, *et al.* Renal involvement in the systemic inflammatory reaction syndrome. *Renal Failure* 1998, (20): 103-116.

32. Brierre S, Kumari R., Deboisblanc BP, The endocrine system during sepsis. *Amer J Med Sci* 2004, 328(4): 238-247.

33. Chambrier C, Laville M, Rhziuoal BK, *et al.* Insulin sensitivity of glucose and fat metabolism in severe sepsis. *Clin Sci* 2000, 99: 321-328.

34. Van den Berghe G, Wouters P, Weekers F, *et al.* Intensive insulin therapy in critically ill patients. *N Engl J Med* 2001, 345: 1359-1367.

35. Van den Berghe G, Wilmer A, Hermans G, *et al.* Intensive insulin therapy in the Medical ICU. *N Engl J Med* 2006, 354:449-461.

36. Brunkhorst FM, Kuhnt E, Engel C, Meier-Hellmann A, Ragaller M, Quintel M, Weiler N, Grundling M, Oppert M, Deufel T, *et al.* Intensive insulin therapy in patients with severe sepsis and septic shock is associated with an increased rate of hypoglycemia – results from a randomized multicenter study (VISEP) [abstract]. *Infection* 2005, 33:19–20

37. Surviving Sepsis Campaign: international guidelines for management of severe sepsis and septic shock: *Crit Care Med* 2008 Jan; 36(1):296-327.

38. Annane, D., Time for a consensus definition of corticosteroid insufficiency in critically ill patients. *Crit Care Med* 2003. 31: 1868-1869.

39. Manlik S, Flores E., Lubarsky L, *et al.* Glucocorticoid insufficiency in patients who present to the hospital with severe sepsis: a prospective clinical trial. *Crit Care Med* 2003. 31: 1668-1675.

40. Annane D, Sebille V, Charpentier C, *et al.* Effect of treatment with low doses of hydrocortisone and fludrocortisone on mortality in patients with septic shock *JAMA* 2002. 288: 862-871.

41. Landry DW, Levin H, Gallant EM, *et al.* Vasopressin deficiency contributes to the vasodilation of septic shock. *Circulation* 1997. 95: 1122-1125.

42. Sharshar T, Blanchard A., Paillard M, *et al.* Circulating vasopressin levels in septic shock. *Crit Care Med* 2003. 31: 1752-1758.

43. Chopra, I., Euthyroid sick syndrome: is it a misnomer? *J Clin Endocrinol Metab* 1997. 82: 329-334.

44. Kellum JA, Kramer D, Lee K, *et al.* Release of lactate by the lung in acute lung injury. *Chest* 1997. 111: 1301-1305.

45. Lee, C., Intensive care unit neuromuscular syndrome? *Anesthesiology* 1995. 83: 237-240.

46. Semmler A, Okulla T, Sastre M, *et al.* Systemic inflammation induces apoptosis with variable vulnerability of different brain regions. *J Chem Neuroanatomy* 2005, 30: 144-157.

47. Procianoy RS, Silveira RC. Association between high cytokine levels with white matter injury in preterm infants with sepsis. *Pediatr Crit Care Med* 2011. [Epub ahead of print]

48. SAFE Study, A comparison of albumin and saline for fluid resuscitation in the intensive care unit. *N Engl J Med* 2004. 350: 2247-2256.

49. Carcillo JA, Davis A, and Zaritsky A, Role of early fluid resuscitation in pediatric septic shock. *JAMA* 1991, 226: 1242-1245.

50. Rozensweig EB, StarcT, Chen JM, *et al.* Intravenous arginine-vasopressin in children with vasodilatory shock after cardiac surgery. *Circulation* 1999. 100 (19 Suppl): 182-186.

51. Rivers E, Nguyen R, Havstad S, *et al.* Early goal-directed therapy in the treatment of severe sepsis and septic shock. *N Engl J Med* 2001. 345: 1368-1377.

52. Sarnaik AP, Lieh-Lai M., Adult respiratory distress syndrome in children. *Pediatr Clin N Amer* 1994. 41: 337-363.

53. ARDS Network, Ventilation with lower tidal volumes as compared with traditional tidal volumes for acute lung injury and the acute respiratory distress syndrome. *N Engl J Med* 2000. 342: 1301-1308.

54. Sarnaik AP, Meert K, Pappas MD, *et al.* Predicting outcome in children with severe acute respiratory failure treated with high-frequency ventilation. *Crit Care Med* 1996. 24: 1396-1402.

55. Wilson DF, Thomas N., Markovitz BP, *et al.* Effect of exogenous surfactant in pediatric acute lung injury. A randomized control trial. *JAMA* 2005, 293: 470-476.

56. Heidemann SM, Sarnaik AP, Blood exchange transfusion improves pulmonary gas exchange and hemodynamic stability in severe septic shock *Pediatr Res* 1997.

57. Busund R, Koukline V, Utrobin U, *et al.* Plasmapheresis in severe sepsis and septic shock: a prospective, randomised, controlled trial. *Intensive Care Med* 2002 Oct; 28(10):1434-9. Epub 2002 Jul 23.

58. Darmon M, Azoulay E, Thiery G, *et al.* Time course of organ dysfunction in thrombotic microangiopathy patients receiving either plasma perfusion or plasma exchange. *Crit Care Med* 2006 Aug; 34(8): 2127-2133.

59. Warren BL, Eid A, Singer P, *et al.* Caring for the critically ill patient. High-dose antithrombin III in severe sepsis: a randomized controlled trial. *JAMA* 2001. 286(15): 1869-1878.

60. Nadel S, Goldstein B, Williams MD, *et al.* Drotrecogin alfa (activated) in children with severe sepsis: a multicentre phase III randomised controlled trial. Researching severe Sepsis and Organ dysfunction in children: a gLobal perspective (RESOLVE) study group. *Lancet* 2007 Mar 10;369(9564):836-843.

61. Honore PM, Jamez J., Wauthier M, Lee PA, *et al.* Prospective evaluation of short-term, high volume isovolemic ultrafiltration on the hemodynamic course and outcome in patients with intractable circulatory failure resulting from septic shock. *Crit Care Med* 2000. 28: 3581-3587.

62. Tonelli M, Manns B, Feller-Kopman D, *et al.* Acute renal failure in the intensive care unit: a systematic review of the impact of dialytic modality on mortality and renal recovery. *Amer J Kidney Dis* 2002. 40: 875-885.

63. Sprung CL, Annane D, Keh D, *et al.* CORTICUS Study Group. Hydrocortisone therapy for patients with septic shock. *N Engl J Med* 2008; 358:111-124.

64. Zimmerman JJ, Williams MD. Adjunctive corticosteroid therapy in pediatric severe sepsis: observations from the RESOLVE study. *Pediatr Crit Care Med* 2011 Jan; 12(1):2-8.

65. Zingarelli B, Sheehan M, Wong H, Nuclear factor-kB as a therapeutic target in critical care medicine. *Crit Care Med* 2003. 31: S105-S111.

66. Huber-Lang MS, Sarma J, McGuire SR, *et al.* Protective effects of anti-C5a peptide antibodies in experimental sepsis. *FASEB J,* 2001. 15: 568-570.

67. Zygun DA, Laupland K., Fick GH, *et al.* Limited ability of SOFA and MOD scores to discriminate outcome: a prospective evaluation in 1,436 patients. *Can J Anaesth* 2005. 52(3): 302-308.

68. Vincent J-L, de Mendonca A, *et al.* Use of the SOFA score to assess the incidence of organ dysfunction/failure in intensive care units: results of a multicenter, prospective study. *Crit Care Med* 1998. 26: 1793-1799.

69. Proulx F, Gauthier M, Nadeau D, *et al.* Timing and predictors of death in pediatric patients with multiple organ system failure. *Crit Care Med* 1994. 22: 1025-1031.

Supportive Care of Critically Sick Children

Sunil Saharan and Rakesh Lodha

The main goal of intensive care is to salvage and resuscitate critically ill patients by utilizing standardized and effective protocols such as Pediatric Advanced Life Support (PALS). The aim is to provide titrated care to each organ system in order to re-establish normal physiology and prevent multiple organ failure, while at the same time balancing therapeutic intervention in terms of benefits and likely complications.

Children have special needs in terms of fluid requirements, temperature control and unique susceptibility of the growing brain to damage due to a variety of offending insults. In critically ill children instability of homeostatic mechanisms, functional immaturity of vital organs and occurrence of multiple problems simultaneously leads to the development of a complex clinical syndrome.

The success of intensive care is dependent on early identification of a critically sick child followed by prompt decision and appropriate intervention. The care of critically sick children in PICU demands regular clinical and technology-based assessment and monitoring to identify whether the patient is stable or unstable and improving or worsening. *However, technology is no substitute for good clinical assessment and one must remember that critical care is highly labor-intensive.* The clinical skills should be effectively harnessed to provide rational care with due compassion and concern.

The primary or precipitating disorder should be the focus of attention and specific intervention. In order to provide holistic care due attention should be focused on homeostasis, fluid and electrolyte balance, temperature control, nutrition, sedation and analgesia along with prevention and control of infection. The decision making in PICU is a continuous cycle of evaluation followed by intervention and re-evaluation. The therapeutic goals should be defined and achieved with simple and safe interventions wherever possible. The dictum of "First Do No Harm" must be followed by keeping in mind the global interests of the patient, family and society.

The assessment and monitoring data should be recorded on a pre-designed simplified chart. In order to reduce the risk of medical errors and improve the quality of care, there is a need to follow evidence-based guidelines[1]. Protocols have been designed to ensure rational management of common problems, like weaning from mechanical ventilation[2,3], strict glucose control[4], and adequate sedation[5]. Guidelines are also available for treatment of complex medical problems like hypovolemia, septic shock, acute lung injury, and ARDS but they are difficult to implement and need to be individualized for each patient[6].

IDENTIFICATION OF A SERIOUSLY ILL CHILD

In order to improve the survival of seriously ill children, it is mandatory to recognize a sick child at the earliest. The early identification of a critically ill child is required both on arrival to the Emergency Department and also, amongst children already admitted in the hospital. It is important to recognize the development of derangements and potential complications, arising either from the disease process or its therapy in critically sick children with known chronic disorders (such as malignancy, renal or hepatic disorders).

At first contact, the ABCs are assessed quickly for patency of **A**irways, adequacy of **B**reathing and **C**irculation. If there is an abnormality in any of these, appropriate life support/resuscitation must be initiated. The important symptoms in seriously ill children are summarized in Table 8.1.

The assessment whether a child is well or ill can also be made by grading the degree of compromise in a variety of age-specific behavioral and activity parameters. Various clinical scoring systems are available for describing the severity of illness. The parameters which are objectively evaluated in some of these scores include respiratory effort, level of activity, color, temperature, playfulness, quality of cry, response

Table 8.1 Salient symptoms in a critically sick child

1. Cold and clammy extremities (particularly in the absence of cold environment)
2. Excessive irritability
3. Decreased activity, lethargy and drowsiness
4. Seizure activity
5. Difficulty in breathing
6. Apneic episodes/ cyanosis
7. Bilious vomiting
8. Decreased feeding/ decreased intake of fluids
9. Decrease in the urine output (e.g. less than 4 wet diapers in the previous 24 hours)
10. Bleeding manifestations

to parental overtures, and hydration status. Some of the scores are Yale Observation Score, Young Infant Observation Scale, and Severity Index Score. These scores help in objective assessment of a sick child but none of these are 100% sensitive and specific.

Examination is conducted to identify abnormalities in various organ systems. As mentioned earlier, the priority should be given to assessment of ABCs. Pulse rate, character of the pulse, respiratory rate and effort, temperature, capillary refill time, and oxygen saturation by pulse oximetry should be accurately measured. In addition, look for pallor, icterus, edema, wasting, and signs of dehydration. Examine the central nervous system for alteration of sensorium, any neurological deficits, and signs of meningeal irritation. Assess the renal function by recording the urine output.

In a sick child, commonly performed investigations include complete blood count, blood glucose, electrolytes, and arterial blood gases. The rest of laboratory work up should be tailored according to the clinical profile of the patient. Once a sick child is identified and assessed completely, appropriate interventions are performed and the child is periodically reexamined to assess the impact of intervention and to identify any complications due to the disease or intervention.

PRINCIPLES OF MONITORING

Monitoring of critically ill children is an essential component of management. The main purposes of monitoring are listed below:

1. To measure key physiologic indices that help in diagnosis and management.
2. To provide guidance to the health care team regarding the important changes that have occurred in the child's condition.

3. To identify and evaluate trends that would help in the assessment of treatment and prognosis of the patient.

The monitoring system should be relevant to the child's underlying disease/involved organ system, and its management. The data should be accurate, easily interpretable, valid and reproducible. Technology used must be sensitive to detect changes in the key parameters. Patient's safety should always be kept in mind while selecting a monitoring device. The parameters to be monitored and the frequency of monitoring should be decided by the treating team on the basis of child's diagnosis, severity of illness, and the organ system involved. While various monitoring equipment based on latest technology are available, the role of physical examination by an astute clinician cannot be overemphasized.

Respiratory Monitoring[7]

Goal of cardiorespiratory monitoring is to provide an assessment of gas exchange, oxygen delivery and oxygen utilization. The child should be observed for rate and pattern of breathing, nasal flaring, use of accessory muscles, audible wheeze and color. On auscultation, look for symmetry of air entry, type of breath sounds and presence of stridor, wheeze, and crepitations. Respiratory rate can also be monitored continuously by impedance pneumography, which measures the impedance to current flow during the respiratory cycle by using three electrodes over the chest. Apnea is defined as any cessation in breathing for more than 20 seconds or any respiratory pause associated with bradycardia, pallor, or cyanosis. One must be aware about the normal range of breathing and heart rates at different ages in order to detect an abnormality (Table 8.2).

Table 8.2 Respiratory rates and heart rates at different ages (mean and range)

Age (years)	Respiratory rate (breaths/min)	Heart rate (beats/min)
1	30 (24- 38)	120 (80- 160)
2	25 (17- 33)	110 (80- 130)
4	23 (17- 27)	100 (80- 120)
6	21 (15- 26)	100 (75- 115)
8	20 (15- 26)	90 (70- 110)
10	18 (15- 25)	90 (70- 110)
12	18 (14- 26)	85 (65- 105)
14	17 (15- 23)	80 (60- 100)
16	17 (12- 22)	75 (55- 95)

Pulse oximetry measures the percent oxygen saturation of arterial hemoglobin with a non-invasive method. The technique is based on Beer-Lambert law. The ratio of oxyhemoglobin to the sum of total hemoglobin (reduced hemoglobin and oxyhemoglobin) is estimated by measuring absorption at wavelengths of 660 nm (red) and 940 nm (infrared)[8]. In last 30 years there have been significant advances in technology in terms of light emitting diodes, spectrophotometry and plethysmography. Pulse oximetry is very safe, portable, accurate and relatively inexpensive. The major advantage of pulse oximetry is early detection of hypoxemia and assessing the effect of the intervention. It is fairly reliable in most settings except in low cardiac output states, the artifacts due to motion, dyshemoglobinemias (methemoglobin, carbon monoxide, and fetal hemoglobin), dyes and pigments (methylene blue), increased venous pulsations, and optical interference due to external light sources.

Transcutaneous blood gas monitoring is now feasible for continuous monitoring of pO_2 and pCO_2. It has been used extensively in newborns for monitoring arterial oxygen tension. But its correlation with arterial oxygen tension is poor in situations with low cardiac output. Moreover, it has the limitations of frequent calibration, high costs, being less useful with increasing age and occasional burns at skin probe site[9].

Capnography provides the graphic waveform depiction of CO_2 concentration variation throughout the respiratory cycle. A side stream or mainstream device can be used to collect a sample of inspired and expired gases from the patient. There are two different types of capnography which are either volume or time-based. The time based capnography is the classical end-tidal CO_2 monitoring. Volumetric capnography has been used to measure the dead space, perfusion of pulmonary capillaries and effective ventilation. Capnography measurements are based upon either infrared spectroscopy or mass spectroscopy. End-tidal CO_2 is used for monitoring adequacy of ventilation, respiratory rate, patency and position of endotracheal tube, detecting mechanical failures, and analysis of respiratory support. In mechanically ventilated children, respiratory mechanics help in better understanding of respiratory pathophysiology.

Apart from these continuous monitoring modalities chest radiography and arterial blood gas analyses are also performed periodically depending upon the clinical situation. Key to successful outcome in respiratory monitoring is integration of physical examination findings with technology-based monitoring data before making a final therapeutic decision.

Hemodynamic and Cardiac Function Monitoring[10, 11]

Hemodynamic monitoring provides vital information regarding the perfusion of different organs. Physical examination is the cornerstone of hemodynamic monitoring with special emphasis on the rate, rhythm and character of all peripheral pulses. The heart rate varies with the age as shown in Table 8.2 and also with the physiologic state (like presence of fever, anxiety, pain, etc.), and one must be aware of these physiological changes to interpret the abnormalities. The capillary filling time is helpful for assessment of the microcirculation. Firm pressure is applied over the sternum or forehead by ball of the thumb or tip of index figure for 5 seconds to blanch the skin. On release of pressure, the color returns and the time taken for complete return of color is noted. The normal capillary filling time is 3 seconds or less. Any prolongation of capillary refill time signifies impairment of microcirculation but it is important to rule out presence of hypothermia (especially in neonates). Prolongation of capillary filling time helps in early diagnosis of hemodynamic compromise than drop in arterial blood pressure. Adequacy of the peripheral perfusion can also be assessed by measuring the gradient between core and peripheral body temperatures. A gradient of more than 3°C indicates either hypoperfusion or low cardiac output.

Blood pressure may be determined non-invasively by using a sphygmomanometer either manually or by use of automated systems. Automated blood pressure monitors measure blood pressure by oscillometric method and can simultaneously measure heart rate, systolic and diastolic blood pressure and mean arterial pressure. Invasive methods rely on placement of a catheter in an artery and pressure measurement by manometer or via electronic transducers. Radial artery is the most frequent site of arterial cannulation. Adequacy of collateral blood flow to hand should be assessed in children by doing Allen's test before the radial artery cannulation. Noninvasive blood pressure monitoring may be inaccurate in children with hemodynamic instability, and critical illness. In children with hemodynamic compromise, blood pressures may not drop significantly until the compromise is severe, due to the presence of effective compensatory mechanisms which attempt to maintain tissue perfusion of vital organs (brain, heart, and kidneys) at all costs.

During physical examination variations in the intensity of the heart sounds and presence of heart murmurs may indicate underlying heart disease. Patients who have peripheral vasoconstriction may be normotensive and yet they may have a low cardiac output. Similarly patients who have peripheral vasodilatation may have a relatively low blood pressure but a clinically adequate cardiac output. In order to recognize low cardiac output state most consistently it is important to assess the combination of clinical signs like heart rate, pulse volume, capillary refill, core-peripheral temperature gradient, urine output, mental status, and additional data like arterial pressure waveforms, metabolic acidosis on blood gas analysis, mixed venous oxygenation, and blood lactate level. Young infants (<3 months), who have a rate dependent circulation with limited capacity to increase stroke volume, may show bradycardia in states of low cardiac output.

In order to detect changes in heart rate and rhythm and to identify the effects of metabolic abnormalities (hypo- or hyperkalemia, hypocalcemia, hypomagnesemia) at the earliest, continuous ECG monitoring is mandatory in critically ill children admitted to the ICU.

Central venous pressures are monitored by placing a catheter through a large vein into the right atrium which provides information about the venous return and the preload. Normal right atrial pressure is less than 6 mm Hg. If the pressures are low in a child with hypotension, it signifies a low intravascular fluid volume. On the other hand, CVP may be increased due to myocardial dysfunction, fluid overload or increased pulmonary artery pressures.

In addition to the above-mentioned monitoring parameters, a number of invasive and complex criteria are assessed in tertiary care PICUs. In pediatric patients with septic shock, maintenance of a normal cardiac index (CI) of 3.3-6.0 l/min/m^2 and normal pulmonary capillary occlusion pressure as per early goal directed therapy has been shown to be associated with improved survival[12]. In contrast to adults with septic shock, mortality in pediatric patients with septic shock is usually due to low cardiac output even among those who are adequately resuscitated with fluids. This low output state may defy early recognition because decrease in blood pressure may not always occur if the systemic vascular resistance (SVR) is high. The lowering of blood pressure may actually be due to low cardiac output, low SVR or both. A low cardiac output (CO) may occur due to many causes including inadequate vascular volume, excessive afterload, poor contractility, myocardial restriction, diastolic dysfunction, valvular stenosis/insufficiency, or an arrhythmia. Any combination of these abnormalities may coexist and severity of abnormality may fluctuate during the course of an illness, so that an appropriate therapy at one point in time may become inappropriate as the patient's clinical status may change to the better or worse. Role of cardiac monitoring encompasses assessment of the initial hemodynamic state, assessing response to therapy, and ongoing evaluation of change in the hemodynamic status as the disease progresses.

Thompson[13] has suggested that cardiac output should be measured in all critically sick children with shock, congenital and acquired heart disease, multiple organ failure, cardiopulmonary abnormalities during mechanical ventilation, and as a clinical research tool for a greater understanding of the disease process. Cardiac output can be monitored by Fick's method, indicator dilution method or by using impedance methods. Assessment of cardiac output by conventional pulmonary artery (PA) catheterization may not be possible in most centers in India. Echocardiography is a non-invasive modality to assess cardiac structure and function by using Doppler ultrasound in conjunction with 2D echocardiography. A study comparing transesophageal echocardiography with femoral artery thermodilution technique in 100 pediatric ICU patients found the former to be an effective and reliable tool to estimate cardiac output across all ages[14]. In addition to measurement of cardiac output, it can also give an assessment of indices of diastolic dysfunction, regional wall abnormalities, valvular regurgitation, pericardial effusion, chamber dilatation, and cardiac chamber interdependence. A small study of 14 patients where end-systolic wall stress analysis was done by echocardiography showed that wall-stress indices reliably detected patient deterioration, recovery, and response to changes due to dopamine infusion[15].

Mixed venous saturation decreases when either there is increase in oxygen consumption or decrease in oxygen delivery. Normal mixed venous saturation is in the range of 65 to 75%. Monitoring of mixed venous saturation is helpful in early goal directed therapy. Some of the newer techniques to measure regional perfusion are optical monitoring methods and tissue PCO_2 monitoring using tonometry. Various optical monitoring methods include laser Doppler flowmetry, near infrared spectroscopy (NIRS), orthogonal polarization spectral imaging, and peripheral perfusion index. Near infrared spectroscopy is based on the principle that by the passage of light at two different wavelengths one can detect changes in concentration of oxyhemoglobin and deoxyhemoglobin, which allows the calculation of percent oxygen saturation in the tissues. The main difficulty with NIRS is the interpretation of oxygen saturation of different regions. Moreover, the oxygen saturation may be falsely normal in certain clinical conditions like mitochondrial dysfunction and brain death.

Renal Functions

Urine output is a reliable and simple marker of renal perfusion and kidney function. Urine output of less than 0.5 ml/kg/hr in a child with normal kidneys signifies either poor renal perfusion or excessive ADH. Poor renal perfusion may be due to depletion of intravascular volume or conditions like congestive cardiac failure. It is important to follow the trends of the urine output; decreasing urine output is an important marker of worsening renal status.

Neurologic Status

The primary goals of cardio-pulmonary-cerebral resuscitation are a to ensure integrity of brain and normal functionality of the patient on recovery. Following return of spontaneous circulation, after a brief initial period of hyperemia, the cerebral blood flow is reduced ("no-reflow phenomenon") as a result of microvascular dysfunction. This reduction occurs even when cerebral perfusion pressure is normal. Neurologic support for the unresponsive patient should include measures to optimize cerebral perfusion pressure by maintaining a normal or slightly elevated mean arterial pressure and reducing intracranial pressure if it is elevated. Because both hyperthermia and seizures increase the oxygen requirements of the brain, hyperthermia should be treated promptly and seizures should be controlled effectively with anticonvulsant therapy. Patients with status epilepticus or traumatic brain injury may require continuous EEG monitoring or intracranial pressure monitoring, if facilities are available. Evidence shows that monitoring the intracranial pressure in children with severe traumatic brain injury improves the outcome. At the same time intraoperative and postoperative monitoring of children with congenital heart disease using NIRS improve their outcome. Recently there have been advances in monitoring the cerebral blood flow by different modalities like

ultrasound, tissue oxygenation, local blood flow, regional oxygenation indices and jugular venous oxygenation. Monitoring the level of sensorium and neurologic status gives useful information about the perfusion of the brain.

Monitoring of other parameters depends on the child's diagnosis and the involvement of organ systems. This would include monitoring of the hepatic, renal, hematologic and biochemical parameters depending upon the organ system involved[16].

ONGOING ASSESSEMENT AND SUPPORT

'FAST HUG'/'STABLE'

Over last few years there has been significant improvements in the quality of health care services along with reduction in medical errors by following evidence-based guidelines. Suggested mechanisms in order to reduce errors and encourage application of the latest clinical study results include implementation of protocols, checklists, and physicians' rounds. Recently a mnemonic 'FAST HUG' has been suggested as a means to identify and check some of the key parameters for the general care of critically ill patients[17]. The components include **F**eeding, **A**nalgesia, **S**edation, **T**hromboembolic prophylaxis, **H**ead-of-bed elevation, stress **U**lcer prevention, and **G**lucose control. In neonates the mnemonic 'STABLE' has been recommended which stands for **S**ugar, **T**emperature, **A**ssisted breathing, **B**lood pressure, **L**ab work, **E**motional support with primary focus on post-resuscitation and pre-transport stabilization of sick newborns.

Glucose Control

The strict maintenance of blood glucose levels between 80-110 mg/dl as recommended by Van den Berghe et al[18] may be difficult to achieve in routine patient care, but it may be feasible to keep blood glucose levels below 150 mg/dl. Another study by the same authors showed that short-term hyperglycemia in the intial phase may be helpful but prolonged hyperglycemia is detrimental[19]. It has been documented that hyperglycemia is common in critically ill children and the peak blood glucose level and the duration of hyperglycemia are independently associated with increased mortality in PICU[20-24]. While further large scale studies (Glucontrol study and NICE-SUGAR study) are awaited, it is recommended to monitor blood glucose regularly in critically ill children and maintain the blood glucose levels below 150 mg/dl. Vlasselaers et al studied the beneficial effects of targeting age adjusted normoglycemia with insulin infusions in critically ill infants and children on outcome[25]. Normoglycemia protected the cardiovascular system, prevented secondary infections, and attenuated inflammatory response, reducing the overall length of stay in ICU. The approach reduced mortality by absolute 3.1% (95% CI 0.2–6.0)[25]. In view of the available evidence, it is beneficial to monitor blood glucose regularly in critically ill children and maintain blood glucose levels below 150 mg/dL; at the same time, it is essential to prevent hypoglycemia. If the blood glucose levels are consistently above 180 mg/dL despite reduction of glucose infusion rates, insulin infusion may be considered.

Pressure Sores

In a prospective study, 27% of PICU patients developed pressure ulcers[26]. The patients at high risk are those supported on mechanical ventilation (especially with high PEEP) and with hypotension. Other risk factors are malnutrition, coma, sensory loss, dependent edema and length of stay above 96 hours. The extrinsic risk factors involved in tissue damage include pressure, shearing and friction. It is important to examine the skin regularly in all children admitted to the PICU. The following maneuvers should not be used as pressure relieving aids i.e. water filled gloves; synthetic or genuine sheepskins and doughnut-type devices. Children who are 'at risk' of development of pressure ulcers should be repositioned frequently depending upon the results of skin inspection and individual needs of the patient and not by a ritualistic schedule. The preventive strategies include adequate nutrition, use of alternating pressure mattresses or other high-technology pressure redistributing systems[27].

Eye Care

In children admitted to ICU abnormalities of the cornea and conjunctiva have been reported in nearly a quarter of patients[28]. The risk factors for corneal erosions include patient's inability to fully close the eyes and use of neuromuscular blocking agents[29]. These complications occur frequently in association with neurological diseases, nocturnal lagophthalmos, coma, infection, and mechanical ventilation. It is beneficial to use lubricating ointments and artificial tears to keep the corneal and conjunctival surfaces wet. In addition, protective eyelid taping is effective in preventing and treating the corneal erosion.

Oral Hygiene

Oropharyngeal colonization is of paramount importance in the pathogenesis of ventilator-associated pneumonia, and prevention of colonization at this site is an effective method for prevention of infection. Several studies have documented benefits of selective oral decontamination in adults but similar studies are not available in children[30-32]. Maintenance of oral hygiene is frequently neglected in critically ill children. Surveys performed in the US and UK suggested that oral care methods in sick children were not consistent with current research and oral care protocols[33, 34]. Results of a prospective study in a British PICU revealed a highly significant increase in plaque accumulation and gingival inflammation between admission to the PICU and discharge[35]. The authors concluded that the prevailing mouth care regimen was not effective in preventing the build up of plaque or maintaining gingival health, thus placing these children at unnecessary risk from local or systemic spread of oral microorganisms. The preventive measures should include regular cleaning of the oral cavity especially in intubated children. Use of chlorhexidine based oral hygiene products may be beneficial.

Prevention of Stress Ulcers

Critically ill patients are at risk of developing stress ulcers in the stomach. Prophylaxis against stress ulcers has been recommended for the prevention of upper gastrointestinal bleeding in critically ill adult patients. Various risk factors for upper gastrointestinal bleeding in critically ill children include thrombocytopenia, prolonged partial thromboplastin time, organ failure, mechanical ventilation and high pressure ventilator settings and severity of illness[36, 37]. Recently, a systematic review and meta-analysis found limited high-quality data to recommend routine use of stress ulcer prophylaxis[38]. Till more evidence is available, stress ulcer prophylaxis using ranitidine, sucralfate, or proton-pump inhibitors may be instituted in children with multiple risk factors for development of stress ulcers.

Thromboembolic Prophylaxis

Venous thromboembolism is being increasingly recognized in the pediatric age group[39]. Children in intensive care unit are at increased risk of venous thromboembolism, either due to the underlying disease or selected therapeutic interventions. Presence of central venous catheter is most common risk factor for venous thromboembolism. Standard unfractionated heparin remains the mainstay of therapy and prophylaxis; but low molecular weight heparins are being increasingly used[40]. Thrombolytic therapy is reserved only for severe, life-threatening, acute thrombosis. There is lack of data on pediatric ICU patients to define clearly the 'at-risk' group and to administer the most 'effective medication'. Also, the benefit of prophylaxis must be weighed against the risk of bleeding complications. The Surviving Sepsis Campaign guidelines recommend the use of deep venous thrombosis (DVT) prophylaxis in all post pubertal children with severe sepsis[41].

Care of Intravenous Lines, Central Lines, Chest Tubes, and PD Catheters

All patients with an IV cannula must be examined at least once per shift for any signs of infusion phlebitis. The cannula site must also be observed whenever bolus injections are administered, IV flow rates are checked or altered and when solution containers are changed. A visual infusion phlebitis (VIP) scale has been devised for objective assessment of the IV sites and appropriate intervention[42] (Table 8.3). The peripheral IV cannula should be replaced at the first indication of infusion phlebitis i.e. stage 2 of VIP score.

Central venous lines and arterial lines are important adjuncts for monitoring and management of children in the intensive care. They should be observed regularly for displacement, bleeding, patency, infection and hematoma at the insertion site. They should preferably be removed as soon as they are no longer necessary and always when a patient develops fever with no other obvious focus of infection.

Chest drains should be assessed periodically for movement of fluid column, amount and nature of drainage, displacement, breath sounds, and for any evidence of subcutaneous emphysema. Peritoneal dialysis catheters should be inserted following thorough asepsis routine, and during the peritoneal dialysis patency and flow rate should be monitored regularly. After completion of dialysis, catheter should be removed as early as possible and the peritoneal dialysis fluid and catheter tip should be sent for culture to look for infection.

Care of a Child with Special Needs

Children with neurologic and neuromuscular disorders have special needs as they are more prone to recurrent aspiration, have poor cough and airway clearance, and may have significant respiratory muscle weakness requiring prolonged ventilatory support and chest physiotherapy. They may require prolonged respiratory support even after extubation, either with nasal mask CPAP or Bi-PAP or tracheostomy. They need regular monitoring of strength of respiratory muscles and lung functions to identify worsening of respiratory status early before they reach the threshold of respiratory failure. They also require special emphasis on nutritional support, regular changing of position and physiotherapy for prevention of contractures and

Table 8.3 Visual infusion phlebitis (VIP) score			
Score	**Features**	**Interpretation**	**Action**
0	Site appears healthy	No signs of phlebitis	Observe cannula
1	**One** of the following is present: slight pain, slight redness	Possible early signs of phlebitis	Observe cannula
2	**Two** of the following are present: pain at iv site, swelling, erythema	Early stage of phlebitis	Remove cannula and change site
3	**All** of the following signs are evident: pain along the path of cannula, induration, and erythema	Medium stage phlebitis	Remove cannula, change site, consider treatment
4	**All** the following are evident and are **extensive**: pain along the path of cannula, induration, palpable venous cord, and erythema	Advanced stage phlebitis	Remove cannula, change site, consider treatment
5	**All** the following are evident and are extensive: Pain along the path of cannula, induration, erythema, palpable venous cord, and **pyrexia**	Advanced stage thrombophlebitis	Remove cannula, change site, initiate treatment

pressure sores. Children with Duchenne muscular dystrophy have sleep disordered breathing and alveolar hypoventilation in addition to underlying cardiac dysfunction which constitutes the second most common cause of death in these children.

NUTRITION OF CRITICALLY ILL CHILD

It is essential to provide adequate nutrition during the course of severe illness in order to improve the outcome as malnutrition increases risk of complications. Many children are already malnourished on admission to the ICU and need adequate and appropriate nutritional support. Unfortunately, there is no specific and reliable laboratory marker of nutritional status. At is not practical to perform indirect calorimetry on all patients, but a clinical assessment including measurement of weight loss is very reliable. It has been observed that children admitted to the ICU accumulate substantial energy and protein deficits which are related to decrease in their anthropometric parameters[43].

Stress leads to increase in resting energy expenditure, proteolysis, gluconeogenesis, urinary nitrogen loss, glucose intolerance and resistance to insulin. In addition there is increased protein breakdown or tissue catabolism which is not entirely suppressed by protein and energy intake. There is also a reprioritization of protein synthesis with an increase in the synthesis of acute phase proteins and decreased production of structural body proteins and an overall increased protein turnover. Provision of glucose alone does not suppress 'auto-cannibalism'. Earlier, children in the PICU were fed according to the predicted energy expenditure (PEE) which was extrapolated from the nomograms of healthy children, leading to overestimation of caloric needs. But studies using indirect calorimetry show that provision of calories in accordance with the resting energy expenditure (REE) may be more physiological[44].

The REE is variable among different patient populations depending upon the degree of illness, level of sedation, analgesia and neuromuscular blockade. Therefore, in order to avoid the complications of delivery of excess calories (like hyperglycemia, hyperinsulinemia, hepatic steatosis) in the initial unstable resuscitative phase of child's illness, 'permissive hypocaloric nutritional support' is recommended with typical caloric intakes ranging from 20-30 kcal/kg/day. In a study on 57 critically ill children, the median resting energy expenditure measured by indirect calorimetry was 37.2 (range 11.9-66.6) kcal/kg/day[45]. However, once the

recovery phase sets in and it is clear that inefficient metabolism has ceased, the caloric supply may be increased to hypercaloric level to promote tissue growth and healing.

Enteral Feeds

Provided the intestines are functioning, enteral route is the preferred one. It is safer and more cost-effective than total parenteral nutrition (TPN). Enteral nutrition also helps in maintaining the gut barrier and reduces the risk of bacteremia and pneumonia[46]. Possible disadvantages of enteral nutrition include exacerbation of gastro-esophageal reflux, risk of aspiration, bacterial overgrowth, and complications related to the feeding tube (necrosis of nasal septum, sinusitis or rarely bowel perforation) or due to its misplacement (esophagitis and esophageal ulceration). Diarrhea may occur because of hyperosmolar formula, infection, or malabsorption. Severely malnourished children and those who haven't received any other form of nutritional support but are given high caloric loads are at increased risk for the development of re-feeding syndrome which is characterized by hyperglycemia, hypokalemia, hypomagnesemia, and hypophosphatemia. Contraindications for enteral nutrition include severe gastrointestinal hemorrhage, recent GI surgery, intestinal obstruction, necrotizing enterocolitis, and severe vomiting or diarrhea.

Intermittent and continuous gastric feeding regimens have been shown to have similar outcomes with respect to the number of stools per day and the prevalence of diarrhea and vomiting in pediatric intensive care patients[47]. Gastroduodenal hypomotility and the presence of a feeding tube at the lower esophageal sphincter may increase the risk of reflux and aspiration in critically ill patients[48]. In children where decreased gut motility is anticipated, such as children on vasoactive agents, neuromuscular blockade, or those with recent major insult (surgery or trauma), nasoduodenal or transpyloric feeding may be considered. Small-bowel feeds may allow a greater amount of nutrition to be successfully delivered to critically ill children but they do not prevent aspiration of gastric contents[49]. A variety of techniques for placing tubes beyond the pylorus have been described including the use of stylets, weighted tube tips, magnets, mechanical manipulations of the tube during placement, and prokinetic drugs including metoclopramide and erythromycin. Small-bowel feeding tubes also have been successfully placed using fluoroscopy or endoscopy, but not without added radiation exposure and/or cost. Patients who have undergone extensive facial or skull trauma or surgery, placement of percutaneous endoscopic gastrostomy (PEG) tube is a viable option for initiation of enteral feeds.

Elemental and non-elemental diets are available. The simplest kind of feed is a milk based feed. The elemental formulae contain carbohydrates as oligosaccharides, maltodextrins or hydrolyzed corn starch; nitrogen as peptides or free amino acid and lipids as various oils or medium-chain triglycerides. In addition, special formulae are also available e.g. low-lactose or lactose-free and gluten-free diets. For children with pulmonary disorders (especially poor ventilatory reserve), it may be preferable to use a formula high in fat, as high carbohydrate content is associated with increased CO_2 production. Similarly for patients with hepatic failure, medium chain triglyceride based formulas are preferred to improve fat absorption. For patients with renal failure it is best to individualize the type and amount of feeds, based on the severity of renal dysfunction and the effectiveness of ongoing renal replacement therapy. Protein intake may be restricted to 0.5-1.0 g/kg/day to suppress catabolism. In infants or neonates who are undergoing dialysis, protein intake may be further liberalized to 1.5-2.0 g/kg/day. Branched chain amino acids have been shown to be of benefit in patients with liver failure and ARDS.

Enteral feeds may be delivered directly into the stomach through nasogastric or orogastric tube. Start with 10-15 ml/kg/d of feeds and increase by 10-15 ml/kg/d till target calories are achieved. It is preferable to advance dilute formula to full strength before advancing the rate of infusion. Supplementation of vitamins and minerals is also important. Even during insertion of transpyloric tube, a single dose of oral or IV erythromycin can facilitate the propagation of the tube tip into the small intestine. However, some pediatric studies have not found any benefit with use of erythromycin[50].

Residual volumes should be checked prior to each feed and the next feed should be withheld if the volume of aspirate is greater than half of the volume of the previous feed. The results of study by Horn et al[51] provided some support for the theoretical definition of delayed gastric emptying when gastric aspirate exceeds 5ml/kg. For continuous transpyloric tube feeding, it is necessary to check residuals every 4 hourly and intolerance should be suspected when the child develops abdominal distension, diarrhea or constipation. It may be necessary to hold the feeds in the latter method if the residual gastric volume is greater than the volume infused during the last two hours.

Total Parenteral Nutrition (TPN)

Parenteral nutrition refers to the delivery of all the nutrients directly into the blood stream; amino acid mixture, lipids, glucose, and trace minerals and vitamins[52]. These may be infused into a peripheral or central vein. The use of peripheral veins is limited by the osmolality of infusate (should be <800 mOsm/l). Therefore, in order to ensure delivery of adequate calories, central venous access is essential. Glucose infusion is started at a rate of 5-6 mg/kg/minute and increased gradually; insulin may be used if there is hyperglycemia. Amino acids are begun at 1g/kg/d; then increased over 2-3 days to 2.5 g/kg/d. Lipids are infused at a rate of 0.5 g/kg on day 1 and increased to 2.0-2.5 g/kg/d over 4-5 days. Appropriate combinations can be achieved on the basis of fluid requirements. Trace elements and vitamin supplements are added.

Use of TPN requires monitoring blood glucose three times a day; serum electrolytes and blood urea twice a week; and serum chemistry, triglycerides, and complete blood counts once a week. Weight is recorded daily, while other anthropometric measurements are recorded once a week. The complications include catheter related infections, liver dysfunction, hyperglycemia, hyperlipidemia, acidosis, and electrolyte imbalance.

Early institution of enteral feeds is desirable as soon as gut function improves. There is growing evidence that TPN is systemically immuno-suppressive and non-use of GI tract not only leads to suppression of GALT and disuse atrophy of gastrointestinal mucosa but also suppresses the immune protection of other epithelial surfaces such as respiratory and genitourinary tracts. Thus there is emergence of the concept of "Total splanchnic resuscitation" which combines the practice of minimal enteral nutrition along with the use of immunonutrients[53].

Immunonutrition

The use of immunonutrients like glutamine, arginine, ω-3 fatty acids, nucleotides, taurine, cysteine, certain complex carbohydrates and probiotics has been demonstrated to modulate gut function, inflammatory and immune responses. Use of immunonutrition has been shown to reduce the length of ICU and hospital stay and decrease the risk of infectious complications in critically ill patients. There is evidence to support use of immunonutrition in critically ill patients, especially adults[54-57]. However, a recent trial comparing the mortality of critically ill adult patients given either enteral feeding with an immune-enhancing formula or parenteral nutrition was terminated after the interim analysis showed that enteral immuno-nutrition, compared to parenteral nutrition, may be associated with excess mortality in patients with severe sepsis[58]. In a systematic review on the utility of immune-modulating diets in critically ill, no consistent benefits were observed[59]. In view of the paucity of data in children use of the immuno-nutrition products is questionable.

SEDATION, ANALGESIA AND PARALYSIS

The goal of sedation is safe and effective control of pain, anxiety, and stress so as to allow a necessary procedure to be performed and to provide appropriate amnesia or decreased aware-ness. The management of acute pain and anxiety in children undergoing therapeutic and diagnostic procedures outside the operating theater has improved substantially over the last 25 years[60-62]. The need for sedation and analgesia is significantly higher in intensive care units. Relatively few units possess clinical guidelines for the sedation of critically ill children, and minority of them formally assesses sedation levels. Where neuromuscular blocking agents are administered, sedation is frequently inadequately assessed and the depth of neuromuscular blockade is rarely estimated.

The American Society of Anesthesiologists (ASA) has issued guidelines for administration of sedation by non-anesthesiologists and has defined four levels of sedation[63]. The state of sedation varies along a continuum, ranging from anxiolysis to moderate sedation to deep sedation to general anesthesia. *Minimal sedation (Anxiolysis)* is a drug-induced state during which patients respond normally to verbal commands. Although cognitive functions and coordination may be impaired, ventilatory and cardiovascular functions are unaffected. *Moderate sedation/analgesia ("Conscious sedation")* is a drug-induced depression of consciousness during which patients respond purposefully to verbal commands, either alone or accompanied by light tactile stimulation. No interventions are required to maintain a patent airway, and spontaneous ventilation is adequate. Cardiovascular functions are usually maintained. *Deep sedation/analgesia* is a drug-induced depression of consciousness during which patients cannot be easily aroused but respond purposefully following repeated or painful stimulation. The ability to independently maintain ventilatory function may be impaired. Patients may require assistance in maintaining a patent airway, and spontaneous ventilation may be inadequate. Cardiovascular function is usually maintained. *General anesthesia* is a drug-induced loss of consciousness during which patients are not arousable, even by painful stimulation. The ability to independently maintain ventilatory function is often impaired. Patients often require assistance in maintaining a patent airway, and positive pressure ventilation may be required because of depressed spontaneous ventilation or drug-induced depression of neuromuscular function. Cardiovascular functions may be impaired.

Table 8.4 ASA physical status of the patient before sedation[63]			
Class	**Description**	**Example**	**Sedation suitability**
1	Healthy patient	Unremarkable past medical history	Excellent
2	Patient with mild systemic disease and no functional limitation	Mild asthma, controlled seizure disorder, anemia, controlled diabetes mellitus	Generally good
3	Patient with severe systemic disease with definite functional limitation	Moderate to severe asthma, poorly controlled seizure disorder, pneumonia, poorly controlled diabetes mellitus, moderate obesity	Intermediate to poor. Consider benefits relative to risks
4	Patient with severe systemic disease that is constant threat to life	Severe bronchopulmonary dysplasia, sepsis, advanced stage of pulmonary, cardiac, hepatic, renal, or endocrine insufficiency	Poor; benefits rarely outweigh risks
5	Moribund patient who is not expected to survive without the procedure or operation	Septic shock, severe trauma	Extremely poor

Presedation assessment

The child should be carefully assessed before sedation. This includes evaluation of underlying medical problems, medication use, allergies and time and nature of last oral intake. For safe sedation, it is mandatory to have skilled personnel capable of rapidly identifying and treating cardio-respiratory complications. This includes evaluation of underlying medical problems, medication use, allergies and time and nature of last oral intake[63]. Table 8.4 summarizes ASA classification of physical status as part of presedation evaluation.

Monitoring

During sedation child's face, mouth and movement of chest wall must be continuously observed. The vital signs should be documented before, after the administration of the drugs, on completion of the procedure, during recovery and at discharge from the hospital. ECG monitoring and pulse oximetry are useful adjuncts. The sedation and procedure room should have all the essential equipment for airway management and the physicians performing procedures under moderate to deep sedation must be proficient at handling airway emergencies.

There are several scoring systems to monitor the depth of sedation and effectiveness of analgesia including the COMFORT scale for pediatric patients[64]. However, these scales do not provide continuous measurements and are subject to significant intra-observer and inter-observer variations. In addition these scores do not differentiate between manifestations of lack of sedation due to delirium or due to pain. Due to these limitations there has been a shift in focus towards use of objective electrophysiologic measures like processed EEG and auditory evoked potentials, in order to monitor level of sedation. The changes in bispectral index have been used for the assessment of depth of sedation[65]. In the absence of BIS, the level of sedation of chemically paralyzed pediatric patients can be better guided by changes in mean arterial pressure (MAP) than heart rate, particularly in patients receiving vasoactive drugs[66]. Table 8.5 lists various clinical scenarios requiring sedation and analgesia.

Table 8.6 summarizes the details of commonly used drugs for sedation and analgesia. For children undergoing mechanical ventilation, continuous infusion of midazolam or diazepam may be used for better control of ventilation. In addition, intermittent doses or continuous infusion of fentanyl or morphine may be used for pain control.

Neuromuscular Blocking Drugs

The use of neuromuscular blocking drugs (NMBD) is common in intensive care units[67]. A large number of drugs are now available to tailor a regimen to child's specific needs. Succinyl choline is the only depolarizing muscle relaxant available. The non-depolarizing drugs include pancuronium, atracurium, vecuronium, doxacurium, mivacurium and rocuronium. Short-acting drugs include succinylcholine and mivacurium; intermediate acting drugs are atracurium, vecuronium and rocuronium while long-acting drugs are pancuronium and doxacurium. NMBDs must always be administered after adequate sedation has been achieved because they do not have any analgesic or sedative effect. The major indications for use of NMBDs in intensive care units are to prevent asynchronous patient ventilator interactions. However with improved ventilator techniques and development of ventilators that can synchronize with child's own inspiratory

Table 8.5 Indications for sedation and analgesia for various procedures		
Procedure	**Examples**	**Sedation strategy**
Non-invasive procedures	CT, echocardiography, EEG, MRI, ultrasonography	Comfort and reassurance to older children. Chloral hydrate PO, triclofos PO, midazolam IV
Procedures associated with low intensity of pain but high anxiety level	Intravenous cannulations, phlebotomy, lumbar puncture, flexible fiberoptic bronchoscopy	Comforting and local anesthesia
Procedures associated with high level of pain and anxiety	Central catheter placement, bone marrow aspiration, endoscopy, abscess- incision and drainage, interventional radiology procedures, intercostal drainage, paracentesis.	Midazolam and fentanyl/morphine IV, ketamine IV or IM

Table 8.6 Commonly used medications for sedation and analgesia

	Drug	Clinical effects	Dose	Onset of action	Duration of action
Sedatives					
1.	Chloral hydrate	Sedation, anxiolysis	25-100 mg/kg PO, maximum dose 2 g	15-30 min	60-120 min
2.	Triclofos	Sedation, no analgesia	20-100 mg/kg PO	30-45 min	4- 6 hours
3.	Midazolam	Sedation, anxiolysis, no analgesia	0.05 mg-0.1 mg/kg IV and adjusted upto 0.4-0.6 mg/kg Infusion: 1- 10 µg/kg/min IV	2-3 min	45- 60 min
4.	Diazepam	Sedation, anxiolysis	0.2- 0.3 mg/ kg IV Infusion: 0.1-0.5 mg/kg/ hr	2-5 min	60-120 min
5.	Lorazepam	Sedation	0.05-0.1 mg/ kg IV Infusion: 0.025-0.05 mg/kg/hr		
6.	Propofol	Sedation, no analgesia	2-3 mg/kg IV Infusion: 5-10 mg/kg/hr	1 min	5-20 min
7.	Dexmedetomidine	Sedation	0.3- 1 mcg/kg IV Infusion: 0.25-0.7 mcg/kg/hr	<1 min	5-15 min
8.	Phenobarbitone	Sedation, no analgesia	5–10 mg/kg IV		
9.	Pentobarbital	Sedation, no analgesia	0.5-1 mg/kg IV Infusion: 1-2 mg/kg/hr IV		
10.	Ketamine	Dissociative anesthesia, analgesia	1-2 mg/kg IV Infusion: 1-2 mg/kg//hr	1-2 min	15-60 min
11.	Thiopentone	Sedation, no analgesia	3–5 mg/kg IV	<1min	10-45 min
Analgesics					
1.	Morphine	Analgesia, sedation	0.1 mg/kg IV		
2.	Fentanyl	Analgesia	1 µg/kg/ dose, may be repeated every 3 min Infusion: 1- 5 ug/ kg/hr	2- 3 min	30- 60 min
3.	Remifentanil	Sedation, analgesia	0.05-0.1 µg/kg/min IV	1-2 min	4-5 min
4.	Ketamine	Dissociative anesthesia, analgesia	1-1.5 mg/kg IV over 1- 2 min 3- 5 mg/kg IM	1-2 min 3- 5 min	15- 60 min 15-150 min

efforts have reduced the need for use of NMBDs. But they may also be required for patients undergoing relatively uncomfortable ventilatory strategies like use of high PEEP, permissive hypercapnia or prone ventilation. Different indications for use of NMBDs are summarized in Table 8.7.

Table 8.8 summarizes the characteristics and doses of various neuromuscular blocking drugs. Children receiving neuromuscular blocking drugs should be monitored very carefully. Particular attention should be paid to the position of artificial airway and adequacy of ventilation. Unlike sedation, it is possible to objectively monitor the depth of neuromuscular blockade using a peripheral nerve stimulator to adjust the dose of neuromuscular blocking drug. Prolonged usage of NMBDs can cause muscle atrophy and joint contractures which can be reduced by passive movements and splinting of joints in functional position. Pressure sores and skin ulcers are likely to develop because of

Table 8.7 Indications for use of neuromuscular blocking drugs

Short term
1. Facilitation of airway instrumentation
2. Facilitation of invasive procedures

Long term
1. Facilitation of mechanical ventilation, to overcome patient-ventilation dyssynchrony, and to facilitate ventilation at high settings especially in patients in whom sedation alone is ineffective in providing necessary condition for effective mechanical ventilation.
2. Reduction of work of breathing/metabolic demand.
3. Treatment of agitation, unresponsive to maximum sedation and analgesia provided the airway has been protected and patient is on respiratory support.
4. Treatment of tetanus.
5. Facilitation of treatment of status epilepticus under continuous EEG monitoring.

immobilization and impaired skin perfusion. Absence of eye blink may lead to corneal drying and abrasions. This can be avoided by use of lubricating ointment and artificial tears and gentle closing of the eyelid. If a child is receiving NMBDs, he/she should simultaneously receive a sedative and analgesic for overcoming anxiety and pain. Some children experience prolonged muscle weakness after discontinuation of NMBD (critical illness myopathy). Use of succinylcholine may lead to vagal-mediated bradycardia, sinus arrest or functional rhythms; larger doses may lead to tachycardia, ventricular arrhythmias and hypertension.

NOSOCOMIAL INFECTIONS

Nosocomial (hospital acquired infections or health care associated infections) are those infections that occur during a patient's stay in the hospital and are not present or incubating at the time of admission[68]. Also any infection that appears to have been acquired in the hospital but does not manifest until after discharge is also judged to be a nosocomial infection. Therefore, all infections diagnosed 48 hours after admission till 72 hours after discharge should be considered as nosocomial in origin.

Nosocomial infections are a significant problem in pediatric intensive care units. The increased risk of infection is accounted for both due to greater severity of the underlying disease process and greater opportunities for the infection because of frequent interventions and use of devices that bypass natural barriers to infection. The estimated rate of nosocomial infection is 10-20 infections per 1000 patient days for pediatric ICUs. The overall nosocomial infection rates in the PICUs are reported to be 6-10%[69, 70]. These rates are lower than those seen in adult intensive care units. The primary blood stream infections are the commonest nosocomial infections (25- 30%) in PICUs followed by the lower respiratory tract infections (20- 25%) and urinary tract infection (15-20%). In adults, UTI is the commonest nosocomial infection followed by post surgical infections and lower respiratory tract infections. *Staphylococcous aureus*, coagulase negative staphylococci, *E.coli*, *Pseudomonas aeruginosa*, Klebseilla, enterococci and Candida are the common pathogens in pediatric ICU.

The risk of nosocomial infection in a PICU is direct consequence of the severity of illness, the level of invasive monitoring, the indiscriminate use of antimicrobials and the nature of diagnostic procedures. The duration of stay in an ICU is an important determinant of nosocomial infection. The use of invasive devices (endotracheal tubes,

Table 8.8 Characteristics and doses of neuromuscular blocking drugs

Drug	Intubation dose (mg/kg)	Onset of action (min)	Duration (min)	Infusion rate (μg/kg/min)
Pancuronium	0.1	2-5	60-120	-
Atracurium	0.1	1-3	30-45	0.4-4
Vecuronium	0.1	1-3	45-90	1
Rocuronium	0.6-1.2	1-3	35-75	3-10
Doxacurium	0.06	4-6	90-150	-
Mivacurium	0.2-0.3	2-3	15-20	3-15
Succinyl choline	1-2	0.5-1	4-5	-

intravascular catheters, urinary catheters) has an important role in development of nosocomial infections. It is observed that about 90% of all blood stream infections occurred in children with central venous lines, 95% of nosocomial pneumonias occurred in those on mechanical ventilation and 75% of UTIs in children with urinary catheters. These figures highlight the role of various devices in the incidence of nosocomial infections.

Nosocomial infections may be caused by organisms that originate from exogenous sources in the hospital or from endogenous sources such as child's own flora. The hospital environment may contribute to acquisition and spread of most endemic nosocomial infections. Even if only environmental surfaces are contaminated with microbes, they can be spread to patients by hand contact. Because of alteration of child's flora associated with the illness and hospitalization, such distinction may not be easy. The altered flora mainly includes Gram-negative bacilli and *Staphylococcus aureus*, which are often resistant to antibiotics. It is estimated that the overall mortality attributed to nosocomial infections is about 10%. Blood stream infections caused by *Klebsiella pneumoniae* or the fungi have mortality risk of 18-20%. The nosocomial infections increase the duration of stay in the hospital and hence cost of therapy.

Strategies to Reduce the Incidence of Nosocomial Infections

For reducing the incidence of nosocomial infections, each PICU should have an infection control program. There should be a written description of the goals, objectives, and structure of the program. Adequate and well trained staff, both nursing staff and physicians, is essential for infection control. Education of the staff about various infection control practices and procedure-specific guidelines has an important role in the reduction of incidence of nosocomial infections. The education program should be on a continuing basis with periodic evaluation of the knowledge and practices. A team of health care professionals should ensure implementation of the policies and compliance on the part of the PICU team. Well-directed infection control activities can reduce the nosocomial infection rates by upto 50%[71].

The policy of hand washing and hand disinfection is of fundamental importance. The appropriate hand washing technique includes wetting the hands, taking soap, rubbing hands to produce a lather, and performing wash movements that include rubbing palm to palm, right palm over left dorsum and *vice versa*, palm to palm with fingers interlocked, backs of fingers to opposing palm with fingers interlocked, rotational rubbing of right thumb clasped in left palm and *vice versa*, rotational rubbing with clasped fingers of right hand in palm of left hand and with changed roles. The whole procedure should not take less than 30 seconds. After washing, hands should be dried with disposable paper or cloth towel. In order to improve compliance, various hygienic hand rubs can be used. Rubbing of 3-5 ml of a fast acting antiseptic preparation on both the hands can be an effective substitute to hand washing. The various preparations available include n-propanol, isopropanol, ethanol, and chlorhexidine diacetate. For various medical devices, proper sterilization/disinfection should be ensured as recommended by the manufacturers; single use devices should not be reused. Aseptic precautions should be followed strictly whenever any invasive procedure is being carried out.

Surveillance of nosocomial infections is an essential element of any infection control program. The most important goal of surveillance is to reduce the risk of acquiring nosocomial infections. This provides useful data for identifying infected patients, determining the site of infection and identifying the factors that contribute to nosocomial infections. Control measures can be evaluated objectively if the surveillance is good.

Specific preventive measures

Prevention of nosocomial pneumonias[68]. The colonization of upper airways by pathogenic microbes and thereby, the risk of nosocomial pneumonia can be reduced by several measures including effective hand washing, chlorhexidine or alcohol containing rubs. The reduction in the number of microorganisms on hands is related to the volume and number of times the antiseptic hand rubs are used. In addition, the hospital workers should comply with hospital infection control policies.

The gastrointestinal tract is an important source for endogenous upper airway colonization. Use of antacids and H_2 blockers raise gastric pH and facilitate gastric microbial colonization. When indicated, instead of H_2 blockers and antacids, sucralfate may be used for prophylaxis against gastric bleeding as the gastric pH remains low with its use. The use of selective decontamination of the gut using antimicrobial such as tobramycin, gentamicin, polymyxin and nystatin is controversial and is not recommended.

Contaminated respiratory therapy equipments have been implicated in nosocomial pneumonias.

Resuscitation bags, ventilator tubings, and nebulizers should be disinfected. Only sterile fluids should be used for nebulization or for use in humidifiers. Personnel taking care of intubated children should wash their hands before and after delivering care. The ventilator circuit tubings should be changed every 48 hours. Care should be taken to prevent contamination during suctioning. Positioning of patients with head end elevation does reduce the risk of aspiration and nosocomial pneumonia.

Prevention of blood stream infections[69]. The major factors associated with development of catheter-related nosocomial infections include (i) the sterility of the technique of insertion and maintenance of the catheter throughout its life, (ii) type of solution being administered through the intravenous line, (iii) number of "break ins" into the catheter system and intravenous tubing, and (iv) the presence of infection elsewhere in the body. The following measures may help in reducing catheter-related infections:

(a) Selection of subclavian, basilic or cephalic vein site rather then femoral or internal jugular vein.
(b) Using maximal aseptic technique for catheter "insertion"
(c) Using cotton gauze rather than transparent dressing.
(d) Having an experienced physician to insert the catheter.
(e) Avoiding the use of TPN catheters for non TPN infusion.
(f) Having adequate staff for management of patients with central venous catheters.

Prevention of urinary tract infections[70, 71]. Urinary catheterization should be kept to a minimum. The need for catheterization must be strictly evaluated and it should be replaced by closed condom drainage whenever possible. Strict asepsis should be maintained during insertion of the catheter using sterile gloves, drapes, and local antiseptics. The catheter should be removed as soon as its purpose has been fulfilled. Closed drainage must be strictly maintained and this has been shown to bring down the rates of infection. The closed drainage must be maintained with the help of a collection tubing and bag kept below the level of the patient's bladder and the tubing must always be above the level of the bag. When in place the closed drainage system must be handled and manipulated as infrequently as possible. Antibiotic prophylaxis does reduce the frequency of infections but is not universally recommended as it may lead to emergence of multidrug resistant strains of pathogens.

A number of new innovative technologies are available to reduce the risk of nosocomial infections, various studies have demonstrated efficacy and cost-effectiveness of simple, non-technologic and educational approaches in reduction of nosocomial infections[72, 73].

BLOOD COMPONENT THERAPY

Blood component transfusion is an integral part of the treatment plan of many children managed in ICU. Blood products are prepared from either collected whole blood or by apheresis. Donated whole blood units can be separated into red blood cells, plasma and platelet components by differential centrifugation. Automated apheresis procedures can be used to collect platelets, granulocytes or plasma only from donor. Cryoprecipitate can be prepared from a plasma unit. Plasma proteins such as albumin, anti-D immune serum globulins, immunoglobulins and concentrated coagulation factors are prepared by processing of large pools of donor plasma obtained from whole blood or plasmapheresis donations.

Donor blood must be screened for HIV, hepatitis B surface antigen, antibodies to hepatitis C, syphilis and malaria. For immunocompromised recipients, it is necessary to ensure that blood products are CMV-negative or irradiated prior to transfusion.

Red Blood Cell Transfusion

Red cell suspensions containing 150-200 ml of red cells with minimal plasma along with a mixture of normal saline, adenine, glucose and mannitol (SAG-M) are used specifically to reduce transfusion reactions caused by donor hemolysins. Units prepared in CPDA-1 usually have a 35 day shelf life with a hematocrit of 70-80%. The indications for RBC transfusion are listed in Table 8.9.

In practice, the available data suggest that all critically ill children with hemoglobin concentration below 5 g/dL should receive an RBC transfusion but if the hemoglobin is above 7 g/dL the transfusion can be withheld. Other factors that should be taken into consideration for blood transfusion other than hemoglobin concentration are age, severity of illness, significant cardiovascular disease, organ dysfunction, and comorbid conditions like sickle cell disease, hemolytic uremic syndrome, and thalassemia.

Table 8.9 Indications for transfusion of RBCs[74, 75]

Neonates and infants

1. Asymptomatic infant with hematocrit ≤20% and reticulocytes <100,000/cu mm.
2. Infant with hematocrit ≤30% and requiring oxygen <35%; CPAP or mechanical ventilation; and significant apnea or bradycardia; heart rate >180/min or respiratory rate >80/min persisting for >24 hours; or weight gain <10 g/day observed over 4 days while on ≥100 cal/kg/d or undergoing surgery.
3. Infant with hematocrit ≤35% if receiving oxygen >35% or on mechanical ventilation.
4. Acute blood loss >10% of blood volume.

Older children

1. Hemoglobin 4 g/dl or less (Hematocrit 12%) irrespective of the clinical status.
2. Hemoglobin 4-6 g/dl (Hematocrit 13-18%) with features of hypoxia, acidosis, altered consciousness, hyperparasitemia in malaria (>20%) and presence of cardiac decompensation.

Transfusion for chronic anemia

Children with chronic anemia usually tolerate hemoglobin levels as low as 4 g/dl and the underlying cause of anemia should be diagnosed for specific management of the patient. The patient should be investigated and examined for any evidence of abnormal physical signs of cardiovascular decompensation. Along with blood transfusion the definitive therapy should also be given to improve the outcome and reduce the need for further transfusions.

Transfusion for acute blood loss

If a patient is not stabilized after 2 boluses of 20 ml/kg of isotonic crystalloid solution and the suspected blood loss is >10% whole blood can be rapidly infused for acute blood loss. Usually stored whole blood is deficient in Factor VIII and Factor V and in patient with active bleeding these factors might have to be transfused.

Amount of transfusion

The quantity of blood transfused depends on the hematocrit of RBC unit, pretransfusion hemoglobin level and patient's weight. If the hemoglobin level is ≥5 g/dl and CPDA-1 RBCs are used (Hematocrit 0.7-0.75), a transfusion of 10 ml/kg usually raises hemoglobin level by 2.5 g/dl. If anemia has developed slowly and hemoglobin level is <5 g/dl, RBC transfusion should be given slowly or in small quantities to avoid precipitating cardiac failure due to circulatory overload. The traditional formula for calculating the amount of blood required is as follows:

(Total blood volume × increment in Hb desired)/ Hb of the donor unit

However, this formula may lead to inadequate increase in the hemoglobin level. Another formula for calculation of transfusion need is:

Volume of packed cells for transfusion (ml) = 4.8 × weight of the patient (kg) × desired rise in Hb (g/dl)[76].

Choice of blood group

The principle for RBC transfusion is that the recipient plasma should not contain antibodies corresponding to donor A and/or B antigens. For plasma and platelet transfusion, donor plasma must not contain A or B antibodies corresponding to recipient's A or B antigens. Patients who are RhD antigen positive may receive RhD positive or negative RBCs but patients who are RhD antigen negative should receive only RhD negative RBCs. Ideally the same blood group RBC which is compatible with the recipient plasma should be transfused. The acceptable choices of ABO blood groups for RBCs, plasma and platelet transfusions are summarized in Table 8.10.

Table 8.10 The choice of ABO blood groups for RBCs, plasma and platelet transfusions

Recipient's blood group	Acceptable ABO group of group blood component to be transfused		
	RBCs	Plasma	Platelets
O	O	O A,B,AB	O A,B,AB
A	A O	A AB	A AB
B	B O	B AB	B AB
AB	AB A,B,O	AB	AB

Use of leukocyte-depleted blood

Leukocyte depleted blood contains $<5 \times 10^6/mm^3$ leukocytes and is used for conditions listed in Table 8.11. Use of leukocyte depleted blood is not recommended merely for prevention of transfusion associated GVHD. For that, gamma-irradiation of blood products is the standard practice. There is at present insufficient evidence regarding use of leukocyte depleted blood products for producing

Table 8.11 Indications for transfusion of leukocyte-depleted blood

Definite indications
1. To prevent non-hemolytic febrile transfusion reactions
2. For reducing graft rejection after hematopoietic cell transplantation
3. For prevention of transmission of viral infections
4. For fetal/neonatal transfusions

Possible indications
1. Platelet refractoriness
2. For kidney transplant recipients

immunomodulatory effects in post-surgical patients (prevention of infection or tumor recurrence) or for delaying the progression of HIV infection.

Washing of RBCs

RBC washing involves the use of sterile saline to remove the plasma that remains in an RBC unit. The procedure removes >98% of the plasma, including plasma proteins, microaggregates, and cytokines. This product is indicated for severe, recurrent allergic reaction to blood components which is not prevented by premedication with antihistamines. Typically, such reactions are caused by allergy to plasma proteins. Patients with severe deficiency of circulatory anti-IgA antibody may develop anaphylactic reactions to the IgA present in blood components. These patients should receive either RBCs from IgA-deficient donors or washed RBCs. Washed RBCs have a shelf life of 24 hours at 1-6°C.

Platelets

Platelet concentrates are usually separated from whole blood either by Buffy coat or by platelet rich plasma method or may be collected by apheresis technique. The platelet bag contains 5.5×10^{10} platelets/unit and about 50 ml of plasma, 0.5 ml of RBCs and varying number of leukocytes (upto 10^8/unit). While apheresis platelet units contain 3×10^{11} platelets, approximately 250-300 ml plasma, trace

Table 8.12 Indications for platelet transfusion

- Platelet count < 10×10^9/l
- Platelet count <20×10^9/l with bone marrow infiltration, severe mucositis, DIC, anticoagulation therapy
- Platelet count < $30-40 \times 10^9$/l and DIC
- Platelet count < $50-60 \times 10^9$/l and major surgical intervention
- Qualitative defects of platelet function with active bleeding irrespective of platelet count

to 5 ml of RBCs and 10^6– 10^9 leukocytes. Platelets can be stored upto 5 days at 20-24°C. The indications for platelet transfusion are summarized in the Table 8.12.

Generally, one unit of platelet concentrate is indicated per 10 kg body weight in children. Rh negative females with child-bearing potential should not receive platelet concentrates from Rh positive donors in order to reduce the risk of iso-immunization.

Plasma

Plasma is either separated from whole blood by centrifugation or collected using automated apheresis technique. A unit of plasma usually contains 150-250 ml. Fresh plasma contains approximately 1 unit/ml of each of coagulation factors. After 24 hours of donation, plasma contains less than 15% of factor V and factor VIII. Plasma collected within 6 hours of donation and rapidly frozen to -25°C or colder contains at least 0.7 U/ml of Factor VIII and is called fresh frozen plasma (FFP)[77]. FFP may be stored for 12 months at temperature -18°C. Once thawed, it should be stored in a refrigerator at +2 to+6°C and should preferably be used within 6 hours. The use of FFP should be limited exclusively for the treatment or prevention of clinically significant bleeding due to deficiency of plasma coagulation factors. Indications for plasma transfusion are summarized in Table 8.13.

Table 8.13 Indications for FFP transfusion

- Use of vitamin K antagonists (e.g. warfarin overdose)
- Severe liver disease
- Disseminated intravascular coagulation (DIC)
- Massive transfusion
- Isolated congenital coagulation factor deficiency

Dosage and administration

Plasma should be ABO compatible with recipient's RBCs. Usually Rh group need not be considered unless in cases where large volume of FFP is needed. FFP may be thawed in a water bath at 30-70°C or in a microwave designed for this purpose. Dose of FFP depends on the clinical situation and the underlying disease. Administration of 10-20 ml/kg of plasma increases the level of coagulation factors by 20%.

Cryoprecipitate

Cryoprecipitate is formed during controlled thawing of FFP at 4°C which is then refrozen within

1 hour in 10-15 ml of the donor plasma and stored at -18°C or less for a period up to one year. Cryoprecipitate contains 80-100 units of Factor VIII, 100-250 mg of fibrinogen, 40-60 mg of fibronectin, 40-70% of VWF and 30% of Factor XIII. Indications for cryoprecipitate administration include hemophilia, von Willebrand disease, and congenital deficiencies of fibrinogen or Factor XIII. Specific factor concentrates like Factor VIII concentrate contains 0.5-20 IU/mg protein. In chronically transfused patients with Factor VIII inhibitors, a heat-treated plasma fraction containing partly activated coagulation factors may be used. Prothrombin complex concentrates and factor IX concentrates are used for treatment of Hemophilia B (Christmas disease) and for correction of prolonged prothrombin time.

Compatibility testing of cryoprecipitate units is not necessary but ABO compatible units should be used irrespective of Rh group. One unit/5-10 kg of recipient weight is transfused rapidly (preferably within 6 hours of thawing) and the duration of transfusion should not exceed 4 hours.

Granulocyte transfusion

Granulocyte transfusions are useful in patients with severe neutropenia and bacterial or fungal infections not improving with therapy especially when bone marrow recovery is expected to be delayed up to 2 to 3 weeks and also in patients with granulocyte dysfunction. Granulocyte transfusions of at least 1×10^{10} must be transfused daily until there is clinical improvement. In a granulocyte product high metabolic activity can deplete glucose, produce lactic acid, and increase cell death. Granulocytes are stored at room temperature because cold storage inactivates the neutrophils. Granulocytes must be transfused within 24 hrs. As granulocytes cannot be leukoreduced, the risk of CMV transmission is significant. Granulocytes must be ABO compatible and crossmatched prior to transfusion. One relative contraindication to granulocyte transfusions is the presence of anti-HLA or anti-granulocyte antibodies in the recipient, due to possibility of developing transfusion-associated acute lung injury.

Risks of blood transfusion

One should always weigh the risks and hazards of transfusion against the possible therapeutic advantages before transfusing blood or blood products. Possible risks of transfusion are serious hemolytic reaction, transmission of HIV, HBV, HCV, syphilis, malaria, CMV, and risk of contamination with bacteria. For whole blood/packed RBCs, the product should be started within 30 minutes of removing the pack from storage temperature (+2°C+6°C) and transfusion should preferably be completed within 4 hours of starting the infusion, if the room temperature is between 22°C to 25°C. In case of high ambient temperature, shorter out-of-refrigeration times should be used. Platelets should be transfused as soon as they have been received and the transfusion of each unit should be completed in about 20 minutes.

The blood products should be infused through a new, sterile blood administration set with an integral 170-200 μm filter. Blood administration set should be changed every 12 hourly if multiple transfusions are required. For platelet transfusion a fresh blood administration set primed with saline should be used. The child should be monitored frequently during infusion of blood or blood products.

Transfusion reactions

Acute and delayed adverse effects of transfusion of blood and blood products are summarized in Tables 8.14 and 8.15.

Massive transfusion

Massive transfusion is defined as replacement of blood loss equivalent to or greater than the patient's total blood volume with stored blood in less than 24 hours (70 ml/kg in adults and 80-90 ml/kg in children/infants). The various complications of massive transfusion include acidosis, hyperkalemia, citrate toxicity, hypocalcemia, depletion of fibrinogen and coagulation factors, depletion of platelets, DIC, hypothermia, reduced 2,3DPG and formation of microaggregates.

Blood substitutes

In order to avoid the risks associated with transfusion of blood and blood products, there has been increasing amount of research on the use of various forms of blood substitutes and introduction of several other alternative strategies for minimizing the need for transfusions, especially in peri-operative period and for patients with chronic anemia (Table 8.16).

In addition several hemoglobin based compounds are being developed as blood substitutes. Free hemoglobin suspensions have poor oxygen delivery because the oxygen dissociation curve is shifted to the left in the absence of 2, 3 DPG, and unless pyridoxylated and polymerized, they have low hemoglobin concentrations. Stable

	Category	Signs	Symptoms	Cause	Treatment
1.	Mild	Urticaria, skin rash	Pruritus	Hypersensitivity reaction	Slow the infusion rate and give antihistaminic (Chlorpheniramine maleate 0.1 mg/kg). If no improvement occur in 30 minutes, treat as category 2
2.	Moderate	Flushing, urticaria, rigors, fever, restlessness and tachycardia	Anxiety, itching, palpitations, mild dyspnea and headache	Hypersensitivity reaction	Stop infusion and replace IV set. Notify the blood bank. Sample from the bag and patient should be sent for repeat cross matching. Give antihistaminic, antipyretic, steroids (IV and bronchodilator if needed. Collect urine sample for hemolysis. If patient improves restart infusion slowly. If no improvement occurs in 15 minutes treat as category 3
3.	Life threatening	Rigors, fever restlessness, hypotension, tachycardia, hemoglobinuria (red urine) and DIC (bleeding)	Anxiety chest pain, pain at IV site, respiratory distress, backache, headache and dyspnea	Hemolysis, bacterial contamination, fluid overload, anaphylaxis, transfusion-associated lung injury and septic shock	Stop infusion and maintain ABC. Change IV set and administer normal saline 20 ml/kg bolus (repeat if needed). Elevate the legs and give adrenaline (1:1000) 0.01 mg/kg IV/SC, steroids IV and bronchodilator (if needed) and ionotropes (if needed) Notify blood bank and send a sample from the bag and patient for repeat cross matching. Collect urine sample for hemolysis. If bleeding (DIC) occurs, give platelets, cryoprecipitate, FFP or factor concentrates. If acute renal failure supervenes check fluid balance, give furosemide (1mg/kg), and undertake dialysis if needed. If bacteremia is suspected, send blood culture and start antibiotics.

Table 8.14 Adverse effects of blood and blood products

Table 8.15 Delayed complications of transfusion of blood and blood products

Type of reaction	Clinical features	Treatment
Delayed hemolytic reaction (5-10 days later)	Fever, anemia and jaundice	If hypotension occurs treat as acute intravascular hemolysis
Post transfusion purpura (5-10 days later)	Increased bleeding tendency and thrombocytopenia	High dose steroids, IVIG, and plasma exchange
Graft vs host disease (GVHD) 10-12 days later	Fever, rash and desquamation, diarrhea, hepatitis, and pancytopenia	Supportive care
Iron overload	Cardiac and liver failure in transfusion dependent patients	Iron chelating agents desferioxamine (subcutaneous infusion) or oral deferiprone

IVIG: Intravenous immunoglobulins

perfluorocarbon emulsions have been tried as they can dissolve more oxygen than water or plasma. Among the various polymerized products that were developed, three polyhemoglobins survived in the phase III clinical trials, namely polyheme (human Hb polymerized with glutaraldehyde), biopure (bovine Hb polymerized with glutaraldehyde), hemolink (raffinose polymerized human Hb)[81]. The clinical trials with Optro (a recombinant hemoglobin) and Hemassist (an intramolecularly crosslinked

Table 8.16 Strategies to minimize the transfusion reactions by use of blood substitutes[78-80]

- Pre-operative autologous transfusions
- Acute normovolemic hemodilution
- Intraoperative autotransfusion
- Autologous blood cell salvage
- Pharmacological agents to reduce surgical bleeding (Aprotinin, desmopressin, tranexamic acid, vitamin K)
- Use of recombinant erythropoietin
- Use of minimally invasive, 'bloodless' surgical techniques

hemoglobin) were abandoned due to adverse effects. A lot of research has been going on in this field ever since world war II but it is likely to take some time before we find the simple and safe alternative to replace human blood for transfusion.

REFERENCES

1. Morris AH. Rational use of computerized protocols in the intensive care unit. *Crit Care* 2001; 5:249-254.

2. Dries DJ, McGonigal MD, Malian MS, *et al*. Protocol-driven ventilator weaning reduces use of mechanical ventilation, rate of early reintubation, and ventilator-associated pneumonia. *J Trauma* 2004; 56:943-951.

3. Ely EW, Baker AM, Dunagan DP, *et al*. Effect on the duration of mechanical ventilation of identifying patients capable of breathing spontaneously. *N Engl J Med* 1996; 335:1864-1869.

4. Malhotra A. Intensive insulin in intensive care. *New Engl J Med* 2006; 354:516–518.

5. Detriche O, Berre J, Massaut J, *et al*. The Brussels sedation scale: use of a simple clinical sedation scale can avoid excessive sedation in patients undergoing mechanical ventilation in the intensive care unit. *Br J Anaesth* 1999; 83:698-701.

6. Carcillo JA, Fields AI. American College of Critical Care Medicine Task Force Committee Members. Clinical practice parameters for hemodynamic support of pediatric and neonatal patients in septic shock. *Crit Care Med* 2002; 30:1365-1378.

7. Cheifetz IM, Venkataraman ST, Hamel DS. Respiratory monitoring. In: Roger's Textbook of Pediatric Intensive Care. Nichols DG (Ed). *Lippincott Williams and Wilkins.* 2008: pp 662-685.

8. Aoyagi T, Miyasaka K. Pulse oximetry: Its invention, contribution to medicine and future tasks. *Anesth Analg* 2002; 94:S1-S3.

9. Berkenbosch JW, Lam J, Burd RS, *et al*. Noninvasive monitoring of carbon dioxide during mechanical ventilation in older children: End-tidal versus transcutaneous techniques. *Anesth Analg* 2001; 92: 1427-1431.

10. Halley GC, Tibby S. Hemodynamic monitoring. In: Roger's Textbook of Pediatric Intensive Care. Nichols DG (Ed). *Lippincott Williams and Wilkins.* 2008: pp 1039-1062.

11. Tibby SM, Murdoch IA. Monitoring cardiac function in intensive care. *Arch Dis Child* 2003; 88:46-52.

12. Ceneviva G, Paschall JA, Maffei F, Carcillo JA. Hemodynamic support in fluid refractory pediatric septic shock. *Pediatrics* 1998; 102: e19.

13. Thompson AE. Pulmonary artery catheterization in children. *New Horiz* 1997; 5:244–250.

14. Tibby SM, Hatherill M, Murdoch IA. Use of transesophageal Doppler ultrasonography in ventilated pediatric patients: Derivation of cardiac output. *Crit Care Med* 2000; 28: 2045-2050.

15. Courand JA, Marshall J, Chang YC, King ME. Clinical applications of wall stress analysis in pediatric intensive care unit. *Crit Care Med* 2001; 29:526-533.

16. Hulst JM, van Goudoever JB, Zimmermann LJ, Tibboel D, Joosten KF. The role of initial monitoring of routine biochemical nutritional markers in critically ill children. *J Nutr Biochem* 2006;17:57-62.

17. Vincent JL. Give your patient a FAST HUG (at least) once a day. *Crit Care Med* 2005; 33:1225-1229.

18. Van den Berghe G, Wouters P, Weekers F, *et al*. Intensive insulin therapy in the critically ill patient. *N Engl J Med* 2001; 345: 1359-1367.

19. Van den Berghe G, Wilmer A, Hermans G, *et al*. Intensive insulin therapy in the medical ICU. *N Engl J Med* 2006; 354:449-61.

20. Srinivasan V, Spinella PC, Drott HR, *et al*. Association of timing, duration, and intensity of hyperglycemia with intensive care unit mortality in critically ill children. *Pediatr Crit Care Med* 2004; 5:329-336.

21. Yung M, Wilking B, Norton L, Slater A. Glucose control, organ failure, and mortality in Pediatric intensive care. *Pediatr Crit Care Med.* 2008; 9:147–152.

22. Ali NA, O'Brien Jr JM, Dungan K, et al. Glucose variability and mortality in patients with sepsis. *Crit Care Med.* 2008;36:2316–2321.

23. Krinsley JS. Glycemic variability: A strong independent predictor of mortality in critically ill patients. *Crit Care Med.* 2008; 36:3008–3013.

24. Rake AJ, Srinivasan V, Nadkarni V, Kaptan R, Newth CJ. Glucose variability and survival in critically ill children: Allostasis or harm? *Pediatr Crit Care Med* 2010; 11: 707-712.

25. Vlasselaers D, Milants I, Desmet L, et al. Intensive insulin therapy for patients in paediatric intensive care: a prospective, randomized controlled study. *Lancet.* 2009; 373:547–556.

26. Curley MA, Quigley SM, Lin M. Pressure ulcers in pediatric intensive care: incidence and associated factors. *Pediatr Crit Care Med* 2003; 4:284-290.

27. http://www.rcn.org.uk/publications/pdf/guidelines/pressure_ulcer_risk_assess_1.pdf

28. Rosenberg JB, Eisen LA. Eye care in the intensive care unit: narrative review and meta-analysis. *Crit Care Med* 2008; 36:3151–3155.

29. Imanaka H, Taenaka N, Nakamura J, *et al.* Ocular surface disorders in the critically ill. *Anesth Analg* 1997; 85: 343-346.

30. Bergmans DC, Bonten MJ, Gaillard CA, *et al.* Prevention of ventilator-associated pneumonia by oral decontamination: a prospective, randomized, double-blind, placebo-controlled study. *Am J Respir Crit Care Med* 2001; 164:382-388.

31. de Jonge E, Schultz MJ, Spanjaard L, *et al.* Effects of selective decontamination of digestive tract on mortality and acquisition of resistant bacteria in intensive care: a randomised controlled trial. *Lancet* 2003; 362:1011-1016.

32. Silvestri L, van Saene HK, Milanese M, *et al.* Prevention of MRSA pneumonia by oral vancomycin decontamination: a randomised trial. *Eur Respir J* 2004; 23: 921-926.

33. Binkley C, Furr LA, Carrico R, McCurren C. Survey of oral care practices in US intensive care units. *Am J Infect Control* 2004; 32:161-169.

34. Jones H, Newton JT, Bower EJ. A survey of the oral care practices of intensive care nurses. *Intensive Crit Care Nurs* 2004; 20:69-76.

35. Franklin D, Senior N, James I, Roberts G. Oral health status of children in a Paediatric Intensive Care Unit. *Intensive Care Med* 2000; 26:319-324.

36. Deerojanawong J, Peongsujarit D, Vivatvakin B, Prapphal N. Incidence and risk factors of upper gastrointestinal bleeding in mechanically ventilated children. *Pediatr Crit Care Med.* 2009;10:91–95.

37. Nithiwathanapong C, Reungrongrat S, Ukarapol N. Prevalence and risk factors of stress-induced gastrointestinal bleeding in critically ill children. *World J Gastroenterol.* 2005;11:6839–6842.

38. Reveiz L, Guerrero-Lozano R, Camacho A, Yara L, Mosquera PA. Stress ulcer, gastritis, and gastrointestinal bleeding prophylaxis in critically ill pediatric patients: a systematic review. *Pediatr Crit Care Med.* 2010; 11:124–132.

39. Donnelly KM. Venous thromboembolic disease in the pediatric intensive care unit. *Curr Opin Pediatr* 1999; 11:213-217.

40. Graziano JN, Charpie JR. Thrombosis in the intensive care unit: etiology, diagnosis, management, and prevention in adults and children. *Cardiol Rev* 2001; 9:173-182.

41. Dellinger RP, Levy MM, Carlet JM, *et al.* Surviving Sepsis Campaign: international guidelines for management of severe sepsis and septic shock: 2008. *Crit Care Med.* 2008; 36:296–327.

42. Jackson A. Infection control—a battle in vein: infusion phlebitis. *Nurs Times* 1998; 94:68- 71.

43. Hulst JM, van Goudoever JB, Zimmermann LJ, *et al.* The effect of cumulative energy and protein deficiency on anthropometric parameters in a pediatric ICU population. *Clin Nutr* 2004; 23:1381-1389.

44. Coss-Bu JA, Klish WJ, Walding D, Stein F, Smith EO, Jefferson LS. Energy metabolism, nitrogen balance, and substrate utilization in critically ill children. *Am J Clin Nutr* 2001; 74: 664-669.

45. Taylor RM, Cheeseman P, Preedy V, Baker AJ, Grimble G. Can energy expenditure be predicted in critically ill children? *Pediatr Crit Care Med* 2003; 4:176-180.

46. DeWitt, RC, Kudsk, KA The gut's role in metabolism, mucosal barrier function, and gut immunology. *Infect Dis Clin North Am* 1999; 13:465-481

47. Horn D, Chaboyer W. Gastric feeding in critically ill children: a randomized controlled trial. *Am J Crit Care* 2003; 12:461-468.

48. Bosscha K, Nieuwenhuijs VB, Vos A, *et al.* Gastrointestinal motility and gastric tube feeding in mechanically ventilated patients. *Crit Care Med* 1998; 26:1510-1517.

49. Meert KL, Daphtary KM, Metheny NA. Gastric vs small-bowel feeding in critically ill children receiving mechanical ventilation: a randomized controlled trial. *Chest* 2004; 126:872-878.

50. Gharpure V, Meert KL, Sarnaik AP. Efficacy of erythromycin for postpyloric placement of feeding tubes in critically ill children: a randomized, double-blind, placebo controlled study. *J Parenter Enteral Nutr* 2001; 25:160-165.

51. Horn D, Chaboyer W, Schluter PJ. Gastric residual volumes in critically ill paediatric patients: a comparison of feeding regimens. *Aust Crit Care* 2004; 17:98-100.

52. Haber BA, Deutschmann CS. Nutrition and metabolism in the critically ill child. In: *Textbook of Pediatric Intensive Care*. Rogers MC (Ed). Baltimore. Williams and Wilkins. 1996: pp 1141-1162.

53. Marik PE. Total splanchnic resuscitation, SIRS and MODS. *Crit Care Med* 1999; 27:257-258.

54. Beale RJ, Bryg DJ, Bihari DJ. Immunonutrition in the critically ill: a systematic review of clinical outcome. *Crit Care Med* 1999; 27: 2799-2805.

55. Heyland DK, Novak F, Drover JW, Jain M, Su X, Suchner U. Should immunonutrition become routine in critically ill patients? A systematic review of the evidence. *JAMA* 2001; 286:944-953.

56. Montejo JC, Zarazaga A, Lopez-Martinez J, Urrutia G, Roque M, Blesa AL, *et al.* Immunonutrition in the intensive care unit. A systematic review and consensus statement. *Clin Nutr* 2003; 22:221-233.

57. Novak F, Heyland DK, Avenell A, Drover JW, Su X. Glutamine supplementation in serious illness: A

systematic review of the evidence. *Crit Care Med* 2002; 30: 2022–2029.

58. Bertolini G, Iapichino G, Radrizzani D, *et al.* Early enteral immunonutrition in patients with severe sepsis: results of an interim analysis of a randomized multicentre clinical trial. *Intensive Care Med* 2003; 29:834-840.

59. Marik PE, Zaloga GP. Immunonutrition in critically ill patients: a systematic review and analysis of the literature. *Intensive Care Med.* 2008; 34:1980–1990.

60. Krauss B, Steven SM. Sedation and analgesia for procedures in children. *N Engl J Med* 2000; 342: 938-945.

61. Young C, Knudsen N, Hilton A, Reves JG. Sedation in intensive care unit. *Crit Care Med* 2000; 28:854-866.

62. Committee on Drugs. American Academy of Pediatrics. Guidelines for monitoring and management of pediatric patients during and after sedation for diagnostic and therapeutic procedures: addendum. *Pediatrics* 2002; 110:836-838.

63. American Society of Anesthesiologists Task Force on Sedation and Analgesia by Non-Anesthesiologists. Practice guidelines for sedation and analgesia by non-anesthesiologists. *Anesthesiology* 2002; 96:1004-1017.

64. De Jonghe B, Cook D, Appere-De-Vecchi C, *et al.* Using and understanding sedation scoring systems: a systematic review. *Intensive Care Med* 2000; 26: 275-285.

65. Crain N, Slonim A, Pollack MM. Assessing sedation in the pediatric intensive care unit by using BIS and the COMFORT scale. *Pediatr Crit Care Med* 2002; 3: 11-14.

66. Trope RM, Silver PC, Sagy M. Concomitant assessment of depth of sedation by changes in bispectral index and changes in autonomic variables (heart rate and/or BP) in pediatric critically ill patients receiving neuromuscular blockade. *Chest* 2005; 128:303-307.

67. Martin LD, Bratton SL, O'Rourke PP. Clinical uses and controversies of neuromuscular blocking agents in infants and children. *Crit Care Med* 1999; 27: 1358-1368.

68. Lodha R, Natchu UCM, Nanda M, Kabra SK. Nosocomial infections in pediatric intensive care units. *Indian J Pediatr* 2001; 68:1063- 1070.

69. Richards MJ, Edwards JR, Culver DH, Gaynes RP. The National Nosocomial Infection Surveillance System. Nosocomial infections in pediatric intensive care units in the United States. *Pediatrics* 1999; 103:e39.

70. Gupta A, Kapil A, Lodha R, Kabra SK, Sood S, Dhawan B, Das BK, Sreenivas V. Burden of healthcare-associated infections in a paediatric intensive care unit of a developing country: a single centre experience using active surveillance. *J Hosp Infect.* 2011 Jun 13. [Epub ahead of print].

71. Haley RW, Culver DH, White JW, *et al.* The efficacy of infection surveillance and control programs in preventing nosocomial infections in US hospitals. *Am J Epidemiology* 1985; 121:182-187.

72. Babcock HM, Zack JE, Garrison T, *et al.* An educational intervention to reduce ventilator-associated pneumonia in an integrated health system: a comparison of effects. *Chest* 2004; 125:2224-2331.

73. Gnass SA, Barboza L, Bilicich D, *et al.* Prevention of central venous catheter-related bloodstream infections using non-technologic strategies. *Infect Control Hosp Epidemiol* 2004; 25:675-677.

74. BCSH guidelines. Transfusion guidelines for neonates and older children. *Br J Haemat* 2004; 124:433–453.

75. Lacroix J, Luban NL, Wong EC. Blood products in PICU. In: Roger's Textbook of Pediatric Intensive Care. Nichols DG (Ed). *Lippincott Williams and Wilkins.* 2008: pp 584-599.

76. Morris KP, Naqvi N, Davies P, Smith M, Lee PW. A new formula for blood transfusion volume in the critically ill. *Arch Dis Child* 2005; 90: 724-728.

77. Ewalenko P, Deloof T, Peeters J. Composition of fresh frozen plasma. *Crit Care Med* 1986; 14:145-146.

78. Goodnough LT, Shander A, Spence R. Bloodless medicine: Clinical care without allogeneic blood transfusion. *Transfusion* 2003; 43:668-676.

79. Weldon BC. Blood conservation in pediatric anesthesia. *Anesthesiology Clin N Am* 2005; 23:347-361.

80. Wong EC. Acute normovolemic hemodilution: A critical evaluation of its safety and utility in pediatric patients. *Transfusion Alternatives Transfusion Med* 2004; 6: 10-21.

81. Chang TMS. Is there a need for blood substitutes in the new millennium and what can we expect in way of safety and efficacy? *Art Cells Blood Sub Immob Biotech* 2000; 28:1-7.

9

Medico-legal Issues in the Emergency Department

TD Dogra and Sanjeev Lalwani

Apart from critical life-saving concerns, the medical team in the emergency department is expected to face several medico-legel issues[1]. Emergency medical practitioner has responsibility not only towards the patient for saving life but also towards the state particularly in medico-legal cases. Priority must be given to the life saving treatment rather than completing the medico-legal formalities, but they should never be ignored. In any emergency situation, patient is examined, treated and stabilized by using all possible medical or surgical interventions at the earliest. However, in the given situation, medical rescue should be carried out by the emergency physician in accordance with the applicable law. The current emergency medico-legal issues may involve both patient and physician related factors specifically targeting optimal and rational patient care and damage claims. Therefore, awareness of these issues could be helpful not only in minimizing medico-legal risk but also in improving the patient care[2].

Medico-legal Cases in the Emergency Department

As per the guidelines prepared in 1983 by the committee constituted by Delhi Government for uniformity in medico-legal work, medico-legal case is defined as "the case of injury or ailment, where an attending doctor after taking history and clinical examination of the patient/s, thinks that some investigations by law enforcing agencies for evident homicides including attempted suicides are essential, so as to fix the responsibility regarding the case in accordance with the law of the land".[3] The following cases are labelled as medico-legal cases and should be handled accordingly.

(i)   Accidents and unnatural mishaps.

(ii) Suspected or evident homicides including attempted homicides.

(iii) Suspected or evident suicides including attempted poisoning.

(iv) Burn injury due to any cause.

(v)   Any injury where foul play is suspected or doctor thinks that the patient is a victim or accused in a crime case.

(vi) Injury cases where there is likelihood of death in the near future.

(vii) Suspected or evident sexual offences.

(viii) Suspected or evident criminal abortion cases.

(ix) Comatosed patients where cause of unconsciousness is not clear.

(x)   Cases brought dead in suspicious circumstances.

(xi) Cases referred by court or otherwise which require age certificate or other medical certificates.

Principles governing medico-legal cases are listed below.

- Even if a patient reports several days after the incident, medico-legal report is prepared.

- Medico-legal report can be prepared in emergency department or ward or intensive care unit depending upon the condition of the patient.

- It is not necessary for the police to accompany medico-legal cases.

- Failure to make medico-legal report is an offence punishable under section 201 and 202 IPC.

Information to the police

Not only as a physician but also as a citizen of India, we must inform the nearby police station in writing about any crime which comes to our knowledge. Information should be given by the hospital regarding all medico-legal cases which are brought for treatment or are admitted and particularly about those where police is not accompanying the victim. Failure to inform the police is a punishable offence (39 Cr PC)[4].

Consent for treatment

The need for consent is based on the fundamental principle of autonomy of an individual. This has been recognised within the right of life and personal liberty (Article 21 of Constitution of India). The important reason for taking consent is respect for human dignity and bodily integrity. Honourable Supreme Court of India has also said that "correctness or appropriateness of the treatment procedure does not make the treatment legal in the absence of consent"[5].

Indian Medical Council (Professional conduct, etiquette and ethics) Regulations 2002 vide regulation no 7.16 states that; "Before performing an operation, physician should obtain in writing the consent from the husband, wife, parent or guardian (in case of minor) or the patient himself as the case may be"[6].

In an emergency situation when a patient arrives for treatment, formal consent to medical examination is not required, as his reporting to the emergency department amounts to implied consent. However, the implied consent cannot be extended to a complex procedure. In such situations written or oral expressed informed consent is taken in the presence of disinterested third party[7].

In case of Dr Prabha Manchanda vs Samira Kohli (2008), the Honourable Supreme Court of India has ruled as follows[8]:

(i) A doctor has to seek and record the consent of the patient before commencing a 'treatment' (the term 'treatment' includes surgery also). The consent so obtained should be real and valid, which means that (a) the patient should have the capacity and competence to consent, (b) his consent should be voluntary, (c) and his consent should be on the basis of adequate information concerning the nature of the treatment or procedure, so that he knows what he is consenting to.

(ii) The 'adequate information' should be furnished by the doctor (or a member of his team) who treats the patient, which should enable the patient to make a balanced judgment as to whether he/she should submit himself/herself to the particular treatment or not. This means that the doctor should disclose (a) the nature of the treatment and procedure and its purpose, benefits and side effects; (b) alternatives if any available; (c) an outline of the likely risks; and (d) adverse consequences of refusing treatment

The physician should be pragmatic and there is no need to explain remote or theoretical risks involved, which may frighten or confuse a patient and result in refusal of consent for the necessary treatment. Similarly, there is no need to explain the remote or theoretical risks of a procedure or treatment which may force a patient to undergo a fanciful or unnecessary treatment. A balance should be achieved between the need for disclosing necessary and adequate information and at the same time avoiding the possibility of the patient being deterred from agreeing to a necessary treatment or offering to undergo an unnecessary treatment.

(iii) The consent given only for a diagnostic procedure, cannot be considered as consent for therapeutic treatment. And a consent given for a specific treatment or procedure will not be valid for conducting some other treatment or procedure. The fact that the unauthorized additional surgery is beneficial to the patient, or that it would save considerable time and expense to the patient, or would relieve the patient from pain and suffering in future, are not grounds of defence in an action in tort for negligence or assault and its consequences. The only exception to this rule is where the additional procedure though unauthorized, was necessary in order to save the life or preserve the health of the patient and it would have been unreasonable to delay such unauthorized procedure until patient regains consciousness to take a decision.

(iv) There can be a common consent for diagnostic and operative procedures when they are contemplated. There can also be a common consent for a particular surgical procedure and an additional or further procedure that may become necessary during the course of surgery.

(v) The nature and extent of information to be furnished by the doctor to the patient to secure the consent need not be of the stringent and high degree. But it should be of a reasonable extent which is accepted as normal and proper by a body of medical men skilled and experienced in the particular field. It will depend upon the physical and mental condition of the patient, the nature of treatment, and the risk and consequences attached to the treatment.

Section 89 IPC mentions that a child less than 12 years of age cannot give a valid consent and in such situations consent of parents or guardian is taken[4]. Any harm caused to patient in good faith, even without the person's consent, is not an offence if the circumstances are such that it is impossible for the person to give consent, and he has no guardian or other person in lawful charge of him from whom it is possible to obtain consent in time (Section 92 IPC)[4]. In an emergency involving children when their parents or guardians are not available, consent is taken from the person who brings the child to the emergency department like teacher, head master, relative etc[7].

Documentation

The documentation or medico-legal report should be prepared by the treating doctor himself in the prescribed format soon after providing life saving treatment to the patient. The report is always prepared in duplicate. One original copy is handed over to the investigating officer and the other duplicate or carbon copy is kept in hospital records. In suspected poisoning cases one copy of the report mentioning signs and symptoms and findings of clinical examination should be provided to the forensic science laboratory.

Every medico-legal report has three components, preamble, body of information and conclusions or inference. Preamble mentions particulars of patient like name, father's name, age, sex, address, religion, identifications marks including thumb impression, date and time of examination and name of person accompanying including relations or police officer with belt number and rank. In body of the report, details of illness like history, complaints, findings of medical/clinical examination including general physical and systemic examination along with vital parameters, details of injuries with nature, size, site and shape, treatment prescribed (both prophylactic and definitive treatment), details of exhibits/evidences (clothings, blood, vaginal slides, vaginal swabs, anal swabs, blood sample, gastric lavage, urine etc.) preserved, investigations suggested (X-rays, CT scan, USG, etc.) and referral made to other specialist should be mentioned. Firearm injuries should mention characteristics of entry wounds like burning, blackening, tattooing, abrasion collar, contusion collar etc. and details of exit wound if any. In conclusion the medical expert should give his opinion regarding nature of injuries whether simple; grievous or dangerous, age of injury and should also opine about probable weapon used. In case immediate opinion cannot be given for want of X-ray report or reports of other investigations, the same should be mentioned as "opinion reserved" with remarks/reasons. The report must be signed by the treating medical expert with full name, designation and address[3,14].

Preservation of Evidence

In medico-legal cases all relevant biological specimens from the body of accused or victim as deemed necessary by medical officer or requested by the investigating officer must be preserved. Important specimens include blood for grouping, bullets/pellets recovered from the body of person, gastric lavage, blood or urine in poisoning cases, vaginal swabs, vaginal slides, anal swabs in cases of sexual offences.

Garments of the accused or victim are also important for further investigation of the case and could give valuable information. In case clothing are stained with wet blood they should be dried first and then sealed and handed over to the investigating officer.

All evidences should be properly preserved and labelled mentioning details about particulars of the patient. They should be properly sealed and handed over to the investigating officer along with sample of the seal. The description of preserved articles should be noted in the medico-legal report.

Pediatric Trauma Cases

The various trauma cases include injury, hurt and assault. As per section 44 of IPC, injury has been defined as any harm caused to person's body, mind, property and reputation. Hurt is causing bodily pain, disease or infirmity caused to any person (319 IPC). Assault is an offer or threat or attempt to apply force to body of another in a hostile manner (351 IPC)[4]. The child may present with accidental or homicidal or suicidal injuries in form of abrasions, bruises, lacerations, sharp weapon injuries, firearm injuries, and explosion related injuries etc.

In medico-legal cases, after examination and treatment of the patient, physician is required to give opinion regarding the nature of injury and type of the weapon that could have caused the injury. The injuries which are not dangerous and do not fulfill the criteria of grievous hurt, are labelled as simple in nature. The opinion of the doctor should be guided by the Section 320 IPC by grading following inquires as grievous in nature[4]:

(i)   Emasculation

(ii)   Permanent privation of sight of either eye

(iii) Permanent privation of hearing of either ear

(iv)   Fracture or dislocation of a bone or tooth

(v)   Permanent disfigurment of the head or face

(vi)   Privation of any limb or joint

(vii) Destruction or permanent impairing of the powers of any limb or joint

(viii) Any hurt which endangers life, or which causes the victim to be in severe bodily pain or unable to follow his ordinary pursuits for a period of 20 days.

However, dangerous injuries are those where there is imminent danger to the life of the patient due to involvement of important vital organs or structures or extensive areas of the body. In case patient fails to receive timely medical or surgical intervention, the injury may prove fatal. Section 324 and 326 of IPC mentions the nature of injuries caused by dangerous weapons[4]. Dangerous weapons or means include any instrument used for shooting, stabbing or cutting or any instrument, which when used as a weapon of offence, is likely to cause death; fire or any heated substance; poison or any corrosive substance; explosive substance or any substance which is harmful to the human body to inhale, to swallow, or to receive into the blood directly or by means of any animal.

All investigations prescribed by the treating physician in the medico-legal cases like X-rays, USG, CT scan, blood or urine examination should be recorded in the proper forms mentioning the particulars of the patient and the label of medico-legal case. The forms should mention the identification marks or thumb impression of the patient.

Special Medico-legal Situations

Sexual abuse

Child sexual abuse may be with or without physical contact. Non-contact abuses include exposure, voyeurism, and child pornography. Contact abuses include fondling a child's genitals, masturbation, oral-genital contact, digital penetration, vaginal and anal intercourse[7].

In cases of rape or forceful sexual activity on female children, the injuries that could be seen on the genitals may include red tender vulva, extensive bruising and laceration on external genitalia. There may be tears involving perineal body, anal canal, vestibular mucosa and on anterior and posterior vaginal wall. Hymen may remain intact as it is deep seated. There may be heavy bleeding or discharge per vaginum. Beside local injuries there may be extensive bodily injuries in form of abrasions, lacerations or bruises. Tearing and soiling of clothings should be looked for[10-12].

In cases of anal penetration or sodomy the local examination may reveal injuries, tears, fissures or scars in anal canal. There may be dilatation of the anal canal with loss of tone and elasticity. Digital examination may be exquisitely tender and painful. Swelling or hematoma on margins of anal canal or tearing and laxity of sphincter ani may be observed. There may be blood stains, seminal stain, fecal matter or signs of venereal infection. Bodily injuries suggestive of struggle are commonly seen[10-12].

The impact of sexual abuse in children is not merely in form of physical injuries but also makes them vulnerable to uunwanted pregnancy, STD's including HIV, menstrual problems and long term behavioral and psychological complications.

Emergency department is frequently the point of first contact for care of sexually abused children and adolescents. Emergency physician may be the first to report such cases. Emergency physician plays an important role by providing mandatory reporting, triage, assessment, treatment and follow-up[13].

Physical abuse

The high index of suspicion and variable or non-consistent history not correlating with physical findings, provide useful leads for the diagnosis of physical abuse in a child. The findings of physical abuse in children may include soft tissue injuries, bruises, abrasions and lacerations. Patterned injuries like pinch marks, butterfly bruises, traumatic alopecia, belt marks, cigarette burns, rail road bruises, black eye, sub-conjunctival hemorrhages, retinal separation, retinal hemorrhages, diminution of vision, visceral injuries like subdural hematoma (40%), skeletal injuries like periosteal hematoma, fractures with retardation of physical growth and mental development are common correlates of child abuse[8,10].

Estimation of age

Sometimes children accused or victims of criminal offences, children rescued from factories and domestic services and trafficked victims are brought to the emergency department for medical examination as well as estimation of age for further legal proceedings. Age is assessed by general physical examination including secondary sexual characteristics, dental examination and radiological examination.

Dealing with a dead patient

When a child patient is declared brought dead on arrival and there is no documentary proof of any illness or treatment or the history given by relatives or accompanying person is not proper, the case may be labelled as medico-legal case and information given to the concerned police station. In the medico-legal report of such cases, personal details like name, age, sex, etc. of the child along with person accompanying should be mentioned. The report must mention that the person was brought dead. In such a situation body is wrapped in shrouds and must be sent to mortuary. In medico-legal cases, after completion of formalities, the dead body is handed over to investigating police officer who after completing the proper inquest into circumstances and cause of death along with autopsy examination hands over the body to relatives.

In case a child patient labelled as medico-legal case is declared dead after treatment in the emergency department, the information regarding his death is given to the concerned police station. In such cases, death certificate and death summary is prepared. Copy of the same is given to the investigating police officer and also kept in hospital records. In such a case the dead body is wrapped in shrouds and must be sent to mortuary for proper inquest into the circumstances and cause of death along with autopsy examination. The body is handed over to the relatives by the investigating police officer.

REFERENCES

1. Rice MM. Medico-legal issues in paediatric and adolescent emergencies. *Emerg Med Clin North Amer* 1991; 9(3): 677-695.

2. Vukmir RB. Medical malpractice: managing the risk. *Med Law* 2004; 23 (3): 495-513.

3. Guidelines for Medico-legal work for various Hospitals of Delhi. Director General of Health Services, Govt of NCT of Delhi 1983.

4. The Criminal Major Acts. PK Gupta (Ed) *Vinod Publishing House, Delhi.*

5. Singh J, Vishnu Bhushan. Medical Negligence and Compensation. *Bharat Law Publications.* 3rd Edition 2004.

6. Indian Medical Council (Professional conduct, etiquettes and ethics) Regulations 2002

7. Child Sexual Abuse, Facts for Families No 9, 2008, American Academy of Child and Adolescent Psychiatry.

8. Reddy KSN. Sexual offences. The Essentials of Forensic Medicine and Toxicology. *K Suguna Devi Hyderabad.* 27th edition 2008.

9. Judgement of Hon'ble Supreme court of India dated 16/1/2008 in case Dr Prabha Manchanda vs Samira Kohli. Civil 1949 of 2004.

10. Vij K. The Textbook of Forensic Medicine and Toxicology, *Elsevier Publications,* 4th Edition, 2008.

11. Paradise JE. The medical evaluation of the sexually abused child. *Pediatr Clin North Amer* 1990; 37(4): 839-862.

12. Newton AW, Vandeven AM. The role of the medical provider in the evaluation of sexually abused children and adolescents. *J Child Sex Abuse* 2010; 19(6): 669-686.

13. Markins PP, Jordan KS. Paediatric sexual abuse: emergency department evaluation and management. *Adv Emerg Nurs J* 2009; 31(2):140-152.

14. Philip SS, Douglas B. Documentation in the paediatric emergency department: A review of resuscitation cases. *Annals of Emerg Med* 1991, 20: 641-643.

Transport of Sick Children

10

Praveen Kumar

A sick child may need to be transported to a higher level facility if the medical infrastructure and expertise required for care are not available locally[1]. Inter-hospital or intra-hospital transport may also be required for a sick child needing a specialized investigation. The third situation where transport is required is return or "back-transport" wherein after the child's condition has improved, he/she is referred back to the parent hospital or another lower level facility for further ongoing care. This helps in decreasing the pressure on the beds in the tertiary care centers making them available for more sick patients and allows families to be closer to their homes.

Organization of the transport program is intimately linked to regionalization of care[2]. One of the major reasons for lack of organized transport services in our country is lack of effective regionalization or tier system. The major constraints in a developing country like ours are that the tertiary care facilities are too few and often too far away. The referral facilities are too distant, overcrowded and often beds are not available. The road network in rural areas is unsatisfactory and of poor quality. Well equipped transport vehicles are usually not available and there are very few trained paramedical/medical personnel available to accompany the patient during the transport. The communication system till recently was very poor though the current mobile revolution seems to be changing that scenario; however, there is poor networking between the referral and referring health facilities.

In the Western world, transport of sick patients is usually managed by specialized transport programs which have the responsibility of providing transport services as well as training and education of the personnel involved in transport. The responsibility of picking up a sick baby or child lies with the transport team of the tertiary care center. This is logical and more cost-effective because the team members of the referral center are better equipped and trained to do this. They are also able to keep their skills upto date because of the frequency of performing such tasks. In our country, majority of the referral centers except for a few in the private sector have not taken up this responsibility. The burden of organizing the transport is on the family and the referring hospital, which makes it more difficult and compromises the outcomes.

Components of Transport Program

The organization of a transport system requires a multidisciplinary team with a director/leader, transport equipment and vehicles, a good communication system and an inbuilt mechanism of quality assurance and improvement[3, 4]. The program must have for a system of ongoing training to update knowledge and skills of the current and new team members.

For effective and smooth functioning, there should be clearly identified and mutually agreed indications for transport, which should be known to both, the referral as well as the referring units. High risk perinatal patients need to be identified during the early prenatal, intrapartum and neonatal periods to provide timely access to appropriate level of care. Despite efforts to identify high risk perinatal patients in the antepartum period, 30-50 % of infants who ultimately require additional neonatal care are not recognized until late intrapartum or early neonatal period[5].

Transport Team

The team members for transport duty should be pre-identified and readily available to leave at short notice. The overall organizational leader of the team is a medical director. The other team members are a medical control physician (can be a consultant or senior resident), nurse and respiratory therapist (for airway and respiratory support). The medical control physician provides necessary care to the child at the referring facility and en-route. He or she may seek additional consultation from subspecialists and should know the local geography and transport environment. He or she should also have good interpersonal skills to maintain cordial and positive attitude during potentially stressful situations. The role of respiratory therapist can be taken over by another nurse or physician in our country as we do not have the cadre of respiratory therapists. A physician may or may not be part of the transport team depending on the complexity of the situation. Nurses can be given specialized training in the discipline of transport to take over the responsibilities of the physician. Knowledgeable, specially trained and experienced vehicle drivers are the other crucial members of the team.

Regardless of the composition, the team must have the combined expertise to resuscitate, stabilize and provide critical care to the child before and during the transport. The team members need to be trained in airway management, vascular access, pathophysiology of pediatric diseases and transport environment. Use of specially trained health care personnel for inter-hospital transport of pediatric patients has been shown to reduce intensive care related adverse events[6].

Equipment and Medications

Apart from the vehicle itself, equipment is required for monitoring of physiological parameters (heart rate, respiratory rate, blood pressure, temperature and oxygen saturation), temperature maintenance, respiratory support and infusion of fluids and drugs. The list of equipment, supplies and medications required is virtually the same both in the NICU and PICU with adaptations[3, 7]. The lists of equipment and their qualities are shown in Tables 10.1 and 10.2 respectively.

Mode of Transport and Transport Vehicle

The transport could be by road or air. The choice depends on the distance, local geography, availability, weather and traffic conditions, safety, cost and disease severity. Of these, the main factor to be considered is transport time. In general, road transport is preferred for distances up to 150 km, helicopter for 150 to 300 km and fixed wing aircraft for longer distances. In our country, road transport is the one most often used and most easily available. It is the least expensive, and universally available. It also has the flexibility that one can stop the

---

Table 10.1 List of essential transport equipment

A. Equipment for thermoregulation
- Transport incubator
- Warming devices/ insulated blankets

B. Resuscitation equipment (with all supplies for different sized neonates and children)

C. Monitoring equipment
- Stethoscope
- Vital signs monitors (HR, SpO_2, RR, temperature, BP)
- ECG monitor/defibrillator
- Glucometer

D. Respiratory equipment
- Oxygen delivery systems (50 psi with alarm system); oxygen and air cylinders
- Oxygen hood
- FiO_2 monitor
- Flowmeter
- Portable ventilator
- Nebulizer
- Nitric oxide tanks and delivery system (if expected to transport infants with pulmonary hypertension)

E. Other equipment
- Suction devices
- Infusion pumps
- Penlight/flashlight
- Transilluminator (cold light)
- Child restraints

F. Drugs and disposables

Table 10.2 Characteristics of transport equipment

- Light weight and portable
- Easy availability of spares and back-up for maintenance
- Easily cleanable
- Capable of running with AC/DC power
- Battery backup to support the entire duration of transport if no other power source is available
- No interference with aircraft/helicopter navigation in case of air transport
- Durable and sturdy in order to withstand mechanical, vibrational, barometric and electric stresses
- Compatible with other equipment, power supplies, oxygen and air supplies

vehicle anytime or divert to another nearest hospital in case of a dire emergency.

Ambulances can be customized and retrofitted for the type of patients likely to be transported[8]. It is better to have an exclusive neonatal/infant transport vehicle. Extensive retrofitting will improve patient care capabilities but will increase the costs and decrease the vehicle usefulness for other services. The ambulance should have adequate earmarked spaces for personnel and securing various equipments. The European Committee for Standardization has published standards for securing of all personnel, items and transport incubators in ambulances[9]. It should have enough power outlets, adequate lighting and temperature control system. There should be an easy communication system between the patient area and the driver, between the transport team and the referral hospital (mobile or walky-talky). The patient area should be sufficiently free of noise and vibration. It should be possible to easily slide and secure the transport incubator or trolley in and out of the transport vehicle.

The speed limit guidelines for the ambulances depend on the traffic and road conditions. In developed countries, a speed of approximately 10 – 20 mph above the permissible speed limits on various roads is allowed. However, considering the poor and bumpy roads and traffic congestion in our country, it may be advisable to keep strictly to permissible speed limits or even lower than that[10]. Higher speeds are associated with higher risk of accidents and destabilization.

Transport Incubator

It is the central piece of the overall neonatal transport equipment. In contrast to a standard incubator, the transport incubator is smaller, can run on DC power and is securable and mountable on a trolley. It should be rugged with strong lockable wheels, IV poles and have facility to attach additional equipments. It should have transparent canopy for observation, portholes for access to the baby and facility to monitor baby's temperature. The baby must be secured properly in the incubator.

In the absence of proper incubators, improvisations have been made utilizing thermocole boxes, electric or chemical heating pads, hot water bottles and phase-change materials (PCM). These products should be used with caution and after conducting safety and efficacy tests. Hot water bottles are known to cause serious burns and are best avoided. Skin-to-skin contact with mother or any other adult (Kangaroo care) can be used effectively to keep the baby warm during transport. In this maneuver, the baby is kept naked except for cap, nappy and socks and is placed facing the mother with direct skin-to-skin contact between breasts. The back of the baby is covered with a gown or light blanket which is affixed with a strap.

Mother's womb is indeed the best transport incubator. If it is anticipated that the neonate would need a level of care which is not locally available, it is best to do in-utero transport and deliver the mother in a tertiary care center having appropriate facilities. In-utero transport is also more economical and associated with better outcome and survival.

Oxygen and Air Tanks

Majority of the sick children requiring transport need supplemental oxygen. Oxygen concentration should be monitored by a FiO_2 analyzer. The concentration is controlled by regulating the proportional flow of air and oxygen if blender is not available. The FiO_2 achieved by different air and oxygen flow rates should be available as a ready-reckoner chart. It can also be calculated by the formula:

$$FiO_2 = \frac{(0.21 \times Vair) + ViO_2}{Vair + ViO_2}$$ where Vair = air flow and ViO_2 is oxygen flow

The capacity and pressure of the tank should be checked to estimate the duration for which it will last. A second back-up tank should also be carried. A ready reckoner chart should be available providing the estimated duration of oxygen flow taking into account the flow rate, cylinder size and pressure.

Communication and Documentation

Besides the vehicle and essential equipment and supplies, effective and reliable communication and documentation is most crucial. There should be a clear and ongoing communication between the referring and referral units. In an organized program, there should be a single central toll-free number for the whole region which should operate 24 hours a day, 7 days a week. At the initial consultation, the medical control physician should discuss and advise the referring team regarding measures to be taken to stabilize the child while transport is being arranged. The physician should be available on telephone for ongoing advice to the referring team depending on the changing condition of the child till the transport can be done.

Telemedicine in the form of real time audiovisual transmission to permit accurate assessment of severity of illness has been tested and shown to be feasible and accurate in pediatric transport[11]. The transport team leader should have a mobile/walky-talky to enable him/her to communicate with the referring team and the medical control physician en-route. At the conclusion of the transport, the referring physician and parents, if not accompanying, should be relayed the information about the safe arrival and condition of the child. The parents should be introduced to and given the names of the contact people and their telephone numbers in the referral hospital. The communication logs should be maintained with clear and accurate documentation. These are very useful for medico-legal purposes as well as audit and quality improvement. Most medico-legal problems result from poor and inadequate communication. The condition of baby, risks involved during transport, financial implications of transport and treatment at the referral centre and realistic expectations should be discussed with family and documented in the case record. An informed written consent should be taken prior to the transport.

Pre-transport Stabilization

The child must be stabilized before the transport is begun. An unstable infant will suffer more harm than benefit from urgent transport[12]. It is a misconception that quicker the transport, better is the outcome. Till the transport team is able to reach the referring hospital, the local care providers must be guided to take actions according to their capabilities. Following parameters must be assessed and corrective actions taken before transport:

(i) *Temperature*. Pre-transport measures should be taken to warm the child if the temperature is subnormal.

(ii) *Airway and breathing*. Patency of airways should be maintained by positioning and clearing the secretions. The breathing efforts should be carefully assessed. Oxygen supplementation and assistance in respiratory efforts may be provided as needed. Although it is safer to transport without a tube in the trachea, it is better to intubate before transport if it appears intubation may be required en-route. If the expertise for intubation is not available or if the attempts are unsuccessful, laryngeal mask airway (LMA) is a very useful alternative. It has been used successfully in the inter-hospital transport of sick children as well as neonates[13, 14]. Placement of LMA does not require manipulation of patient's head, neck and jaw, is not influenced by anatomic factors and does not require laryngoscopy. It is particularly useful in patients with airway malformations.

(iii) *Circulation*. Check pulse volume, blood pressure and capillary filling time and take corrective measures.

(iv) *Fluids and glucose*. Check blood glucose. Estimate the travel time and plan for feeding en-route if required. If enteral feeding is contraindicated, dextrose infusion must be started.

(v) *Medications*. Give vitamin K to newborn babies. Administer a dose of antibiotics if sepsis is suspected. All administered drugs must be documented in the referral record.

(vi) *Emotional support*. The transport team on arrival must communicate with the child and his/her parents and family intimating the medical condition, the transport process and realistic expectations.

The components of pre-transport stabilization can be remembered by an acronym S.T.A.B.L.E. – **S**ugar, **T**emperature, **A**irway, **B**lood pressure, **La**b work, **E**motional support[15]. Apart from stabilizing the medical condition of the child, many other arrangements related to transport need to be checked in a systematic manner (Table 10.3).

Table 10.3 Pre-transport check
• Write a precise referral note.
• Careful and complete assessment of the child.
• Check temperature and other vital signs.
• Stabilize the child.
• Administer vitamin K (neonates).
• Give first dose of antibiotics if sepsis is suspected.
• Compile and send lab reports and imaging studies along with the child.
• Take informed consent and provide emotional support to the family.
• Check all equipment, disposables and supplies.
• Check oxygen and air tanks to ensure that they will last during the whole duration of transport.
• Encourage mother to accompany for breast feeding and for providing supportive care. If it is not possible, send a blood sample of the mother along with for cross-matching.
• Communicate and counsel the family about the condition of the child and expected course, location of the referral hospital and contact names/numbers, costs involved, etc.

Care during Transport

Close monitoring of all vital parameters should be carried out and a record maintained. Ensure open airway by proper neck positioning and removal of secretions. Ensure adequacy of spontaneous or supported breathing. Special precautions should be taken to maintain the temperature of small babies. Ensure normoglycemia either by feeding or an uninterrupted infusion of dextrose. If there are new developments, contact should be made with the medical control physician to take advice. The referral unit should also be contacted to give the estimated time of arrival. In case the baby deteriorates, the vehicle should be stopped for any interventions or procedures. It could also be diverted to the nearest health facility.

Adverse events during transport of sick children can be categorized into two: mishaps related to intensive care (e.g. lead disconnection, loss of battery power, accidental extubation, exhaustion of oxygen supply) and physiologic deterioration related to critical illness (e.g. worsening of hypotension or hypoxemia).

Post-transport Checklist

At the end of each transport, all equipment should be placed back in their respective positions and checked. The batteries should be put to charging and supplies re-stocked. The malfunctioning equipment should be repaired or replaced. A check-list of these activities should be kept along with the transport equipment.

Quality Assurance and Quality Improvement

These should be an integral part of the transport program. The guidelines of national societies for pediatric and neonatal transport should be followed to ensure quality and as a safeguard against medico-legal issues. American Academy of Pediatrics has its guidelines for transport of sick children and newborns[3]. National Neonatology Forum of India has also published guidelines for neonatal transport[10]. Various mechanisms like periodic audit of all transport logs and use of scoring systems like Transport Risk Index of Physiologic Stability (TRIPS) or Mortality Index of Neonatal Transport (MINT) can be utilized to achieve this[16-19]. TRIPS is a risk-weighted neonatal transport score and comprises of 4 empirically weighted items (temperature, blood pressure, respiratory status, and response to noxious stimuli) and is able to predict 7-day NICU mortality and

overall NICU mortality (Table 10.4)[16]. The MINT score is a 7 variable score (Apgar score at 1 minute, birth weight, presence of a congenital anomaly, infant's age, pH, partial pressure of oxygen, and intubation at the time of the call) which is recorded on receiving the first call and is a good predictor of neonatal or perinatal mortality (Table 10.5)[18]. The TRIPS is derived from data collected by the transport team immediately after arrival at the referring hospital and again after arrival at the destination hospital. In contrast, MINT score uses that data pertaining to the condition of the child when the referring hospital first contacts the transport team via telephone. A simplified assessment of 4 parameters at admission-**T**emperature, **O**xygenation, capillary refill time (proxy for **P**erfusion) and blood **S**ugar (TOPS) has also been shown to be a good predictor of mortality in transported neonates[20]. In the pediatric age group, four pre-transport variables viz. systolic blood pressure, oxygen requirement, altered mental status and respiratory rate have been shown to predict post-transfer in-hospital mortality and can be used to compare various transport sytems[19].

Table 10.4 Transport risk index of physiologic stability (TRIPS) score[16]		
Variable	**Finding**	**Score**
• Temperature	<36.1°C	8
	36.1 – 36.5°C	1
	36.6 – 37.1°C	0
	37.2 – 37.6°C	1
	>37.6°C	8
• Respiratory dysfunction	Severe (apnea, gasping, intubated)	14
	Moderate (respiratory rate >60 breaths per minute and /or SpO_2 <85%)	5
	None or mild (respiratory rate ≤60 breaths per minute and SpO_2 ≥85%)	0
• Systolic blood pressure	<20 mm Hg	26
	20 – 40 mm Hg	16
	>40 mm Hg	0
• Response to noxious stimuli	None, seizures, muscle relaxant	17
	Lethargic response, no cry	6
	Withdraws vigorously, cries	0

Adapted from Lee SK *et al.* Transport risk index of physiologic stability: A practical system for assessing infant transport care. *J Pediatr* 2001; 139:220-226.

Table 10.5 Mortality index for neonatal transportation (MINT) score[18]		
Variable	**Finding**	**Score**
1. Birth weight	<750 g	5
	751-1000 g	2
	1001-1500 g	1
	>1500 g	0
2. 1-min Apgar score	0	8
	1	5
	2	2
	3	2
	>3	0
3. Age	0-1 hr	4
	> 1 hr	0
4. Congenital abnormality	Yes	5
	No	0
5. pH	<6.9	10
	6.9-7.1	4
	>7.1	0
6. PaO_2	≤3 kPa	2
	>3 kPa	0
7. Intubated at time of call	Yes	6
	No	0

Broughton et al.Neonatal Intensive Care Study Group. The mortality index for neonatal transportation score: a new mortality prediction model for retrieved neonates. *Pediatrics* 2004; 114:e424-8.

Recent developments in our country

In the recent years, the government has developed a network of modern transport vehicles under public-private partnership in several states. These ambulances are well equipped and reach the patient within 20 to 30 minutes by calling a central toll free number 108. They are free of cost and are available even for transporting laboring women to the hospital as well as back-transport after discharge. However, there is an acute shortage of trained para-medics to man these ambulances as well as there is a shortage of hospital beds providing specialized acute care[20]. Although transport facilities have become available, there is an urgent need for coordinated transport network programs, wherein the bed status of all hospitals in a geographic area is inter-linked and the patient can be taken directly to a place where facilities are available.

Conclusions

Till recently, organized transport programs in our country have been virtually non-existent. The most important reason for that is lack of effective regionalization. Development of reliable and model transport system requires cooperative efforts of the apex institutions, district hospitals, private hospitals, government and the professional associations of pediatricians. With the currently available technology, it should not be difficult to develop a good communication module and establish networking between the referring and referral units. The organization of the transport program would need training of multidisciplinary teams of physicians, nurses and other paramedical staff. When transport is required, the referral unit must be contacted without any delay for seeking prompt consultation and help. The transport team should rush to referring unit. The patient must be stabilized before the start of journey and the process of transport should be steady and smooth and handled with confidence and due expertise.

REFERENCES

1.   Insoft RM. Neonatal transport. In: Manual of Neonatal Care. Cloherty JP, Eichenwald EC (Eds.) 6th edition 2008. *Lippincott Williams and Wilkins, Philadelhphia.* pp 147-153.

2.   Rojas MA, Shirley K, Rush MG. In: Merenstein and Gardner's Handbook of Neonatal Intensive Care. Gardner SL, Carter BS, Enzman-Hines MI, Hernandez JA. (Eds.) *Mosby St. Louis,* 7th edition 2011, pp39-51.

3.   American Academy of Pediatrics. Guidelines for Air and Ground Transport of Neonatal and Pediatric Patients. *Elk Grove Village Ill.: American Academy of Pediatrics* 2006.

4.   American Academy of Pediatrics, Committee on Pediatric Emergency Medicine, American College of Critical Care Medicine, Society of Critical Care Medicine: Consensus Report on Regionalization of Services for Critically ill or Injured Children. *Pediatrics* 2000; 105:152-155.

5.   Kinsella JP, Schmidt JM, Abman SH. Inhaled nitric oxide treatment for stabilization and emergency medical transport of critically ill newborns and infants. *Pediatrics* 1995; 92:773-776.

6.   Edge WE, Kanter RK, Weigle CG, Walsh RF. Reduction of morbidity in inter-hospital transport by specialized pediatric staff. *Crit Care Med* 1994; 22:1186-1191.

7.   Lupton BA, Pendray MR. Regionalized neonatal emergency transport. *Semin Neonatol* 2004; 9:125-133.

8. Vos GD, Buurman WA, van Waardenburg DA, Visser TP, Ramsay G, Donckerwolcke RA. Inter-hospital paediatric intensive care transport: a novel transport unit based on a standard ambulance trolley. *Eur J Emerg Med* 2003; 10:195-199.

9. BS EN 1789:2007. Medical vehicles and their equipment. Road ambulances. *British Standards Institute London:* 2007.

10. Saluja S, Malviya M, Garg P. Transport of sick neonate. In: Evidence Based Clinical Practice Guidelines. Kumar P, Jain N,Thakre R, Murki S, Venkataseshan S (Eds.) *National Neonatology Forum , India* 2010. P 303-327.

11. Kofos D, Pitetti R, Orr R, Thompson A. Telemedicine in pediatric transport: A feasibility study. *Pediatrics* 1998; 102:e58.

12. Han YY, Carcillo JA, Dragotta MA, Bills DM, Watson RS, Westerman ME, Orr RA. Early reversal of pediatric-neonatal septic shock by community physicians is associated with improved outcome. *Pediatrics* 2003; 112:793-799.

13. Trevisanuto D, Verghese C, Doglioni N, Ferrarese P, Zanardo V. Laryngeal mask airway for the inter-hospital transport of neonates. *Pediatrics* 2005; 115:e109-111.

14. Berry AM, Brimacombe JR, Verghese C. The laryngeal mask airway in emergency medicine, neonatal resuscitation and intensive care medicine. *Int Anesthesiol Clin* 1998; 36:91-109.

15. Taylor RM, Price-Douglas W. The S.T.A.B.L.E. Program: Postresuscitation/Pretransport stabilization care of sick infants. *J Perinatal Neonatal Nursing* 2008;22:165-171.

16. Lee SK, Zupancic JAF, Pendray M, Thiessen P, Schmidt B, Whyte R, Shorten D, Stewart S, *et al.* The Canadian Neonatal Network. Transport risk index of physiologic stability: a practical system for assessing infant transport care. *J Pediatr* 2001; 139:220-226.

17. Gunnarsson B, Heard CM, Rotta AT, Heard AM, Kourkounis BH, Fletcher JE. Use of a physiologic scoring system during interhospital transport of pediatric patients. *Air Med J* 2001; 20:23-26.

18. Broughton SJ, Berry A, Jacobe S, Cheeseman P, Tarnow-Mordi WO, Greenough A. Neonatal Intensive Care Study Group. The mortality index for neonatal transportation score: a new mortality prediction model for retrieved neonates. *Pediatrics* 2004; 114:e424-428.

19. Orr RA, Venkataraman ST, McCloskey KA, Janosky JE, Dragotta M, Bills D, King WD. Measurement of pediatric illness severity using simple pretransport variables. *Prehosp Emerg Care* 2001; 5:127-133.

20. Mathur NB, Arora D. Role of TOPS (a simplified assessment of neonatal acute physiology) in predicting mortality in transported neonates. *Acta Paediatr* 2007 ;96(2):172-175.

21. David SS, Vasnaik M. Emergency medicine in India: why are we unable to 'walk the talk'? *Emerg Med Australia* 2007 ;19(4):289-295.

2

Symptom-related Emergencies

The Crying Infant and Toddler

11

Meharban Singh

In infants and young children who cannot speak, cry is the only signal to express their needs and draw attention to their discomfort, hunger, and painful or unpleasant conditions. Certain amount of crying is physiological and desirable and is believed to be akin to "exercise period" and "letting off the steam" to give vent to their anger, frustration and to seek attention. Crying may even serve an important development purpose. Healthy infants cry for 2-3 hours on an average every day during first 8 weeks of life[1,2]. Periodic crying in infants is most commonly due to hunger, thirst, uncomfortable environment, over clothing or under clothing, wet nappies, and boredom. Most infants cry and fret while falling asleep. An intelligent and perceptive mother can readily differentiate between the cry due to hunger and cry as a signal of discomfort[3]. A large number of disorders during infancy can be diagnosed on the basis of nature, quality and character of crying[4]. Most parents are quite used to episodic crying of their infants but *persistent or protracted and inconsolable crying* is frightening and presents as one of the common disorders in the emergency department. Excessive crying, especially in the absence of any predisposing conditions and localizing features, poses a great diagnostic challenge to a pediatrician[5-7]. The majority of cases of infants with excessive crying are due to nonserious conditions but at times crying babies may have illnesses that may be life-threatening.

CAUSES

Excessive crying and restlessness most commonly occurs due to a painful condition originating in any of the body systems (Table 11.1). Hypoxia due to cardio-respiratory disorders and shock is an important cause of restlessness and crying but the clinical picture is dominated by underlying condition and infant looks critically sick. Visceral pain occurs due to sudden distension of viscera and stretching of their serosal coverings because internal body organs *per se* are not supplied by pain fibers.

Table 11.1 Causes of excessive crying in infants

Central nervous system
Raised intracranial pressure
- Meningitis/encephalitis
- Reye's syndrome
- Intracranial bleeding
- Space occupying lesion
- Pseudotumor cerebri
- Brain damaged infant

Cardiovascular system
- Congestive heart failure
- Myocarditis
- Pericarditis
- Arrhythmias (paroxysmal supraventricular tachycardia)
- Vaso-occlusive disorders (sickle cell disease, vasculitis, thrombophlebitis, and acrodynia)
- Abnormal left coronary artery from pulmonary artery (ALCAPA)

Respiratory system
- Blocked nose
- Acute suppurative otitis media
- Pneumonia
- Bronchospasm
- Foreign body in the air passages
- Pleural effusion and empyema

Gastrointestinal system
- Aphthous stomatitis
- Herpangina
- Teething
- Intestinal colic (evening colic)
- Lactose intolerance
- Cow's milk allergy
- Mesenteric adenitis
- Appendicitis
- Gastroesophageal reflux disease (GERD)
- Intussusception
- Henoch-Schönlein syndrome
- Acute intermittent porphyria
- Constipation
- Anal fissure
- Foreign body ingestion
- Pinworms

(Table Contd.)

Table 11.1 Causes of excessive crying in infants (Contd.)

Genitourinary system
- Urinary tract infection
- Urinary retention
- Renal colic
- Torsion of testis
- Incarcerated hernia

Musculoskeletal system
- Unrecognised trauma
- Fracture
- Dislocation (elbow, shoulder)
- Osteomyelitis/arthritis
- Bone pains (acute leukemia)
- Scurvy
- Caffey's disease
- Battered baby syndrome

Emotional causes
- Over stimulation or neglect
- Tension in the family dynamics
- Over anxious mother or grandmother
- Post-partum depression

Miscellaneous conditions
- Temper tantrum
- Over covered or exposed baby
- Foreign body in the eye or nose
- Insect bites
- Open diaper pin
- Hair tourniquet syndrome
- Scared or frightened infant
- DTwP vaccine
- Poisoning
- Drugs

Night Crying
- ☐ Evening colic
- ☐ Nasal congestion
- ☐ Over clothing or under clothing
- ☐ Teething
- ☐ Pinworms
- ☐ Diaper rash
- ☐ Insect bites (mosquitoes, bed bugs, mites)
- ☐ Excessive light or noise
- ☐ Gastroesophageal reflux disease (GERD)
- ☐ Bronchospasm
- ☐ Bone pains (growing pains, acute leukemia)

wriggle into the vaginal orifice[12, 13]. Episodes of crying spells with arching of back, vomiting and poor feeding due to esophagitis and heart burn are suggestive of gastro-esophageal reflux disease (GERD). There may be sleeplessness, difficulty in burping, gagging, ear infection and coughing at night due to aspiration into lungs[14].

Some infants with perinatal distress factors, and neuromotor retardation have increased incidence of unexplained crying possibly due to cerebral irritability. Infants with acute gastroenteritis often cry due to thirst but it is often misinterpreted as colic. Crying or fussiness while feeding should alert to the possibility of nose block, aphthous stomatitis and herpangina. Biting of gums, rubbing of ears, refusal of feeds and drooling of saliva during second semester of infancy in a fretful infant are suggestive of discomfort of teething which hardly ever poses as a medical emergency. Infants cannot vocalize to indicate the site of pain, which may be suggested by certain gestures like flexion of thighs over abdomen with passage of flatus (intestinal colic), head banging (head ache), poking fingers or pulling at ears (ear ache), touching or rubbing genitals (UTI or balanitis), inability to move a limb (pseudoparalysis due to scurvy, osteomyelitis, congenital syphilis, fracture and dislocation etc.), blinking, rubbing and watering of an eye due to foreign body and conjunctivitis.

HISTORY

Detailed history should be elicited to identify preceding events and associated symptoms[8]. Episodes of crying, fretfulness and fussiness in the evening in infants between 2-16 weeks of age with characteristic periodicity is highly suggestive of evening colic[9-11]. Night crying is common during infancy (Box). It is apparent rather than real because infants are not aware of day and night, even physiological whimpering due to hunger or wet napkin appear too loud during the quietness and solitude of night. Night crying is more disturbing and troublesome to tired parents and neighbours because it interferes with their relaxation and sleep. Abnormal and excessive crying at night should alert to the possibilities of exposure to cold or hot environment, wet napkin, nappy rash, insect bites due to mosquitoes and bed bugs. Pinworms though uncommon in infants may cause crying at night due to perianal itching. Sudden episodes of crying at night may occur in female infants when pinworms

Most crying infants are quietened when picked up or gently rocked. When episodes of crying are precipitated or aggravated when the baby is picked up, it is suggestive of a painful condition in the musculoskeletal system. Sudden pulling of a resisting toddler by forearms may lead to severe pain and inconsolable crying due to subluxation of the radial head (annular ligament displacement) which is commonly called as "nursemaid's elbow". Chronic constipation and crying while defecating are suggestive of anal fissure. *When an infant with acute gastroenteritis develops sudden constipation with passage of currant-jelly stools and episodes of inconsolable crying due to abdominal colic, it is highly suggestive of acute intussusception*[15]. Rarely, intussusception may occur following administration of rotavirus vaccine. Unexpalined episodes of severe abdominal pain and bone pains may occur due to vaso-occlusive crises of sickle cell disease and in children with acute leukemia. The conditions may at times be confused with surgical abdomen and osteomyelitis. Presence of fever is suggestive of an infective condition and in these cases the cause of crying can be usually established. Attempt should be made to look for symptoms referable to various systems of the body; central nervous system (head banging, vomiting, photophopia), cardio-respiratory system (cough, breathing and feeding difficulty), gastrointestinal system (vomiting, constipation, diarrhea, colic) and genitourinary system (dysuria, frequency, urinary retention, abnormalities in urinary stream). Most healthy infants may cry before passing urine due to the unpleasant sensation of full bladder. However, they become quiet, relaxed and dazed while passing urine and start crying again after having passed urine due to wet napkins.

Specific history should be asked for inhalation or ingestion of a foreign body. Sudden episode of choking and crying in an infant who was seen to be fiddling and mouthing some objects (peanut, coin, beads, toys with loose or sharp components etc.) is highly suggestive of inhalation or ingestion of a foreign body. Detailed enquiry should be made regarding the medications being taken. Excessive irritability and restlessness may occur due to intake of atropine derivatives, pseudoephedrine, antispasmodics and xanthine derivatives. Some infants are known to become restless following intake of sedatives, which are also known to precipitate abdominal colic in patients with acute intermittent porphyria. Excessive crying due to pseudotumor cerebri is a recognized side effect of excessive or prolonged intake of nalidixic acid, norfloxacin, tetracyclines, corticosteroids, and vitamin A. Prolonged and excessive local application of topical anesthetic (lignocaine hydrochloride) over perianal area in an infant with anal fissure may lead to excessive irritability, restlessness and even seizures. Excessive and inconsolable crying is a recognised adverse effect due to pertussis component of DTwP vaccination. History of accidental and intentional trauma should be elicited with tact and ingenuity. Inconsolable crying of an infant is a challenge and frustrating experience for parents and may lead to infant abuse and "shaking" of a crying infant. Changes in the emotional milieu

like change of environment, visit by guests, change in type and mode of feeding, tension among parents, inappropriate response on the part of mother to meet the needs of her infant are important causes of fretfulness and fussiness[16].

PHYSICAL EXAMINATION

A detailed physical examination of a nude infant from "top-to-toes" remains the cornerstone of evaluation of the crying infant. Special emphasis should be placed on general physical examination. External marks of injuries, insect bites, swellings, fracture and dislocation should be looked for. Presence of papules and wheals over the exposed parts is suggestive of mosquito or insect bites. Watch for range and strength of spontaneous movements of all the extremities. Infants with "pulled elbow" (subluxation of radial head) are unable to use the arm which is kept semiflexed and supinated (nursemaid's position or Indian lady supporting her saree). Look at toes and fingers to exclude strangulation due to hair tourniquet. The diaper must be removed to exclude torsion of testis, incarcerated hernia, strangulation of penis, diaper rash and injury by diaper pin. Unilateral scrotal swelling with suffusion or blueness of overlying skin with absence of cremasteric reflex are suggestive of torsion of testis. Exclude anal fissure and look for perianal redness as a marker of pin worm infestation. Entrapment of the penis in the zipper of the trousers is easy to diagnose but at times extremely difficult to extricate. Vital signs should be recorded to exclude fever, hypothermia, shock and hypotension, tachypnea and dyspnea, tachycardia and dysrhythmia which provide useful clues to the involvement of major organ systems.

Eyes should be examined for pupillary size and eyelids must be everted to look for any evidence of a foreign body. Oral examination should be conducted to exclude aphthous ulcers, swelling of gums due to teething, and angina of throat. Otoscopy is mandatory to visualize tympanic membrane to exclude acute otitis media. Fundus examination should be done to look for retinal hemorrhages (as an evidence of battering and vigorous shaking) and papilledema. Bulging anterior fontanel is suggestive of raised intracranial tension. Neck stiffness may be absent or insignificant in young infants with meningitis.

Systemic examination should be conducted to exclude potentially life-threatening conditions. During the bout of screaming, heart (to exclude tachyrhythmia like PSVT) and abdomen (to look for borborygmi due to intestinal obstruction and colic) should be carefully auscultated. Evidences of congestive heart failure point to the underlying cardiac problem while tachypnea with intercostal and subcostal retractions are suggestive of pneumonia and bronchospasm. In young infants excessive and inconsolable crying may be the sole manifestation of septicemia[17]. ALCAPA (abnormal origin of left coronary artery from pulmonary artery) is a rare cause of sudden episodes of inconsolable crying with sweating which is followed by lethargy and extreme exhaustion. The infant is likely to have evidences of cardiac failure with findings of anterolateral myocardial infarction on EKG i.e. deep Q waves in lead 1, aVL and V1-V4. History of sudden choking, stridor and unilateral wheezing are diagnostic of a foreign body in the air passages. Look for abdominal distension and persistaltic movements to exclude intestinal obstruction. When indicated, rectal examination should be done to exclude intussusception. Urinary retention should be excluded by percussing the suprapubic area and by palpating for a distended urinary bladder.

Wessel et al[7] has proposed "the rule of three" to define infantile colic i.e. irritability, fussing or crying lasting for more than 3 hours in a day, occuring on more than 3 days in a week and lasting for at least 3 weeks. Evening colic is the most common cause of unexplained crying in infants. It occurs in about 20 percent of "normal" infants and is characterized by paroxysmal episodes of inconsolable crying during the evening in infants between 2 to 16 weeks of age[1, 5, 14]. The spell of crying occurs everyday at the same time in a clockwise regularity. The infant appears in severe discomfort, cries loudly, often flexes the legs over the abdomen, boxes the arms and may pass wind to obtain temporary relief. The condition is seen in equal frequency in both breast and bottle fed babies. The episodes of crying abort spontaneously and none of the therapeutic interventions seem to offer any definite relief. The condition disappears after the age of 12 weeks. The etiology is unknown but various postulations include intestinal colic ("blocked" wind), milk allergy, lactose intolerance, altered flora of gut, immaturity of intestinal tract or central nervous system, oversensitive wiry infant, excessive stimulation, parental anxiety, abnormal emotional tension in the environment, and inappropriate response on the part of mother to serve the needs and desires of the infant[14,18,19].

INVESTIGATIONS

Careful history, detailed physical examination and close observation are most crucial to identify the cause of inconsolable crying in an infant. In about two-thirds of cases, cause of excessive crying can be identified by good history and detailed physical examinaton[20]. No routine investigations are needed for an afebrile crying infant with no signs of illness. Investigations should be planned depending upon the clues obtained on clinical assessment[21]. No uniform plan of investigations can be recommended for all crying infants. In the absence of any localizing symptoms and signs, abdominal colic, urinary tract infection, sepsis, episodic cardiac arrhythmia or angina equivalent and emotional causes should be seriously considered. Urine examination (routine and culture) is recommended in all infants to exclude UTI and acute intermittent porphyria. When tachypnea and dyspnea are associated, detailed cardio-respiratory workup is indicated to diagnose underlying pulmonary and cardiac disorders. In infants with bulging anterior fontanel or retinal hemorrhages, exclude meningitis and intracranial bleeding by CSF examination and CT scan of brain. When abdominal distension is present or UTI is documented, skiagrams of abdomen should be taken and ultrasonography done. Skeletal survey is indicated if there are any clinical evidences of scurvy, osteomyelitis/arthritis, trauma and Caffey's disease. When corneal foreign body is suspected, flourescein staining is indicated to delineate it.

MANAGEMENT

Excessive crying in the first months of life is usually benign and self limiting. The specific management depends upon the nature of underlying disease process. Symptomatic relief should be attempted when serious life threatening conditions have been excluded. Analgesics like paracetamol, and ibuprofen are useful for relief of pain due to inflammatory and traumatic conditions affecting musculoskeletal system. Antispasmodics (dicyclomine hydrochloride, oxyphenonium bromide, pipenzolate mythylbromide) are useful for relief of colicky visceral pain. Nothing seems to offer consistent benefit to infants with evening colic. Temporary relief is obtained by rhythmic rocking, crib vibrator, playing some soft music, positioning the baby prone on the thighs and patting on the back, giving lift in a car or producing a continuous sound with an alarm clock, hair dryer, an electric shaver or a washing machine. Mother should not follow the policy of 'cry it out' (CIO) to manage a cranky infant because it does not work and may lead to insecurity, behavior disorder and distributed parent-child relationship. Mother must respond promptly to a child in discomfort by picking and cuddling him without any fear of spoiling the child. Diaper should be checked for soiling and feed given if child is hungry. Application of *hing* (asfoetida) dissolved in warm water over the periumbilical area and giving decoction of *ajwain* (carom seeds) and *sonf* (anethi seeds) provides prompt relief against intestinal colic[20]. Gripe water formulated without alcohol may be given. Dicyclomine hydrochloride (2-3 mg/dose) 30 minutes before the anticipated time of evening colic may offer relief to some infants but it is not without side effects. In a randomized placebo-controlled, double-blind study, administration of probiotics (*Lactobocillus reuteri*) for 21 days was associated with reduction in the severity and duration of colic[20]. There is no need to change the type and mode of feeding and attempts should be made to reduce environmental tension and decrease stimulation to the child. Excessive crying and sleep disturbances have been treated by chiropractice practices like gentle touch, pressure and spinal manipulations[22]. The condition gradually resolves and spontaneously disappears by the age of 3 months.

Use of mosquito net and mebendazole for pinworms may relieve spells of night crying. Night crying due to GERD can be managed by positioning the infant with head raised, administration of proton pump inhibitor (ranitidine, lansoprazole) and prokinetics (domperidone, metoclopramide) before feeds[23]. Lansoprazole is given in a dose of 1.0 mg/kg q 12 hr for 8-12 weeks. Excessive crying during acute gastroenteritis is often due to thirst and promptly responds to administration of ORS. Fussiness and discomfort of teething can be relieved by use of a mild sedative (triclofos sodium 10-20 mg/kg/dose) or administration of paracetamol and application of anesthetic gel over the gums. Infants who continue to cry excessively during the prolonged period of observation are likely to have a serious cause for crying[24]. Some of the conditions listed in Table 11.1 would need urgent surgical intervention.

Anal fissure is managed by local application of anesthetic cream and relief of constipation by use of fruit juice, honey, milk of magnesia and dietary advise. Subluxation of radial head can be readily corrected in the emergency department by "hand shake" or "supination-flexion" maneuver[25]. In the former procedure, child's hand is held as if to shake it and the affected elbow is enclosed by the physician in the other hand. Abruptly the forearm is pronated while increasing flexion at the elbow. Alternatively, hold the affected elbow of the child in your left hand by placing thumb over the radial head. With your right hand, quickly supinate the forearm while slightly flexing the elbow. The subluxation is promptly corrected and a palpable click may be felt by your thumb. There is no need to take any skiagrams before and after the procedure. Recurrence of nursemaid's elbow may occur in 5%–39% cases and has been successfully treated by giving instructions on telephone[26].

Crying due to raised intracranial tension caused by medications responds promptly on discontinuation of the offending drug. Restlessness and crying due to cerebral irritability in brain damaged children may be treated by administration of diphenhydramine hydrochloride (5 mg/kg/day q 8 hr). For management of life-threatening disorders associated with excessive inconsolable crying refer to the appropriate sections of the book.

REFERENCES

1. Brazelton TBA. Crying in infancy. *Pediatrics* 1962; 29:579-588.

2. St. James-Roberts I, Halil T. Infant crying patterns in the first year: Normative and clinical findings. *J Child Psychol Psychiatry* 1991; 32: 951-968.

3. Nash C, Morris J, Goodman B. A study describing mother's opinions of the crying behaviour of infants under one year of age. *Child Abuse Review* 2008, 17: 191-200.

4. Corwin MJ, Lester BM, Golub HL. The infant cry: What can it tell us? *Curr Prob Pediatr* 1996; 26:325-334.

5. Barr RG, Rotman A, Yaremko J, *et al*. The crying infant with colic: A controlled empirical description. *Pediatrics* 1992; 90:14-21.

6. St. James-Roberts I. Persistent infant crying. *Arch Dis Child* 1991; 66:653-655.

7. Wessel MA, Cobb JC, Jackson EB, *et al*. Paroxysmal fussing in infancy, sometimes called "colic". *Pediatrics* 1954; 14:421-434.

8. Valman HB. The first year of life: crying babies. *Brit Med J* 1980; 280:1522-1555.

9. Illingworth RS. Three months colic. *Arch Dis Child* 1954; 29:165-174.

10. Illingworth RS. Crying in infants and children. *Brit Med J* 1955; 1: 75.

11. Illingworth RS. Infantile colic revisited. *Arch Dis Child* 1985; 60: 981-985.

12. Ferber R. Sleeplessness, night awakening and night crying in the infant to toddler. *Pediatr Rev* 1987; 9:69-82.

13. Bruce JW. Infantile colic. *Pediatr Clin North Amer* 1961; 8:143-145.

14. Bhatia J, Parish A. GERD or not GERD: The fussy infant. J Perinatol 2009, 29 (Suppl 2): S7-S11.

15. Singh M. Main dangers of diarrhea In: A Manual of Essential Pediatrics. *Thieme Medical and Scientific Publishers Private Limited, New Delhi* 2nd edition 2013, p 334.

16. St. James Roberts I. Persistent crying in infancy. *J Child Psychol Psychiatry* 1989; 3:189-195.

17. Ruis-Conteraras J, Urquio L, Bastero R. Persistent crying as predominant manifestation of sepsis in infants and newborns. *Pediatr Emerg Care* 1999; 15:113-115.

18. McKenzile S. Troublesome crying in infants: effect of advice to reduce stimulation. *Arch Dis Child* 1991; 66:1416-1420.

19. Taubman B. Parental counselling compared with elimination of cow's milk or soy milk protein for the treatment of infant colic syndrome: a radomized trial. *Pediatrics* 1988; 3:189-195.

20. Singh M. The 'windy' baby. In: The Art and Science of Baby and Child Care. *CBS Publishers & Distributors Pvt Ltd, New Delhi,* 4th edition 2015; p 65.

21. Freedman SB, Al-Harthy N, Thull-Freedman J. The crying infant: Diagnostic testing and frequency of serious underlying disease. *Pediatrics* 2009, 123: 841-848.

22. Huhtala V, Lehtonen L, Heinonen R, Korvenrant H. Infant massage compared with crib vibrator in the treatment of colicky infants. *Pediatrics* 2000, 105 (6): E84.

23. Lee JH, Kim MJ, Lee JS, Chol YH. The effects of three alternative treatment strategies after 8 weeks of proton pump inhibitor therapy for GERD children. *Arch Dis Child* 2011, 96: 9-13

24. Poole SR. The infant with acute unexplained excessive crying. *Pediatrics* 1991; 88:450-455.

25. Schunk JE. Radial head subluxation: epidemiology and treatment of 87 episodes. *Ann Emerg Med* 1990; 19:1019-1023.

26. Kaplan RE, Lillis KA. Recurrent nursemaid's elbow (annular ligament displacement) treatment via telephone. *Pediatrics* 2002; 110:171-174.

Section 2

12

Acute Abdomen

Sandeep Agarwala and Ankur Mandelia

The term acute abdomen is applied to any condition that gives rise to acute abdominal pain. Abdominal pain is one of the most frequent complaints in children and adolescents for seeking consultation with a physician. The evaluation of abdominal pain is a challenging clinical problem in pediatric medical or surgical practice.[1,2] In children with acute abdomen, pain may often be overshadowed by other symptoms like vomiting, abdominal distension, obstipation, diarrhea, fever, hematemesis or melena. Occasionally these latter associated symptoms may be the only presenting symptoms of an acute abdominal pathology. The clinician evaluating the child with acute abdominal pain must decide whether the child has a "surgical abdomen", a medical problem which needs admission to the hospital or one which can be managed on an outpatient basis. Though surgical causes account for only about 10 percent of all causes of abdominal pain in children but they have the potential of being fatal if untreated[3].

Abdominal pain is classified as visceral, parietal and referred. The parietal peritoneum is derived from the somatopleural mesoderm, while the splanchnopleural mesoderm gives rise to the visceral peritoneum. Because of this different derivation, the parietal peritoneum shares its neurovascular and lymphatic connections with the musculoskeletal abdominal wall, while the visceral peritoneum shares its connections with the associated visceral organs.

Visceral pain is perceived through neuronal pathways from the lower thoracic and lumbar splanchnic nerves and the parasympathetic pathways of the vagus and sacral plexus. Sensation of pain from the viscera is produced in response to streching or distension of the wall of a hollow organ or capsule of a solid organ, inflammation or ischemia. It may also occur due to pull on or twisting of the mesentry as in torsion of the pedicle of different organs such as ovary or testis. Visceral pain is usually dull aching, when it is because of inflammation, or colicky (griping) when due to distension of a hollow viscus. When hyperperistalsis is the cause of pain, as in the initial phases of mechanical obstruction of the bowel or the ureters, the pain is intermittent and griping and is synchronous to each bout of hyperperistalsis. Mild pressure on the abdomen at times is reported to give some relief to the pain due to spasm. Nausea, vomiting and sweating commonly occur in association with visceral pain. Visceral pain is poorly localized in the epigastric, periumbilical or hypogastric regions depending upon the dermatomes that innervate the organ. Pain from the liver, pancreas, biliary tree, stomach or proximal small intestine (T5 to T8) is felt in the epigastrium. Pain from the distal small intestine, right colon and appendix (T9-T10) is felt in the periumbilical region while that from the left colon, rectum, urinary tract and genital organs (T11, T12, L1, L2) is usually felt over the suprapubic region.

The neuronal innervation to the parietal peritoneum is derived from the somatic nerves supplying the adjacent abdominal wall structures and skin. Therefore, *parietal pain* is more steady, localized, intense and of a burning character. Parietal pain (or somatic pain) is because of the peritoneal inflammation or irritation by blood, inflammatory exudate or contents of a hollow viscus. It is usually associated with voluntary guarding or rigidity with or without rebound tenderness. Pressure over the area usually aggravates the pain. Pain beginning as a dull poorly localized pain of visceral origin may become sharp and localized because of localized peritoneal inflammation. Subsequently when this pain becomes more diffuse and severe it suggests that a hollow viscus has perforated leading to generalized peritonitis

Referred pain has many of the characteristics of parietal pain but is felt in remote areas supplied by the same dermatome as the diseased organ. It results from shared central pathways for afferent neurons from different sites. A classic example is a patient with pneumonia who presents with abdominal pain because the T9 dermatome distribution is shared by the lung and the abdomen.[4] The common extra-abdominal primary sites which may cause referred pain to the abdomen include thorax, spine, hips and pelvis.

Approach to a Child with Acute Abdomen

Accurate history is of paramount importance but is dependent on the ability and willingness of the child to communicate and on the observational skills of the parents. Most children above the age of 4-5 years will give a useful history if obtained in a relaxed environment. Depending upon his age the child should be kept in the parents lap or seated comfortably besides the parent. Historical data may be non-specific in infants and children too young to verbalize their complaints. Often children may be placed in day care centers, and a reliable history may not be available from the parents. In such situations physical examination is more important.

It is necessary to record the age of the patient as many conditions are common in certain age groups (Table 12.1). Acute abdominal conditions in infants, children and adolescents are often different from those in adults. Certain diseases are more frequent in infants than in older children and adolescents. In infants, acute abdomen is commonly due to incarceration of hernia, obstruction from intussusception or volvulus and necrotizing enterocolitis. Older children are more likely to have abdominal symptoms from appendicitis, mesenteric adenitis, intestinal obstruction (as in severe ascaris infestation or in tubercular abdomen), urinary tract infection and viral syndromes. In the prepubertal children and adolescents the diseases seen in adults become more common. These include gallstones, pancreatitis, inflammatory bowel disease and appendicitis. One must not forget the pain of mittleschmirz, pelvic inflammatory disease, ectopic pregnancy, ovarian neoplasms, cysts and their torsion in adolescent girls.

Four main symptoms which need to be critically evaluated are *pain, vomiting, bowel function and urinary symptoms* in addition to general systemic features and the past medical history.

Table 12.1 Common causes of acute abdominal pain at various age groups[3]
Neonates (upto 28 days)
• Evening or infantile colic
• Necrotizing enterocolitis
• Intestinal obstruction
• Malrotation with volvulus
Infants (< 2 years)
• Incarcerated hernia
• Intussusception
• Urinary tract infection
• Gastroenteritis
• Intestinal obstruction
• Malrotation with volvulus
• Trauma
• Lower lobe pneumonitis
Children (2-18 years)
• Appendicitis
• Gastroenteritis
• Constipation
• Helmenthiasis
• Trauma
• Hepatitis
• Peptic ulcer disease
• Abdominal tuberculosis
• Pancreatitis
• Lower lobe pneumonia
• Abdominal tumors
• Gall stones
• Inflammatory bowel disease
• Pyelonephritis/ cystitis
• Incarcerated hernia
• Testicular or ovarian torsion
• Amebic typhlitis
• Pharyngitis/ tonsillitis
• Meckel's diverticulitis
• Mesenteric adenitis
• Spontaneous bacterial peritonitis
• Pelvic inflammatory disease
• Ectopic pregnancy
• Ovarian cyst
• Henoch-Schonlein purpura
• Sickle cell crisis
• Porphyria
• Lead poisoning
• Dietary indiscretion
• Idiopathic

Pain

Time of onset of pain. Pain of less than 6 hours duration, accompanied by nonspecific findings would require further observation to determine the nature of illness. Pain lasting for more than 6 hours is more likely to have a serious underlying surgical or medical cause.

Mode of onset. The pain is sudden in onset in visceral colic, perforation and torsion of pedicles. In acute intestinal obstruction the pain may be mild initially, but soon increases in intensity.

The location of pain. This is of great help in arriving at a diagnosis. Pain of parietal character indicates affliction of the underlying organ. On being asked to indicate the location of pain, a child more than 4-5 years of age would point with a finger to a localized area in a case of localized pain. They generally tend to use vaguely the flat of the palm over the abdomen in case the pain is of more diffuse or nonspecific character. Pain that is migratory or fleeting in character is seldom suggestive of a surgical problem and is more likely to be due to gastroenteritis, typhlitis, constipation or flatulence.

Shifting of pain. The typical example being that of acute appendicitis in which the initial dull, poorly localized pain because of the distension of the appendix is perceived in the periumbilical region. This then shifts to become a more continuous, sharp pain localized to the right iliac fossa because of the inflammation of the parietal peritoneum over the appendix. Later if there is perforation and generalized peritonitis, the pain becomes generalized all over the abdomen with other signs like guarding and rigidity.

Migration of pain. This generally occurs in spreading peritonitis. In pancreatitis pain migrates to the back while pain due to renal colic migrates or is referred towards the groin and inner side of thigh.

Referral of pain. This is because of the dual identical innervation of a viscera and somatic site. The diaphragm is supplied by the phrenic nerve (C4) which also has cutaneous distribution over the shoulder through the supraclavicular nerves. Therefore, any irritation of the underside of the diaphragm, causes referred pain to the corresponding shoulder. Pain of renal colic is referred to the groin, testis and the inner side of the thigh i.e. the distribution of the genitofemoral

nerve (L1 & L2) which supplies the ureter also. Biliary colic is often referred to the tip of the right scapula and the pancreatic pain is typically referred to the back. The irritation of the parietal pleura may occur in children with basal pneumonia, resulting in pain in abdomen.

Character of pain. This is important to distinguish visceral from parietal pain but is often difficult for a child to describe. The character of pain cannot be ascertained in infants and toddlers but the observant parents can determine whether the discomfort is constant or intermittant. In colicky pain because of intussusception the child characteristically draws up the thighs on to the abdomen and cries for 2-5 minutes after which it is spontaneously relieved, only to recur after a varying period of 15-30 minutes. It is also important to note any change in character of pain. For example, the colicky pain of acute intestinal obstruction may change to constant burning pain of peritonitis. Decrease in the severity of pain after the above sequence should not be mistaken for resolution of the disease process because some relief may occur due to dilution of the irritant intestinal contents with the peritoneal exudate. In such a situation, though the pain has decreased, the child deteriorates, looks sicker, becomes apathetic, with a rising pulse rate, increasing abdominal distension, labored breathing and other features of septic shock. The major causes of obstruction in children are abdominal tuberculosis, intussusception, malrotation, congenital webs and stenosis, congenital bands and adhesions, incarcerated hernias, helminthiasis and Hirschsprung's disease.[5]

Child's activity level. This is an important indicator of the severity of underlying disease. A pain sufficiently severe to awaken a child from sound sleep is more significant than the pain that occurs just before going to school or when coaxed to drink milk but never on weekends. A child with renal colic, gallstone or gastroenteritis may toss and turn during the discomfort while a child with peritonitis or appendicitis prefers to lie motionless. A child who can jump down the examination table is unlikely to have appendicitis.

Whether the pain is related to a natural act like defecation, micturition or respiration. Pain during the act of defecation may be because of anal fissure leading to severe constipation. Pain during micurition is commonly seen in children suffering from urinary tract infection. It may also be seen in cases of lower ureteric calculi, urethral calculi, pelvic abscess and pelvic appendix with appendicitis.

How is the pain relieved? The pain may be relieved spontaneously (as in intussusception) or with antispasmodics (as in renal colic). Temporary relief in colics may be obtained by applying pressure or hot fomentation over abdomen while the pain of pancreatitis is classically relieved on sitting-up and bending forward.

Vomiting

Pathophysiology. Despite the frequency of vomiting as a chief complaint in many illnesses, its pathophysiology is not well understood. Afferent inputs from the chemoreceptor trigger zone, vestibular apparatus, cerebral cortex, and GI tract result in the release of multiple neurotransmitters, including dopamine, acetylcholine, serotonin, and histamine. Afferent inputs arrive at the vomiting center, a nucleus of cells located in the medulla, where efferent impulses are sent to the salivation, and respiratory centers, abdominal muscles, and cranial nerves.[6]

Its relationship with pain. In acute surgical conditions, such as intestinal obstruction, acute appendicitis, biliary and renal colics, pancreatitis etc., the pain always occurs before or during vomiting. If the vomiting has occurred before the onset of pain, one must suspect gastroenteritis or other non-specific causes of pain. In high intestinal obstruction at the level of duodenum or upper jejunum, the vomiting appears almost simultaneously with pain, even before the onset of any significant distension. In contrast, in low small bowel obstruction, vomiting occurs a few hours after the onset of pain by which time there is significant abdominal distension with or without visible peristalsis. In colonic obstruction vomiting is absent or a very late feature while distension is predominant.

Frequency and quantity. In acute appendicitis one or two episodes of vomiting may occur in the early stages but may cease later on only to reappear in case generalized peritonitis sets in. Vomiting is invariable, frequent and profuse in acute intestinal obstruction and pancreatitis. Assessment of the frequency and the quantity would also help in proper assessment of the fluid and electrolyte losses.

Character of the act. In high intestinal obstruction, vomiting is forceful or projectile. In peritonitis and paralytic ileus the vomiting is usually effortless regurgitation of mouthfuls. It is this type of vomiting which places an obtunded child at a great risk of aspiration which presents in the postoperative period as severe chest infection.

Nature of vomitus. Bilious vomiting always indicates intestinal obstruction unless proved otherwise. Dark green vomitus indicate an obstruction lower down which is of longer duration. In peritonitis and distal intestinal obstruction the vomitus is often feculent or dark brown and may be mixed with altered blood. Dark brown altered blood or fresh blood in the vomitus indicates gastritis or other conditions like peptic ulcer disease or portal hypertension.

Bowel functions

Diarrhea occurs commonly in intestinal diseases of viral or bacterial etiology. These agents cause diarrhea by adherence, mucosal invasion, enterotoxin production, and/or cytotoxin production. These mechanisms result in increased fluid secretion and/or decreased absorption. This produces an increased luminal fluid content that cannot be adequately reabsorbed, leading to dehydration and the loss of electrolytes and nutrients. In these conditions the stool volume is usually large and accompanied with cramping abdominal pain which is alleviated by passage of diarrheal stools. Semi-loose or soft stools mixed with mucus and blood, which tends to stick to the pan is indicative of amebiasis. In intussusception the initial episode of diarrhea may be replaced with frequent passage of mucus and later by currant-jelly stools. In pelvic appendicitis, pelvic abscess, pelvic inflammatory disease and tubo-ovarian masses the irritation of the rectum leads to tenesmus i.e. constant urge to defecate with ineffectual and painful straining at stools. The stools in such instances are of small volume but frequently passed. Enterocolitis due to Hirschsprung's disease may present with loose watery, foul smelling stools accompanied by features of systemic toxemia. The diagnosis of Hirschsprung's disease, in such cases is suspected because of the long-standing history of chronic constipation usually dating back to birth.

Absolute *constipation (obstipation)* is characterized by absence of passage of both feces and flatus and is the usual accompaniment of acute intestinal obstruction or peritonitis. Even in complete obstruction, the child may pass feces a couple of times, after the onset of pain, but this would cease once the distal bowel becomes empty.

Urinary symptoms

Frequency, hematuria, and dysuria are suggestive of genitourinary pathology. Inflammed pelvic appendix lying on the ureter is known to cause dysuria and pain which may radiate down to the groin and may be a cause of confusion in clinical diagnosis. Genitourinary diseases generally present as chronic problems but a few like acute pyelonephritis, urinary calculi and occasionally severe urinary tract infection may present in the form of an acute abdominal emergency with symptoms of infection and obstruction. Renal angle tenderness may be present in pyelonephritis in addition to high grade unrelenting fever and pain in the flanks. The diagnosis can be suggested by an ultrasound examination which will usually show hydronephrosis with debris in the pelvicalyceal system. Obstruction due to urinary calculi also presents primarily as pain abdomen which classically radiates depending on the location of the stone. There may or may not be gross hematuria but microscopic hematuria is invariably present and the diagnosis in such cases is confirmed on a X-ray and ultrasound evaluation of entire kidney-ureter-bladder regions.

History of systemic illness

Presence of headache, sore throat, and generalized aches and pains with fever and malaise are suggestive of an acute viral illness. Some of the systemic illnesses may present as acute abdominal pain and must be seriously considered (Table 12.2). The common systemic conditions include pharyngitis, epiglottitis, mumps, measles, and pneumonia. Other systemic disorders like acute

Table 12.2 Systemic causes of acute abdominal pain
Metabolic and hematologic
• Acute porphyria
• Hereditary angioneurotic edema
• Sickle cell crisis
• Leukemia
• Lymphoma
• Acute hemolytic states
• Diabetic ketoacidosis
• Hemolytic uremic syndrome
• Addison disease
• Electrolyte imbalance
• Hyperparathyroidism-hypercalcemic states (urolithiasis, pancreatitis)
• Hypertriglyceridemia (pancreatitis)
Musculo-skeletal
• Arthritis, discitis
• Osteomyelitis
• Thoracic nerve root dysfunction
• Trauma/child abuse
• Hernia
Neurologic
• Abdominal epilepsy
• Abdominal migraine
• Brain tumor
• Multiple sclerosis
• Radiculopathy
• Neuropathy
• Herpes zoster
Drugs, toxins and heavy metal poisoning
• Lead
• Arsenic
• Mercury
• Mushroom ingestion
• Narcotic withdrawal
Infectious/inflammatory
• Acute rheumatic fever
• Infectious mononucleosis
• Measles
• Mumps
• Pneumonia
• Pericarditis/endocarditis
• Pharyngitis
• Epididymitis/orchitis
• Henoch-Schönlein purpura
• Systemic lupus erythematosus

porphyria, sickle cell crisis, leukemia, diabetic ketoacidosis, hemolytic uremic syndrome, and Henoch-Schonlein purpura must always be kept in mind to avoid unnecessary laparotomy (Table 12.3).

Table 12.3 Medical history that may suggest the cause of acute abdomen	
Historical factor	**Cause of pain**
• Sickle cell anemia	Vaso-occlusive disease, cholelithiasis, hepatitis, hemolytic crisis, renal infarction, splenic sequestration
• Diabetes mellitus	Pancreatitis, gastric neuropathy
• Cirrhosis, nephrotic syndrome	Primary bacterial peritonitis
• SLE and other autoimmune disorders	Vasculitis, serositis, pancreatitis, infarction
• Corticosteroids	Gastric ulceration, pancreatitis
• NSAIDs	Gastric ulceration, ileal perforation, renal papillary necrosis
• HIV	Gastroenteritis, hepatitis, pancreatitis, esophagitis, lymphoma
• Infectious mononucleosis	Hepatitis, splenic rupture
• Cystic fibrosis	Pancreatitis, diabetes mellitus, meconium ileus equivalent, appendicitis, intussusception, biliary or urinary stones
• Henoch-Schonlein purpura	Mucosal hemorrhages, intussusception
• Hemolytic uremic syndrome	Colitis
• Upper respiratory tract infection	Mesenteric adenitis, pneumonia
• Prior history of surgery	Abscess, adhesions, obstruction, stricture, pancreatitis, ectopic pregnancy
• Inborn errors of metabolism	Pancreatitis due to hypertryglyceridemia, Hypercalcemia

Gynecologic history

In girls, a thorough gynecologic history, including menstrual history and history of sexual activity and contraception, is essential. Purulent vaginal discharge suggests salpingitis. Amenorrhea may indicate pregnancy. Sudden onset of midcycle pain of short duration suggests mittelschmerz.[7]

Past illnesses

A history of surgery not only can eliminate certain diagnoses but also can increase the risk of others, such as intestinal obstruction from adhesions. A history of a similar pain in the past may suggest a recurrent problem. A detailed history of drug intake is important, because certain drugs (eg. erythromycin, salicylates, NSAIDs) may cause abdominal pain and dyspepsia. Abdominal discomfort is the commonset side effect of a large number of drugs.

Family history

A family history of sickle cell anemia or cystic fibrosis may indicate the likely diagnosis. The patient's ethnic background is important because sickle cell anemia is most common in blacks of African origin and tribal communities.

PHYSICAL EXAMINATION

Physical examination actually begins as soon as the child enters the consultation chamber of the physician. Does the child appear ill? Is the child lethargic and appears detached from the surroundings or is he alert but lying very still? Is the child constantly rolling or wriggling due to pain. A listless, lethargic child who is un-interested in the surroundings is probably severely dehydrated, toxemic and in shock and is very ill due to advanced peritonitis.

A child who is alert but lying very still, in a somewhat flexed posture, may be suffering from an inflammatory process like appendicitis. A child who is intermittently crying loudly due to colic may be suffering from gastroenteritis, typhlitis or a more serious surgical problem like intussusception or other forms of intestinal or other luminal obstruction.

Once the history taking is complete the school going child is asked to lie on the examination table by himself. When the child can climb to the examination table without any assestance, it rules out any serious condition including generalized peritoneal irritation. If the child keeps the hips flexed when lying supine it indicates the presence of psoas spasm which may occur due to appendicitis, psoas abscess or a perinephric abscess. The outer bulky clothing must be removed, specially in winter, but it is not essential to completely undress the child.

Examination should be performed in a relaxed and friendly manner. The outcome of the examination depends on the child's trust and cooperation. The attention of the child should be diverted during palpation of abdomen. As a young child may be frightened and apprehensive, it may be helpful to examine the child in the parent's lap where they feel more secure and comfortable. It is usually best to examine the region of suspected abdominal pathology last, as this may be painful and will make the child more apprehensive thereby precluding further meaningful evaluation.

Examination of the head and neck, chest and extremities must precede the abdominal examination. In infants unable to verbalize complaints and accurately localize pain, an otitis media may be sufficiently painful to cause incessant crying, and may be confused with abdominal pain. Streptococcal pharyngitis is sometimes accompanied by severe abdominal pain. Such children have significant fever, appear ill, have tender cervical adenopathy, and obvious tonsillitis or pharyngitis[2]. Decreased breath sounds/and or rales in the lower lobe specially on the right side may indicate pneumonia. Abdominal examination must progress in a systematic manner.

Inspection

Before the examiner actually touches the abdomen it must be carefully observed. Inspect all hernial sites including the saphenous opening to avoid missing a femoral hernia.

Contour of the abdomen. Distension of abdomen in acute obstruction occurs gradually and may not be evident till quite late. The more distal is the site of obstruction the more severe and global is likely to be abdominal distension. The distension is central in small bowel obstruction, peripheral in large bowel obstruction and absent in biliary and renal colics. This classic distribution of distension may not be evident in infants and small children.

Respiratory movements. The movements of the abdomen as well as the chest are noted to see if there is any alteration in the normal abdomino-thoracic rhythm (during inspiration both the abdomen and the chest expand). If the abdomen does not expand during inspiration it is indicative of generalized peritoneal irritation. Localized limitation of respiratory movements occur in localized peritoneal inflammation.

Peristaltic movements. If present, the character and direction must be noted. Peristaltic activity is rarely observed in children with acute abdomen though it may sometimes be seen in children suffering from acute on chronic abdomen. This may be seen in children with chronic subacute intestinal obstruction as in tubercular involvement or Hirschsprung's disease.

Skin. Tense shiny skin with distension is indicative of ascites which is infected. In neonates and small infants, edema and erythema of the skin of the abdominal wall indicates serious intra-abdominal problem with probably necrotic intestine. Patches of ecchymosis in the loin (Grey-Turner sign) or bluish hue around the umbilicus (Cullen's sign) may be found in cases of acute pancreatitis or rupture of ectopic pregnancy.

Palpation

Palpation should begin far away from the site of abdominal pain and it should be done with the flat of the hand. It is important to place a warm hand on the abdomen otherwise there is voluntary contraction of the abdominal muscles which may be interpreted as guarding and it will make palpation of intra-abdominal organs difficult. Because of the apprehension, voluntary guarding usually starts before the palpation begins and this can be overcome by asking the child to take deep breaths or by distracting the child by various maneuvers appropriate for his age[2]. A positive Murphy's sign (interruption of deep inspiration by pain when the physician's fingers are pressed beneath the right costal margin) suggests acute cholecystitis. In young children and adolescents, another helpful maneuver is to distract the child during examination by talking. During abdominal palpation it is more useful to look at the child's face rather than the abdomen. The palpation of the painful area should be gentle and should be just deep enough to elicit a grimace on the face or a verbal complaint of pain.

In children who are very apprehensive, palpating the abdomen with the help of a stethoscope is another useful tool. This may be done in continuation of the auscultation of the chest where the stethoscope is placed on the various areas of the abdomen and used both for auscultation and palpation.

Hyperesthesia. This is elicited by gently picking up the skin and subcutaneous fat and drawing it away from the abdominal wall or by stroking it with a pin. Hyperasthesia in the Sherren's triangle (formed by lines joining the umbilicus, right anterior superior iliac spine and symphysis pubis) may be observed in early cases of acute appendicitis.

Tenderness. This is assessed on palpation over the inflamed organ. In acute appendicitis the point of maximum tenderness is over the McBurney's point. The degree and extent of tenderness is indicative of the severity and spread of the disease. In acute appendicitis the spread of tenderness from the right iliac fossa to the left indicates spread of peritonitis. Rebound tenderness is indicative of peritoneal irritation. It occurs when an inflamed focus within the abdomen is compressed and then suddenly released resulting in severe pain. Although this sign is helpful in diagnosing peritonitis it is often not necessary and should be avoided as this maneuver may make a cooperative child totally uncooperative. In lieu of this the tenderness over the inflamed organ can be elicited by gentle percussion or palpation with the stethoscope. Appearance of this sign in a case of acute intestinal obstruction indicates strangulation of the gut.

In referred pain due to thoracic diseases like basal pneumonia, the patient may wince as soon as the abdomen is touched (like in hyperasthesia) but when the pressure on the abdomen is increased there is no corresponding increase in pain and there is never any rebound tenderness. In acute appendicitis there are some indirect ways of eliciting tenderness. Rovsing's sign is eilicited when a sharp pressure on the left iliac fossa elicits pain in the right iliac fossa because of shift of coils of intestine which then impinge on the inflamed appendix. Cope's psoas test is positive in cases of retrocecal appendix. The inflamed appendix is lying on the psoas major muscle which when stretched by extending the hip joint causes pain. Cope's obturator test is positive in cases of pelvic appendix which is lying on the obturator internus. Stretching this muscle by flexing and medially rotating the thigh causes pain.

Abdominal guarding and rigidity. Finer degrees of guarding can be appreciated by "pill rolling" movements of the fingers over various regions of the abdomen. Guarding may be voluntary or involuntary (rigidity). Voluntary guarding may be present in an apprehensive child, or when a cold hand is placed on the abdomen or when the fingers are pushed deeply into the abdomen. Voluntary guarding disappears during expiration and is always bilateral. Involuntary guarding (rigidity) is constant and is localized to one segment of the abdominal wall which corresponds to the inflamed organ. Irritation of the parietal peritoneum from any cause such as inflammatory exudate, blood, bile, or intestinal contents will give rise to rigidity. Rigidity will be absent when there is no cause of irritation of the parietal peritoneum as in a case of abdominal colic. In acute intestinal obstruction the appearance of rigidity is indicative of strangulation or perforation. In late cases of perforation with severe toxemia as in enteric perforation, the rigidity may be absent because of exhaustion of the protective mechanism.

Swelling and organomegaly. When a lump or tumor is felt it should be thoroughly examined to ascertain its origin and whether it is the cause of acute abdomen. Sudden increase in size of an intra-abdominal tumor, especially due to hemorrhage, is known to present like an acute abdomen. Sudden organomegaly such as hepatomegaly in cases of congestive cardiac failure, or in viral hepatitis can also be the cause of acute pain due to stretch of the pain sensitive capsule. In acute appendicitis a vague lump may be palpable in the right iliac fossa. In acute intestinal obstruction when the flat of the hand is gently placed on the abdomen for a few minutes the underlying coils of intestine may be felt to harden and soften alternatively. The classic sausage shaped lump of intussusception is felt to harden under the palpating finger synchronously with the bout of pain. The doughy feel of the abdomen in cases of tubercular abdomen is something one learns by experience and is often helpful in establishing the cause of acute intestinal obstruction.

Groin and external genitalia. Examination of the groin and external genitalia is an integral part of the abdominal examination in every child with acute abdomen. Important causes of abdominal pain like an obstructed or incarcerated inguinal hernia, testicular torsion, epididymo-orchitis, imperforate hymen with hematometra or foreign body in the vagina may otherwise go undetected. Foul smelling vaginal discharge may be found in girls with primary peritonitis.

Percussion

Shifting dullness. This is present when there is free fluid in the abdominal cavity. It may be falsely positive when there is massive dilatation of the intestines as in chronic obstruction. In such situations the shifting of fluid inside the grossly dilated colon may be picked up as a shifting dullness even in the absence of free intraperitoneal fluid.

Obliteration of liver dullness. This indicates the presence of free gas in the abdomen in a case of intestinal perforation. Though the obliteration of liver dullness confirms perforation of bowel its absence does not rule it out.

Auscultation

Bowel sounds are usually non-specific in children with acute abdomen but they are helpful in certain situations. To appreciate various types of abnormal sounds one must be aware of the frequency and character of normal bowel sounds. Normal intestinal sounds are heard as clicks or gurgles at well spaced intervals. The silent abdomen of diffuse peritonitis or due to other causes of paralytic ileus is easily appreciated and differentiated from the noisy abdomen of early intestinal obstruction. In cases of obstruction there are frequent high pitched tinkles or rushes. Bowel sounds in gastroenteritis may also be very active and loud. In advanced cases of ileus with silent abdomen, the respiratory or cardiac sounds may be surprisingly well heard.

Rectal and pelvic examination

A complete abdominal examination includes a rectal examination but if the diagnosis is already obvious it can be avoided, although this should not be made a common practice. The bulging anterior wall of the rectum with tenderness is diagnostic of pelvis abscess. This is often accompanied with a history of diarrhea (spurious) or frequency of stools or tenesmus. The right wall of the pelvis is extremely tender in appendicitis specially when it is a pelvic appendix. A common finding in acute abdomen with paralytic ileus is ballooning of the rectum which is completely empty. In intussusception the finger stall may be smeared with mucus and blood (red currant-jelly) with absence of stool. In rare cases of advanced intussusception, the intussusceptien may actually be palpated rectally.

INVESTIGATIONS

The aim of investigations in a child with acute abdomen is two fold; to confirm clinical suspicion when the diagnosis is not possible on the basis of history and examination. It will also help in assessing the general condition of the child as regards anemia, dehydration, electrolyte and acid-base imbalance. The investigations do help in establishing the diagnosis but cannot and should not replace clinical judgement.

Laboratory studies

These include estimation of complete blood count, serum sodium and potassium, blood urea and urinalysis. Other specific investigations like arterial blood gases, serum amylase, lipase, creatinine, liver function tests, Widal, and blood culture should be ordered when indicated. The hemoglobin levels will reveal anemia due to acute or chronic blood loss as in peptic ulcer disease, inflammatory bowel conditions, Meckel's diverticula and massive hook worm infestation. A low hemoglobin level may also suggest an underlying hematologic abnormalities, such as sickle cell disease. It must be remembered that a large number of Indian children may have a base line anemia because of nutritional deficiencies. The level of dehydration must also be kept in mind as in the presence of dehydration the hemoglobin values may be falsely elevated. A repeat hemoglobin estimation after correction of dehydration will reveal the true hemoglobin status.

An elevated white blood count suggests the presence of an inflammatory pathology. In uncomplicated acute appendicitis blood counts may be normal to elevated in the range of 15,000-16,000/mm^3. But a normal or mildly elevated blood count should not be taken against the diagnosis of acute appendicitis if the clinical picture is otherwise suggestive. A very high blood count (>18,000/mm^3) usually indicates intestinal gangrene, perforation or abscess formation. A high blood count may also be obtained in acute gastroenteritis, streptococcal disease, pyelonephritis, pelvic inflammatory disease and pneumonia. In enteric fever classically there is relative leukopenia but by the time these children present with acute abdomen due to perforation and peritonitis they usually have leukocytosis. Striking lymphocytosis may indicate some form of viral gastroenteritis or other viral pathology.Urinalysis can help identify urinary tract pathology, such as infection or stones.

Radiologic investigations

Radiologic evaluation in children with acute abdomen usually consist of a plain abdominal radiographs in erect and supine positions, and if indicated special investigations like ultrasound evaluation, barium GI studies and computerized tomography.

Plain radiographs. Plain X-ray chest, X-ray abdomen in an erect position including both domes of diaphragm and the bladder area must be obtained.

The chest X-ray helps to assess the presence of pneumonia. The X-ray abdomen may confirm the presence of intestinal obstruction and the pattern of air-fluid levels in conjunction with the history will indicate a pyloric (Figure 12.1), duodenal (Figure 12.1B), proximal small bowel (Figure 12.1C) or a distal bowel obstruction (Figure 12.1D). In a neonate with acute abdomen pneumotosis intestinalis is suggestive of necrotizing enterocolitis (Figure 12.2). The X-rays may show the presence of biliary or renal calculi. Gas under the diaphragm (Figure 12.3) will indicate the presence of

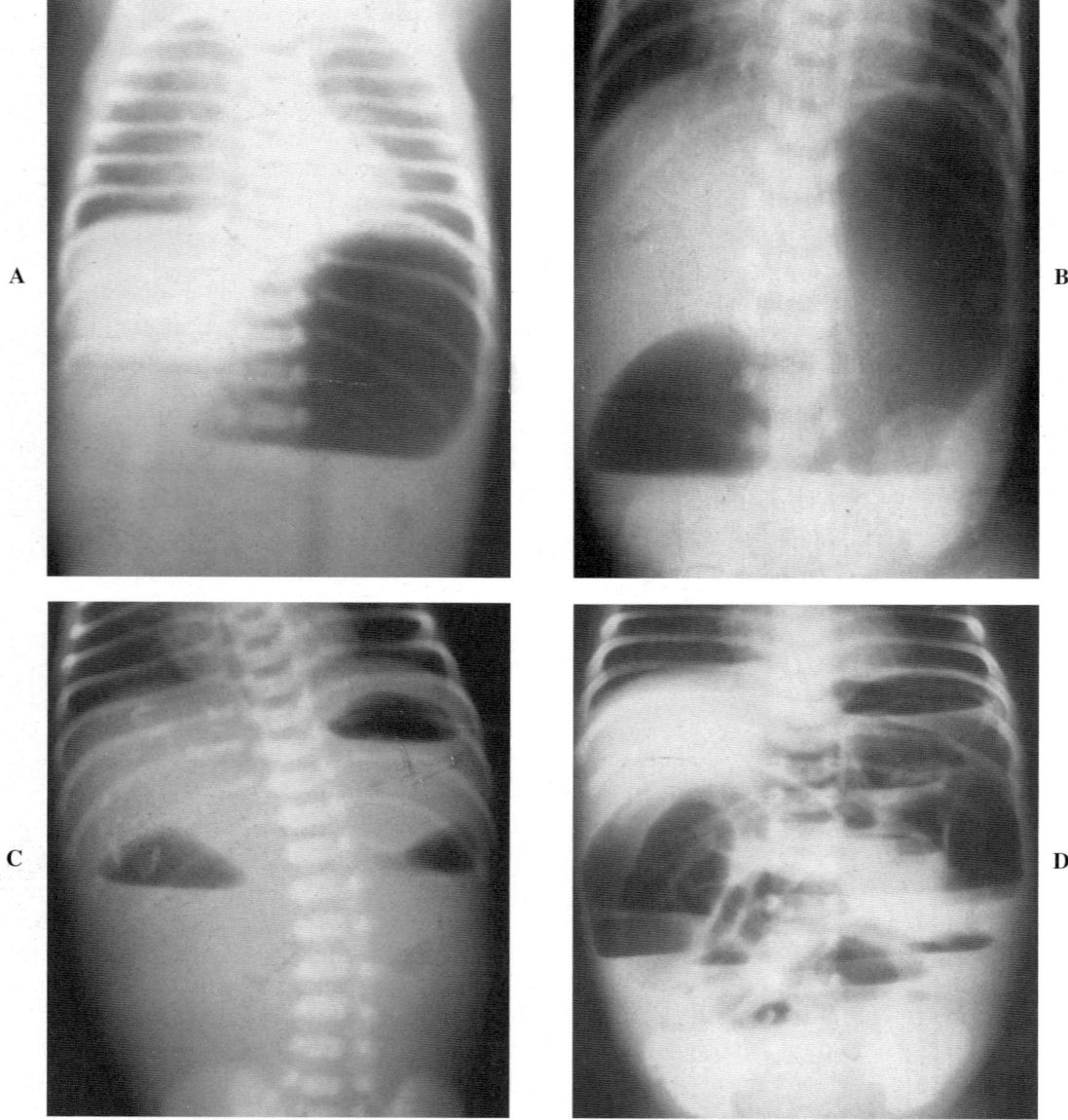

Figure 12.1 Erect x-ray showing a single bubble (A), double bubble (B), few air-fluid levels (C), and multiple air-fluid levels (D) indicative of pyloric obstruction, duodenal obstruction, proximal small bowel obstruction and distal bowel obstruction respectively. In addition there are scattered calcification (C) in the right upper quadrant (arrow) suggestive of meconium peritonitis as the cause of obstruction in this particular case

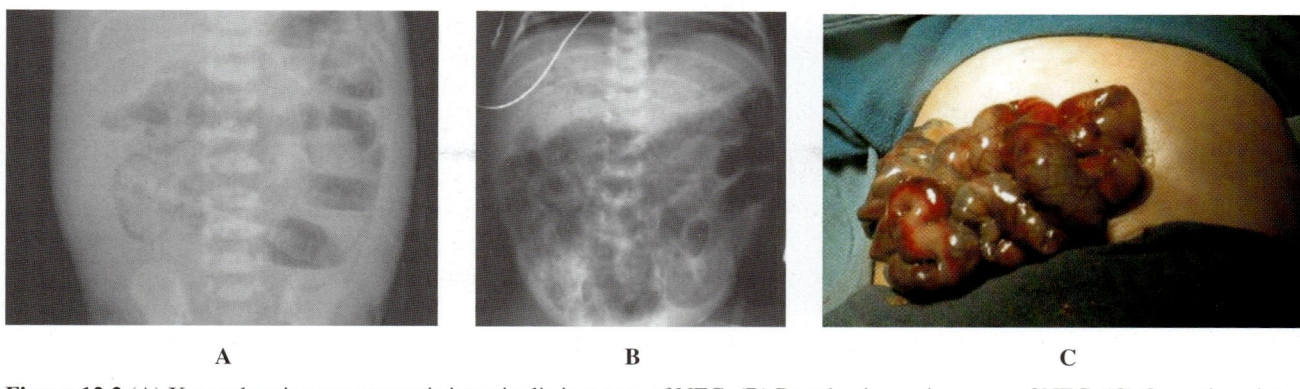

A   **B**   **C**

Figure 12.2 (A) X-ray showing pneumotosis intestinalis in a case of NEC; (B) Portal vein gas in a case of NEC; (C) Operative picture of NEC

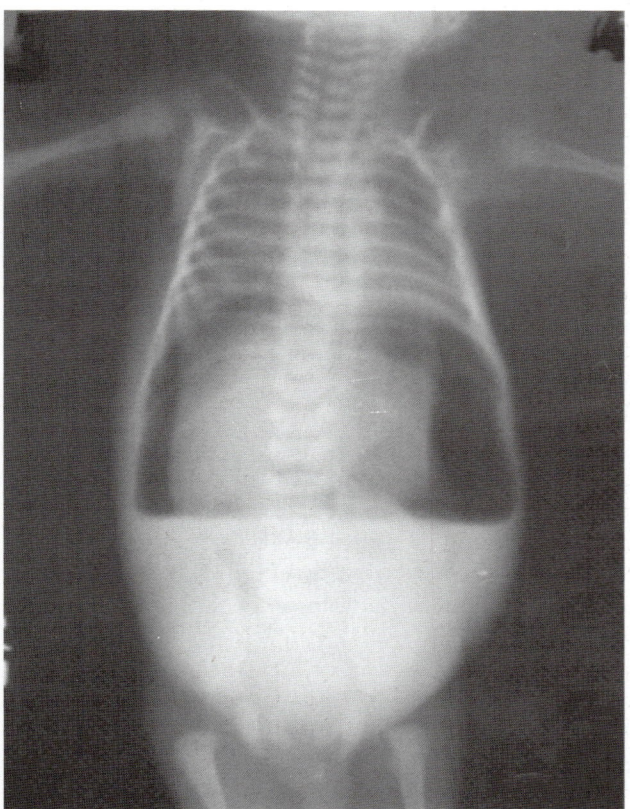

Figure 12.3 Erect x-ray showing free gas in the peritoneum indicative of bowel perforation

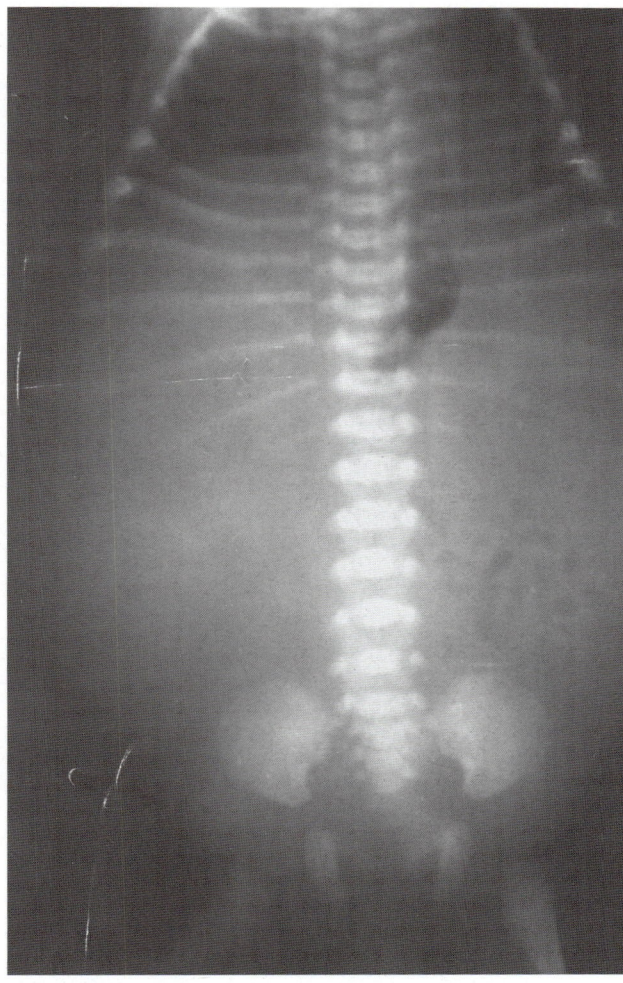

Figure 12.4 Ground glass appearance due to peritoneal fluid collection as in ascitic phase of meconium peritonitis

pneumoperitoneum because of intestinal perforation. Ground glass appearance with paucity of air-fluid levels indicates the presence of peritoneal fluid (Figure 12.4). Displacement of bowel loops to one side with a ground glass appearance on the other side may indicate the presence of a mass like a duplication cyst, meconium cyst (Figure 12.5) or encysted ascites. The plain X-rays will also reveal the presence of any bony abnormalities like vertebral anomalies in patients with duplication cyst (Figure 12.6).

Barium GI studies. Upper GI and follow-through barium studies are rarely required in acute abdomen and may actually be detrimental in cases of intestinal obstruction. Sometimes in cases of recurrent abdominal pain associated with bilious vomiting and clinical features of duodenal or gastric

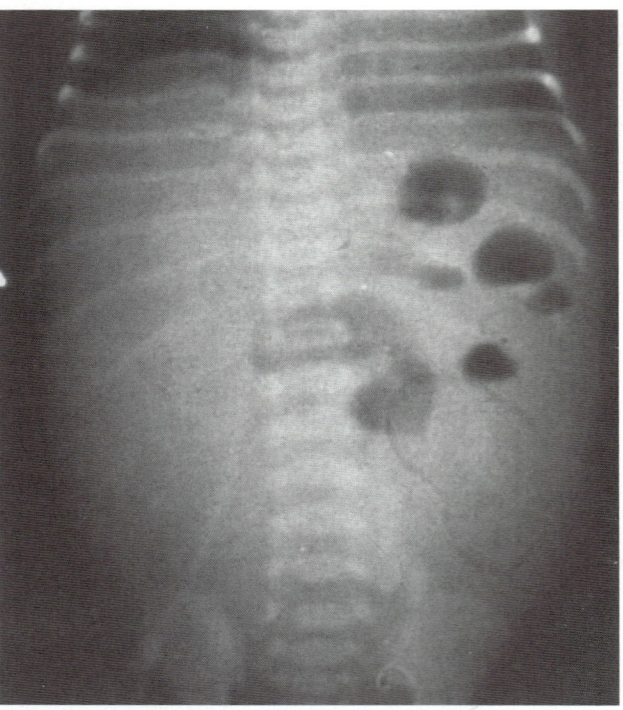

Figure 12.5 X-ray abdomen showing multiple air fluid levels with loops displaced to the left and a homogenous opacity in the right lower quadrant (arrow) due to meconium cyst

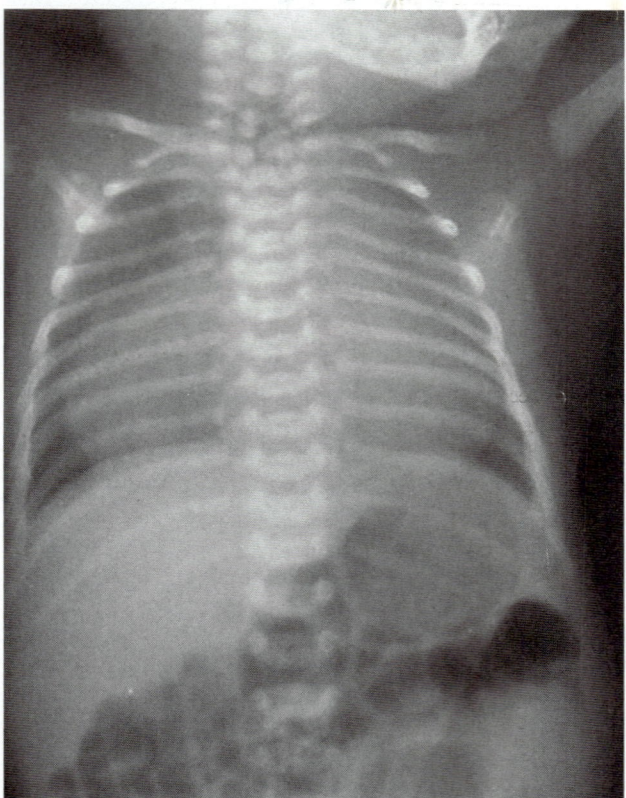

Figure 12.6 Chest X-ray showing a homogenous mass in the left hemithorax with associated vertebral anomalies that suggest that the thoracic mass is a foregut duplication cyst

outlet obstruction, barium upper GI study may clinch the diagnosis by revealing malrotation with or without volvulus (Figure 12.7) or an intrinsic duodenal obstruction (Figure 12.8). Barium meal and follow through may occasionally show displaced bowel loops as in a case of duplication cyst of the bowel (Figure 12.9). Barium enema may be required in suspected cases of Hirschspurng's disease, specially those presenting with features of enterocolitis (Figure 12.10). In such cases the enema should be performed after achieving hemodynamic stability. Another condition where barium enema is both diagnostic and therapeutic is intussusception where hydrostatic reduction is a well established procedure for management (Figure 12.11).

Ultrasound examination. Ultrasound examination is ideal for children as it is usually painless, requires no radiation or intravenous/ oral contrast and can usually be performed without sedation. The main limitation of US examination is the presence of excessive bowel gas. It is the most useful investigation in defining the character of an abdominal mass. It can delineate the mass of an intussusception which is characteristically seen as a target lesion (Figure 12.12.). It can sometimes define the bulky pancreas of pancreatitis but this is often not possible because of the overlying gas filled bowel loops. Ultrasound examination can easily pickup a pseudocyst, appendicular mass or intussusception. Definition of biliary or renal calculi is also very good. An ultrasound is the investigation of choice for pelvic pathology specially in adolescent girls.

Special tests. Contrast enhanced CT scans or MRI may occasionally be needed specially when conditions like chronic pancreatitis and pseudocyst (Figures 12.13 and 12.14), intra-abdominal tumor is suspected or in case of an equivocal diagnosis. Technetium labeled radionuclide scan to pick-up ectopic gastric mucosa may be helpful in suspected cases of duplication cysts or bleeding Meckel's diverticulum.

SUPPORTIVE/PRE-OPERATIVE MEDICAL MANAGEMENT

A child with acute abdomen needs as excellent pre-operative management to stabilize him hemodynamically. This is essential for reducing the operative morbidity and mortality. Except in life-threatening rare situation, surgical intervention should only be undertaken when the child is

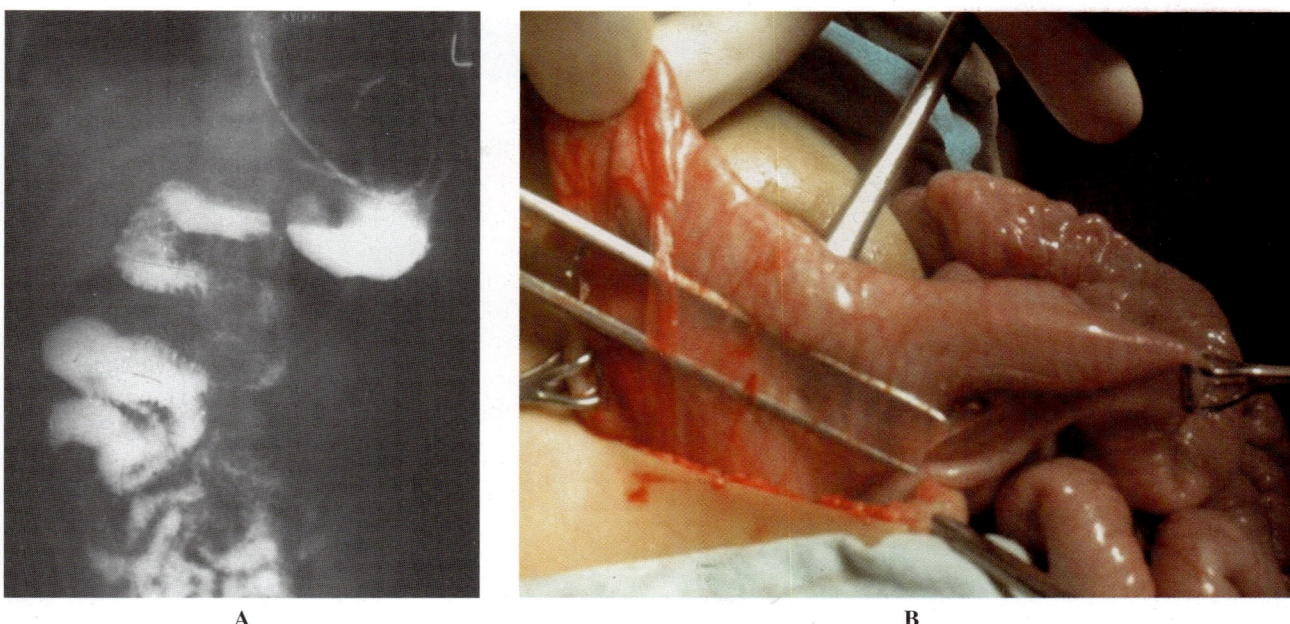

A   B

Figure 12.7 (A) Barium meal follow through showing duodeno-jejunal junction on the right of the vertebral margin and corkscrew appearance of the proximal small bowel indicating malrotation with small bowel volvulus. (B) Operative picture showing the Ladd's bands across the second part of the deuodenum (arrow) in a case of malrotation

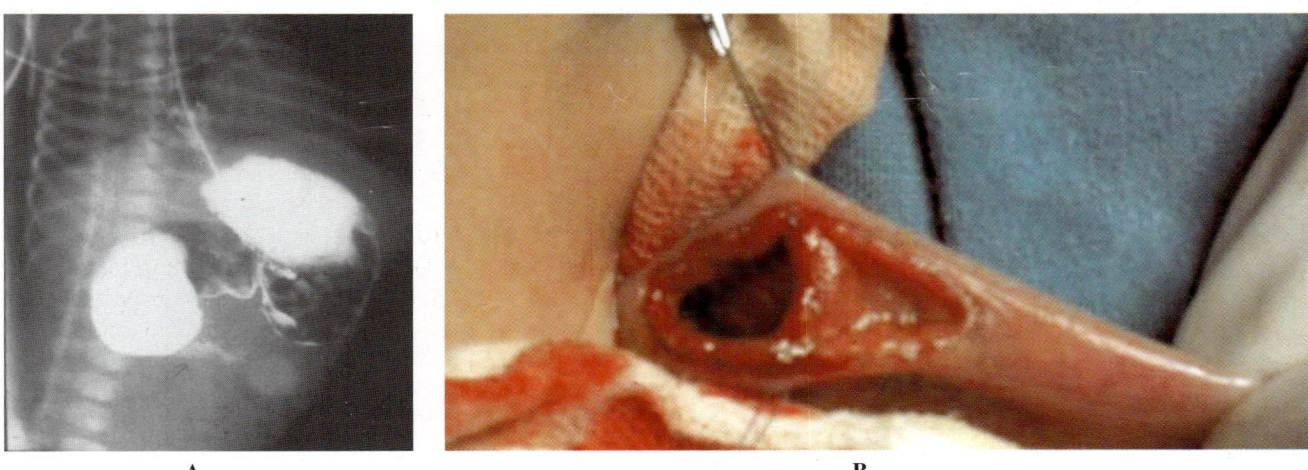

A   B

Figure 12.8 (A) Barium meal follow through showing grossly dilated first and second parts of duodenum with little distal passage of contrast indicative of a duodenal web with a hole. (B) Operative picture showing the duodenal web (arrow)

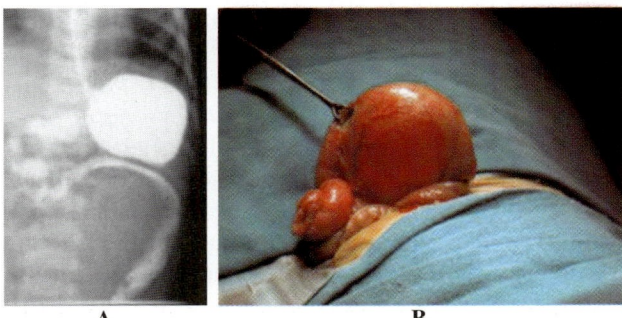

A   B

Figure 12.9 (A) Barium meal follow through showing anteriorly displaced and stretched out small bowel loop in a case of duplication cyst of the small bowel (arrow). (B) Operative picture showing the duplication cyst

adequately hydrated and has an adequate urine output and normal serum electrolytes.

An intravenous access of adequate caliber should be established at the earliest and this opportunity should be taken to draw blood samples for hemoglobin, total and differential leukocyte counts, serum electrolytes and blood urea estimations in addition to any other specific investigation as the condition demands. Sample for grouping and cross matching should also be taken and blood and other blood products arranged. Initial intravenous fluids should be started as detailed below. A good caliber nasogastric tube is positioned

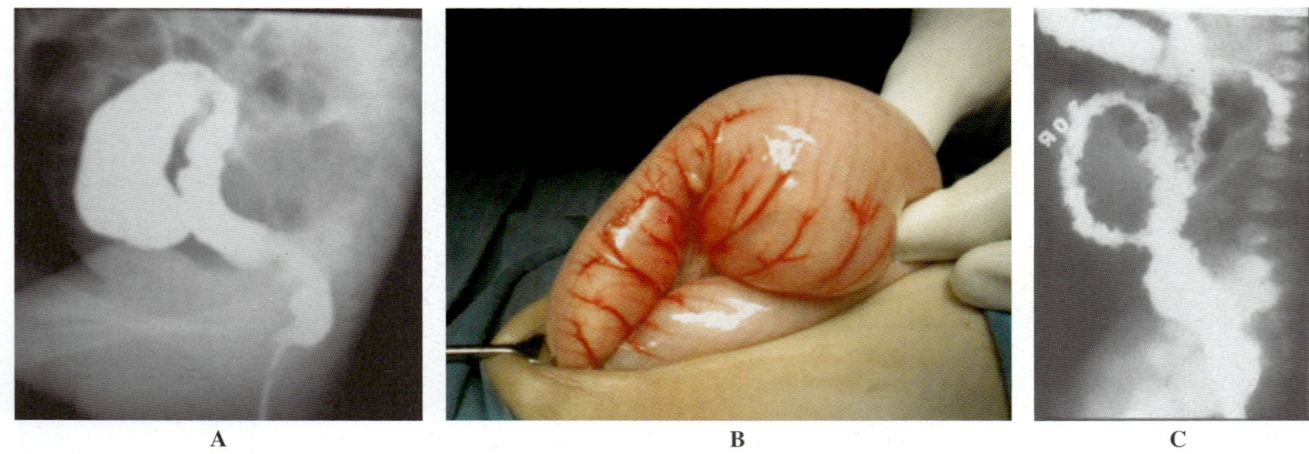

Figure 12.10 (A) Barium enema in a case of Hirschsprung's disease showing the narrow aganglionic segment, the funneling of the transition zone and the proximal dilated ganglionic colon. (B) Operative picture depicting the same. (C) Barium enema in a case of Hirschsprung's disease with enterocolitis

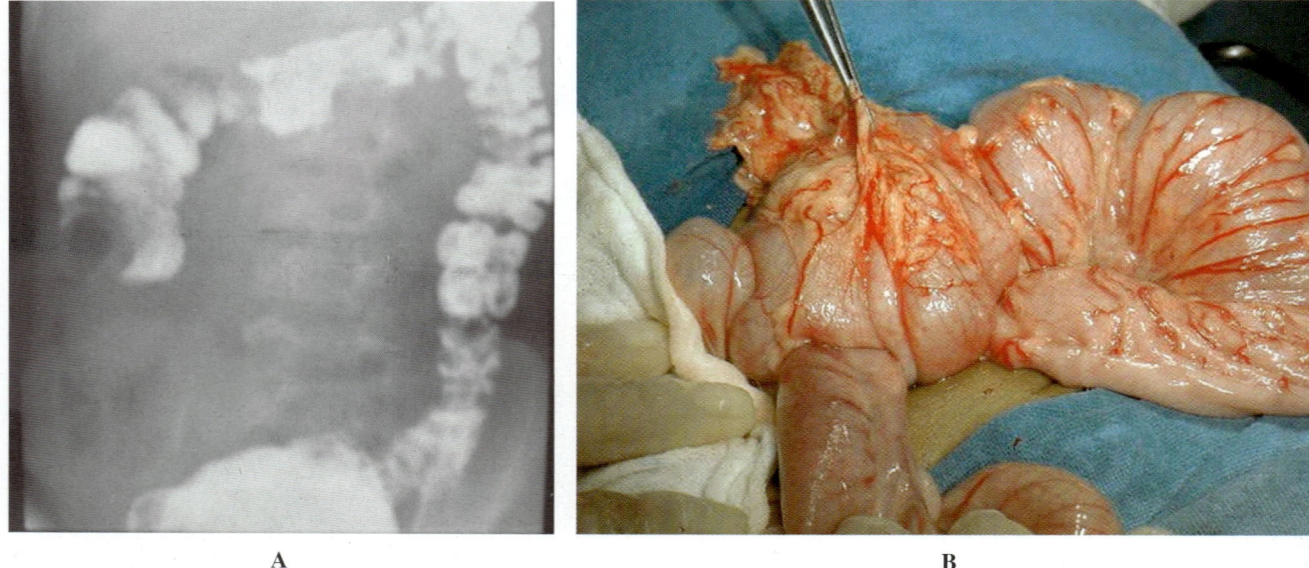

Figure 12.11 (A) Barium enema in a case of ileocolic intussusception. (B) Operative picture depicting the same

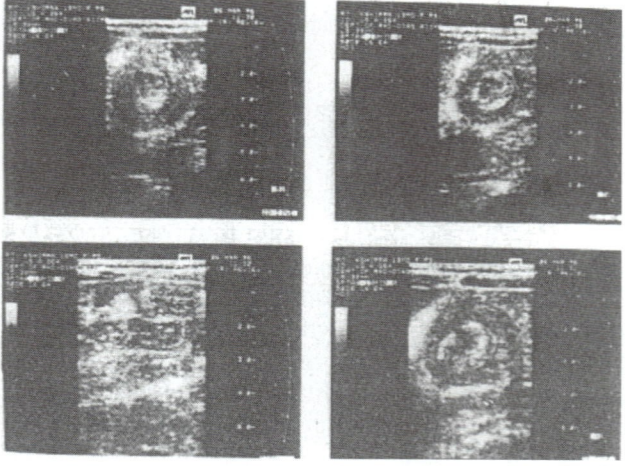

Figure 12.12 Ultrasound examination of abdomen showing the target sign in a case of intussusception

and on hourly aspiration is done along with continuous drainage. Since the aspirate from the upper gastrointestinal tract contains 60-75 mEq/L of sodium and 2 mEq/L of potassium, the nasogastric aspirate should be replaced volume for volume every 4 hourly with N/2 saline in 5% dextrose plus 1 ml/100 ml of 15% potassium chloride.

A Foley's catheter should be placed in the urinary bladder to accurately monitor the urine output on an hourly basis. After measuring the initial amount of urine obtained after placing the catheter, the urine output should be considered normal if it is at least 1-2 ml/kg/hour. If the child is severely dehydrated or has been anuric for the past several hours or if the initial urine obtained is very small in quantity and of high color, the child should be started on intravenous normal saline (without any

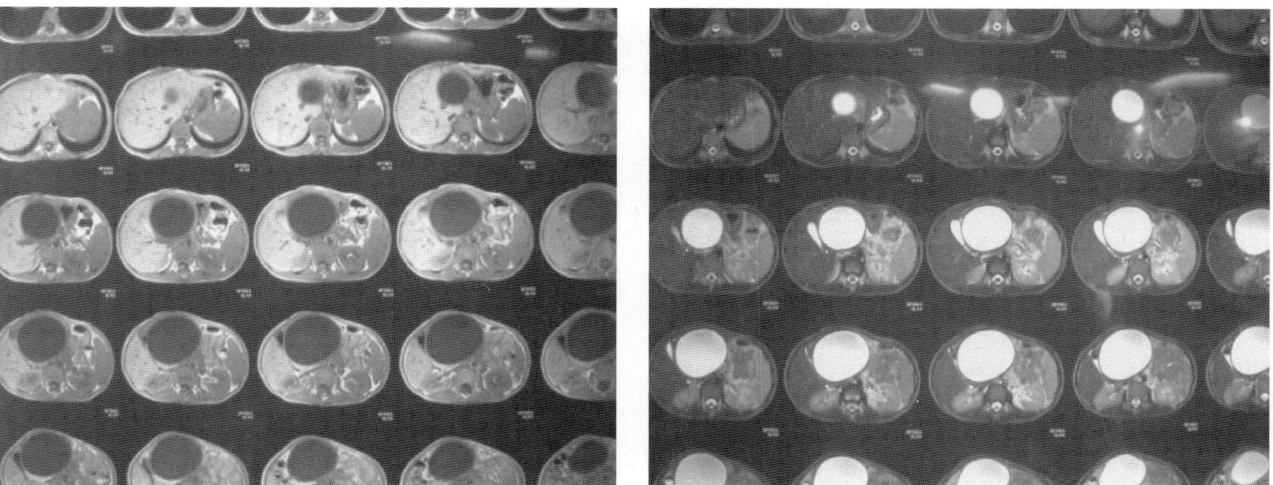

Figure 12.13 MRI findings in a case of pseudocyst of the pancreas

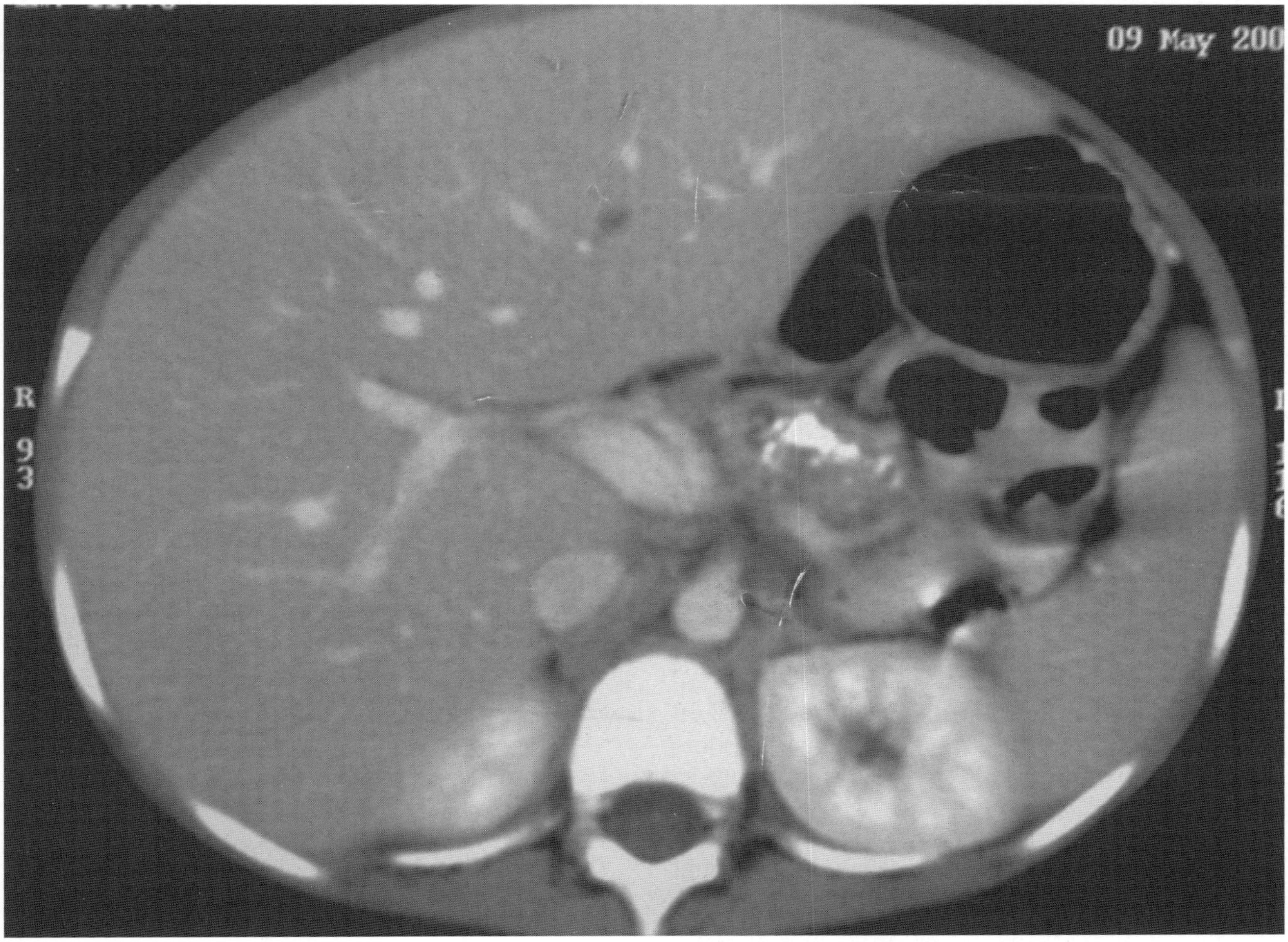

Figure 12.14 Contrast enhanced CT scan in a case of chronic calcific pancreatitis with a pseudocyst

potassium) at a rate of 20 ml/kg/hour in the first hour. If no urine is produced within one hour then the fluid bolus is repeated again in the next hour. If still no urine output is obtained then intravenous furosemide is administered in a dose of 0.5-1.0 mg/kg. If still no urine output is obtained then the child should be considered to be in acute renal failure and the further fluid management should be done accordingly. If urine flow is established, the child is started on intravenous fluids which are calculated by computing the maintenance requirements along with fluid deficit and concurrent aspiration losses. The daily maintenance requirements in children is normally adequately met with N/3 saline in 5% dextrose (N/5 saline in 5% or 10% dextrose in neonates) in a volume calculated as below.

- Infants upto 10 kg: 100 ml/kg.
- Children between 11-12 kg: 1000 ml + 50 ml/each kg above 10 kg.
- Children > 21 kg: 1500 ml + 20 ml/each kg above 20 kg.

The rough estimation of fluid deficit is calculated depending upon the clinical assessment of degree of dehydration:

- Mild dehydration: 10-30 ml/kg
- Moderate dehydration: 30-80 ml/kg
- Severe dehydration: 80-120 ml/kg.

The total deficit is calculated and 50% of this volume is infused during the first 8 hours along with the maintenance fluids for those 8 hours. The remaining 50% of the deficit correction is done over the next 16 hours. It must be remembered that the ongoing losses from the NG aspiration/vomiting must also be concurrently replaced as detailed previously. It is important to remember that potassium is added to the fluids only after the urine output is established. If excessively low serum sodium or potassium levels are obtained then the constitution of the fluids may be changed accordingly. Many a times one does not get 24 hours for correction of fluid and electrolyte abnormalities and the aim should be to achieve reasonable hydration and electrolyte balance as soon as possible in approximately 6-8 hours and then operate and continue the hydration process intra- and post-operatively. Most children with acute abdomen are also started on broad spectrum antibiotics to cover Gram-positive, Gram-negative bacteria and also for anerobes. Most physicians prefer a combination of a third generation cephalosporin, an aminoglycoside and metronidazole.

These children need to be closely monitored both clinically and biochemically. The regular pre-operative monitoring include hourly charting of pulse rate, respiratory rate, blood pressure, abdominal girth, intake and output. When facilities are available the patient should preferably be attached to a multi-channel vital sign monitor and pulse oximeter. In a very sick and unstable child it is advisable to put a central venous catheter and monitor the central venous pressure so that fluids can be given fast without overloading the system and causing pulmonary edema. It is also important to remember that a large number of Indian children are anemic and hypoproteinemic and therefore will have low oxygen carrying capacity and low oncotic pressure. Therefore, they need to be supported with packed cell transfusions and supplemental oxygen with a hood, mask or nasal catheter. The plasma oncotic pressure should be normalized by pre-operative transfusion of plasma or albumin. Those children who are septicemic need infusions of fresh frozen plasma and platelet-rich plasma to avoid excessive bleeding during surgery. All these infusions must be accounted for in the total intravenous fluid calculations. Newborn babies should be given vitamin K before surgery.

The supportive medical management should be started immediately when acute abdomen is suspected and continued during the ongoing investigative procedures like ultrasound abdomen. The medical pre-operative management should never be deferred till a definite diagnosis is reached. The administration of analgesics in children with suspected appendicitis is controversial. Withholding analgesia from patients with acute abdominal pain and suspected appendicitis is common. This practice, however, is not supported by published literature. Although a few trials have noted some changes in abdominal examination with analgesia, this has not been associated with any adverse outcome. Larger multicenter trials are needed to establish practice guidelines.[8]

COMMON CONDITIONS PRESENTING AS ACUTE ABDOMEN IN CHILDREN

Infantile Colic

This is characterized by an unexplained paroxysms of irritability, fussing or crying in an infant. The crying is intense and often inconsolable. Such episodes usually start by about 2-3 weeks of age and subside spontaneously by 3 to 4 months of life. Pain is sudden in onset and recur generally at the same time each day. The episodes typically occur in the late afternoon or evening (Evening colic). At other times of the day, the infant has normal activity, feeding and appearance. The episodes are intermittent, occurring more than three times a week and each episode lasting for about three hours.[9] The physical examination and laboratory investigations are invariably normal but it is essential to carefully rule out other causes of a crying infant (Refer to Chapter 11).

Acute Appendicitis

In cases of acute appendicitis pain is invariably present and is nearly always the first symptom. Occasionally there may be some mild gastrointestinal symptoms before the onset of pain in the form of indigestion, "gastritis" or subtle changes in bowel habits. In the presence of severe GI symptoms before the onset of pain, one must strongly consider alternative diagnosis. The early visceral pain of appendicitis is non-specific and localized to epigastric or umbilical region which shifts and gets localized to the right lower quadrant at the McBurney's point. Occasionally the pain may start at this point without the earlier visceral component. In cases of retrocecal appendix, the somatic pain is often delayed and may be more in the flank or the mid back. A pelvic appendix near the ureter or the testicular vessels can cause urinary frequency, testicular pain or both. Inflammation of the ureter or the bladder in such situations may cause pain on micturition (which is different from the dysuria of urinary tract infection). Anorexia, nausea and vomiting usually follows the onset of pain within a few hours. Anorexia is a very important sign and any child who is hungry could hardly be harboring an inflamed appendix. Vomiting is usually mild and occur once or twice at the beginning but does not persist. Constipation or obstipation is rare but there may be tenesmus specially in cases of pelvic appendicitis. Diarrhea in the initial few hours is not uncommon in children and is probably occurs due to irritation of the terminal ileum and the cecum.

Clinical features. Children with appendicitis tend to lie still in bed as movement increases pain. On walking they may limp a little because of the flexion at the right hip joint due to spasm of the psoas muscle. Cutaneous hyperasthesia may be there in the Sherren's triangle but this is not easily elicitable in children. Localized tenderness in the right iliac fossa elicited by deep palpation or percussion is the corner stone for the diagnosis of acute appendicitis. In retrocecal appendix this point

of maximum tenderness is in the flank or the back, midway between the 12th rib and the posterior superior iliac spine. In pelvic appendicitis there is marked rectal tenderness specially in the right fornix. With progression of the disease there may be perforation followed by peritonitis with signs becoming more generalized and the general condition becoming worse. Generalized peritonitis due to perforated appendix is commoner in infants and small children while a localized appendicular abscess is more common in older children and adolescents.

When the diagnosis is unclear, serial examinations by the same person is important in clinching the diagnosis.[10] It is important that during this period of observation the child should be kept nil orally and on intravenous fluids, antibiotics and analgesics. There is no evidence to support the notion that early pain relief for patients with suspected appendicitis will interfere with diagnosis.

Investigations. Total leukocyte count and neutrophil count may be elevated.[11,12] The sensitivity of an elevated leukocyte count ranges from 52-96 percent.[11-14] A plain radiograph of the abdomen may rarely show a fecolith in the region of the right iliac fossa. There may be lumbar scoliosis away from the right and obliteration of the psoas shadow. A chest X-ray is a must to rule out basal pneumonia. Ultrasonography in skilled hands is a useful investigation modality in all cases. Ultrasound is reported to have an excellent specificity (>90%) in most series but a variable sensitivity.[15] CT scan has a higher sensitivity and specificity (>95%) than ultrasound in most pediatric series for the diagnosis of acute appendicitis.[16] However, a contrast enhanced CT (CECT) scan is more expensive, requires contrast injection and may require sedation in small children. Also there is risk of radiation exposure. Some workers have also reported excellent accuracy with unenhanced CT scans in children.[17] MRI has been reported to have 100% sensitivity for the diagnosis of acute appendicitis in children[18] but this is even more expensive and time consuming than a CT scan. Despite the availability of these investigations, most clinicians still believe that these radiological investigations offer no significant improvement in the diagnostic accuracy of appendicitis achieved on the basis of careful history, physical examination and routine laboratory investigations.[19,20] These investigations are usually indicated in clinically equivocal cases to confirm or exclude the diagnosis

Section 2

Irreducible Hernia

An incarcerated hernia is one in which the contents of the sac cannot be easily reduced into the abdominal cavity. In strangulated hernia there is a tight constriction in its passage through the inguinal canal and the hernial contents have become or are likely to become gangrenous. The incidence of incarcerated hernia is 12-17 percent[21,22] and two-thirds of these occur in the first year of life.[21] Presentation is usually with irritability, pain in the groin, abdominal pain and vomiting. Examination would reveal a tense, non-fluctuant mass in the inguinal region which may extend down into the scrotum. The mass is tender and irreducible. With the onset of ischemic changes, the pain intensifies, and vomiting becomes bilious or feculent. Blood may be noted in the stools. There is often edema and reddening of the overlying skin with other evidences of intestinal obstruction. The testis is usually normal but in some cases of prolonged strangulation, the testis may become swollen and hard because of venous congestion and compression of spermatic vessels and lymph channels. The main differential diagnoses include torsion of the testis, inguinal or femoral lymphadenitis and a hydrocele of the cord. The treatment is surgical correction.

Intussusception

Intussusception (Figure 12.11) is a disease primarily of infants and toddlers and 80-90 percent of the cases of intussusception occur in children between 3 months and 3 years of age.[23] Most of the cases are idiopathic and only 2-12 percent of all pediatric cases have an identifiable lead point[23] and the frequency increases with age so that in children above 4 years of age the incidence of an identifiable lead point is about 57 percent.[24] Typical history is that of a male infant above the age of 3 months, suddenly suffers from bouts of crying, often drawing his knees up with abdominal discomfort. Frequently this is associated with vomiting. The discomfort lasts briefly, after which the infant is quiet and may appear well. The episodes of crying are repetitive, typically occurring every 15-30 minutes intervals. The child may pass stools once or twice at the beginning of the episode but later develops obstipation. Frequent passage of small amounts of mucus with or without blood may be mistaken for passage of liquid stools and these children get labeled as gastroenteritis. As time passes, the child becomes increasingly ill, with increasing dehydration, vomiting, abdominal distension with appearance of red currant-jelly stools. There is usually severe tachycardia and hypotension. A sausage shaped mass may be palpated in the right upper quadrant and careful examination may reveal the absence of cecum in the right lower quadrant (sign of Dance). Rarely in advanced cases there may be prolapse of the intussusception from the anus. In 60-90 percent of cases there is gross or occult blood on the finger following rectal examination.[25]

Plain upright abdominal films will show non-specific features of distal small bowel obstruction (Figure 12.1D). Ultrasound examination is helpful in diagnosis and will show the classical target lesion (Figure 12.12. Ultrasonography is now routinely used as a screening investigation to evaluate a child with suspected intussusception.[26,27] The findings of a "target sign" on a transverse scan or a "pseudo-kidney sign" on a longitudinal scan are quite characteristic. The target sign consists of two rings of low echogenicity separated by a hyperechoic ring. This effective screening modality may reduce the number of unnecessary contrast enemas and therefore exposure to ionizing radiation. Barium enema is confirmatory and may be helpful to achieve hydrostatic reduction (Figure 12.11). Hydrostatic or pneumatic reduction under fluoroscopy or ultrasound guidance may be attempted if the history is of less than 24 hours and the child is relatively stable. If such manipulations are unsuccessful or not indicated, the surgical correction is the only option left but this must be undertaken after a reasonable hemodynamic stability is achieved. Non-operative reduction of intussusception can now be achieved under sonographic guidance using 10% meglumineioxitamalate enema in balanced salt solution or pneumatic pressure.[28,29] In a child presenting within 24 hours of onset of symptoms, with classical findings of colic, an abdominal mass or currant-jelly stools and without evidence of peritonitis, a contrast enema still remains the gold standard for diagnosis and reduction and is considered safe[22]. CT scans have been found to be useful in the diagnosis of transient small bowel intussusceptions.[30]

Meckel's Diverticulum

Meckel's diverticulum occurs in about 2 percent of the population, making it the most prevalent congenital abnormality of the gastrointestinal tract. Meckel's diverticulum is a true intestinal diverticulum that results from the failure of the vitelline duct to obliterate during the fifth week of fetal development. In addition to the normal layers of the intestinal wall, approximately 50 percent of diverticula contain ectopic tissue. Gastric and pancreatic tissue predominate, with an incidence of 60 to 85 percent and 5 to 16 percent respectively.[31-33] Meckel's diverticulum arises from the antimesenteric border of the intestine. Ninety percent of the diverticula are within 90 cm of the ileocecal valve.[32]

Diagnosis. The diagnosis of Meckel's diverticulum must be considered in a child with unexplained abdominal complaints, nausea and vomiting, or intestinal bleeding. There is a 4 to 6 percent life time risk of developing a complication.[32] The major complications include hemorrhage, obstruction, intussusception, diverticulitis and perforation. Meckel's diverticulum can mimic a variety of more common ailments, such as peptic ulcer disease, gastroenteritis, biliary colic, colonic diverticulitis and milk allergy. Appendicitis is the most common preoperative diagnosis in cases of complicated Meckel's diverticulum. Contrast studies such as upper gastrointestinal series with small bowel follow-through are of limited value because the layers of barium-filled intestine will obstruct the view of the diverticulum.[1] Computed tomographic scans are often nonspecific but occasionally helpful.[34-36] The most useful method of detection of a Meckel's diverticulum is technetium-99m pertechnetate scanning. However, the technetium scan depends on uptake by heterotopic gastric mucosa.

Treatment. The approach to treatment of a Meckel's diverticulum depends on whether it was discovered incidentally or as a result of symptoms. A physician can choose to leave the incidentally discovered diverticulum or perform a simple diverticulectomy or an ileal resection. Some physicians have voiced concern that ectopic tissue may be left behind if ileal resection is not performed. However, because the ectopic tissue is generally found at the distal end of the diverticulum, it will usually be included in the excised diverticulum. If the diverticulum is left intact, any fibrous bands attached to the diverticulum must be excised to prevent any future torsion or obstruction. Laparoscopy is useful in the diagnosis and treatment of Meckel's diverticulum. In addition, the laparoscope can be used to remove an incidentally discovered diverticulum. Reports are available regarding the successful use of laparoscopic diverticulectomy in infants with bleeding Meckel's diverticulum.[37,38]

Malrotation and Volvulus

Malrotation occurs when the normal process of rotation is arrested or deviated at any stage. The most frequent association of malration is when the cecum has failed to reach the right iliac fossa and lies in a subhepatic or central position. This may also be associated with anomalous fixation of the gut, usually with dense fibrous bands extending from the cecum and right colon across the duodenum to the retroperitoneum of the right upper quadrant.

Presentation. The pathologic effects of anomalies of rotation arise from excessive mobility, compression, or kinking of bowel and predisposition to torsion, volvulus, and intussusception. Most cases present in infancy but up to 20% develop symptoms after 1 year of age. The most frequent symptom being bile-stained vomitings. The clinical features in the neonate are indistinguishable from those of duodenal stenosis with vomiting, which is usually green or yellow in color, and upper abdominal distension, which resolves on aspiration by nasogastric tube. Pain or irritability is not a prominent common feature in the neonate, but is a common feature in the toddler and older child. The abdomen is soft and nontender to palpation until strangulation of bowel has developed, when it becomes distended and tender and stools are blood stained. In an older child, the most frequent symptoms are persistent vomitings and intermittent colicky abdominal pain.

Diagnosis. Abdominal radiographs may show a dilated duodenum with a fluid level and some gas in the distal bowel. Volvulus of the midgut is often characterized by a "gasless" abdomen. Assessment of the position, relative relationship of the superior mesenteric vessels by ultrasound and Doppler flow characteristics, may be useful adjuncts but are not sufficiently accurate to confidently exclude malrotation or volvulus. An upper GI contrast study with careful delineation of the duodenojejunal course is now the preferred study (Figure 12.7). The position of the duodeno-jejunal junction is assessed relative to the midline or center of the vertebral body and the level of gastric outlet. A normal finding is defined as the duodeno-jejunal junction to the left of the vertebral body and at the level of the gastric outlet. Malrotation is described by many pediatric radiologists as "typical" if the ligament is to the right of midline or absent, and "atypical" if the duodeno-jejunal junction is midline or to the left and below the gastric outlet. Cecal position is classified as either right lower quadrant (normal) or somewhere other than right lower quadrant (abnormal).[39,40]

Section 2

Treatment. Infants with suspected midgut volvulus and vomiting may be dehydrated and show signs of hypovolemia and hypochloremia and require rapid intravenous resuscitation with a physiologic salt solution. Additional measures, including placement of a nasogastric tube, satisfactory intravenous access, and administration of parenteral antibiotics, should be accomplished as quickly as possible. The Ladd procedure corrects the fundamental abnormalities associated with malrotation with or without midgut volvulus. This procedure consists of the following important steps, which must be carried out in the proper sequence: (a) Evisceration of the bowel and inspection of the mesenteric root; (b) counter clockwise derotation of the midgut volvulus; (c) lysis of Ladd's peritoneal bands, with straightening of the duodenum along the right abdominal gutter; (d) appendectomy; and (e) placement of the cecum in the left upper quadrant.[39,40]

Pancreatitis

Acute pancreatitis is defined as a single or recurrent episodes of severe abdominal pain with protracted vomitings associated with an elevated serum pancreatic enzyme levels.[41] It is an important but an uncommon cause of abdominal pain in children.[42] The causes of acute panceratitis in children include trauma, biliary tract stone disease, choledochal cyst, biliary duct anomalies, drugs (corticosteroids, valproic acid), metabolic derangements and infections. Most commonly no cause can be pinpointed and most cases are labeled as idiopathic. Systemic illness and metabolic conditions such as cystic fibrosis, with inspissation of pancreatic secretions in the ducts, Reye's syndrome, Kawasaki's disease, hyperlipidemias and hypercalcemia may cause pancreatitis. Infections with viruses (Coxsackie virus and rotavirus) and generalized bacterial sepsis can also cause pancreatitis.[43]

Clinical features. These children present with severe abdominal pain, tenderness, ileus and guarding. The pain is epigastric in location and of constant character with radiation to the mid back or the flanks. Fever, nausea and vomiting often accompanies the discomfort. On examination there is abdominal distension and tenderness. Rarely a vague abdominal mass may be palpable. In some cases of necrotizing or hemorrhagic pancreatitis, hemorrhage may dissect from the pancreas along the tissue planes, appearing as ecchymosis either in the flanks (Grey-Turner sign) or at the umbilicus (Cullen's sign).

Diagnosis. Elevated levels of amylase in serum or urine are diagnostic.[44] Although amylase is elevated in other abdominal conditions such as intestinal perforation or obstruction, appendicitis and acute cholecystitis, the levels reached are usually not as high as those found in acute pancreatitis.[45] In cases where the serum amylase is not elevated, the amylase-creatinine ratio is calculated and if found to be more than 5, it is suggestive of pancreatitis. In addition investigations may reveal hemoconcentration, leukocytosis, hypocalcemia, coagulopathy, hypergylcemia and altered liver function tests. Plain radiographs of the chest and abdomen are done to exclude perforation.[46] Occasionally a gas filled right colon or a distended loop of small intestine (sentinel loop) may be seen. Left basal pleural effusion is common. Mottling of lung field is a sign of systemic cytokine release. Ultrasound examination may be difficult because the overlying bowel gas may interfere with the adequate visualization of the parenchymal edema and ductal dilatation. In such cases CT scan is useful in defining the degree of parenchymal destruction or pseudocyst/abscess formation. Ultrasound/ CT examination are also helpful in delineating any other pancreatic pathology.[47] Magnetic resonance cholangiopancreatography (MRCP) is a new non-invasive technique, requiring no contrast injection and is now the initial imaging modality in children with unexplained or recurrent pancreatitis.[48,49]

Primary Peritonitis

This is an infectious process of the peritoneal cavity that has no intra-abdominal source[50] and is synonymous with idiopathic or spontaneous peritonitis. Presentation is often with acute abdominal pain associated with febrile illness.[51] It may be associated with nausea, vomiting and diarrhea. The pain is diffuse without any localization and occurs due to irritation of both the visceral and parietal peritoneal surfaces. There is diffuse retroperitoneal tenderness. Sometimes if the child is on systemic steroids as in cases of nephrotic syndrome, there may be complete suppression of all signs and symptoms. Primary peritonitis is more common in children suffering from nephrotic syndrome, hepatic dysfunction, adrenogenital syndrome, cystic fibrosis, post splenectomy, long term steroid administration or chronic renal failure on continuous ambulatory peritoneal dialysis. Primary peritonitis may occur in otherwise healthy girls. The source of infection, however, is unclear in most of the times. The common micro-organisms implicated in primary peritonitis are *Streptococcus pneumoniae, E.coli, beta Hemolytic sreptococci, and Klebsiella pneumoniae.*

Enterocolitis due to Hirschsprung's Disease

This manifests clinically as explosive diarrhea, abdominal distension, fever, vomiting and lethargy and the mortality rates vary between 6-30 percent.[52] There is usually a past history of severe constipation, requiring enemas for evacuation, dating back to neonatal period or early infancy. Examination reveals severe abdominal distension with explosive evacuation of foul smelling liquid stools following per rectal examination (Blast sign). Erect abdominal X-ray may show features of distal bowel obstruction (Figure 12.1D) or the "intestinal cut-off sign" which is highly sensitive (74%) and specific (86%) for enterocolitis.[53] Barium enema performed during an episode of enterocolitis may reveal jejunisation of the sigmoid colon which has a typical spiculated appearance (Figure 12.10 C).

Liver Abscess

Children suffering from liver abscess present with high grade fever with chills, nausea, right upper quadrant pain, abdominal distension and anorexia.[54] Jaundice may or may not be present. Most would appear ill and have a tender hepatomegaly. Breath sounds are often decreased in the lower right chest and right pleural effusion is common. Blood tests would reveal abnormalities in leukocyte count, liver enzymes and bilirubin levels. More than 50 percent of the children are under 5 years of age[55] and multiple abscesses are more common than a solitary abscess.[56] The diagnosis is confirmed by an ultrasound or a contrast enhanced CT scan[57, 58]. The diagnosis may sometimes be suspected on a plain X-ray chest which may show raised right dome of diaphragm with basal atelectasis and minimal pleural effusion (Figure 12.15). Pyogenic abscesses are commoner than an amebic abscess in children. The most common organisms found in liver abscesses are *Staphylococcus aureus, Streptococcus pyogenes, E. coli and Klebsiella pneumoniae.*[58] More than 20 percent cases would also have anerobic organisms[58], therefore the initial antibiotics must provide coverage against Gram-positive, Gram-negative and anerobic organisms. The preferred treatment of pyogenic abscess is systemic antibiotics and closed continuous percutaneous ultrasound or CT guided drainage. Surgical drainage is indicated if percutaneous drainage is not feasible or has failed.

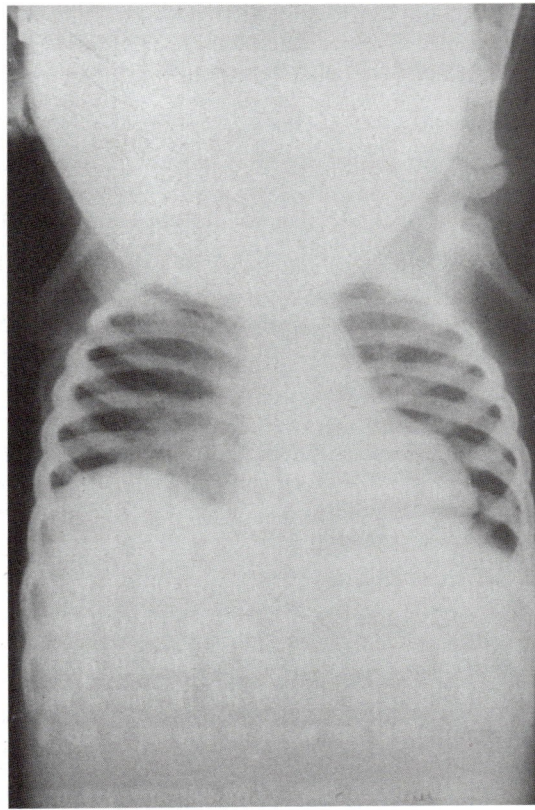

Figure 12.15 Chest X-ray in a case of hepatic abscess in the right lobe showing raised dome of diaphragm with minimal pleural effusion

REFERENCES

1. Barkin RM. Acute abdominal pain. In: Emergency Pediatrics. Barkin RM (ed.). St Louis. *The CV Mosby Co.* 1984; p 142-144.

2. Smith M. Gastroenterological emergencies and abdominal pain In : Pediatric Emergency Medicine. Brennan PO (ed.). *BIOS Scientific Publishers Ltd,* 2003: p 87-102.

3. Hrabovsky E. Acute and chronic abdominal pain. In: Practical Strategies in Pediatric Diagnosis and Therapy. Kliegman RM (ed) *WB Saunders Company, Philadelphia,* 1996; p 258-278.

4. Ravichandran D, Burge DM. Pneumonia presenting with acute abdominal pain in children. *Br J Surg* 1996; 83:1707-1708.

5. Hajivassiliou CA. Intestinal obstruction in neonatal/pediatric surgery. *Sem Pediatr Surg* 2003, 12:241-253.

6. Gregory RE, Ettinger DS. 5-HT3 receptor antagonists for the prevention of chemotherapy induced nausea and vomiting: a comparison of their pharmacology and clinical efficacy. *Drugs* 1998; 55(1):173-189.

7. Leung AK, Sigalet DL. Acute abdominal pain in children. *Am Fam Physician* 2003; 67:2321-2326.

Section 2

8. Bromberg R, Goldman RD. Does analgesia mask diagnosis of appendicitis among children? *Can Fam Physician* 2007 Jan; 53(1):39-41.

9. Petrack ME. The irritable infant. In: Practical Strategies in Pediatric Diagnosis and Therapy. Kliegman RM (ed), *WB Saunders Company, Philadelphia,* 1996; p 518-525.

10. Smink DS, *et al.* Diagnosis of acute appendicitis in children using a clinical practice guideline *Pediatr Surg* 2004, 39:458-463.

11. Bolton JP, Craven ER, Croft RJ, *et al.* An assessment of the value of white cell count in the management of suspected acute appendicitis. *Br J Surg* 1975; 62:906-908.

12. Wang LT, Prentiss KA, Simon JZ, Doody DP, Ryan DP The use of white blood cell count and left shift in the diagnosis of appendicitis in children. *Pediatr Emerg Care* 2007 Feb; 23(2):69-76.

13. Cardall T, Glasser J, Guss DA Clinical value of the total white blood cell count and temperature in the evaluation of patients with suspected appendicitis. . *Acad Emerg Med* 2004 Oct; 11(10):1021-1027.

14. Pearl RH, Hale DA, Molloy M, *et al.* Pediatric appendectomy. *J Pediatr Surg* 1995; 30:173.

15. Hahn HB, Hoepner FU, Kalle, *et al.* Ultrasound in suspected acute appendicitis in children: 7 years experience. *Pediatr Radiol* 1998; 28:147-151.

16. Sivit CJ, Applegate KE, Stallion A, *et al.* Imaging evaluation of suspected appendicitis in a pediatric population: effectiveness of sonography versus CT. Am *J Roentgenol* 2000; 175:977-980.

17. Lowe LH, Penny MW, Stein SM, *et al.* Unenhanced limited CT of the abdomen in the diagnosis of appendicitis in children: comparison with sonography. *Am J Roentgenol* 2001; 176:31-35.

18. Horman M, Paya K, Eibennerger K, *et al.* MR imaging in children with nonperforated acute appendicitis: value of unenhanced MR imaging in sonographically selected cases. *Am J Roentgenol* 1998; 171:467-470.

19. Stephen AE, Segev KL, Ryan DP, *et al.* The diagnosis of appendicitis in a pediatric population: To CT or not to CT. *J Pediatr Surg* 2003; 38:367-371.

20. Patric DA, Janik JE, Janik JS, *et al.* Increased CT scan utilization does not improve the diagnostic accuracy of appendicitis in children. *J Pediatr Surg* 2003; 8: 659-662.

21. Gholoum S, Baird R, Laberge JM, Puligandla PS. Incarceration rates in pediatric inguinal hernia: do not trust the coding. . *J Pediatr Surg* 2010 May; 45(5): 1007-1011.

22. Stephens BJ, Rice WT, Kouchy CJ, *et al.* Optimal timing of elective indirect inguinal hernia repair on healthy children: clinical considerations for improved outcome. *World J Surg* 1992; 16:952-956.

23. Doody P Daniel. Intussusception. In: Surgery of Infants and Children: Scientific Principles and Practice. Oldham KT, Colombani PM, Fogila RP (eds). *Lippincort-Raven Publishers, Philadelphia* 1997; p 1241-1252.

24. Ong NT, Beasley SW. The lead point in intussusception. *J Pediatr Surg* 1990; 25:640-643.

25. Losek JD, Fiete RL. Intussusception and the diagnostic value of testing stool for occult blood. *Am J Emerg Med* 1991; 9:1-3.

26. Smith DS, Bonadio WA, Losele JD, *et al.* The role of abdominal X-rays in the diagnosis and management of intussusception. *Pediatr Emerg Care* 1992; 8:325-327.

27. Daneman A, Navarro O. Intussusception, Part I: a review of diagnostic approaches. *Pediatr Radiol* 2003; 33:79-85.

28. Crystal P, Hertzamm Y, Fraber B, *et al.* Sonographically guided hydrostatic reduction of intussusception in children. *J Clin Ultrasound* 2002; 30:343-348.

29. Gu L, Zhu H, Wang S. Sonographic guidance of air enema for intussusception reduction in children. *Pediatr Radiol* 2000; 30:339-342.

30. Strouse PJ, DiPietro MA, Saez F. Transient small bowel intussusception in children on CT. *Pediatr Radiol* 2003; 33:316-320.

31. Mackey WC, Dineen P. A fifty-year experience with Meckel's diverticulum. *Surg Gynecol Obstet* 1983; 156:56-1564.

32. Cullen JJ, Kelly KA, Moir CR, Hodge DO, Zinsmeister AR, Melton LJ. Surgical management of Meckel's diverticulum. An epidemiologic, population-based study. *Ann Surg* 1994; 220:564-569.

33. Artigas V, Calabuig R, Badia F, Rius X, Allende L, Jover J. Meckel's diverticulum: value of ectopic tissue. *Am J Surg* 1986; 151:631-634.

34. Simms M, Caldwell J, Lundgrin D. Inverted Meckel's diverticulum diagnosed with computed tomography: case report. *Canad Assoc Radiol* J 1999; 50:17-19.

35. Daneman A, Lobo E, Alton DJ, Shuckett B. The value of sonography, CT and air enema for detection of complicated Meckel diverticulum in children with nonspecific clinical presentation. *Pediatr Radiol* 1998; 28:928-932.

36. Hughes JA, Hatrick A, Rankin S. Computed tomography findings in an inflamed Meckel diverticulum. *Br J Radiol* 1998; 71:882-883.

37. Sanders LE. Laparoscopic treatment of Meckel's diverticulum. Obstruction and bleeding managed with minimal morbidity. *Surg Endosc* 1995; 9:724-727.

38. Huang CS, Lin LH. Laparoscopic Meckel's diverticulectomy in infants: report of three cases. *J Pediatr Surg* 1993; 28:1486-1489.

39. Millar AJ, Rode H, Cywes S. Malrotation and volvulus in infancy and childhood. *Semin Pediatr Surg* 2003 Nov; 12(4):229-236.

40. Smith SD. Disorders of intestinal rotation and fixation. In: Pediatric Surgery. Grosfeld JL (ed) . *Mosby Inc.* 6th ed. 2006.

41. Miyano T. The pancreas. In: Pediatric Surgery O'Neill JA (Jr), Rowe MI, Grosfeild JL, Fonkalsrud EW, Coran AG (eds) 5th edition. Mosby, St Louis, 1998; p 1527-1544.

42. Weiman Z, Durie PR. Acute pancreatitis in childhood. *J Pediatr* 1988; 113:24.

43. Weizmann Z. An update on diseases of the pancreas in children. *Curr Opin Pediatr* 1997; 9:494-497.

44. Gwozdz GP, Steinberg WM, Werner M, *et al.* Comparative evaluation of the diagnosis of acute pancreatitis based on serum and urine enzyme assays. *Clin Chim Acta* 1990; 187:243-254.

45. Pieper-Bigelow C, Strocchi A, Levitt MD. Where does serum amylase come from and where does it go? *Gastroenterol Clin North Am* 1990; 19:793-810.

46. Clancy TE. Management of acute pancreatitis. In: Maingot's Abdominal Operations Zinner MJ, Ashley SW (eds). *McGraw-Hill* 11th Ed. 2006.

47. Badea R. Ultrasound of acute pancreatitis – an essay in images. *Rom Gastroenterol* 2005: 14; 83-89

48. Neblett WW III, O'Neill JA Jr. Surgical management of recurrent pancreatitis in children with pancreas divisum. *Ann Surg* 2000; 231:899-908.

49. Arcement CM, Meza MP, Arumanala S, *et al.* MRCP in the evaluation of pancreatobiliary disease in children. *Pediatr Radiol* 2001; 31:92-97.

50. Cãruntu FA, Benea L. Spontaneous bacterial peritonitis: pathogenesis, diagnosis, treatment. *J Gastrointest Liver Dis* 2006 Mar; 15(1):51-56.

51. Kimber CP, Hutson JM. Primary peritonitis in children. *Aust N Z J Surg* 1996 Mar; 66(3):169-170.

52. Vieten D, Spicer R. Enterocolitis complicating Hirschsprung's disease. *Semin Pediatr Surg* 2004 Nov; 13(4):263-272.

53. Elhalaby EA, Teitbaum DH, Coran AG, *et al.* Enterocolitis associated with Hirschsprung's disease: A clinical-radiological characterization based on 168 patients. *J Pediatr Surg* 1995; 30:76.

54. Breurer CK, Vacanti JP. Surgical liver disease. In: Surgery of Infants and Children: Scientific Principles and Practice. Oldham KT, Colombani PM, Fogila RP (eds) *Lippincott-Raven publishers, Philadelphia* 1997; p 1385-1394.

55. Holcomb GW III, Pietsch JB. Gall bladder disease and hepatic infections. In: Pediatric Surgery O'Neill JA (Jr), Rowe MI, Grosfeild JL, Fonkalsrud EW, Coran AG (eds) 5th edition. *Mosby, St Louis,* 1998; p 1495-1504.

56. Branum GD, Tyson GS, Branum MA, *et al.* Hepatic abscess. Changes in etiology, diagnosis and management. *Ann Surg* 1990; 212:655-662.

57. Brook I, Fraizer EH. Role of anaerobic bacteria in liver abscesses in children. *Pediatr Infect Dis* J 1993; 12:743.

58. Sharma MP. Liver abscesses in children. *Indian Pediatr* 2006, 73:813-817.

13

Acute Fever without a Focus

Meharban Singh

> *"Humanity has but three great enemies; fever, famine and war. Of these, by far the greatest, by far the most terrible, is fever".*
> — *Sir William Osler*

Fever is the commonest symptom or signal of an illness in children. Depending upon the site of infection or focus of disease, generally there are localising symptoms and signs due to the underlying disease process. At times, because of host characteristics and the nature of the disease process, there may be no localizing features to suggest the site of infection. Fever is usually a protective response on the part of the body to fight an infection. However, in young children (6-36 months), fever may cause convulsions. Moreover, during an episode of fever the requirements of fluids, food and oxygen go up due to rise in the metabolic rate of the body[1].

BODY TEMPERATURE

The normal oral body temperature is maintained between a narrow range of 98.2°F ± 0.7°F (36.8°C ± 0.4°C). There are normal variations in body temperature, it is lowest in the morning and highest in the evening (upto 99.9°F oral temperature in summer). Rectal temperature is the gold standard but should be recorded by a trained nurse in a health care facility. Rectal thermometer (round short bulb) should be inserted gently in a non-struggling infant upto a depth of 2-3 cm by directing it posteriorly as a safeguard against rectal perforation[2]. Skin temperature can be recorded with the help of a digital thermometer, thermocrystal strips or infrared technology. The axilla or groin should be swiped dry and thermometer kept *in-situ* for at least 2 minutes. In ambulatory practice, the infra red thermoscan is often used by the busy clinician to record the temperature of tympanic membrane as it gives a read-out within one second. Oral temperature is the reference or standard body temperature but cannot be recorded in pre-school children. Rectal or core body temperature (including tympanic) is generally 0.75°F (0.5°C) higher than the oral temperature and oral temperature is 0.75°F (0.5°C) higher than the skin temperature[3].

DEFINITION

In young children fever is defined as an elevation of rectal temperature above 100.4°F (38°C). A number of studies have shown that skin and tympanic temperatures are unreliable in children. When fever of acute onset and short duration (< 1 week) occurs without any localizing symptoms on history or any clinical signs on carefully conducted physical examination, it is called fever without focus (FWF) or fever without source (FWS)[3]. When fever without focus continues beyond one week and no cause is identified despite carefully conducted observations and laboratory investigations for another week, the condition is called as pyrexia of unknown origin (PUO) or fever of unknown origin (FUO) which is not the focus of discussion in this chapter. There is an overlap between these two conditions and FWF way gradually progress and evolve to become FUO. The occurrence of acute fever without a focus is a medical emergency and it poses a great challenge to the clinical acumen and diagnostic capabilities of the pediatrician.

ETIOLOGIC SPECTRUM

In clinical practice, no other symptom has such a large spectrum of diagnostic possibilities than fever.[4] A large number of host-related conditions may lead to FWF. Immunocompromised children such as preterm infants, children with severe protein-energy malnutrition, nephrotic syndrome, asplenia, sickle cell disease, lymphoreticular malignancy and HIV infection are unable to localize infection and produce non-specific features of bacteremia and septicemia. Children on immuno-suppressive drugs like corticosteroids and antimitotic agents are unable to produce localizing symptoms and signs of infection. Apart from lack of localizing symptoms and signs, many a time, immuno-compromised children may not even produce any febrile reponse. It is well known that preterm babies with septicemia may actually manifest with hypothermia rather than fever[5].

Viral infections are the leading cause of self-limited fever of acute onset and short duration at all age groups[6]. The common causes of fever of acute onset and without any focus are listed in Table 13.1. When infection is blood-borne and not localized to any body organ, it does not produce any localizing symptoms or signs.

Table 13.1 Common causes of fever without a focus
❑ Vaccine-associated fever
❑ Viral fever
❑ ENT infections: Streptococeal pharyngitis; acute otitis media (AOM), mastoiditis or sinusitis
❑ Malaria
❑ Bacteremia or septicemia
❑ Enteric or typhoid fever
❑ Urinary tract infection
❑ Pneumonia
❑ Hyperthermia

The introduction of vaccines to prevent *Haemophilus influenzae type b* (Hib) and pneumococcal disease (PCV-13) has reduced the incidence of occult bacteremia and serious bacterial infections from 10% to 1% in children below 36 months[7]. The infective diseases which may present as FWF of a relatively long duration include tuberculosis, bacterial endocarditis, brucellosis, infectious mononucleosis, cytomegalovirus infections, toxoplasmosis, viral hepatitis, occult abscesses in the bones and joints, liver, subphrenic and perinephric areas and injection sites should be looked for in all patients with FWF. Fungal infections should be seriously considered specially among immuno-compromised or neutropenic children receiving broad spectrum antibiotics and parenteral nutrition.

Non-infective inflammatory conditions which may manifest as FWF include allergic disorders, drug fever, serum sickness, immunization reaction, and hyperthermia (anhidrotic ectodermal dysplasia, diabetes inspidus, faulty thalamic thermostat, excessively clothed or swaddled baby, high environmental temperature). In hyperthermia, hypothalamic set point is not elevated and fever occurs due to excessive environmental temperature or inability to lose body heat. There is no role of antipyretics in the treatment of hyperthermia which is managed by cooling measures and hydrotherapy. Fever may occur because of hypersensitivity or autoimmune disorders (inflammatory bowel disease, juvenile rheumatoid arthritis), lymphoblastic leukemia, lymphoma or due to an unknown cause (Kawasaki disease).

HISTORY

The posibility of finding useful leads on history and clinical examination depends upon the experience, expertise and thoroughness of the pediatrician. Even after taking detailed history and doing a thorough physical examination, it is not possible to identify the cause of fever in one out of five acutely ill non-toxic children[7]. A detailed history should be taken to identify subtle markers of common conditions which are associated with fever of short duration. Viral infections are the leading cause of FWF of short duration. History of viral fever in other family members, siblings, or care takers, is highly suggestive that the fever is most likely to be viral in origin. The positive history of viral fever in the recent past among the family members or close contacts is reassuring that the patient is likely to be suffering from a self-limited viral disease[8].

Intermittent fever with chills and rigors is suggestive of malaria but typical picture may be absent. The diagnostic utility of chills is limited because it is difficult to evaluate in pre-school children and may ocur in a large number of infective conditions like viremia, bacteremia or sepsis, brucellosis, rickettsiosis, leptospirosis, urinary tract infection, and cholangitis. Excessive and inconsolable crying in an infant with fever is suggestive of a painful condition such as acute otitis media, pyogenic meningitis, arthritis, osteomyelitis. A detailed systematic review of all the body systems should be made by asking leading questions to elicit any localizing symptoms. History of lethargy, inactivity, irritability and poor feeding or refusal to take feeds are ominous symptoms suggestive of a serious infection.

PHYSICAL SIGNS

> *"Most errors in clinical practice are made by taking incomplete history and making a cursory, incomplete examination than due to lack of knowledge and skills".*
>
> *— Henry Cohen*

A detailed physical examination should be conducted under good light by adequate exposure of the child. A repeat assessment of the child after 48 hours is useful because the localizing symptoms and signs are usually absent during first 24–48 hours of onset of fever. The presence of toxemia, poor activity, lethargy, refusal of feeds and unstable vital signs are ominous indicating a serious disorder[9]. In infants and immunocompromised children, the classical features of malaria, typhoid fever and urinary tract infection are not seen and they are likely to have non-specific or atypical manifestations. Meningeal signs may be absent in children below 6 months and seizures may occur due to non-CNS or metabolic causes in young children. Bulging of anterior fontanel in a quiet infant is a useful sign of raised intracranial tension due to meningitis. Skin should be examined for any rash, petechiae, ecchymoses and gangrenous patches which provide useful clues for the underlying condition which is discussed in detail in Chapter 14. A detailed ear, nose and throat examination is mandatory to exclude upper respiratory tract infection, acute otitis media and sinusitis. Urinary tract infection may not produce any specific symptoms and signs in young children and must be ruled out. In boys, tight prepuce and meatitis or balanitis are useful markers of urinary tract infection[10].

Table 13.2 Correlates of viral infection in infants

- History of viral fever in a family member or close contact (maid, creche, play school)
- Coryza or nasal congestion
- Gingivostomatitis or aphthous ulcers (Herpes)
- Pharyngeal vesicles (Coxsackie)
- Stridor
- Papules and vesicles over the hands, feet and mouth (Hand-foot-and-mouth disease)
- Viral exanthemata
- Normal WBC count with elevation of lymphocytes or monocytes
- CRP may be elevated but procalcitonin is not raised

A number of clinical markers are suggestive of a viral infection and should be diligently looked for (Table 13.2). Generalized lymphadenopathy and hepato-splenomegaly in febrile children may be seen due to a variety of infections like tuberculosis, infectious mononucleosis, toxoplasmosis, cytomegalovirus infection, lymphoreticular malignancy and collagen vascular disorders. Kawasaki disease, which is associated with vasculitis of medium sized vessels, is usually characterized by moderate duration of fever with marked irritability, suffusion or redness of eyes, unilateral cervical lymphadenopathy, fissured red lips, strawberry tongue, skin rash, swelling of hands and feet with periungual desquamation of palms and soles.

Attempt should be made to look for any swelling and tenderness over the bones and joints which may occur in patients with arthritis,

osteomyelitis, collagen vascular disorder and lymphoreticular malignancy. Tenderness and swelling over the site of occult abscess and renal angles suggest underlying inflammatory condition. The fever due to drugs is characterized by skin rash, eosinophilia and ''flat temperature'' between 100°F-102°F without any hectic fluctuations characteristic of bacteremia or septicemia. The fever resolves after 2-3 days of stopping the drug/s.

LABORATORY INVESTIGATIONS

Most cases of fever without focus are viral in etiology and no investigations are required. The choice of investigations should be individualized depending upon the vital clues obtained on history and carefully conducted physical examination. When there are no clinical correlates of a viral infection as listed in Table 13.2, complete blood count (CBC), thick and thin blood smears for malarial parasites, erythrocyte sedimentation rate (ESR), C-reactive protein (CRP) and procalcitonin (PCT) levels should be checked. Leukopenia ($\leq$ 5000/mm^3) with increase in lymphocytes and monocytes is suggestive of viral infection but may occur in immuno-compromised children with bacterial infection. In children with bacteremia and/or sepsis, there is leukocytosis ($\geq$ 15,000/mm^3), elevation of absolute neutrophil count ($\geq$10,000/mm^3), absolute band cell count of $\geq$ 1500/mm^3, ratio of unsegmented (band cells) to segmented neutrophils of more than 0.2, thrombocytopenia ($\leq$ 100,000/mm^3), elevated erythrocyte sedimentation rate ($\geq$ 30 mm in 1st hour), elevated C-reactive protein ($\geq$10 mg/dl) and procalcitonin ($\geq$ 2 ng/ml)[11-16]. C-reactive protein may be elevated both in viral and bacterial infections but procalcitonin is a more useful marker of bacterial infection but its utility is limited by cost and availability. In collagen vascular disorders, ESR may be markedly elevated while CRP is usually normal.

Urine for routine examination (including leukocyte esterase or nitrite) and culture, colony count and antibacterial sensitivity pattern should be obtained in all infants having fever without a focus. Urine for culture studies can be collected by a clean catch method or preferably by catheterization which should be conducted under strict aseptic conditions. Urine may be collected by suprapubic puncture in infants if there is tight phimosis or severe labial adhesions. In a male infant urine sample can be collected by affixing a sterile test tube over the penis. Bag sample is unsuitable for culture studies and is not recommended.

In a sick infant, whenever occult bacteremia is suspected, blood sample should be taken for culture studies. The blood sample should be collected under strict aseptic conditions. The ratio of blood to volume of the culture medium should be 1:10 i.e. 1.0 ml blood should be poured in a culture bottle containing 10 ml of the medium. Bact/Alert and BACTEC automated culture system should be used because it is associated with lower risk of contamination, shorter incubation period and higher isolation rates. Availability of PCR for identification of viruses helps in their early diagnosis and serves to decrease the unnecessary use of antibiotics. PCR technology is also useful for identification of bacterial antigens but is available only in advanced centers[17]. Lumbar puncture should be done in critically sick children or whenever indicated. It should be interpreted with care taking into account the wide variations in various indices in healthy infants[18]. Skiagram of chest is taken whenever, there is suspicion of pneumonia, presence of high grade fever or when there is marked leukocytosis ($\geq$20,000/mm^3)[19,20].

MANAGEMENT

Symptomatic Therapy

The child with fever should be kept in a cool, well-ventilated room. The patient should not be covered with a blanket and should wear light cotton clothes. The child should be given plenty of fluids and good nutritious diet without any restrictions. Antipyretic should be given if oral temperature exceeds 38.5°C (101°F) or for relief of associated discomfort due to headache and body aches. Fever is a protective response on the part of the body to fight infection and no attempts should be made to treat mild fever or use a strong antipyretic agent. There is no correlation between the response to antipyretics and cause of the fever[21].

According to WHO, paracetamol (15 mg/kg/dose q 4-6 hr) is the antipyretic of first choice because of its assured efficacy and safety. The recommended dose should be administered accurately with the help of a graduated dispenser provided by the manufacturer. Ibuprofen (10 mg/kg/dose q 6-8 hr) can be used as an alternative second line drug. No other NSAID or antipyretic agents are licensed for use in children by US FDA[1]. *Acetylsalicylic acid should not be used as an antipyretic agent in children due to potential risk of development of life-threatening Reye's syndrome.* When body temperature goes above 104°F, despite use of an antipyretic agent, body sponging with tap water is recommended while keeping the child under a fan. Cold or chilled water should not be used for hydrotherapy as it may cause discomfort and rigors with further elevation of body temperature.

Specific Therapy

Ambulatory care

Many children with acute fever may provide significant clues for the possible cause of fever during observation and they can be managed on ambulatory basis.[22] Viral fever is managed by good supportive and symptomatic care because antiviral therapy is not available for most non specific viral infections. *Unnecessary administration of antibiotics in children with viral infections is not only useless but it is potentially harmful both for the patient and community*[23].

When peripheral blood smear examination shows malarial parasites or blood is positive for malarial antigens, oral chloroquine phosphate is given in a dose of 10 mg of base /kg stat followed by 5 mg/kg after 6 hr, 24 hr and 48 hr. In falciparum malaria and in regions with high incidence of chloroquine resistance, quinine sulphate 10 mg of base/kg/dose is given 3 times/day for 3 days followed by administration of pyrimethamine and sulfadoxine on the third day. Alternatively, a combination of artemether and lumefantrine can be given. Acute otitis media is managed by administration of an analgesic, amoxycillin or macrolides or cefuroxime axetil for 7 days and saline nose drops to relieve nasal congestion.

Most pneumonias are viral in origin but in clinical practice, they are treated by antibacterial agents because of difficulty in making etiologic diagnosis and life-threatening nature of the disease. Community acquired pneumonia is treated by oral administration of amoxycillin or cefaclor or macrolides for 5-7 days. The useful second line antibiotics for ambulatory treatment of pneumonia include amoxycillin-clavulanic acid, cefuroxime axetil and cefdinir. Administration of antihistaminics and sedatives are contraindicated in patients with pneumonia. Typhoid fever can be managed on ambulatory basis if child is not critically sick and is accepting feeds. The antibiotics of choice include oral cefixime (10 mg/kg/dose q 12 hr) or ofloxacin (10 mg/kg/dose q 12 hr) because of high prevalence of multidrug resistant strains of *S.typhi*. Azithromycin (10 mg/kg/dose q 12 hr) is also effective against *S. typhi* and is credited to reduce the risk of relapse. Recent observations suggest that several isolates of *S.typhi* have become sensitive to amoxycillin and chloramphenicol. The antibiotic therapy should be continued for at least 4-5 days after complete resolution of fever to prevent risk of relapse.

Children with Possible Bacterial Infection

Infants with acute bacterial infection, who are effectively immunized, can be treated on an ambulatory basis if they are able to accept feeds. Early and effective parenteral antibiotic therapy to cover the likely pathogens i.e. *S.pneumoniae, S. aureus*, or *N. meningitidis* and *H. influenzae type b*, is associated with good outcome. The management of occult bacterial infection in children below 36 months of age is shown in the algorithm (Figure 13.1)[6].

Neonates

Every neonate ($\leq$ 28 days) with fever but without any markers of viral infection like family contact, coryza or nasal congestion, should be admitted in the hospital and subjected to complete sepsis work-up and managed accordingly. Neonatal HSV infection should be considered if there are high risk factors like genital herpes in the mother, vaginal delivery and use of fetal scalp electrodes.

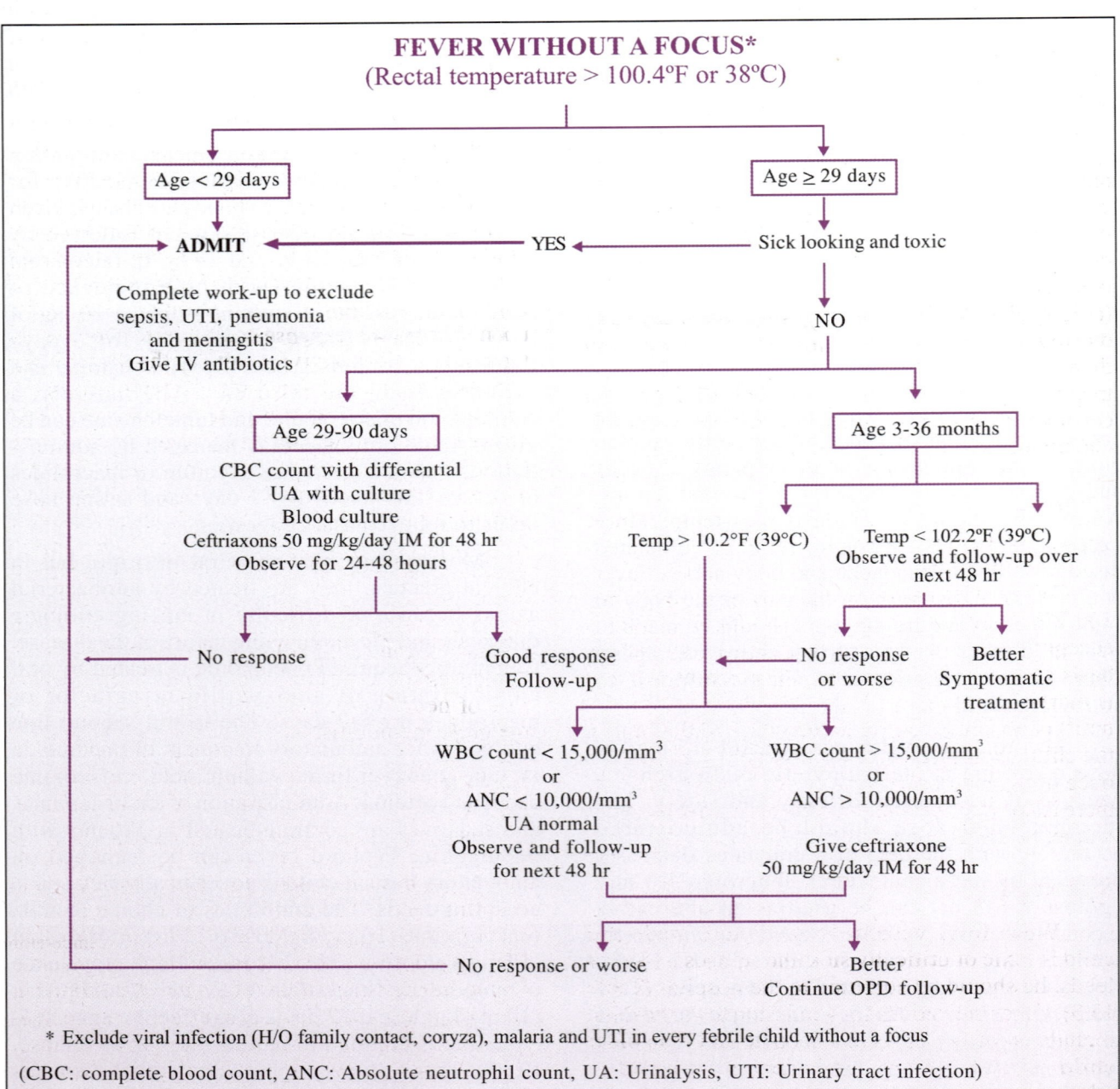

Figure 13.1 Algorithm for treatment of a child with fever without any source

The presence of vesicles over the skin, mouth or eyes of the baby, CSF pleocytosis and lack of response to antibiotic therapy are highly suggestive of HSV infection[24].

Infants between 29-90 days

They are also at an increased risk to develop occult bacteremia or sepsis. A complete work-up for bacterial infection should be undertaken before starting antibiotic therapy. They can be managed on ambulatory basis if child is not toxic and accepting feeds. It is advised to administer ceftriaxone 50 mg/kg IM once daily and child reassessed after 24-48 hours. The therapy may be continued if child is showing good response or modified on the basis of laboratory reports. A meta-analysis of four randomized controlled trials of 7899 children, between 3-36 months age, who had fever $\geq 39.0°C$ ($\geq 102.2°F$), found that treatment of occult bacteremia with a single dose of intramuscular ceftriaxone reduced the chances of serious bacterial infection by 75 percent while oral amoxycillin had no protective effect[25]. When urinary tract infection is diagnosed on the basis of positive urine culture (colony count of 10^5 or more), it is most commonly due to *E.coli* and pyelonephritis is far more common than cystitis in infants below one year. It is best treated by parenteral administration of amikacin and cefriaxone for 7 days followed by oral amoxycillin-clavulanic acid or cefixime for another week.

Children between 3-36 months

Well child

When child is having rectal temperature below 102.2°F (<39°C) and is not sick looking and is accepting feeds, he can be manged on ambulatory basis *vide-supra*. If the condition worsens or there is marked elevation of leukocyte count ($\geq 15,000/$ mm^3) or absolute neutrophil count ($\geq 10,000/$mm^3), the child should be given ceftriaxone 50 mg/kg IM once daily and observed over next 24–48 hours. If there is no significant improvement or child becomes worse, he should be admitted in the hospital.

Sick child

When fever without focus is high grade and child is toxic or critically sick and refuses to accept feeds, he should be admitted to the hospital (Table 13.3). Other indications for admission to the hospital include bacterial sepsis in a neonate and if an older child is unresponsive or becomes worse after administration of single dose of ceftriaxone. Samples of urine, blood and CSF should be collected

---

Table 13.3 Criteria for toxic and sick-looking infant

- ☐ High grade fever $\geq 102.2°F$ ($39.0°C$)
- ☐ Lethargy, drowsiness, irritability, moaning, high-pitched or inconsolable crying
- ☐ Poor feeding or refusal to feed
- ☐ Bradypnea, tachypnea, respiratory distress, stridor, cyanosis or $SaO_2 \leq 95\%$
- ☐ Seizures or bulging anterior fontanel
- ☐ Abdominal distension
- ☐ Bleeding manifestations, petechiae, necrotic or gangrenous skin lesions
- ☐ Cellulitis, abscess, swelling of bone or joint
- ☐ Evidences of dehydration
- ☐ Cold and pale, sallow, mottled skin of extremities or poor tissue perfusion

---

for culture studies before starting antibiotic therapy. The child should be hooked to a vital sign monitor. Intravenous access should be established for administration of fluids and antibiotics. Initial antibiotic therapy includes administration of amikacin (20 mg/kg/d q 12 hr) and cefotaxime (200 mg/kg/d q 12 hr) or ceftriaxone (100 mg/kg/d q 12 hr) which is continued for 7-10 days. Depending upon the clinical response and bacterial isolates and their antibiotic sensitivity pattern, the therapy may be modified. In children with pyogenic meningitis or when antibiotic resistant pneumococci or MRSA are suspected as the likely pathogens, vancomycin (60 mg/kg/d q 6-8 hr) is administered intravenously. The intravenous administration rate of vancomycin should not exceed 15 mg/kg per hour to minimize the risk of "red-man syndrome", and hypotension. Antibiotic therapy is continued for at least 10-14 days in children with meningitis. According to Cochrane data base, administration of dexa-methasone (one dose before starting antibiotics and two doses subsequently) is associated with reduced risk of neuromotor sequelae and deafness due to pyogenic meningitis.

REFERENCES

1. Singh M. Fever of acute onset and short duration. In: A Manual of Essential Pediatrics, *Thieme Medical and Scientific Publishers Pvt Ltd, New Delhi,* 2nd edition, 2013, pp. 233-240.

2. Craig JV, Lancaster GA, Taylor S, *et al.* Temperature measured at the rectum in children and young people: a systematic review. *BMJ* 2000, 141: 1174-1178.

3. Ishimine P. Fever without source in children 0-36 months of age. *Pediatr Clin Amer* 2006, 53: 167-194.

4. Irwin AD, Drew RJ, Marshall P et al. Etiology of childhood bacteremia and timely antibiotics adminis-tration in the emergency department. *Pediatrics* 2015, 135:635.

5. Singh M. Neonatal septicemia. In: Care of the Newborn. *CBS Publishers & Distributors Pvt Ltd, New Delhi,* 8th edition, 2015, pp. 285-294.

6. Sur DK, Bukont EL. Evaluating fever of unidentifiable source in young children. *Am Fam Physician* 2007, 75(12): 1805-1811.

7. Manzano S, Bailey B, Gervaix A, Cousineau J, Delvin E, Girodias JB. Markers for bacterial infections in children with fever without source. *Arch Dis Child* 2011, 96(5): 440-446.

8. Craig JC, Williams GJ, Jones M, *et al.* The accuracy of clinical symptoms and signs for the diagnosis of serious bacterial infection in young febrile children: Prospective cohort study of 15,781 febrile illnesses. *BMJ* April 20, 2010, 340: C1594.

9. Bonadia WA. The history and physical assessment of the febrile infant. *Pediatr Clin North Amer* 1998, 45(1): 65-77.

10. Galletto-Larcour A, Zamora SA, Andreola B, *et al.* Validation of a laboratory risk index score for the identification of severe bacterial infection in children with fever without source. *Arch Dis Child* 2010, 95 (12): 968-973.

11. Mintegi S, Beuto J, Pijoan JI, *et al.* Occult pneumonia in infants with high fever without source: a prospective multicenter study. *Pediatr Emerg Care* 2010, 26 (7): 470-474.

12. Gilsdorf JR. C-reactive protein and procalcitonin are helpful in diagnosis of serious bacterial infections in children. *J Pediatr* 2011, 160:173.

13. Vander Bruel A, Thompson MJ, Haj-Hassan T, et al. Diagnostic value of laboratory tests in identifying serious infections in febrile children: Systematic review. *BMJ* 2011, 342:d 3082.

14. Andreola B, Bressam S, Callegaro S, *et al.* Procalcitonin and C-reactive protein as diagnostic markers of severe bacterial infection in febrile infants and childen in the emergency department. *Pediatr Infect Dis J* 2007, 26 (8): 672-677.

15. Lacour AG, Zanora SA, Cervaix A. A score identifying serious bacterial infections in children with fever without source. *Pediatr Infect Dis J* 2008, 27(7): 654-656.

16. Manzano S, Bailey B, Gervaix A, Cousineau J, Delvin E, Girodias J-B. Markers of bacterial infection in children with fever without source. *Arch Dis Child* 2011, 96: 440-446.

17. Antonyrajah B, Mukundan D. Fever without apparent source on clinical examination. *Pediatrics* 2008, 20(1): 96-102.

18. Byrington CL, Kendrick J, Sheng X. Normative cerebrospinal fluid profiles in febrile infants. *J Pediatr* 2011, 158 (1): 33-37.

19. Olaciregni I, Hernandez U, Munoz JA, *et al.* Markers that predict serious bacterial infection in infants under 3 months of age presenting with fever of unknown origin. *Arch Dis Child* 2009, 94 (7): 501-505.

20. Hsias AL, Baker MD. Fever in the new millenium: A review of recent studies of markers of serious bacterial infection in febrile children. *Curr Opin Pediatr* 2005, 17: 56-61.

21. Farrar H, Sullivan JE. Fever and antipyretic use in children. *Pediatrics* 2011, 127: 580-587.

22. Jhaveri R, Byington CL, Klein JO, Shapiro ED. Management of the nontoxic–appearing acutely febrile child: A 21st century approach. *J Pediatr* 2011, 159:181.

23. Baroff LJ. Management of fever without source in infants and children. *Ann Emerg Med* 2000, 36 (6): 602-614.

24. Massin MM, Montesanti J, Lepage P. Management of fever without source in young children presenting to an emergency room. *Acta Paediatr* 2006, 95 (11): 1446-1450.

25. Bullock B, Craig WR, Klassen TP. The use of antibiotics to prevent serious sequelae in children at risk of occult bacteremia: a meta-analysis. *Acad Emerg Med* 1997, 4 (7), 679-87.

14

Acute Fever with a Skin Rash

Surjit Singh

INTRODUCTION

Acute fever with a skin rash is a common clinical presentation of children visiting the emergency room[1-3]. While most of these children would turn out to have a benign self-limiting illness, occasionally one comes across patients with a life-threatening condition. In many of these patients, the diagnosis can be established on clinical grounds alone and appropriate treatment initiated before the laboratory results are available[2-6]. It is incumbent upon the attending pediatrician to identify patterns of illnesses presenting mainly with fever and skin rash. These illnesses may be infectious or non-infectious[1,2].

Apart from the time honored tools of a good clinical history and detailed physical examination, the site of onset, morphology and evolution of the rash provide important diagnostic clues regarding the underlying etiology[1]. The clinical history should focus on the immunization status of the child, drug intake in the recent past, contact with pets, history of insect bites and exposure to sick individuals[2-6].

Acute fever with a skin rash may be secondary to an underlying systemic disease or it may be a primary skin eruption that may be associated with fever. These skin eruptions may be in the form of cellulitis (infection of deep subcutaneous tissues), erysipelas (infection of superficial subcutaneous tissues), folliculitis (pustular swelling of hair follicles), furuncles (development of a deep inflammatory nodule in established folliculitis) or carbuncles (extensive involvement of subcutaneous fat producing multiple abscesses separated by fibrous septa). Majority of the latter lesions are clinically obvious and it is not difficult to arrive at a diagnosis. An intravenous cannula that has been left in place for long can present with fever and localized rash but here again the diagnosis is straight forward[1-3]. However, the systemic illnesses presenting with fever and skin rash create the most

diagonostic difficulties. Some familiarity with the mode of presentation, pathophysiology and treatment of these conditions enables the practitioner to successfully manage these children[1,2].

TERMINOLOGY

'Rash' is a common nonspecific term used for first hand description of a cutaneous lesion[1]. The morphology and distribution of a rash is of great clinical help in arriving at the correct underlying diagnosis. The common descriptive terms applied for cutaneous lesions are described below:

(a) *Macular.* These are flat and nonpalpable areas of color change (e.g. measles, rubella, Kawasaki disease, toxin-mediated strepto-coccal and staphylococcal infections).

(b) *Papular.* Circumscribed and elevated skin lesions of less than 0.5 cm in diameter (e.g. Henoch-Schonlein purpura).

(c) *Maculopapular.* When the cutaneous lesions have both macules and papules.

(d) *Vesicular.* When the rash consists of circumscribed, elevated lesions that are filled with clear fluid (e.g. varicella, herpes simplex, candidiasis).

(e) *Pustular.* Elevated skin lesions that are filled with purulent material or pus (impetigo, varicella with super added infection).

(f) *Hemorrhagic.* There are large areas of extra-vasated blood and they cannot be blanched on pressure (e.g. Dengue fever, meningo-coccemia).

(g) *Petechiae.* Pin-head sized macules of extra-vasated blood (viral hemorrhagic fevers, Rickettsial infections).

(h) *Target lesions.* The skin lesions have three well defined zones: (i) central zone of dusky

erythema; (ii) middle paler zone of edema and (iii) an outer ring of erythema with well defined edges. Target lesions are less than 3 cm in diameter and are typically seen in Stevens-Johnson syndrome and herpes simplex virus infection.

The site of onset, evolution and distribution of rash can provide important clinical clues. Skin rash with a predominant central distribution is seen in measles, rubella, erythema infectiosum, exanthem subitum, dengue fever and typhus fever. Non-infectious conditions with a centrally distributed macular rash include acute rheumatic fever (erythema marginatum), systemic lupus erythematosus (in addition to the malar rash on the face) and juvenile rheumatoid arthritis[1-3,6]. In contrast, there are clinical conditions where the skin rash begins in the periphery and then spreads centripetally. These include erythema multiforme; hand-foot-and-mouth disease; secondary syphilis and Rocky Mountain spotted fever[1-3,6]. A diffuse erythematous rash may be seen in patients with Kawasaki disease, dengue fever toxin-mediated streptococcal and staphylococcal infections, staphylococcal scalded skin syndrome and scarlet fever. Desquamation is a pathognomonic clinical feature of this group of conditions[1-3,6]. One of the most important determinants of cause of fever with skin rash is the age of the patient. Children presenting with acute fever and skin rash can be classified as shown in Table 14.1.

Table 14.1 Common causes of acute fever with skin rash	
A. NEWBORN PERIOD	
(i) Macular, erythematous rash. Early stages of staphylococcal/streptococcal infection.	
(ii) Vesicular rash. Varicella or herpes simplex infection and late stages of staphylococcal infection.	
B. INFANTS AND YOUNG CHILDREN	
Fever of short duration *(i.e. less than 5-7)*	**Fever of long duration** *(i.e. more than 5-7 days)*
(i) *Macular, erythematous rash* Viral exanthemata (including measles, rubella, roseola infantum), toxic shock syndrome, Rickettsial infections, staphylococcal scalded skin syndrome, drug rash	Kawasaki disease, JRA, graft-versus-host disease
(ii) *Vesicular rash* Varicella	Varicella with superadded bacterial infection
(iii) *Hemorrhagic rash* Meningococcemia, viral hemorrhagic fevers, leukemia, hemorrhagic edema of infancy, septicemia with disseminated intravascular coagulation, purpura fulminans.	Viral hemorrhagic fevers
(iv) *Pustular* Pyoderma, systemic candidiasis	
C. OLDER CHILDREN	
(i) *Macular, eythematous rash* Viral exanthemata (including measles, rubella, dengue fever, infectious mononucleosis, erythema infectiosum), scarlet fever, rickettsial infections, Lyme disease, drug rash	Enteric fever, Kawasaki disease, systemic-onset JRA, systemic lupus erythematosus, Stevens-Johnson syndrome, graft-versus-host disease, pityriasis rosea
(ii) *Vesicular rash* Varicella, herpes zoster; hand-foot-and-mouth disease, herpes simplex infection	Varicella with secondary infection
(iii) *Hemorrhagic rash* Meningococcemia, viral hemorrhagic fever, Henoch-Schönlein purpura, leukemia, leptospirosis, Rickettsial infections, septicemia with disseminated intravascular coagulation, purpura fulminans	Viral hemorrhagic fevers

NEWBORN BABIES

Isolated skin rash is common in the newborn period and it is usually self-limiting. The combined presence of fever and skin rash should never be ignored. It may be a simple condition like staphylococcal impetigo (which presents as isolated pustular lesions and is treated with oral antimicrobials) or it can be a pointer towards a more serious underlying infection like staphylococcal toxin mediated disease (e.g. staphylococcal scalded skin syndrome—SSSS)[1-3]. Any delay in recognition and initiation of specific therapy for the latter can be fatal. Infants with SSSS present with sudden onset of fever and irritability. The rash can be in the form of macular, erythematous lesions associated with characteristic cutaneous tenderness. Erythema is often accentuated in flexural areas and skin denudation may begin at these sites. This is followed by conjunctival inflammation, perioral erythema, fissuring in the lips but typically without any intraoral mucosal lesions. The erythematous lesions then evolve to form blisters and erosions within 24-48 hours. Large areas of the epidermis may peel off. Treatment is with antistaphylococcal antimicrobials along with general measures like skin compresses and adequate fluid replacement. Some viruses that can occasionally present with fever and a macular skin rash in the neonatal period include influenza and enteroviruses[1,2].

When a neonate presents primarily with a vesicular eruption, the differential diagnosis includes neonatal varicella and herpes simplex virus infection[1-3]. The former classically presents with "dewdrop vesicular lesions" at various stages of evolution. The skin lesions are most prominent on the trunk and there may be a history of recent maternal varicella (i.e. onset of eruption within a week prior to or soon after delivery). In the herpes simplex infection, the vesicles are distributed along a dermatome and the mother may have evidences of genital herpes. Neonatal varicella as well as herpes simplex are both treated with acyclovir. Delay in therapy is associated with high mortality.

Other uncommon infectious causes of vesiculo-bullous lesions in the newborn include Gram-negative sepsis (eg. Klebsiella, *Pseudomonas aeruginosa*), listeriosis, syphilis and intrauterine candidiasis. However, fever is not a common symptom in these conditions[1-3].

INFANTS AND YOUNG CHILDREN

It is a common misconception among parents and pediatricians that the most common cause of fever and skin rash in a young child is measles. With the widespread use of measles vaccine in our country, the disease has become relatively less common[1,2,5,7,8]. A number of other medical conditions may simulate the clinical features of measles[1-3]. The list of causes include both infectious and non-infectious conditions (Table 14.1). Important clinical clues can be obtained from the morphology and evolution of skin rash and the duration of fever[8]. Table 14.2 lists the clinical features of the important conditions seen in this age group.

Table 14.2 Characteristic features of common febrile conditions with skin rash seen in infants and young children				
Condition	**Type of fever**	**Characteristics of rash**	**Other clinical features**	**Treatment**
1. **Measles** (IP: 10-12 days; POI: 3 days before and 4 days after rash)	Peristent high grade fever for 2-3 days precedes the rash; fever is accompanied by coryza, cough, conjunctivitis and Koplik' spots; fever peaks with appearance of rash	Pink in color, macular/ maculopapular; starts behind the ears (along the hairline) and on the face and then spreads down but spares palms and soles; lesions are confluent in upper part of body and more discrete lower down; rash fades after 2-3 days leaving a brownish coppery desquamation; pruritis is uncommon	Prodromal illness mimics an upper respiratory catarrh; Koplik spots seen on buccal mucosa opposite the molars and look like salt grains on an erythematous base. Child is irritable and unwell; conjunctivitis and photophobia is invariably present; severity of disease is directly related to the extent and confluence of rash; modified measles may occur in a host partially immune from prior vaccination	Symptomatic; vitamin A may decrease the morbidity and mortality in the severely mal-nourished.

Table 14.2 contd.

Table 14.2 Characteristic features of common febrile conditions with skin rash seen in infants and young children
(Contd.)

Condition	Type of fever	Characteristics of rash	Other clinical features	Treatment
2. **Rubella (German measles)** (IP: 14-21 days; POI: 7 days before and 5 days after the rash)	Usually mild and seen only on first day of rash; may be accompanied by asymptomatic adenopathy; prodrome more common in adolescents	Faintly pink macular rash, starts on face and neck; much less prominent than in measles; progresses cephalocaudally and clears from previously affected areas as it migrates; does not desquamate	Petechial lesions may be seen on soft palate (Forschheimer sign); lymph nodes may be enlarged in occipital, post-auricular and posterior cervical region. Some children may complain of characteristic pain behind the eyes or on eye movement. The infection may be asymptomatic in 50% cases.	Symptomatic
3. **Varicella** (IP: 10-21 days; POI: 2 days before and 5 days after the rash) *"Dew drop rash"*	May be mild to moderate with minimal or no coryza, often occurring in winter and spring	Papular rash first seen on the trunk and proximal limbs; rash progresses rapidly from papules to vesicles; umbilication begins shortly thereafter. Crops of vesicles appear over the next 3-7 days; enanthem may be prominent in some; pruritus is common	Rash usually appears without a prodromal illness; new lesions occur every 2-4 days; each crop may be associated with a fever spike; lesions are in various stages of development. Infection is considered severe if there are > 500 lesions; time to crusting 2-12 days; time to healing 16 days; infants with atopic dermatitis can develop severe disease (Kaposi's varicelliform eruption)	Drug therapy (aciclovir*) is required for perinatally acquired varicella. Children with immune deficiency or those with varicella pneumonitis; and children above 13 years of age or those with chronic skin disorder
4. **Meningo-coccemia**	Fever is present in 70% but may be deceptively mild	Transient faint blanching erythematous macular rash followed by a non-blanching rash which may be petechial or purpuric; may be seen anywhere on the body	Initial symptoms (fever, vomiting, headache, abdominal pain and myalgia) may mimic a viral illness; disease may progress rapidly over hours; meningitis may or may not be present	Intravenous fluids; benzyl penicillin; hydro-cortisone
5. **Kawasaki disease** *"Irritability is out of proportion to the degree of fever; no coryza"*	High grade fever lasting more than 5-7 days; not accompanied by coryza (i.e. dry fever); fever is unresponsive to antimicrobials	May be macular, maculo-papular or urticarial but is never vesicular; morphology and distribution can be very variable; lesions can be discrete or confluent; membranous desquamation, beginning periungually is seen in the third week	Characteristic irritability out of proportion to degree of fever; associated unilateral non-purulent cervical adenopathy, non-purulent conjunctival injection and redness/swelling of hands and feet (i.e. indurative edema) is usually present; thrombocytosis is characteristic in the third and fourth weeks	Intravenous immung-lobulin; high dose aspirin for first 1-2 weeks; low dose aspirin for the following few weeks
6. **Systemic onset JRA** *"Quotidian fever with salmon rash"*	High grade fever with twice daily spikes; temperature may be normal in between; fever often occurs at the same time each day	Evanescent, faintl erythematous macular rash may be seen on the trunk and proximal extremeties and does not spread ; rash is more prominent at the time when fever spikes; mild dermographism may be demonstrable; target lesions can be seen	Child usually looks ill during the fever; arthritis may or may not be clinically obvious; infections and acute leukemia need to be ruled out	Systemic steroids with nonsteroidal anti-inflammatory drugs followed by low dose tapering predniso-lone; some children may require metho-trexate

Table 14.2 contd.

Table 14.2 Characteristic features of common febrile conditions with skin rash seen in infants and young children *(Contd.)*

Condition	Type of fever	Characteristics of rash	Other clinical features	Treatment
7. **Roseola infantum (Exanthem subitum)** (IP- 9 days) *"3 days fever and 3 days rash- most prominent on the trunk"*	High grade short duration fever (usually of 3 days) precedes the rash; fever disappears abruptly as the rash appears	Generalized erythematous maculopapular rash of short duration; most prominent on the trunk and may spread to neck and proximal extremities; lesions are discrete and fade within 24-48 hours; no desquamation or hyperpigmentation	Child appears well; children are usually between 6-18 months of age; total duration of disease is 3-6 days; febrile convulsions commonly associated; ulcers may be seen at the uvulopalatoglossal junction (Nagayama spots)	Symptomatic
8. **Rickettsial diseases** *"Fever like typhoid and rash like measles"*	Acute onset high grade fever with chills; prominent headache, malaise and prostration	Macular rash around the 4th-5th day of fever; rash is usually more prominent on the trunk; punched out ulcer covered with a blackened scab at the site of arthropod bite	Pyrexia falls by lysis around the 3rd week in untreated cases; generalized adenopathy and lymphocytosis are common	Doxycycline; azithromycin; and chloramphenicol are effective
9. **Toxic shock syndrome**	Fever is variable- some children may have abrupt onset of high grade fever	Diffuse erythematous blanching rash; may be more prominent on chest and spreads to arms and legs; accentuated in the flexures; desquamates on recovery by peeling of hands and feet	Usually associated with multisystem involvement; clinical features include vomiting, diarrhea, headache; and hypotension Disease may progress over hours; unlike KD, there is no cervical adenopathy and no thrombocytosis	Intravenous fluids; antimicrobials; high dose steroids; and intravenous immunoglobulins
10. **Gianotti-Crosti syndrome**	Usually mild	Characteristic monomorphic flat lentil sized lesions; symmetrically distributed on the face, buttocks and limbs. Trunk, antecubital and popliteal surfaces are spared. The skin rash may became papulovesicular	Mucous membranes are not affected	Symptomatic
11. **Viral hemorrhagic fever**	Variable	Variable petechial rash; ecchymoses may be present	History of travel to areas endemic for arboviruses and arenaviruses should be sought	Symptomatic; intravenous fluids; and blood transfusion

(IP- Incubation period; POI - Period of infectivity; *Famciclovir and valaciclovir have better gastrointestinal absorption)

Enteroviruses (e.g. Coxsackie, Echo) can cause nonspecific syndromes of fever and rash that may appear like measles or rubella[1-3]. Roseola infantum (exanthem subitum) is another well recognized entity seen in this age group but hardly ever recognized clinically in our country. It is caused by human herpes virus 6 infection[8,9]. It presents with a short duration of high grade fever followed by a pathognomonic skin rash on subsidence of fever. Some children may develop febrile seizures at the peak of fever. A recent study reports that up to one-third of young children with febrile seizures may have evidence of HHV6 infection[1-3].

Kawasaki disease (KD) also presents in this age group[11-12]. This condition is recognized by the temporal sequence of a constellation of clinical findings, which appear sequentially over a couple of weeks[11-14]. None of the findings is pathognomonic by itself. KD remains essentially a clinical diagnosis, there being no confirmatory laboratory test (Figure 14.1). It is believed to be

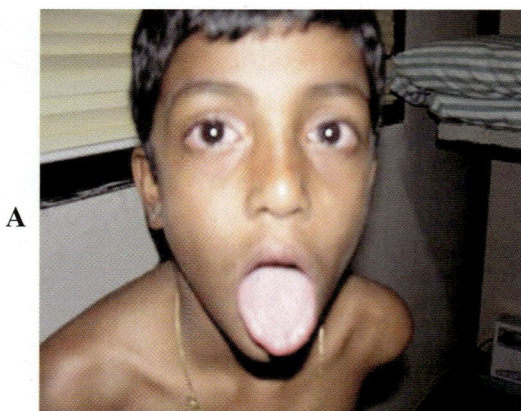

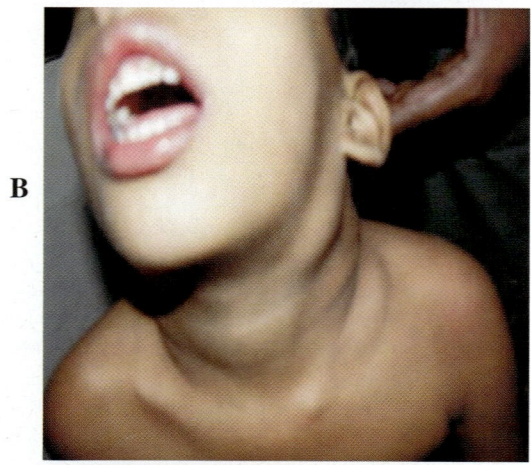

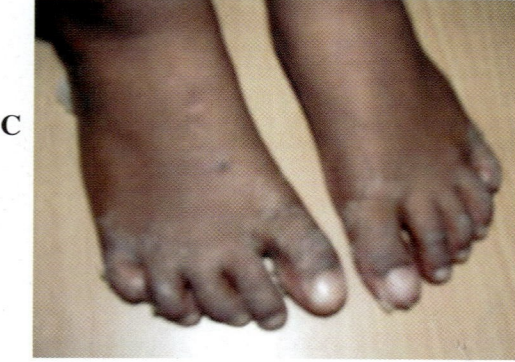

Figure 14.1 Clinical features during various stages of Kawasaki disease. A marked congestion of eyes and strawberry tongue. B. Cervical lymphadenopathy on left side of the neck C. Periungual desquamation of feet during recovery

the commonest vasculitic disorder in children. There is evidence to suggest that KD may, in fact, be more common than Henoch-Schönlein purpura! If one is not familiar with the clinical features and evolution of KD, it can be easily confused with drug reactions, Stevens-Johnson syndrome and streptococcal/ staphylococcal toxin-mediated diseases like scarlet fever and toxic shock syndrome. It would appear that the diagnosis of KD is often missed in our country[13-14].

Rickettsial infections are occasionally seen in specific geographical regions of our country (eg. Himachal Pradesh, Jammu & Kashmir) and are usually not considered in the differential diagnosis at most other places[1-3,15]. However, there is evidence to suggest that these infections are, in fact, more widespread in India than what is usually believed[15]. For instance, murine typhus and Indian tick typhus have been reported from Central (Nagpur, Jabalpur, Sagar), Western (Pune, Mumbai) and Southern (Bangalore) parts of our country[15].

Hemorrhagic edema of infancy is an uncommon condition with a benign prognosis but failure to recognize this entity can lead to unnecessary investigations. It is believed to be a variant of Henoch-Schönlein purpura. When the fever is more prolonged, the differential diagnosis should also include noninfectious conditions like systemic-onset juvenile rheumatoid arthritis[16,17].

OLDER CHILDREN AND ADOLESCENTS

Most of the aforementioned conditions listed above can also present in older children and adolescents. However, there are some exceptions. For instance roseola infantum is usually not seen in older children[1-3]. Similarly Kawasaki disease is more common in the pre-school age group than in older children[1-3,12,13]. Conditions which are preferentially seen in older children and are uncommon in infants include enteric fever (rash may be barely discernible in dark skinned individuals), varicella, infectious mononucleosis and erythema infectiosum[1-4,18-21].

Table 14.3 lists the clinical features of the important conditions seen in this age group. Drug rash is a relatively common clinical phenomenon and is often associated with fever[1,2,22.] Some children with drug fever may develop organ dysfunction i.e. drug hypersensitivity syndrome. The latter may be very difficult to differentiate from infectious mononucleosis. Children with drug rash can present with maculopapular, urticarial and erythema multiforme like lesions. Erythema multiforme is characteristic of Stevens-Johnson syndrome and toxic epidermal necrolysis (TEN). The term SJS is used when the area of involved skin is 10-30% of the body surface area and at least two mucosal surfaces are affected while the term TEN is used when the area of involved skin is > 30% of the body surface area. TEN connotes more serious and life-threatening disease[1,2,22].

Table 14.3 Characteristic clinical features of febrile conditions with skin rash in older children and adolescents**

Condition	Type of fever	Characteristics of rash	Other clinical features	Treatment
1. **Dengue fever** (IP: 2-7 days) *"Break bone fever"*	Sudden onset of high grade fever, continuous or saddle back; fever comes down by lysis and profuse sweating	Transient macular or maculopapular rash appears around 3rd-4th day of the fever; usually starts from the trunk; rash spreads centrifugally but spares palms and soles; rash fades as the fever subsides (around day 7)	Patients with thrombocytopenia may develop petechiae; backache (break bone fever), headache, arthralgia and pain on eye movements may be present; swelling on dorsum of hands and feet is seen occasionally	Symptomatic, intravenous fluids; platelet transfusions
1. **Infectious mononucleosis** (IP: 4-5 weeks)	Mild to moderate; may be associated with adenopathy	Non-specific diffuse macular or maculopapular rash	Rash may become more prominent on intake of ampicillin/amoxycillin; associated features may include pharyngeal inflammation, palatal petechiae, hepatitis and splenomegaly; extreme fatigue is characteristic; disease may last from weeks to several months	Symptomatic
3. **Herpes simplex infection** *"Vesicular lesions around mucocutaneous junctions"*	Variable fever for 2-7 days	Papulovesicular lesions around mucocutaneous junctions, spread on to lips, gingivae, palate, buccal mucosa and tongue; gingivo-stomatitis may be prominent and may present as dribbling of saliva in young children; children with eczema may have widespread involvement (eczema herpeticum)	Associated clinical features may include keratitis and paronychia (herpetic whitlow); crops of lesions may appear over several days; unlike chicken pox all lesions are in the same stage of development	Drug therapy (aciclovir*) indicated for perinatally acquired HSV and HSV in immunocompromised patients
4. **Herpes zoster** *"Vesicular lesions along dermatomes – not crossing the midline"*	May be mild	Grouped papulovesicular lesions over background of erythema; lesions seen over contiguous dermatomes, peripheral or cranial nerves; lesions do not cross the mildline; last for 10-14 days; lesions undergo central necrosis and crust formation	Associated clinical features in adolescents include burning sensation/excruciating pain – neuralgia is uncommon in young children. Herpes zoster may be the first manifestation of HIV infection in a subject who previously had chicken pox; noncontiguous dermatomal involvement and disseminated lesions may be seen in immunocompromized subjects	Drug therapy (aciclovir*) is necessary in immunocompromised patients, individuals with lesions over the face (V & VII cranial nerve involvement) and those with disseminated disease; drug therapy is believed to decrease both early and late onset pain.
5. **Enteric fever**	High grade stepladder pattern	Faint macular rose-red spots which fade on pressure may be seen at the end of first week	Child looks ill; rash may be more prominent in paratyphoid fever; other clinical features include malaise, coated tongue, relative bradycardia	Ceftriaxone, ciprofloxacin, chloramphenicol, azithromycin are effective
6. **Drug rash**	Variable, flat and non hectic pattern	Variable macular or maculopapular rash; usually central in distribution; may be pruritic	Temporal association between introduction of drug and appearance of rash may be obvious	Withdrawal of concerned drug; antihistaminics and steroids

Table 14.3 contd.

Section 2

Table 14.3 Characteristic clinical features of febrile conditions with skin rash in older children and adolescents *(Contd.)*

Condition	Type of fever	Characteristics of rash	Other clinical features	Treatment
7. **Stevens Johnson syndrome** *"Target lesions & mucosal involvement – bandit appearance"*	Variable	May start as edema and swelling of the face followed by erythema and itching; target lesions symmetrically distributed on the limbs; may later spread on to the trunk; mucosal involvement may be prominent; conjunctival and corneal involvement is common	Associated infections (e.g. Mycoplasma/Herpes simplex) may be present; children get a characteristic "bandit appearance" with involvement around the eyes and on the hands and feet; internal organ involvement may occur as late as 1-2 weeks; commonly implicated drugs include antiepileptics, sulphonamides, nonsteroidal anti-inflammatory and antitubercular drugs	Symptomatic; withdrawal of suspected drug; steroids may be useful if started in the first week of illness but their role remains controversial; intravenous immunoglobulins?;
8. **Henoch-Schonlein purpura** *"Palpable purpura with gravity dependent extensor distribution"*	Usually mild	Edema over the ears, scalp, sacrum and on the hands/feet is a common early finding; palpable purpuric lesions usually most prominent over extensor aspect of legs and buttocks; tend to occur in successive crops; eruption is said to be "pressure dependent" and "gravity dependent"	Associated clilnical features include arthritis, nephritis and gastrointestinal involvement (volvulus, colic, intussusception); HSP is rare in dark skinned individuals!	Symptomatic; steroids may be indicated for children with severe gastrointestinal involvement or seizures; nephritis requires prolonged therapy
9. **Hand-foot-and -mouth disease** (IP:4-6 days) *"Typical distribution – other body areas spared"*	Usually mild fever precedes the rash; may be accompanied by sore mouth	Papulovesicular ulcerative lesions are seen over the buccal mucosa and tongue; these are then followed by characteristic grey-white vesiculopustules on the palmoplantar surfaces of hands and feet; erythematous papular rash may be seen on the buttocks and thighs	Most other body areas are spared; disease occurs in epidemics	Symptomatic
10. **Erythema infectiosum (Fifth disease)** (IP:4-28 days) *"Slapped cheek appearance with 3 stage rash – trunk not involved"*	Usually mild and precedes the rash; minimal prodrome	Characteristic 3 stage rash: (a) Red and flushed cheeks (slapped cheek appearance) with circumoral pallor (b) Maculopapular rash over proximal extremities after a few days; more prominent over extensor surfaces (c) Central clearing of rash thereby giving a reticulated and lace-like appearance as it fades Trunk is not involved; the rash can recur over the next 4-6 weeks after exercise, warm bath or exposure to sunlight	Child does not look ill; arthralgia may be seen in early stage; other clinical associations include vasculitis, anemia and thrombocytopenia; at least 50% infections are completely asymptomatic; unlike many other exanthems, patients are not infectious at the time of eruption; Koplik spots have been described!	Symptomatic; intravenous immunoglobulins and steroids have been used for children with systemic involvement

Table 14.3 contd.

Table 14.3 Characteristic clinical features of febrile conditions with skin rash in older children and adolescents** *(Contd.)*

Condition	Type of fever	Characteristics of rash	Other clinical features	Treatment
11. **Scarlet fever** *"May mimic Kawasaki disease"*	Usually high grade; always subsides within 5-7 days; may be accompanied by vomiting, headache and sore throat	Diffuse, dark red punctate rash most prominent on neck, face and axillae; lesions have sandpaper like texture; oral mucosa may appear red; petechial lesions may be seen on palate; characteristic circumoral pallor; punctate, papular rash spreads to involve the hands and feet; prominent desquamation	Asssociated clinical features include a red, strawberry tongue; transverse red streaks due to capillary fragility seen in skin folds (Pastia's lines); unlike KD, there is no conjunctival involvement	Penicillin
12. **Lyme Disease** *"Erythema migrans"*	Variable	Characteristic erythema migrans – red macular or maculopapular lesions that enlarge peripherally and show central clearing; mildly pruritic and tender	Associated clinical features may include neurologic involvement (meningitis, cranial nerve palsies, neuropathies); cardiac involvement (heart blocks); arthritis may mimic JRA	Ceftriaxone
13. **Purpura fulminans** *"Sharply demarcated necrotic lesions"*	Mild to moderate	Starts with erythematous discoloration; sharply demarcated areas of purpura with bullae formation in overlying skin followed by gangrene of skin; associated involvement of deeper tissues may also be present	Laboratory evidences of disseminated intravascular coagulation may be seen; thrombosis can spread rapidly	Transfusion of fresh frozen plasma in the acute stage; long term anticoagulation; activated Protein C/ Antithrombin III for respective deficiency; tissue plasminogen activator may have a role
14. **Systemic lupus erythematosus** *"Butterfly rash with painless oral ulcers"*	Mild to moderate	Macular, erythematous rash is seen in a butterfly distribution over the bridge of nose and cheeks ; a diffuse macular/maculopapular rash may also be seen	Associated clinical features include oral ulcers (which are painless), photosensitivity and systemic involvement (nephritis, carditis hepatitis, CNS involvement); discoid rash is rare in children; vasculitis of skin is not uncommon	High dose steroids followed by low dose maintenance therapy; hydroxychloroquine and other immunosuppressants are often added in the regimen
15. **Acute rheumatic fever** *"Erythema marginatum"*	Usually mild to moderate	Annular, reddish macules that spread rapidly and may attain a size of up to a few centimetres; most prominent on the trunk and proximal extremities; margins may merge; there may be prominent central clearing; lesions fade centrally and are characteristically evanescent— may completelly disappear within a few hours	Erythema marginatum lesions are often most prominent in the afternoon; recurrent crops may occur at weekly intervals; associated clinical features inclulde subcutaneous nodules, arthritis and carditis	Aspirin in high doses; prophylactic benzathine penicillin

IP- Incubation period; POI- Period of infectivity; *Famciclovir and valaciclovir have better gastrointestinal absorption; ** Several conditions included in Table 14.2 can occur in this age group as well eg. varicella, rubella, Rickettsial infections, meningococcal infection and viral hemorrhagic fevers, Kawasaki disease and systemic onset JRA

Section 2

Drug rash must be considered in the differential diagnosis of older children presenting with fever and skin rash even though it may be very difficult to confirm the diagnosis. Drug fever is usually flat (non-remittent), skin rash may be associated with itching and eosinophilia. Failure to recognize this relatively common entity, in our experience, can often result in unnecessary investigations and therapeutic misadventures. The clinical variables which may be of some help to the clinician are listed below.[1-3]

(i)   *Nature of drug.* It is known that up to 30-40% of patients with HIV infection may develop a skin rash when exposed to sulfa-drugs (e.g. trimethoprim-sulphamethoxazole). Similarly, more than half of patients with infectious mononucleosis may present with a macular erythematous eruption on exposure to ampicillin/amoxicillin. Drug eruptions are common following administration of multiple antibiotics, antitubercular and antiepileptic agents.

(ii)   *Temporal association.* Most adverse cutaneous reactions occur within 1-2 weeks of initiation of therapy. However, drug hypersensitivity syndromes (commonly seen with antiepileptics) may have a delayed onset and may be very difficult to diagnose.

(iii)   *Withdrawal and rechallenge.* While most adverse cutaneous reactions remit on withdrawal of the drug, rechallenge provides the most definitive clue to the diagnosis. However, the latter may not be feasible in patients with severe reactions like SJS and TEN.

Other noninfectious causes of fever with skin rash in this age-group include Henoch-Schonlein purpura (HSP), systemic onset JRA and systemic lupus erythematosus (SLE). HSP is a relatively common entity[23-25]. Most children present in the autumn and winter months. In majority of cases the diagnosis is quite straightforward but problems may arise when the rash is atypical or the child presents late (Figure 14.2). Children with SLE can often present for the first time with fever and skin rash. The latter can be very variable in distribution and morphology[24,25]. Purpura fulminans is a life-threatening disorder due to homozygous Protein C or Protein S deficiency. It presents with widespread disseminated intravascular coagulation. Delay in initiation of specific therapy may result in loss of limb and can also be life-threatening. Hand-foot-and-mouth disease is a self-limited viral infection

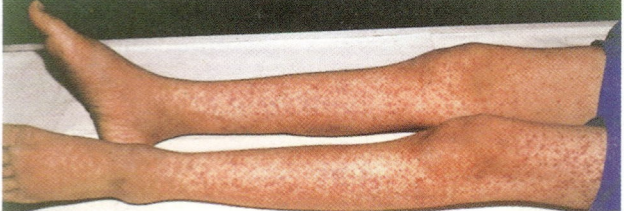

Figure 14.2 The characteristic purpuric skin rash which is slightly raised above the surface (due to vasculitis) gives a flea-bitten appearance in a patient with Henoch-Schonlein syndrome. The rash is distributed over the extensor surfaces of legs, buttocks and elbows

caused by Coxsackie A 16 and manifests with fever, mucosal lesions and painful erythematous vesicles over the palms, soles and buttocks (Figure 14.3).

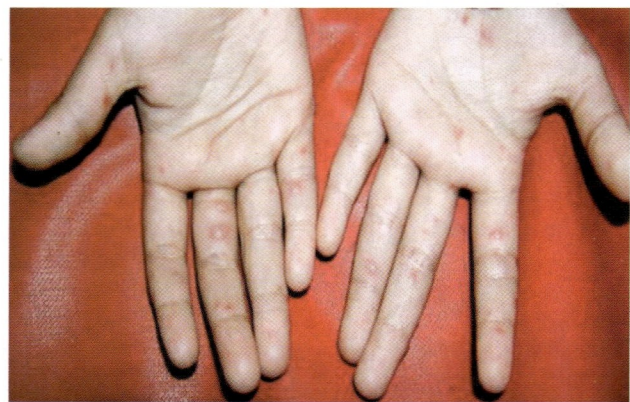

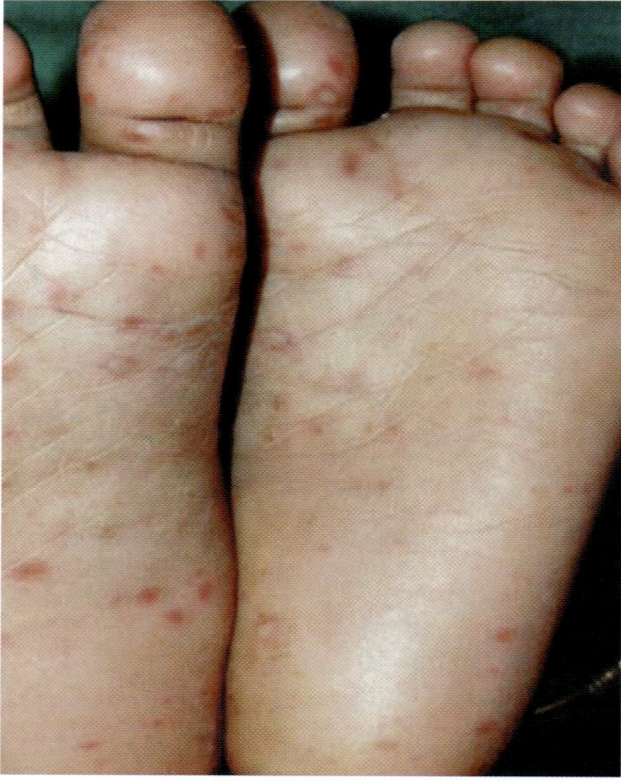

Figure 14.3 Typical vesicular lesions over the palms and soles in a child with hand-foot-and-mouth disease.

REFERENCES

1. Schlossberg D. Fever and rash. *Infect Dis Clin Amer* 1996; 10(1): 101-110.

2. Aber C, Alvarez Connelly E, Schachner LA. Fever and rash in a child: when to worry? *Pediatr Ann* 2007; 36(1):30-38.

3. Drago F, Rampini E, Rebora A. Atypical exanthems: morphology and laboratory investigations may lead to an aetiological diagnosis in about 70% of cases. *Br J Dermatol* 2002; 147(2):255-260.

4. Dyer JA. Childhood viral exanthems. *Pediatr Ann* 2007; 36(1):21-29.

5. Koch WC. Parvovirus B19. In: Nelson Textbook of Pediatrics, Kliegman RM, Behrman RE, Jenson HB, Stanton BF. (Eds.) *Saunders Elsevier, Philadelphia,* 18th edition, 2008, pp. 1357-1360.

6. Mason WH. Measles. In: Nelson Textbook of Pediatrics, Kliegman RM, Behrman RE, Jenson HB, Stanton BF (Eds.). *Saunders Elsevier, Philadelphia,* 18th edition, 2008, pp. 1331-1337.

7. Brogan PA, Raffles A. The management of fever and petechiae: making sense of rash decisions. *Arch Dis Child* 2000; 83:506-509.

8. Ely JW, Stone MS. The generalized rash: diagnostic approach. *Amer Fam Phys* 2010; 81(6):735-739.

9. Sommer A. Vitamin A, infectious diisease, and childhood mortality: a solution? *J Infect Dis* 1993; 167: 1003-1007.

10. Jones CMV, Dunn HG, Thomas EE, *et al.* Acute encephalopathy and status epilepticus associated with human herpes virus 6 infection. *Dev Med Child Neurol* 1994; 36: 646-650.

11. Breese Hall C, Long CE, Schnabel KC, *et al.* Human herpesvirus-6 infection in children. A prospective study of complications and reactivation. *N Engl J Med* 1994; 331: 432-428.

12a. Tizard EJ, Suzuki A, Dillon MJ. Clinical aspects of 100 patients with Kawasaki disease. *Arch Dis Child* 1991; 66: 185-188.

12b. Singh S, Bansal A, Gupta A, Manoj Kumar R, Mittal BR. Kawasaki disease – a decade of experience from north India. *Int Heart J* 2005; 46(4):679-89.

13. Singh S, Aulakh R, Bhalla AK, Suri D, Manoj Kumar R, Narula N, Burns JC. Is Kawasaki disease incidence rising in Chandigarh, north India? *Arch Dis Child* 2011; 96:137-140.

14. Singh S, Kawasaki T. Kawasaki disease – an Indian perspective. *Indian Pediatr* 2009; 46(7): 563-571

15. Park K. Rickettsial zoonoses. In: Park's Textbook of Preventive and Social Medicine, 17th. Edition. Banarsidas Bhanot Publishers, Jabalpur, 2002, pp. 229-232.

16. Singh S, Salaria M, Kumar L, Datta V, Sehgal S. Clinico-immunological profile of juvenile rheumatoid arthritis at Chandigarh. *Indian Pediatr* 1999, 36: 449-454.

17. Singh S. Chronic arthritis : current perspectives. (Editorial). *Indian Pediatr* 2003, 40: 393-397.

18. Preblud S. Age-specific risks of varicella complications. *Pediatrics* 1981; 68: 14-17.

19. Anderson LJ, Torok TJ. Human Parvovirus B19. *N Engl J Med* 1989; 321: 536-538.

20. Evans LM, Grossman MC, Gregery N. Koplik spots and a purpuric eruption associated with Parvovirus B19 infection. *J Am Acad Dermatol* 1992; 27: 466-467.

21. Dass R, Ramesh P, Ratho RK, Saxena AK, Singh S. Parvovirus B19 induced multisystem disease simulating systemic vasculitis in a young child. *Rheumatol Int* 2005, 25 (2): 125-129.

22. Shear NH, Landau M, Shapiro LE. Hypersensitivity reactions to drugs. In: Textbook of Pediatric Dermatology. Harper J, Oranje A, Prose N. (Eds.). *Blackwell Science, London,* 2000 , pp1743-52.

23. Kumar L, Singh S, Goraya JS, Uppal B, Kakkar S, Walker R and Sehgal, S. Henoch Schonlein Purpura: Chandigarh experience. *Indian Pediatr* 1997; 35: 19-25.

24. Singh S, Aulakh R. Kawasaki disease and Henoch Schonlein purpura: changing trends at a tertiary care hospital in north India (1993-2008). *Rheumatol Int* 2010; 30(6):771-774.

25. Singh S, Kumar L, Khetarpal R, Aggarwal P, Marwaha RK, Minz RW, Sehgal S. Clinical and immunological profile of SLE : some unusual features. *Indian Pediatr* 1997, 34: 979-986.

Section 2

15

Hyperpyrexia, Heat Exhaustion and Heat Stroke

Sourabh Dutta and Subodh Ganu

The ability of the body to regulate core body temperature depends on a host of factors, including ambient temperature, acclimatization, humidity, wind, clothing, pre-existing medical conditions, and use of medications. The normal core body temperature for humans, measured rectally, depends on the environmental climate and internal metabolic function. When the core body temperature rises, the basal metabolic rate increases significantly. For every 0.6°C increase in core temperature, there is a 10 percent elevation in the basal metabolic rate. Core temperature can increase as a result of elevated ambient temperature or through work-related activities and physical exertion due to sport activities that increase metabolic rate. Hyperpyrexia can occur due to heat stroke *per se*, or due to conditions such as malaria, central nervous system infections, atropine poisoning, pontine hemorrhage and malignant hyperthermia. Heat exhaustion is a clinical syndrome characterized by salt and/or water depletion that occurs under conditions of heat stress. Patients with heat exhaustion generally do not have hyperpyrexia or major neurological dysfunction. Heat stroke is a state of acute thermoregulatory failure characterized by hyperpyrexia, disturbance of the central nervous system and generalized anhidrosis. Heat stroke could occur either because of extreme ambient heat, or because the mechanisms to control body temperature are overwhelmed by endogenous heat production[1-3]. Data from the US suggests that patients aged less than 19 years account for 47.6% of exertional heat related injuries.[4]

Temperature Regulation

Human beings, like all warm-blooded mammals, are homeothermic creatures. The human enzymatic and biological processes function optimally within a narrow range of temperature. Thermoregulation is controlled by the hypothalamus. The parasympathetic system controls sweating, with the sympathetic nervous system regulating increase in skin blood flow and vasodilatation for heat dissipation. Normally, thermoregulation is highly efficient, for every 25°C to 30°C change in the ambient temperature there is only 1.0°C elevation in core body temperature[1]. The hypothalamus receives inputs from thermoreceptors in the skin and the body core. It integrates this information and uses various efferent pathways to either increase body heat or promote heat loss, depending on whether the body temperature is below or above the set thermostat temperature. Bodily heat can be increased either by increasing endogenous heat production or by conserving the heat produced. Endogenous heat production is increased either by muscular activity (shivering, exercise) or by metabolic activity (catabolism of fat). Assuming a flexed posture to decrease the surface area, vasoconstriction, and pilo-erection or by the insulation provided by subcutaneous fat and clothing can conserve heat.

There are four processes by which the body rids itself of excess heat; conduction, convection, radiation, and evaporation. Conduction occurs when the body comes in direct contact with something cold or hot, allowing heat to be transferred to the cooler object, such as when one applies cold packs to the body. Convection takes place when air passes over the body, lifting heat away, as occurs on a windy day or through the use of fans. Infrared dissipation of heat from the body to the environment, is called radiation. Finally, the evaporation of sweat from the skin plays a major role in heat dissipation during exercise and is the primary thermoregulatory mechanism when the ambient temperature is high. Heat loss is promoted by vasodilatation, sweating or rapid breathing. Vasodilatation brings warm blood to the skin, from where the warmth is lost to the environment. Sweating is mediated through the autonomic nervous system, and the evaporation of the sweat cools down the body. Evaporation of each gram of water results in loss of 1.7 calories. Rapid breathing results in heat being lost from the warm blood brought to the lungs by the pulmonary circulation.

The latter is a relatively unimportant mechanism in humans (unlike dogs)[1-3].

The thermostat of the hypothalamus can be reset to a higher level by pyrogens released by infectious agents or by inflammatory cells. To a certain extent this is a protective and beneficial response on the part of the body to fight infection. However, when the response is excessive as in hyperpyrexia there is a danger that it may cause deleterious effects on the central nervous system.

Children deserve special consideration in the diagnosis and management of heat-related illnesses. Compared with adults, children produce proportionately more metabolic heat, have a core temperature that rises faster during dehydration, and have smaller organ systems, allowing for less efficient heat dissipation. Thus, caution should be exercised with children when conditions are right for heat illness. Close observation of an active child is important, because a fatal event can occur within 20 minutes if normal heat loss mechanisms are overwhelmed[2].

CLASSIFICATION OF HEAT ILLNESSES

(i) **Minor heat illnesses**
   (a) Prickly heat
   (b) Heat cramps
   (c) Heat edema
   (d) Heat syncope

(ii) **Major heat illnesses**
   (a) Heat exhaustion
   (b) Heat stroke

Minor Heat Illnesses

Prickly heat is an acute inflammatory condition seen in tropical climates, characterized by intensely pruritic vesicles on an erythematous base, which ultimately evolve to white non-pruritic papules. This disorder results from blockade of sweat pores by macerated stratum corneum and secondary staphylococcal infection. Frequent bathing of skin, application of chlorhexidine lotion, 1% salicylic acid and oral erythromycin have been used for treatment.[3]

Heat cramps are brief muscular cramps that occur in fatigued muscles after exercise. Heat cramps occur due to salt deficiency in individuals who produce large amounts of sweat, but drink salt–free water. Stretching the affected muscles and maintaining good hydration status are important. Liberal intake of water is recommended, but this may induce hyponatremia if lost salt is not replaced. Commercial electrolyte solutions may help to prevent excessive salt loss, and a home made formula of 1 tea spoon of salt in 500 ml of water may also be used. There are no systemic symptoms in these patients[5].

Heat edema is a minimal pitting pedal edema seen in non-acclimatized individuals. It probably occurs due to vasodilatation, orthostatic pooling and hyperaldosteronism. It does not require any treatment.

Heat syncope occurs in individuals who stand for protracted periods in a hot environment. The intense vasodilatation causes redistribution of blood to the skin at the expense of thoracic blood volume; and this combined with pooling of blood in the lower limbs and evaporative water loss results in a drop in cardiac output and consequently a decrease in cerebral perfusion. The problem can be prevented by contracting calf muscles frequently, consuming enough fluids and avoidance of protracted standing in a hot environment[5].

Major Heat Illnesses

The two major heat illness syndromes are heat exhaustion and heat stroke. They are different entities, with different etiologies and clinical presentations. The salient differences between these conditions are summarized in Table 15.1. If heat exhaustion is not adequately managed it may lead on to heat stroke.

Table 15.1 Differences between heat exhaustion and heat stroke		
Parameters	**Heat exhaustion**	**Heat stroke**
♦ Core temperature	May be normal; if elevated, it is usually less than 40°C	Almost always greater than 41°C
♦ Thermoregulatory mechanisms	Intact	Failed
♦ CNS functions	Essentially normal	Invariably deranged
♦ Dehydration	Common	Uncommon
♦ Anhidrosis	Not seen	Common
♦ Hepatic transaminases	Normal	Markedly elevated

HEAT EXHAUSTION

Heat exhaustion occurs as two types, water depleted and sodium depleted, although in reality they often overlap. Potentially dangerous clinical manifestations include circulatory collapse and raised body temperature. Core body temperature is usually higher than 38°C (100.4°F) but below the cutoff for heatstroke, which is 40°C (104°F). The signs and symptoms are variable and non-specific. They include weakness, fatigue, frontal headache, impaired judgment, vertigo, orthostatic hypotension and nausea. Sweating is profuse and the core temperature is only marginally elevated. The temperature never crosses 40.6° C. The signs of severe CNS damage, such as coma or seizures, are not present[6,7].

Water depletion heat exhaustion results from inadequate water intake in a hot environment. This may occur in young infants or in individuals without free access to water. Even mild dehydration impairs thermoregulation, making it difficult for the body to loose heat. Thus the patient develops pyrexia, and if left untreated, water depletion and heat exhaustion progresses to heat stroke.

Salt depletion heat exhaustion takes longer to develop as compared to water depletion. It occurs when large quantities of thermal sweat are replaced by water with too little or no salt[8]. It differs from heat cramps because it is associated with systemic symptoms. Clinical features are similar to water depletion, except that temperature usually remains near normal. These patients have hyponatremia and hypochloremia and low urinary sodium and chloride. In clinical situations most cases have mixed water and salt depletion.

Treatment

Patients with heat exhaustion should be allowed to rest in a cool environment. The volume depletion is treated with fluids. The electrolyte composition of the fluid depends on the serum sodium, blood urea and evidences of hemodynamic compromise. Mild cases can be treated with oral fluids. Patients with hemodynamic compromise should receive isotonic saline intravenously. Those patients who have hypernatremia should receive low sodium fluids over 48 hours to correct the fluid deficit. In some cases it may be difficult to differentiate heat exhaustion from heat stroke, because the temperature may be around 40°C and there may be evolving CNS manifestations. The two conditions may be differentiated on the basis of elevated hepatic transaminases. Heat stroke causes transaminases to be raised to tens of thousands by 24 hours[9]. However, if laboratory values are not accessible immediately or if there is any doubt about the diagnosis, it is prudent to treat the victim as a case of heat stroke because a delay in the treatment of heat stroke may prove fatal.

HEAT STROKE

The afore mentioned conditions discussed so far do not affect the thermoregulatory mechanisms. Heat stroke, on the other hand, is a catastrophic life-threatening emergency that occurs when these mechanisms fail[10]. Heat stroke is a much more severe entity than heat exhaustion. The diagnosis of heat stroke rests on two critical factors: hyperthermia and central nervous system dysfunction. Heat stroke is a medical emergency, and mortality can approach 10 percent. It is essential that clinicians recognize the signs of heat stroke and initiate cooling rapidly. Heat stroke is seen more often among adults than children because adults are more likely to be exposed to a hot outdoor environment. However, given the same conditions, children are more susceptible to heat stroke than adults[11,12]. Children have less efficient thermoregulation due to slower acclimatization, delayed or inefficient sweating mechanism and greater impairment of thermoregulation by dehydration.

Types of Heat Stroke

Patients of heat stroke may have either of two forms of presentation; classic heat stroke or exertional heat stroke. The differences are summarized in Table 15.2.

Table 15.2 Differences between classic and exertional heat stroke		
Parameter	**Classic**	**Exertional**
◆ Age group	Younger children	Older children, adolescents
◆ Activity	Sedentary	Strenuous exercise
◆ Sweating	Absent	Present in 50%
◆ Rhabdomyolysis	Uncommon	Severe
◆ Acute renal failure	<5% cases	25% cases
◆ DIC*	Mild	Severe
◆ Lactic acidosis	Usually absent	Common
◆ Hyperuricemia	Moderate	Severe
◆ Creatinine phosphokinase	Mild elevation	Markedly elevated
* DIC: Disseminated intravascular coagulopathy		

Classic heat stroke occurs during periods of high environmental temperature and humidity e.g. summer heat wave. It usually affects infants or invalid children, who are dependant on adults for intake of water and for moving to cooler surroundings. Infants are particularly vulnerable to classic heat stroke because of the immaturity of their thermoregulatory mechanisms and their propensity to water depletion by virtue of their renal immaturity. Classic heat stroke is also commoner among unacclimatized subjects, those who receive drugs that inhibit sweating (such as anticholinergic drugs, antihistaminics, phenothiazines and beta-blockers), those who have intercurrent febrile illness and those patients who have one of the rare skin diseases which retard sweating (such as congenital ectodermal dysplasia, hyperkeratosis and ichthyosis). Sweating is found to be totally absent in 84 to 100% of patients with classic heat stroke[9]. A unique cause of classic heat stroke is enclosure of the child in an unattended vehicle.[13]

In contrast, patients with *exertional heat stroke* are usually healthy children and adolescents who engage in strenuous exercise. The sweating mechanism is impaired in 50% of patients but what is more important is that the endogenous heat production overwhelms the mechanisms for dispelling heat. Certain complications are commoner among patients with exertional heat stroke; such as rhabdomyolysis, renal failure, hypoglycemia and coagulopathy. Exertional heat stroke can also be produced by cocaine and amphetamine abuse and as a result of status epilepticus[14]

PATHOGENESIS

The basic mechanism of heat stroke is still speculative. The most plausible hypothesis envisages that there is a rise in intracellular sodium in a hyperthermic patient. This rise in intracellular sodium is partly attributable to the increased Na^+-H^+ pump activity, that serves to decrease the intracellular acidity in patients with hyperthermia; and partly attributable to the sweating and dehydration. As a result the Na^+-K^+-ATPase activity increases to pump out the extra sodium, and this generates more heat. Thus a vicious cycle is created because the heat generated results in further intracellular Na^+ accumulation, secondary to dehydration and acidity. The energy depletion finally leads to a situation where there is insufficient energy to sustain thermoregulatory mechanisms. This causes a dramatic increase in the core temperature of the body and consequently the pathological changes of heat stroke[15].

To understand the pathogenesis of heat stroke, the systemic and cellular responses to heat stress must be appreciated. These responses include thermoregulation (with acclimatization), an acute-phase response, and a response that involves the production of heat-shock proteins.

Thermoregulation and Acclimatization

Body heat is gained from the environment and is produced by metabolism. This overall heat load must be dissipated to maintain a body temperature of 36.8°C + 0.4°C (98.2°F + 0.7°F), a process called thermoregulation. A rise in the temperature of the blood by less than 1°C activates peripheral and hypothalamic heat receptors that signal the hypothalamic thermoregulatory center and the efferent response from this center increases the delivery of heated blood to the surface of the body. Active sympathetic cutaneous vasodilation increases blood flow to the skin by up to 8 liters per minute. An increase in the blood temperature also initiates thermal sweating. If the air surrounding the surface of the body is not saturated with water, sweat will vaporize and cool the body surface. At maximal efficiency in a dry environment, sweating can dissipate upto 600 kcal per hour. The thermal gradient established by the evaporation of sweat is critical for the transfer of heat from the body to the environment. As blood is shunted from the central circulation to the muscles and skin to facilitate heat dissipation, visceral perfusion is reduced, particularly in the intestines and kidneys.

Losses of salt and water by sweating, which may amount to 2 liters or more per hour, must be balanced by generous salt supplementation to facilitate thermoregulation. Dehydration and salt depletion impair thermoregulation. Acclimatization is a process of adaptation that eventually allow a person to work safely at levels of heat that were previously intolerable or life-threatening. The process of acclimatization to heat takes several weeks and involves enhancement of cardiovascular performance, activation of the renin–angiotensin–aldosterone axis, salt conservation by the sweat glands and kidneys, an increase in the capacity to secrete sweat, expansion of plasma volume, an increase in the glomerular filtration rate, and an increase in the ability to resist exertional rhabdomyolysis[15]. It is important to appreciate the concept of a thermal maximum, the temperature and duration of exposure that cells can encounter without sustaining damage. The human ambient thermal maximum has been established at 42°C (107.6°F) for a period of 45 to 480 min[16].

Acute-phase Response

The acute-phase response to heat stress is a coordinated reaction that involves endothelial cells, leukocytes, and epithelial cells which try to provide protection against tissue injury and promote repair. The interleukin-6 produced during heat stress modulates local and systemic acute inflammatory responses by controlling the levels of inflammatory cytokines. Interleukin-6 also stimulates hepatic production of antiinflammatory acute-phase proteins, which inhibit the production of reactive oxygen species and the release of proteolytic enzymes from activated leukocytes. Other acute-phase proteins stimulate endothelial-cell adhesion, proliferation, and angiogenesis, thus contributing to repair and healing. The increased expression of the gene encoding interleukin-6 in human muscle cells, but not in blood monocytes, during the acute-phase response to exercise suggests that the onset of inflammation is local. The systemic progression of the inflammatory response is secondary and involves other cells, such as monocytes. A similar sequence of events has been shown to occur in sepsis[15, 17].

Heat-shock Response

Nearly all cells respond to sudden heating by producing heat-shock proteins or stress proteins. Expression of heat-shock proteins is controlled primarily at the level of gene transcription. During heat stress, one or more heat-shock transcription factors bind to the heat-shock element, resulting in an increased rate of transcription of heat-shock proteins. Increased levels of heat-shock proteins in a cell induce a transient state of tolerance to a second, otherwise lethal, stage of heat stress, allowing the cell to survive. Blocking the synthesis of heat-shock proteins either at the gene-transcription level or by specific antibodies renders the cells extremely sensitive to a minor degree of heat stress. The protection conferred against heat-stroke injury correlates with the level of heat-shock protein 72, which accumulates in the brain after the priming heat-shock treatment. The mechanism by which heat-shock proteins protect cells may relate to their function as molecular chaperones that bind to partially folded or misfolded proteins, thus preventing their irreversible denaturation. Another possible mechanism involves heat-shock proteins that act as central regulators of the baroreceptor-reflex response during severe heat stress, preventing development of hypotension and bradycardia and conferring cardiovascular protection[17].

Progression from Heat Stress to Heat Stroke

Thermoregulatory failure, exaggeration of the acute-phase response, and alteration in the expression of heat-shock proteins may contribute to the progression from heat stress to heat stroke.

Thermoregulatory Failure. The normal cardiovascular adaptation to severe heat stress is an increase in cardiac output by up to 20 liters per minute and a shift of heated blood from the core circulation to the peripheral circulation. An inability to increase cardiac output because of salt and water depletion, cardiovascular disease, or a medication that interferes with cardiac function can impair heat tolerance and result in increased susceptibility to heat stroke.

Exaggeration of the Acute-phase Response. It is possible that the gastrointestinal tract fuels the inflammatory response. During strenuous exercise or hyperthermia, blood shifts from the mesenteric circulation to the working muscles and the skin, leading to ischemia of the gut and intestinal hyperpermeability. There is abundant evidence of hyperpermeability during heat stress in animal models but much less evidence of this phenomenon in humans. In rats, heat stress leads to increased metabolic demand and reduced splanchnic blood flow, which in turn induce intestinal and hepato-cellular hypoxia; the hypoxia results in the generation of highly reactive oxygen and nitrogen species that accelerate mucosal injury[17,18].

Alteration of Heat-shock Response. Increased levels of heat-shock proteins protect cells from damage by heat, ischemia, hypoxia, endotoxins, and inflammatory cytokines. In persons who are subjected to heat stress, examination of muscle tissue, blood monocytes, and serum reveals that such a heat-shock response occurs in vivo. Attenuation of the heat-shock response during heat stroke suggests that this adaptative response is protective. Conditions associated with a low level of expression of heat-shock proteins include aging, lack of acclimatization to heat, and certain genetic polymorphisms which may favor the progression from heat stress to heat stroke.[17-19]

CLINICAL MANIFESTATIONS

Patients suffering from heat stroke would generally have a core temperature above 41°C (105°F) or more. Some patients may have already received some form of cooling therapy prior to arrival at the hospital, and their temperature at admission may be misleading. Most patients with classic heat stroke and about half the patients with exertional heat stroke have dry and hot skin.

CNS dysfunction

Heat stroke is invariably associated with signs of serious CNS dysfunction. Delirium or coma are almost universal. Convulsions occur in 75% patients. Other CNS manifestations include opisthotonos, hallucinations, decerebate rigidity, cerebellar dysfunction, dystonia and tremors. Pupils may be fixed and dilated and the electro-encephalogram may be flat, but these changes are potentially reversible, and hence they do not constitute a basis for withholding intensive care. Permanent neurological damage may be seen in severe cases. Neurological dysfunction is a cardinal feature of heat stroke[20]. The neurological deficits are common to both classical and exertional heat stroke, although the latter are likely to have more transient dysfunction.

Cardiovascular dysfunction

Patients with heat stroke have a hyperdynamic circulation because of the vasodilatation. However, myocardial injury and pulmonary hypertension combine to cause a raised central venous pressure and signs of right heart failure. Thus they have clinical signs of a wide pulse pressure and congestive heart failure. Hypovolemia is more pronounced in heat stroke victims. Interestingly, signs of peripheral vasoconstriction are observed more often in patients with heat stroke while heat exhaustion patients are more likely to demonstrate peripheral vasodilatation. There may be marked changes in all components of the ECG. Rhythm disturbances, including sinus tachycardia, atrial fibrillation and supraventricular tachycardia, have been reported. These may settle with cooling or require cardioversion. Conduction defects include right bundle branch block and intraventricular conduction defects, which tend to persist for at least 24 hours. Prolongation of the Q–T interval is the most commonly observed ECG finding, and may be related to hypocalcemia, hypoklemia or hypomagnesemia[21,22].

Muscle features

Although rhabdomyolysis is not always a feature of heat stroke, but it is a serious complication that may lead to development of renal failure because of the myoglobinuria.

Hematological manifestations

Heat stroke results in widespread derangements of the hemostatic processes through various mechanisms including hepatic damage, vascular endothelial damage, thermal activation of clotting factors, platelet dysfunction and heat induced fibrinolysis. Various bleeding manifestations have been reported involving all parts of the body. Bleeding diathesis is a poor prognostic factor[23].

Immunological abnormalities

When blood is redistributed from the splanchnic circulation to the periphery in an attempt to lose heat and supply skeletal muscle, there is a risk of gut ischemia. This facilitates the absorption of bacterial endotoxins. Inflammatory mediators, which appear in the circulation in response to endotoxemia, are soluble tumor necrosis factor, interleukins 1, 2, 6 and 8, platelet-activating factor, vasoactive amines and arachidonic acid metabolites.

Hepatic damage

Hepatic damage is a consistent feature of heat stroke, and the absence of raised transaminases virtually rules out the possibility of this diagnosis[24,25]. Transaminases are elevated ten thousand-fold and reach peak levels at about 24 hours after onset. Survivors usually don't have any signs of permanent loss of hepatocellular function. Hepatic failure is an important contributor to paediatric mortality. Liver damage can lead to jaundice, encephalopathy, hypoglycemia, consumptive coagulopathy.

Renal damage

Acute oliguric renal failure is a common complication. Splanchnic vasoconstriction, rhabdomyolysis, disseminated intravascular coagulation and thermal injury contribute to the development of renal damage. Hypotension due to cardiac injury and urate nephropathy may aggravate renal damage. The initial urine sample in a patient with heat stroke is usually scanty, brownish and turbid. Microscopic examination often reveals proteinuria, red blood cells and casts. The renal damage is completely reversible[26-28].

Metabolic derangements

Hypoglycemia is frequent in exertional heat stroke. Lactic acidosis is a common metabolic problem. Interestingly, severe lactic acidosis is fairly common in patients with exertional heat stroke, and is not associated with any adverse long-term outcome. In contrast, among patients with classic heat stroke, moderate lactic acidosis is associated with severe neurological damage, and severe lactic acidosis is associated with a high mortality. Disturbances of sodium and potassium may occur, with hypo- and hypernatremia and hypo- and hyperkalemia. Respiratory alkalosis is a physiological response to hyperthermia and may be severe enough to cause tetany and hypocalcemia. Tissue breakdown may result in hyperuricemia. Both hypophosphatemia and hyperphosphatemia have been described, of which latter is more common[29].

Acid-base disturbances are well described in exertional heat stroke. Lactic acidosis may occur even as a normal response to severe exertion, but lactate is rapidly cleared by the liver and converted to glucose. In heat stroke the patient is shocked, this mechanism is less efficient, and restoration of the circulating blood volume may lead to worsening of lactic acidosis as skeletal muscle is reperfused. The body compensates with acute respiratory alkalosis secondary to increased respiratory effort. This may in itself lead to heat-induced tetany. After several hours, the situation changes from a mixed picture of acidosis and alkalosis to predominant metabolic acidosis because of sustained tissue damage.

Because anhidrosis is such a prominent finding in many patients with heat stroke, it had been widely believed that cessation of sweating due to "sweat gland fatigue" is the primary cause of heat stroke. However, not only is sweating seen in early stages of some patients of classic heat stroke, it is also seen in about 50% of patients with established exertional heat stroke. Hence this hypothesis is no longer widely accepted.[15]

DIFFERENTIAL DIAGNOSIS

Due to changes in the mental status, it is difficult to obtain a reliable history of the patient. Whenever possible, information about prodromal symptoms such as weakness and dizziness should be elicited. Prescription medications such as diuretics and antihypertensives, can decrease the body's ability to thermoregulate. Differential diagnoses should be considered only after rapid and effective cooling has been achieved, because any delay resulting from attempts to find out alternative diagnoses, may be fatal, if the underlying condition happens to be heat stroke.[22] A rapid improvement in sensorium with effective cooling virtually rules out other possibilities. A history of shaking chills at admission may provide a clue that the hyperthermia is due to a raised hypothalamic thermostat rather than due to heat stroke.[30,31]

Meningitis and encephalitis may closely mimic heat stroke. A cerebrospinal fluid examination can differentiate these conditions. In heat stroke the spinal fluid is usually clear, with occasional lymphocytes, but proteins may be elevated to 150 mg/dl[30,32].

Cerebral malaria is also a close differential in endemic areas. Several clinical features, such as encephalopathy, lactic acidosis, renal failure, hypoglycemia and hepatic injury overlap between cerebral malaria and heat stroke. Hence in India it is essential that a thick and thin blood films are examined in all cases of heat stroke. In case of doubt, treatment for both the conditions may be started empirically[3,33].

Thyroid storm resembles exertional heat stroke because it causes hyperthermia by increased endogenous heat production. Rapid cooling is an important step in the initial treatment of both the conditions. Fortunately thyroid storm is rare in children.

Drug-induced heat illness is another important condition in the differential diagnosis. Both heat stroke and anticholinergic poisoning can produce hyperpyrexia, dry and hot skin, tachycardia and altered sensorium. However, anticholinergic poisoning is typically associated with pin-point pupils, unlike the situation in heat stroke.

Typhoid fever and *hypothalamic lesions* can also produce symptoms similar to heat stroke. If a diagnosis cannot be made on purely clinical grounds, a measurement of hepatic transaminases is helpful. Heat stroke would invariably have dramatically high levels of these enzymes.

The hemorrhagic shock encephalopathy syndrome has several features similar to heat stroke, and it has been postulated that the two conditions have the same etiopathogenesis, although there is usually no history of overt overheating in this syndrome[34].

TREATMENT

Initial evaluation of a patient with suspected heatstroke should include an assessment of the airway, breathing, and circulation[35,36]. Tachycardia, tachypnea, and normotension are common in heat stroke. Rectal temperature should be measured immediately without any delay[37]. Core temperatures in patients with heat stroke typically range from 40°C to 44°C (104°F to 111.2°F), with reports as high as 47°C (116.6°F), and should be monitored rectally or with a bladder or esophageal probe. However, elevated temperatures are not necessary for the diagnosis of heat stroke. Peripheral temperature measurements may be as much as 1°C lower than core readings, and cooling by emergency medical technicians may falsely decrease peripheral temperatures further. *Cooling the patient takes precedence over all other interventions[38]*. The important investigations that should be done alongside the treatment are summarized in Table 15.3.

Cooling

Prompt reversal of hyperthermia is the cornerstone of heat stroke treatment. Patients who present with suspected heat stroke in a community environment should be stabilized in a cool, shady area and transferred to a health care facility as soon as heat stroke is considered as the most likely diagnosis. Immediate initiation of rapid and effective cooling is crucial in a patient with heat stroke. If feasible, cooling should be initiated while the patient is awaiting transport. Blood should be drawn for biochemical parameters and abnormalities addressed once the cooling process has begun[38].

Cooling methods generally are categorized as external or internal. External methods include evaporative and immersion cooling, but evaporative methods are most commonly used in the field. In evaporative cooling, a mist of cool water (15°C or 59°F) is sprayed on the patient's skin, while warm air (45°C or 113°F) is fanned over the body. Cooling rates with this technique have been found to be around 0.31°C (0.56°F) per hour[39].

The most widely used method of cooling is to immerse the patient in a tub of ice water. Vigorous skin massage is advocated to maintain skin circulation, otherwise it is felt that vasoconstriction and shivering may defeat the whole purpose of cooling. Immersion cooling can be achieved with an ice bath, or by using cooling blankets in conjunction with ice packs placed on the axilla, groin, neck, and head. Although immersion methods are thought to be less effective than evaporative cooling,

direct comparison studies are lacking. An alternative method of cooling uses the principle of evaporative cooling. In this method the patient is suspended on a net while being sprayed with atomized water and warmed air (45°C to 48°C) is blown over the skin surface. This method maximizes evaporative cooling by maintaining vasodilatation and preventing shivering. Immersion in ice cold water or cool water reduces core temperature at the rate of 0.13°C to 0.16°C/min, whereas the evaporative cooling method reduces it at the rate of 0.31°C/min[15]. The core temperature should either be monitored continuously using a rectal probe or at least every 5 minutes by a thermometer to ensure that overshoot hypothermia does not occur. Active cooling techniques can be discontinued once the core temperature is 38.3°C to prevent iatrogenic hypothermia.

Internal cooling methods are more effective in rapidly decreasing temperature[39]. Gastric, bladder, and rectal cold water lavage can be accomplished with minimal invasion. Peritoneal and thoracic lavage are performed only in extreme cases. Cardiopulmonary bypass is rarely used but is an effective cooling method[40].

The use of antipyretics and dantrolene have been studied but have not been found to be efficacious in the management of heat stroke. They may actually be harmful by predisposing to development of bleeding manifestations.

Fluid management

If the patient is hypotensive he must initially receive a bolus of isotonic saline or Ringer's lactate. Hypoglycemia is common and dextrose boluses and continuous dextrose infusion is indicated. Patients with heat stroke are hypotensive more often because of vasodilatation rather than severe dehydration. Cooling itself causes vasoconstriction

Table 15.3 Investigations in patients with heat stroke	
Investigations	**Expected results**
● Complete blood counts	Raised hematocrit, leucocytosis, thrombocytopenia
● Arterial blood gases	Respiratory alkalosis, metabolic acidosis
● Serum electrolytes	Hyperkalemia, hypernatremia, hypocalcemia, hypophosphatemia
● Blood glucose	Hypoglycemia
● Renal function tests	Raised urea, creatinine
● Urinalysis	Proteinuria, hematuria, casts, myoglobinuria
● Liver function tests	Markedly elevated liver enzymes
● ECG	Conduction abnormalities, ST-T wave changes
● Coagulation studies	Deranged coagulogram, elevated fibrin degradation products
● Peripheral smear	No malarial parasites
● CSF examination	No cells, elevated protein

and hence plays an important role in the correction of the hypotension. Fluids should be administered cautiously because these patients often have co-existing cardiac and renal compromise. Dobutamine may have a role in patients with raised central venous pressure, especially because it maintains peripheral vasodilatation. Drugs that can cause intense vasoconstriction, like norepinephrine, should not be used before effective cooling is established, because they interfere with heat exchange without improving cardiac contractility. Ideally patients of heat stroke must have the benefit of central venous pressure and pulmonary artery wedge pressure monitoring[15]. Muscle damage can lead to hyperkalemia, hypocalcemia and hypophosphatemia. Calcium replacement and treatment with potassium lowering resins may be required. Rhabdomyolysis is treated with administration of large amounts of intravenous fluids, alkalinization of the urine and osmotic diuresis.

Respiratory management

Patients with heat stroke may need to be intubated if they are comatose or are seizuring. Supplemental oxygen should be provided, because the markedly increased metabolic rate results in a steep rise in oxygen consumption. Arterial blood gases should be monitored.

Management of convulsions

Diazepam should be used to control convulsions. Phenobarbitone can be used for intermediate long-term management, taking care that its metabolism may be affected by hepatic dysfunction. Mannitol has a role in the management of cerebral edema. Steroids have no role in the treatment of heat stroke[15].

Renal failure

The urine output and renal function tests must be monitored. The urine must be alkalinized with bicarbonate to prevent renal shutdown secondary to myoglobinuria and urate nephropathy. The indications of dialysis are the same as in any other case of acute renal failure.

Management of coagulopathy

Disturbances in hemostasis primarily occur on the second or third day of the illness. Fresh frozen plasma and platelet concentrates should be used to replace the deficits. The use of ε-amino caproic acid is contraindicated in heat stroke because this drug can itself cause rhabdomyolysis. Recombinant activated protein C has been considered for use in heat stroke associated with DIC.[15] Data is still lacking.

Care of a comatose patient

The patient should be nursed in a lateral position with the head end low and should be turned to either side at regular intervals. A ripple bed should be used to prevent bedsores. The pressure points should be kept clean and dry. It is important to keep the air passages patent by suctioning the oropharynx frequently and using an oral airway. Nutrition should be provided by a nasogastric tube. Bladder and bowel care must be ensured.

SEQUELAE

50% of all patients who recover from heat stroke have some neurological sequelae. Of these the vast majority are minor problems and disappear over a period of a few weeks to 2 years. Only 1% patients have long-term sequelae. The commonest problem is persistent headache. Psychological complaints include non-specific limb pains, vertigo, insomnia, amnesia and personality changes. The commonest neurological deficit is ataxia. Other neurological deficits include aphasia, cerebellar dysfunction, monoplegia, hemiplegia, epilepsy, and various cranial nerve palsies. All these patients require symptomatic treatment and physiotherapy[15].

PROGNOSIS

The most important factors influencing prognosis are the time taken by the patient to seek medical help and the rapidity with which the patient is cooled. Duration of symptoms of heat stroke has an important bearing on the degree of disability. Effective cooling is defined as any method by which the rectal temperature is reduced below 39°C within one hour, regardless of the initial temperature. Rapid fall in core temperature, with restoration of consciousness by 4 hours is a good prognostic sign. Circulatory failure, bleeding diathesis, persistent coma, severe lactic acidosis, shock, liver failure and a waxing and waning sensorium are all poor prognostic factors. Mortality for heat stroke ranges from 17% to 70%, depending on the severity of heat stroke and age of the patient[15,24,30]. Serum procalcitonin has been found to be elevated in heat stroke survivors but not in those who died[41].

PREVENTION

Heat illnesses can be prevented if environmental temperature, humidity and air movement are controlled. During hot weather the clothing should be cotton, loose fitting and minimum. Adequate fluid and salt intake should be ensured. The children should be kept indoors during hot summer months. The sports activities and physical training program should be restricted to early morning or late evening during summer. *Infants and toddlers should never be left unattended in a car during shopping sprees.*

REFERENCES

1. Tek D, Olschaker JS. Heat illness. *Emerg Med Clin North Amer* 1992; 10: 299-309.

2. Squire DL. Heat illness. Fluid and electrolyte issues for pediatric and adolescent athletes. *Pediatr Clin North Amer* 1990; 37:1085-1109.

3. MacPherson RK, O'Brien JP. Effects of heat. In: Tropical Medicine. Hunter G, Swartzwelda JC, Clyde DF (Eds.). *WB Saunders. Philadelphia* 5th Ed., 1976.

4. Nelson NG, Collins CL, Comstock RD, McKenzie LB. Exertional heat-related injuries treated in emergency departments in the U.S., 1997-2006. *Amer J Prev Med* 2011; 40(1):54-60

5. Ladell WSS. Heat cramps. *Lancet* 1949; 2:836.

6. Shibolet S, Lancaster MC, Danon Y. Heat stroke: a review. *Aviat Space Environ Med* 1976; 47:280.

7. Convertino VA, Greenleaf JE, Bernauer EM. Role of thermal and exercise factors in the mechanism of hypervolemia. *J Appl Physiol* 1980; 48: 657.

8. McCance RA. Experimental sodium chloride deficiency in man. *Proc Royal Soc London Biol* 1936; 119:245.

9. Shibolet S, Coll R, Gilat T, Sohar E, *et al*. Heat stroke: its clinical picture and mechanism in 36 cases. *Q J Med* 1967; 36:525.

10. Petersdorf RG. Disturbances of heat regulation. In: Harrisons Principles of Internal Medicine 12th ed. *McGraw Hill International Book Company* 1991; p 50-57.

11. Bar-Or O. Children and physical performance in warm and cold environments. In: Advances in Pediatric Sports Sciences. Volume I: Biological issues. *Champaign, Illinois, Human Kinetic Publishers,* 1984, pp 117-129.

12. Bar-Or O. Climate and the exercising child: a review. *Int J Sports Med* 1980; 1:53-65.

13. McLaren J, Null J, Quinn J. Heat stress from enclosed vehicles: moderate ambient temperatures cause significant temperature rise in enclosed vehicles. *Pediatrics* 2005; 116:109-12

14. Helman RS. Heat stroke 2007. Available at HTTP://WWW.emedicine.com/med/topic956.htm

15. Bouchama A, Knochel JP. Heat stroke. *N Engl J Med* 2002; 346(25):1978-88.

16. Glazer JL. Management of heat stroke and heat exhaustion. 2005; 71:2133-40

17. Bouchama A, Hammami MM, Haq A. Evidence for endothelial cell activation/injury in heatstroke. *Crit Care Med* 1996; 24(7):1173-8.

18. Yang YL, Lin MT. Heat shock protein expression protects against cerebral ischemia and monoamine overload in rat heatstroke. *Am J Physiol* 1999; 276:H1961-H1967.

19. Hubbard RW, Matthew CB, Durkot MJ, Francesconi RP. Novel approaches to the pathophysiology of heatstroke: the energy depletion model. *Ann Emerg Med* 1987; 16(9):1066-75

20. Malamud N, Haymaker W, Custer RP. Heat stroke. A clinico-pathological study of 125 fatal cases. *Milit Surg* 1946; 99:397-449.

21. Akhtar MJ, al-Nozha M, al-Harthi S, Nouh MS. Electrocardiographic abnormalities in patients with heat stroke. *Chest* 1993; 104(2):411-4.

22. Milvy P (Ed.). The Marathon: Physiological, Medical, Epidemiological and Psychological Studies, *New York Academy of Medical Sciences,* 1977.

23. Bouchama A, Bridey F, Hammami MM, *et al*. Activation of coagulation and fibrinolysis in heat stroke. *Thrombosis and Hemostasis* 1996; 76: 909-915.

24. Kew M, Bersohn I, Setfel H. The diagnostic and prognostic significance of the serum enzyme changes in heat stroke. *Trans Royal Soc Trop Med Hyg* 1971; 65:325.

25. Kew M, Bersohn I, Seftel H, Kent G. Liver damage in heat stroke. *Am J Med* 1970; 49:192.

26. Herman RH, Sullivan BH. Heat stroke and jaundice. *Am J Med* 1959; 27:154.

27. Vertel RM, Knochel JP. Acute renal failure due to heat injury: an analysis of ten cases associated with a high incidence of myglobinuria. *Am J Med* 1967; 43:435.

28. Castenfars J. Renal function during exercise. *Acta Physiol Scand* 1967; 70:7.

29. Costrini AM, Pitt HA, Gustafson AB, Uddin DE. Cardiovascular and metabolic manifestations of heat stroke and severe heat exhaustion. *Am J Med* 1979; 66:296.

30. Austin MG, Berry JW. Observations on one hundred cases of heat stroke. *JAMA* 1956; 161:1525.

31. Danks DM, Webb DW, Allen J. Heat illness in infants and young children. *Brit Med J* 1962; 2:287-291.

Section 2

32. Ferris EB, Blankenhorn MA, Robinson HW, *et al*. Heat stroke: clinical and chemical observations on 44 cases. *J Clin Invest* 1938; 17:249.

33. Leithead CS and Lind AR. Heat stroke and heat hyperpyrexia. In: Heat Stroke and Heat disorders. *Cassell and Company Ltd., London* 1964; 195-236.

34. Bacon CJ, Hall SM. Hemorrhagic shock encephalopathy syndrome in the British Isles. *Arch Dis Child* 1992; 67:985-993.

35. Barger AC. Venous pressure and cutaneous reactive hyperemia in exhausting exercise and certain other circulatory stresses. *J Appl Physiol* 1949; 2:81.

36. Spring CL. Heat stroke: modern approaches to an ancient disease. *Chest* 1980; 77:461.

37. Ash CJ, Cook JR, McMurry TA, Auner CR. The use of rectal temperature to monitor heat stroke. *Military Med* 1992; 89(5):283-288.

38. Kumar P, Rathore CK, Nagar AM, *et al*. Hyperpyrexia with special reference to heat stroke: on analysis of 108 cases. *J Indian Med Assoc* 1964; 43:213-219.

39. Weiner JS, Khogali M. A physiological body-cooling unit for treatment of heat stroke. *Lancet* 1980; 1:276.

40. Bynum GD, Patton JF. The use of peritoneal dialysis for the rapid reduction of core temperature in heat stroked dogs. *Presented at the 59th Annual Meeting of the Federation of American Society for Experimental Biology., Atlanta City, NJ,* April 13-18, 1975.

41. Nylen ES, Arifi AA, Becker KL, Snider RH, Alzeer A. Effects of classic heat stroke on serum procalcitonin. *Crit Care Med* 1997; 25:1362-1365.

Acute Respiratory Distress and Respiratory Failure

16

Sunit Singhi

Acute respiratory illnesses are one of the most important causes of morbidity and mortality in children. Most often these children present with acute respiratory distress and/or respiratory failure. Early recognition of children at risk of respiratory failure and institution of supportive and specific therapy at the earliest, depending upon the underlying cause of the respiratory distress, can save many lives.

In general, any child having difficulty in breathing may be considered as suffering from respiratory distress. Children rarely complain of dyspnea and parents generally notice shortness of breath or distress. Objectively, respiratory distress is said to be present if any of the following signs are present: altered breathing pattern (fast, slow, feeble or absent), forced breathing efforts or obstructed breathing, and chest wall indrawing during breathing. Table 16.1 outlines the criteria to grade the severity of respiratory distress.

Table 16.1 Grading of acute respiratory distress

Mild
1. Tachypnea (< 50 breaths/min)
2. Dypsnea or shortness of breath

Moderate
1. Tachypnea (50-70 breaths/min)
2. Minimal chest wall retractions
3. Flaring of alae nasi

Severe
1. Tachypnea (> 70 breaths/min)
2. Apneic episodes, bradypnea or irregular breathing
3. Severe chest wall retractions
4. Head bobbing (use of sternocleidomastoid muscles)
5. Cyanosis

Respiratory failure
1. Respiratory distress + cyanosis with CNS* and/or cardiovascular** signs of hypoxemia

* CNS signs of hypoxemia: restlessness, obtunded sensorium, somnolence, seizures, coma.
** Cardiovascular signs of hypoxemia: marked tachycardia, bradycardia, hypotension, and cardiac arrest.

Respiratory failure denotes inadequacy of pulmonary functions to deliver sufficient oxygen to meet demands of the body and inability to eliminate carbon dioxide. Any child with respiratory distress has a potential to progress to respiratory failure. Presence of severe respiratory distress, with clinical evidences of hypoxemia, namely cyanosis with hypoxic central nervous system (CNS) changes such as somnolence or depressed level of consciousness, seizures and coma, or hypoxic cardiovascular manifestations such as bradycardia or marked tachycardia and hypotension are suggestive of acute respiratory failure. Arterial blood gas analysis in these cases shows a $paCO_2$ >50 mm Hg and/or a paO_2 < 60 mm Hg while breathing 40 percent oxygen.

PATHOPHYSIOLOGY AND ETIOLOGY

The normal process of respiration is a net function of the following pulmonary mechanics:

(i) Mechanical work of breathing (contraction of diaphragm and intercostal muscles; and generation of negative intrapleural pressure).
(ii) Expansion of lungs-alveolar ventilation.
(iii) Alveolar gas exchange through diffusion.
(iv) Transport of oxygen in the blood to various tissues.

In a healthy individual, coordinated action of muscles of respiration and movements of chest wall, patent airways, compliant lungs, open alveoli and adequate perfusion of ventilated alveoli by circulating blood with normal central control mechanisms, ensures effective respiratory functions. Impairment of any of the above functions can lead to inefficient respiration, and cause respiratory distress.

The etiology of respiratory distress thus, may be classified as follows:

1. **Central nervous system disturbances** with altered central regulation of respiration. This may occur due to impaired consciousness,

raised intracranial pressure, intracranial bleeding, depression of respiratory center due to barbiturate or opiate poisoning; or stimulation of respiratory center by acidosis and salicylate intoxication.

2. **Neuromuscular problems** associated with paralysis or weakness of respiratory muscles. This can occur in acute paralytic poliomyelitis, Guillain-Barre syndrome, organophosphate poisoning etc. Lung expansion is inadequate which may lead to progressive atelectasis, and increased intrapulmonary shunting.

3. **Interference with air entry** can occur due to the following conditions:

(i) Obstruction in the upper airways because of acute laryngitis, laryngotracheitis, diphtheria and foreign body aspiration or in the lower airways caused by bronchiolitis and asthma. Depending on the site and degree of obstruction, this leads to increased resistance to airflow to and from the lungs distal to obstruction, reduction in total volume of air entering and leaving the lungs during each breath (tidal volume) and hence areas of atelectasis and air trapping. This results in marked heterogeneity of gas exchange, and decreased lung compliance. In addition, to overcome the obstruction, mechanical work of breathing increases. This manifests as dyspnea, forced breathing, intercostal retractions, etc. Eventually, hypoxemia and fatigue lead to inadequate gas exchange and respiratory failure.

(ii) Compression of lungs by large pleural effusion, pneumothorax, tumors and elevated dome(s) of diaphragm because of massive ascites, diaphragmatic hernia and lobar emphysema in infants.

(iii) Thoracic wall injuries with hemo or pneumothorax and flail chest.

4. **Interference with alveolar gas exchange** is caused either by failure of alveolar ventilation such as occurs in pneumonia, pulmonary edema, pulmonary hemorrhage, pulmonary fibrosis etc. or from failure of diffusion of gas across alveolo-capillary membrane which also occurs in pneumonia, pulmonary edema, pulmonary fibrosis and pulmonary embolism. In parenchymal lung disease, which includes pneumonia, there is edema of interstitial spaces, alveoli are fluid filled, and there is progressive narrowing of small airways leading to atelectasis. Thus, a large number of alveoli remain non ventilated and alveolar diffusion of gas is impaired. This causes ventilation perfusion inequality, impaired gas exchange and hypoxemia. Additionally, inflammatory edema of interstitium and atelectasis makes lungs more stiff and reduces pulmonary compliance. Thus, a greater negative intrapleural pressure must be generated to expand a less compliant lung, and the patient's work of breathing increases. The child responds to this by breathing faster with a reduced tidal volume causing further alveolar collapse. Progressively, gas exchange becomes less efficient with further increase in shunt and dead space ventilation.

5. **Cardiovascular problems** such as congestive cardiac failure, arrhythmias, myocarditis and pericarditis affect alveolar perfusion and cause ventilation perfusion inequality or pulmonary edema. Right-to-left shunts which create a hypoxic state also clinically manifests with respiratory distress.

6. **Insufficient oxygen supply to tissues and/ or increased oxygen demands** from any etiology such as sepsis, severe anemia, high altitude, carbon monoxide exposure, smoke inhalation etc. can cause respiratory distress.

Anatomic and Physiologic Characteristics of Respiratory Tract

Several anatomic and physiological characteristics of respiratory tract, predispose infants and children to greater risk of respiratory distress and failure. Most important of these are listed below:

1. The diameter of the airways is smaller in children as compared to adults. Flow of air through the airways is reciprocal to the resistance offered which in turn is inversely proportional to the radius of the airways raised to the fourth power. Airway resistance is, therefore, higher in children and any further decrease in airway diameter is likely to increase the resistance to air flow markedly.

2. The average value for airway resistance in infants is 18 cm of water/L/second (compared to 13 cm of water/L/second in adults). Upto 50% of this resistance is in the small airways ($\leq$ 2mm in diameter) as compared to only 20% in adults. Infants and children upto 5 years of age are, therefore, particularly severely affected by diseases involving small airways.

3. In early infancy, the chest wall is soft and compliant, pleural pressure at end expiration

is zero and the alveolar diameter is small. A combination of these factors lead to increased tendency to alveolar collapse and difficulty in their re-expansion.

4. In infants the ribs are located horizontally, the sternum is softer and intercostal muscles are poorly developed; thus the usual 'bucket handle' action during respiration is less efficient than in older children and adults.

5. Diaphragm does not have the same curvature as in the adult, and hence works at a mechanical disadvantage.

6. There are incoordinated movements of the rib cage and abdominal wall in infants, which are more prominent during REM sleep.

In pre-term infants, lung development and surfactant production is often limited. This results in higher surface tension within alveoli, making them less distensible. Such infants present with the classical idiopathic respiratory distress syndrome.

The common causes of respiratory distress in children are pneumonia, bronchiolitis, asthma, upper airway obstruction due to laryngo-tracheo-bronchitis, diphtheria, foreign body aspiration, pleural effusion and empyema, and congestive heart failure. Less common causes include pneumothorax, acute meningitis and encephalitis, neuromuscular diseases such as acute paralytic poliomyelitis and Guillain-Barre syndrome, and accidental kerosene and barbiturate poisoning.

IMMEDIATE CARE

Any child who is brought with respiratory distress must be rapidly assessed for clinical signs of adequacy of gas exchange and circulatory status. Patency of the airways, respiratory rate, rhythm, depth and efforts, groaning, stridor, wheezing, chest indrawing, signs of pneumothorax etc. should be looked for. If ventilation or oxygenation is impaired, as evident from signs of severe distress and low arterial oxygen saturation (SaO_2), immediate respiratory support is needed. Most cardiac arrests in children are preceded by respiratory insufficiency; it takes only a few minutes for a child to worsen from complete apnea to cardiac arrest. Early intervention at this stage could be life-saving.

1. **Airway patency.** Rapid restoration of airways is mandatory in a child with respiratory distress, apnea, cyanosis, stridor or clinical signs of hypoxemia. Properly position the child; extend the neck and pull the mandible forward, thereby lifting the tongue away from the posterior pharyngeal wall. Oropharynx should be cleaned of any secretions, manually if necessary, follwed by insertion of an oro-pharyngeal airway. If spontaneous breathing efforts are feeble or absent, endotracheal intubation is indicated.

Presence of stridor, dysphagia and drooling suggest upper airway obstruction. An emergency endotracheal intubation or tracheostomy may be necessary. In a near complete obstruction, patency can be achieved rapidly by percutaneous insertion of a wide bore cannula (eg. medicut size 12, pneumothorax trocar, or 12-15 gauge needle) into trachea through cricothyroid membrane (cricothyrotomy). It should be followed by a tracheostomy after stabilizing the child.

2. **Ensure breathing/respiration.** If spontaneous normal breathing is absent even after establishing a clear airway, the patient needs assisted rescue breaths. Any form of breathing: mouth to mouth, mouth to tube, or bag and mask ventilation can deliver adequate oxygen. *Resuscitation must never be delayed just because a tube or bag is not available. Such a delay is known to be a common reason for death of the patient.*

Bag and mask or tube ventilation with maximal concentration of oxygen must be provided as soon as possible. In practice most children can be managed with bag and mask ventilation using 100% oxygen. The method is effective even when airway obstruction is caused by infection.

3. Feeble or absent femoral pulse is a sufficient indication to commence **external cardiac compressions.** (Refer to Chapter 3 on cardiopulmonary resuscitation).

4. If **pneumothorax** is detected, a needle thoracotomy in the second intercostal space for immediate decompression is life saving. It should be followed by a chest tube drainage connected to an under water seal.

5. **Establish IV access.** An intravenous access must be obtained in every child with severe respiratory distress. If a vein is not available, intraosseous access may be used in children under 6 years. Metabolic acidosis is invariably present with respiratory failure. Empiric use of sodium bicarbonate should be avoided. It may be administered after arterial blood gas analysis, if pH is <7.20, effective ventilation must be established before administration of sodium bicarbonate.

DIAGNOSTIC EVALUATION

After resuscitation and stabilization, it is essential to identify the cause of respiratory distress so that specific therapy can be instituted. A good history and a thorough physical examination will usually provide clues to the diagnosis. Not only the respiratory system but also other systems, particularly cardiovascular and central nervous systems should be evaluated. Further evaluation for the cause and severity of respiratory distress may require laboratory and radiological data. An outline of diagnostic evaluation is given in Table 16.2.

History

If respiratory distress is acute, the history of cough, fever, skin rash, ingestion/inhalation of foreign body, aspiration, trauma or accident, exposure to fire or smoke etc. should be sought. Sudden choking and coughing spell suggests inhalation of a foreign body in the upper airways. History of trauma or accident indicates a need to look for chest wall injury, traumatic pneumothorax or head injury. If the present episode is a recurrence of previous illness or an acute exacerbation of a chronic illness such as asthma, history of similar attacks and previous diagnosis are helpful. History of medications before reaching the hospital must always be obtained. Family history of exposure to an acute infection, tuberculosis or recurrent pulmonary problems should be sought.

Physical Examination

This must include all the parameters listed in Table 16.2.

Respiratory rate counted for one full minute is a useful indicator. However, it may be difficult to evaluate breathing rate in a crying infant. Rhythm, depth and character of breathing should be looked for. A respiratory rate of >60/minute is a good indicator of hypoxia (SaO$_2$ <90%) in infants under 2 months of age[1].

Audible noise in the form *of stridor and wheezing* suggests upper or lower airway obstruction respectively. *Grunting* is produced by expiration against a partially closed glottis in an attempt to maintain positive airway pressure during expiration. It indicates an alveolar disease that has caused widespread loss of functional residual capacity; such as pulmonary edema, diffuse pneumonia *etc.*

Table 16.2 Diagnostic evaluation of respiratory distress

A. History
1. Acute, recurrent or chronic and nature of progression.
2. Associated symptoms: Cough, fever, rash and chest pain
3. Preceding events: Foreign body inhalation, trauma/accident, and exposure to chemical or environmental irritants.
4. Family history: Exposure to infections, tuberculosis, atopy.

B. Physical examination
1. To assess stability of the airways, and ventilatory status.
    * Respiratory rate, rhythm, depth and work of breathing.
    * Color, level of activity and playfulness.
    * Chest movements, indrawing of chest wall
    * Stridor, wheezing, grunting
2. Tracheal position
3. Segmental percussion
4. Auscultation: Air entry, type of breath sounds, wheeze, rhonchi and crepitations
5. Assessment of CVS and CNS

C. Diagnostic work-up
1. Direct laryngoscopy, if there is upper airway obstruction
2. Skiagrams of chest, lateral neck, and decubitus views
3. Arterial blood gas analysis, and SaO$_2$ monitoring
4. Sepsis work-up: Blood counts and culture studies

Tracheal position and adequacy and symmetry of chest wall movements should be recorded.

Segmental percussion and auscultation. Attention should be given to air entry, type of breath sounds in inspiration and expiration, and presence of rales and rhonchi. Auscultation should be carried out not only during quiet breathing but also during crying, deep breathing, and forced expiration, after coughing and nasal suctioning whenever possible.

Extrapulmonary manifestations such as cervical and axillary lymphadenopathy, clubbing of nails etc., should be looked for. Evaluation of cardiovascular system for presence of heart disease and CNS examination for evidences of infection, raised intracranial pressure and paralytic illness should be looked for.

The clinical signs that help in the assessment of severity of *hypoxemia and hypercarbia* should be critically assessed. A child's spontaneous level of activity is a useful guide to oxygenation. Easy fatiguability suggests increased work of breathing and hypoxia.

Depending upon the diagnostic possibilities the following laboratory studies may be required:

Radiological studies (X-ray chest PA, lateral decubitus views, lateral view of neck and contrast studies) should be undertaken for confirmation of the diagnosis.

Oximetry (SaO_2 measurement) *and arterial blood gas (ABG)* studies should be obtained in all children with moderate to severe distress to assess efficacy of alveolar gas exchange.

ABG provides the most important data in assessing the severity of respiratory failure. Blood is usually obtained either from radial, posterior tibial or dorsalis pedis artery. Three major alterations may be noted; hypoxemia (paO_2 <60 mm Hg), hypercarbia ($paCO_2$ >40 mm Hg) and alterations in pH (acidosis or alkalosis). Arterial oxygen tension (paO_2) reflects the state of alveolar ventilation and perfusion of lungs, and depends on the ambient concentration of oxygen.

Microbiological studies. Complete blood counts, blood culture, culture of sputum, nasopharyngeal secretions, transtracheal aspirate, or lung aspirate must be obtained in febrile toxic children.

DIFFERENTIAL DIAGNOSIS

After clinical evaluation children with respiratory distress can be easily categorized depending on the predominant symptoms and signs, in the following six groups:

1. Stridor
2. Cough, fever and breathing difficulty/fast breathing.
3. Wheezing
4. Mediastinal shift with severe distress
5. Slow or irregular breathing in the absence of any pulmonary signs.
6. Respiratory distress with cardiac findings.

Stridor

Stridor is a harsh crowing sound usually heard during inspiration. It indicates upper airway obstruction (pharynx to trachea). Inspiratory stridor is usually supraglottic, while expiratory stridor emanates from the trachea. Supraglottic stridor may be associated with muffled voice and dysphagia while subglottic stridor is accompanied by hoarseness of voice or cry and barking cough. Any patient with a persistent stridor of acute onset must be hospitalised for treatment and observation.

Evaluation. Check other symptoms, such as voice change and fever, history of trauma to head or neck, and history of choking, which could lead to foreign body aspiration.

(i) Throat should be examined for evidence of acute inflammation, exudates and membrane.

(ii) In the neck look for any swelling, extrinsic mass, evidence of trauma and tracheal position.

(iii) If the patient's condition permits, consider a laryngoscopic examination and obtain a lateral X-ray of neck in children with severe distress. Laryngoscopy or any procedure that may agitate the patient is postponed till an emergency airway is established. Visualization of epiglottis in a suspected case of epiglottitis should be attempted only after making preparations for immediate intubation or tracheostomy

The common diagnostic possibilities in a child with stridor are discussed below:

Acute laryngotracheitis (viral croup) usually occurs in children between 3 months to 3 years of age. There is usually a preceding history of mild URI followed by brassy or barking cough, hoarseness of voice followed by stridor. Signs of severe respiratory distress are commonly present. Lateral X-ray of neck shows narrowing of subepiglottic airway and normal epiglottis and aryepiglottic folds and mild distension of hypopharynx.

Bacterial tracheitis should be suspected when a clinical picture similar to that of viral croup is complicated by high grade fever, toxicity and copious purulent tracheal secretions[2]. *Staphylococcus aureus*, Streptococci and *H. influenzae* are common etiologic agents.

Foreign body in the trachea/larynx. An acute episode of coughing, choking or gagging followed by stridor in infants and toddlers while eating nuts or playing with small objects is typical of a foreign body aspiration. In 30% of patients below 3 years of age, however, such a history may not be available. Besides stridor, aphonia, dysphagia and severe air hunger are the predominant signs of laryngeal and tracheal foreign bodies.

Diphtheria has a gradual onset, with a mild sore throat and moderate fever. A grayish membrane forms over the tonsils, which may extend to affect the larynx. This results in harsh cough, hoarse voice, stridor and increasing difficulty in breathing. By this time, the child is severely toxic and death may occur due to laryngeal obstruction unless an emergency tracheostomy is performed.

Acute epiglottitis is a rare cause of stridor in India. It usually occurs in children between 2 to 7 years of age but may occur below 2 years of age. *H. influenzae type b* is the commonest pathogen. Characteristically there is sudden onset of high grade fever (39°C), rapidly progressing rattling or snoring stridor, toxic appearance, extreme sore throat, muffled voice, and difficulty in swallowing. The child assumes a characteristic 'airway protective' posture i.e. sitting and leaning forward, with protrusion of jaw and open mouth with drooling of saliva. Examination of pharynx may reveal a cherry red epiglottis. When the diagnosis is not clear, lateral X-ray of neck may be useful. This shows a grossly distended hypopharynx, swollen epiglottis and aryepiglottic folds, and a normal subglottic airway.

Retropharyngeal abscess is an uncommon cause of stridor. It occurs in infants and young children because of secondary infection of retropharyngeal space and lymph nodes following an upper respiratory infection. The infection is most often a mixed one caused by Streptococci, *Staphylococcus aureus* and anerobic organisms. Typically, there is high grade fever, sore throat, inspiratory stridor and difficulty in swallowing. The neck is generally hyper extended so as to achieve maximum airway. A lateral X-ray of the neck is diagnostic[3]. It shows airway narrowing and widening of retropharyngeal space. Presence of air lucencies indicates perforation.

Acute severe tonsillitis superimposed on *tonsillar and adenoidal hypertrophy* is an important cause of severe upper airway obstruction. Inflammatory edema extending down to larynx may further aggravate obstruction of the airway.

The less common causes of acute stridor include hypocalcemic laryngeal tetany and angioneurotic edema. Chronic stridor is seen with congenital malformations such as laryngomalacia, tracheomalacia, laryngeal web, and vascular rings. It may worsen in the presence of an upper respiratory tract infection.

Cough, Fever and Fast or difficult Breathing

Cough, fever and fast and/or difficult breathing in the absence of signs of airway obstruction are suggestive of pneumonia[4]. Cough may sometimes be absent in very young infants. Presence of grunting, chest wall indrawing and inability to feed normally are signs of severe disease. Examination frequently reveals fine crepitations distributed all over the chest and occasionally classic signs of lobar or segmental consolidation (dullness on percussion, diminished air entry and bronchial breathing). Chest signs may be difficult to elicit in very young infants and malnourished children.

Measles pneumonia should be considered in the presence of generalized erythematous, maculopapular rash preceding the onset of fast breathing. A history of paroxysms of cough followed by a 'whoop' suggests whooping cough. In very young infants (below 6 months) whooping cough may present with cough and apneic episodes. In a child who develops cough, choking and respiratory distress while feeding or vomiting especially during sleep or in a state of depressed consciousness, aspiration pneumonia must be suspected. Chemical pneumonia may occur following ingestion of hydrocarbons such as kerosene. In all cases of suspected pneumonia with moderate or severe respiratory distress, if feasible, an X-ray chest should be obtained to confirm the diagnosis.

Wheezing

Wheezing is a high pitched, musical sound caused by partial obstruction of the lower airways (from lower part of trachea to terminal airways) and is most often expiratory. There is often an associated suppression of breath sounds and overall decrease in the air entry. When it is audible over the entire lung fields, the commonest diagnostic possibility is bronchiolitis in young infants or bronchial asthma after infancy. Other important possibilities are aspiration of foreign body in lower airway, bronchitis and pneumonia. Rarely, stridor and wheezing may coexist. The common underlying diagnoses in these patients include gastroesophageal reflux disease (GERD), congenital lesions pressing the airway, tracheal stenosis, foreign body in the airway or esophagus, or a combination of croup and bronchiolitis[5].

Bronchiolitis should be considered in any child less than 2 years of age with first episode of wheezing and respiratory distress. It is a viral infection (respiratory syncytial virus in 60-70% cases) that causes inflammation of bronchioles with edema, loss of cilia, necrosis of epithelial cells and patchy obstruction of lumen by cellular debris and thick secretions. The patchy obstruction results in scattered areas of atelectasis and hyperinflation with marked ventilation perfusion inequalities and respiratory distress. There is usually a history of coryza 2-3 days preceding the onset of irritating cough, wheezing and respiratory distress. The chest may appear 'barrel shaped'. Auscultation reveals reduced air entry with bilateral fine crepitations and sibilant rhonchi. Skiagram of chest typically shows hyperlucent lung fields and flattening of diaphragm, peribronchial thickening, patchy atelectasis and perihilar infiltrates.

Acute asthma is the most common cause of wheezing in children. A family history of allergy, a history of similar attacks in the past, intractable cough, expiratory wheeze and multiple adventitious sounds (rhonchi, whistles, crackles, snaps, pops etc.) on auscultation are characteristic. Attacks are frequently precipitated by exposure to allergens, infection, exercise, and sometimes by emotional disturbances. Life threatening complications of asthma include pneumothorax, cardiac dysrhythmia, bronchial plugging and respiratory failure.

Bronchitis and pneumonia may be associated with wheezing and can be confused with the first attack of asthma. Wheezing occurs secondary to airway edema and mucous production. An element of irritative bronchospasm may be present. A clinical picture consistent with infection and a chest X-ray are helpful for its differentiation from asthma.

Foreign body aspiration[6]. There is usually a *sudden onset with cough, choking and onset of stridor and wheezing.* Stridor may occur initially but once the foreign body slips below the level of carina, stridor disappears and wheezing predominates. A foreign body in one of the main stem bronchus may cause signs of collapse and mediastinal shift to the same side. Secondary infection usually occurs. A partial obstruction to the bronchus produces obstructive emphysema with displacement of the mediastinum to the opposite side due to ball valve effect of the foreign body. The acute episode of choking may be ignored or forgotten and child may present with episodes of recurrent respiratory infections. For detailed discussion on clinical features, diagnosis and management of foreign bodies in the air passages refer to Chapter 48.

Uncommon causes of wheezing in children include enlarged mediastinal lymph nodes, tumors, anaphylaxis, congestive heart failure, tracheo-bronchomalacia, gastro-esophageal reflux with aspiration and vascular anomalies such as pulmonary vascular rings.

Mediastinal Shift

A shift in the position of trachea to one side with diminished chest wall movements, stony dull percussion and suppression of breath sounds on the opposite side, indicates a large pleural effusion or empyema. X-ray chest in upright position and a pleural tap will confirm the diagnosis. On the other hand, a mediastinal shift with diminished or absent breath sounds on the same side and lobar or segmental impaired percussion note, is indicative of underlying atelectasis. Most often this is caused by compression of adjacent bronchi by enlarged hilar and mediastinal lymph nodes. This can occur in tuberculosis or lymphoreticular malignancy. Frequently, collapse may occur secondary to an intrabronchial obstruction caused by a foreign body lodged in the main stem bronchus. The most valuable tool to confirm the diagnosis is the X-ray of the chest and bronchoscopy. A shift in the position of trachea to one side with hyperresonant percussion note, and diminished breath sounds on the opposite side is suggestive of a tension pneumothorax. On the side of the pneumothorax, the chest wall movements are diminished, intercostal spaces may be bulging, and subcutaneous emphysema may appear.

Bradypnea and/or Irregular Breathing

In the absence of history or physical findings suggestive of a primary respiratory illness, bradypnea and/or irregular breathing is most likely to be due to depression of central nervous system. Accompanying generalized muscular weakness or paralysis of limbs suggest acute poliomyelitis or Guillain-Barre syndrome.

Associated Findings of Congestive Heart Failure

The presence of significant auscultatory findings on examination of heart in association with congestive heart failure generally indicate underlying heart disease. Moreover, acute respiratory infection commonly supervenes in a child with congenital heart disease with left-to-right shunt. Sometimes, it is indeed very difficult to differentiate between respiratory distress due to congestive heart failure and pulmonary infection while at times both may coexist. Chest X-ray, ECG, and hyperoxia test may be helpful in differentiating the two.

GENERAL MANAGEMENT AND RESPIRATORY SUPPORT

Respiratory support is essential for all patients with respiratory distress. It is directed towards relieving hypoxemia by providing support to the respiratory functions until specific therapy for the underlying disease becomes effective.

(i) Allow the child to assume a *position of maximum comfort* and administer *oxygen* without agitating the child. Relief of the concomitant hypoxia will benefit respiratory distress due to any cause.

(ii) *Minimize handling and procedures.* There is no urgency to agitate the child for blood sampling if diagnosis is obvious e.g. immediate arterial blood gas analysis may be unnecessary in a cyanosed child or if SaO_2 is normal.

(iii) *Ensure adequacy of circulation and normal temperature and hydration.* Subsequently, repeated clinical and laboratory assessments may be undertaken to monitor the progression of the illness and adequacy of therapy.

Oxygen Therapy

Oxygen plays a vital role in checking the progress of incipient respiratory failure and for management of the established failure. Addition of oxygen to inspired air improves hemoglobin saturation only slightly but it increases concentration of oxygen dissolved in plasma. This provides an appreciable additional source of oxygen for the tissues, when considered in relation to the total amount of oxygen uptake by the tissues from the blood. Most of the conditions characterised by hypoxemia respond well to increased ambient oxygen. A*ny child who is cyanosed or has wheezing or stridor or a respiratory rate of >50/ min with intercostal recessions needs oxygen.* Infants under 2 months with a respiratory rate of >60/min should also receive oxygen[1].

Oxygen can be given by an intranasal catheter or nasal prongs at a flow rate of 1-3 L/min; too high a flow rate is wasteful. The catheter should be inserted one half of the distance between the tip of nose and tip of the ear. If the catheter is inserted too far it may enter the esophagus and cause gastric dilatation and further respiratory embarrassment. However, to deliver higher concentration of oxygen, an oxygen tent, a face mask, or a head box will be required. For children less than 18 months oxygen is best given in an oxygen tent and for those over 5 years with a facemask. Venturi face mask usually provides 25 to 40 percent oxygen. Some of the masks may provide upto 50 percent oxygen concentration in inspired air at a flow rate of 8-10 L/min, while >80% oxygen concentration can be achieved in a head box. There should be no interruption in oxygen therapy unless it is for a therapeutic reason.

Humidification

Ordinarily the inspired air gets saturated with water vapour during its passage through upper airway. When this process is disturbed or is bypassed such as with the use of endotracheal or tracheostomy tubes, inspired air or oxygen is no longer humidified. As a result, the epithelium of the respiratory passages gets dried up, ciliary functions are paralysed and mucous becomes viscid. This obstructs airways and causes atelectasis and intrapulmonary shunting. Humidification of inspired air and oxygen is, therefore, necessary. It may be achieved with the help of a condenser humidifier, heated water bath, or by nebulization[7].

Endotracheal Intubation

In children with severe respiratory distress, cyanosis or impending respiratory failure, endotracheal intubation is the preferred treatment. It protects the airways and permits the delivery of high concentration of oxygen and application of PEEP. A proper sized endotracheal tube should be used for optimal benefit.

Continuous Positive Airway Pressure (CPAP)

In the CPAP system, the child breathes spontaneously from a continuous flow of humidified gases, and exhales against a desired pressure resistance. This positive pressure prevents airway collapse and maintains patency of alveoli at the end of expiration. CPAP facility can be easily established in any emergency room. The air-flow (or air + oxygen mixture) during CPAP should be 2 to 3 times that of patient's minute volume. It can be given by a facemask for a short period of time. The problem with this method is inability to obtain a reliable tight fitting seal. There is also a danger of pressure necrosis of eyes and face. When CPAP is required for a long duration, it is preferable to use nasal prongs or endotracheal tube and T-piece.

The optimal CPAP requirements vary widely among different patients; it ranges from 5 to 20 cm H_2O. It is best to start CPAP with 5 cm H_2O or less; because all children with respiratory compromise will tolerate it. CPAP can be gradually stepped up in increments of 2 cm H_2O while monitoring paO_2 and $paCO_2$. At higher levels of CPAP (>10 cm H_2O) cardiac output may get compromised and should be monitored.

Mechanical Ventilation

Serious respiratory depression or paralysis causing hypoventilation or apnea is a recognized indication for artificial ventilation. Mechanical ventilation should also be considered in any severely distressed, cyanosed patient, whose hypoxemia (paO_2 < 60 mmHg) persists inspite of maximal oxygen therapy and who has a reversible disease such as pneumonia, aspiration syndrome, pulmonary edema, laryngotracheitis, bronchiolitis and asthma etc.

Any mode of ventilation is effective, as long as it allows adequate volume adjustment to make small changes that may be necessary for an infant. Volume limited ventilator continues to deliver a preset tidal volume even when the compliance of the lung decreases. In such a situation, airway pressure increases, and sometimes may be high enough to rupture the lung. On the other hand, pressure limited ventilator delivers a tidal volume till preset pressure limit is reached. The tidal volume is, therefore, variable. Any increase in the compliance may decrease the tidal volume and hence the alveolar ventilation. However, with careful monitoring the changes in pressure and compliance can be taken care of. Generally, it is more convenient to utilise pressure preset ventilators with variable flow rate in infants and young children (<10 kg), whereas volume preset ventilators are used most commonly in older children (>10 kg). For further details concerning assisted ventilation refer to Chapter 57.

SPECIFIC MANAGEMENT OF PNEUMONIAS

Bacterial Pneumonia

WHO has classified pneumonias in three categories; non severe pneumonia, severe pneumonia and very severe pneumonia, to streamline case management strategy at a small hospital and primary health center level. This classification and management strategies have been found useful at all levels (Table 16.3).

Most cases of severe and very severe pneumonia in developing countries are caused by *Streptococcus pneumoniae, H.influenzae, Staphylococcus aureus* and *Klebsiella* species. All children diagnosed to have pneumonia should, therefore, receive antibiotics because it is not possible to differentiate between viral and bacterial pneumonia with certainty.

Assess the severity of illness. Chest indrawing, cyanosis and inability to feed are reliable signs of severity of the disease process. Presence of any of the latter two signs is associated with

higher risk of mortality despite treatment[8]. Degree of fever and toxic appearance are less reliable indicators of severity of pneumonia. Severely malnourished children and infants below 3 months of age should be considered as severely ill and treated after admission to the hospital.

Non-severe pneumonia

Non-severe pneumonia is treated on ambulatory basis with oral antibiotics for 5 days. Oral amoxycillin is given in a dose of 15-20 mg/kg/dose every 8 hours. There is now sufficient evidence showing that three days of amoxycillin therapy is as effective as five days[9-11]. Co-trimoxazole is an effective alternative[12]. Mother should be advised to give extra fluids and adequate food to the child. Frequent feeding, continuation of breast feeding and oral fluid intake should be encouraged. Anorexia is common and child should not be forced but encouraged to eat. A review after 48 hours and after completion of antibiotic course is advised.

If the child has persistent raised respiratory rate but no indication for admission to the hospital, change to amoxycillin-clavulanic acid (80-90 mg/kg/day of amoxycillin) in 2 divided doses for 5 days or add azithromycin 5-10 mg/kg once daily for 5 days if clinical and radiological features suggest atypical pneumonia in an older child.

Cough medicines like expectorants, cough suppressants, and decongestants are not recommended because they are ineffective and associated with adverse effects.

Severe and very severe community acquired pneumonia (CAP)

Patients with signs of severe pneumonia (chest indrawing) or very severe pneumonia (cyanosis or inability to drink) need hospitalization and respiratory support. Humidified oxygen therapy should be started after clearing the airways with gentle suction and an IV line should be established. Oxygen may be delivered either by nasal catheter or prongs; both are equally effective[13]. An X-ray chest and septic work up (including lumbar tap if indicated) are mandatory.

Antibiotics must be administered parenterally, preferably intravenously. In severe pneumonia start therapy with amoxicillin (50 mg/kg/day in 3 divided doses) IV/IM For severe pneumonia without hypoxia, oral amoxicillin may be given instead of injectable ampicillin/amoxicillin when patient can be closely observed. When child has improved

Table 16.3 Classification of pneumonia and standard case management as proposed by WHO

No pneumonia	Pneumonia	Severe pneumonia	Very severe pneumonia
2 MONTHS – 5 YEARS OF AGE			
SIGNS			
No chest indrawing No fast breathing	No chest indrawing Fast breathing present (2-12 months >50/min, 1-5 yr >40/min)	Chest indrawing, nasal flaring, grunting and cyanosis	Not able to drink, convulsions, abnormally sleepy or difficult to wake, stridor in a calm child, severe malnutrition
TREATMENT			
Symptomatic treatment of cough and cold	Start oral amoxycillin Reasses after 48 hr. Give antibiotics for 5 days	Treat fever/wheeze and give any one of the following antibiotics: <ul><li>C. Penicillin 50,000 u/kg per dose 6 hourly IM</li><li>Ampicillin 50 mg/ kg/dose 6 hourly IM</li><li>Chloramphenicol 25 mg/kg/dose IM</li></ul> *After 48 hrs** Oral ampicillin or amoxycillin therapy for 5 days	Treat fever/wheeze If cerebral malaria is a possibility, give antimalarials <ul><li>Oxygen, IV fluids</li><li>Ampicillin 50 mg/ kg/dose 6 hourly IM/IV plus gentamicin 7.5 mg OD, IM/ IV for 7-14 d. Change to oral ampicillin or amoxicillin after 4-5 days when child starts accepting orally and has no chest indrawing</li></ul>

No pneumonia	Severe pneumonia	Very severe pneumonia		
LESS THAN 2 MONTHS				
SIGNS				
No chest indrawing No fast breathing	Severe chest indrawing or fast breathing > 60/min	Refusal of feeds, convulsions, abnormally sleepy or difficult to wake, stridor in a calm child, fever/ low body temperature, wheezing		
			< 7d	>7d
TREATMENT				
<ul><li>Keep infant warm</li><li>Breast feed</li><li>Frequently clear the nose</li></ul>	Refer urgently to a hospital after giving 1st dose of antibiotic: Ampicillin and gentamicin	C. Penicillin 50,000 iu/kg/dose +	12 hr	6 hr
		Ampicillin 50 mg/kg/dose +	12 hr	8 hr
		Gentamicin 2.5 mg/kg/dose	12 hr	8 hr

*If no response in 48 hours: Change to cloxacillin plus gentamicin in very severe pneumonia and ampicillin plus chloramphenicol in severe pneumonia.

significantly and chest indrawing has settled (usually after 2 to 3 days) oral amoxycillin 15 mg/kg/dose 8 hourly is substituted. In infants below 2 months of age and in those with very severe pneumonia a combination of ampicillin (100-200 mg/kg/day) and gentamicin (5.0 7.5 mg/kg/day) or amikacin is recommended for 10 days. Early switch over from parenteral to oral therapy decreases cost of care due to reduced duration of hospitalization[14]. For children with severe and very severe community-acquired pneumonia, ampicillin with gentamicin is superior to chloramphenicol[15]. The other alternative drugs for such patients include ceftriaxone, levofloxacin, amox-clavulanate and cefuroxime axetil[11].

If staphylococcal pneumonia is suspected (presence of a large dense areas with one or more pneumatoceles on chest X-ray), cloxacillin (25-50 mg/kg/dose 6 hourly IV) plus gentamicin (5.0-7.5 mg/kg once a day IV) or amikacin (15 mg/kg single dose daily) should be used. If child does not improve within 24-48 hours, consider administration of antibiotics to cover Gram-negative organisms. Ceftriaxone (50 mg/kg/dose q 8 hr IV) is useful for management of life-threatening pneumonia. Our protocols for treatment of community acquired pneumonia are available elsewhere[16].

Supportive Care

(a) **Fluid therapy**. Dehydration if present should be corrected by intravenous infusion of 0.18% (N/5) saline in 5% glucose solution. There is no evidence that liberal fluid intake will loosen the pulmonary secretions. On the other hand, it may cause over hydration because of high levels of circulating ADH. Intravenous line should be maintained for first 3 to 4 days for administration of antibiotics. Since hyponatremia and inappropriate ADH secretion is common in pneumonia, it is wiser to restrict maintenance fluids to about two third of the normal maintenance requirements during first 2-3 days of hospital stay while closely monitoring the hydration status of the patient.[17]

(b) **Warmth**. It is important to avoid over heating or exposing a child with pneumonia, because both can increase the oxygen consumption of the child by two to three folds and precipitate respiratory failure. Therefore, patient should be nursed in a comfortable warm room (25-28°C).

(c) **Humidification and steam inhalation** is generally practiced but it has not been shown to influence recovery or shorten the duration of respiratory distress and hospitalisation in children with pneumonia[7].

(d) **Antipyretics**. Moderate elevation of body temperature (upto 38°C) improves body's defenses against infection. High fever increases oxygen consumption and may cause convulsions and should be controlled by use of paracetamol (15 mg/kg/dose every 4-6 hourly). Cold or tepid water sponging is usually uncomfortable, not very effective and greatly increases oxygen consumption due to shivering, which may precipitate respiratory failure in a child with severe pneumonia.

(e) **Avoid the use of sedatives** especially those which are known to cause depression of respiratory center. The irritability and restlessness is a sign of hypoxia, which should be managed by improving oxygenation. If necessary small doses of trichlophos or chloral hydrate may be used with caution.

Monitoring

(i) *If child worsens* as evidenced by increasing severity of distress; consider a change in antibiotics. Septic work-up should be repeated and lung aspiration obtained for etiological diagnosis. Radiograph of chest should be repeated to look for development of empyema, pleural effusion or air leaks.

(ii) *When respiratory failure* supervenes consider a trial of CPAP, and if it fails switch over to mechanical ventilation.

(iii) *When there is no improvement or child worsens during the treatment* reassess for possible diagnosis of pulmonary tuberculosis, undiagnosed asthma, foreign body aspiration, presence of congestive cardiac failure, and unusual pathogens like chlamydiae and *Pneumocystis carinii*. Further diagnostic work-up and appropriate therapy to cover the unusual pathogens is recommended[18].

Measles pneumonia

Children with measles pneumonia are generally severely ill. Pneumonia early in the course of the illness with rash is usually of interstitial type due to measles virus. Pneumonia appearing after disappearance of rash or after several days of onset of illness is generally due to secondary bacterial infection. The most common etiologic agent in such cases is S. *aureus*; therefore, severely ill patients are best treated with amoxicillin-clavulanic acid or a combination of cloxacillin (25 50 mg/kg/dose 6 hourly) and gentamicin (5 mg/kg once daily) intravenously. Supportive therapy and monitoring should be ensured as described above.

Mortality in measles is by and large related to superadded bacterial pneumonia. Use of prophylactic antibiotics like penicillins or co-trimoxazole can significantly reduce the burden of pneumonia, and reduce the morbidity and mortality as shown in a meta-analysis[20]. Although there is some evidence to suggest that vitamin A supplementation reduces the severity of respiratory infection and other systemic complications of measles, the WHO Programme for the Control of Acute Respiratory Infections did not find unequivocal evidence for this benefit[20]. A recent Cochrane review found no overall significant reduction is mortality with vitamin A therapy for children with measles, however two doses reduced overall and pneumonia specific mortality in children aged less than 2 years. No trials directly compared a single dose with two doses of vitamin A[21].

Whooping cough

Typically the child with whooping cough has upper respiratory tract symptoms, progressing to irritating cough within a few days and to paroxysms of cough within 2-3 weeks. Any child below 6 months of age with a probable diagnosis of whooping cough or with a history of convulsions or signs of respiratory distress and pneumonia should be hospitalised.

(i) The patency of airways should be maintained by gentle suctioning

(ii) Oxygen should be administered if child becomes cyanosed while coughing.

(iii) Erythromycin (10-15 mg/kg/dose 8 hourly), is first line drug. It is effective in reducing the infectivity of the patient and to treat superadded pneumonia. Other macrolides such as azithromycin and clarithromycin are equally effective and have fewer side effects[22-23]. In infants under one month of age azithromycin is the drug of choice for treatment or prophylaxis[24]. An effective alternative for patients above 2 months of age who can not tolerate macrolides is trimethoprim-sulfamethoxazole; it eradicates *B. pertussis* and may be better tolerated by some patients[24].

(iv) The morbidity in whooping cough is related to the paroxysmal nature of the cough. Various interventions have been tried to control cough including corticosteroids, salbutamol, anti-histamines (diphenhydramine) and pertussis-specific immunoglobulin. However, a systematic review to assess their effectiveness concluded that the available data was insufficient to demonstrate a clear benefit from any of these interventions[25].

(v) If convulsions occur, phenobarbitone (10 mg/kg loading dose, followed by 5 mg/kg/day) therapy is recommended for 2 weeks.

(vi) The supportive therapy should be provided. Special emphasis should be given to feeding after paroxysms of cough and vomiting. It is important to remember that pertussis is highly contagious and 70 to 100 percent of susceptible household members and 50 to 80 percent of susceptible school contacts become infected following exposure[27.] The antimicrobial agents and dosages used for chemoprophylaxis of contacts are the same as that recommended for treatment of the patient[26].

Aspiration pneumonia

Children with altered state of consciousness, mental retardation, impaired gag reflex, cough or swallowing, esophageal reflux, hiatus hernia or tracheoesophageal fistula are at increased risk of aspiration pneumonia. Aspiration of nasopharyngeal or gastric contents introduces a large inoculum of bacteria into the respiratory tract. The acidic nature of the gastric contents, in addition may cause alveolar injury, pulmonary edema and reflex bronchospasm. The common end result is a gravity-dependent pneumonia, or necrotising pneumonia and less often, lung abscess and empyema as sequelae. Bacterial culture from transtracheal aspirate in such cases in one series showed an average of 4.9 isolates per specimen with equal preponderance of anerobes and aerobes. Common anerobes were *Bacteroides, Peptococcus,* and *Peptostreptococcus while aerobes included Hemolytic streptococci, Pseudomonas aeruginosa, S. pneumoniae, E. coli, Klebsiella pneumoniae and Staphylococcus aureus.* Antimicrobial therapy in these children should, therefore, be adequate to cover above organisms. Gram-negative organisms are more likely under 2 years of age. In a previously healthy immunocompetent child, a a beta-lactam penicillin with a beta-lactamase inhibitor (amoxicillin-clavulanate or piperacillin tazobactum) or clindamycin is adequate. In a previously unwell hospitalised child, gentamicin (5.0 mg/kg single dose daily) or amikacin (15 mg/kg single dose daily) with a third generation cephalosporin (cefotaxime, ceftriaxone) is recommended. If *Pseudomonas aeruginosa* is suspected, or the patient is immunocompromised, piperacillin-tazobactum or ceftazidime should be added to the regimen[27].

SPECIFIC MANAGEMENT OF UPPER AIRWAY OBSTRUCTION

The modalities of treatment are summarized in Table 16.4.

Laryngotracheitis (Viral croup)

The management is mainly supportive and directed at relieving mucosal edema.

(i) The child with mild croup can be managed at home if stridor and recessions disappear at

Table 16.4 Specific treatment priorities for management of upper airway obstruction	
Diagnosis	**Therapy**
• Mild laryngotracheitis	Observation at home, mist or steam
• Moderate laryngotracheitis	Admission to hospital, observation, inhaled budesonide and mist
• Severe laryngotracheitis	Close observation, oxygen, intravenous dexamethasone and nebulized adrenaline; may require intubation
• Spasmodic croup	Usually nebulized budesonide, may need adrenaline nebulization
• Acute epiglottitis	Elective intubation (preceded by minimal disturbance) and intravenous antibiotics
• Bacterial tracheitis	Usually require intubation, antibiotics to treat S. *aureus and H. influenzae*
• Foreign body	Removal by rigid bronchoscopy
• Tonsillar obstruction	Antibiotics if bacterial cause, steroids unproven in EBV infection. Occasionally require nasopharyngeal airway, or endotracheal intubation
• Retropharyngeal abscess	Surgical drainage and antibiotics
• Diphtheria	Antitoxin and penicillin. Usually require tracheostomy
• Acute angioneurotic edema	Adrenaline IM

Section 2

rest. The patient should be hospitalized if stridor is present at rest and there is moderate to severe respiratory distress.

(ii) Avoid unpleasant and traumatic investigations.

(iii) Give oxygen and cold nebulised mist or steam. Warm or cold humidified air remains the mainstay of therapy[7]. Owing to lack of scientific evidence of its efficacy, the practice of humidification of inspired air has been abandoned in many countries[28-29].

(iv) To relieve severe symptoms, adrenaline (epinephrine) 3-5 ml of 1:1000 solution or racemic epinephrine as nebulised aerosol (2.25% solution in 1:8 dilution) is recommended. The therapy is more effective when given with intermittent positive pressure breathing (IPPB) by using a facemask. This reduces the need for intubation in severe cases. The effect lasts for upto 45 minutes. Treatment may be repeated 2 hourly if stridor recurs. Clinical evaluation, pulse oximetery, ECG and cardiac monitoring should be done while using this therapy.

(v) Corticosteroids in some form are needed for sustained relief of symptoms. A detailed systematic review comprising 31 studies with over 3700 subjects concluded that dexamethasone and budesonide are effective in relieving symptoms of croup and are associated with decreased rate of hospitalization, shorter duration of hospital stay if admitted, reduced incidence of endotracheal intubation and fewer return visits to the hospital[30].

Nebulized dexamethasone or budesonide (1,000 μg given 30 minutes apart) or oral dexamethasone provides prompt and significant clinical improvement in children with mild to moderate croup and reduces the need for hospitalization[30,31]. Nebulized budesonide is as effective as nebulised adrenaline in moderately severe croup[32]. Oral dexamethasone in combination with racemic epinephrine and mist is generally effective as outpatient treatment[33].

(vi) Severe cases should receive hydrocortisone 10 mg/kg or dexamethasone 0.3-0.6 mg/kg/ dose IV; repeated 6 hourly for 4 doses. A high single dose of dexamethasone upto 1.0-1.5 mg/ kg has also been used. Higher doses are associated with earlier improvement and better outcome.

(vii) Consider endotracheal intubation if severe distress persists, or signs of respiratory failure appear ($paCO_2$ >50 mmHg). Use a smaller endotracheal tube size than normally recommended to negotiate obstruction and avoid trauma. As a guideline, use 3.5 mm diameter tube for children between 3 months to 3 years, 4.0 mm for 3-5 years and 4.5 mm for above 5 years. If intubation fails tracheostomy is indicated.

Bacterial Tracheitis

If bacterial tracheitis is suspected, antibiotics that cover *S. aureus, Streptococcus, Moraxella (Brahamnella) catarrhalis* and *H. influenzae* are administered. A combination of cloxacillin (100-200 mg/kg in 4 divided doses per day) and ceftriaxone

(50-100 mg/kg/day single dose) is recommended. Early intubation is necessary for effective clearing of the airways.

Acute Epiglottitis

Sudden death may occur if diagnosis and treatment is delayed. The following guidelines should be followed:

(i) If epiglottitis is strongly suspected, do not disturb the child, and do not examine the throat in a hurry. All cases need admission to PICU and urgent attention.

(ii) Provide humidified oxygen with a bag and mask, if this does not agitate the child.

(iii) If indicated, establish an emergency airway (Bag and mask, cricothyrotomy).

(iv) Electively intubate all patients. Intubation in a controlled situation, under general anesthesia is preferable. If intubation fails, do a tracheostomy.

(v) Obtain blood culture and complete blood counts.

(vi) Give intravenous ceftriaxone (100 mg/kg stat, maximum 2 g, then 50 mg/kg /dose 12 hourly).

(vii) Nasotracheal tube can be removed after 48-72 hours in most cases, as recovery is usually very rapid.

Foreign Bodies

(i) Assess the child for severity of respiratory distress and give resuscitative or supportive therapy accordingly.

(ii) Establish the location of the foreign body by taking X-ray chest PA and lateral views, and both inspiratory and expiratory films.

(iii) If it is suspected in the upper airways, remove it as early as possible. Place the child face downward across your knees and give 3 to 4 blows to the back. If this fails, proceed with rapid compressions of chest four times as if performing external cardiac massage to raise intrathoracic pressure. In children over one year of age, Heimlich maneuver may be performed. It is most easily performed from behind the patient, by placing one's hands on the upper abdomen and rapidly squeezing it towards epigastrium. Sudden compression of upper abdomen forces the diaphragm up and propels the object out of the airway.

(iv) If these procedures fail, it may be possible to remove the foreign body by visualization under direct laryngoscopy and use of a Magill's forceps. An emergency airway with wide bore cannula inserted through cricothyroid membrane in trachea must be established before the procedure.

(v) If this fails urgent bronchoscopic removal is indicated. While some institutions routinely perform rigid bronchoscopy for removal, it is possible to do this with a flexible fiber-optic bronchoscope as well.

(vi) If the child is breathing and able to cough, give oxygen and leave in position of comfort. Arrange for bronchoscopy as soon as possible, even if there is complete relief of symptoms. It is especially true of peanut aspiration because symptoms are likely to aggravate due to omotic swelling of the nut. This is one situation where a negative endoscopy is preferable to missing the foreign body.

Angioneurotic Edema

The condition is best treated by intramuscular administration of adrenaline (1:1000), 0.01 ml/kg (maximum 0.3 ml), hydrocortisone 10 mg/kg IV and antihistamines such as chlorpheniramine maleate.

Retropharyngeal Abscess

The following steps of management should be followed:

(i) Antibiotics: Cloxacillin (100 mg/kg/day q 6 hr) and gentamicin (5-7.5 mg/kg/day q 8 hr) IV.

(ii) Active management of airways. Endotracheal intubation should be done in any child with a significant degree of obstruction even if air exchange appears adequate initially. Orotracheal intubation is preferred because of the risk of rupture of the abscess[34].

(iii) Surgical drainage.

Diphtheria

Although uncommon, diphtheria can kill and should be managed promptly using the following protocol:

(i) Send throat swab for bacteriological studies (Albert's stain and culture) to confirm the diagnosis.

(ii) If signs of severe airway obstruction (stridor, severe distress and cyanosis) are present, establish emergency airway and *consider an early tracheostomy,* which is usually required.

(iii) Give diphtheria antitoxin 80,000-120,000 units preferably IV or IM.

(iv) Administer procaine penicillin 50,000 u/kg/day IM for 7-10 days.

Acute Asthma Exacerbation

Asthma is a reversible obstructive airway disease; the obstruction is caused by a combination of bronchospasm and inflammation (mucosal edema, and excessive secretions causing mucous plugging). The goal of therapy in acute asthma, therefore, is to rapidly and safely reverse airway obstruction. Bronchodilator drugs and cortico-steroids as anti-inflammatory agents are the mainstay of therapy in reversing acute severe asthma along with supportive respiratory care. For details regarding the pathophysiology and management of acute severe asthma refer to Chapter 30.

Evaluation

The evaluation should include information on duration of wheezing, medications used and time of their administration, any precipitating factors such as infection, allergens, drugs or exercise, oral fluid intake, course of previous episodes and outcome. The severity of attack (Table 16.5), especially signs of hypoxemia and exhaustion, air entry in the lungs, peak expiratory flow rate (PEFR) and presence of pulsus paradoxus should be assessed and recorded. Marked tachypnea, chest wall indrawing, use of accessory muscles of respiration, diminished or absent breath sounds, PEFR <50% of expected, cyanosis, and pulsus paradoxus of 20 mmHg or more indicate a severe or life-threatening attack. Fatigue, somnolence, disorientation and air hunger indicate impending respiratory failure.

Initial Treatment

(i) Administer oxygen by face mask and a rapid acting bronchodilator (β_2 agonist) by nebulization. Give nebulized salbutamol (0.5% solution, 0.15-0.30 mg/kg/dose diluted in 2 3 ml normal saline) every 20 minutes for a maximum of 3 doses.

(ii) Inhaled salbutamol using a spacer device may be used as an alternative in mild and moderate exacerbation. One can use adrenaline (epinephrine) 1: 1000 solution, 0.01 ml/kg/dose (maximum dose 0.3 ml), subcutaneously or intramuscularly every 15-20 minutes for a maximum of 3 doses if inhaled or nebulised salbutamol cannot be given.

(iii) Inhaled budesonide (800 µg/dose) either by MDI or nebulization at 20 min intervals and a

Table 16.5 Clinical signs useful for assessment of severity of acute asthma

Clinical manifestations of severe acute asthma
- Tachycardia >120 beats/min
- Tachypnea >30 breaths/min
- Dyspnea
- Inability to speak
- Use of accessory muscles of breathing
- Pulsus paradoxus >15 mmHg

Signs of a life-threatening attack
- A silent chest on auscultation
- Cyanosis
- Altered consciousness
- Respiratory muscle fatigue (e.g. abdominal paradox)
- Pneumothorax

single dose of oral predinsolone or along with salbutamol improves initial response and reduces the need for hospitalization[36-37].

(iv) After each dose assessment should include the respiratory status and heart rate. If there is significant clearance of wheeze with improved air entry and PEFR is >70% of the expected, the child may be sent home on salbutamol therapy and called for review after 48 hours.

Severely distressed patients and those who fail to respond to initial emergency treatment

These children should be admitted to the hospital and managed with following protocol.

(i) Continue humidified oxygen by facemask or nasal prongs.

(ii) Obtain ABGs and chest X-ray to rule out pneumothorax, pneumonia, and pulmonary edema.

(iii) Maximize nebulised salbutamol; give 0.15-0.3 mg/kg every hourly, or by continuous nebulization. Continuous nebulization is safe and results in more rapid clinical improvement than intermittent nebulization. A systematic review addressed the question of whether continuous rather than intermittent nebulization is more beneficial and concluded that continuous delivery of beta-2 agonist was a better option in severe exacerbation and those not responding to intermittent nebulization[38].

(iv) Give intravenous hydrocortisone 5-10 mg/kg or methyl prednisolone 2 mg/kg every 4-6 hourly. Oral prednisolone should be substituted when acute attack is subsiding and tapered off over next 5-7 days. There is no benefit of adding inhaled corticosteroids to systemic steroids[39]. Any child who had required hospitalization for a previous attack of asthma or is on long-term corticosteroid therapy should also receive intravenous corticosteroids. Early administration of corticosteroids is vital because there is delay of several hours before measurable relief in airway obstruction is achieved.

(v)   Ipratropium bromide by nebulization 250-500 ug every 20 minutes for 3 doses may reduce the need for hospitalization[40]. Single dose of anticholinergic is not effective for the treatment of mild and moderate exacerbations and is insufficient for the treatment of severe exacerbations. Adding multiple doses of anticholinergics to beta-2 agonists appears safe, improves lung function and would avoid hospital admission in 1 of 12 such treated patients. However, there is no conclusive evidence for using multiple doses of anticholinergics in children with mild or moderate exacerbations[40].

(vi) Intravenous aminophylline by continuous infusion: Use of intravenous aminophylline in acute severe asthma has gradually gone out of favour because of a narrow therapeutic index and availability of other therapeutic options. However, IV aminophylline may be used in patients who have fail to respond to above treatment[41]. If patient has not received any rapidly absorbable theophylline preparation in the last 4 hours, or a slow release preparation in the last 12-18 hours, a loading dose is required (5-6 mg/kg slowly over 20 minutes). It is followed by continuous infusion of 0.65-0.8 mg/kg/hr in children above 1 year of age. If theophylline medications have been taken recently, then a lower loading dose of 2-3 mg/kg is used. A systematic review on the use of aminophylline in children concluded that addition of intravenous aminophylline should be considered early in the treatment of acute severe asthma with suboptimal response to the initial inhaled bronchodilator therapy. There is increased risk of vomiting following administration of aminophylline through any route.

(vii) In patients with acute moderate and severe asthma who have failed to respond to initial treatment, magnesium sulfate (50-75 mg/kg or 0.1 ml of 50% sol/kg) IV infusion over 20 minutes is a useful modality[42, 43]. It may be repeated every 6 hourly for 3-4 doses.

(viii) Acidosis should be corrected if pH is <7.15. with slow intravenous infusion of sodium bicarbonate 1-2 mEq/kg diluted with double volume of 5% dextrose. This reduces myocardial irritability and enhances bronchodilator responsiveness.

(ix) The patient should be monitored for respiratory status, heart rate, blood pressure, SpO_2, PEFR and arterial pH and blood gases. Cardiac monitoring is desirable in patients receiving aminophylline infusion. Complications such as pneumothorax, mucous plugs and pulmonary edema should be looked for when stepping up the therapy. Respiratory failure should be suspected if the patient has poor air exchange, low SpO_2, persistent cyanosis or depressed level of consciousness. If there is refractory hypoxemia (paO_2 < 60 mmHg), severe hypercapnia ($paCO_2$ >50 mmHg) or continuing rise in $paCO_2$ by 5 mmHg per hour, the patient should be admitted to the intensive care unit.

(x)   Infusion of β_2 sympathomimetics like terburaline or salbutamol may avoid the need for assisted ventilation[44]. It is recommended to administer IV salbutamol 5 µg/kg over 10 min, followed by infusion of 0.1-0.4 µg/kg/min (maximum 4 µg/kg/min) or terbutaline 10 µg/kg over 30 min, followed by infusion at 0.1 mg/kg/min gradually increased to 0.4 mg/kg/min (maximum of 4 mg/kg/min). A separate intravenous line and an infusion pump should be used for its administration.

In a recently completed study at our centre, magnesium sulphate infusion was superior to terbutaline and aminophylline infusion in children who had failed to respond to one hour treatment with salbutamol, ipratropium and inhaled and systemic corticosteroids[45]. Sedation with ketamine and inhalation of anesthetic gases like isoflurane may be tried.

Mechanical ventilation is indicated if signs of life-threatening attack appear or respiratory failure supervenes despite aggressive medical therapy. Stabilize the patient on 100% oxygen by bag and mask. Clear the airways of secretions, aspirate the stomach, do a nasotracheal intubation and connect to a volume preset ventilator, to give a tidal volume of 8 ml/kg. Inspiratory expiratory ratio should be kept at 1:3 and PIP of <30 cm of H_2O. Bronchodilator therapy should be continued during ventilation. Sedation with morphine 0.1-0.2 mg/kg or pethidine 1-2 mg/kg and neuromuscular blockade may be required.

Fluid and electrolyte therapy. These children are generally mildly dehydrated. The deficit should be corrected gradually over 24 hours period. The maintenance fluid should be 0.45% saline (N/2 saline) in 5% dextrose solution with 40 mEq/L of potassium. Hypokalemia may occur because of salbutamol nebulization[46] or increased urinary potassium loss due to steroids and theophylline induced diuresis. Hydration status should be closely monitored; over hydration should be avoided, as renal water excretion capacity is impaired in status asthmaticus.

Antibiotics may be used when superadded bacterial infection is suspected. Cough expectorants do not have any proven role.

ACUTE BRONCHIOLITIS

The management is mainly supportive[47]. It is directed at assessment of respiratory status and prevention of respiratory failure. Mild illness may be treated on an ambulatory basis by advising adequate intake of fluids and providing steam inhalation and humidity. Children over one year of age may be administered salbutamol though its role is doubtful. Antibiotics are not indicated unless there is superadded bacterial infection. The following treatment protocol should be followed in infants with severe illness.

(i) **Hospitalize.** Avoid agitating the child. A mild sedative like trichlophos may be used to pacify a crying infant. Set up an IV line.

(ii) Administer humidified oxygen to relieve hypoxia. This is the most important therapeutic modality. Humidified oxygen 30-40% may be given through a venturi facemask or through a head box. Oxygen levels inside the head box should be monitored.

(iii) Get an X-ray chest, blood counts and blood culture and arterial blood gas measurement.

(iv) Give steam inhalation every 4-6 hourly, for about 20 30 minutes in a tent. Most babies respond within 24 hours[7].

(v) *β₂-agonist inhalation*. Nebulized salbutamol (0.5 ml of 0.5% solution + 1.5 ml saline) or l-epinephrine may be used in an emergency situation[48,49]. Adrenaline subcutaneously in the same doses as for asthma can be tried if child is over one year of age. There is some evidence that adrenaline (epinephrine) is more effective[50]. If no beneficial response is achieved, β₂-agonist inhalation should be discontinued. In general bronchodilators produce modest short term improvement in clinical features of mild or moderately severe bronchiolitis and are not recommended for routine management of first time wheezers.

(vi) *Nebulised hypertonic saline*. It may help in making secretions less viscous and promote their excretion, resulting in clinical improvement. However, nebulized hypertonic saline has a limited role in bronchiolitis.

(vii) *Corticosteroids*. A recent RCT concluded that combined therapy with dexamethasone 1 mg/kg (maximum dose 10 mg) once daily IM or IV for 5 days and epinephrine nebulization (3 ml of 1:1000 solution) may significantly reduce hospital stay[51].

(viii) *Antibiotics* are not indicated but if there is a suspicion of bronchopneumonia, provide a broad-spectrum antibiotic coverage.

(ix) *Ribavirin aerosol therapy* (20 mg/ml) for 12-18 hours per day for 3-5 days may be used in selected high-risk groups with RSV infection namely infants with congenital heart disease, bronchopulmonary dysplasia, immuno-deficiency disorder or respiratory failure. Nonetheless, it is very expensive and offers only marginal benefit. Current evidence suggests that in children and infants admitted to hospital with RSV bronchiolitis, ribavirin did not significantly reduce mortality, respiratory deterioration, or duration of hospital stay compared with placebo but it significantly reduced the duration of ventilation compared with placebo[52].

(x) *Monitor* the progress by recording vital signs.

(xi) *Consider CPAP* using facemask, nasal catheters or ET tube if there are any apneic attacks or paCO₂ >60 mmHg, or if signs of exhaustion appear. A recent randomized controlled trial (n=31) compared the use of nasal CPAP with standard treatment. CPAP improved ventilation and hypercapnia[53].

(xii) *Intubation and ventilation* is required if apnea is recurrent and signs of respiratory failure are observed.

(xiii) *Fluid therapy*. In most of the seriously ill infants, adequate oral fluid intake cannot be maintained; and intravenous hydration is required. Inappropriate secretion of antidiuretic hormone is common, body water is increased and renal water excretion is impaired in acute phase of bronchiolitis[54]. It is, therefore, wise to give two-thirds of normal maintenance fluid requirements and monitor clinical signs of over hydration.

(xiv) Lately surfactant and intravenous immuno-globulins (IVIG) have been shown to be of some benefit. However, the indication for their use and doses need to be defined.

(xv) Physiotherapy of chest may be useful if the child is not critically ill.

PNEUMOTHORAX

A tension pneumothorax is seen commonly following rupture of a pneumatocele in staphylococcal pneumonia, rupture of an emphysematous bulla or a pulmonary cyst or trauma. Once the clinical diagnosis is made, rapid decompression is indicated without waiting for a confirmatory chest X-ray. A needle aspiration in the second or third intercostal space just lateral to mid clavicular line followed by an intercostal tube connected to under water seal drainage with mild suction (5 to 10 cm H_2O) should be undertaken urgently (Figure 16.1A). A chest X-ray should be obtained after the evacuation of the air to assess the reexpansion of the lungs. In most instances the drainage will be required for a few days.

In case of a post traumatic open pneumo-thorax, which is a life-threatening emergency, occlude the chest wall defect by a bulky sterile dressing and convert this open pneumothorax to a tension pneumothorax. Simultaneously, establish a pleural decompression by closed intercostal tube drainage (Figure 16.1B). Definitive repair of the defect can be undertaken at a later stage.

MONITORING

Monitoring the clinical status of an acutely ill child with respiratory distress is mandatory. Although it is possible to monitor some parameters such as respiratory rate, heart rate and blood pressure by an electronic multichannel vital sign monitor, but human observations are indispensable. The information is vital for continuing therapy and for early diagnosis of respiratory failure. The following data should be recorded on a flow sheet:

1. *Vital signs.* Breathing (rate, rhythm, depth, use of accessory muscles), heart rate, blood pressure and core body temperature.

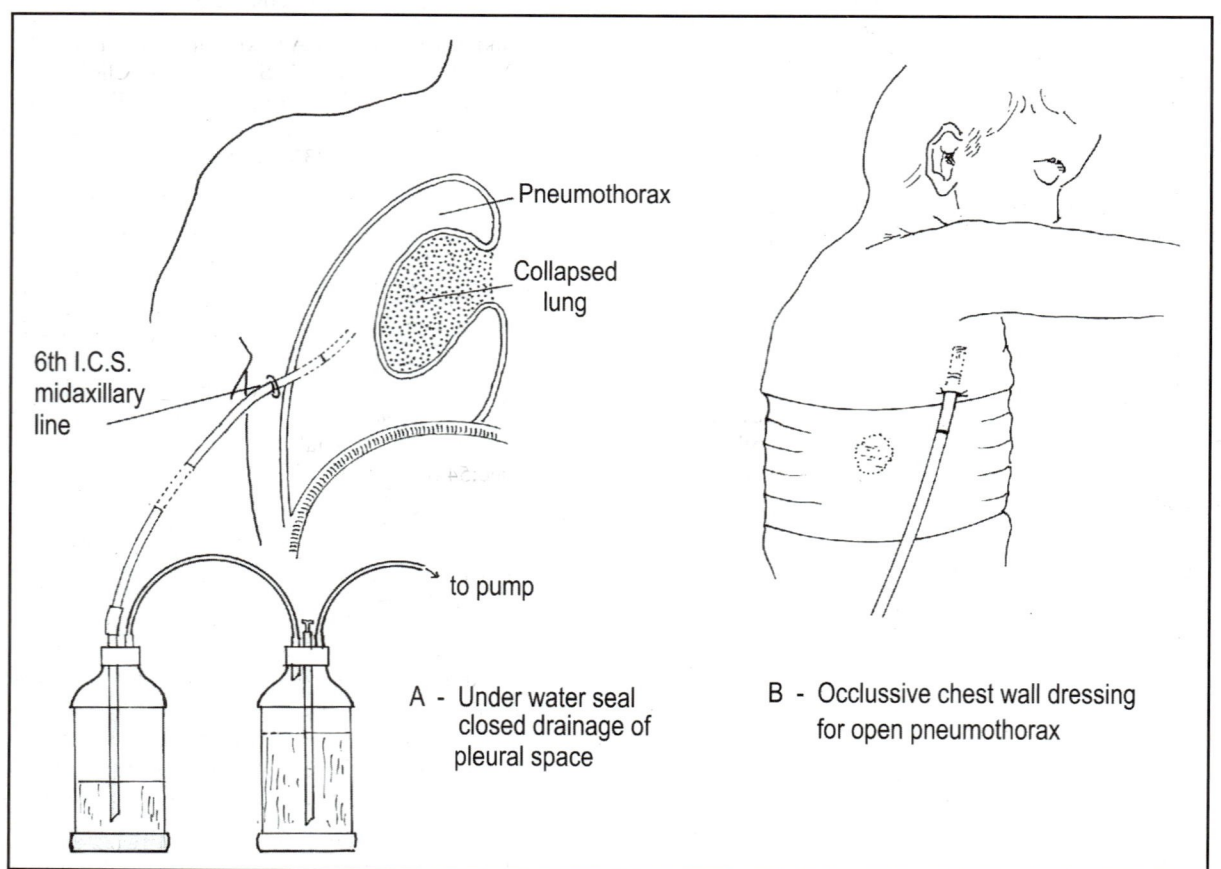

Pneumothorax

Collapsed lung

6th I.C.S. midaxillary line

to pump

A - Under water seal closed drainage of pleural space

B - Occlussive chest wall dressing for open pneumothorax

Figure 16.1 Underwater seal drainage is essential to avoid entry of atmospheric air into the pleural cavity. Gentle constant negative pressure of 5-10 cm H_2O facilitates the drainage of air and pus (A). In open pneumothorax following chest trauma, the chest wall should be dressed tightly to seal the external wound (B)

2. Presence/absence of cyanosis

3. Use of accessory muscles, flaring of alae nasi and chest wall retractions, and degree of the distress.

4. Air entry in both lungs. In case an endotracheal tube has been passed, check its position and patency and need for suction.

5. Signs of exhaustion such as somnolence, confusion, and seizures.

6. Non invasive monitoring. Oxygen saturation (pulse oximetry) is a very useful noninvasive parameter of oxygen requirement. It also helps in quick recognition of hypoxia before baby turns blue. SaO_2 of < 90% indicates hypoxemia. Similarly end tidal CO_2 (Et CO_2) is helpful to estimate CO_2 levels.

7. Arterial blood gases (ABGs). Blood gas measurement is the best objective determinant of ventilation. This must be interpreted together with the clinical data of the patient.

Arterial pH gives information regarding ventilatory and metabolic status of the patient. $paCO_2$ reflects the adequacy of alveolar ventilation while paO_2 reflects alveolar gas exchange. paO_2 may also be affected by inadequate perfusion or increased metabolic demands. Determination of paO_2 in room air and in 100% oxygen can help to distinguish between ventilation/perfusion inequality and large left-to-right shunt. The paO_2 in 100% oxygen will be greater than 100 mmHg if ventilation/perfusion abnormality is present.

In severely distressed children and those on mechanical ventilation, frequent monitoring (every half to one hour intervals) may be needed. Whenever there is any change in clinical signs or settings of ventilator, ABGs must be checked. In moderately distressed children, or those who have improved and have a stable clinical picture, monitoring may be required less frequently. Monitoring of ambient oxygen concentration, reliability and functionality of the electronic equipment should also be checked regularly.

REFERENCES

1. Rajesh VT, Singhi S, Katariya S. Tachypnea is a good predictor of hypoxia in acutely ill infants under 2 months. *Arch Dis Child* 2000; 82: 46-49.

2. Singhi S, Singh RP, Kumar L, Walia BNS. Bacterial tracheitis. *Indian Pediatr* 1989; 26:390-396.

3. Morrison JE, Pashley NRT. Retropharyngeal abscess in children: A 10-year review. *Pediatr Emerg Care* 1988; 4:9-11.

4. WHO Programme for the Control of Acute Respiratory Infections. *Technical Basis for the WHO Recommendations on Management of Pneumonia in Children at first level health facilities.* WHO/ARI/91.20. 1991; 12-16.

5. Poole SR, Mauro RD, Fan LL and Broks J. The child with simultaneous stridor and wheezing. *Pediatr Emerg Care* 1990; 6:33-37.

6. Day RL, Gelin ES, Dubois B. Choking. The Heimlich abdominal thrust vs back blows, an approach to measurement of inertial and aerodynamic forces. *Pediatrics* 1982, 70:113-119.

7. Singh M, Singhi S, Walia BNS. Evaluation of steam therapy in acute lower respiratory tract infections: a pilot study. *Indian Pediatr* 1990; 27:945-951.

8. WHO Programme for the Control of Acute Respiratory Infections. Acute respiratory infections in children: Case management in small hospitals in developing countries. *A Manual for Doctors and Other Senior Health Workers.* WHO/ARI/90.5 1990: 5-11.

9. Agarwal G, Awasthi S, Kabra SK, Kaul A, Singhi S, Walter SD; ISCAP Study Group. Three day versus five day treatment with amoxicillin for non-severe pneumonia in young children: a multicentre randomised controlled trial. *BMJ* 2004; 328(7443):791.

10. Pakistan Multicentre Amoxicillin Short Course Therapy (MASCOT) Pneumonia Study Group. Clinical efficacy of 3 days versus 5 days of oral amoxicillin for treatment of childhood pneumonia: a multicentre double-blind trial. *Lancet* 2002: 360; 835-841.

11. Kabra SK, Lodha R. Pandey RM, Antibiotics for community acquired pneumonia in children. *Cochrane Database Syst Rev.* 2010 Mar; Issue 3, Art.No. CD004874.

12. Awasthi S, Agarwal G, Singh JV, Kabra SK, Pillai RM, Singhi S, *et al.* Effectiveness of 3-day amoxicillin vs 5 day cotrimoxazole in the treatment of non-severe pneumonia in children aged 2-59 months of age: A multicentric open labeled trial. *J Trop Pediatr* 2008 Dec;54 (6): 382-389.

13. Muhe L, Degefu H, Worku B, Oljira B, Mulholland EK. Comparison of nasal prongs with nasal catheters in the delivery of oxygen to children with hypoxia. *J Trop Pediatr* 1998; 44:365-368.

14. Castro-Guardiola A, Viejo-Rodriguez AL, Soler-Simon S, Armengou-Arxe A, Bisbe-Company V, Penarroja-Matutano G, Bisbe-Company J, Garcia-Bragado F. Efficacy and safety of oral and early-switch therapy for community-acquired pneumonia: a randomized controlled trial. *Am J Med* 2001; 111: 367-374

15. Asghar R, Banajeh S, Egas J, Singhi S, *et. al,* Severe Pneumonia Evaluation Antimicrobial Research Study Group. Chloramphenicol versus ampicillin plus gentamicin for community acquired very severe pneumonia among children aged 2-59 months in low

resource settings: multicentre randomised controlled trial (SPEAR study). *BMJ* 2008 Jan, 12;336(7635):80-84.

16. Dekate PS, Mathew JL, Jayashree M, Singhi SC. Acute community acquired pneumonia in emergency room. *Indian J Pediatr* 2011 Sep; 78 (9): 1127-1135

17. Dhawan A, Narang A, Singhi S. Hyponatremia and the inappropriate ADH syndrome in pneumonia. *Annals Trop Pediatr* 1992; 12: 455 462.

18. Singhi S, Sharma A, Majumdar S. Body water and plasma volume in severe community acquired pneumonia in children: implications in fluid therapy. *Annals Trop Pediatr* 2005 Dec; 25 (4) : 243-252.

19. Kabra SK, Lodha R, Hilton DJ. Antibiotics for preventing complications in children with measles. *Cochrane Database Syst Rev.* 2008, Issue 3. Art.No.: CD001477.

20. The Vitamin A and Pneumonia Working Group. Potential interventions for the prevention of childhood pneumonia in developing countries: a meta-analysis of data from field trials to assess the impact of vitamin A supplementation on pneumonia morbidity and mortality. *Bull WHO* 1995; 73:609-619.

21. Yang HM, Mao M, Wan C. Vitamin A treating measles in children.*Cochrane Data Syst Rev:* 2005, Issue 4. Art. No. : CD001479

22. Lebel MH, Mehra S. Efficacy and safety of clarithromycin versus erythromycin for the treatment of pertussis: a prospective, randomized, single blind trial. *Pediatr Infect Dis J* 2001; 20:1149-1154.

23. Bamberger ES, Srugo I. what is new in pertussis? *Eur J Pediatr* 2008;167:133-139.

24. American Academy of Pediatrics Pertussis (Whooping cough). In: Red Book: 2009 Report of the Committee on Infectious Diseases. 28th ed. Pickening LK, Baker CJ, Kimbalin DW, Long SS, (eds). *E&K Grove Village, IL: American Academy of Pediatrics;* 2009: 504-519.

25. Pillay V, Swingler G Symptomatic treatment of the cough in whooping cough (Cochrane Review). In: The Cochrane Library, Issue 1, 2004. *Chichester, UK: John Wiley & Sons, Ltd.*

26. Altunaiji SM, Kukuruzovic RH, Curtis NC, Massie J. Antibiotics for whooping cough (Pertussis) *Cochrane Database Sys Rev* 2007, Issue 3. Art.No.: CD004404.

27. Brook I. Anaerobic pulmonary infection in children. *Pediatr Emerg Care* 2004 Sep, 20: 636-640.

28. Neto GM, Kentab O, Klassen TP, Osmond MH. A randomized controlled trial of mist in the acute treatment of moderate croup. *Acad Emerg Med* 2002; 9:873-879.

29. Moore M, Little P. Humidified air inhalation for treating croup (Protocol for a Cochrane Review). In: The Cochrane Library, Issue 1, 2004. *Chichester, UK: John Wiley & Sons, Ltd.*

30. Russell K, Wiebe N, Saenz A, Ausejo Segura M, Johnson D, Hartling L, Klassen TP. Glucocorticoids for croup (Cochrane Review). In: *The Cochrane Library*, Issue 1, 2004. *Chichester, UK: John Wiley & Sons, Ltd.*

31. Luria JW, Gonzalez-del-Rey JA, DiGiulio GA, McAneney CM, Olson JJ, Ruddy RM. Effectiveness of oral or nebulized dexamethasone for children with mild croup. *Arch Pediatr Adol Med* 2001; 155:1340-1345.

32. Donaldson D, Poleski D, Knipple E, Filips K, Reetz L, Pascual RG, Jackson RE. Intramuscular versus oral dexamethasone for the treatment of moderate to severe croup: a randomized, double-blind trial. *Acad Emerg Med* 2003; 10:16-21.

33. Fitzgerald D, Mellis C, Johnson M, *et al.* Nebulized budesonide is as effective as nebulised adrenaline in moderately severe croup. *Pediatrics* 1996; 97:722-725.

34. Ledwith CA, Shea LM, Mauro RD. Safety and efficacy of nebulized racemic epinephrine in conjunction with oral dexamethasone and mist in the outpatient treatment of croup. *Ann Emerg Med* 1995; 25:331-337.

35. Shargorodsky J, Whittemore KR, Lee GS. Bacterial tracheitis: A therapeutic approach. *Laryngoscope 2010*; 120(12): 2498-501.

36. Singhi S, Banerjee S, Nanjundaswamy H. Inhaled budesonide in acute asthma. *J Paediatr Child Hlth* 1999 Oct;35(5):483-487.

37. Devidayal, Singhi S, Kumar L, *et al.* Efficacy of nebulized budesonide compared to oral prednisolone in acute bronchial asthma. *Acta Paediatr* 1999 Aug; 88(8): 835-840.

38. Camargo CA Jr, Spooner CH, Rowe BH. Continuous versus intermittent beta-agonists for acute asthma (Cochrane Review). In: The Cochrane Library, Issue 1, 2004. *Chichester, UK: John Wiley & Sons, Ltd.*

39. Smith M, Iqbal S, Elliott TM, Rowe BH. Corticosteroids for hospitalised children with acute asthma (Cochrane Review). In: The Cochrane Library, Issue 1, 2004. *Chichester, UK: John Wiley & Sons, Ltd.*

40. Plotnick LH, Ducharme FM. Combined inhaled anticholinergics and beta 2-agonists for initial treatment of acute asthma in children (Cochrane Review). In: The Cochrane Library, Issue 1, 2004. *Chichester, UK: John Wiley & Sons, Ltd.*

41. Mitra A, Bassler D, Ducharme FM. Intravenous aminophylline for acute severe asthma in children over 2 years using inhaled bronchodilators (Cochrane Review). In: The Cochrane Library, Issue 1, 2004. *Chichester, UK: John Wiley & Sons, Ltd.*

42. Devi R, Kumar L, Singhi S, *et al.* Intravenous magnesium sulfate in acute severe asthma not responding to conventional therapy. *Indian Pediatr* 1997; 34:389-397.

43. Rowe BH, Bretzlaff JA, Bourdon C, *et al.* Magnesium sulphate for treating exacerbations of acute asthma in the emergency department. *Cochrane Database Syst Rev* 2000; (2): CD001490.

Section 2

44. Kambalapalli M, Nischani S, Upadhyayula S. Safety of intravenous terbutaline in acute severe asthma: a retrospective study. *Acta Paediatr* 2005; 94(9):1214-1217.

45. Singhi S, Bansal A, Chopra K, Grover S. Randomized comparison of magnesium sulfate, terbutaline and aminophylline infusion in acute severe asthma in children . *Crit Care Med* 2010;38:371. (Abstract).

46. Singhi SC, Jayashree K, Sarkar B. Hypokalemia following nebulized salbutamol in children with acute attack of bronchial asthma. *J Pediatr Child Hlth* 1996 Dec; 32(6): 495-497.

47. Grover S, Mathew J, Bansal A, Singhi SC. Approach to a child with lower airway obstruction and bronchiolitis. *Indian J Pediatr* 2011 Nov;78(11):1396-400.

48. Gadomski AM, Bhasale AL. Bronchodilators for bronchiolitis. *Cochrane Database Syst Rev* 2006, 3: CD001266.

49. Hartling L, Russell KF, Patel H, et al. Epinephrine for bronchiolitis. *Cochrane Database of Systematic Reviews* 2004, (1): CD003123.

50. Mathew JL. Hypertonic saline nebulization for bronchiolitis. *Indian Pediatr* 2008; 45: 987-989.

51. Plint AC, Johnson DW, Patel H, *et al.* Epinephrine and dexamethasone in children with bronchiolitis. *New Eng J Med* 2009;360:2079-89.

52. Randolph AG, Wang EEL. Ribavirin for respiratory syncytial virus infection of the lower respiratory tract (Cochrane Review). In: The Cochrane Library, Issue 1, 2004, *Chichester, UK: John Wily and Sons, Ltd.*

53. Thia LP, McKenzie SA, Blyth PB, *et al.* Randomised controlled trial of nasal continuous positive airways pressure (CPAP) in bronchiolitis. *Arch Dis Child* 2008; 93: 45-47.

54. Poddar U, Singhi S, Ganguli NK, Sialy R. Water electrolyte homeostasis in acute bronchiolitis. *Indian Pediatr* 1995; 32:59-65.

Section 2

17

The Comatose Child

Pratibha D Singhi and Sunit Singhi

Coma is a life-threatening pediatric emergency caused by a multitude of conditions that affect the central nervous system directly or indirectly. The comatose child warrants urgent life saving measures coupled with a systematic approach towards diagnosis and appropriate definitive management.

DEFINITIONS

Coma is a state of deep, unarousable, sustained pathologic unconsciousness with the eyes closed. The patient has no awareness of self and surroundings and cannot be woken up by stimulation. Coma is an acute condition that usually requires the period of unconsciousness to persist for at least one hour to distinguish it from states of transient loss of consciousness.[1,2]

Persistent vegetative state is a condition in which the patient wakes up with eyes open, and sleeps with eyes closed but has complete lack of awareness of self and the environment. There is no language comprehension or expression and no voluntary movement. Patients have sleep-awake cycles with either complete or partial preservation of hypothalamic and brain-stem autonomic functions including breathing and circulation.[1,2]

Minimally conscious state is a state of severely altered consciousness in which patients show minimal but definite behavioral evidence of awareness of themselves or their environment by following simple commands, gesturers or verbal yes/no responses, intelligible speech, or purposeful behavior in response to a stimulus (e.g., sustained visual fixation or tracking, appropriate smiling or crying to stimuli, appropriate verbal or gestural responses to questions, reaching for an object, or using it appropriately).[1,2,3]

Brain death is defined as the permanent absence of all brain functions including those of the brainstem.[4]

PATHOPHYSIOLOGY

Consciousness is a state of awareness of self and environment. It has two dimensions, wakefulness and awareness[3]. Wakefulness requires ascending stimuli emanating from reticular activating system (RAS) which extends from the medulla to the midbrain. It receives collaterals from every major somatic and special sensory pathway. Awareness is determined by cerebral cortical neurons and their reciprocal projections to and from the major subcortical nuclei. Awareness requires wakefulness, but wakefulness can be present without awareness. Unconsciousness implies global or total unawareness and is characteristic of both coma and vegetative state. Patients in a coma are unconscious because they lack both wakefulness and awareness. Patients in a vegetative state are unconscious because, although they are wakeful, they lack awareness.[1] Coma occurs with dysfunction of either (i) both cerebral hemispheres or (ii) the brain stem. This may occur due to (a) structural lesions (b) metabolic or toxic effects at molecular level, or both.[2] Disease states causing coma are also associated with changes in intracranial pressure (ICP) and cerebral blood flow (CBF).

APPROACH TO A CHILD IN COMA

A child in coma must be regarded as a medical emergency, and certain urgent measures should be undertaken to salvage the life of the child. Simultaneously a diagnostic work up should be done and subsequent definitive treatment instituted. Ideally the child should be managed in a Pediatric Intensive Care Unit.

Emergency Measures

These should be undertaken immediately even before doing a complete clinical examination. First of all one should ensure that the child has stable airway, breathing and circulation (ABC). Measures to establish these should be instituted like in any emergency situation (Table 17.1).

Table 17.1 Emergency measures to be taken in a comatose child
1. Check airway patency: Intubate if Glasgow coma score <8; or there is pooling of secretions, shock, or evidence of herniation.
2. Check breathing: Give 100% oxygen to keep oxygen saturation above 92%; use bag and mask/tube ventilation if breathing efforts are unsatisfactory
3. Check circulation: Start IV normal saline or Ringer's lactate 20 ml/kg to maintain blood pressure and peripheral perfusion. Give inotropic support if needed. Hypertension if present , could be both cause and effect of coma, so reduce it slowly.
4. Seizures: Control with benzodiazepines (lorazepam 0.1 mg/kg or diazepam 0.3 mg/kg IV, or midazolam followed by phenytoin 20 mg/kg IV.)
5. Raised ICP or impending herniation: Head elevation 15-30°, manual hyperventilation, mannitol 0.25-0.5g/kg IV over 20 min.
6. Metabolic support: 2 ml/kg of 25% dextrose IV if blood sugar is < 60 mg/dl.
7. If the child is febrile, give empiric first dose of IV ceftriaxone 100 mg/kg IV and acyclovir/artesunate if indicated.
8. Administer specific antidotes in case of known poisoning

Simultaneously a quick neurological assessment should be performed to (i) evaluate the level of consciousness and (ii) assess for any evidence of raised ICP and impending herniation. If there is any evidence of raised ICP, immediate steps should be instituted for its management (Table 17.2). One should not wait for signs of herniation to appear. It is better to assume that central herniation is imminent and one must take appropriate measures to prevent it.

The neurological assessment helps in (i) determining the severity of the neurological injury and planning the type of intervention measures needed and (ii) recording important baseline information before certain drugs are administered. It is ideal to use an objective tool for assessment of severity and evolution of coma. The Glasgow Coma Scale (with its modification for children) is a simple and useful tool which is widely used for this purpose (Table 17.3). If there is a suspicion of trauma either by history or on physical examination, the child should be evaluated by a trauma team (which

Table 17.2 Measures to reduce raised intracranial pressure
1. Position head in neutral position with 30° elevation.
2. Ensure oxygenation and maintain normal mean arterial blood pressure.
3. Provide hyperventilation with a bag and mask or ventilator. Maintain $PaCO_2$ between 30-35 mm Hg. Use it for a short period of 10-15 minutes only.
4. Osmotic diuretics like mannitol 0.5g/kg or 0.25 g/kg IV over 20 minutes, may be repeated, 4-6 hourly for 3-4 doses.
5. Hypertonic saline (3%) 5-10 ml/kg may be used in place of mannitol particularly if patient is in shock.
6. Dexamethasone 1-2 mg/kg IV q 6 hr is useful in cytotoxic cerebral edema eg. in brain abscess, granuloma and tumor.
7. Rarely thiopental or pentobarbital may be needed in refractory cases.
8. CSF drainage in children with obstructive hydrocephalus.
9. Ensure excellent supportive care viz. reduction of fever, avoidance of pain, loud noise and noxious stimuli.

includes a neurosurgeon and general surgeon) and managed appropriately. In this chapter we shall discuss the approach to a child with non-traumatic coma. Coma due to head inqury is discussed in detail in Chapter 54.

THE DIAGNOSTIC APPROACH

After ensuring that the child is stabilized, the following questions should be asked:

1. Where is the lesion?
2. Is it progressive?
3. What is the specific etiology?
4. What is the specific treatment?

A systematic approach involving a carefully taken history, physical and neurological examination, along with some important investigations are needed for answering these questions.

History

The following points in history are often helpful to identify the cause of coma.

1. *Onset.* A gradual onset indicates a slowly progressive cause such as a space occupying

Table 17.3 Modified Glasgow Coma Scale		
Eye opening		
Score	**>1 year**	**< 1 year**
4	Spontaneously	Spontaneously
3	To verbal command	To shout
2	To pain	To pain
1	No response	No response
Best motor response		
Score	**>1 year**	**< 1 year**
6	Obeys	Spontaneous
5	Localizes pain	Localizes pain
4	Flexion withdrawal	Flexion withdrawal
3	Flexion abnormal (decorticate rigidity)	Flexion abnormal (decorticate rigidity)
2	Extension (decerebrate rigidity)	Extension (decerebrate rigidity)
1	No response	No response

Best verbal response			
Score	**>5 years**	**2-5 years**	**< 2 years**
5	Oriented and converses	Appropriate words and phrases	Smiles, coos appropriately
4	Disoriented and converses	Inappropriate words	Cries, consolable
3	Inappropriate words	Persistent cries and screams	Persistent inappropriate or inconsolable crying or screaming
2	Incomprehensible sounds	Grunts	Grunts, agitated or restless
1	No response	No response	No response

or a destructive lesion, a subacute onset is generally seen with metabolic or an inflammatory process, whereas a sudden onset often indicates a vascular event. A tumor or an abscess may at times have a sudden onset of coma particularly if there is a bleed into the tumor or rupture of abscess into the ventricle.

2. *Fever.* Fever generally indicates an infectious cause viz. meningitis, encephalitis, cerebral malaria etc. Fever may, however, precipitate coma of a metabolic nature and cause ketoacidosis.

3. *Associated symptoms.* A viral prodrome often suggests viral encephalitis. A biphasic illness with the child going into altered sensorium while apparently recovering from a viral illness suggests Reye's syndrome or acute disseminated encephalomyelitis (ADEM). An awareness of seasonal variations, and epidemics of certain illnesses like Japanese encephalitis and cerebral malaria is helpful.

4. *Ingestion of toxic substances.* Accidental or deliberate intake of tablets, liquids and poisonous products lying at home may give a clue to poisoning. At times direct history may not be available, and one has to actively enquire into circumstantial history eg. an empty bottle found near the comatose child.

5. *Bite/sting.* History of snake bite or scorpion sting may be forthcoming or there may be circumstantial evidence like presence of a bite mark.

6. *Past illness.* Children with a known illness such as diabetes mellitus, epilepsy, renal disease, heart disease etc. may develop coma because of associated complications.

7. *Trauma.* History of trauma at times may not be forthcoming because it is unnoticed or self

inflected. Information may be deliberately withheld for fear of 'charge of negligence' or 'abuse'. In an infant with unexplained afebrile coma the possibility of non-accidental head injury must be kept in mind and other signs looked for.

Physical Examination

The following physical and neurological findings should be actively looked for:

1. *Fever.* Fever, specially when associated with irritability, and seizures often points to a CNS infection (meningitis/encephalitis) which is the commonest cause of coma in children in developing countries. Some poisons and post epileptic states may be associated with mild elevation of temperature but these can be differentiated by history. Rarely, a brain stem lesion may cause fever due to disturbance of temperature regulating center.

2. *Skin rash* may be seen with meningo-coccemia, dengue, measles, arboviral and rickettsial diseases

3. *Petechiae* may be seen with meningo-coccemia, dengue and hemorrhagic fevers.

4. *Elevated blood pressure.* The presence of hypertension may indicate raised ICP or hypertensive encephalopathy. In hypertensive encephalopathy there will be diastolic hypertension, with associated findings of left ventricular hypertrophy (ECG, ECHO) and there may be changes in retina suggestive of hypertensive retinopathy.

5. *Peculiar odor.* The presence of fruity odor is suggestive of diabetic ketoacidosis, and urine-like smell of uremia and fetor hepaticus of hepatic coma. The diagnosis of a specific poisoning may be suspected by characteristic odor of breath.

6. *Jaundice and hepatomegaly* are suggestive of a primary hepatic cause. However, malaria, dengue, rickettsial disease, enteric fever and leptospirosis are other important differential diagnoses.

7. *Splenomegaly and anemia* in a child with high grade fever is suggestive of cerebral malaria particularly in endemic areas. Mild hepatomegaly is commonly seen in Reye syndrome.

8. *Cardiac findings.* Cardiac arrhythmias and congestive heart failure may suggest a hypoxic-ischemic cause.

9. *Signs of trauma.* The presence of bruising and bleeding are indicative of associated or underlying traumatic cause.

10. *Neurological impairment or developmental delay.* Unexplained coma in such children may be due to an underlying inborn error of metabolism.

Neurological Examination

In addition to the standard neurological examination in a comatose child, the important components include (i) signs of raised ICP and brainstem herniation, (ii) examination of eyes, (iii) posture and motor responses, (iv) the breathing pattern and (v) meningeal signs (Tables 17.4, 17.5 and 17.6).

Signs of raised ICP and brainstem herniation. These include headache, bulging anterior fontanel, bradycardia, hypertension, irregular breathing, papilledema and evidences of 3rd or 6th cranial nerve compression. Brainstem herniation proceeds from higher to lower brain centers. Coma is followed by decorticate rigidity (flexion and adduction of upper and lower extremities), small pupils, and Cheyne-Stokes breathing. As the midbrain and pons get involved, child develops decerebrate rigidity (hyperextension and inversion of upper and lower limbs with opisthotonos), pupils become midposition and non-reactive with hyperpneic breathing pattern. When medulla is compromised or compressed, there is marked flaccidity with wide fluctuations in blood pressure and heart rate and breathing becomes apneic or irregular. Unilateral uncal lobe herniation is characterized by ipsilateral anisocoria, loss of pupillary reflexes and ptosis due to involvement of 3rd cranial nerve.

Examination of the eyes. The eyes must be examined carefully as this gives useful and most important information in comatose patients.

(i) *Position and movements of the eyes.* Normally the eyes at rest are in midposition and aligned straight forward. In a comatose child the eyes are usually in midposition or slightly divergent. Conjugate deviation of the eyes suggests either an ipsilateral cerebral hemispheric lesion or a contralateral pontine lesion. Dysconjugate deviation of the eyes either at rest or evoked by head turning or caloric stimulation, indicates a brainstem lesion. Abnormalities of lateral gaze result from structural rather than metabolic disturbance, while impairment of upward gaze may be produced by either. Tonic upward gaze indicates bilateral hemispheric damage.

(ii) *The pupils.* Pupillary size and reaction to light gives valuable clues to the diagnosis (Table 17.4). Pupils may be affected variably in metabolic coma, but generally remain reactive. Anticonvulsants like phenobarbitone and phenytoin may abolish ocular movements but the pupillary reflexes remain intact. Absence of pupillary reaction is strongly suggestive of structural involvement of optic pathways.

(iii) *Corneal reflex* is often lost in children with deep coma. Unilateral absence of corneal reflex may suggest a hemispheric or pontine lesion.

(iv) *The oculocephalic reflex (Doll's eyes).* This is tested in the comatose child who does not have any spontaneous eye movements. The head with eyes open is suddenly turned to one side. If the eyes deviate to the opposite side, this is called the positive oculocephalic or Doll's eye reflex. The positive reflex indicates an intact brainstem. The reflex is retained in children with diffuse hemispheric disease and patients with supratentorial coma while it is lost in children with brain stem lesions. *The*

Table 17.4 Pupillary size and their reaction to light

Pupils	Lesion/dysfunction
• Pinpoint (<2 mm)	Pontine, cerebeller lesions, poisoning (opiates, organo-phosphates)
• Small (2-3 mm)	Medullary lesion, metabolic cause due to poisonings (opiates, organophosphates, barbiturates, phenothiazines)
• Midsize (5-7 mm) midposition and non-reactive	Midbrain or below this level
• Dilated non-reactive	Diffuse damage, postictal states, botulism, and drugs (amphetamine, atropine, barbiturates)
• Unilateral dilated non-reactive	Ipsilateral uncal herniation

reflex should never be tested in children with suspected cervical injuries.

The same information can be obtained by oculovestibular reflex (cold caloric response). This reflex can be tested even in patients with cervical injuries. The head is positioned in midline and raised 30° from the horizontal. Ice cold water (about 50 ml), is slowly injected through a catheter into auditory canal. In an awake person, nystagmus is produced with the slow component in the opposite direction. In children with supratentorial lesions and an intact brain stem, tonic deviation of the eyes occurs towards the side of cold stimulus. Absence of the reflex indicates brain stem damage. Certain drugs like sedatives, antiepileptics, anticholinergics and aminoglycosides may depress or even abolish the caloric response.

(v) *Fundus.* Papilledema with or without retinal hemorrhages indicates raised ICP. Subhyaloid hemorrhage may occur with subarachnoid hemorrhage, subdural hematoma, and trauma. Retinal hemorrhages are commonly seen in "shaken baby" syndrome. They may be seen in children with severe falciparum malaria. It must be remembered that most children with raised ICP secondary to acute CNS infections and metabolic causes do not have papilledema.

Posture and motor responses. The comatose child may be lying in an abnormal posture, which may indicate the site of lesion and/or severity and at times etiology of coma.

Decorticate posture. Flexion and adduction of upper and lower limbs occurs with lesions above pontine and midbrain regions, bilateral hemispheric lesion, or severe hypoxemia. Decerebrate posturing is seen in children with lesions in the mid brain or upper pontine area.

The motor response which is elicited by a painful stimulus like pressure over nail bed or deep pressure over supraorbital region may be either appropriate, inappropriate or absent. *An appropriate response* implies withdrawal from the painful stimulus. Purposeful withdrawal and/or vocalization suggests preservation of cortical function. *Inappropriate response* may be in the form of decorticate or decerebrate posturing. *Asymmetric response* occurs with hemiplegia, and other focal deficits. Flaccidity with absence of motor response suggests a ponto-medullary or lower brainstem lesion. Dystonia may be seen with Japanese encephalitis and certain inborn errors of metabolism.

Table 17.5 Focussed clinical examination and localisation in coma		
Respiratory pattern	Normal	Brainstem intact
	Cheyne- Stokes	Diencephalic
	Hyperventilation	Midbrain/upper pontine
	Ataxic, shallow	Lower pontine
	Gasping, slow, irregular	Medullary
Posture	Normal	Brainstem intact
	Hemiparesis	Uncal herniation
	Decorticate	Diencephalic
	Decerebrate	Midbrain/upper pontine
	Flaccid	Lower pontine or medulla
Response to pain	Flexion to supraocular pain	Diencephalic
	Extension to supraocular pain	Midbrain/upper pontine
	None	Lower pontine
Tone, reflexes and plantars	Normal	Brainstem intact
	Unilateral pyramidal	Uncal herniation
	Bilateral pyramidal	Diencephalic
	Flaccidity/extensor plantars	Lower pontine
Oculocephalic reflex (doll's eye) Exclude cord injury before testing dolls' eyes Turn head from side to side, and watch the eyes	Saccadic eye movements	Normal forebrain control
	Full deviation of eyes away from the movement	Diencephalic
	Minimal deviation of eyes	Midbrain/upper pontine
	No movement of eyes	Lower pontine
Pupil size	Normal midpoint	Midbrain/upper pontine
	Small	Diencephalic
	Unilaterally large	Uncal herniation
	Bilaterally large	Lower pontine
Pupillary response to bright light	Brisk	Brainstem intact
	Unresponsive pupils	Midbrain/upper pontine

Breathing pattern. The pattern of respiration forms an important part of the neurological examination. Most children with involvement of cerebral hemispheres and with impending transtentorial herniation, have Cheyne-Stokes breathing. Neurogenic hyperventilation may be seen with involvement of midbrain and pons.

Meningeal signs. The presence of meningeal signs is suggestive of meningitis, meningo-encephalitis, ADEM or subarachnoid bleed. Meningismus may be seen in children with enteric fever and cerebral malaria. The presence of meningismus with focal signs is suggestive of brain abscess, epidural hemorrhage, cerebrovascular accident, tumors including tuberculoma and cerebellar herniation. *Meningeal signs are often absent in infants and severely malnourished children and may be lost in deeply comatose children.*

After a proper history, physical examination and neurological assessment, one should be able to decide whether the comatose child has (i) an infectious or metabolic disorder or (ii) a structural lesion (supratentorial/infratentorial).

Infections and metabolic abnormalities generally affect the nervous system diffusely. The onset of coma is gradually progressive. The

Table 17.6 Clinical signs suggestive of various herniation syndromes	
Uncal	*Unilateral fixed dilated pupil* *Unilateral ptosis* *Minimal deviation of eyes on oculocephalic/oculovestibular testing* *Hemiparesis*
Diencephalic	*Small or midpoint pupils reactive to light* *Full deviation of eyes on oculocephalic/oculovestibular testing* *Flexor response to pain and/or decorticate posturing* *Hypertonia and/or hyperreflexia with extensor plantars* *Cheyne–Stokes respiration*
Midbrain/upper pontine	*Midpoint pupils, unresponsive to light* *Minimal deviation of eyes on oculocephalic/oculovestibular testing* *Extensor response to pain and/or decerebrate posturing* *Hyperventilation*
Lower pontine	Midpoint pupils, fixed and unrespnsive to light No response on oculocephalic/oculovestibular testing No response to pain or there is only flexion of legs Flaccidity with extensor plantars Shallow or ataxic respiration
Medullary	Pupils dilated and fixed to light Slow, irregular, or gasping respiration Respiratory arrest with adequate cardiac output
Italics refers to clinical signs of potentially reversible cerebral herniation	

neurological findings in metabolic coma are usually symmetrical. Asymmetry if present, is never marked, and may alternate from side to side. The pupillary light reflex and spontaneous eye movements are preserved. Infections are sometimes associated with focal signs e.g. herpes encephalitis, infarcts associated with meningitis, and brain abscess etc. Scattered neurological findings in a child with history of viral illness or immunization in the recent past suggest ADEM.

Structural lesions. These may either be supratentorial or subtentorial.

(i) *Supratentorial lesions.* Coma is usually produced by bilateral supratentorial lesions. Unilateral lesions may cause coma either by compressing the contralateral hemisphere or the brain stem by affecting the RAS. They are characterized by (i) initial asymmetric findings eg. hemiparesis, hemisensory deficit or aphasia, (ii) deterioration occurs characteristically in a rostral caudal manner with rapid changes in clinical findings. At times supratentorial lesions may present with symmetric findings.

(ii) *Subtentorial (brain stem) lesions.* As these lesions involve the RAS and the cranial nerves, they cause early coma and cranial nerve palsies. The rostrocaudal progression of CNS findings is not seen. Evaluation of eye movements is very useful and *when all the eye movements are preserved it virtually excludes a brain stem lesion.* Any child with findings of brain stem involvement should be considered to have a structural lesion unless proved otherwise.

CAUSES OF COMA

The common causes of non-traumatic coma are shown in Table 17.7. The most important cause of non-traumatic coma in developing countries is CNS infections.[5,6] In a study of 100 consecutive cases of non-traumatic coma in children, we found CNS infections in 60 percent cases, with tubercular meningitis, pyogenic meningitis and encephalitis almost equally common.[5] The other common causes were toxic-metabolic conditions (19%), status epilepticus (10%), and non-traumatic intracranial bleeds.

INVESTIGATIONS

Initial diagnostic work up. The usual initial laboratory studies include a complete and differential blood count, blood glucose, electrolytes, liver and renal functions, blood ammonia and lactate level and arterial blood gas studies (ABG). Urine must be examined for glucose and ketones (Table 17.8). The priority of investigations is determined by the suspected cause. Stomach aspirate should be sent

Table 17.7 Common causes of non-traumatic coma in children

Infections

- Meningitis (bacterial, tubercular)
- Encephalitis, acute disseminated encephalomyelitis (ADEM)
- Sepsis (particularly Gram-negative)
- Cerebral malaria
- Enteric and shigella encephalopathy
- Brain abscess
- Subdural/epidural empyema
- Dyselectrolytemia*

Metabolic

- Hyperglycemia and diabetic ketoacidosis
- Hyperosmolar states
- Hypoglycemia
- Reye's syndrome
- Acidosis, alkalosis
- Hepatic failure
- Uremia
- Hypercapnia
- Hyperammonemia

Drugs and poisons

- Opiates
- Barbiturates
- Salicylates
- Sedatives
- Organophosphates
- Snake bite

Miscellaneous conditions

- Postictal (status epilepticus)
- Hypoxic-ischemic (shock, post-cardiac arrest, pulmonary edema)
- Hypertensive encephalopathy
- Mass lesions in brain· Demyelinating disorders of CNS

* Hyponatremia, hypomagnesemia, hypermagnesemia, hypocalcemia, hypercalcemia

to the poison control laboratory and toxicology screen done in suspected cases. Lumbar puncture is indicated when meningitis is suspected provided it is not contraindicated due to clinical or radiological features of raised ICP, focal signs, thrombocytopenia, local infection or hemodynamic instability. It is best avoided in the deeply comatose child and

is generally done when the child shows signs of recovery from coma. Broad-spectrum antibiotics and acyclovir are given to cover for suspected bacterial and herpetic encephalitis until results of LP become available. If the child is resident of *P. falciparum* endemic area, and has hypoglycemia, anemia, or absent meningeal signs then empiric IV artesunate/quinine may be given. In intractable cases when diagnosis is elusive, 5 ml heparinized blood and urine should be saved for metabolic studies.

Neuroimaging studies. A CT scan is often needed as an emergency investigation particularly in children with suspected trauma, structural lesion, raised ICP and focal neurological deficits. The comatose child should be stabilized and intubated before getting a CT scan. The CT scan reveals the site and often the nature of the lesion and helps in ruling out lesions that are likely to cause cerebral herniation. In children with diffuse involvement of CNS with raised ICP, CT may show signs of cerebral edema with loss of gray-white matter differentiation and chinking of ventricles. A normal CT does not, however, rule out raised ICP. If the CT scan is normal and if one is suspecting ADEM or lesions in the posterior fossa, an MRI should be done. MRI is also better than CT in demonstrating lesions in children with Japanese and herpes encephalitis.

EEG. The EEG has a diagnostic as well as prognostic role in a comatose child.[7-10] Serial EEGs are more useful than single isolated EEG. Portable EEG facility is an asset for evaluation of comatose children. At times EEG may be the only clue in a child having ongoing epileptogenic activity as there may not be any clinical seizures. Typical EEG findings in some conditions causing coma are shown in Table 17.9.

EEG pattern of burst suppression, monorhythmical alpha like activity, electrocerebral silence or very low amplitude and monotonous 0.5-3 hz high voltage activity are associated with poor outcome.[7,9] Our study showed that non-discernible posterior basic rhythm and very low amplitude waves are associated with poor outcome.[7] EEG findings suggestive of poor outcome do not always correlate with the clinical assessment of depth of coma. The appearance of sleep spindles is indicative of a good prognosis, even in the presence of delta waves.

Table 17.8 Laboratory investigations in a comatose child		
Investigations	**Findings**	**Interpretation**
Blood film	Malarial parasites	Cerebral malaria
Urine (catheter specimen)	Ketones, sugar, protein	Diabetes mellitus, renal hypertension
Dextrostix/blood biochemistry	Elevated or reduced blood glucose electrolytes, elevated blood urea	Diabetic ketoacidosis, hypoglycemic coma, hyponatremia, uremia
Lumbar puncture	Increased cells, hypoglycorrachia, elevated protein, RBCs	Meningitis, encephalitis, subarachnoid hemorrhage
Blood culture	Positive	Sepsis
Viral serology	Positive	Viruses like herpes, enteroviruses
PCR (Blood,CSF)	Positive	Identification of various pathogens
X-ray skull	Fracture	Trauma
Gastric contents	Drugs/poisons	Poisoning

Table 17.9 EEG findings and cause of coma	
EEG findings	**Interpretation**
• High voltage focal slow waves	Underlying supratentorial lesion
• Periodic lateralized epileptiform discharges (PLEDS)	Herpes encephalitis (Rarely other encephalitis)
• Paroxysmal seizure discharges	Status epilepticus
• Slowing of alpha-rhythm progressing to diffuse slowing	Metabolic coma
• Bilateral triphasic paroxysmal waves 2-4 hz/sec	Hepatic or other causes of metabolic coma

Evoked potentials are useful in monitoring and assessment of brain stem functions in patients with coma.[11,12] The absence of all waveforms is associated with severe neurological damage or brain death. Somatosensory evoked potentials (SEPs) are most sensitive and reliable for evaluation of the neurological outcome in the comatose child. Normal SEPs during the course of coma predict a favourable outcome in 100 percent cases. The presence of asymmetrical SEPs is typically associated with neurological sequelae such as hemiparesis. Abnormalities in motor evoked potentials (MEPs) during the acute phase of coma have been shown to accurately predict motor deficits during follow up.[12] Also P-300 event related potentials have been found to be predictive of recovery from coma[11].

MANAGEMENT

After initial stabilization in the emergency room as outlined in Table 17.1, the comatose child should be shifted to the Pediatric Intensive Care Unit and managed as follows:

General Measures and Monitoring

(i) The vital signs and neurological parameters should be monitored to detect any life-threatening events like raised ICP, or herniation syndrome. Intracranial pressure monitoring may be warranted in some children and the cerebral perfusion pressure (CPP = Mean systemic arterial pressure – ICP) should be ideally maintained above 50 mm Hg in infants and above 60 mmHg in children and adolescents.

(ii) Maintain patency of airways and provide oxygenation.

(iii) Optimal fluid intake and output management. Fluid restriction is advised if there is hyponatremia due to syndrome of inappropriate antidiuretic hormone (SIADH) secretion. In SIADH urine osmolality is often higher than serum osmolality. Patients with SIADH are usually normotensive and non-edematous in contrast to patients with

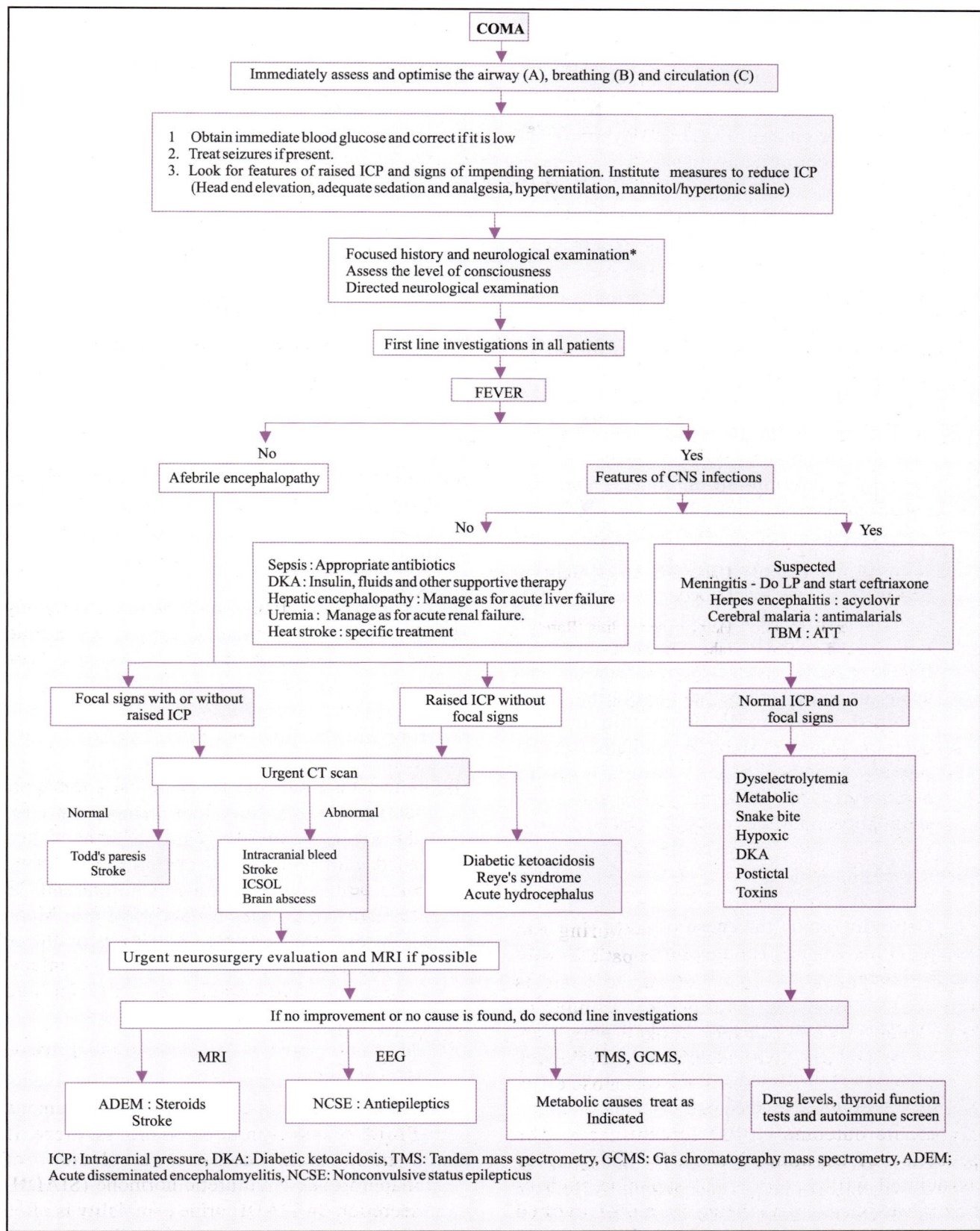

Figure 17.1 Algorithmic approach to a child with coma

hyponatremia due to cardiac, hepatic, and renal failure or adrenal insufficiency.

(iv) Correction of acid base and electrolyte disturbances.

(v) Temperature control. Fever and hypothermia should be appropriately managed.

(vi) Nursing care. The patient should be nursed on the side and his position should be regularly changed, cleanliness and hygiene of oral cavity and skin should be maintained. The eyes should be protected. Urinary catheterization is often required to guide fluid therapy and prevent stasis. Ensure deloading of colon with use of laxatives as bowel distension may also cause surge in ICP.

(vii) Maintenance of nutrition. Adequate nutrition should be maintained by nasogastric feeding in children with prolonged coma. Parenteral nutrition may be required in rare occasions when enteral nutrition is not tolerated.

(viii) Monitor vital signs continuously (at least hourly), changing level of consciousness (GCS hourly), neurological status, brainstem signs, ICP, cerebral perfusion pressure, SpO_2, or $EtCO_2$ or ABG, assess adequate sedation and analgesia, input and output monitoring daily, weigh the child daily if possible and not contraindicated (raised ICP, ventilated), check bowel sounds, blood counts, serum electrolytes, blood sugar, serum and urine osmolality and EEG.

Specific Management

Depending upon the cause of coma, specific therapy is life saving. The measurement steps are summarized in Figure 17.1.

1. Antibiotics are given for treatment of meningitis (refer to Chapter 27). If lumbar puncture is contraindicated because of raised ICP, antibiotics should be started on the basis of clinical suspicion of meningitis.

2. Antiviral drugs like acyclovir is indicated for management of herpes encephalitis. Acyclovir is given in a dose of 20 mg/kg every 8 hr intravenously (as 20 mg/ml solution slowly over one hour) for 21 days (refer to Chapter 37).

3. Methylprednisolone (30 mg/kg once daily for 5 days) is used in children with ADEM.

4. Antimalarials (Artesunate/Quinine by IV infusion) for proven or strongly suspected case of cerebral malaria (refer to Chapter 28).

5. Anticonvulsants for status epilepticus (refer to Chapter 38).

6. Antidotes for specific poisonings and insect bites (refer to Chapters 55 and 52).

7. Antihypertensives for management of hypertensive encephalopathy .

8. Insulin and fluids and electrolytes for management of diabetic ketoacidosis (refer to Chapter 41).

PROGNOSIS

The prognosis of coma mainly depends upon its etiology, duration and depth. Recovery is best in children with coma due to primary epilepsy, whereas anoxia has the worst outcome. In our study survival was significantly better in children with CNS infections (63%) as compared to toxic metabolic causes and intracranial bleed[5]. We found a poor outcome in children presenting with shock, hypothermia, Glasgow coma score of <6, non reacting pupils, absent corneal reflexes and decerebrate or decorticate posturing. None of the children with apnea or ataxic respirations survived. Fixed dilated pupils for more than two hours, decerebration, flaccidity and areflexia are associated with poor outcome. Cardiorespiratory arrest occurring any time in a comatose child and absent brain stem reflexes have a grave prognosis. Longer the duration and greater the depth of coma, poorer is the outcome.

CONCLUSION

Prompt management of life-threatening events followed by a systematic approach and meticulous neurological assessment is mandatory in all comatose children. Further management in a Pediatric Intensive Care Unit with adequate monitoring is warranted till the child improves. Appropriate investigations are required to find the specific cause, which can be treated definitively by medical or surgical methods.

REFERENCES

1. Cavanna AE, Cavanna SL, Servo S, Monaco F. The neural correlates of impaired consciousness in coma and unresponsive states. *Discov Med* 2010 May; 9 (48):431-438.

2. Medical aspects of the persistent vegetative state (1). The Multi-Society Task Force on PVS. *N Engl J Med* 1994 May 26; 330(21):1499-1508.

3. Posner JB, Plum F, Saper CB. Plum and Posner's Diagnosis of Stupor and Coma. *Oxford University Press;* 2007.

4. Nakagawa TA, Ashwal S, Mathur M, Mysore M. The Society of Critical Care Medicine; section on critical care and section on neurology of the american Academy of Pediatrics; the Child Neurology Society. Clinical Report: Guidelines for the Determination of Brain Death in Infants and Children: An Update of the 1987 Task Force Recommendations. *Pediatrics* 2011 Aug 28. [Epub ahead of print].

5. Bansal A, Singhi SC, Singhi PD, Khandelwal N, Ramesh S. Non traumatic coma. *Indian J Pediatr* 2005 June; 72(6):467-473.

6. Melka A, Tekie-Haimanot R, Assefa M. Aetiology and outcome of non-traumatic altered states of consciousness in north western Ethiopia. *East Afr Med J* 1997 Jan; 74(1):49-53.

7. Singhi PD, Bansal A, Ramesh S, Khandelwal N, Singhi SC. Predictive value of electroencephalography and computed tomography in childhood non-traumatic coma. *Indian J Pediatr* 2005 June; 72(6):475-479.

8. Hirsch LJ. Classification of EEG patterns in patients with impaired consciousness. *Epilepsia* 2011 Oct; 52 Suppl 8:21-24.

9. Schomer DL, Silva FL da. Niedermeyer's Electroencephalography: Basic Principles, Clinical Applications, and Related Fields. Sixth Edition. *Lippincott Williams & Wilkins;* 2010.

10. Boccagni C, Bagnato S, Sant Angelo A, Prestandrea C, Galardi G. Usefulness of standard EEG in predicting the outcome of patients with disorders of consciousness after anoxic coma. *Clin Neurophysiol* Vol, 28, N. 5, October 2011.

11. De Giorgio CM, Rabinowicz AL, Gott PS. Predictive value of P300 event-related potentials compared with EEG and somatosensory evoked potentials in non-traumatic coma. *Acta Neurol Scand* 1993 May; 87(5):423-427.

12. Rohde V, Irle S, Hassler WE. Prediction of the post-comatose motor function by motor evoked potentials obtained in the acute phase of traumatic and non-traumatic coma. *Acta Neurochir* (Wien) 1999; 141(8):841-848.

Section 2

18

Raised Intracranial Pressure

Naveen Sankhyan

Raised intracranial pressure (ICP) is a common neurological complication in critically ill children. The cause of raised ICP may be either an increase in brain volume, cerebral blood flow, or cerebrospinal fluid (CSF) volume. The most common causes of raised ICP in children include severe traumatic brain injury, hydrocephalus, neuroinfections, brain tumors, hypoxic-ischemic brain injury, intracranial hemorrhage and metabolic encephalopathies (Table 18.1). Despite being a relatively common problem, there are few systematically evaluated treatments for raised ICP. Most management protocols are based on clinical experience and research done on patients with traumatic brain injury.

Intracranial pressure is the total pressure exerted by the brain, blood and CSF in the intracranial vault. The Monroe-Kellie hypothesis states the sum of the intracranial volumes of brain ($\approx 80\%$), blood ($\approx 10\%$), and CSF($\approx 10\%$) is constant. When there is an increase in any one of these components, it must be offset by an equal decrease in another, or else the intracranial pressure would increase. The ICP varies with age and the normative values for children are not well established. Normal values are less than 10 to 15 mm Hg in adults and older children, 3 to 7 mm Hg for young children, and 1.5 to 6 mm Hg for term infants.[1] ICP values greater than 20 to 25 mm Hg require treatment in most circumstances. Sustained ICP values of greater than 40 mm Hg indicate severe, life-threatening intracranial hypertension[2]. If facilities for ICP monitoring are available it is prudent to target an ICP of <15 mmHg for infants, <18 mmHg for children 1-8 years, <20 mmHg for children older than 8 years.

Cerebral perfusion pressure (CPP) is a major factor that affects cerebral blood flow to the brain. CPP measurement is expressed in millimeters of mercury and is determined by measuring the difference between the mean arterial pressure (MAP) and ICP (CPP = MAP – ICP). It is apparent from the formula that, CPP can reduce as a result of reduced MAP or raised ICP, or a combination of these two. CPP measurements reflect the amount of blood volume present in the intracranial space. It is used as an important clinical indicator of cerebral blood flow and hence adequate oxygenation. Normal CPP values for children are not clearly established, but the following values are generally accepted as the minimal pressure necessary to prevent ischemia: adults CPP > 70 mm Hg; children CPP > 50–60 mm Hg; infants/toddlers CPP > 40–50 mm Hg[3].

CAUSES OF RAISED ICP

The various causes of raised ICP can occur individually or in various combinations (Table 18.1). Based on the Monroe-Kellie hypothesis, raised ICP can result from increase in volume of brain, blood, or CSF. Frequently it is a combination of these factors that result in raised ICP. The causes of raised ICP can also be divided into primary or secondary depending upon the underlying pathology. In primary causes of increased ICP, normalization of ICP depends on rapidly addressing the underlying brain disorder. In secondary causes of raised ICP the underlying systemic or extracranial cause has to be managed.

Table 18.1 Important causes of raised intracranial pressure (HIT-TEARS)	
H	Hydrocephalus, hematoma (intracranial), hepatic encephalopathy
I	Ischemic encephalopathy (drowning, post cardiac arrest)
T	Traumatic brain injury
T	Tumors
E	Encephalitis and other neuroinfections (meningitis, ventriculitis), encephalopathies due to enteric, shigella, cerebral malaria, and metabolic conditions
A	Abscess (brain)
R	Reye's syndrome
S	Stroke (arterial/venous)

ASSESSMENT AND MONITORING

> *Bradycardia with hypertension and irregular breathing/apnea, tonic posturing or flaccidity, rapidly worsening sensorium, unequal or dilated non-reactive pupils are signs of dangerously elevated ICP requiring immediate intervention*

Children who are at risk to develop raised ICP include head trauma, neuro-infections or intracranial mass lesions (hemorrhage, large vessel stroke, posterior fossa mass). Raised ICP usually manifests as headache, vomiting, irritability, squint, tonic posturing or worsening sensorium. However, the symptoms depend on the age, cause, and evolution of the raised ICP (Table 18.2).

Primary assessment

Assess the child for patency and maintenance of the airway, breathing and circulatory function, and level of consciousness. The evidences of a systemic disorder, CNS infection, trauma and bleeding manifestations should be looked for. An immediate priority is to look for potentially life-threatening signs of herniation (Table 18.3). If these signs are present, the measures to decrease intracranial pressure should be immediately instituted.

Neurological assessment

After the initial stabilization, a thorough history and clinical examination is performed to determine the possible etiology and further course of management. Pupillary abnormalities and abnormalities in ocular movements as determined by spontaneous, doll's eye or cold caloric testing are important clues to the localization of brainstem dysfunction. The fundus is examined for detection of papilledema, keeping in mind that its absence does not rule out raised ICP. The motor system examination focuses on identifying posturing or flaccidity due to raised ICP or focal deficits. Findings on the general physical and systemic examination may provide clues to the underlying cause for raised ICP (e.g. signs of meningeal irritation in CNS infections, evidences of sepsis, jaundice/hepatomegaly in hepatic encephalopathy, rash in viral encephalitis, etc).

Neuroimaging

The imaging study of choice for the patient with suspected raised intracranial pressure presenting to the emergency room is a computed tomography (CT) scan. A contrast study is helpful to identify features of infection (meningeal enhancement, brain abscess etc) and tumors. If CT is normal, and the patient has clinical features of raised ICP, an MRI with MR venogram must be obtained when the patient is stabilized. MRI can pick up early stroke, venous thromboses, posterior fossa tumors and demyelinating lesions which may be missed on CT.

Intracranial Pressure Monitoring

Intracranial pressure (ICP) monitoring can be done both invasively and non-invasively. The non-invasive methods like transcranial Doppler, brain stem auditory and visually evoked responses are

Section 2

Table 18.2 Signs and symptoms of raised intracranial pressure[7]	
Early signs and symptoms	**Late signs and symptoms**
■ Headache	■ Further decrease in level of consciousness/GCS
■ Vomiting	■ Bulging anterior fontanel
■ Sensorial changes	■ Decreasing spontaneous movements
■ Decrease in Glasgow come score (GCS)	■ Tonic posturing
■ Irritability	■ Papilledema
■ Sun-setting sign (infants)	■ Dilatation of pupils with decreased or no light response
■ Decreased eye contact (infants)	■ Bradycardia
■ Pupil dysfunction	■ Irregular respirations
■ Cranial nerve dysfunction	■ Increased blood pressure
■ Seizures	■ Cushing's triad* (Late and ominous sign)
* Bradycardia, increase in blood pressure, slow irregular breathing.	

Table 18.3 Clinical recognition of herniation syndromes

Type of herniation	Clinical manifestations
Subfalcine herniation (medial to the cingulate gyrus)	Impaired consciousness, *monoparesis of the contralateral lower extremity**
Central transtentorial	Impaired consciousness, abnormal respirations, *symmetrical small reactive** or midposition fixed non-reactive pupils, *decorticate** posture evolving to decerebrate posturing
Lateral transtentorial (downward and medial of uncus and parahippocampal gyrus)	Impaired consciousness, abnormal respirations, *third nerve palsy** (unilateral dilated pupil, ptosis), *hemiparesis**
Upward transtentorial (upward of the cerebellar vermis and midbrain)	Prominent brainstem signs, downward gaze deviation, upgaze palsy, decerebrate posturing
Transforaminal (downward of cerebellar tonsils and medulla)	Impaired consciousness, neck rigidity, opisthotonos, decerebrate rigidity, vomiting, irregular respirations, apnea, bradycardia

* Clinical signs of potentially reversible brain herniation

available but are rarely used for this purpose. The primary methods for direct ICP monitoring involve the use of a intracranialy placed device. Guidelines for ICP monitoring are available for traumatic brain injury[4]. ICP monitoring is indicated for a patient with GCS score of 3-8 (after resuscitation) with either an abnormal head CT on admission or motor posturing and hypotension. Other indications may include massive hemispheric strokes, diffuse cerebral edema, fulminant hepatic failure, neurological examination[5,6]. In other brain injuries, such as hypoxic and ischemic encephalopathy, monitoring of ICP has not been shown to improve the outcome[3].

Invasive ICP monitoring devices. The primary methods for direct ICP measurement include ventriculostomy, subdural bolt and fiberoptic catheter. Each device has advantages and disadvantages. The intraventricular catheter remains the gold standard for ICP monitoring, due to a high quality, reliable ICP wave-form, and the ability to drain CSF[7]. Disadvantages of this method include high risk of infection, bleeding, and technical difficulties in placement of catheter in some patients. The parenchymal (Camino) monitor provides a good quality ICP waveform, but it does not allow for CSF drainage. The parenchymal catheter cannot be recalibrated after placement, and may give inaccurate readings with prolonged use. The subarachnoid, subdural, and epidural monitors have lower risks of infection and hemorrhage, but provide lower quality of ICP waveforms. Malfunction and obstruction can occur with these devices. The subarchanoid device is the least expensive of the commonly used devices.

Intracranial pressure waveforms. In 1960, Lundberg described the characteristic ICP wave forms (A,B,C) that bear his name[8]. Lundberg A waves (plateau waves) are the most ominous, and may signal impending herniation and brain death. The duration of Lundberg A waves is 5 to 20 minutes, with amplitude > 50 mmHg. Lundberg B waves last 2 to 5 minutes, have an amplitude of >20 mmHg. The clinical significance of B waves is less certain compared with A waves; however, they may represent decreased intracranial compliance. Type C waves (Hering-Traube waves) are short, low amplitude waves (<20 mmHg) with unknown clinical significance. In addition to the periodic waveform patterns described by Lundberg, each individual waveform contains three superimposed consecutive peaks (P1, P2, and P3) related to the cardiac cycle. The first wave, P1 (percussion wave), represents the arrival of arterial blood into the intracranial vault. The second wave, P2 (tidal wave), is thought to reflect the status of intracranial elastance. The significance of the P3 (dicrotic wave) is unknown. Normally, the amplitude of P1 is greater than P2; however, with decreasing intracranial compliance, P2 increases in magnitude relative to P1.

MANAGEMENT

The goals of management are to reduce ICP and treat the underlying condition causing it. The stepwise management of ICP is shown in the algorithm (Figure 18.1). It is important not to delay treatment, in situations where identifying the underlying cause will take time. When elevated ICP is clinically evident, the situation is urgent and requires immediate reduction in ICP. Avoidance of

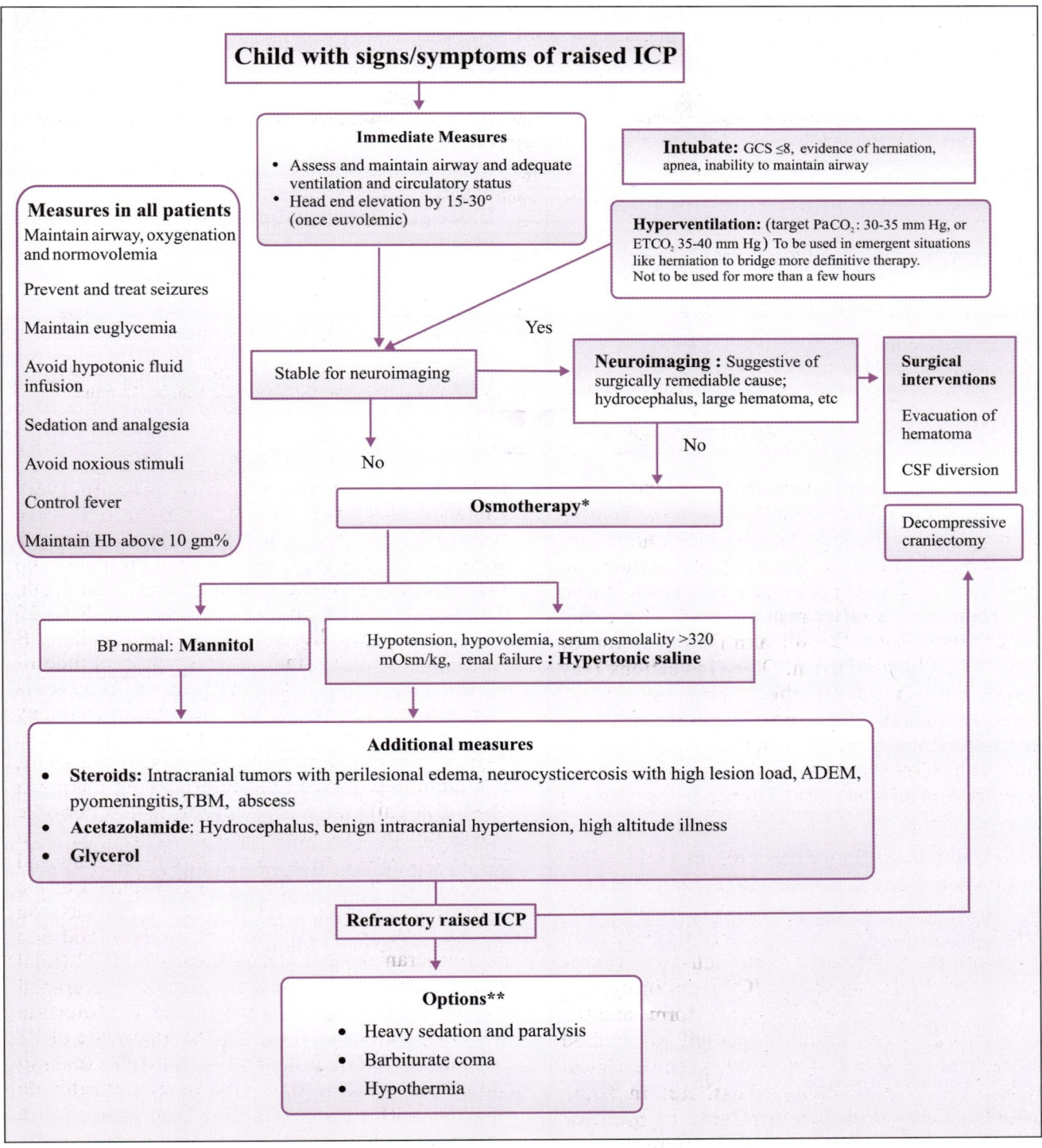

Figure 18.1 Algorithmic approach to a child with raised ICP (adapted)[53]

factors aggravating or precipitating raised ICP is an important goal for all children with intracranial hypertension. The ICP monitors are invasive and not readily available and it should not come in the way of urgent management of raised ICP. The management of the child with raised intracranial pressure is summarized in Table 18.4.

ABCs

The assessment and management of the airway, breathing and circulation (ABCs) should be accorded priority. Early endotracheal intubation should be considered for those children with GCS ≤ 8, evidences of herniation, apnea or inability to

Table 18.4 Summary of therapeutic measures to manage raised intracranial pressure

1. Assessment and management of Airway, Breathing and Circulation: Ensure adequate oxygenation and ventilation; target PaO_2 >60 mmHg, SpO_2 >90%, $PaCO_2$ 30-35 mmHg. Prevent and treat hypotension.

2. Early intubation if GCS <8, evidence of herniation, apnea, and inability to maintain airway.

3. Nurse in supine position with head in midline and slight elevation of 15-30^0 (Ensure that the child is euvolemic prior to positioning).

4. Hyperventilation : Target $PaCO_2$ 30-35mm of Hg (suitable for acute, sharp increases in ICP or when there are signs of impending herniation).

5. Mannitol: Initial bolus 0.25-1g/ kg, then 0.25-0.5g/ kg, q 2-6 hours as per requirement, upto 48 hours.

6. Hypertonic saline: Preferable in the presence of hypotension, hypovolemia, serum osmolality >320 mOsm/kg and renal failure. Dose: 0.1-1ml/kg/hr infusion, target Na^+ 145-155 mEq/L.

7. Steroids: Dexamethasone 0.4-1.5 mg/kg/day, q 6 hr. *Indications:* Intracranial tumors with perilesional edema, neurocysticerocosis with high lesion load, acute disseminated encephalomyelitis, pyogenic meningitis, tuberculous meningitis, brain abscess.

8. Acetazolamide (20-100 mg/kg/day q 8 hr, maximum 2 g/ day). Hydrocephalus, benign intracranial hypertension, high altitude illness.

   Glycerol 0.5-1 ml/kg/day, q 6 hr as an additional oral agent for control of ICP.

9. Drain CSF in hydrocephalus.

10. Adequate sedation and pain relief.

11. Prevention and treatment of seizures: Use lorazepam or midazolam followed by phenytoin as initial choice.

12. Avoid noxious stimuli and minimize their effect: Use lignocaine prior to ET suctioning (nebulized 4% lidocaine mixed in 0.9% saline) or intravenous (1-2 mg/kg as 1% solution) given 90 seconds prior to suctioning.

13. Control fever: Use antipyretics and cooling measures

14. Maintain euvolemia: Use isotonic or hypertonic fluids for maintenance (Ringer lactate, 0.9% saline, 5% dextrose in 0.9% NS). Avoid hypotonic fluids(e.g. Isolyte P, N/5 5% dextrose).

15. Maintain euglycemia. Target blood sugar 80-120 mg/dL.

16. Refractory raised ICP
    - Heavy sedation and muscle paralysis
    - Barbiturate coma
    - Hypothermia
    - Decompressive craniectomy

maintain airway. Intubation should proceed with administration of medications to reduce impact on ICP during the procedure. The useful medications include lidocaine, thiopental and a short-acting non depolarizing neuromuscular blockade agent (eg.vecuronium, atracurium)[9]. Appropriate oxygenation should be ensured. If there is evidence of circulatory failure, fluid bolus should be given. Blood samples should be drawn for investigations as guided by history and physical examination.

Positioning

The child's head is positioned midline with the head end of the bed elevated to 15-30^0 to encourage jugular venous drainage[10]. Sharp head angulations and tight neck garments or taping should be avoided[11]. *One has to ensure that the child is euvolemic before elevating the head.*

Hyperventilation

Using hyperventilation to decrease the $PaCO_2$ to 30-35 mm of Hg is an effective and rapid measure to reduce ICP[9,12]. Hyperventilation acts by constriction of cerebral blood vessels and lowering of CBF. The vasoconstrictive effect on cerebral arterioles lasts only 10 to 20 hours because the pH of the CSF rapidly equilibrates to the new $PaCO_2$ level. Moreover, aggressive hyperventilation can dramatically decreases the CBF, causing or aggravating cerebral ischemia[13,14]. Hence the most effective use of hyperventilation is for management of acute or dramatic increase in ICP or signs of impending herniation[15]. During ongoing care of a child with raised ICP, one should be alert to avoid both hypercapnia and excessive CO_2 washout. In ventilated children arterial blood gases should be monitored every 12 hourly.

Osmotherapy

Mannitol has been used as the osmotherapy of choice for treatment of raised ICP. Recently hypertonic saline has been used for the same purpose. Both are effective regardless of the pathophysiology and the distribution of edema[44].

Mannitol. Mannitol functions by virtue of two main mechanisms of action, osmotic diuresis that produces a gradient, drawing fluid from the brain tissue into the vascular space to be excreted via kidneys. This effect occurs in 15-30 minutes and lasts up to 6 to 8 hours. Mannitol decreases blood viscosity and hematocrit and increases CBF and cerebral oxygen delivery. There is a subsequent reduction in cerebral blood volume due to autoregulatory vasoconstriction[16, 17]. In addition mannitol has immunomodulatory effects. It is believed to cause free radical scavenging and inhibition of apoptosis[18, 19].

Autoregulation of CBF must be intact for the effects of mannitol to work. This autoregulation is adversely affected in many conditions associated with brain edema[20]. There is a lack of data on the optimal dosing of mannitol. A reasonable approach would be to use an initial bolus of 0.25-1g/kg (the higher dose for more urgent reduction of ICP) followed by 0.25-0.5g/kg boluses every 2-6 hours as per requirement. Attention has to be paid to replace fluid lost by diuresis, to maintain the child in euvolemic state. There is a concern of possible leakage of mannitol into the damaged brain tissue potentially leading to "rebound" rise in ICP[21]. For this reason, mannitol should not be suddenly stopped and it should be tapered to prevent a rebound in cerebral edema and ICP. Apart from hypotension and rebound rise in ICP, mannitol may also lead to hypokalemia, hemolysis and renal failure.

Hypertonic saline. Recently the use of hypertonic saline for lowering ICP has received renewed attention. As with mannitol, use of hypertonic saline is believed to act through similar mechanisms. Hypertonic saline reduces ICP predominantly through marked osmotic shift of fluid from the intracellular to the interstitial and intravascular space[22]. There is normalization of endothelial cell volume, increased capillary diameter and reduced resistance to blood flow[23, 24]. The plasma viscosity is reduced and there is a direct relaxant effect on vascular smooth muscle with resultant arteriolar dilatation. The increase in intravascular volume is believed to lead to an autoregulatory reduction in intracerebral blood volume. There is enhanced cardiac output and to a lesser extent increase in mean arterial pressure[25]. Hypertonic saline blunts the neutrophil activation and alters the cytokine production and promotes a more balanced inflammatory response to hemorrhagic shock[26].

Hypertonic saline has a clear advantage over mannitol in children who are hypovolemic or hypotensive. Other situations where it may be preferred are renal failure or serum osmolality of greater than 320 mOsmol/Kg[27]. Hypertonic saline administration may cause hematologic and electrolyte abnormalities, such as bleeding (secondary to decreased platelet aggregation and prolonged coagulation time), rebound rise in ICP, hypokalemia, and hyperchloremic acidosis[28]. Rapid changes in serum osmolarity may lead to central

pontine myelinolysis, acute volume overload, renal failure, cardiac failure or pulmonary edema[29,30]. Despite these concerns, current evidence suggests that hypertonic saline is effective and safe and does not result in major adverse effects[31]. In different studies the concentration of hypertonic saline used has varied from 1.7% to 30%. The method of administration has also varied and hence evidence based recommendations are not available. It would be reasonable to administer hypertonic saline as a continuous infusion at 0.1 to 1.0 ml/kg/hr. It is postulated that slow infusion of saline will cause gradual changes in the serum sodium with reduced risk of intracranial bleed or osmotic myelinolysis. Serum sodium and neurological status should be closely monitored during therapy. When the hypertonic saline therapy is no longer indicated, serum sodium should be slowly corrected to normal values (0.5-1.0 mEq/L/hour) to avoid complications due to sudden fluid shifts. It would be reasonable to target a serum sodium level of 145-155 mEq/L[32,33] during hypertonic saline therapy. Serum sodium and serum osmolality should be closely monitored till target level is reached and then followed up with 12 hourly estimations. Using careful monitoring protocol hypertonic saline has been safely used for upto seven days[34].

Other agents

Acetazolamide. This drug is a carbonic anhydrase inhibitor and is credited to reduce the production of CSF. It is useful in patients with hydrocephalus, high altitude sickness and benign intracranial hypertension. It is used in a dose of 20-100 mg/kg/day (maximum 2g/day), q 8 hr.

Furosemide. Its a loop diuretic which is administered either alone or in combination with mannitol or hypertonic saline, with variable success[35,36]. It is used in a doses of 1 mg/kg/day, q 8 hr. Excessive diuresis may lead to hypovolemia and dyselectrolytemia.

Glycerol. It is an alternative osmotic agent for treatment of raised ICP. It is used in a oral dose of 0.5-1 ml/kg/day q 6 hr. Intravenously it reduces ICP with immediate effect which lasts for about 70 minutes without any prolonged effect on serum osmolality[37]. There is concern of rebound rise in ICP with its use which needs to be studied further.

Steroids. Glucocorticoids are very effective in ameliorating the vasogenic edema that accompanies tumors, inflammatory conditions, infections and other disorders associated with increased permeability of blood brain barrier, including surgical manipulations[38]. They are used in reducing ICP in intracranial tumors with perilesional edema, neurocysticercal encephalitis, acute demyelinating encephalomyelitis, tubercular meningitis, tuberculoma, and brain abscess. Dexamethasone is the preferred agent due to its very low mineralocorticoid activity. It is given in a dose of 0.4-1.5 mg/kg per day q 6 hr PO or IV. Steroids are not routinely indicated in individuals with traumatic brain injury[39]. Steroids have not been found to be useful and may be detrimental in children with ischemic lesions, cerebral malaria and intracranial hemorrhage[40, 41].

General Measures

> **Ongoing care of a child with raised ICP**
>
> - *Seizure control*
> - *Adequate analgesia*
> - *Sedation*
> - *Avoiding noxious stimuli*
> - *Normothermia*
> - *Euglycemia*
> - *Euvolemia*
> - *Avoid hypotonic fluids*
> - *Prevent and treat anemia*

Sedation and analgesia. Raised ICP is worsened due to agitation, pain, and patient-ventilator asynchrony[11]. Adequate analgesia, sedation and occasionally neuro-muscular blockade are useful adjuvants in the management of raised ICP. Appropriate analgesia and sedation is usually preferred over neuromuscular blockade, as it is quickly reversible and allows for neurological monitoring. It is preferable to use sedative agents with minimal effect on blood pressure. Short acting benzodiazepines (eg. midazolam) are useful for sedation in children.

Minimization of stimuli. Attempt must be made to reduce the number of unnecessary interventions that are likely to be painful. Lidocaine instilled into endotracheal tube has been shown to prevent the endotracheal suctioning-induced ICP increase and CPP reduction in adults with severe traumatic brain injury[42]. Lidocaine can be nebulized (usually 4% lidocaine mixed in 0.9% saline) or given intravenously (1-2 mg/kg as 1% solution) 90 seconds prior to suctioning.

Fluids. In a child with raised ICP, the main goal of fluid therapy is to maintain euvolemia, normoglycemia and prevent hyponatremia. Children with raised ICP should receive fluids at a daily maintenance rate, as well as fluid boluses as indicated for correction of hypovolemia, hypotension, or decreased urine output. Maintenance fluids usually consist of normal saline with daily requirements of potassium chloride based on body weight. All fluids administered must be isotonic or hypertonic (eg. Ringer lactate, normal saline) and hypotonic fluids must be avoided (e.g. 0.18% saline in 5% dextrose, Isolyte P).

Euglycemia. Blood glucose must be maintained between 80-120 mg/dL in a child with raised ICP[11]. Studies in children with traumatic brain injury have shown that hyperglycemia is associated with poor neurological outcome and increased mortality[43]. On the other hand hypoglycemia is known to induce a systemic stress response and cause disturbances in CBF, increasing the regional CBF by as much as 300% in severe hypoglycemia. Hypoglycemia can also lead to neuronal injury. Dextrose (5%) in 0.9% saline solution is used if the blood glucose falls below 80 mg/dL.

Temperature regulation. Normothermia should be maintained by frequent measurements of body temperature and correcting any fluctuations by using antipyretics assisted cooling or heating as per needs.

Prevention and treatment of seizures. Children with significant head injury and neuroinfections are at risk to develop seizures. Seizures can increase CBF and cerebral blood volume leading to increased ICP. They can also increase the metabolic needs of the brain and predispose to ischemia[9]. Seizures, when clinically evident, must be treated. It is reasonable, and a common practice to use prophylactic anticonvulsants for short term in children with raised ICP, unless contraindicated[9, 44]. If facilities are available, it is prudent to use continuous electroencephalography (EEG) to identify subclinical seizure activity in children with increased risk for seizures.

Prevention and treatment of anemia. Theoretically, anemia would increase CBF and secondarily raise ICP. There have been case reports of patients with severe anemia presenting with symptoms of raised ICP and papilledema[45]. Though not prospectively studied, it is a common practice to maintain hemoglobin level above 10 g/dL in patients with traumatic brain injury and raised ICP.

Surgical Therapy

Cerebrospinal fluid drainage. CSF drainage using an external ventricular drainage (EVD) or ventriculoperitoneal shunt provides for an immediately effective means to lower ICP. In addition EVD provides a method for continuously monitoring ICP. CSF drainage is particularly useful in the presence of hydrocephalus. Its effectiveness in lowering ICP has been shown to be comparable to intravenous mannitol or hyperventilation[46]. However, it is of limited utility in diffuse brain edema with collapsed ventricles.

Resection of mass lesion. Surgery should be undertaken when a lesion amenable to surgical intervention is identified as the primary cause of raised ICP. Common situations where this neurosurgical intervention is preferentially employed are acute epidural or subdural hematomas, brain abscess, or brain tumor.

Targets of therapy

The end points of management of raised ICP include an adequate CPP (Infants/toddlers 40-50 mmHg and children 50-60 mmHg) and ICP within normal range (Infants < 15 mmHg, 1-8 yr < 18 mmHg, > 8 years < 20 mmHg). The other end points of management are normal core body temperature (36°C-37°C), hematocrit 30%, right atrial pressure 5-10 mmHg, SpO2 > 90%, $PaCO_2$ 35-40 mmHg, $EtCO_2$ 35-40 mmHg and osmolality <320 mOsm/L.

Other Therapies for Refractory Raised ICP

Barbiturates. Use of barbiturates is generally reserved for cases with raised ICP which is refractory to conventional treatment. Thiopentone can be used for this purpose and the dosing of the drug is adjusted to a target ICP as monitored on an ICP monitor. The drug is titrated to a 90% burst suppression (2-6 bursts per minute) using an EEG monitor. Monitoring a child in barbiturate coma should include EEG, ICP monitoring, invasive hemodynamic monitoring (arterial blood pressure, central venous pressure, $SjvO_2$) and frequent assessment of oxygenation status. The complication rate of barbiturate therapy is high and includes hypotension, hypokalemia, respiratory complications, infections, hepatic and renal dysfunction[47].

Hypothermia. Evidence from carefully conducted studies in adults do not show any improvement in the neurologic outcome of patients with head injury with the use of therapeutic hypothermia[48, 49]. However, studies do suggest a lowered ICP during hypothermia therapy in children[48, 50]. Therefore, in children with refractory raised ICP, controlled hypothermia may be considered.

Decompressive craniectomy. On rare occasions, when all other measures fail, decompressive craniectomy with duraplasty may be a valuable procedure. Reports of its use in children with traumatic brain injury have shown benefit[51, 52]. It may offer an alternative treatment option in uncontrolled ICP refractory to other measures.

REFERENCES

1. Welch K. The intracranial pressure in infants. *J Neurosurg* 1980; 52:693–699.

2. Castillo LR, Gopinath S, Robertson CS. *Neurol Clin* 2008; 26: 521-541.

3. Goldstein B, Aboy M, Graham A. Neurologic monitoring. In: Rogers textbook of Pediatric Intensive Care, Nichols DG, (Ed.), *Lippincott Williams & Wilkins,* 4th edition, 2008.

4. Adelson PD, Bratton SL, Carney NA, *et al.* Guidelines for the acute medical management of severe traumatic brain injury in infants, children, and adolescents: Indications for intracranial pressure monitoring in pediatric patients with severe traumatic brain injury. *Pediatr Crit Care Med* 2003; 4: S19-S24.

5. Lee KR, Hoff JT. Intracranial pressure. In: Neurological Surgery. Youmans JR, (ed) *Philadelphia; Saunders*; 1996; pp.491-518.

6. Jordan KG. Neurophysiologic monitoring in the neuro-science intensive care unit. *Neurol Clin* 1995; 13(3): 579-626.

7. Lang EW, Chesnut RM. Intracranial pressure. Monitoring and management. *Neurosurg Clin N Amer* 1994; 5(4): 573-605.

8. Lundberg N. Continuous recording and control of ventricular fluid pressure in neurosurgical practice. *Acta Psychiatr Scand Suppl* 1960; 36(149): 1-193.

9. Marcoux KK. Management of increased intracranial pressure in critically ill child with acute neurological injury. *AACN Clinical Issues* 2005; 16: 212-231.

10. Feldman Z, Kanter MJ, Robertson CS, *et al.* Effect of head elevation on intracranial pressure, cerebral perfusion pressure, and cerebral blood flow in head-injured patients. *J Neurosurg* 1992; 76:207-211.

11. Layon JA, Gabrielli A. Elevated intracranial pressure. In: Textbook of Neurointensive Care. Layon JA, Gabrielli A, Friedman WA (Eds.). 1st edition, *Saunders, Pennsylvania* 2004: 709-732.

12. Marsh ML, Marshall LF, Shapiro HM. Neurological intensive care. *Anesthesiology* 1997; 47:149-163.

13. Skippen P, Seear M, Poskitt K, Kestle J, *et al.* Effect of hyperventilation on regional cerebral blood flow in head-injured children. *Crit Care Med* 1997; 25: 1275-1278.

14. Robertson CS, Valadka AB, Hannay HJ, Contant CF, *et el*. Prevention of secondary ischemia insult after severe head injury. *Crit Care Med* 1992; 27: 2086-2095.

15. Miller JD, D Earden NM, Piper IR, *et al*. Control of intracranial pressure in patients with severe head injury. *J. Neurotrauma* 1992; 9: S 317.

16. Muizelaar JP, Lutz HA III, Becker DP. Effect of mannitol on ICP and CBF and correlation with pressure autoregulation in severely head injured patients. *J Neurosurgery* 1984; 61: 700-706.

17. Rosner MJ, Coley I. Cerebral perfusion pressure: a hemodynamic mechanisms of mannitol and post-mannitol hemogram. *Neurosurgery* 1987; 21: 147-156.

18. Alvarez B, Fereer-Sueta G, Radi R. Slowing of peroxynitrite decomposition in the presence of mannitol and ethanol. *Free Radic Biol Med* 1998; 24: 1331-1337.

19. Korenkov AI, Pahnke J, Frei K, Warzok R, Schroeder HW, Frick R, Muljana L, Piek J, Yonekawa Y, Gaab MR. Treatment with nimodipine or mannitol reduces programmed cell death and infarct size following focal cerebral ischemia. *Neurosurg Rev* 2000; 23: 145-150.

20. Diringer MN, Zazulia AR. Osmotic therapy, fact or fiction? *Neurocrit Care* 2004; 1:219-234.

21. Kaufmann AM, Cardoso ER. Aggravation of vasogenic edema by multiple-dose mannitol. *J Neurosurg* 1992; 77: 584-589.

22. De Carvalho WB. Hypertonic solutions for pediatric patients. *J Pediatr* 2003; 79: S187-S194.

23. Thompson R, Greaves I. Hypertonic saline-hydroxyethyl starch in trauma resuscitation. *J R Army Med Corps* 2006; 152: 6-12.

24. Zhao L, Wang B, You G, Zhou H. Effects of different resuscitation fluids on the rheologic behavior of red blood cells, blood viscosity and plasma viscosity in experimental hemorrhagic shock. *Resuscitation* 2009; 80:253-258.

25. Tseng MY, AI-Rawi PG, Pickard JD, Rasulo FA, Kirkpatrick PJ. Effect of hypertonic saline on cerebral blood flow in poor-grade patients with subarachnoid hemorrhage. *Stroke* 2003; 34: 1398-1396.

26. Rizoli SB, Rhind SG, Shek PN, Inaba K, Filips D, Tien H, Brenneman F, Rotstein O. The immunomodulatory effects of hypertonic saline resuscitation in patients sustaining traumatic hemorrhagic shock: a randomized, controlled, double-blinded trial. *Ann Surg* 2006 243: 47-57.

27. Ziai WC, Toung TJ, Bhardwaj A. Hypertonic saline: first-line therapy for cerebral edema? *J Neurol Sci* 2007; 261:157-166.

28. Doyle JA, Davis DP, Hoyt DB. The use of hypertonic saline in the treatment of traumatic brain injury. *J Trauma* 2001; 50: 367-383.

29. Himmelseher S. Hypertonic saline solutions for treatment of intracranial hypertension. *Curr Opin Anaesthesiol* 2007; 20: 414-428.

30. Suarez JI. Hypertonic saline for cerebral edema and elevated intracranial pressure. *Cleve Clin J Med* 2004; 71: S9-S13.

31. Strandvik GF. Hypertonic saline in critical care: a review of the literature and guidelines for use in hypotensive states and raised intracranial pressure. *Anaesthesia* 2009; 64: 990-1003.

32. Larive LL, Denise H. Rhoney DH, Dennis Parker D, Coplin WM, Carhuapoma JR. Introducing hypertonic saline for cerebral edema. *Neurocrit Care* 2004; 1: 435-440.

33. Qureshi A, Suarez J, Bhardwaj A, *et al*. Use of hypertonic saline/acetate infusion in the treatment of cerebral edema: effect on intracranial pressure and lateral displacement of the brain. Crit Care Med 1998; 26: 440-446.

34. Peterson B, Khanna S, Fischer B, Marshall L. Prolonged hypernatremia controls elevated intracranial pressure in head injured pediatric patients. *Crit Care Med* 2008; 28: 1136-1143.

35. Thenuwara K, Todd MM, Brain JE, *et al*. Effect of mannitol and furosemide on plasma osmolality and brain water. *Anesthesiology* 2002; 96: 416-421.

36. Tornheim PA, McLaurin RL, Sawaya R. Effect of furosemide on experimental traumatic cerebral edema. *Neurosurgery* 1979; 4: 48-52.

37. Berger C, Sakowitz OW, Kiening KL, Schwab S. Neurochemical monitoring of glycerol therapy in patients with ischemic brain edema. *Stroke* 2005; 36: e4-6.

38. French LA, Galicich JH. The use of steroids for control of cerebral edema. *Clin Neurosurg* 1964; 10: 212-223.

39. Edwards P, Arango M, Balica L, *et al*. Final results of MRCCRASH, a randomised placebo-controlled trial of intravenous corticosteroids in adults with head injured outcomes at 6 months. *Lancet* 2005; 365: 1957-1959.

40. Feigin VL, Anderson N, Rinkel GJ, et al. Corticosteroids for aneurysmal subarachnoid haemorrhage and primary intracerebral haemorrhage. *Cochrane Database Syst Rev* 2005; CD004583.

41. Hoffman SL, Rustama D, Punjabi NH, *et al*. High-dose dexamethasone in quinine-treated patients with cerebral malaria: a double-blind, placebo-controlled trial. *J Infect Dis* 1988; 158-325-331.

42. Bilitta F, Branca G, Lam A, Cuzzone V, Doronzio A, Rosa G. Endotraceal lidocaine in preventing endotracheal suctioning induced changes in cerebral hemodynamics in patients with severe head trauma. *Neurocrit Care* 2008; 8: 241-246.

43. Cochran A, Scaife ER, Hansen KW, Downey EC. Hyperglycemia and outcomes from pediatric traumatic brain injury. *J Trauma* 2003; 55: 1035-1038.

44. Rabinstein AA. Treatment of cerebral edema. *The Neurologist* 2006; 12: 59-73.

45. Biousse V, Rucker JC, Vignal C, et al. Anemia and papilledema, *Am J Ophthalmol* 2003; 135: 437-446.

46. Fortune JB, Feustal PJ, Grace L, et al. Effect of hyperventilation, mannitol, and ventriculostomy drainage on cerebral blood flow after head injury. J *Trauma* 1995; 39:1091-1099.

47. Schalen W, Sonesson B, Messeter K, *et al.* Clinical outcome and cognitive impairment in patients with severe head injuries treated with barbiturate coma. *Acta Neurochir* (Wien) 1992; 117-153-159.

48. Hutchison JS, Ward RE, Lacroix J, *et al.* Hypothermia therapy after traumatic brain injury in children. *N Engl J Med* 2008; 358: 2447-2456.

49. Clifton GL, Miller ER, Choi SC, Levin HS, *et al.* Lack of effect of induction of hypothermia after acute brain injury. *N Engl J Med* 2001; 344: 556-563.

50. Adelson PD, Ragheb J, Kanev P, et al. Phase II clinical trial of moderate hypothermia after severe traumatic brain injury in children. *Neurosurgery* 2005; 56: 740-754.

51. Berger S, Schwarz M, Huth R. Hypertonic saline solution and decompressive craniectomy for treatment of intracranial hypertension in pediatric severe traumatic brain injury. *J Trauma* 2002; 53-558-563.

52. Taylor A, Butt W, Rosenfeld J, et al. A randomized trial of very early decompressive craniectomy in children with traumatic brain injury and sustained intracranial hypertension. *Child's Nerv Syst* 2001; 17: 154-162.

53. Sankhyan N, Vykunta Raju KN, Sharma S, Gulati S. Management of raised intracranial pressure. *Indian J Pediatr* 2010; 77: 1409-1416.

Section 2

Neonatal Emergencies

Neonatal Emergencies in the Delivery Room

Ramesh Agarwal and Meharban Singh

Birthing is believed to be the most dangerous period in one's life. The process of transition from fetal to extrauterine life may be complicated by a number of life-threatening conditions, which have bearing on immediate survival as well as long term neurological outcome. Every birth must be considered as a medical emergency and in India we should be prepared to handle 26 million emergencies every year. It is, therefore, essential for all health professionals caring for newborns to be aware of and be prepared to deal with these emergencies arising in the delivery room (DR), many of which respond favorably with appropriate timely intervention. The first step for effective management of neonatal emergencies in DR is to be adequately equipped with functional equipment, protocols, supplies and availability of skilled healthcare professionals.

The preparation to deal with emergencies in DR, should start from prenatal period itself, as the timely recognition of many of these problems can be made by fetal ultrasound and other diagnostic modalities. When there is reasonable anticipation for the likely emergency to be faced at birth, adequate preparations should be made to manage it effectively at birth. Prenatal interventions exist for some disorders such as antenatal steroids for extremely preterm babies and tracheal plugging for management of diaphragmatic hernia. New NRP guidelines recommend simulation based training program for health professionals to effectively deal with DR emergencies, which significantly improves the teamwork that requires effective communication, coordination and skills[1]. The common neonatal emergencies which may be faced in DR are listed in Table 19.1.

RESUSCITATION OF AN ASPHYXIATED BABY

The most common emergency that a pediatrician confronts everyday is the infant failing to breathe and/or maintain an effective breathing (perinatal asphyxia; birth asphyxia) with devastating

Table 19.1 Neonatal emergencies which can present in the labor room

- Failure to initiate or maintain effective breathing
- Multiple births
- Shock and/or hypovolemia
- Severe anemia
- Pneumothorax
- Hydrops, ascites, or pleural effusion
- Convulsions
- Birth of extremely preterm baby
- Maternal conditions/drugs affecting the fetus and neonate
- Life-threatening malformations
  - (a) Airways
  - (b) Lungs
  - (c) Heart
  - (d) Other organ systems: Neural tube defects, intestinal, and GU anomalies, and skeletal dysplasias
- Birth trauma
  - (a) Injuries to body organs
  - (b) Peripheral nerve injuries

consequences in terms of survival and subsequent neuromotor disability. As per the latest estimates, perinatal asphyxia accounts for 9% of total under-5 mortality worldwide, being one of the three most common causes of neonatal deaths along with prematurity and bacterial infections[2]. Apart from neonatal deaths, asphyxia is responsible for lifelong disability in a large number of children.

Resuscitation Alert

The existence of certain high risk factors during pregnancy and labor serve to forewarn and alert the DR staff that they should be fully prepared to meet the challenge of an asphyxiated baby[3] (Table 19.2). Several time honored clinical parameters of fetal distress offer useful guidelines to an experienced obstetrician.

Exaggerated Fetal Movements. The asphyxiated fetus behaves like a strangulated individual and makes desperate physical efforts

Table 19.2 Conditions demanding resuscitation alert

Antepartum risk factors

- Bad obstetrical history
- Young (<16 yr) or elderly (>35 yr) mother
- Maternal systemic disease or poor nutritional status
- Pregnancy-induced hypertension
- Multiple gestation
- Rhesus-isoimmunization
- Fetal malformations
- Polyhydramnios or oligohydramnios
- Fetal size to gestation discrepancy i.e. undersized or oversized baby
- Prolonged rupture of membranes (>18 hours) and chorioamnionitis
- Drug therapy: Reserpine, lithium carbonate, magnesium sulfate, adrenergic blocking agents, maternal drug abuse etc.

Intrapartum risk factors

- Fetal distress
- Premature or post-term gestation
- Malpresentation
- Large or macrosomic fetus
- Cord prolapse or tight nuchal cord
- APH: Placenta previa or abruptio placentae
- Prolonged labor (>24 hours) or prolonged second stage of labor (>2 hours)
- Maternal narcotics, analgesics and anesthetics
- Meconium-stained amniotic fluid
- Difficult or instrumental (forceps or vacuum-assisted) or operative (emergency cesarean section) delivery

Table 19.3 Apgar scoring system

Criteria	Score		
	0	1	2
1. Respiration	Nil	Slow, gasping	Crying
2. Heart rate /min	Nil	Upto 100	More than 100
3. Muscle tone	Flaccid	In-between	Flexed
4. Reflex response	Nil	Grimace	Cough, sneeze, cry
5. Color	Pale or blue	Peripheral cyanosis	Completely pink

followed by reduced or absent physical movements terminally.

Fetal Heart Rate. Due to release of catecholamines, initially there is tachycardia followed by bradycardia and slow-irregular heart beats. Bradycardia is a compensatory mechanism that allows longer coronary blood flow and ventricular filling because of prolonged diastole. The heart rate should be assessed during the later phase of uterine contraction.

Visceral Overactivity. The passage of meconium in a vertex presenting baby is an important and ominous sign of fetal hypoxia. It is fraught with the risk of aspiration of meconium by the gasping fetus. In preterm babies fetal diarrhea as a result of listeriosis is an uncommon cause of meconium staining of the liquor in the absence of fetal hypoxia.

Evaluation of the Infant at Birth

Despite its limitations, the Apgar scoring system is conventionally used for assessing the condition of the newborn baby at 60 seconds after birth (Table 19.3). The respiratory effort and heart beat per minute are critical components of Apgar scoring system because muscle tone, response to reflex stimulus and color are dependent upon the cardio-respiratory status of the baby.

Apgar scoring system ignores the time of cry after birth which is important to identify and differentiate between primary and terminal apnea. The peripheral cyanosis is awarded a score of one, although majority of healthy normally breathing babies are never totally pink at 1-minute. Tone and response to reflex stimulus are dependent upon gestational maturity. Moreover, centrally blue (asphyxia livida) and totally pale (asphyxia pallida) babies are given an identical score, although latter are more gravely sick due to the combined effect of cardio-respiratory failure. *Apgar scoring system is no longer used for initiating various steps of resuscitation.* However, Apgar score at 5-minutes after birth or subsequently is a useful correlate of future mental prognosis of asphyxiated babies[4-6].

Resuscitation Kit

It is a sad fact that most delivery rooms in developing countries are not adequately equipped for the resuscitation of an asphyxiated newborn baby. The procedure of carrying the newly born baby from the delivery room to another room for resuscitation is most unsatisfactory. Each delivery room must have a well-lighted and warm microenvironment to receive the newly born infant. The resuscitation kit must be checked by the staff nurse of every duty shift and rechecked by the physician before each delivery. The pencil-handle laryngoscope with infant (0 and 1) straight blade is preferred. Its light source and batteries should be in working condition. Gamma-irradiated disposable endotracheal tubes with internal diameters of 2.5 mm, 3.0 mm and 3.5 mm and mounted with adapters should be available. The electrical points and suction machine should be in working order. Press-type rubber bulb or oral suction mucus trap must be available to meet the exigencies of electrical failure (Figure 19.1). Oxygen cylinder should be checked for its contents. Ambu bag and mask is extremely useful and handy to resuscitate an apneic baby. The self inflatable bags are easy to use but provide only 40% to 50% oxygen. The attachment of a corrugated tube provides a reservoir for oxygen and can deliver upto 80% oxygen to the infant. The kit should contain disposable sterile endotracheal tube and suction catheters, plastic oral airway, syringes and needles, 7.5% sodium bicarbonate, atropine, epinephrine 1:10,000, calcium gluconate 10%, neonatal nalorphine (1.0 mg/ml), naloxone hydrochloride (0.4 mg/ml), ampoules of distilled water, physiological saline, albumin 5% solution and 5% dextrose. Sterile neonatal delivery packs containing bowl, scissors, cotton swabs and umbilical ties should be available for each delivery. The bassinet on which the baby is to be received should be kept warm and provided with an over head radiant heat source and a stopclock to accurately time the sequence of events after birth (Figure 19.2). Pulse oximetry is being increasingly used in most centers for continuous monitoring of oxygen saturation during resuscitation.

It is desirable that equipment for resuscitation should be maintained in sterile condition and baby received in sterile warm sheets with due aseptic precautions. Above all, the physician must be adept in the art of cardio-pulmonary resuscitaton. The art of endotracheal intubation should be learnt and perfected by continued practice on the still born and dead neonates. Several life support neonatal training simulators and modules are available to learn

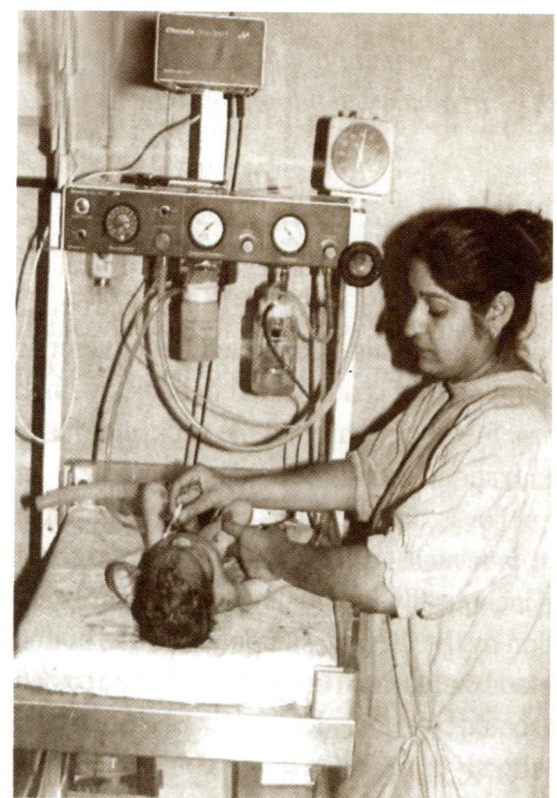

Figure 19.2 Resuscitator with overhead warmer and in-built facilities for suction, oxygen supply and intermittent positive pressure ventilation

the skills of external cardiac massage and artificial ventilation. The retention of cardio-pulmonary skills is shortlived unless they are constantly revised and practiced.

Initial Steps in Resuscitation

The resuscitation kit should be checked before the baby is born. The radiant warmer should be put on and plenty of sterile prewarmed linen should be available. Due to increasing prevalence and risk of AIDS it is desirable that the pediatrician resuscitating the baby wears the gloves. The baby should be received in a warm sheet and head kept slightly low (Figure 19.3). The conventional practice of holding the baby upside down from its feet is undesirable. The baby should be placed under the radiant warmer and both hypothermia as well as hyperthermia should be prevented. The baby should be placed supine or on its side, with the head in a neutral or slightly extended position. The infant's mouth, oropharynx, hypopharynx and nose are sucked, in that order, using thick 10 Fr suction catheter with gentle intermittent suction. The nose should not be sucked first as it would lead to reflex breathing with the risk of aspiration of secretions

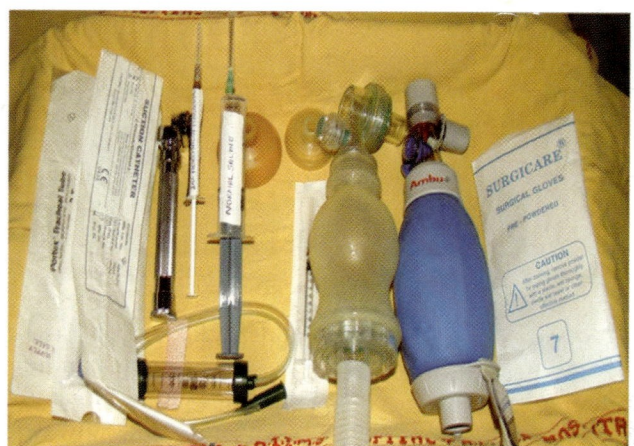

Figure 19.1 Resuscitation kit. Note corrugated tube attached at the inlet of Ambu bag to enhance concentration of oxygen delivered to the infant

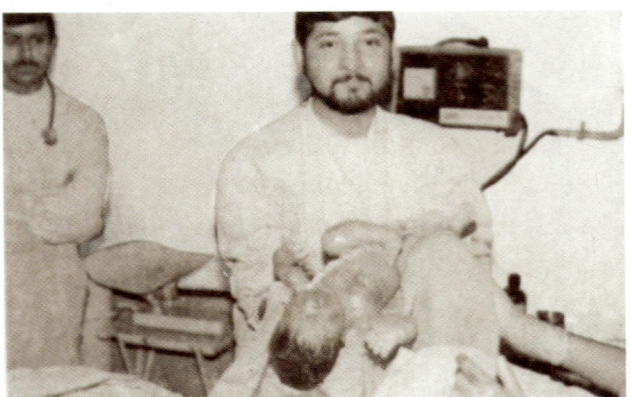

Figure 19.3 The correct method of holding the baby at birth

contained in the oral cavity. After suction, the baby should be dried effectively and wet linen should be removed. Head constitutes a large surface area of the baby and must be effectively dried. The process of drying and suction produce enough stimulation to initiate effective respiration in most newly born babies. If an infant is not breathing or his breathing efforts are sluggish, he should be stimulated by flicking the soles or rubbing the back. The tactile stimulation should not be continued beyond 3 to 4 flicks and when it is ineffective the baby should be promptly ventilated with a bag and mask. *Evaluate the infant every 30 sec by simultaneously observing respirations, heart rate and color to decide the need for further steps in resuscitation[7-9].* Availability of a stop clock mounted on the resuscitator is essential to accurately time the sequence of events after birth.

Approach to a Meconium-stained Baby

About 10-15 percent pregnancies are complicated by passage of meconium in-utero during labor. It is a reliable sign of fetal distress with additional risk of respiratory morbidity due to meconium aspiration syndrome. The detection of in-utero passage of meconium may be delayed if membranes are intact. Thick meconium staining of liquor (pea-soup appearance) is ominous. Yellow staining of skin, umbilical cord and nails indicate that meconium has been passed at least 4-6 hours before delivery. It is associated with increased risk of birth asphyxia and meconium aspiration syndrome. When amniotic fluid is meconium stained, the baby should be promptly delivered either by cesarean section or by forceps if cervix is adequately dilated. The practice of suctioning the oral cavity by obstetrician as soon as the head is delivered is no longer recommended. Recent multicentric study has shown that intrapartum suctioning does not reduce the risk of meconium

aspiration syndrome because babies breathe in-utero and aspirate meconium before head is delivered.

After delivery, thorough suction of oral cavity, oropharynx and glottic area should be done under direct vision with the help of a laryngoscope. When a meconium-stained baby is depressed as evidenced by poor cry, flaccidity, or bradycardia (heart rate <100 bpm), it is recommended that endotracheal intubation should be done. The need for intubation is not based on consistency or thickness of meconium. The endotracheal tube is attached directly to a gentle intermittent suction source to suck out the meconium. The endotracheal tube is gradually withdrawn while suction is being applied. The infant may have to be intubated 2 to 3 times till all the meconium has been sucked out. At times saline lavage may be required to remove thick tenacious meconium. The meconium cannot be sucked by inserting a suction catheter through the endotracheal tube. The practice of sucking the endotracheal tube with oral negative pressure of the resuscitator, is not recommended due to the potential risk of HIV infection. The meconium stained baby should not be ventilated or bagged till air passages have been effectively cleared of all possible meconium. However, if the infant's heart rate or respiration is severely depressed, it is desirable to institute positive-pressure ventilation despite the presence of some meconium in the airway. If a meconium stained baby is vigorously crying at birth, there is no need to do endotracheal intubation. There is a potential risk of injury to the vocal cords while trying to intubate a vigorous and crying term infant. When the baby is stable, stomach wash is recommended to reduce the risk of vomiting and aspiration of meconium-stained gastric contents. Infant should be closely watched for development of respiratory distress due to meconium aspiration syndrome and onset of persistent pulmonary hemorrhage.

Resuscitation of an Asphyxiated Baby

American Academy of Pediatrics (AAP) and Americal Heart Association (AHS) along with several other organizations have formalized a partnership with International Liaison Committee on Resuscitation (ILCOR) to update and revise recommendations for neonatal resuscitation program (NRP). The recent Consensus On Science and Treatment Recommendations (COSTR) published in 2010 provides the latest NRP guidelines which are considered as gold standard.[1]

Most babies have a smooth transition from fetal to neonatal life and establish spontaneous breathing at birth without any active assistance. About 5.0% to 7.5% babies are likely to have difficulty in initiating spontaneous breathing at birth and need active resuscitation. At every delivery, there should be at least one person, who is adequately trained in the art of neonatal resuscitation, to look after the needs of the newly born baby. When the delivery is high risk, at least two trained personnel are required to perform complete resuscitation including bag and mask ventilation, endotracheal intubation, chest compressions and administration of medications. When a mother is having multiple gestations, separate teams of trained personnel and equipment should be available to handle and resuscitate each baby. The procedure of neonatal resuscitation must be carried out by skilled and experienced person with a sense of urgency but without any panic. The revised neonatal resuscitation program (NRP) guidelines of the Technical Committee of National Neonatology Forum of India recommends that the newly born baby should be assessed by asking the following question[10].

Is baby breathing or crying?

When answer to the above question is YES, the baby needs routine care. But when answer is NO, the baby is provided initial steps for resuscitation. During the initial steps, the baby is correctly positioned, airway is cleared and he is effectively dried and kept warm. When a baby is breathing but is cyanosed, he is administered free-flow oxygen at a rate of 5 liters/min till he becomes pink. Free-flow oxygen is administered through an oxygen mask or flow-inflating bag or a hand cupped around the oxygen tubing. If a baby is not breathing or having gasping breaths, he is provided tactile stimulation by flicking the soles or rubbing the back to promote breathing. Avoid prolonged tactile stimulation in an apneic baby, as this will waste valuable time. The baby is simultaneously assesed for respiration, heart rate and color to take further decisions for resuscitation (Figure 19.4).

Bag and mask ventilation

If despite stimulation, the baby is still apneic or having ineffective ventilations as evidenced by heart rate of less than 100 beats per minute, he should be given bag and mask ventilation. Position the infant supine by placing a small roll of towel under the shoulders inorder to extend the neck and open the airways (Figure 19.5). Thorough suctioning of oral cavity, hypopharynx and nose is mandatory before starting bag and mask ventilation. The mask should tightly fit on the face enclosing nose and mouth of the baby (Figure 19.6). Supplemental oxygen (30-40%) can be given during bag and mask ventilation but there is no need to attach the oxygen reservoir to the bag to increase the concentration of oxygen. *In community setting, when oxygen is not available infant can be successfully ventilated with room air (21% oxygen) with the help of bag and mask or tube and mask*[10]. The infant should be ventilated at a rate of 40-60 breaths per minute. To avoid alveolar rupture and pneumothorax, the operator should train himself or herself to deliver 15-20 cm H_2O pressure with the help of a manometer. To open up the collapsed alveoli, few initial inflatory pressures of 30-40 cm H_2O pressure are recommended. There should be a noticeable rise and fall of the chest during each ventilation. Naloxone hydrochloride 0.1 mg/kg should be administered intravenously through umbilical vein if mother had received pethidine or morphine within 4 hours before delivery. If needed it can be repeated after every 2-3 minutes. During bag and mask ventilation heart rate should be closely monitored after every 30 seconds. Heart rate is assessed by auscultating the precordium or feeling pulsations at the base of the umbilical cord. To save time, heart rate is counted for 6 seconds and multiplied by 10 to get the heart rate per minute. If despite effective bag and mask ventilation, heart rate is not coming up or it further slows down and drops below 60 per minute, the infant should be intubated. *A large majority of asphyxiated babies can be effectively revived and resuscitated by using bag and mask ventilation alone and intubation is usually not required.*

In Indian setting, the use of laryngeal mask airway is currently not recommended due to the expense involved and lack of training and expertise in this procedure. In preterm neonates, a T-piece resuscitator is more useful as it can provide PEEP. There is no role of dexamethasone, atropine, calcium and respiratory stimulants like nikethamide and lobeline during resuscitation. The Apgar scoring system is not taken into consideration while taking management decisions during resuscitation of a newborn baby. The management is guided by the status of breathing, heart rate and color of the baby. Apgar score may be recorded at 1-minute, 5-minutes and subsequently (till it is more than 7) to serve as a prognostic indicator of the outcome of an asphyxiated baby. For details of bag and mask ventilation, techniques of tracheal intubation and external cardiac massage refer to Chapter 58.

Section 3

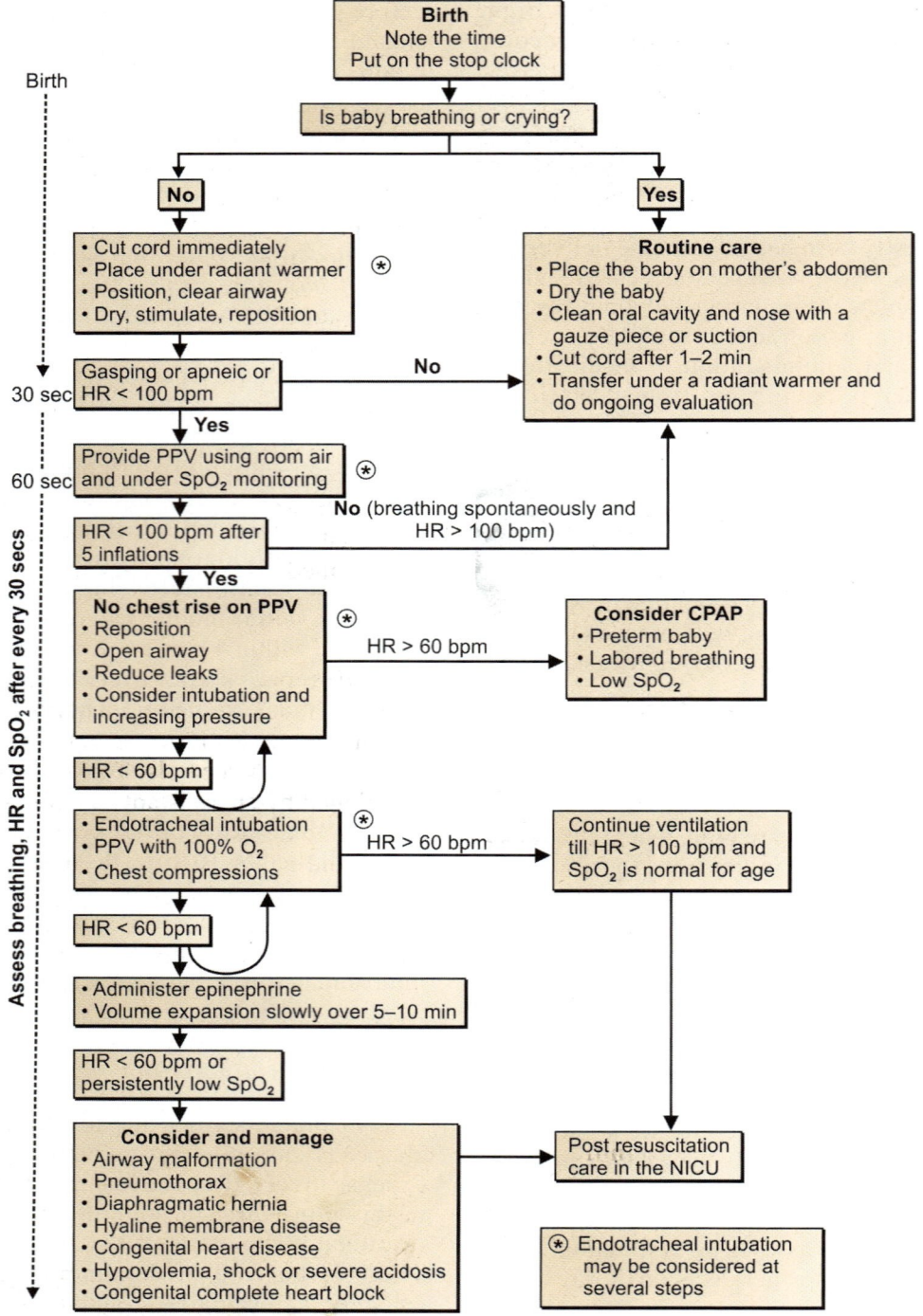

Figure 19.4 Algorithm for resuscitation of an asphyxiated newborn baby. Adapted from NRP–India guidelines.

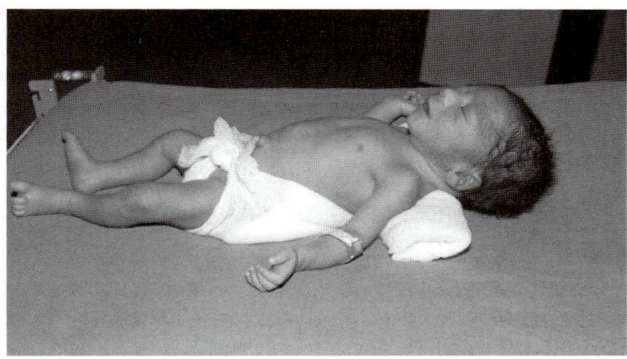

Figure 19.5 Positioning the newborn baby to maintain the patency of airways. Note the folded sheet under the shoulders to extend the neck

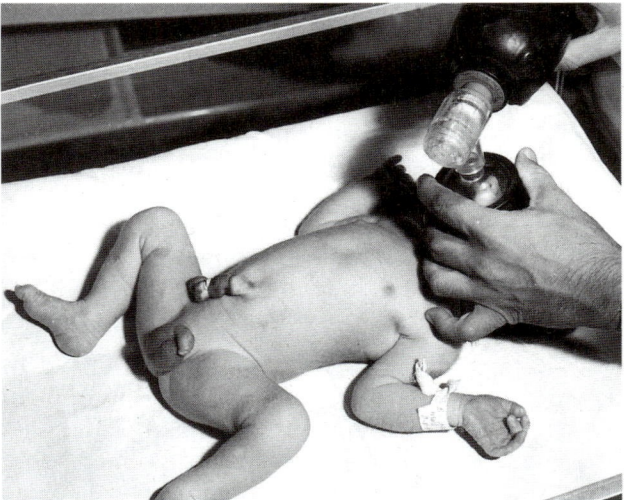

Figure 19.6 Bag and mask resuscitation. Most of the asphyxiated infants can be successfully resuscitated by this technique.

Endotracheal intubation

Endotracheal intubation is indicated in following situations[7,8].

- When tracheal suctioning is required in a meconium-stained depressed baby.

- If bag and mask ventilation is ineffective (heart rate remains <80 bpm) or it is prolonged.

- When chest compressions are performed.

- Extremely preterm babies and neonates requiring administration of surfactant.

- Infants with airway anomalies, diaphragmatic hernia, and hydrops fetalis.

The art of intubation cannot be taught and must be learnt by practicing on stillborn babies, neonates dying in the nursery and baby simulators. The appropriate sized (4.0 mm in a term baby and 2.5

mm in a tiny baby) endotracheal tube should be prepared by shortening it to 13 cm and attaching a connector. Proper length of insertion of ET tube from lips can be calculated by weight of the infant in kg + 6 cm. It is easy to intubate an asphyxiated baby with some practice because of lack of resistance and hypotonia. The endotracheal tube should be suctioned before starting positive pressure ventilation with a bag or machine. The laryngeal mask airway may serve as an effective alternative for establishing an airway if bag-mask ventilation is ineffective or attempts at intubation have failed. In preterm babies (< 32 weeks) T-piece resuscitator with inbuilt PEEP are useful for resuscitation. In preterm babies, availability of an oxygen blender and pulse oximeter is useful for resuscitation. The ventilation can be stopped as soon as the baby establishes spontaneous breathing and heart rate is maintained above 100 beats per minute.

External cardiac massage

External cardiac massage is indicated in babies in whom heart rate drops below 60 per minute despite effective ventilation with 100% oxygen for 30 seconds. The ventilation should be continued by an assistant and simultaneously heart should be massaged either by using two fingers of one hand or encircling the chest of the baby with both the hands and applying sternal compressions with two thumbs (Figures 19.7 and 19.8). Available data suggest that the 2 thumb-encircling hand technique is more convenient and effective in generating peak systolic and coronary perfusion pressures.

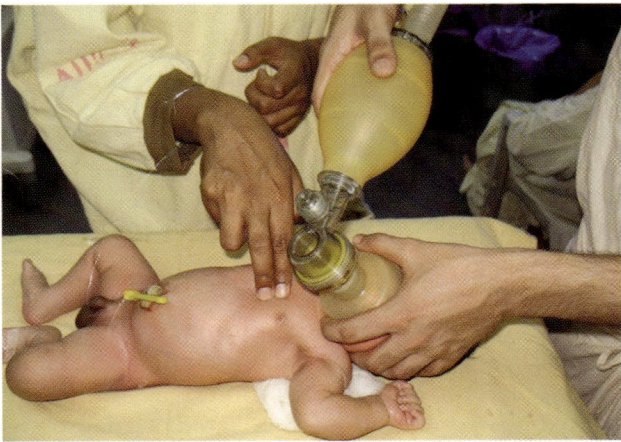

Figure 19.7 External cardiac massage with two fingers. Index and middle fingers are placed vertically over the lower third of sternum to provide cardiac compressions at a rate of 120/min. Bag and mask or bag and endotracheal tube ventilation should continue during chest compressions

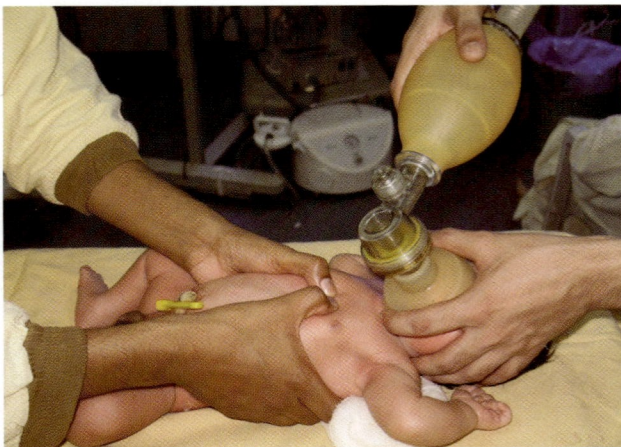

Figure 19.8 External cardiac massage with thumbs. The chest is enclosed within both hands and thumbs opposed over the lower one-third of mid sternal region for providing compressions. In extremely low birth weight baby one thumb can be placed over the other (instead of side by side) because of small size of the precordial area. Two-thumb technique is more effective in generating peak systolic and coronary perfusion pressures

Press the lower part of the sternum just above the xiphoid cartilage to a depth of one-third of the anterior-posterior diameter of the chest at a rate of 90 compressions and 30 ventilations (3:1 ratio) per minute. The thumbs and tips of fingers (depending upon the method used) should remain in contact with the sternum all the time and they should not be lifted off after each compression. Check the heart rate after every 30 seconds and chest compressions may be stopped when heart rate goes above 60 bpm.

Medications

Epinephrine is indicated when the heart rate remains below 60 bpm despite 30 seconds of assisted ventilation and another 30 seconds of coordinated chest compressions and assisted ventilation. Administer 0.1-0.3 ml/kg of 1.10,000 solution (0.01-0.03 mg/kg) of epinephrine through the umbilical vein or 0.3-1.0 ml/kg through endotracheal tube[7]. Intracardiac route is dangerous and should be avoided due to risk of damage to the coronary vessels and development of hemo-pericardium. The dose of epinephrine may be repeated after every 3-5 minutes as indicated. Naloxone hydrochloride is indicated in a depressed infant whose mother received narcotics within 4 hours of delivery. Adequate ventilation must be established before administration of naloxone. The recommended dose of naloxone is 0.1 mg/kg (0.4 mg/ml solution) and can be given IV, IM or

SC. If a baby is in shock, consider the use of plasma expander (ORh-negative RBCs, normal saline or Ringer's lactate) in a dose of 10 ml per kg slow intravenous push over 5 to 10 minutes. The fluids of choice for volume expansion is an isotonic crystalloid solution like physiological saline or Ringer's lactate. 5% albumin is no longer recommended for volume expansion.

Effective ventilation is followed by sponta-neous correction of acidosis and alkali therapy should be guided by monitoring blood acid base parameters. When blood gasometry facilities are not available, sodium bicarbonate 5-10 ml of 7.5% solution (adequately diluted with equal volume of distilled water or double volume of 5% dextrose) should be administered intravenously slowly at a rate of 1.0 ml/minute to infants in whom effective ventilation is not established even by 10 minutes or later (Apgar score of less than 7 at 10 minutes). Bolus administration of sodium bicarbonate should be avoided due to the risk of development of intraventricular hemorrage in preterm babies. Effective ventilation must be established before administration of sodium bicarbonate.

When to deny or stop CPR at birth?

Resuscitation at birth may be denied or abandoned when it is considered futile in terms of survival or survival is likely to be associated with gross neuromotor disability with extremely poor quality of life. It is justified and ethical to deny resuscitation to infants with gross non-correctable lethal congenital malformations and micropremies (<750 g in developing countries). The resuscitation efforts may be abandoned in fresh still born babies (zero apgar score at one minute) if there are no signs of life at 10 minutes or if spontaneous breathing is not established by 30 minutes.

Intractable Birth Asphyxia

The conditions listed in Table 19.4 should be suspected if ventilation remains unsatisfactory even after 10 minutes of birth. Effective and thorough suctioning, endotracheal intubation and assisted ventilation are mandatory in these infants. Skiagram of chest should be taken for further management of such an infant. Blood gases, acid-base parameters, electrolytes, glucose, BUN and lactate should be monitored. Drainage of ascites and thoracentesis would improve respiration in hydropic infants. Removal of air from pleural cavity in an infant with tension pneumothorax would be life saving. It can be promptly diagnosed in the labor room with the help of fiber optic cold light. Oral airway facilitates

Table 19.4 Causes of intractable birth asphyxia
♦ Meconium aspiration or tracheal plug
♦ Congenital malformations of airways namely choanal atresia, laryngeal web, diaphragmatic hernia, esophageal atresia with tracheo-esophageal fistula, lobar emphysema or cyst, and asphyxiating thoracic dystrophy
♦ Pneumothorax and pneumomediastinum
♦ Intracranial hemorrhage
♦ Shock (cardiogenic or hypovolemic)
♦ Profound metablioc alterations
♦ Congenital pneumonia
♦ Hydrops fetalis
♦ Severe immaturity (< 28 weeks gestation)
♦ Paralysis of respiratory muscles or malformation of brain
♦ Pulmonary hemorrhage
♦ Excessive maternal sedation

breathing in infants with choanal atresia. When congenital diaphragmatic hernia is suspected, stomach should be decompressed with an orogastric catheter and infant should be ventilated after endotracheal intubation. Many centers advocate routine elective intubation of extremely preterm babies to support ventilation and administer surfactant. Bolus administration of volume expanders or hyperosmolar solutions should be avoided due to potential risk of causing intraventricular hemorrhage.

Whole Body or Selective Brain Cooling

There is an experimental and clinical evidence to suggest that mild to moderate whole body or selective brain cooling with a cold cap is neuro-protective against the adverse effects of birth asphyxia[11-17]. Cerebral hypothermia reduces ATP production and lowers metabolic rate of the brain with increase in the levels of inhibitory neuro-modulators like glycine, taurine, GABA and adenosine which are neuroprotective[13]. There is reduced alterations in ion flux and preservation of blood brain barrier. Cooling is begun within 1-6 hour after hypoxic insult by maintaining brain or core body temperature between 33-34°C for 48-72 hours.

Whole body cooling is recommended in term infants (>36 weeks), if three of the following five inclusion criteria are fulfilled.

(i) Apgar score ≤5 at 10 minutes.

(ii) pH of cord blood or infant's blood ≤7.0 within one hour of age.

(iii) Base deficit of cord blood or infant's blood within one hour age of ≥16 mEq/l.

(iv) Need for continued assisted ventilations at birth for at least 10 minutes.

(v) History of seizures or CNS abnormalities suggestive of grade 3 or more hypoxic-ischemic encephalopathy (HIE).

These infants should be given adequate sedation and excellent supportive care. There is evidence to suggest that neuroprotective effect of moderate hypothermia can be enhanced by co-administration of topiramate. However, inadvertent excessive cooling with fall in core body temperature is associated with adverse metabolic and physiologic effects with higher risk of morbidity and mortality. It would appear that hypothermia and selective cooling of brain after perinatal asphyxia still is an experimental intervention and cannot be recommen-ded for routine clinical use till more data is available regarding its safety and efficacy in developing countries.

Systemic Manifestations of Severe Birth Asphyxia

Seeds of neonatal morbidity and neuromotor disability are sown in the labor room. A variety of clinical problems are encountered during early neonatal period among babies who are severely asphyxiated at birth (Table 19.5). Hypoxia can

Table 19.5 Systemic manifestations of severe birth asphyxia	
Organ/ system	Features
Brain	Hypoxic-ischemic encephalopathy, intracranial hemorrhage, apneic attacks, seizures and neuromotor disability
Heart	Persistent fetal circulation, dysrhythmias, myocardial damage, tricuspid regurgita-tion, and congestive cardiac failure
Lungs	Meconium or liquor aspiration, hyaline membrane disease, transient tachypnea, persistent pulmonary hypertension, pulmonary hemorrhage, pneumonia, pneumothorax, and shock lung
Kidneys	Hematuria, renal failure, acute tubular necrosis, and renal vein thrombosis
Hematologic	Coagulopathy (DIC), thrombocytopenia, hyperbilirubinemia, and sepsis
Gastro-intestinal	Necrotizing enterocolitis, GI bleeding, para-lytic ileus and and hepatic dysfunction
Endocrinal	Syndrome of inappropriate secretion of antidiuretic hormone, adrenal hemorrhage, and transient hypoparathyroidism
Immunologic	Septicemia
Metabolic	Acidosis, hypoglycemia, hypocalcemia, hyponatremia and hyperkalemia

cause damage to almost every tissue and organ of the baby. During hypoxia, series of protective mechanisms collectively called as 'diving sea reflex' attempt to redistribute available blood flow from lesser to more vital organs. The blood flow to brain, heart and adrenal glands of the newborn is preserved at the expense of reduction of perfusion to kidneys, lungs, gastrointestinal tract, liver, spleen and skeletal muscles.

Prognosis

Severe birth asphyxia is the commonest cause of death on the first day of life. Depending upon the gestational maturity and quality of newborn care facilities, 15% to 50% of neonates exhibiting manifestations of HIE die during neonatal period. Effective management of the baby at birth with early establishment of breathing, prevention of hypothermia and hypotension are associated with improved survival and outcome[18, 19.] The brain of a newborn baby, especially that of a preterm, is relatively resistant to the damaging effects of hypoxia and can withstand oxygen lack upto 5 to 7 minutes without any apparent sequelae[20]. In an individual baby it is difficult to prognosticate for future mental development. It is amazing that several severely asphyxiated babies achieve fairly normal development without any neurological handicaps[21]. Therefore, as a general policy, a guarded rather than hopeless prognosis should be communicated to the parents to cushion the anxiety and to avoid deliberate neglect of the child.

Following severe birth asphyxia 25% infants are likely to develop evidences of HIE. Relatively adverse outcome is anticipated if the infant was in terminal apnea especially when heart beats were absent at birth or 10-minute Apgar score was less than 3. Arterial blood pH of less than 7.0, plasma lactate level of more than 60 mg/dl, hypoglycemia, occurrence of neonatal convulsions, brain stem signs (poor sucking, pooling of oral secretions, pupillary changes etc.) or abnormal neurological behavior for more than 5 days and multiple diffuse chaotic spike pattern or isopotential amplitude integrated electroencephalogram (a-EEG) are associated with unfavorable outcome[22-24]. Multi-organ failure especially development of acute renal failure is associated with poor outcome.

The American Academy of Pediatrics has proposed that the terminology of perinatal or birth asphyxia should be reserved to describe an infant who manifests all of the following features: (i) Cord umbilical artery pH >7.0 with a base deficit of >10mEq/L; (ii) neonatal neurologic manifestations suggestive of hypoxic-ischemic encephalopathy (HIE); (iii) Evidences of multisystem organ dysfunction involving cardiovascular, renal, gastrointestinal, hematologic or pulmonary system.

The incidence of cerebral palsy following birth asphyxia varies between 6.5-18.5 percent. Infants with evidences of intraventricular or parenchymal hemorrhage and extensive areas of infarction (hypodensity) on CT scan during early neonatal period are often associated with neurological handicaps on follow-up. Brain stem auditory, visual and somatosensory evoked responses by and large are of limited prognostic utility. Inferior colliculi which are credited to produce wave V are specially damaged by hypoxia. In normal infants, wave V obtained during brain stem auditory evoked response is bigger in amplitude as compared to wave 1. The ratio of wave V (actually waves IV and V which are often merged) to wave 1 gets reversed when there is hypoxic damage to the inferior colliculi which is associated with increased mortality and poor late neuromotor outcome among the survivors.

SHOCK AND HYPOVOLEMIA

Shock in neonates in DR setting can occur either because of acute blood loss, myocardial dysfunction or a cardiac rhythm disorder such as complete congenital heart block (CCHB). Acute blood loss may occur because of placenta previa, vasa previa, placental abruption, tight nuchal cord (preferential occlusion of low pressure umbilical vein compared to the umbilical arteries resulting in loss of blood to placenta), or traumatic cord bleeding. Myocardial dysfunction can occur as a result of severe asphyxia, in extremely preterm babies because of inability of the left ventricular myocardium to bear the load of high resistance systemic circulation and rarely in certain cardiomyopathies.

Attempts should be made to promptly search for signs of shock if an infant shows poor response to resuscitative measures. Shock manifests as tachycardia or bradycardia, fast and labored breathing, low pulse volume, pale or mottled skin, cyanosis, low mean arterial pressure and metabolic acidosis.

Shock should be treated with normal saline or Ringer lactate bolus in a dose of 10 ml/kg, infused through umbilical vein over 5 to 10 minutes. The same dose can be repeated if hypovolemia is the likely cause of shock, and there has been inadequate response to the previous bolus. Randomized controlled trials in neonates have shown that isotonic crystalloid is as effective as albumin for the treatment of hypovolemic shock[25]. One may infuse O-Rh negative blood (without any cross matching) to correct for volume loss in acute hemorrhagic shock. Dopamine (5 to 20 µg per kg per min) and dobutamine (5 to 20 µg per kg per min) infusion should be considered, if the response to crystalloid bolus(es) has been suboptimal[26].

MULTIPLE BIRTHS

Birth of multiple babies (twins, triplets or higher order) can present as an emergency, because these babies are usually preterm, at higher risk of asphyxia, birth injury and inter-twin transfusion. The key to management is timely antenatal detection and delivery at a center equipped with independent neonatology teams with dedicated sets of equipment and supplies (Figure 19.9).

SEVERE ANEMIA

Anemia at birth constitutes an emergency requiring urgent intervention and may occur either due to acute or chronic blood loss or immune hemolysis. The common causes of acute blood loss have been mentioned *vide supra*. Chronic blood loss can occur due to twin-to-twin transfusion syndrome (TTTS), feto-maternal or feto-placental bleeding. Immune hemolysis occurs commonly as a result of Rh and ABO blood group incompatibility, autoimmune hemolytic anemia, or rarely due to intrauterine infection with parvovirus, bone marrow hypoplasia or disorders such as hereditary spherocytosis[27]. Long standing severe anemia can precipitate hydrops in the baby (Figure 19.10), creating a major challenge for resuscitation. Severe anemia impairs postnatal adaptations in the infant and there may be congestive heart failure.

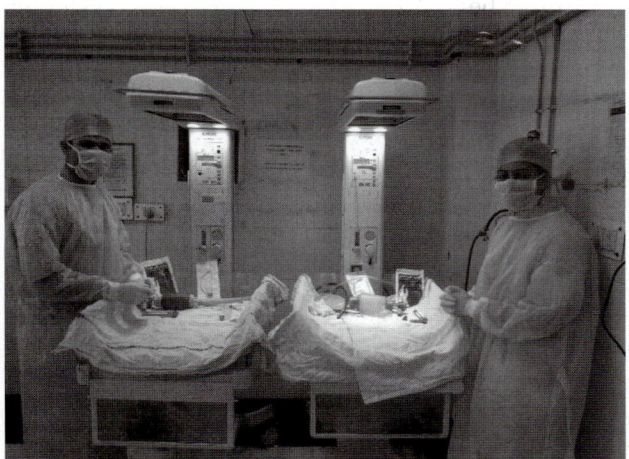

Figure 19.9 Delivery room equipped with two radiant warmers, team of health professionals, equipment and supplies to deal with a twin delivery

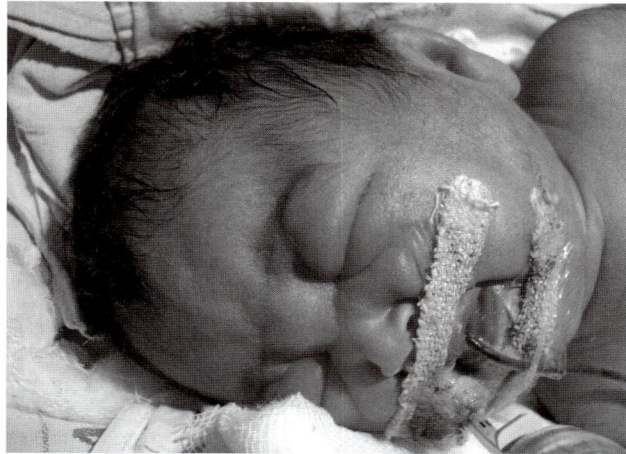

Figure 19.10 Immune hydrops secondary to severe Rh isoimmunisation. Note marked edema of eyelids and moon facies. The baby required thoracocentesis and ascitic tap for effective ventilation and partial exchange transfusion for correction of anemia

After establishing the airway and breathing by appropriate means, partial exchange blood transfusion using ORh-negative packed red blood cells should be undertaken to quickly improve the oxygen carrying capacity and general condition of the baby. Appropriate blood samples should be preserved before exchange transfusion to carry out investigations (Hemoglobin, reticulocyte count, DCT, peripheral smear, infection screen, as indicated) to find out the cause of anemia.

PNEUMOTHORAX

Air leak into the pleural cavity (pneumothorax) can occur spontaneously in up to 3% of neonates, but often it is a complication of positive pressure ventilation (PPV). The risk is higher when the infant has been born through meconium stained amniotic fluid (MSAF) or has pulmonary hypoplasia. Small airleaks may be innocuous and can resolve on its own. However, significant amount of air can cause ventilation failure and shock because of flutter of the mediastinum and the heart, mandating immediate intervention to save life.

Pneumothorax is an important differential diagnosis in an unstable baby, particularly when there is an acute deterioration in the condition of the baby or when the baby has received positive pressure ventilation. It manifests as failure to resuscitate, desaturation, bradycardia with or without poor perfusion. A discerning physician would be able to pick up decreased chest movements, bulging and decreased breath sounds on auscultation on the affected side.

Section 3

Transillumination of the chest wall on the affected side with fiberoptic cold light is useful to make a quick diagnosis, particularly in infants with significant pneumothorax and thin chest wall. Confirmation can be done by X-ray chest, but the treatment should not be delayed. An 18-20 G angiocath should be inserted on the affected side in 4th intercostal space, just above the lower rib, in anterior axillary line (Figure 19.11)[28]. The catheter should be attached through a three way to a 20 ml saline filled syringe. Air escaping through the saline into the syringe would confirm the diagnosis of pneumothorax and would result in quick improvement of the baby. As a definitive measure, the infant requires placement of intercostal drainage (ICD) tube for continuous drainage of air until the pleural rupture gets healed.

HYDROPS, ISOLATED ASCITES OR PLEURAL EFFUSION

Birth of a hydropic infant is a life threatening situation in the delivery room. Hydrops can result because of chronic anemia due to immune hemolysis as a result of blood group incompatibility or autoimmune hemolysis, or from a variety of other conditions such as chromosomal anomalies, congenital malformations, and developmental syndromes (non-immune hydrops)[28].

Hydrops is characterized by widespread subcutaneous edema thus distorting the anatomy that makes airway management including intubation difficult. Presence of ascites and pleural and/or pericardial effusion interferes in establishing successful ventilation and hemodynamic sufficiency. In addition, there may be severe anemia necessitating urgent transfusion of ORh-negative red blood cells for successful postnatal transition from fetal life.

Adequate preparations are needed in DR to resuscitate a hydropic baby and this includes availability of at least three health care professionals adequately trained in neonatal resuscitation, ORh-negative red blood cells and supplies for urgent thoracocentesis, pericardiocentesis and ascitic tap. These infants should be intubated in case of respiratory failure using a smaller calibre endotracheal tube rather than attempting PPV using a bag and mask. One should be prepared to perform urgent thoracocentesis, pericardiocentesis and/or ascitic tap, as the need may be. No more than 20 ml/kg of fluid should be aspirated in one sitting. Partial exchange blood transfusion using ORh-negative red blood cells should be performed to correct anemia.

CONVULSIONS

The infant may rarely manifest convulsions in DR as a result of severe hypoxic-ischemic encephalopathy (HIE), opioid withdrawal following naloxone injection, cerebral dysgenesis, inadvertent injection of local anesthetic into fetal scalp, or pyridoxine dependency[29]. Immediate management involves securing airway and breathing by administration of glucose, calcium and anti-convulsants especially phenobarbitone. The details of management are discussed in Chapter 23.

EXTREMELY PRETERM BABY

Birth of an extremely preterm baby presents an emergency in DR and requires a coordinated teamwork for optimum outcome (Figure 19.12). Extremely low gestational age (ELGA) babies are at risk of hypothermia and respiratory failure as they have stiff and immature lungs combined with

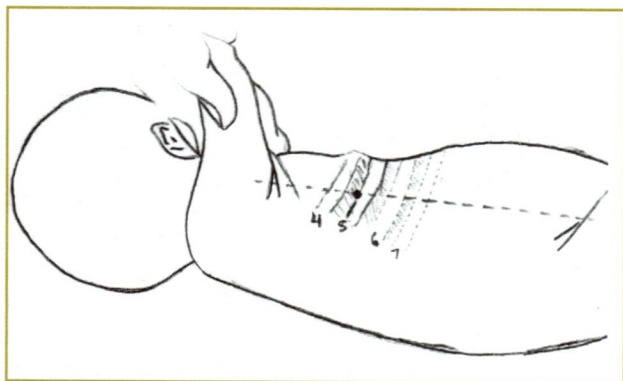

Figure 19.11 The site for needle thoracostomy or intercostal drainage (ICD) tube insertion for pneumothorax

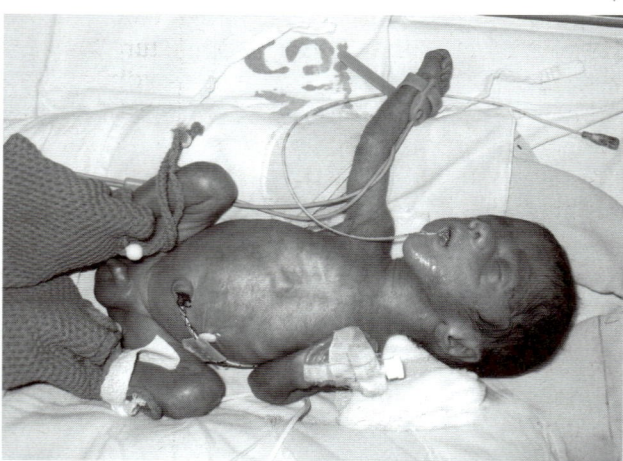

Figure 19.12 Extremely low gestational age (ELGA/ELBW) baby on day 10 of life. The baby required early positive pressure ventilation, rescue surfactant therapy and CPAP for one week

poor CNS drive for effective breathing, brain injury because of intracranial bleed and periventricular leucomalacia, hypotension and healthcare associated infections.

Survival of ELGA babies is inversely proportional to gestational age of the baby, and is dependent upon the capabilities and availability of the optimal infrastructure of the neonatal unit. Apart from high death rates, these babies are at a substantial risk of ongoing physical morbidities as well as adverse neurodevelopmental outcome[30]. Each neonatal unit should review its own survival and neuromorbidity data of ELGA babies, taking into consideration their capabilities and formulate a policy of non-initiation of resuscitation in those ELGA/ELBW babies who are unlikely to survive with the available infrastructure and expertise. Parental wishes must be taken into consideration in making such decision in an individual case. At AIIMS, we take a decision of non-initiation/discontinuation of resuscitation if the baby is less than 25 weeks or less than 700 gm.

The risk of hypothermia is greatest in ELGA babies owing to their large surface area to body weight ratio, thin permeable skin and high transepidermal water loss (TEWL). Usual precautions to prevent hypothermia such as rapid drying, removing wet linen, placing baby under radiant warmer and using warm equipment and supplies are generally insufficient. There is a need for additional measures to protect the infant from hypothermia such as wrapping the baby in plastic sheet to reduce TEWL and using warm and humidified oxygen for resuscitation.

These babies, owing to stiff and immature lungs coupled with poor respiratory drive, often require positive pressure ventilation (PPV). However, PPV can damage the immature lungs as a result of excessive tidal volumes (volutrauma), high inflating pressures (barotrauma) and high oxygen concentration (oxytrauma) culminating into acute lung injury and chronic lung disease (CLD). Therefore, babies should be provided with PPV using small volume breaths (low tidal volume) with positive end-expiratory pressure (PEEP). Since conventional resuscitation bag does not have the facility to provide PEEP or effectively control inflating pressures, it is preferable to use special devices (such as Neopuff, Fisher and Paykel) to deliver PPV to such babies.

It is important to avoid hyperventilation as this may produce hypocarbia with attendant risk of reducing cerebral perfusion and hyperoxia. Monitoring oxygen saturations by using pulse oximetry is recommended in ELGA babies to minimize the risk of high oxygen saturations. New resuscitation guidelines recommends use of intermediate concentration of oxygen (60%) and then titrate it to achieve the desired oxygen saturations.

Prophylactic surfactant replacement therapy (SRT) in such babies has been shown to improve the survival. However, recent evidence suggests that it is more beneficial to put these babies (particularly those treated with antenatal steroids) on nasal CPAP immediately after birth (delivery room CPAP) and use early rescue SRT only if the baby develops moderate to severe respiratory distress. These infants need utmost gentle handling, avoiding unnecessary fluid boluses and fiddling to prevent brain injuries like IVH and PVL.

MATERNAL CONDITIONS/DRUGS AFFECTING THE FETUS OR NEONATE

1. ***Inadvertent injection of lidocaine into fetal scalp.*** It can occur accidentally while injecting the drug to the mother for paracervical and pudendal block or for producing anesthesia for episiotomy. Lidocaine toxicity in the neonate would manifest as bradycardia, apnea, hypotonia and as a depressed baby. The condition closely mimics hypoxic ischemic encephalopathy (HIE) because apart from the aforementioned manifestations, there may be tonic seizures that occur within minutes to hours of birth[31]. The condition can be differentiated from HIE by presence of fixed dilated pupils and absence of doll's eye reflex, which is rarely seen in initial stages of HIE. In addition, lidocaine toxicity would improve within 24 to 48 hours of supportive care while HIE often shows clinical deterioration during the same period.

   Infants affected with lidocaine toxicity require optimum supportive care including effective ventilation. Inducing diuresis and acidification of urine promotes excretion of the drug. Exchange blood transfusion has a limited therapeutic value. The prognosis is excellent with good supportive care.

2. ***Maternal myasthenia gravis*** can produce a similar illness in the infant as a result of transplacentally transferred antibodies. It is a self-limiting illness, which can last a for few days to weeks, and manifests as hypotonia, areflexia, respiratory depression and bulbar involvement. The management is supportive by taking care of ventilation and ensuring optimum nutrition.

Section 3

3. ***Magnesium sulfate toxicity*** may occur in neonates born to mothers treated with magsulf for pre-eclampsia or arrest of preterm labor. It manifests as lethargy, apnea, respiratory depression and poor reflexes. There is no specific antidote, intravenous 10% calcium gluconate 2 ml/kg over 10 minutes may be tried. It requires supportive care including assisted ventilation at times.

4. ***Opioid toxicity*** can occur in infants born to mothers treated with opioids such as morphine within 4 hours of delivery. The affected neonates show respiratory depression in the presence of normal heart rate and color. After ensuring optimum ventilation, naloxone can be administered to reverse the effect of the drug.

LIFE-THREATENING MALFORMATIONS

Anomalies of Airways

A variety of airway anomalies, can present as an emergency in DR and include bilateral choanal atresia, pharyngeal abnormalities such as Pierre-Robin syndrome, laryngeal anomalies like bilateral vocal cord palsy, congenital laryngeal atresia, laryngo-tracheo-esophageal (LTE) cleft, and tracheal anomalies such as agenesis of trachea. These infants can be provided with temporary airway support with the help of laryngeal mask airway (LMA).

1. **Bilateral choanal atresia**

   Congenital choanal atresia occurs as result of abnormal persistence of bucco-nasal membrane. There is a female preponderance and nearly half of them are bilateral. It can occur as an isolated anomaly or as a part of Treacher-Collins syndrome or CHARGE (colobomas of eyes, heart anomalies, atresia of choanae, retardation of physical and mental growth, genital and ear abnormalities) association.

   As the neonates are preferential nose breathers, the infant manifests with cyanosis that gets relieved on crying and reappears when baby stops crying (cyclic cyanosis). Diagnosis is suspected by inability to pass a catheter through nostrils and confirmed by CT scan. The affected neonate is treated with placement of an oral airway, as an emergency measure, and surgical reconstruction of the airways within first few days, as the definitive measure. Following surgical correction, polyvinyl tubes are sutured in the nasal passages to prevent re-stenosis and they can be removed after 6 weeks.

2. **Pierre Robin syndrome**

   The primary abnormality in Pierre Robin syndrome is mandibular hypoplasia (micrognathia) that sets in a deformation sequence resulting in posterior falling of tongue (glossoptosis), and cleft palate in 60% of cases. The narrowing of pharyngeal airway results in respiratory distress, cyanosis and apnea that gets worse in supine posture.

   It is managed with tracheal intubation or placement of a tracheal tube through the nose into the hypopharynx to relieve the obstruction. The infant should be kept in prone position to minimize the airway obstruction due to glossoptosis.

3. **Bilateral vocal cord palsy**

   A variety of central nervous system disorders such as HIE, intracranial hemorrhage, Arnold-Chiari malformation and brainstem dysgenesis may be associated with bilateral vocal cord palsy. It manifests as inspiratory stridor and breathing difficulty but cry is normal. The condition can be suspected on direct laryngoscopy, which can be confirmed by inspecting adducted and non-mobile vocal cords on flexible bronchoscopy. It requires tracheal intubation to maintain the patency of airway, and ultimate prognosis is determined by the underlying/associated conditions.

4. **Congenital laryngeal atresia (congenital high airway obstruction syndrome; CHAOS)**

   The larynx is completely obstructed by a web in this condition. Typical presentation includes a resident getting frustrated by repeated failure of intubation attempts in a cyanotic baby. In most cases, a number of malformations are associated with laryngeal atresia (Figure 19.13). The condition can be suspected on antenatal ultrasound by enlarged lungs, dilated trachea and abdominal displacement of the diaphragm. There may be associated hydrops in the baby.

   At times one may be able to push the tracheal tube across the obstruction, but often it requires emergency cricothyrotomy to establish the airway. Prognosis is generally poor, because laryngeal reconstruction is extremely difficult.

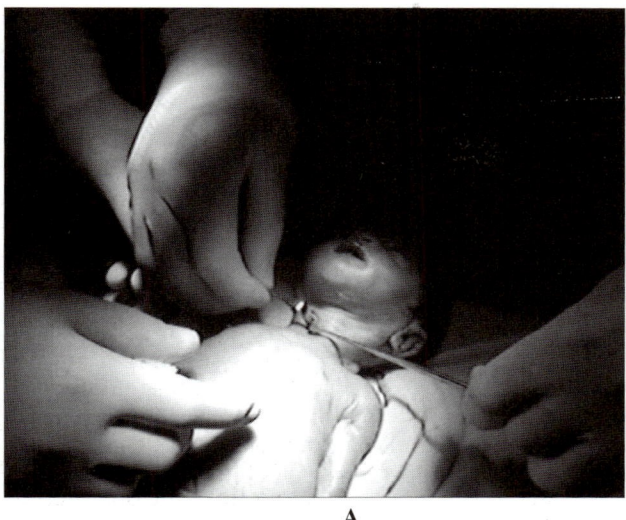

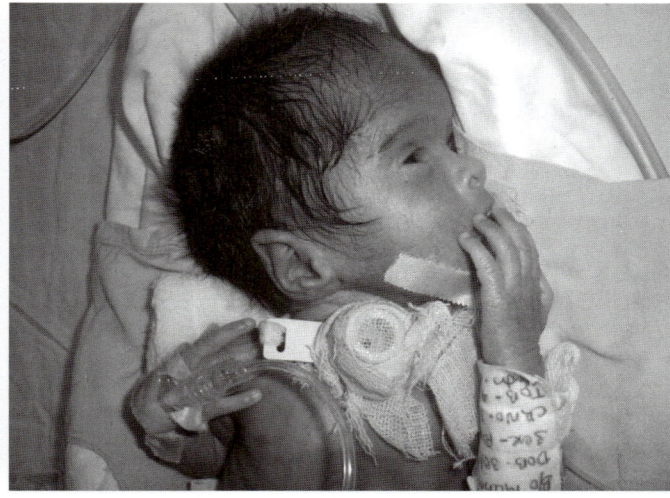

A   B

Figure 19.13 Congenital high airway obstruction syndrome (CHAOS). **A.** The neonate is being tracheostomized immediately after birth, while the placental circulation is maintained by oxygenation and ventilation; **B.** Baby is doing well after a couple of weeks

5. **Laryngotracheoesophageal (LTE) cleft**

    The abnormality occurs as the airway and the esophagus fail to separate leaving a wide communication between two structures extending from larynx to as far down to trachea. Affected infants develop respiratory distress, stridor and cyanosis. The condition requires securing airway by tracheal intubation, as an emergency measure, followed by surgical repair. The prognosis is poor.

6. **Agenesis of trachea**

    In this condition, the trachea is completely atretic, resulting in severe respiratory distress and cyanosis. Associated tracheo-esophageal fistula makes it possible to achieve some ventilation through esophageal intubation. The nature of anomaly and associated malformations often lead to poor prognosis in this condition.

Anomalies of Lung Parenchyma

A variety of lung malformations can present as an emergency in DR and include congenital diaphragmatic hernia (CDH), esophageal atresia (EA) with and without tracheoesophageal fistula (TEF), bronchogenic, neurenteric and pulmonary cysts, congenital cystic adenomatoid malformation (CCAM), bronchopulmonary sequestration, lobar emphysema, unilateral pulmonary agenesis, hemangiomatosis and pulmonary hypoplasia.[32]

These conditions are rare and manifest during later part of neonatal period, infancy or even childhood but sometimes these can be severe enough to present at birth as fetal non-immune hydrops because of pressure effect on surrounding vessels.

1. **Congenital diaphragmatic hernia**

    Many cases of CDH may present as barrel shaped chest, scaphoid abdomen and with respiratory distress soon after birth. Most CDH are on the left side but condition may occur rarely on the right side (Figure 19.14). One may be able to auscultate bowel sounds in the chest on affected side. Nearly 40% babies have associated malformations.

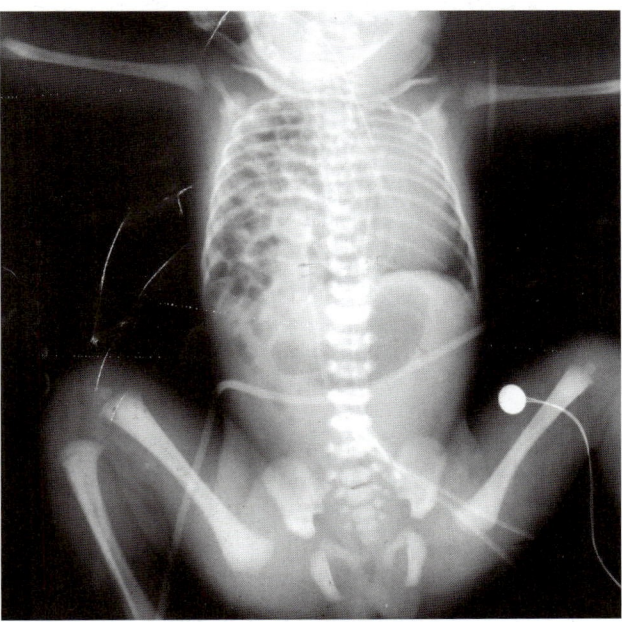

Figure 19.14 Right sided diaphragmatic hernia, detected in a baby who failed to breathe at birth and had a scaphoid abdomen

If required, infants with CDH should be intubated and ventilated with endotracheal tube and bag. *Bag and mask ventilation should never be attempted to prevent gut distension with air and worsening of dyspnea.* Concomitant pulmonary hypoplasia makes lung stiff requiring high inflating pressures for ventilation, but care should be taken to ventilate gently by limiting pressure, and using higher rates, to avoid lung injury and pneumothorax. Orogastric tube should be inserted to decompress the gut in the thoracic cavity inorder to allow the compressed lung to expand. After achieving hemodynamic stability, the defect should be corrected surgically. The condition is often complicated with PPHN and is associated with poor outcome.[33]

2.   Esophageal atresia (EA)

Esophageal atresia can occur in isolation, but often co-exists with tracheoesophageal fistula (TEF) in most cases. The most common variety is characterized by proximal EA and distal TEF, and babies present with respiratory distress and excessive salivation. Infants with distal EA and proximal TEF are at greatest risk of aspiration and present with severe respiratory distress due to aspiration and right upper lobe pneumonitis. Apart from initial resuscitation, these babies should be nursed in supine position with mild head elevation to prevent gastric acid aspiration into the lungs. The upper pouch of esophagus requires frequent or continuous suctioning to prevent aspiration.

3.   Cysts

Bronchogenic, neurenteric and pulmonary cysts are duplication cysts of variable sizes occurring as an aberration in fetal foregut development. They may be fluid or air filled and large enough to produce mass effect. Pulmonary cyst may be confused with tension pneumothorax, but can be differentiated by the presence of lung markings.

4.   Congenital cystic adenomatoid malformation (CCAM)

CCAM occurs due to abnormal overgrowth of the terminal airways leading to formation of cysts of varying sizes, precluding normal alveolarization in the affected lobe, and producing mass effect. There may be associated malformations in about quarter of cases.

5.   Bronchopulmonary sequestration

Sequestration is characterized by abnormal lung tissue mass deriving its blood supply from systemic rather than pulmonary circulation, and does not take part in normal gas exchange process. The anomalous mass may be wrapped within the main pleural cavity (intrapulmonary) or may have its own pleural covering (extra-pulmonary).

6.   Unilateral pulmonary agenesis and pulmonary hemangiomatosis

In this condition there is abnormal proliferation of vessels and may present in DR with severe respiratory distress.

7.   Pulmonary hypoplasia

It is a relatively common condition and occurs as a deformation sequence secondary to compression of lung tissue from early fetal life by an underlying malformation such as CDH, other mass lesions described above, or by chronic drainage of amniotic fluid starting early in fetal life and continuing for a prolonged period. Pulmonary hypoplasia may also occur in a variety of skeletal dysplasias such as thanatophoric dwarfism or severe myopathy, neuropathy or muscular dystrophy.

The affected neonates present with respiratory distress. The hypoplastic lungs require high pressures for ventilation. The chest may be bell shaped and the babies are at risk of developing pneumothorax.

Heart Defects

Most heart defects whether cyanotic or acyanotic do not manifest at the time of birth. However, some cardiac malformations can manifest with severe cyanosis that is unresponsive to routine resuscitative measures. A neonate should be suspected to have a cyanotic heart defect if the cyanosis does not respond to oxygen and/or ventilation. Sometimes additional clues to the diagnosis such as cardiac murmur, abnormal heart sounds or associated congenital defects can be found. Some rhythm abnormalities can also present at birth namely complete congenital heart block (CCHB) as bradycardia, or supraventricular tachycardia with cardiac failure. Severely affected babies may have hydrops at birth.

The neonates with congenital heart defects may require assisted ventilation in the event of severe hypoxemia and/or respiratory distress.

Prostaglandin E$_1$ therapy may be required to maintain the patency of duct. Bradyarrhythmias may require isoprenaline infusion to augment heart rate, while preparations are made for pacemaking. Supraventricular tachycardia may require reflex vagal maneuvers or adenosine injection to control the heart rate.

Defects of other Organ Systems

A variety of developmental defects pertaining to other organ systems may pose significant challenge in the DR. The common ones are meningomyelocele and neural tube defects (NTDs), anterior abdominal wall defects, massive tumors such as sacrococcygeal teratomas, hydronephrosis, hydrocephalus and conjoined infants.

Babies with NTDs should be provided nursing care to preserve the meningeal sac and prevent further injury and infection. The lesion should be covered with sterile saline moist gauze. Contact with latex gloves should be avoided in case of open lesions to avoid any risk of hypersensitivity and anaphylaxis.

Anterior abdominal wall defects such as omphalocele and gastroschisis would require extreme care in resuscitation and preventing further injury to the gut. Unusual situations such as massive sacrococcygeal teratoma (Figure 19.15), conjoined twins (Figure 19.16), massive hydrocephalus, and obstructive uropathy with consequent urinary ascites are other important life-threatening conditions that require a coordinated approach by trained personnel.

BIRTH TRAUMA

Birth trauma may at times be serious enough to present as an emergency in DR and these include

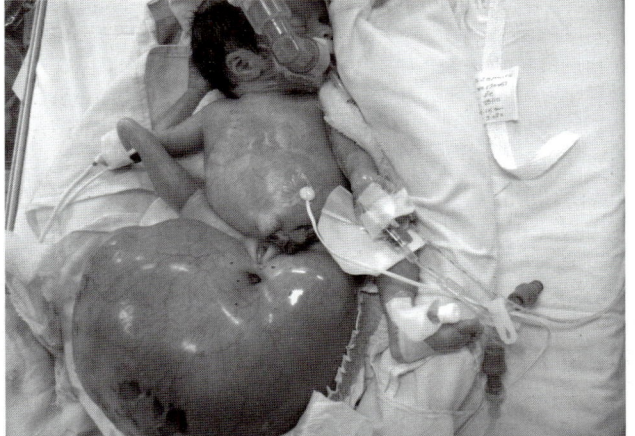

Figure 19.15 Massive sacrococcygeal teratoma leading to severe congestive heart failure in the infant

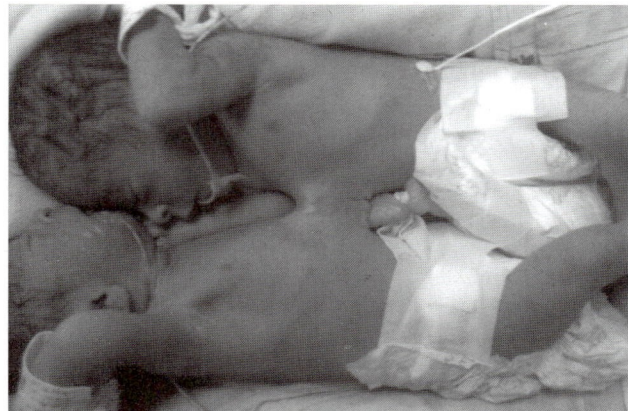

Figure 19.16 Conjoined twins can pose a major challenge to access the airway for resuscitation

spinal cord injury, subdural hemorrhage, brachial plexus injury involving C4 roots (phrenic nerve), injury to the liver or spleen, and facture of facial bones. The factors responsible for birth trauma may coexist with hypoxic-ischemic encephelopathy.

Spinal cord injury may occur following complicated breech delivery due to longitudinal, lateral or rotational traction of the neck. Often the lesion is akin to complete transection of cord and presents with marked hypotonia, weak respiratory efforts and areflexia (spinal shock), and carries a poor prognosis. Management is essentially supportive and good nursing care.

Subdural hemorrhage (SDH) results from sheer forces acting during labor and tearing apart of the dural sinuses in falx cerebri and falx cerebelli. of SDH evolves rapidly with signs of blood loss, brainstem herniation and raised intracranial pressure. The management consists of supportive care including effective ventilation and replacing blood loss. A minority of affected infants require neurosurgical intervention.

CONCLUSIONS

Delivery room (DR) emergencies are common and can be managed effectively and carry good prognosis in many cases if managed adequately. The common DR emergencies include inability to initiate or maintain breathing, shock, anemia or multiple births. However, a variety of other developmental conditions can manifest as an emergency in DR and may require specific treatment in addition to ensuring optimum airway, oxygenation and circulation. The key to success in management of DR emergencies is adequate preparedness in terms of skilled manpower, functional equipment, supplies and ability to respond with a sense of urgency.

Section 3

ACKNOWLEDGEMENTS

Photographs have been provided by the kind courtesy of DM residents Kamal Arora, Oleti Tejopratap, Aparna Chandra Sekaran and Arun Sasi.

REFERENCES

1. Kattwinkel J, Perlman JM, Aziz K, Colby C, Fairchild K, Gallagher J, *et al.* American Heart Association. Neonatal resuscitation: 2010 American Heart Association Guidelines for Cardiopulmonary Resuscitation and Emergency Cardiovascular Care. *Pediatrics* 2010; 126(5): e1400-13. Epub 2010, Oct 18.

2. Black RE, Cousens S, Johnson HL, Lawn JE, Rudan I, Bassani DG, *et al.* Child Health Epidemiology Reference Group of WHO and UNICEF. Global, regional and national causes of child mortality in 2008: a systematic analysis. *Lancet* 2010 June 5; 375 (9730): 1969-1987. Epub 2010 May 11.

3. Molteno CD, Malan AF, Heese HDV. Neonatal complications and conditions associated with asphyxia neonatorum. *South Africa Med J* 1974; 48:2259.

4. American Academy of Pediatrics. American Collge of obstetricians and Gynecologists, use and abuse of the Apgar score. *Pediatrics* 1996; 98:141-142.

5. Marlow N. Do we need an Apgar score? *Arch Dis Child* 1992; 67: 765-767.

6. McDonald JW, Silverstein FS, Johnston MW. Neuroprotective effects of MK-801, TCP, PCP and CPP against N-methyl-D-aspartate-induced neurotoxicity in an in-vivo perinatal rat model. *Brain Res* 1989; 490:33-40.

7. Kattwinkel J. Textbook of Neonatal Resuscitation. Elk grove village, *Illinois, American Heart Association* 2000.

8. International Guidelines for Neonatal Resuscitation: An Excerpt from the Guidelines 2000 for Cardiopulmonary Resuscitation and Emergency Cardiovascular Care: International Consensus on Science. *Pediatrics* 2000; 106:1-16.

9. Deorari AK. Newer guidelines for neonatal resuscitation: How my practice needs to change? *Indian Pediatr* 2001; 38:496-499.

10. Neonatal Resuscitation: India. *National Neonatology Forum of India,* second edition, 2014.

11. Gunn AJ, Gluckman PG, Gunn TR. Selective head cooling in newborn infants after perinatal asphyxia: a safety study. *Pediatrics* 1998, 102: 885-892.

12. Thoresen M. Cooling the newborn after asphyxia: physiological and experimental background. *Semin Neonatal* 2000; 5:61-73.

13. Blackmon LR, Stark AR, and The Committee on Fetus and Newborn, American Academy of Pediatrics. Hypothermia: A neuroprotective therapy for neonatal hypoxic-ischemic encephalopathy. *Pediatrics* 2006; 117:942-948.

14. Higgins R, Raju T, Perlman J, *et al.* Hypothermia and perinatal asphyxia: executive summary of NICHD workshop. *J Pediatr* 2006; 148:170-175.

15. Eicher DJ, Wagner CL, Katikaneni LP, *et al.* Moderate hypothermia in neonatal encephalopathy: efficacy outcomes. *Pediatr Neurol* 2005; 32:18-24.

16. Gluckman PD, Wyatt JS, Azzopardi D, *et al.* Selective head cooling with mild systemic hypothermia after neonatal encephalopathy: multicentre randomized trial. *Lancet* 2005; 365:663-670.

17. Wilkinson DJ, Singh M, Wyatt J. Ethical challenges in the use of therapeutic hypothermia in Indian neonatal units. *Indian Pediatr* 2010, 47:387-393.

18. Ekert P, Perlman M, Steinlin M, *et al.* Predicting the outcome of post-asphyxial hypoxic-ischemic encephalopathy within 4 hours of birth. *J Pediatr* 1997; 131:613-617.

19. Scott H. Outcome of very severe birth asphyxia. *Arch Dis Child* 1976; 51:712.

20. Grausz JP, Heimler R. Asphyxia and gestaional age. *Obstet Gynecol* 1983; 62:175.

21. Paneth N, Raymond IS. Cerebral palsy and mental retardation in relation to indicators of perinatal asphyxia. *Amer J Obstet Gynecol* 1983; 147:960.

22. D'souza SW, Black P, Cadman J, *et al.* Umbilical venous blood pH: a useful aid in the diagnosis of asphyxia at birth. *Arch Dis Child* 1983; 58:15.

23. Lauener PA, Calame A, Janelek P, *et al.* Systematic pH measurements in the umbilical artery: causes and predictive value of neonatal acidosis. *J Perinatal Med* 1983; 11:278.

24. Vanden Berg PP, Nelen WL, Jongsma HW, *et al.* Neonatal complications in newborn with an umbilical artery pH<7.0. *Am J Obstet Gynecol* 1996; 175:1152-1157.

25. Oca MJ, Nelson M, Donn SM. Randomized trial of normal saline versus 5% albumin for the treatment of neonatal hypotension *J Perinatol* 2003, 23: 473-476.

26. AIIMS Protocols in Neonatology. Paul VK, Deorari AK, (Eds.) 3rd edition, 2011. *Indian Journal of Pediatrics, New Delhi.*

27. Taeusch HW, Ballard RA, Gleason CA. Avery's Diseases of Newborn. 8th Ed. *Philadelphia: Saunders;* 2005.

28. Bahrami KR, MacDonal MG, Eichelberger MR. Throacostomy tubes. In: Procedures in Neonatology. MacDonald MG, Ramesethu J, 4th Ed. *Philadelphia: Lippincott Williams & Wilkins;* 2007, pp. 261-284.

29. Avery GB, Fletcher MA, Macdonald MG. Neonatology: Pathophysiology and Management of the Newborn. *Philadelphia: Lippincott Williams & Wilkins;* 2008.

30. Watts JL, Saigal S. Outcome of extreme prematurity: as information increases so do the dilemmas. *Arch Dis Child Fetal Neonatal Ed* 2006; 91: F221-F225.

31. Volpe JJ. Neurology of the Newborn. 5th Ed. *Philadelphia: Elsevier;* 2005.

32. Sarkar N, Agarwal R, Das AK, Deorari AK. Congenital airway abnormalities in neonates. *Indian J Pediatr* 2002, 69(11): 993-995.

33. Logan JW, Rice HE, Goldberg RN, Cotten CM. Congenital diaphragmatic hernia: A systematic review and summary of best-evidence practice strategies. *J Perinatol* 2007, 27:535.

34. Levine MG, Holroyde J, Woods JR Jr, et al. Birth trauma: incidence and predisposing factors. *Obstet Gynecol* 1984, 63(6): 792-795.

Respiratory Distress in Newborn Babies

Arun K Pramanik

Respiratory disorders are the most frequent cause of admission to the special care nursery in both term and preterm infants. Significant advances have been made in our understanding of the pathophysiological mechanisms and in the care of critically ill neonates with respiratory failure during the last two decades. These include surfactant therapy, newer modalities of ventilation, extracorporeal membrane oxygenation and inhaled nitric oxide, or a combination of these therapies[1-8]. Often the need for tertiary care for these patients with acute respiratory failure can be predicted prior to birth by fetal ultrasound examination and lung maturity tests. Ideally these infants should be delivered in institutions with staff skilled in the care of high-risk mothers, fetuses and infants. However, in reality most infants are not identified prior to birth, or their mothers cannot be transferred to a tertiary care facility. Thus the physician responsible for care of newborn infants with respiratory failure must be able not only to stabilize them, but also evaluate and manage the underlying disease. This chapter gives an overview of the evaluation, diagnosis and management of newborn infants with respiratory distress. For an in-depth understanding of specific causes and management of neonatal respiratory distress, the reader is referred to several excellent reviews on the subject[1-3, 5, 8].

CLINICAL EVALUATION

Infants with respiratory distress present with tachypnea, grunting, nasal flaring, chest retractions, and central cyanosis. Tachypnea in neonates is usually defined as a respiratory rate of greater than 60 breaths per minute in a quiet baby. The central cyanosis (cyanosis of the mucous membranes) is clinically detected when there is 5g/100 ml or more of unsaturated hemoglobin. Because of the high percentage of fetal hemoglobin, cyanosis may not be observed until the arterial oxygen tension (paO_2) is less than 30 to 40 mm Hg, thus, pulse oximetry and blood gases should be done.

Maternal History

This should include birth of previous premature infants and their outcome, diabetes mellitus, hypertension, antenatal care including ultrasound examination (e.g. oligohydramnios suggests hypoplastic lungs, diaphragmatic hernia, congenital anomalies of lungs, heart and abdomen, hydrops fetalis), lung maturity profiles in the amniotic fluid (e.g. premature fetuses, infants of diabetic mothers), evidence of chorioamnionitis, trauma and/or bleeding. Placenta previa or placental abruption increases the likelihood of hypovolemia and anemia, which in turn may lead to acute respiratory distress. Reviewing the history of labor and delivery may give a clue about the etiology of acute respiratory distress, e.g. transient tachypnea of newborn (TTN) which occurs more often in term infants born after cesarean section, pneumothorax in infants requiring resuscitation or receiving positive pressure ventilation, chorioamnionitis suggests pneumonia, meconium staining of amniotic fluid may lead to meconium aspiration syndrome and persistent pulmonary hypertension of newborn.

The age of onset may be helpful in the differential diagnosis of neonates with acute respiratory distress. When signs of respiratory distress develop immediately after birth in a premature infant, one should consider respiratory distress syndrome, also known as hyaline membrane disease, and pneumonia (bacterial or viral). In a full term infant, respiratory distress soon after birth may be due to pneumonia (bacterial or viral), aspiration of meconium, blood or amniotic fluid, transient tachypnea of newborn, congenital heart disease, anemia and hypoglycemia. In contrast, when respiratory distress develops several hours or days after birth, septicemia with pneumonia, cardiac disorders (e.g. coarctation of aorta, hypoplastic left heart syndrome, large ventricular septal defect, complex cardiac disease), inborn errors of metabolism (e.g. urea cycle disorders, aminoacidurias, adrenal insufficiency, galactosemia and primary lactic acidosis), and intracranial hemorrhage should be considered.

Physical Examination

Physical examination should include frequent evaluation of vital signs (respiratory and heart rate, capillary refill, blood pressure and temperature). Hypothermia or hyperthermia suggests infection. Tachycardia may be due to hypovolemia, fever or pneumonia. Asymmetry of breath sounds may indicate pneumothorax, pleural effusion (chylothorax), congenital diaphragmatic hernia or atelectesis. In congenital diaphragmatic hernia, the abdomen may be scaphoid. Low blood pressure or weak pulses may be due to hypovolemia, septicemia or congenital heart disease. Weak pulses or low-blood pressure in the lower extremities suggests coarctation of aorta or hypoplastic left heart syndrome. Hepatosplenomegaly suggests erythroblastosis fetalis, congenital infection, congestive heart failure or maternal diabetes mellitus.

LABORATORY STUDIES

These include chest roentgenogram, hematocrit, blood glucose concentration, arterial blood gases (pH, paO$_2$, paCO$_2$), and blood cultures. *The chest X-ray film is the single most useful test in establishing the diagnosis of respiratory distress and should be taken promptly.* The blood gases are also helpful in evaluating the severity of respiratory distress (hypoxia, respiratory or metabolic acidosis), and thus should be undertaken immediately. An infant who presents with mild respiratory distress in the first few hours of life may be a diagnostic dilemma for the physician. In the majority of such term infants, it is due to transient tachypnea of the newborn (TTN) and resolves spontaneously. However, other infants may have septicemia and/or pneumonia or persistent pulmonary hypertension or spontaneous pneumo-thorax. Therefore, X-ray chest and other laboratory tests listed above should be undertaken, and the diagnosis of TTN should be made after excluding other causes of respiratory distress.

CAUSES OF RESPIRATORY DISTRESS

The causes of respiratory distress in newborn infants are listed in Table 20.1. It is occasionally difficult to distinguish respiratory causes from cardiovascular or sepsis on the basis of clinical signs alone. Hence, in addition to a prompt history and physical examination, laboratory tests as indicated and listed above should be undertaken in all infants with respiratory distress.

Table 20.1 Causes of respiratory distress
◆ **Upper Airway Obstruction**
(a) *Nasal or nasopharyngeal*: Choanal atresia, nasal edema, encephalocele.
(b) *Oral cavity:* Macroglossia, micrognathia (Pierre-Robin syndrome)
(c) *Neck:* Congenital goiter, cystic hygroma
(d) *Larynx:* Web, subglottic stenosis, hemangioma, cord paralysis, laryngomalacia.
(e) *Trachea and bronchi:* Tracheomalacia, tracheo-esophageal fistula, tracheal stenosis, bronchomalacia and bronchial stenosis.
◆ **Lung Parenchymal Diseases**
(a) Respiratory distress syndrome (Hyaline membrane disease)
(b) Transient tachypnea of newborn
(c) Aspiration syndromes (meconium, gastric contents, amniotic fluid, blood)
(d) Pneumonia (bacterial, viral, protozoal, fungal)
(e) Atelectasis
(f) Air leaks (pnemothorax, pneumomediastinum, pnemopericardium, interstitial air)
(g) Persistent pulmonary hypertension of the newborn
(h) Bronchopulmonary dysplasia
(i) Pulmonary hemorrhage
(j) Acute respiratory distress syndrome (secondary to shock or sepsis)
◆ **Development Disorders**
(a) Diaphragmatic hernia, pulmonary hypoplasia or agenesis, congenital lobar emphysema
(b) Chylothorax or pleural effusion
(c) Congenital cystic adenomatous malformation of lungs, other cysts and tumors
(d) Pulmonary sequestration
(e) Tracheoesophageal fistula
◆ **Nonpulmonary Causes**
(a) *Cardiac causes:* Congenital heart disease, cardiomyopathy, congestive heart failure.
(b) *Central nervous system* lesions
(c) *Metabolic causes:* Acidosis, hypothermia, and hypoglycemia

Section 3

I. Upper Airway Obstruction

Newborns with upper airway obstruction may have apnea, cyanosis or inspiratory stridor soon after birth. Choanal atresia may be suspected by failure to pass a soft No. 5 F catheter through each nostril, and confirmed by CT scan. It may be unilateral or bilateral. In infants with Pierre-Robin syndrome (micrognathia, retrognathia, glossoptosis and cleft palate), the posterior displacement of the tongue obstructs the airway and results in respiratory distress; which can be treated by placing the infant in a prone position, fixing the tongue anteriorly by stitches, or by nasopharyngeal intubation.

Stridor may occur due to laryngomalacia, laryngeal cyst, vocal cord paralysis, laryngeal web, subglottic hemangioma, congenital subglottic stenosis, intubation trauma, vascular ring, lymphangiectasis or aspiration of stomach contents. When stridor and respiratory distress is associated with feeding, one should consider gastroesophogeal reflux, central nervous system anomaly or injury, and rarely laryngeal cleft.

II. Lung Parenchymal Diseases

Common causes of respiratory distress in newborn infants include: respiratory distress syndrome (also known as hyaline membrane disease), transient tachypnea of the newborn, aspiration (meconium, blood or amniotic fluid) syndromes, bacterial pneumonia, persistent pulmonary hypertension and bronchopulmonary dysplasia. On rare occasions, morphologic abnormalities of the lung parenclyma may present with respiratory distress. Hence, one must have a high index of suspicion.

RESPIRATORY DISTRESS SYNDROME

Respiratory distress syndrome (RDS), also known as hyaline membrane disease (HMD), occurs almost exclusively in premature infants resulting from surfactant deficiency. Human surfactant is a complex lipoprotein, comprising of six phospholipids and four apoproteins. Functionally, dipalmitoyl phosphatidylcholine (DPPC) or lecithin is the principal phospholipid, which along with apoproteins SP-B and SP-C, or by addition of other substances lowers the surface tension at the alveolar air-fluid interface in-vivo. The components of pulmonary surfactant are synthesized in the Golgi apparatus of the endoplasmic reticulum of the type II alveolar cell (Figure 20.1), packaged in multilamellar vesicles in its cytoplasm, and secreted by a process of

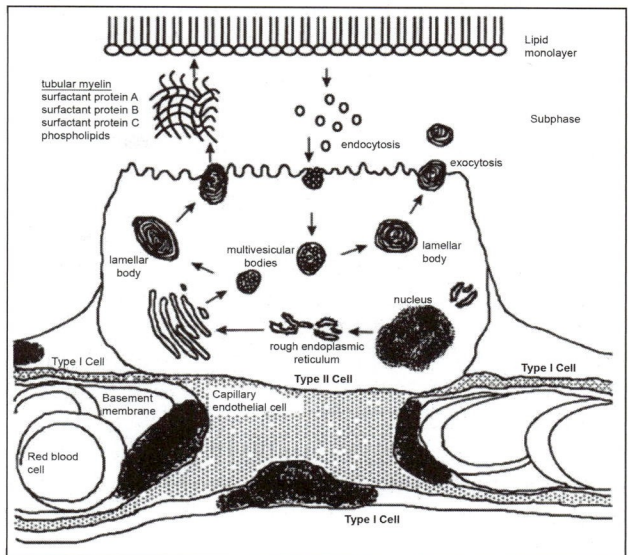

Figure 20.1 Surfactant phospholipids are synthesized in the endoplasmic reticulum, transported through the Golgi apparatus to multivesicular bodies, and ultimately packaged in lamellar bodies before secretion. After exocytosis of the lamellar bodies, surfactant phospholipids are organized into a complex lattice called tubular myelin that provides material for monolayer at the air-liquid interface in the alveolus. Surfactant phospholipids and proteins are taken up by the type II cells, and transported to lamellar bodies for recycling. Surfactant proteins are synthesized in polyribosomes and extensively modified in endoplasmic reticulum, Golgi apparatus, and multivesicular bodies. Surfactant proteins are detected within lamellar bodies or in secretory vesicles closely associated with lamellar bodies before secretion into the alveolus.

exocytosis, the daily rate of which may exceed the weight of the cell itself. Once secreted, the vesicles unwind to form bipolar monolayers of phospholipid molecules that appear to be dependent on one or more of the smaller, hydrophobic apoproteins (SP-B and SP-C) to configure properly in the alveolus. Tubular myelin stores surfactant and may depend on SP-B. Corners of the myelin lattice appear to be "glued" together with the larger apoprotein SP-A, which also may have an important role in phagocytosis. Hypoxia, hypothermia and hypotension may impair surfactant production and/or secretion.

Hyaline membranes that line the alveoli are formed within half hour after birth[9]. In premature infants with less severe HMD, at 36 to 72 hours, the epithelium begins to heal, and surfactant synthesis begins. The proposed mechanism of formation of hyaline membranes and the complex set of factors including oxidant injury, positive pressure ventilation and inflammation resulting in chronic lung disease due to bronchopulmonary dysplasia is outlined in Figure 20.2.

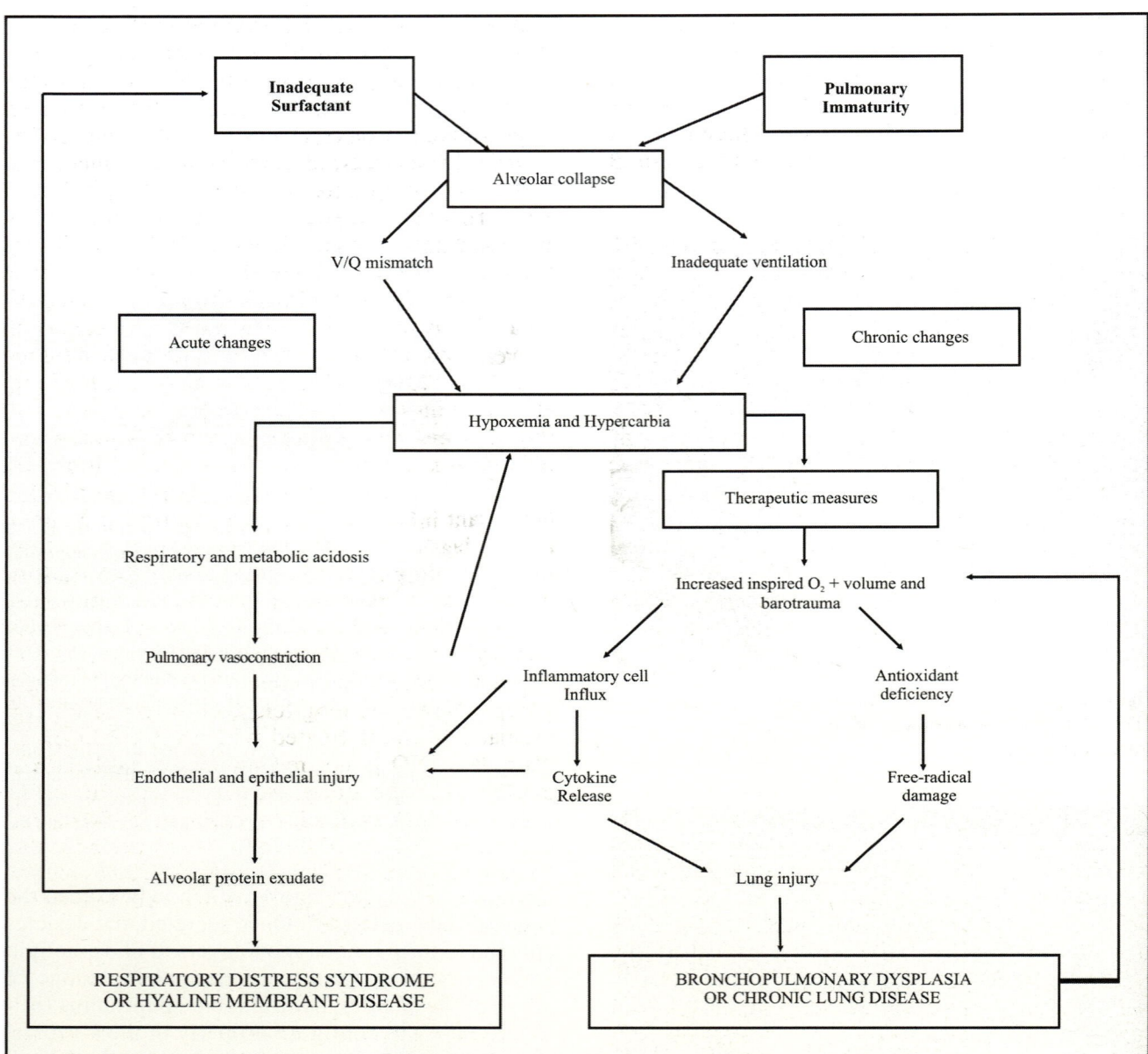

Figure 20.2 Schematic outline of series of events that occur in respiratory distress syndrome or cause lung injury leading bronchopulmonary dysplasia

Risk Factors for the Development of RDS

They include prematurity, maternal diabetes mellitus, and history of HMD in previous siblings, male Caucasian infants, second-born twins, and neonates born by cesarean delivery without trial of labor. Secondary surfactant deficiency occurs due to perinatal asphyxia, pulmonary infections, hemorrhage and meconium aspiration.

Prenatal Prevention and Prediction of RDS

Mothers of infants at risk for RDS as described previously should be managed by experienced obstetricians, preferably at a tertiary perinatal center. HMD may be prevented by: (i) strategies to prevent premature birth, e.g. bed rest, tocolysis, or use of antibiotics; and (ii) by using antenatal corticosteroids to enhance the maturity of the lungs. Fetal lung maturity can be predicted by estimating phosphatidylglycerol and/or lecithin/sphingomyelin ratio in the amniotic fluid.

Diagnosis of RDS

Clinically, these premature infants present soon after birth with symptoms of respiratory distress. Blood gases are indicative of respiratory and metabolic acidosis, along with hypoxia. Chest x-ray shows reticulogranular appearance, air-bronchogram, poor expansion (Figure 20.3), and in severe cases it shows "ground-glass" (haziness or white-out) appearance (Figure 20.4). These findings may coexist with pneumonia due to *group B hemolytic streptococci.*

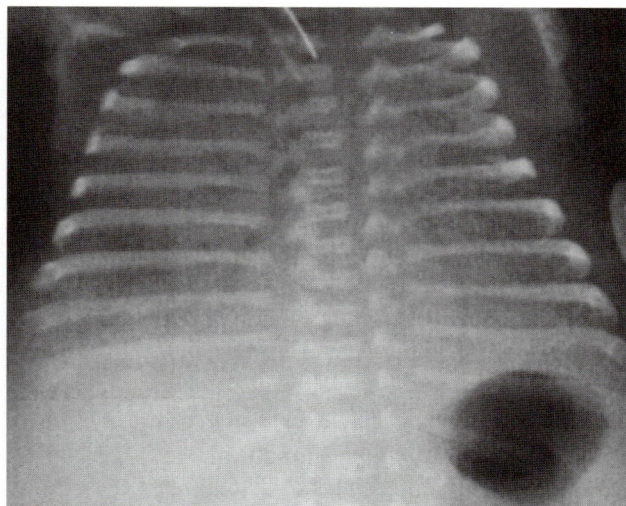

Figure 20.3 Chest roentgenogram of a premature infant with RDS. Note poor expansion, air bronchogram and reticulogranular appearance

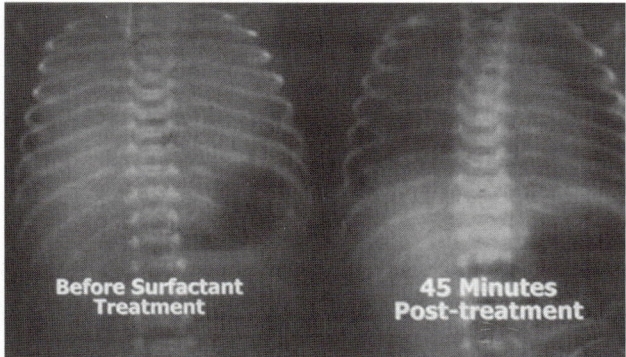

Figure 20.4 X-ray chest after surfactant therapy showing improved aeration. This indicates improved lung compliance, hence positive pressure should be decreased if there is hyperexpansion (i.e. >8 ribs in chest X-ray) or expired tidal volume is greater than 8 ml/kg

Management

It comprises (i) surfactant replacement therapy; (ii) CPAP and assisted ventilation; (iii) supportive therapy which includes fluid and acid-base balance, trophic feeding and nutrition, correction of anemia, hypotension, hypothermia and clinically significant coagulopathy; (iv) treatment of patent ductus arteriosus (v) antibiotic therapy because pneumonia

may exist concurrently or supervene following ventilation and (vi) use of prophylactic fluconazole. In a retrospective analysis of the NICHD neonatal network study centers, the most dramatic improvement in survival and respiratory morbidity in RDS have occurred coincident with increased surfactant use since its availability in 1990[10]. There were further improvements coincident with increased antenatal steroid use in 1994. However, these improvements have shown a plateau since 1998[10]. Recently, two large placebo controlled trials with inhaled nitric oxide (iNO) have been conducted in premature infants with RDS with birth weights of 500 to 1250 g, who were at high risk for lung and brain injury[11, 12]. In the trial of Kinsella *et al* iNO at 5ppm was used at less than 48 hours of age in infants receiving mechanical ventilation[11]. In contrast, Ballard *et al* used iNO on ventilator-dependant infants at 7-21 days, starting at 20 ppm and gradually weaned[12]. There was slight reduction in BPD in the Ballard study, and in the trial of Kinsella *et al*, a secondary outcome i.e. ultrasonographic evidence of brain injury (severe intracranial hemorrhage, periventricular leukomalacia, or ventriculomegaly) was reduced in the iNO treated group. However, long-term follow-up results of premature infants treated with iNO are lacking. Currently, iNO is not recommended until further evaluations are done, because it is the most expensive drug available for children ($300.00 per day and up to $12,000.00 for a 30-day period in the United States), and it is therefore, difficult to justify its routine use in RDS until unequivocal long-term benefits are proven[13].

Surfactant Replacement Therapy

Infants diagnosed with RDS who require more than 0.30 to 0.40 FiO_2 should receive intratracheal surfactant as soon as possible, preferably within 2 hours after birth[7, 9, 14-16]. Since surfactant is protective to these delicate lungs, some investigators have used it prophylactically after resuscitating extremely premature infants[1, 3, 7, 9]. However, surfactant is expensive and 40 to 60 percent of these infants do not have surfactant deficiency or have only mild RDS due to prophylactic use of antenatal steroids or if the infant is stressed in-utero and is growth retarded. Thus these infants would be intubated unnecessarily with its inherent risks[6]. Hence, prediction of RDS by the microbubble stability test on gastric aspirates in newborns less than 32 weeks' gestation has been suggested, but has not been widely accepted due to technical difficulties and because it is not readily available[17]. Routine elective intubation for administration of surfactant to preterm infants $\geq$ 1250 grams with mild to moderate RDS is not recommended[18]. Premature infants with surfactant deficiency and RDS have an alveolar pool size of approximately 5 mg/kg. The dose of clinically available surfactant preparations ranges from 50 to 200 mg/kg, in order to approximate the surfactant sufficient pool of term newborn lungs. While the use of multiple doses of surfactant appears to be more effective than a single dose, some studies suggest that a large initial dose may be equally effective[7]. Rapid bolus administration of surfactant after adequate lung recruitment may lead to a more homogenous distribution. Guidelines for surfactant replacement therapy for respiratory distress syndrome has been developed by the American Academy of Pediatrics[14]. Each institution should modify them to meet their needs, and also evaluate their outcome data. The source, composition and dosages of various surfactant preparations are listed in Table 20.2. The endotracheal tube should be suctioned, preferably using a closed system, surfactant delivered without disconnecting the ventilator and vital signs monitored during and immediately after surfactant administration. If expired tidal volume increases to more than 8 ml/kg, peak inspiratory pressure should be gradually decreased and blood gases measured after 20 to 30 minutes. The choice of surfactant preparation remains controversial. We prefer Curosurf® with greater initial concentration of DPPC delivered through a small volume with rapid improvement in blood gases with faster weaning of oxygen, positive pressure ventilation, and thus minimizing the lung damage.

Surfactant therapy has also been used with limited success in lung diseases with secondary surfactant deficiency e.g. pneumonia (meconium aspiration, bacterial), pulmonary hemorrhage, congenital diaphragmatic hernia, lung hypoplasia and acute respiratory distress syndrome[1, 3, 19-22].

Continuous Positive Airway Pressure (CPAP)

It is a technique with which a sustained continuous pressure is applied to the airways throughout both the inspiratory and expiratory cycles, thereby decreasing right-to-left pulmonary shunt. The mortality and morbidity in infants with RDS has been significantly reduced since the introduction of CPAP by Gregory in 1971[23]. CPAP may be administered either via an endotracheal tube, nasal prongs, mask or nasopharyngeal tube[2-3]. It

Type	Source	Composition	Dosage	Comment
Beractant (Survanta®)	Bovine lung mince	DPPC, tripalmitin SP (B<5%, SP-C 99% of TP wt/wt)	4 ml (100 mg)/kg., 1 to 4 doses q 6 hr	8 ml vials, refrigerate
Bovactant (Alveofact TA®)	Bovine lung lavage	As above	45 mg/ml	German product
Infasurf®	Calf lung lavage	DPPC, tripalmitin, SP (B 290 µg/ml 360 mg/ml)	3 ml (105 mg)/kg, 1-4 doses, q 6 to 12 hr	4 & 8 ml vials, refrigerate
Poractant alpha (Curosurf ®)	Minced pig lung	Phospholipids (DPPC, phosphatidyl glycerol, neutral lipids, fatty, SP-B and SP-C)	2.5 ml (200 mg)/kg stat followed by 1.25 ml (100 mg)/kg q 12 hr	1.5 & 3 ml vials
Colfosceril palmitate (*Exosurf ®)	Synthetic	85% DPPC, 9% hexadecanol, 6% tyloxapol,	5 ml (67.5 mg)/kg, 2-4 doses, q 12 hr	Lyophilized, dissolve in 8 ml
Lucinactant (Surfaxin®)	Synthetic	DPPC, synthetic peptide, protein KL4	175 mg/kg/dose	Not licensed by FDA
Artificial lung expanding compound (*ALEC®)	Synthetic	70% DPPC, 30% unsaturated PG	–	–

Table 20.2 Type, source, composition and dosage of some surfactant preparations

* Exosurf® and ALEC® have been withdrawn from the market.

has also been used following surfactant therapy, and after extubation to prevent de-recruitment of alveoli. The optimum level of CPAP can be defined as the airway pressure at which oxygen saturation and PaO$_2$ are optimized without adverse effects on the cardiac output[2]. Nasal prongs and masks have been used to deliver CPAP without resorting to endotracheal intubation[3]. As the popularity of CPAP has increased, and concerns are being raised about the consequences of endotracheal intubation, the technique of delivering CPAP is gaining renewed interest. A recent review in the Cochrane Database suggests that early surfactant therapy followed by nasal CPAP is associated with a reduced need for mechanical ventilation and decreased utilization of exogenous surfactant therapy[16]. Furthermore, data from two major university centers in the NICHD neonatal network in the United States, showed that Columbia University hospital in New York had one-third less incidence of chronic lung disease in premature infants with RDS, compared to two other NICUs in Boston because Cloumbia hospital care providers placed RDS infants on early "bubble" CPAP, and accepted "borderline" blood gases[24].

Assisted Ventilation

Mechanical ventilation was introduced more than three decades ago when it was shown to decrease mortality due to RDS; however morbidity due to BPD and pulmonary air-leaks had increased. Volutrauma and/or barotrauma may contribute significantly to lung inflammation in premature infants, leading to bronchopulmonary dysplasia

(Figure 20.2). Therefore, newer modalities of ventilation have been introduced, which include patient triggered ventilation and high frequency ventilation. The reader is referred to a comprehensive review on these subjects[2-5, 25, 26]. Currently in the United States most neonatal intensive care units use synchronous intermittent mandatory ventilation (SIMV), and measure expired tidal volumes and monitor "on-line" pulmonary function tests to minimize "volutrauma". If expired tidal volume is greater than 8 ml/kg, the peak inspiration pressure should be decreased. RDS is a self limited disease, hence, many NICUs accept borderline blood gases, i.e. pH >7.25, paO$_2$ 50-60 mm Hg or SaO$_2$ 88 to 93%, and pCO$_2$ 50-55 mm Hg (i.e. permissive hypercapnia). In the acute stage of RDS, blood gases are estimated frequently to adjust the FiO$_2$ and ventilator settings to minimize lung injury. High frequency ventilation has also been used early to minimize lung damage in extremely immature infants with limited success[2, 4, 9, 25, 26]. Complications of CPAP or assisted ventilation in infants with RDS include pneumothorax, interstitial air leak and pneumopericardium (Figures 20.5 and 20.6). Extensive intra alveolar pulmonary hemorrhages has been described in infants dying following surfactant therapy[27]. If pulmonary hemorrhage occurs in premature infants, an echocardiogram should be done to exclude patent ductus arteriosus with right-to-left shunt, because it could be indicative of hemorrhagic pulmonary edema. This should be diagnosed promptly and treated aggressively to improve the outcome. Apnea, bradycardia and desaturation have also been

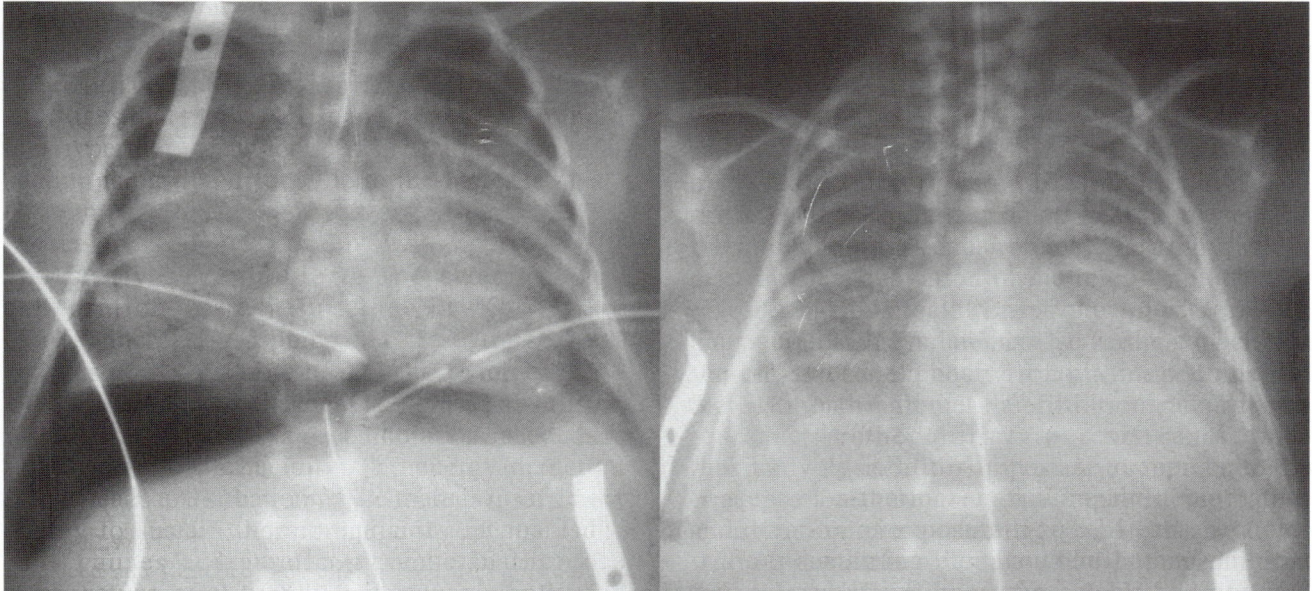

Figure 20.5 Chest roentgenogram of a neonate with pneumothorax and bilateral chest tubes, and after complete resolution four days later

Section 3

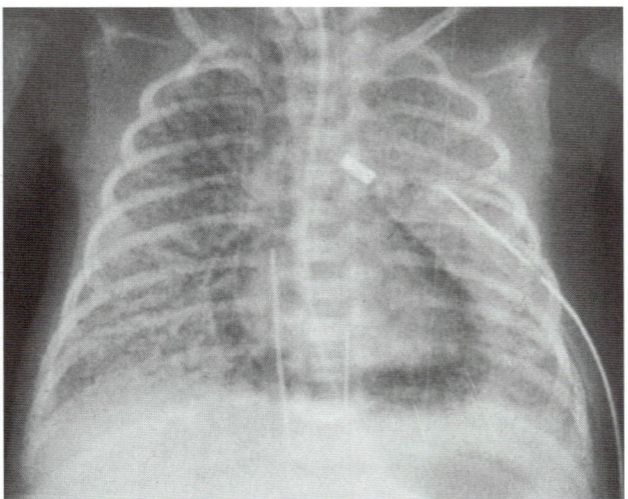

Figure 20.6 Chest roentgenogram of a premature infant with RDS on high ventilator settings showing pulmonary interstitial air and pneumopericardium resulting in cardiac tamponade. The latter must be relieved immediately by placement of a small catheter, and interstitial air is managed by decreasing the mean airway pressure and/or using high frequency jet ventilation if available

described in infants with RDS receiving surfactant therapy, and has been attributed to early extubation. Hence, tiny premature infants should be treated with caffeine prior to extubation. The long-term significance of persistent apnea, bradycardia or desaturation is unclear. In an editorial, Martin and Fanaroff concluded that prevailing data suggest that this should not be considered sinister and is not predictive of either sudden infant death syndrome or adverse neurodevelopmental outcome[28].

In a longitudinal 15-year follow-up of children born at less than 29 weeks' gestation at a single center between 1985 to 1987, who received surfactant therapy, 19% had cerebral palsy and attended regular class, wheras 29% were placed in special classroom[29]. Fifty one children (41%) had no physical or educational impairment, whereas 24 (19%) had at least one severe disability. In these children severe intraventricular hemorrhage and low socioeconomic status were the strongest predictors of adverse outcome[29]. Recent studies have shown that as neonatal care has improved during the last two decades, smaller and sicker premature infants with RDS are surviving with better long-term pulmonary and neurodevelopmental outcomes[29, 30].

Surfactant Protein B and C deficiency

The hydrophobic surfactant proteins B and C are essential for lung function and pulmonary homeostasis after birth[1, 3, 31, 32]. These proteins enhance the spreading absorption and stability of surfactant lipids required for the reduction of surface tension in the alveolus. Surfactant proteins B and C also participate in the regulation of intracellular and extracellular processes critical for the maintainence of respiratory structure and function. Mutations in the gene encoding surfactant protein B and surfactant protein C (*SFTPB* and *SFTPC*, respectively) are associated with acute respiratory failure and interstitial lung disease[32]. The current knowledge regarding the structure and functions of surfactant protein B and C and their roles in the pathogenesis of acute and chronic lung disease in children and adults has been reviewed recently[32]. Nogee *et al* identified a mutation of the *SFTPB* gene, which is a rare and fatal cause of respiratory failure in full-term newborn infants that is refractory to standard therapies including surfactant replacement, and is managed by lung transplant[31]. More than 22 distinct mutations in the *SFTPB* gene that cause respiratory failure have been identified[32]. Most infants present with progressive respiratory failure in the first 24 to 48 hours of life. The disorder is usually inherited as an autosomal recessive condition. Uncommon mutations that cause partial deficiency of surfactant protein B have been associated with interstitial lung disease in childhood. Transient surfactant protein B deficiency with respiratory failure has also been reported[33]. Several recent studies have also associated both deficiency of surfactant protein C and mutations in the *SFTPC* gene with severe familial interstitial lung disease in humans. Mutations of other genes that cause protein misfolding and misrouting may contribute to the pathogenesis of chronic interstitial lung disease by similar mechanisms, namely, intracellular accumulation of injurious proteins, extracellular deficiency of bioactive surfactant peptides or both.

Complications

A large number of acute and chronic complications (due to the disease or therapeutic interventions) may occur. They include (i) alveolar rupture, (ii) nosocomial infections, (iii) intracranial hemorrhage and periventricular leukomalacia, (iv) patent ductus arteriosus, (v) pulmonary hemorrhage, (vi) necrotizing enterocolitis and/or GI perforation (vii) apnea of prematurity, (viii) bronchopulmonary dysplasia, (ix) retinopathy of prematurity and (x) neurologic sequelae. They should be prevented, identified early and managed appropriately.

TRANSIENT TACHYPNEA OF THE NEWBORN

Transient tachypnea of newborn (TTN), also referred to as wet lung syndrome or respiratory distress type II, is thought to be due to delayed resorption of normal fetal lung fluid. The lung fluid accumulates in the peribronchial lymphatics and bronchovascular spaces.

Diagnosis

Prolonged labor with a high incidence of failure to progress and greater likelihood of cesarean section has been associated with transient tachypnea. Maternal administration of hypotonic fluids can occur in this situation and reduce the osmotic gradient that favors resorption of lung fluid in the neonate. Respiratory distress is observed within the first thirty minutes of birth, and comprise of rapid shallow breaths, and rarely grunting, retractions and/or central cyanosis. Arterial blood gases show varying degree of hypoxemia, although respiratory failure is uncommon. Although in most infants the distress resolves within 24 hours, rarely, it may last for seven to ten days. The chest roentgenogram may show increased lung volume, accentuated vascular markings, or fluid in horizontal fissure (Figure 20.7). These findings must be distinguished from those seen in pneumonia (*Group B streptococcus*), and persistent pulmonary hypertension.

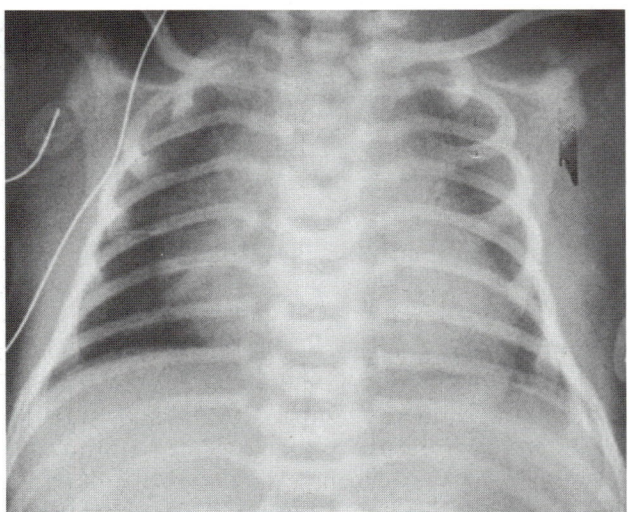

Figure 20.7 Chest roentgenogram of an infant born at term via cesarean section showing transient tachypnea of the newborn. Note fluid in the horizontal fissure and the streaky densities

Management

The diagnosis of TTN is made by excluding other causes of respiratory distress in term infants, such as sepsis, pneumonia, persistent pulmonary hypertension of newborn, congenital heart disease and aspiration syndromes. A course of antibiotics therapy can be begun, depending on the history and clinical status of the infant, and can be terminated after 48 to 72 hours if cultures are negative. The infant is supported with oxygen and assisted ventilation as indicated by blood gases.

ASPIRATION SYNDROMES

Meconium Aspiration Syndrome (MAS) is the commonest and the most important entity in this group[1, 3, 34]. The presence of meconium in the amniotic fluid or the staining of the fetus in a vertex delivery suggests that the infant may have been asphyxiated[34]. Meconium passage *in-utero* occurs in 8 to 20% of all deliveries and is noted more often in infants who are post-mature, have intrauterine growth retardation or have umbilical cord compression. In a healthy fetus, fluid moves from the lungs into the amniotic cavity. In contrast, in fetal distress, amniotic fluid and particulate matter is inhaled into the large airways. Meconium and squames may be detected in the airways of still born infants thereby indicating that meconium aspiration can occur antenatally. After birth with air breathing, especially if it is accompanied by gasping respirations, there is rapid distal migration of meconium within the lung. Thick meconium, fetal tachycardia, and heart rate variability on intrapartum monitoring may identify the infant at-risk for MAS. Its prevalence has decreased significantly with fetal monitoring and prompt resuscitation, which includes suctioning of the oropharynx and nasopharynx prior to delivery of the head when the amniotic fluid is stained with meconium, visualization of vocal cords after delivery and if necessary suctioning under direct vision[34, 35]. Despite these measures, meconium may be aspirated into the lungs after 34 weeks of gestation. Particulate meconium may produce bronchial obstruction with subsequent atelectasis mixed with areas of air trapping which may lead to air leaks, such as, pneumothorax and pneumomediastinum. The bile salts, pancreatic enzymes and other components of meconium may result in chemical pneumonitis. Chronic intrauterine hypoxia and /or acidosis may result in abnormal muscularization of the acinar arteries and the pulmonary vessels, resulting in persistent pulmonary hypertension of the newborn (PPHN)[34] (Figure 20.8).

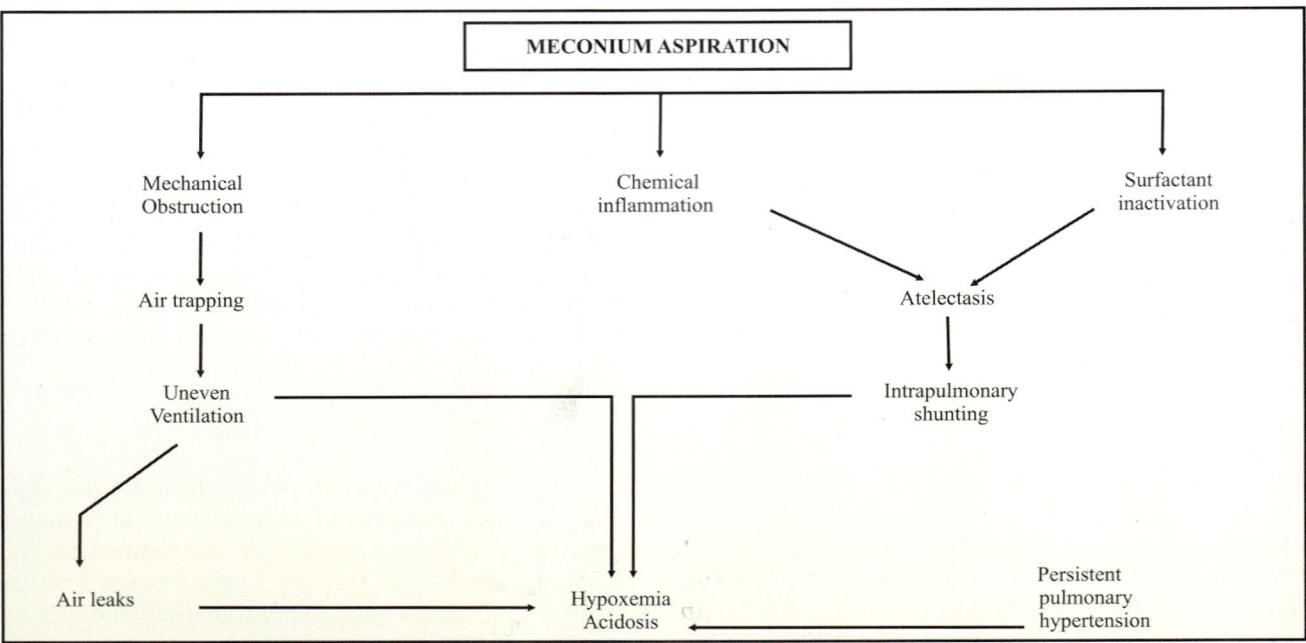

Figure 20.8 Pathophysiology of cardiorespiratory problems accompanying meconium aspiration syndrome

Diagnosis

The diagnosis is made with the history of the presence of meconium at or prior to delivery in a post-term, term or near term infant with respiratory distress. The infant with meconium aspiration syndrome often shows clinical signs of intrauterine growth retardation or post-maturity with yellow staining of nails, skin and umbilical cord. Clinically they may have respiratory distress and hypotonia. Chest roentgenogram demonstrates bilateral coarse patchy infiltrates (Figure 20.9), with subsequent air trapping and hyperexpansion, pneumomediatinum and/or pneumothorax. Blood gases show combined acidosis with hypoxia due to right-to-left shunting, which may lead to PPHN. Therefore, cord blood pH should be obtained and if acidosis is present, they should be managed aggressively.

Management

Efforts should be made by the obstetrician to prevent MAS by suctioning the oro and nasopharynx prior to the delivery of the chest. This is followed by prompt resuscitation of the baby by personnel trained in neonatal advanced life support (NALS). Therapy includes administration of oxygen, correction of acidosis and assisted ventilation (including high frequency or oscillation jet ventilation), which is often life saving[34, 35]. Since meconium is a potent inhibitor of surfactant, lung lavage with dilute surfactant has been advocated, particularly if extracorporeal membrane oxygenation (ECMO) is unavailable[19-21]. However, risk-benefit rates of lung lavage with surfactant therapy awaits further clinical trials. The management of PPHN associated with MAS including inhaled nitric oxide and ECMO therapy are described under PPHN. In infants presenting with severe respiratory failure, surfactant therapy has also been tried successfully[19, 20, 35, 36]. Supportive treatment of hypoglycemia, thermal regulation, antibiotic prophylaxis, fluid and electrolyte imbalance and seizures are also of paramount importance in the overall long-term outcome of these infants.

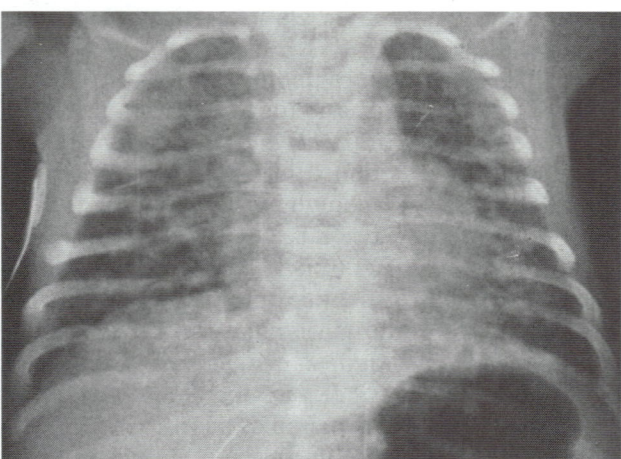

Figure 20.9 Chest X-ray of a full-term newborn with meconium aspiration pneumonia. Note bilateral coarse infiltrates, and fluid in the horizontal fissure which may also be seen in transient tachypnea of newborn

PNEUMONIA

The newborn infant is compromised immunologically, hence, more susceptible to infections, which are often associated with pneumonia. The mortality and morbidity of pneumonia and septicemia is high, particularly in premature infants[1, 3]. Asphyxia, hypoxemia and acidosis may impair the immune response of infants who already have an immature immune system. Because most episodes of early-onset sepsis begins before birth, the first sign of neonatal sepsis may be that of fetal distress, including fetal tachycardia in the second stage of labor and low 5-minute apgar scores. Pneumonia has been reported in 40% of infants with fetal heart rates (FHR) greater than 180 beats per minute (BPM), 20% with FHR of 160 to 180 BPM, but is uncommon with lower fetal heart rates. Although in the United States, *Group B streptococcus* remains an important pathogen for pneumonia and/or septicemia, one must consider other Gram-positive (e.g. staphylococci), Gram-negative (e.g. *E. coli*) pathogens, viruses, fungi and spirochetes (pneumonia alba) depending on the time of presentation and epidemiology in a community. In hospitalized infants in India, *Klebsiella pneumoniae* is the predominant organism, followed by *Staphylococcus aureus*, *E. coli* and Enterobacter which are also common causes of septicemia.

Diagnosis

The diagnosis is suggested by history of maternal fever, chorioamnionitis and other risk factors predisposing these infants to infections. The early signs and symptoms of septicemia may be subtle, e.g. poor feeding, temperature instability, although its diagnosis must be entertained in all patients with respiratory distress. Jaundice, hepatosplenomegaly, lethargy, irritability, anorexia, vomiting, diarrhea and abdominal distension may also be noted. Screening tests, e.g. white blood cell count (total and differential), C-reactive protein, procalcitonin, erythrocyte sedimentation rate for sepsis may be helpful, but they are low in sensitivity and specificity. One should not wait for leukocytosis, leukopenia, thrombocytopenia or isolation of an organism in blood and other body fluids to commence treatment. Chest X-ray may show mild to moderate pulmonary infiltrates (Figure 20.10), or extensive infiltrates, or pneumatoceles and effusion.

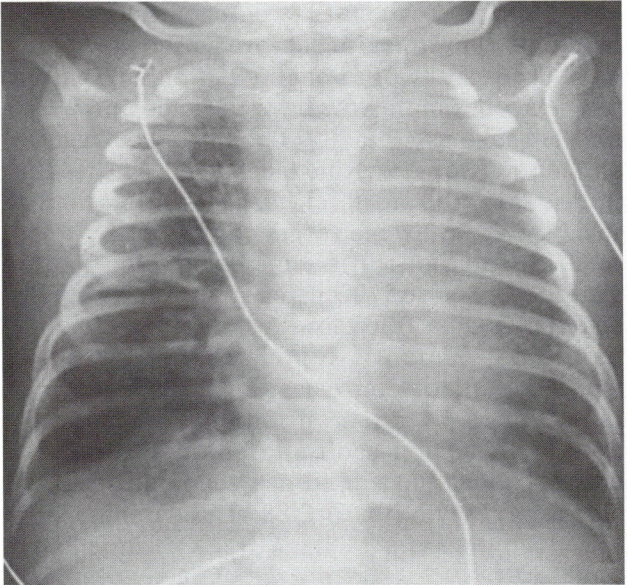

Figure 20.10 Chest roentgenogram of a term infant with respiratory distress secondary to pneumonia. Note the infiltrates in the right upper lobe

Management

The management comprises administration of appropriate antibiotics along with supportive measures. For further details refer to Chapter 24 for treatment of neonatal sepsis.

PERSISTENT PULMONARY HYPERTENSION OF THE NEWBORN (PPHN)

If the normal fetal pulmonary vascular resistance remains high after birth, successful transition from fetal to the neonatal circulation does not occur. Shunting of blood from right-to-left through the ductus arteriosus and/or foramen ovale, and with decreased pulmonary blood flow resuling in severe hypoxemia, which further worsens the existing pulmonary vasoconstriction. This clinical entity is known as persistent pulmonary hypertension of the newborn (PPHN), previously known as persistent fetal circulation[1, 3].

Diagnosis

The diagnosis of PPHN should be suspected in infants with perinatal asphyxia, meconium and other aspiration syndromes, shock, pneumonia/sepsis and HMD. Structural anomalies of the pulmonary vessels are observed in lung hypoplasia with or without congenital diaphragmatic hernia, which increases pulmonary vascular resistance leading to PPHN. Infants with "idiopathic" PPHN are usually born at or near term or are post-term and have respiratory distress within the first few hours of life. Findings on cardiac examination may be indistinguishable from those of congenital cyanotic heart disease. Poor myocardial contractility due to increased right ventricular load may result in tricuspid insufficiency and may have a cardiac murmur. After placing the infant in 100% oxygen concentration, paO_2 measured in blood samples obtained simultaneously from the right radial artery (preductal) may be greater than 10 mm Hg compared to that from the descending aorta (postductal); or a similar SaO_2 gradient of greater than 5% suggests a right-to-left shunt via the ductus arteriosus, which is present in approximately 50 percent of PPHN patients. Placing infants with "ductal-dependent" congenital cyanotic heart disease in 1.0 FiO_2 is not recommended unless intravenous prostacyclin drip is kept ready and a pediatric cardiologist is readily available for consultation. The diagnosis of PPHN is confirmed by echocardiogram after excluding other causes of congenital cyanotic heart disease, particularly infra-diaphragmatic anomalous pulmonary venous return.

Management

The principles of management of PPHN are to increase the infant's paO_2 by administering 1.0 FiO_2, inducing alkalosis by hyperventilation (best achieved by high frequency oscillation), and sodium bicarbonate infusion. Some patients with lung disease may respond to surfactant therapy after adequate lung recruitment.[19-22] Inhaled nitric oxide therapy (iNO), is known to selectively decrease pulmonary vascular resistance[1, 3, 8, 37, 38]. These measures also decrease the need for ECMO in PPHN patients[38]. The role of iNO in neonates with hypoxemia, and it's mechanism of action is shown in Figure 20.11. Oxygenation improves in approximately 50% of infants receiving inhaled nitric oxide, whether they have echocardiographic evidence of PPHN or not does not appear to affect the outcome[8]. Meta-analysis of control studies in infants with respiratory failure and PPHN in term and near term infants suggest use of 20 ppm of inhaled nitric oxide[8]. iNO concentration may be adjusted according to the patient's response and should be weaned by 1 ppm after decreasing to 5 ppm.

BRONCHOPULMONARY DYSPLASIA

In 1967, Northway and colleagues originally described the manifestations of chronic lung disease

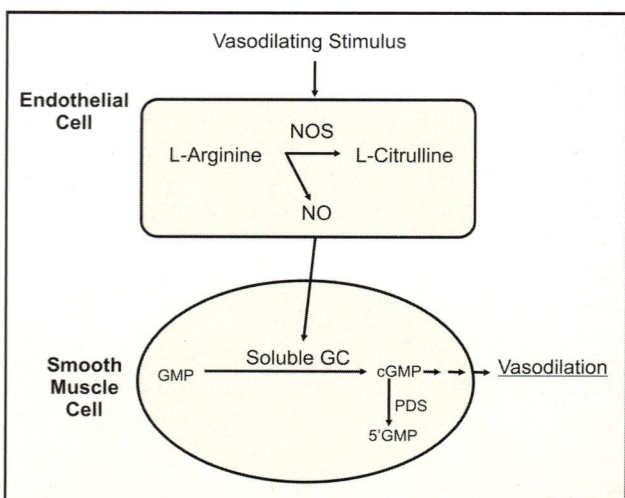

Figure 20.11 Mechanism of action of endogenous nitric oxide (NO). Endothelial-dependent stimuli "activate" NO synthetase (NOS) leading to increased production of NO by the endothelial cells. NO freely diffuses into the underlying smooth muscle cell and stimulates production of the second messenger cyclic GMP (cGMP), resulting in vasodilatation. cGMP is hydrolyzed by cGMP-specific phosphodiesterase enzymes (PDE5) to the inactive metabolite 5GMP. GC = guanylate cyclase

in survivors of hyaline membrane disease with use of assisted ventilation and high concentration of oxygen, and called this disorder bronchopulmonary dysplasia (BPD)[39]. With the advent of surfactant therapy, gentler modes of ventilation, and prudent use of antenatal and postnatal steroids, management of fluids, patent ductus arteriosus (PDA) and perinatal infections, mild to moderate forms of BPD remain the leading cause of chronic lung disease in infancy, because more smaller and sicker premature infants are surviving[3, 40-42]. Pathologically, there is an arrest in lung development and lung inflammation is followed by scarring of the alveoli, airways and finally leading to corpulmonale[43-46]. A recent study suggested that there is an association between increased fluid intake, weight loss during the first 10 days of life and the risk of BPD in extremely low birth weight infants[47].

Diagnosis

BPD is suspected in premature infants requiring oxygen and positive pressure ventilation. Earlier it was arbitrarily defined as oxygen requirement at 28 days (postnatal age), but currently, most neonatologists diagnose BPD if the infant is oxygen dependent at a corrected gestational age beyond 36 weeks[40]. The chest radiographic sequence first described by Northway is no longer commonly seen, and stage I is essentially indistinguishable from uncomplicated RDS[39]. Dense parenchymal opacification, as seen in stage II BPD, may commonly simulate another process, such as congestive heart failure due to PDA, fluid overload, or pulmonary hemorrhage. The bubbly pattern (Figure 20.12) or dense streaky opacification is seen in stage III BPD and may be difficult to differentiate from pneumonia, both often coexist. Finally, stage IV, may be insidious, and is characterized by hyperinflation, dense non-homogenous opacities and streaky densities extending to periphery[39]. The pathophysiology is outlined in the schematics in Figure 20.2. Abnormal pulmonary function is characterized by decreased lung compliance resulting from areas of fibrosis, over distension, atelectasis, and increased pulmonary vascular resistance resulting from airway damage. Some BPD infants may develop wheezing, which may be episodic and contribute to the increased work of breathing and oxygen requirement. Although it has been speculated that lung growth may be affected in the new BPD,[43,44] it has been shown that most BPD patients have normal pulmonary functions with age[30]. The wheezing may be due to reactive airway disease or asthma. Often chronic respiratory acidosis is accompanied by elevated bicarbonate and close to normal pH, which increases serum bicarbonate, and may be worsened with chronic diuretic therapy. Cardiovascular findings by echocardiogram in very low birth weight school going children who had BPD is comparable to those without BPD[48].

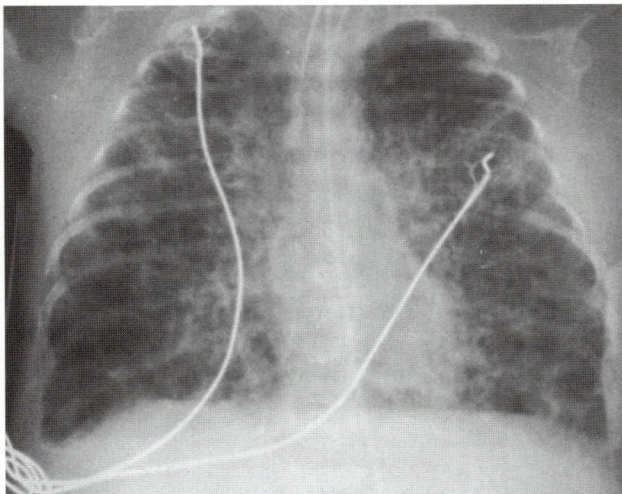

Figure 20.12 Chest X-ray of an infant with bronchopulmonary dysplasia (stage III)

Management

BPD requires skillful adjustment of FiO_2 to keep SaO_2 between 88% and 95%, fluid restriction, prudent use of steroids, diuretics, and bronchodilators.

If corticosteroids are used, it should be used for a short duration (14 to 21 days) at the lowest possible dosages[41]. The use of corticosteroid remains controversial because it may affect neurodevelopmental outcome. Hydrocortisone is preferred over dexamethasone due to reduced risk of causing neuromotor disability. Steroid use does not affect lung growth. Inhaled nitric oxide has also been used in some patients who are ventilator-dependant to decrease pulmonary vascular resistance[49], however its long-term effects are unclear and the cost may be prohibitive. A few patients with severe BPD and ventilator-dependence have been successfully treated with sildenafil, which is a pulmonary vasodilator. However, no controlled studies have been undertaken. Vitamin A supplementation has been recommended and routinely used at a number of centers to minimize oxidant lung injury[50]. These infants are at increased risk of developing reactive airway disease due to passive smoke inhalation and other pollutants, hence appropriate measures should be undertaken to prevent their exposure. Since BPD patients are susceptible to viral infections, particularly respiratory syncytial virus, they should be immunized with palivizumab[51]. Appropriate chest physiotherapy to prevent atelectasis, and adequate nutrition intake for somatic growth and development of new alveoli in these infants who have high oxygen consumption is equally important to improve their outcome.

DEVELOPMENTAL DISORDERS OF THE LUNGS AND AIRWAYS[1,3]

Congenital Diaphragmatic Hernia (CDH)

CDH is a defect of the diaphragm, and is caused by failure of the pleuroperitoneal canal to close at 9 to 10 weeks of gestation. This results in severe pulmonary hypoplasia from compression of the developing lungs by the herniated viscera. The incidence of CDH is estimated to be 1 in 2,200 when intrauterine fetal deaths and stillbirths are included. The etiology of CDH is unknown. Associated anomalies are seen in 25% to 57% by fetal sonogram, and include congenital heart defects, hydronephrosis, renal agenesis, intestinal atresias, extralobar sequestrations, and neurological defects including hydrocephalus, anencephaly and spina bifida. Chromosomal anomalies, including trisomy 21, 18, and 15, occur in association with CDH in 10% to 20% of cases diagnosed prenatally. It usually presents as a life-threatening emergency although occasionally infants are asymptomatic at birth. Prompt diagnosis must be made, preferably in-utero, and the infant delivered at a tertiary center and managed by a skilled team of perinatologists, surgeons, nurses and respiratory therapists. These infants should not be resuscitated with a bag and mask ventilation, because gas pushed down through the esophagus into the intrathoracic intestines, further compromises the ventilation and circulation. The clinical course and the survival of an infant with isolated CDH depends entirely on the degree of pulmonary hypoplasia. The extent of hypoplasia depends on the timing of herniation during development, the volume of viscera herniated, and the duration of herniation. It is better to delay the repair of CDH until the infant has stabilized, which may take days. Chest x-ray should be obtained as soon as possible, and shows herniation of viscera in the hemithorax (Figure 20.13). If the infant's condition detiorates during the "honeymoon period", then ECMO should be initiated. The infant can undergo repair of CDH while on ECMO and should be weaned from the circuit postoperatively. Adequate ventilatory support, while minimizing the risk of tension pneumothorax is often difficult. Sedation and/or paralysis is sometimes helpful in these difficult situations. Tension pneumothorax frequently occur and can be life-threatening; hence, one should be vigilant and prompt diagnosis by transillumination of the chest or chest X-ray should be made and thoracotomy tubes placed. Cardiac support with catecholamines and pulmonary vasodilators such as inhaled nitric oxide is necessary. Some infants may respond to surfactant

therapy, but CDH patients do not respond to inhaled nitric oxide. Extracorporeal membrane oxygenation is undertaken perioperatively. The outcome is not only determined by the degree of lung hypoplasia, but also by the increase in pulmonary vascular resistance, degree of lung damage from chronic ventilatory support, and the experience of the skilled team caring for such infants. Neurological problems including seizures, developmental delay or sensorineural hearing loss have been reported in 20% to 30% of CDH patients. Hence, they should be followed closely and appropriate interventions initiated early to improve long-term outcome.

Fetal Hydrothorax (FHT)

It is either unilateral or bilateral, and is chacterized by a pleural effusion in the fetus that may be primary, as a result of chylous leak; or secondary as a consequence of a generalized fluid retention associated with immune or nonimmune hydrops. Chylothorax is the commonest cause of pleural effusion in the newborn. Secondary FHT may be due to chromosomal anomalies, infections, neoplasms, cardiovascular, hematologic, gastrointestinal, pulmonary, metabolic, placental, and umbilical cord malformations. Fetal hydrothorax (secondary) has been reported in association with congenital diaphragmatic hernia, cystic adenomatous malformation of lung and bronchopulmonary sequestration with mortality rate greater than 90%. The development of hydrops in primary FHT is a poor prognostic sign. These infants should be delivered at a tertiary care setting where appropriate resuscitation is administered promptly. Fluid is removed by thoracentesis, followed by thoracotomy, and residual fluid or pneumothorax is assessed by chest X-ray. In infants with chylothorax, after the infant is stable, feeding is commenced with a formula high in medium chain triglycerides, which bypasses the lymphatics by direct absorption into the blood stream.

Congenital Cystic Adenomatous Malformation (CCAM)

It is a rare malformation of the lung characterized by a multicystic mass of pulmonary tissue with proliferation of bronchial structures. There is a connection between the CCAMs and the normal tracheobronchial tree, although it is a minute tortuous passage. By fetal level 2 ultrasound examination, type I and type II CCAM appear as cystic or echoluscent pulmonary masses. Type III CCAM typically appears as a large, solid,

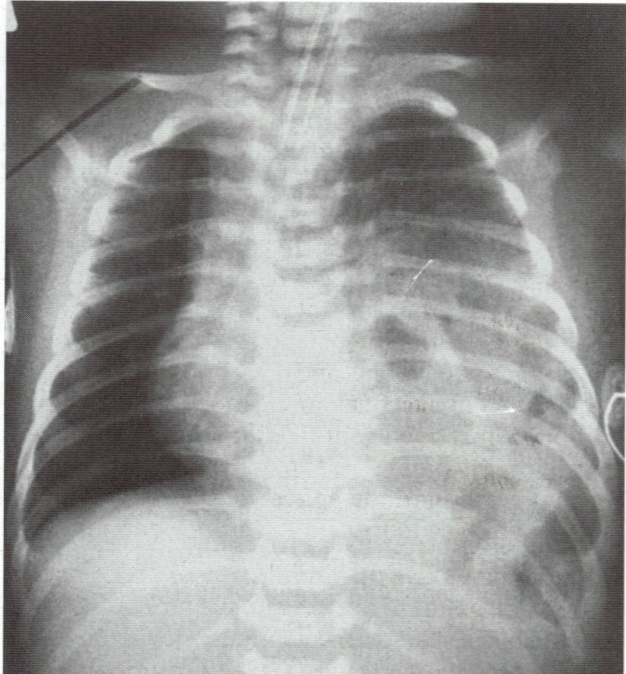

Figure 20.13 Chest roentgenogram of an infant with congenital diaphragmatic hernia

hyperechogenic mass, often with mediastinal shift and hydrops. CCAMs derive their arterial blood supply and venous drainage from normal pulmonary circulation, but anomalous arterial and venous drainage of CCAM can occur. The differential diagnosis of fetal thoracic masses includes CDH, bronchogenic or enteric cysts, bronchopulmonary sequestration, mediastinal cystic hygroma, bronchial atresia, neuroblastoma and brain heterotopia. About 80% of CCAM patients present at birth with severe cardiorespiratory compromise from severe pulmonary hypoplasia. Hence, these infants should be delivered at a center with an intensive care nursery and appropriate staff to resuscitate an infant with pulmonary hypoplasia. Some infants may be at significant risk for air trapping and worsening respiratory status, which may be temporized by selective intubation of the contralateral bronchus, until surgical resection. Pneumothorax is an additional concern in type I or II lesions, requiring thoracotomy. CCAM is usually confined to a single lobe, although rare cases have been reported of multilobar involvement of one lung, wherein lobectomy is the treatment of choice. In cases of extensive involvement of nearly the entire lung, resection of multiple lobes or pneumonectomy may be necessary.

Bronchopulmonary Sequestration (BPS)

It is a cystic mass of nonfunctioning pulmonary tissue that lacks an obvious communication with the tracheobronchial tree and receives all or most of its blood supply from anomalous systemic vessels. There are two forms of BPS: intralobar and extralobar. In infants and children, intralobar BPS is seen in 75% of cases, and shares the same pleura with the normal lung; wheras the 25% of extralobar BPS has a separate pleura from the lung, and may be either intrathoracic or subdiaphragmatic in location. In the fetus, BPS is a solid, highly echogenic mass with a clearly defined systemic feeding vessel. A wide range of severity occurs with BPS, the degree of pulmonary hypoplasia will be the primary determinant of outcome. Hence, these infants should be delivered at a center which is able to provide resuscitation, and uses high frequency ventilation, inhaled nitric oxide therapy and ECMO. Large pleural effusions should be treated immediately by tube thoracotomy. Surgery should be deferred until the infant is stable. The surgical approach to BPS is straight forward with the exception of the management of anomalous blood supply. These blood vessels are often large thin-walled, elastic (rather than muscular) arteries

that are subdiaphragmatic in origin 20% of the time, 15% of the time more than one vessel is present. The subdiaphragmatic origin of the vessels is more common with right-sided lesions. These vessels can retract into the mediastimun or diaphragm and continue to bleed. Intraoperative death has been reported as a result of hemorrhage from unrecognized anomalous vessels. The importance of preoperative assessment of venous drainage as well as arterial supply is underscored by the reports of post operative fatalities from ligation of anomalous veins that constitute the sole or major venous drainage or the entire ipsilateral lung.

REFERENCES

1. Whitsett JA, Pryhuser GS, Rice WR, *et al*. Acute respiratory disorders in neonatology. In: Pathophysiology and Management of the Newborn, Avery GB, Fletcher MA and MacDonald MG (ed) *Lippincot, William and Wilkins, Philadelphia, PA, USA* 5th Edition 1999; pp 485-531.

2. Harris TR, Wood BR. Physiology and principles. In: Assisted Ventilation of the Neonate. Goldsmith JP, Karotkin EH (ed), *4th ed. Philadelphia: W B Saunders,* 2004.

3. The Respiratory System. In: Neonatal-Perinatal Medicine, Diseases of the Fetus and Infant. Martin RJ, Fanaroff AA and Walsh MC (ed.) Vol. 2. *Mosby & Elsevier Co., Philadelphia, PA, USA,* 8th edition, pp 1069-1194.

4. Clark RH. High frequency ventilation. *J Pediatr* 1994; 124:661-670.

5. McGettigan MC, Adolph VR, Ginsberg HG, *et al*. New ways to ventilate newborns in acute respiratory failure. *Pediatr Clin North Am* 1998; 45: 475-509.

6. Pramanik AK, Holtzman RB, Merritt TA. Surfactant replacement therapy for pulmonary diseases. *Pediatr Clin North Am* 1993; 40:913-936.

7. Engle WA. The committee on Fetus and Newborn: Surfactant-replacement Therapy for Respiratory Distress in the Preterm and Term Neonate. *Pediatrics* 2008, 212: 419-432.

8. Finer NN and Barrington KJ. Nitric oxide for respiratory failure in infants born at or near term. *Cochrane Database Sys. Rev* 2001; CD000399.

9. Pramanik AK. Respiratory distress syndrome. In: *eMedicine Pediatrics* 2006; 7(6):1-33.

10. Murphy KE, Hannah ME, Willan AR, *et al*. Multiple courses of antenatal corticosteroids for preterm births (MACS): A randomized controlled trial. *Lancet* Dec 2008, 372:2143-2151.

11. Kinsella JP, Cutter GR, Walsh WF, *et al*. Early inhaled nitric oxide therapy in premature newborns with respiratory failure. *N Engl J Med* 2006; 355:354-364.

12. Walch MC. NOCLD Study Groups. Two year neurodevelopmental outcomes of ventilated preterm infants treated with inhaled nitric oxide. *J Pediatr* 2010, 156:556-561

13. Kinsella JP, Abman SH. Inhaled nitric oxide in the premature newborn. *J. Pediatr* Jul 2007, 151(1): 10-15.

14. Lemons JA, Blackmon LR, Kanto WP, *et al*. Committee on Fetus and Newborn. Surfactant replacement therapy for respiratory distress syndrome. *American Academy of Pediatrics* 1999; 103:684.

15. Kresch MJ, Lin WH, Thrall RS. Surfactant replacement therapy. *Thorax* 1996; 51:1137-1154.

16. Stevens TP, Blennow M, Soll RF. Early surfactant administration with brief ventilation vs selective surfactant and continued mechanical ventilation for preterm infants with or at risk for respiratory distress syndrome. *Cochrane Database Syst Rev* 2004; CD003063.

17. Verder H, Ebbesen F, Linderholm B, *et al*. Prediction of respiratory distress syndrome by the microbubble stability test on gastric aspirates in newborns of less than 32 weeks' gestation. *Acta Paediatr* 2033; 92:728-733.

18. Escobedo MB, Gunkel JH, Kennedy KA, *et al*. Early surfactant for neonates with mild to moderate respiratory distress syndrome: a multicenter, randomized trial. *J Pediatr* 2004; 144:804-808.

19. Lam BCC and Yeung CY. Surfactant lavage for meconium aspiration syndrome: A pilot study. *Pediatrics* 1999; 103:1014-1018.

20. Soll RF and Dargaville P. Surfactant for meconium aspiration syndrome in full term infants. *Cochrane Database of Sys Rev* 2000; 2:CD002054.

21. Findlay RD, Taeusch HW, Walther FJ. Surfactant replacement therapy for meconium aspiration syndrome. *Pediatrics* 1996; 97:48-52.

22. Moya F, Maturna A. Animal-derived surfactants versus past and current synthetic surfactants: Current status. *Clin in Perinatol* 2007, 34:145-177.

23. Gregory GA, Kitterman JA, Phibbs RH, *et al*. Treatment of idiopathic respiratory distress syndrome with continuous airway pressure. *N Engl J Med* 1971; 284:1333.

24. Van Marter LJ, Allred EN, Pagano M, *et al*. Do clinical markers of barotrauma and oxygen toxicity explain interhospital variation in rates of chronic lung disease? *Pediatrics* 2000; 105:1194-1201.

25. Gerstmann DR, Minton SD, Stoddard RA. The Provo multicenter early high-frequency oscillatory ventilation trial: improved pulmonary and clinical outcome in respiratory distress syndrome. *Pediatrics* 1996; 89:1044-1057.

26. McGettigan MC, Adolph VR, Ginsberg HG, *et al*. New ways to ventilate newborns in acute respiratory failure. *Pediatr Clin North Am* 1998; 45:475-509.

27. Pappin A, Shenker N, Hack M, *et al*. Extensive intra-alveolar pulmonary hemorrhage in infants dying after surfactant therapy. *J Pediatr* 1994; 124:621-626.

28. Martin RJ and Fanaroff AA. Neonatal apnea, bradycardia, or desaturation: Does it matter? *J Pediatr* 1998; 132:758-759.

29. D'Angio CT, Sinkin RA, Stevens TP, *et al*. Longitudinal, 15-year follow-up of children born at less than 29 weeks' gestation after introduction of surfactant therapy into a region: Neurologic, cognitive, and educational outcomes. *Pediatrics* 2002; 110:1094-1102.

30. Robin B, Kim YJ, Huth J, *et al*. Pulmonary function in bronchopulmonary dysplasia. *Pediatr Pulmonol* 2004; 37:236-242.

31. Nogee LM, deMello DE, Dehner LP, *et al*. A mutation in the surfactant protein B gene responsable for fatal neonatal respiratory disease in multiple kindreds. *J Clin Invest* 1994; 93:1860-1863.

32. Whitsett JA and Weaver TE. Hydrophobic surfactant proteins in lung function and disease with singletons. *Am J Obstet Gynecol* 2004; 91:271-276.

33. Klein JM, Thompson MW, Snyder JM, *et al*. Transient surfactant protein B deficiency in a term infant with severe respiratory failure. *J Pediatr* 1998; 132:244-248.

34. Peng TCC, Gutcher GR and Van Dorsten JP. A selective aggressive approach to the neonate exposed to meconium stained amniotic fluid. *Am J Obstet Gynecol* 1996; 175:296-303.

35. Cleary GM, Wiswell TE. Meconium-stained amniotic fluid and the meconium aspiration syndrome, an update. *Pediatr Clin North Am* 1998; 45:511-529.

36. Lotze A, Mitchell BR, Bulas DI, *et al*. Multicenter study of surfactant (beractant) use in the treatment of term infants with severe respiratory failure. *J Pediatr* 1998; 132:40-47.

37. Kinsella JP and Abman SH. Clinical approach to inhaled nitric oxide therapy in the newborn with hypoxemia. *J Pediatr* 2000; 136:717-726.

38. Kennaugh JM, Kinsella JP, Abman SH, *et al*. Impact of new treatments for neonatal pulmonary hypertension on extracorporeal membrane oxygenation use and outcome. *J Perinatol* 1997; 17:366-369.

39. Northway WH, Rosan RC, Porter DY. Pulmonary disease following respiratory therapy of hyaline membrane disease. *N Engl J Med* 1967; 276:357-368.

Section 3

40. Farrell PA, Fiascone JM. Bronchopulmonary dysplasia in the 1990s: a review for the pediatrician. *Current Probl Pediatr* 1997; 27:129-163.

41. Blackmon LR, Bell EF, Engle WA, *et al.* Postnatal corticosteroids to treat or prevent chronic lung disease in preterm infants.*Pediatrics* 2002; 109:330-338.

42. Smith VC, Zupancic JAF, McCormick MC, *et al.* Trends in severe bronchopulmonary dysplasia rates between 1994 and 2002. *J Pediatr* 2005; 146:469-473.

43. Jobe AJ. The new BPD: an arrest of lung development. *Pediatr Res* 1999; 46:641-643.

44. Jobe AH. An unknown lung growth and development after very preterm birth. *Am J Respir Crit Care Med* 2002; 166:1529-1530.

45. Jobe AH. Antenatal associations with lung maturation and infection. *J Perinatol* 2005; 25:S31–S35.

46. Kallapur SG, Jobe AH. Contribution of inflammation to lung injury and development. *Arch Dis Child Fetal Neonatal Ed* 2006; 91:F132-F135.

47. Oh W, Poindexter BB, Perritt R, *et al.* Association between fluid intake and weight loss during the first 10 days of life and risk of BPD in ELBW infants. *J Pediatr* 2005; 147:786-790.

48. Korhonen P, Hyödynmaa E, Lautamatti V, *et al.* Cardiovascular findings in very low birthweight schoolchildren with and without bronchopulmonary dysplasia. *Early Hum Dev* 2005; 81:497-505.

49. Peter M. Mourani, D. Dunbar Ivy, Dexiang Gao, and Steven H. Pulmonary vascular effects of inhaled nitric oxide and oxygen tension in bronchopulmonary dysplasia. *Am J Respir Crit Care Med* 2004; 170:1006-1013.

50. Tyson JE, Wright LL, Oh W, *et al.* Vitamin A supplementation for extremely low birth weight infants. *N Engl J Med* 1999; 340:1962-1968.

51. Abramson JS, Baker CJ, Baltimore RS, *et al.* Revised indications for the use of palivizumab and respiratory syncytial virus immune globulin intravenously for the prevention of respiratory syncytial virus infections. *Pediatrics* 2003; 112:1442-1446.

Section 3

Neonatal Jaundice

Srinivas Murki and Praveen Kumar

INTRODUCTION

Neonatal jaundice is the most common clinical condition requiring evaluation and treatment in the newborn and is a common cause for hospital readmission during the first week of postnatal life. In adults, sclera appears jaundiced (icteric) when serum bilirubin exceeds 2 mg/ dl but evaluation of sclera is difficult in neonates because of physiological photophobia. In neonates jaundice becomes apparent on the skin of the face when serum bilirubin reaches 5 mg/dl. Sixty percent of term and 80% of preterm infants are likely to have serum bilirubin greater than 5 mg/ dl in the first week of life and about 6% of term infants will have levels exceeding 15 mg/ dl. Neonatal jaundice should be considered as a medical emergency because elevation of unconjugated bilirubin in high risk infants may cause irreversible brain damage (kernicterus).

PATHOPHYSIOLOGY

Bilirubin is produced in the reticuloendothelial system from the breakdown of heme proteins which are present in hemoglobin, myoglobin and certain heme containing enzymes such as peroxidases and catalases. The catabolism of 1.0 gram of hemoglobin results in the production of 34 mg of bilirubin. A normal term newborn baby produces about 6-10 mg/kg/ day of bilirubin. Bilirubin is bound to albumin for transport in the blood and each gram of albumin binds nearly 8 mg of bilirubin. The free or unbound bilirubin crosses the blood brain barrier and is toxic to the central nervous system.

Upon reaching the liver, bilirubin enters the liver cells and gets bound to ligandin which helps to transport it to the site of conjugation. Conjugation occurs with glucuronic acid to produce mono- and diglucuronides which are water soluble. The conjugated bilirubin is excreted in the bile and discharged into the gut. In the sterile newborn gut, there is an enzyme called beta-glucuronidase which converts bilirubin glucuronide back to unconjugated bilirubin which is reabsorbed through entero-hepatic

circulation. When baby is fed early and frequently, colonization of gut occurs with friendly bacteria. These bacteria deconjugate bilirubin glucuronide into stercobilin which is excreted in the stool, thus inhibiting the enterohepatic circulation (Figure 21.1). Jaundice can occur in newborn babies due to increased production of bilirubin (hemolysis) or defective conjugation (hepatic immaturity) or due to increased enterohepatic circulation (delayed and infreqnent feedings).

Hemolysis, blood collections, decreased albumin or defective binding capacity of albumin to bilirubin, decreased uptake of bilirubin into the liver or decreased conjugation of bilirubin would all result in increased free bilirubin in the blood. Elevated levels of free bilirubin, altered blood brain barrier and increased intrinsic susceptibility of neonatal brain can result in bilirubin encephalopathy. Certain risk factors like low birth weight, prematurity, intrauterine growth restriction, presence of hemolysis, low serum albumin, acidosis, sepsis or meningitis and asphyxia etc. increase the probability of bilirubin encephalopathy at lower serum bilirubin levels[1]. When bilirubin crosses the blood-brain barrier, it predominantly affects the reticular system, globus pallidus, subthalamus (basal ganglia), brain stem, cranial nerve nuclei and hypothalamus.

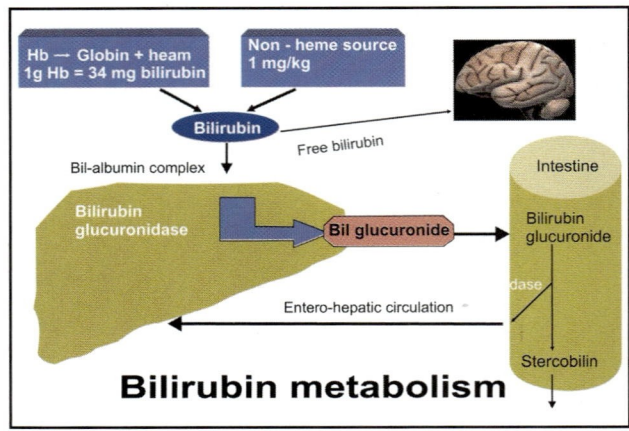

Figure 21.1 Pathophysiology of jaundice

ETIOLOGY

Physiological jaundice is the most common form of jaundice in newborns. This jaundice usually has its onset on day 2 or 3 of life, peaks on day 4 or day 5 and disappears by 7-10 days of life. It occurs due to a large number of predisposing factors.

(i) Shorter RBC life span (90 days versus 120 days in adults)

(ii) Increased RBC mass

(iii) Ineffective erythropoeisis

(iv) Decreased uptake of bilirubin into the liver due to low ligandin levels

(v) Decreased hepatic conjugation secondary to decreased uridine di-phosphoglucuronide transferase (UDPGT) activity. At birth the activity of UDPG-glucuronyl transferase is 5% of adult activity but increases significantly after 24 hours to handle the bilirubin load. In north Indian population, polymorphism (UGT1A1) in the promoter sequence of UDP-glucuronyl tansferase is associated with increased risk of hyperbilirubinemia[2].

(vi) Increased enterohepatic circulation due to decreased gut motility and increased β glucuronidase activity in the gut.

Neonates with physiological jaundice do not require any treatment but should be provided with early and frequent feeds. Jaundice in the newborn that requires evaluation, workup and management is called "pathological" and should be considered in the following situations:

❑ Appearance of jaundice within first 24 hours of life

❑ Icterus of palms and soles

❑ Rapid rise of bilirubin (> 5 mg/dl/day)

❑ Serum bilirubin > 15 mg/dl

❑ Lethargy, decreased activity, poor sucking and / or seizures

❑ Jaundice lasting more than 2 weeks in term and 3 weeks in preterm babies

If the jaundice is associated with clay or white colored stools, high or yellow-colored urine and if conjugated bilirubin is > 2 mg/dl or >20% of the TSB, one should investigate for cholestatic jaundice.

A detailed history regarding the age at onset, high risk factors and physical findings provide useful clues to the possible cause of jaundice (Table 21.1). Etiology can be broadly categorized into that due to increased bilirubin load, defective conjugation and increased enterohepatic circulation. Jaundice having onset within the 24 hours of life, clinical pallor, splenomegaly and hepatomegaly are useful clinical

Section 3

Table 21.1 Etiology of jaundice on the basis of history and physical examination	
History	**Possible etiology**
Previous sibling with neonatal jaundice, family history of anemia, splenectomy	Blood group incompatibility (Rh, ABO), G6PD deficiency, hereditary spherocytosis, Criggler-Najjar syndrome
Maternal fever and rash during pregnancy	Intrauterine infections
Labor and delivery events	Asphyxia, trauma, oxytocin-induced labor, delayed cord clamping
Maternal drugs	Sulphonamides, nitrofurantoin and antimalarials may cause hemolysis in G6PD deficient infant
Liver disease in the family	Galactosemia, Alpha-1-antitrypsin deficiency
Prolonged parenteral nutrition	Cholesatic jaundice
Physical Examination	**Possible etiology**
Small-for-dates baby	IU infections, polycythemia
Microcephaly	IU infections
Pallor	Hemolysis, extravasation of blood
Petechiae	IU infection, Rh iso-immunization, sepsis
Hepatosplenomegaly	IU infections, hemolytic jaundice, liver disease
Chorioretinitis	IU infections
Urine diaper staining and acholic stools	Cholestatic jaundice

markers of hemolysis. Increased bilirubin load occurs in cephalhematoma or subgalael bleeds, immune hemolysis due to ABO or Rh-isoimmunisation and non-immune hemolysis as in RBC membrane and enzyme defects. Defective conjugation is seen in babies with Criggler-Najjar syndrome, Gilbert's syndrome and infections. Enterohepatic circulation is increased in neonates with intestinal obstruction.

The age of onset of jaundice provides useful clues to the possible etiology of jaundice (Table 21.2). Infection must be ruled out when jaundice appears any time after the third day of life. Neonatal jaundice may be multifactorial in origin. Even after extensive investigations, cause may remain uncertain in nearly half of the cases. Hyperbilirubinemia in the first week of life is usually of the indirect variety and common causes in our country include exaggerated physiological jaundice, ABO or Rh iso-immunization, G6PD deficiency, infections, bruising, cephalhematoma and breast milk jaundice.

CLINICAL ASSESSMENT

The clinical evaluation of a jaundiced infant is directed towards assessing the severity of jaundice, identifying the etiology and looking for the signs of bilirubin encephalopathy. The skin over the sternum or the forehead is blanched and visual assessment of jaundice (yellow color) is done in natural day light. Intensity of jaundice in newborns follows cephalo-caudal progression. Mild jaundice affects only the face while severe jaundice spreads to palms and soles. Deep staining of trunk and yellow staining of palms and soles is ominous and indicates that serum bilirubin has exceeded 15 mg/dl. Clinical assessment of bilirubin even by an experienced person is only a rough estimate and must be confirmed by laboratory methods. Transcutaneous bilirubin (TcB) level can be checked over the skin of sternum with the help of hand-held BiliCheck which is a reliable non-invasive method. Total serum bilirubin (TSB) estimation is the gold standard for assessing the severity of jaundice.

Pallor and onset of jaundice within first 24 hours of life and spleno-hepatomegaly are suggestive of hemolysis. Cephalhematoma, bruising or subgaleal bleeds indicate blood collection as the cause of jaundice. IUGR, skin rash, petechiae and hepatomegaly are useful clues to intrauterine infection. Affected previous sibling, rapid rise of bilirubin and geographic origin from northwest states of India are useful pointers towards G6PD deficiency. Lethargy, poor feeding, fever, poor or

Table 21.2 Cause of jaundice on the basis of age of onset
❑ **Appearing within 24 hours of age**   • Hemolytic disease of newborn: Rh, ABO and minor blood group incompatibility   • Infections: Intrauterine viral or bacterial   • G6PD deficiency;   • Congenital malaria
❑ **Appearing between 24-72 hours of life**   • Physiological   • G6PD deficiency   • Sepsis   • Polycythemia   • Concealed hemorrhage: Cephalhematoma, subarachnoid bleed, IVH   • Increased entero-hepatic circulation
❑ **Appearing after 72 hours**   • Sepsis   • Neonatal hepatitis   • Extra hepatic biliary atresia   • Breast milk jaundice   • Metabolic disorders

incomplete Moro's reflex, opisthotonos and seizures suggest bilirubin encephalopathy. The severity of bilirubin encephalopathy is assessed as shown in Table 21.3.

LABORATORY INVESTIGATIONS

Investigations are required for assessing the severity of jaundice, to differentiate conjugated from unconjugated jaundice, to identify the etiology and to predict the risk of bilirubin encephalopathy. Total serum bilirubin with direct and indirect fraction is estimated to assess severity and to differentiate between conjugated and unconjugated or indirect jaundice. Packed cell volume or hemoglobin, reticulocyte count and peripheral smear examination are done to identify hemolysis. Anemia, reticulocytosis (> 5% after day 3), peripheral smear showing marked anisopoikiloctyosis, heterochromia and nucleated RBC's suggest hemolysis. The presence of microspherocytes in the peripheral smear are suggestive of ABO incompatibility. A positive indirect Coombs' test (ICT) in the mother or positive direct Coombs' test (DCT) in the baby are indicative of immune hemolysis. G6PD screening is necessary in endemic areas and when the bilirubin rise is very rapid. When sepsis is suspected, a sepsis screen (C-reactive protein, procalcitonin, blood counts), cultures of urine and blood are recommended. In Rh-isoimmunized mothers, cord blood should be screened for total serum bilirubin, hematocrit, blood grouping and DCT. If the jaundice lasts for more than 2 weeks in term and 3 weeks in preterm infants, a thyroid

Clinical	Non specific, subtle	Progressive toxicity	Advanced toxicity
Table 21.3 Clinical staging of acute bilirubin encephalopathy			
Score for a clinical sign in each column	1	2	3
Ranges of score	1 to 3	4 to 6	7 to 9
Mental status	Sleepy + poor feeding	Lethargy + irritability	Semi-coma and/or seizures
Muscle tone	Slightly decreased	Hyper- or hypotonia depending on arousal state, or mild nuchal/truncal arching	Markedly increased (opisthotonos), or decreased tone, or bicycling movements
Cry	High-pitched	Shrill	Inconsolable

Note: Individual score is assigned to each clinical sign to obtain a maximum score of 9. Infants with scores of 4 to 6 usually have reversible bilirubin encephalopathy. Progression to a higher score is indicative of worsening kernicterus.

profile, urine culture and galactosemia screen are mandatory. Any additional workup will be dictated by the infant's age, additional signs and symptoms, pregnancy events, and family history.

MANAGEMENT

Most jaundiced neonates do not require any treatment. At-risk infants should be identified, jaundice requiring treatment should be differentiated from the more common physiological jaundice and phototherapy should be started at the earliest. The danger signs suggesting bilirubin encephalopathy should be monitored; exchange transfusion when required should be done in a timely manner to avoid bilirubin encephalopathy and its long term sequelae. It should be remembered that once acute bilirubin encephalopathy occurs, the changes may not be reversible even with treatment. The treatment decisions for jaundice are currently based on the total serum bilirubin and the age of the infant in hours, at which TSB was estimated. The direct fraction is not subtracted from the TSB for making management decisions.

Identification of the at-risk Infant

Risk factor based approach, pre-discharge bilirubin and cord bilirubin levels are often used to predict the likely severity of jaundice during first week of life. Risk factor approach consists of assessing the perinatal distress factors associated with clinically significant hyperbilirubinemia. As the risk factors are common and the risk of severe jaundice is relatively low, a combination of risk factors are used to predict the severity of jaundice (Table 21.4). The perinatal risk factors which may aggravate jaundice or predispose to development

of acute bilirubin encephalopathy include birth asphyxia, acidosis, hypothermia, hypoglycemia, dehydration, sepsis and hypoalbuminemia. In healthy term and late preterm infants (gestation 34-36 weeks), hour specific serum bilirubin nomograms predict the development of subsequent severe jaundice in the first week of life[3]. If the TSB value at any age is falling in the high risk zone (>95th centile) or in the intermediate risk zone (40th to 95th centile) the chance of subsequent hyperbilirubinema is 39.5% and 6.4% respectively. If the hour specific TSB is in the low risk zone (<40th centile), there is no measurable risk of subsequent development of severe jaundice. However, these nomograms have been derived from American population and their validity for our populations needs to be established. In term healthy neonates if serum bilirubin at 24 ± 8 hours is < 6 mg/dl, the risk of subsequent hyperbilirubinemia is almost negligible[4].

If the infant is being discharged prior to 72 hours of age, it should be subjected to either a TSB or a transcutaneous bilirubin (TcB) estimation. The risk of subsequent hyperbilirubinemia can be estimated by plotting this value on the hour specific nomogram *vide supra*. When a pre-discharge bilirubin is not feasible or is not done, a day 3 or a day 4 follow-up visit for assessment of jaundice is mandatory. The complete absence of jaundice provides an excellent prediction of an infant's low risk with a 99% negative predictive value (NPV). It is reasonable to defer bilirubin measurement when an infant is not visibly or clinically jaundiced.

Treatment Decisions

Phototherapy and exchange blood transfusion form the mainstay for reducing serum bilirubin

Risk factors (Circle all that apply)	Major risk	Minor risk	Decreased risk
Visible jaundice (Dark skin pigmentation may obscure visualization)	First 24 hrs	Before discharge	None
Gestational age	35-36 wk	37-40 wk	≥ 41 wk
Previous sibling history	Received phototherapy	Jaundiced, no phototherapy	No jaundice
Blood group incompatibility	Coombs positive hemolytic disease	--	--
Physical examination	Cephalohematoma or significant bruising	Macrosomic IDM, male, or mother ≥ 25 years	No risk factor
Feeding	Exclusively breastfed with delayed, infrequent feeding with excessive weight loss	Exclusive but effective breast feeding	Exclusively formula fed
Race	East Asian*	--	Black

Table 21.4 Risk factors for severe jaundice

* 12% risk of G6PD deficiency

levels. In the current practice, American Academy of Pediatrics (AAP) charts are most commonly used for taking decisions regarding treatment in cases of pathological jaundice[5]. The decision to start treatment is based on the total serum bilirubin (TSB), age of the infant in hours and its risk category. Infants are divided into 3 risk categories.

1. Low risk : $\geq$ 38 weeks and "well"
2. Medium risk : $\geq$ 38 weeks with risk factors or 35 to 37 weeks infants who are "well"
3. High risk : 35 to 37 weeks infants with risk factors

The risk factors which are known to increase the severity of jaundice or risk of acute bilirubin encephalopathy include immune hemolysis, G6PD deficiency, asphyxia, significant lethargy, temperature instability, sepsis, acidosis and serum albumin < 3 g/dl.

There are 3 lines in the AAP chart. The top most line is for low risk infants, the middle line is for medium risk and the lower line is for high risk infants. It important to remember that defining a "well" infant is not that simple. In our country, where most deliveries take place at home or small hospitals, an accurate record of birth and postnatal events is not available. The diagnosis of acidosis and asphyxia may not be known. Moreover, G6PD deficiency can be diagnosed only on laboratory testing. Serum albumin of Indian neonates is likely to be low because of their lower birth weights and poor maternal nutrition. Hence, many units in our country consider all infants at a higher risk compared to American infants and use only the medium and high risk lines of the AAP charts. Similar decision charts have been published by National Institute for health and clinical excellence (NICE –UK)[6].

AAP charts are not applicable for preterm infants (gestation <35 weeks) and for infants with intrauterine growth restriction. Serum bilirubin (mg/dl) > 0.75% and > 1% of the birth weight respectively are the routine thresholds for phototherapy and exchange transfusion in premature infants (gestation <35 weeks or birth weight <1500 g). National Neonatology Forum of India recommend birth weight based criteria for management of jaundice in premature infants (Table 21.5). Algorithm summarizes the steps for management of a neonate with jaundice (Figure 21.2).

Phototherapy

Phototherapy involves exposure of the naked baby to blue, or green light of wave length 450-460 nm. The light waves convert the bilirubin to water soluble nontoxic forms which are easily excreted without the need of conjugation. The advantages of phototherapy are that it is noninvasive, effective,

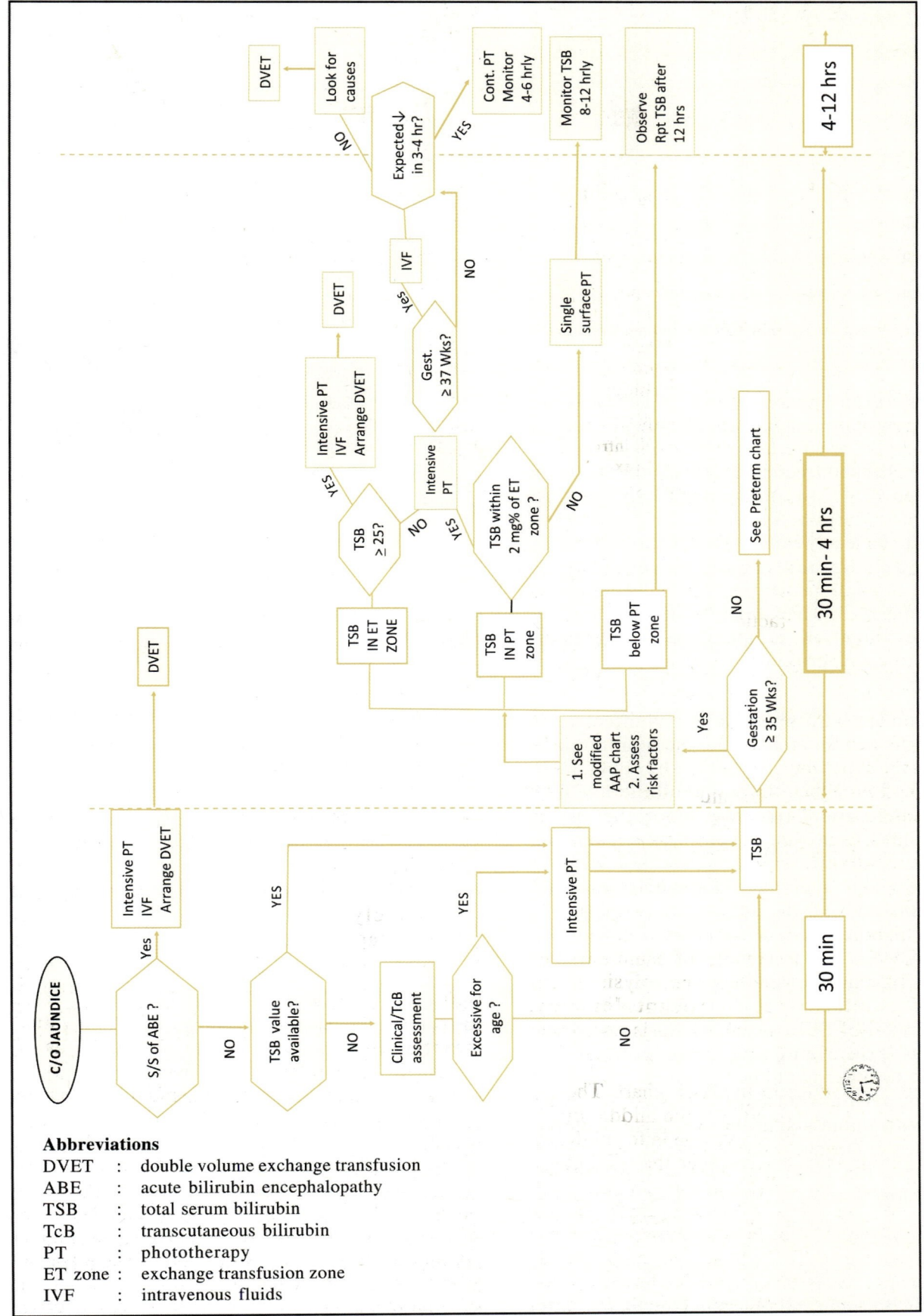

Abbreviations

DVET : double volume exchange transfusion
ABE : acute bilirubin encephalopathy
TSB : total serum bilirubin
TcB : transcutaneous bilirubin
PT : phototherapy
ET zone : exchange transfusion zone
IVF : intravenous fluids

Figure 21.2 Algorithm for management of neonatal jaundice

Table 21.5 Criteria for phototherapy and exchange blood transfusion in premature infants*			
Birth weight (Gram)	Guidelines for PT (mg/dl)		Consider EBT (mg/dl)
	Healthy infant	Sick infant	
<1000	5-7	4-6	10-12
1000-1500	7-10	6-8	12-15
1501-2000	10-12	8-12	15-18
2001-2500	12-15	10-12	18-20

* Martin & Fanaroff. Neonatal-Perinatal Medicine, 8th Edition, p 1450.

inexpensive and easy to use. Conventional phototherapy unit is equipped with 4 to 6 special blue tube lights or CFL lamps. The flux of the unit should be checked frequently and ideally it should be between 12-15 µw/cm^2/nm; preferably as high as possible. The tubelights and CFL lamps are expected to have a life of 1000-2000 hours but this is very variable and cannot be relied upon. Exposure to sunlight for treatment of jaundice is not recommended as it exposes the infant to harmful ultraviolet radiation, temperature disturbances, dehydration and provides a variable degree of irradiance.

Treatment with phototherapy is effective in most infants and on an average, the bilirubin falls by 2 to 3 mg/dl per day. Higher the bilirubin, more rapid is the fall. When the serum bilirubin is near the exchange zone, intensive phototherapy is recommended. It involves exposing the maximum area of the infant's skin to light and with an irradiance >30 µw/cm^2/nm. Phototherapy may fail if the lights are old, the area of skin exposure is minimal, treatment is delayed, infant is dehydrated or if jaundice is due to hemolysis. Light emitting diodes (LED) are newer mode of phototherapy. They are as effective as conventional or CFL phototherapy[7]. LEDs have a much longer lamp life, need less power and are more compact as compared to other phototherapy units. Fiberoptic phototherapy blankets can be placed in direct contact with infant's skin but has lesser efficacy because lesser surface area is covered. Table 21.6 summarizes the technique and side effects of phototherapy.

Exchange Blood Transfusion

Exchange transfusion removes much of the circulating bilirubin and sensitized red blood cells,

Table 21.6 Technique of giving phototherapy

1. Baby is placed naked as close to the lights as possible provided the infant does not get overheated
2. Eyes are covered with eye-patches to prevent damage to the retina by the bright lights; gonads should also be covered in male infants
3. Baby is turned every two hours or after each feed
4. Temperature is monitored every two to four hours
5. Serum bilirubin is monitored at least every 12 hours and more frequently (4 to 6 hourly) during acute phase. Clinical assessment of bilirubin level should not be relied upon in an infant under phototherapy because skin in bleached by phototherapy
6. Weight is taken at least once a day
7. Urine frequency is monitored daily
8. More frequent breast feeding and at times 10-20% extra feeds are recommended. Additional oral intake of plain water or glucose water is neither recommended nor necessary.
9. Phototherapy is discontinued when two serum bilirubin values are < 12 mg/dl or below the treatment threshold
10. Rebound bilirubin is measured 6-8 hours after stopping phototherapy.

Side effects

1. Increased insensible water loss
2. Loose green stools
3. Skin rashes
4. Bronze baby syndrome if baby has conjugated hyperbilirubinemia. Phototherapy should be discontinued
5. Hypo-or hyperthermia
6. Opening of ductus and increased cerebral blood flow in preterm babies
7. Hypocalemia due to secretion of melotinin from pineal gland
8. Impaired maternal infant bonding

replacing them with red cells compatible with mother's antibodies and providing fresh albumin with adequate binding sites for bilirubin. After an exchange, the low levels of serum bilirubin may increase rapidly for several hours as bilirubin in tissues migrates back into the circulation. The decision for an exchange transfusion is based on charts like those provided by AAP as mentioned above, depicting the TSB, age in hours and the risk category. In the presence of signs of acute bilirubin encephalopathy, an exchange transfusion should be performed even in case of borderline TSB values. In addition, exchange transfusion in an infant with Rh-isoimmunization is recommended for the following situations:

(i) Hydrops fetalis (initially only partial exchange may be done to increase hematocrit if baby cannot tolerate double volume exchange)

(ii) History of previous sibling requiring exchange blood transfusion because of Rh-isoimmunization in a baby born with pallor, hepato-splenomegaly and positive DCT

(iii) Cord Hb < 11 g/dl and cord TSB > 5 mg/dl

(iv) Rate of rise of TSB > 1 mg/dl/hour despite phototherapy

(v) Rate of rise of TSB > 0.5 mg/dl despite phototherapy if Hb is between 11 -13 g/dl

(vi) Any TSB > 12 mg/dl in first 24 hours and any TSB > 20 mg/dl subsequently in a at-risk infant are also indications for exchange transfusion.

A 'two-volume' exchange is performed, i.e. the volume of blood exchanged equals twice the infant's blood volume, i.e. 2×80 ml/kg = 160 ml/kg. This replaces 87% of the infant's blood volume with new blood. The *in-out method* is the commonest method but is being used less often now. Aliquots of 5 to 15 ml of infant blood (3% to 5% of birth weight in smaller infants) are withdrawn via an umbilical venous catheter and replaced by an equal volume of donor blood via a three- way tap. This method has higher incidence of complications. *The continuous flow method* is being increasingly preferred. Peripheral arterial and venous lines are inserted. Donor blood is infused at a constant rate via the vein and the baby's blood is withdrawn at the same rate via the artery. It is essential to balance the rate of withdrawal with the infusion rate. Complications are lower with this method. No matter which method is used, a two-volume exchange should take 45-75 minutes to complete. In smaller and sick babies a slower rate should be used. The choice of blood and technique of exchange blood transfusion are given in detail in Chapter 58.

Adjuncts in Management

Intravenous immunoglobulins (IVIG)

Hyperbilirubinemia in both Rh and ABO-sensitized infants results from the destruction of neonatal red blood cells that have been coated by transplacentally acquired maternal iso-antibodies causing extravascular erythrocyte destruction. Fc receptor bearing cells within the reticuloendothelial system probably mediate this red cell destruction. IVIG therapy may alter the course of immune hemolytic disease by blocking Fc receptors, resulting in inhibition of hemolysis and subsequent reduction of bilirubin formation. High dose IVIG in a single dose (1 g/kg) or two doses of 500 mg/kg early in the course of jaundice is effective in decreasing the need for exchange transfusions and in preventing significant hyperbilirubinemia in babies with isoimmune hemolytic anemia[9]. For maximum efficacy IVIG needs to be given as soon as possible after birth in all iso-immunized neonates. Neonates treated with IVIG are likely to develop late-onset anemia. When exchange blood transfusion is planned at birth, IVIG should be given after the procedure.

Fluid supplementation

In neonates presenting to the emergency department with severe jaundice, when the TSB is approaching exchange level, intravenous fluid supplementation with N/5 in 5% dextrose or NS in 5% dextrose over 8 hours; decreases the need for exchange transfusion and the duration of phototherapy[10].

Phenobarbital

Phenobarbital in a dose of 5 to 8 mg/kg every 24 hours induces microsomal enzymes, increases bilirubin conjugation and excretion and increases bile flow. However, it takes 3 to 5 days to induce the liver enzymes. Hence, it is not a useful drug for treatment of acute jaundice but can be effective as a prophylactic agent in very low birth weight infants and chronic cases like hyperbilirubinemia due to Criggler-Najjar syndrome Type II and direct hyperbilirubinemia associated with hyperalimentation[11]. Phenobarbital given antenatally to the mother is also effective in lowering bilirubin levels in erythroblastic infants. It is neither effective for prevention of severe jaundice in G6PD deficient neonates nor for augmenting the efficacy of phototherapy[12].

Albumin

In plasma, bilirubin binds to albumin which prevents its entry into the tissues including CNS. Infusion of albumin 0.5 to 1g/kg 1 to 4 hours prior to exchange transfusion may potentially increase the removal of bilirubin by the exchange, by chelating out bilirbuin from the tissues. This may decrease the duration of phototherapy and need for subsequent exchange transfusions. However, the current evidence is not strong enough for routine recommendation of albumin infusion[13].

Clofibrate

Clofibrate, an anti-lipidemic agent, is an activator of peroxisome proliferator activated receptors. It can increase bilirubin conjugation and excretion within 6 to 16 hours. A single oral dose of 100 mg/kg was shown to be effective in decreasing the duration of phototherapy in some neonates[14]. Gastrointestinal disturbances, muscle cramps, leucopenia, altered lipid and glucose metabolism are known side effects. Gemfibrozil, a newer drug of the same class has not been found to be effective in a double blind controlled trial[15].

Metalloporphyrins

Synthetic metalloporphyrins limit the production of bilirubin by competitively inhibiting heme oxygenase, the rate-limiting enzyme in bilirubin synthesis. In experimental trials they have been used to treat hyperbilirubinemia in Coombs positive ABO hemolytic disease of the newborn and in Criggler-Najjar type I patients. Although the initial results are promising, metalloporphyrins are not yet approved for use in newborn infants, because of concerns of serious toxicity[16].

Other therapies

Agars, activated charcoal, cholestyramine and polyvinyl pyrolidine have been used to bind bilirubin in the gut and to prevent enterohepatic circulation. Minimal benefit has been documented in association with phototherapy. In the case of cholestyramine the benefits are outweighed by potential side effects including hypercholeremic acidosis. These medications are of doubtful utility and are not recommended. Cephalhematoma should be aspirated when it is associated with critical hyperbilirubinemia i.e. serum bilirubin of 15 mg/dl or more[17].

Long term Follow-up

Jaundiced infants with serum bilirubin of more than 20 mg/dl, those who receive exchange transfusion, those with clinical evidences of encephalopathy and with co-morbid conditions such as asphyxia or sepsis or VLBW at birth, should be followed up in a neurodevelopmental clinic. A brain stem evoked audiometry is recommended at discharge or at 3 months of age to identify hearing impairment. Hearing loss is generally more severe in high frequencies and is usually bilateral. The hearing deficit even when severe may often escape clinical detection for several months and may be reflected as delay in speech. In high risk infants (*vide supra*) MRI brain at discharge may identify the typical abnormal T1-weighted image hyper-intensity in the globus pallidus and subthalamus, but normal T2-weighted image intensity in the same regions. The typical tetrad of kernicterus includes superior gaze palsy, sensorineural hearing loss, dental dysplasia and extrapyramidal abnormalities. During infancy, the affected, infants feed poorly, develop high pitched cry, have persistent and obligatory atonic neck reflex, are hypotonic with brisk deep tendon reflexes. Athetosis (involuntary, sinuous, writhing movements) may develop as early as 18 months or may be delayed as late as 8 to 9 years. Affected children may also have dysarthria, facial grimacing, drooling and difficulty in chewing and swallowing.

REFERENCES

1. Murki S, Kumar P, Marwaha N, Majumdar S, Narang A. Risk factors for kernicterus in term babies with non hemolytic jaundice. *Indian Pediatr* 2001;38:757-762

2. Agarwal SK, Kumar P, Rathi R, Sharma N, Das R, Prasad R, Narang A. UGT1A1 gene polymorphism in North Indian neonates presenting with unconjugated hyperbilirubinemia. *Pediatr Res* 2009; 65: 675-680

3. Bhutani VK, Johnson L, Sivieri EM. Predictive ability of a predischarge hour specific serum bilirubin for subsequent significant hyperbilirubinemia in healthy term and near term newborns. *Pediatrics* 1999; 103: 6-14

4. Agarwal R, Kaushal M, Aggarwal R, Paul VK. Deorari AK. Early neonatal hyperbilirubinemia using first day serum bilirubin level. *Indian Pediatr* 2002; 39:724-730

5. American Academy of Pediatrics Subcommittee on Hyperbilirubinemia. Management of hyperbilirubinemia in the newborn infant 35 or more weeks of gestation. *Pediatrics* 2004; 114:297-316

6. National Collaborating Centre for Women's and Children's Health. Neonatal jaundice. London: NICE, 2010.http://guidance.nice.org.uk/CG98. (31 May 2011)

7. Kumar P, Murki S, Malik GK, Chawla D, Deorari AK, Karthi N, Subramanian S, Sravanthi J, Gaddam P, Singh SN. Light emitting diodes versus compact fluorescent tubes for phototherapy in neonatal jaundice: a multi center randomized controlled trial. *Indian Pediatr* 2010; 47(2):131-137.

8. Murki S, Kumar P. Blood exchange transfusion for infants with severe neonatal hyperbilirubinemia. *Semin Perinatol* 2011; 35 (3): 192-197

9. Alcock GS, Liley H. Immunoglobulin infusion for isoimmune hemolytic jaundice in neonates. Cochrane Database Syst Rev. 2002; (3): CD003313

10. Mehta S, Kumar P, Narang A. A randomized controlled trial of fluid supplementation in term neonates with severe hyperbilirubinemia. *J Pediatr* 2005; 147:781-5.

11. Kumar R, Narang A, Kumar P, Garewal G. Phenobarbitone prophylaxis for neonatal jaundice in babies with birth weight 1000-1499 grams. *Indian Pediatr* 2002; 39(10):945-51.

12. Murki S, Dutta S, Narang A, Urmi S, Garewal G. A randomized, triple-blind, placebo-controlled trial of prophylactic oral phenobarbital to reduce the need for phototherapy in G6PD-deficient neonates. *J Perinatol* 2005; 25:325-330.

13. Ahlfors CE. Pre exchange transfusion administration of albumin: an overlooked adjunct in the treatment of severe neonatal jaundice? *Indian Pediatr* 2010; 47(3):231-2.

14. Mohammadzadeh A, Farhat A, Iranpour R. Effect of clofibrate in jaundiced term newborns. *Indian J Pediatr* 2005; 72:123-126

15. Jaikrishan, Kumar P, Narang A. Gemfibrozil in late preterm and term neonates with moderate jaundice: a randomized controlled trial. *Indian Pediatr* 2009; 46(12):1063-9

16. Suresh GK, Martin CL, Soll RF. Metalloporphyrins for treatment of unconjugated hyperbilirubinemia in neonates. Cochrane Database Syst Rev. 2003; (2):CD004207

17. Singh M. Jaundice. In: Care of the Newborn. *Sagar Publications, New Delhi* 7th Edition, 2010, pp 254-274.

Section 3

The Bleeding Neonate

Arun K Pramanik

The newborn infant is particularly susceptible to bleeding and clotting complications due to a variety of reasons; physiologic deficiencies of coagulation factors (quantitative and qualitative), antenatal influences such as maternal diseases or drugs, immaturity of blood vessels, vulnerability to birth trauma, placement of vascular catheter, invasive procedures, hereditary diseases, congenital malformations and other conditions associated with bleeding such as sepsis and asphyxia[1-8].

Local or diffuse hemorrhage and thrombosis are common causes of morbidity and mortality during the newborn period. Using ultrasound examination and micro-coagulation tests, diseases that cause thrombosis and/or bleeding in neonates are being recognized with increasing frequency in intensive care units[9-12]. Physicians caring for such infants should have a high index of suspicion and be conversant in managing them. Thus, it is crucial not only to diagnose the underlying disease(s) in these "sick" infants, but also delineate the underlying coagulation defect(s) because they require aggressive therapy for the underlying disorders to control the bleeding, as well as vigorous support with blood products[3, 6, 7]. On the other hand, physicians caring for "well" neonates may encounter laboratory abnormalities in coagulation without obvious bleeding. These infants usually have primary coagulation defects that are either hereditary or immune-mediated, and their therapy is directed towards correcting the specific coagulation defect. Some patients have bleeding or thrombosis with normal coagulation panel[13-15].

PHYSIOLOGY OF NEONATAL COAGULATION AND HEMOSTASIS

The mechanism of hemostasis is a complex physiological and biochemical process in which blood vessels, platelets, procoagulant and anticoagulant proteins, and fibrinolytic system interact sequentially and simultaneously to prevent excessive bleeding following tissue injury. Tissue injury triggers a number of host defense responses whose goal is to maintain blood vessel integrity while more permanent repair process is under way. Failure in this intricate process manifests itself in bleeding, and conversely, pathologic hyperactivity of this natural defense mechanism results in thrombosis and thromboembolism. The initial defense mechanism against bleeding is the vascular endothelium, which is inadequate in the premature infant compared to that in term infants. A series of events is set in motion when the vascular endothelium is damaged (Figure 22.1)[1-9]. Subendothelial tissue exposed to the blood attract

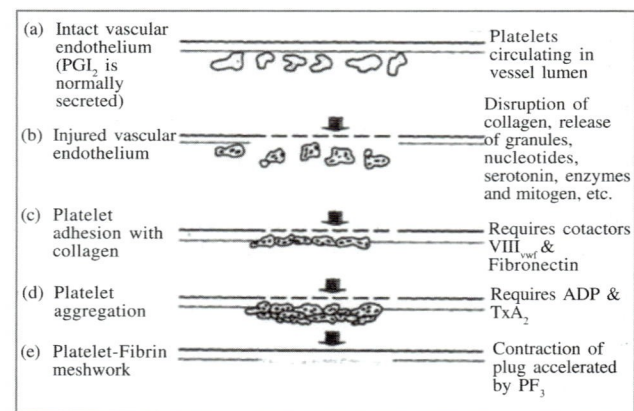

Figure 22.1 Schematics of the sequence in the formation of platelet-fibrin meshwork as "temporary" hemostatic plug. (a) Endothelial cells normally secrete the antithrombotic substance prostacyclin (PGI_2) which prevents platelet activation; (b) Injured vascular endothelium with disruption of collagen and release of granules, nucleotides, serotonin, enzymes and mitogen from platelets occur; (c) Platelet adhesion requires the interaction of factor VIII, von Willebrand factor (VIII vwf) and fibronectin; (d) Platelet aggregation or cohesion of platelets to each other in clumps results from secretion of ADP from its dense granules and generation of thromboxane A_2 (TxA_2), both of which recruit more platelets into the expanding hemostatic plug; and finally; (e) Platelet factor 3 (PF_3), a phospholipid intrinsic to platelet membranes, accelerates the blood coagulation mechanism, promoting the deposition of fibrin strands within the platelet plug. Contractile protein then retracts the plug and complete healing of the injury occurs

platelets (produced in the bone marrow from megakaryocytes and circulating as minute granular fragments with an average life span of 9 days) and induce them initially to adhere and later to aggregate reversibly. Activation or disruption of the endothelial cell lining of blood vessel promotes adhesion of platelets to the site. The platelets become activated and promote activation of additional platelets and other cells in the viscinity. Thrombin is then formed on this mass of loosely interacting platelets. Once platelet lysosomal enzyme is produced from zymogen (enzyme precursor), it generates insoluble cross-linked fibrin and causes irreversible aggregation of platelets. The resulting platelet-fibrin meshwork forms a primary hemostatic plug and acts as a rapid and effective barrier against egress of blood from the vascular system.

The ability of the platelets to selectively adhere to collagen is a unique platelet property and requires two plasma cofactors, one associated with the factor VII molecule (called the von Willebrand factor or VII vwf), and fibronectin. vWF is a multimeric glycoprotein synthesized by megakaryocytes and endothelial cells, secreted by activated platelets, is found in the subendothelial matrix, and also circulates in the plasma as a carrier for coagulation factor VIII. It binds platelet glyco-protein Ib/V/IX complex and promotes platelet adhesion in the subendothelium (Figure 22.2). The primary hemostatic plug also requires various energy-dependent biochemical reactions within the platelets. Aggregation of platelets involves secretion of the zymogen granules with generation of labile prostaglandin intermediates including the vasoconstrictor, thromboxane A2 (TXA$_2$), and release of adenosine-i-phosphate (ADP). This

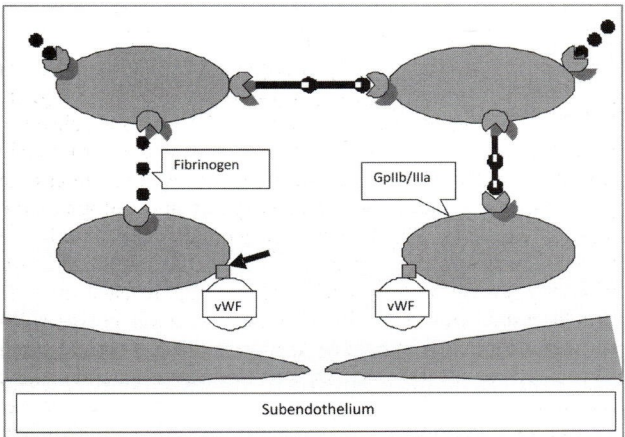

Figure 22.2 Schematic representation of the interaction of platelets with the subendothelium (See text for details) Gp: glycoprotein; vWF: von Willebrand factor

release phenomenon is blocked by a variety of commonly used drugs, notably acetylsalicylic acid (ASA) which can cross the placenta and affect the fetus[7, 11]. Also, premature infants have altered membrane reactivity and diminished TxA$_2$ generation, even though they have similar number of platelets as term infants[1-5]. Although its physiological significance is unclear in healthy premature infants, it may play an important role in bleeding disorders in sick premature infants.

Coagulation Factors

More than a dozen soluble proteins, commonly known as clotting factors, designated with Roman numerals have been identified. The letter "a" is added after the Roman numeral to indicate the activated state. The nomenclature, normal values of clotting factors and the commonly performed coagulation tests in healthy full-term and premature infants during the first 6 months of life are shown in Tables 22.1 and 22.2 respectively[16, 17]. Most of these are decreased in neonates. The reference values for inhibitors of coagulation are shown in Table 22.3[17].

The earliest theories about coagulation postulated that clot formation was initiated when tissue injury resulted in exposure of a critical substance, tissue thromboplastin (later purified and renamed tissue factor), to plasma. With the development of the prothrombin time assay, in which large amount of tissue factor is added to induce coagulation, it was observed that hemophiliac plasma clotted normally. This observation coupled with clinical severity of hemophilia, suggested the existence of a coagulation pathway independent of tissue factor that was probably more important. Thus, in 1964, the coagulation cascade-waterfall hypothesis was introduced (Figure 22.3a). This theory proposed two pathways leading to activation of factor X, and factor IX. Factor IXa, with factor VIIIa, calcium, and phospholipids could cleave factor X. The extrinsic pathway begins when extrinsic factor forms complex with factor VII, VIIa, calcium, phosphpolipids, and activated factor X. Factor Xa would then proceed through the common pathway until fibrin was produced.

The extrinsic and intrinsic pathways are tested separately by the prothrombin time (PT) and the activated partial prothrombin time (aPTT) respectively. Although PT and aPTT have proved

Age	DAY 1	DAY 5	DAY 30	DAY 90	DAY 180	ADULT
Tests	Mean ± SD	Mean ± SD	Mean ± SD	Mean ± SD	Mean ± SD	Mean ± SD
PT (sec)	13.0 ± 1.43	12.4 ± 1.46	11.8 ± 1.25	11.9 ± 1.15	12.3 ± 0.79	12.4 ± 0.78
aPTT (sec)	42.9 ± 5.80	42.6 ± 8.62	40.4 ± 7.42	37.1 ± 6.52	35.5 ± 3.71	33.5 ± 3.44
TCT (sec)	23.5 ± 2.38	23.1 ± 3.07	24.3 ± 2.44	25.1 ± 2.32	25.5 ± 2.86	25.0 ± 2.66
Fibrinogen (g/mL)	2.83 ± 0.58	3.12 ± 0.75	2.70 ± 0.54	2.43 ± 0.68	2.51 ± 0.68	2.78 ± 0.61
Factor II (u/ml)	0.48 ± 0.11	0.63 ± 0.15	0.68 ± 0.17	0.75 ± 0.15	0.88 ± 0.14	1.08 ± 0.19
Factor V (u/ml)	0.72 ± 0.18	0.95 ± 0.25	0.98 ± 0.18	0.90 ± 0.21	0.91 ± 0.18	1.06 ± 0.22
Factor VII (u/ml)	0.66 ± 0.19	0.89 ± 0.27	0.90 ± 0.24	0.91 ± 0.26	0.87 ± 0.20	1.05 ± 0.19
Factor VIII (u/ml)	1.00 ± 0.39	0.88 ± 0.33	0.91 ± 0.33	0.79 ± 0.23	0.73 ± 0.18	0.99 ± 0.25
vWF (u/ml)	1.53 ± 0.67	1.40 ± 0.57	1.28 ± 0.69	1.18 ± 0.44	1.07 ± 0.45	0.92 ± 0.33
Factor IX (u/ml)	0.53 ± 0.19	0.53 ± 0.19	0.51 ± 0.15	0.67 ± 0.23	0.86 ± 0.25	1.09 ± 0.27
Factor X (u/ml)	0.40 ± 0.14	0.49 ± 0.15	0.59 ± 0.14	0.71 ± 0.18	0.78 ± 0.20	1.06 ± 0.23
Factor XI (u/ml)	0.38 ± 0.14	0.55 ± 0.16	0.63 ± 0.13	0.69 ± 0.14	0.86 ± 0.24	0.97 ± 0.15
Factor XII (u/ml)	0.53 ± 0.29	0.47 ± 0.18	0.49 ± 0.16	0.67 ± 0.21	0.77 ± 0.19	108 ± 0.27
Prekallikrein (u/ml)	0.37 ± 0.16	0.48 ± 0.14	0.57 ± 0.17	0.73 ± 0.16	0.86 ± 0.15	1.12 ± 0.25
HMW-K (u/ml)	0.54 ± 0.24	0.74 ± 0.28	0.77 ± 0.22	0.82 ± 0.32	0.82 ± 0.23	0.92 ± 0.22
Factor XIIIa (u/ml)	0.79 ± 0.26	0.94 ± 0.25	0.93 ± 0.27	1.04 ± 0.34	1.04 ± 0.29	1.05 ± 0.25
Factor XIIIb (u/ml)	0.76 ± 0.23	1.06 ± 0.37	1.11 ± 0.36	1.16 ± 0.34	1.10 ± 0.30	0.97 ± 0.20
Plasminogen (u/ml)	1.95 ± 0.35	2.17 ± 0.38	1.98 ± 0.36	2.48 ± 0.37	3.01 ± 0.40	3.36 ± 0.44

Table 22.1 Reference values for coagulation tests and factors in healthy full-term infants during the first 6 months of life

All factors except fibrinogen and plasminogen are expressed as units per milliliter where pooled plasma contains 1 u/ml. Plasminogen units are those recommended by the American Society of Hematology Committee on Thrombolytic Agents (CTA). All values are expressed as mean ± 1 SD. aPTT, activated partial thromboplastin time; HMWK, high molecular weight kininogen; PT, prothrombin time; TCT, thrombin clotting time; vWF, von Willebrand factor. From Andrew M *et al*. The development of the human coagulation sytem in the full-term infant. *Blood* 70:165, 1987[16].

invaluable for evaluation of coagulation factor deficiencies; a number of clinical and laboratory observations could not be explained by the cascade-waterfall theory. A physiological activator of the intrinsic pathway contact factor has not been found and individuals deficient in these contact activation factors, factor XI, prekallikrein, or high molecular-weight kininogen have prolonged aPTT assay but do not bleed abnormally. Patients with hemophilia A (factor VIII deficiency) or hemophilia B (factor IX deficiency) have severe clinical bleeding abnormalities. In contrast, those with deficiency of another intrinsic pathway clotting protein, factor XI do not bleed spontaneously, but only after surgery or trauma. Severe factor VII deficiency results in hemorrhagic abnormalities. In the laboratory, Factor VIIa and tissue factor activate both factor IX and X, suggesting a more important clinical role of factor VII. Renewed interest in the factor VIIa-tissue factor pathway inhibitor (TFPI), along with reports that thrombin could activate factor XI and possible auto-activate factor XI inspired a revised theory of coagulation. In 1991, a revised hypothesis of coagulation was proposed (Figure 22.3b), where in clotting is initiated when subendothelial tissue factor is exposed to circulating factor VII or VIIa. The factor VIIa-tissue factor complex associates with calcium on a phospholipid surface to form the extrinsic tenase complex, which activates factor X and factor IX. Factor IXa in combination with factor VIIIa, calcium, and a phosholipid membrane, forms the intrinsic tenase complex and activates additional

Table 22.2 Reference values for coagulation tests and factors in healthy premature infants (30 to 36 weeks' gestation) during first 6 months of life

Age	Day 1		Day 5		Day 30		Day 90		Day 180		Adult	
Tests	Mean	(Range)	Mean	(Range)	Mean	(Range)	Mean	(Range)	Mean	(Range)	Mean	(Range)
PT (sec)	13.0	(10.6-16.2)	12.5	(10.0-15.3)	11.8	(10.0-13.6)	12.3	(10.0-14.6)	12.5	(10.0-15.0)	12.4	(10.8-13.9)
aPTT (sec)	53.6	(27.5-79.4)	50.5	(26.9-74.1)	44.7	(26.9-62.5)	39.5	(28.3-50.7)	37.5	(21.7-53.3)	33.5	(26.6-40.3)
TCT (sec)	24.8	(19.2-30.4)	24.1	(18.8-24.4)	24.4	(18.8-29.9)	25.1	(19.4-30.8)	25.2	(18.9-31.5)	25.0	(19.7-30.3)
Fibrinogen (g/l)	2.4	(1.50-3.73)	2.8	(1.60-4.18)	2.5	(1.50-4.14)	2.5	(1.50-3.52)	2.3	(1.50-3.60)	2.8	(1.56-4.00)
Factor II (u/ml)	0.5	(0.20-0.77)	0.6	(0.29-0.85)	0.6	(0.36-0.95)	0.7	(0.30-1.06)	0.9	(0.51-1.23)	1.1	(0.70-1.46)
Factor V (u/ml)	0.9	(0.41-1.44)	1.0	(0.46-1.54)	1.0	(0.48-1.56)	1.0	(0.59-1.39)	1.0	(0.58-1.46)	1.1	(0.62-1.50)
Factor VII (u/ml)	0.7	(0.21-1.13)	0.8	(0.30-1.38)	0.8	(0.21-1.45)	0.9	(0.31-1.43)	1.0	(0.47-1.51)	1.1	(0.57-1.46)
Factor VIII (u/ml)	1.1	(0.50-2.13)	1.2	(0.53-2.05)	1.1	(0.50-1.99)	1.1	(0.58-1.88)	1.0	(0.50-1.87)	1.0	(0.50-1.49)
vWF (u/ml)	1.4	(0.78-2.10)	1.3	(0.72-2.19)	1.4	(0.66-2.16)	1.1	(0.75-1.84)	1.0	(0.54-1.58)	0.9	(0.50-1.58)
Factor IX (u/ml)	0.4	(0.19-0.65)	0.4	(0.14-0.74)	0.4	(0.13-0.80)	0.6	(0.25-0.93)	0.8	(0.50-1.20)	1.1	(0.55-1.63)
Factor X (u/ml)	0.4	(0.11-0.71)	0.5	(0.19-0.83)	0.6	(0.20-0.92)	0.7	(0.35-0.99)	0.8	(0.35-1.19)	1.1	(0.70-1.52)
Factor XI (u/ml)	0.3	(0.08-0.52)	0.4	(0.13-0.69)	0.4	(0.15-0.71)	0.6	(0.25-0.93)	0.8	(0.46-1.10)	1.0	(0.67-1.27)
Factor XII (u/ml)	0.4	(0.10-0.66)	0.4	(0.09-0.69)	0.4	(0.11-0.75)	0.6	(0.15-1.07)	0.8	(0.22-1.42)	1.1	(0.52-1.64)
Prekallikrein (u/ml)	0.3	(0.09-0.57)	0.5	(0.26-0.75)	0.6	(0.31-0.87)	0.8	(0.37-1.12)	0.8	(0.40-1.16)	1.1	(0.62-1.62)
HMW-K (u/ml)	0.5	(0.09-0.89)	0.6	(0.24-1.00)	0.6	(0.16-1.12)	0.8	(0.32-1.24)	0.8	(0.41-1.25)	0.9	(0.50-1.36)
Factor XIIIa (u/ml)	0.7	(0.32-1.08)	1.0	(0.57-1.45)	1.0	(0.51-1.47)	1.1	(0.71-1.55)	1.1	(0.65-1.61)	1.1	(0.55-1.55)
Factor XIIIb (u/ml)	0.8	(0.35-1.27)	1.1	(0.68-1.58)	1.1	(0.57-1.57)	1.2	(0.75-1.67)	1.2	(0.67-1.63)	1.0	(0.57-1.37)
Plasminogen (u/ml)	1.7	(1.12-2.48)	1.9	(1.21-2.61)	1.8	(1.09-2.53)	2.4	(1.58-3.18)	2.8	(1.91-3.59)	3.4	(2.48-4.24)

All factors except fibrinogen and plasminogen are expressed as units per milliliter where pooled plasma contains 1 u/ml. Plasminogen units are those recommended by the Committee on Thrombolytic Agents (CTA). All values are given as a mean and lower and upper boundary encompassing 95% of the population. Between 40 and 96 samples were assayed for each value for newborns. aPTT, activated partial thromboplastin time; HMWK, high molecular weight kininogen; PT, prothrombin time; TCT, thrombin clotting time; vWF, von Willebrand factor.

From Andrew M *et al.* Development of the human coagulation system in the healthy premature infant. *Blood* 72:1651, 1988[17].

Section 3

Table 22.3 Reference values for inhibitors of coagulation in healthy infants during first 6 months of life

Age / Tests	Day 1		Day 5		Day 30		Day 90		Day 180		Adult	
	Mean	(Range)	Mean	(Range)	Mean	(Range)	Mean	(Range)	Mean	(Range)	Mean	(Range)
AT III (U/ml)	0.4	(0.14-0.62)	0.6	(0.30-0.82)	0.6	(0.37-0.81)	0.8	(0.45-1.21)	0.9	(0.52-1.28)	1.1	(0.79-1.31)
a2-M (U/ml)	1.1	(0.56-1.82)	1.3	(0.71-1.77)	1.4	(0.72-2.04)	1.8	(1.20-2.66)	2.1	(1.10-3.21)	0.9	(0.52-1.20)
a2-AP (U/ml)	0.8	(0.40-1.16)	0.8	(0.49-1.13)	0.9	(0.55-1.23)	1.1	(0.64-1.48)	1.2	(0.77-1.53)	1.0	(0.68-1.36)
C1-INH (U/ml))	0.7	(0.31-0.99)	0.8	(0.45-1.21)	0.7	(0.40-1.24)	1.1	(0.60-168)	1.4	(0.96-2.04)	1.0	(0.71-1.31)
a2-AT (U/ml)	0.9	(0.36-1.44)	0.9	(0.42-1.46)	0.8	(0.38-1.12)	0.8	(0.49-1.13)	0.8	(0.48-1.16)	0.9	(0.55-1.31)
HC II (U/ml)	0.3	(0.00-0.60)	0.3	(0.00-0.69)	0.4	(0.15-0.71)	0.6	(0.20-1.11)	0.9	(0.45-1.40)	1.0	(0.66-1.26)
Protein C (U/ml)	0.3	(0.12-0.44)	0.3	(0.11-0.51)	0.4	(0.15-0.59)	0.5	(0.23-0.67)	0.6	(0.31-0.83)	1.0	(0.64-1.28)
Protein S (U/ml)	0.3	(0.14-0.38)	0.4	(0.13-0.61)	0.6	(0.22-0.90)	0.8	(0.40-1.12)	0.8	(0.44-1.20)	0.9	(0.60-1.24)

All values are expressed in units per milliliter, where pooled plasma contains 1.0 u/ml. All values are given as a mean followed by lower and upper boundary encompassing 95% of the population. Between 0 and 75 samples were assayed for each value for the newborn. AP, antiplasmin; AT, antithrombin; C1-INH, C1 esterase inhibitor; HC, heparin cofactor; M macroglobulin: From Andrew M et al: Development of the human coagulation system in the healthy premature infant. *Blood* 72:1651, 1988[17].

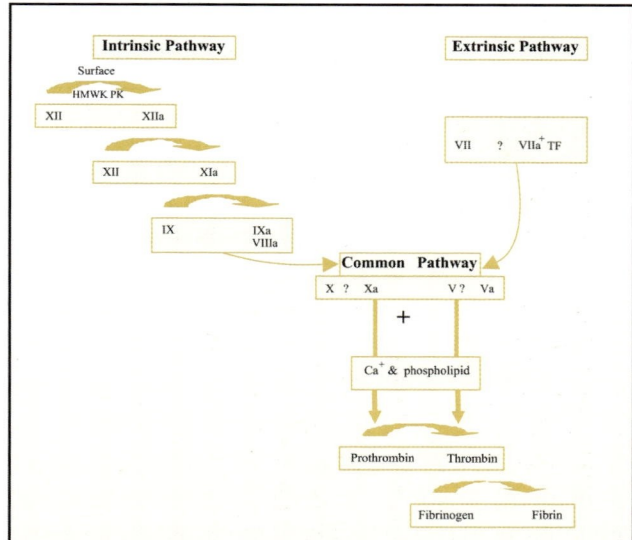

Figure 22.3a The cascade-waterfall hypothesis of blood coagulation. In this scheme, coagulation may be 'initiated by the extrinsic or intrinsic pathway, either of which can lead to thrombin-mediated formation of a fibrin clot via a common pathway involving factor Xa, factor Va, and phospholipid. (PK = prekallikrein, HMWK = high molecular weight kininogen, TK = tissue factor).

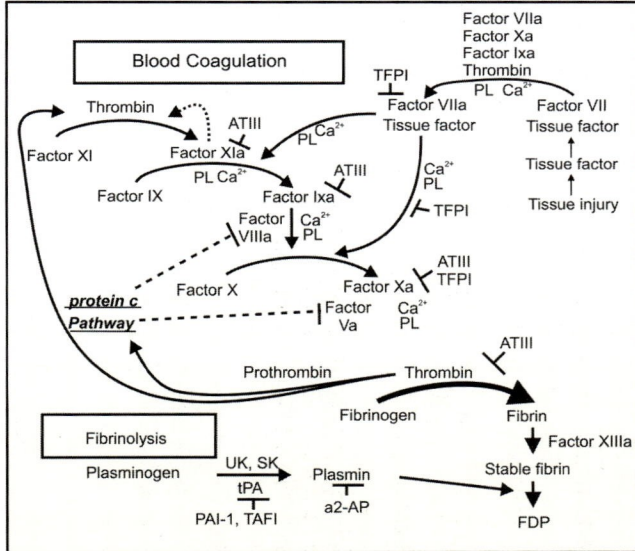

Figure 22.3b Revised hypothesis of blood coagulation. Coagulation is initiated by factor VIIa- and tissue factor (TF)-mediated activation of factors VIIIa and X, sustained through the participation of factors VIIIa and IXa, and consolidated by factor XIa. Tissue factor pathway inhibitor (TFPI) inhibits factor Xa, and in a factor Xa dependent fashion, feeds back and inhibits the factor VIIa-tissue factor complex.

factor X. Some of the factor Xa complexes with factor Va, calcium, and phospholipid (the prothrombinase complex) and cleaves prothrombin to thrombin. Thrombin can cleave fibrinogen to fibrin, leading to production of fibrin clot. The rest

of factor Xa can combine with TFPI/Factor Xa complex produces feedback inhibition of the factor VIIa-tissue factor complex. In this way, initial clot formation requires factors VIIa, IXa, and VIIIa. Additional factor Xa can be generated by 'thrombin-mediated activation or autoactivation of factor XI. In instances of ongoing bleeding or fibrinolysis, deficiency of factor XI would result in clinical bleeding. In this scheme, the contact activation system is not required, accounting for the absence of bleeding in deficient individuals. Fibrin monomers spontaneously polymerize into strands, but covalent bonding of the strands into a stable clot is accomplished by the transglutaminase, factor XIII. Factor XIII-deficient patients exhibit umbilical cord bleeding, delayed post-traumatic bleeding, and breakdown and wound dehiscence. Factor XIII is not measured by the PT, aPTT, or bleeding time tests and must be assessed with a factor XIII assay or by assessing clot stability in a 5M urea solution.

The vitamin K-dependent factors, (II, VII, IX, X) are also physiologically depressed in the premature and term infant which results in prolongation of one-stage prothrombin time. Surprisingly, however, few patients with congenital procoagulant deficiencies have bleeding manifestations during the neonatal period despite relatively decreased plasma procoagulant factors in normal neonates[1-6, 18, 19].

Pathophysiology of anticoagulation systems and proteins. In pathologic states (e.g., acidosis, hypoxia or Gram-negative bacteremia with endotoxin release), diffuse activation of the cellular participants in hemostasis can occur, resulting in systemic thrombosis. In a normal individual, as the activated coagulation factors drift away from the site of clot formation, they are inactivated by the anticoagulant proteins. Thrombin, a necessary component of clot formation also serves to localize and limit the process by complexing with thrombomodulin on the endothelial surface and promoting protein C activation. Activated protein C with its cofactor, protein S proteolytically inactivates factors Va and VIIIa. Circulating antithrombin III (ATIII) inactivates a number of proteases, the most important of which is factor IIa (thrombin), as well as factors XIa, Xa, IXa and plasmin. The anticoagulant drug heparin and naturally occurring cell endothelial cell surface heparin sulfate greatly accelerates the activity of AT III. The anticoagulant activity of heparin is largely due to enhancement of inhibition of thrombin and factor Xa[1-6, 20].

Fibrinolysis. When repair of injured tissue is complete, the fibrin clot is dissolved by the enzyme plasmin[1-6, 21]. The fibrinolytic system is composed of zymogen, plasminogen and its activated counterpart, plasmin; the plasminogen activators (PAs) urokinase type (u-PA) and tissue type (t-PA), and their inhibitors, plasminogen-activator inhibitors PAI-1 and PAI-2 and α2 antiplasmin (Figure 22.4). Inhibition of the action of plasmin can occur via the activator inhibitors PAI-1 or PAI-2 or by inhibition of the enzyme itself with α2–antiplasmin. u-PA is active in the extravascular compartment, whereas t-PA functions to activate plasminogen within the vasculature. Defects in the fibrinolytic system have been associated with excessive thrombosis or bleeding[1-6, 22]. Akin to the normal coagulation system, the fibrinolytic system is normally balanced by inhibitors present in the blood.

Physiologic alterations of coagulation and fibrinolysis in the neonate. Neonatal coagulation system differs from adults. However, understanding of neonatal hemostasis is hampered by lack of adequate number of healthy control infants, and because the values of coagulation factors change rapidly at various gestational and postnatal ages[1-6, 16]. Coagulation and fibrinoytic factors do not cross

the placenta and begin to appear in fetal blood by 10 weeks gestational age[1-4, 23]. Normal ranges of coagulation factors and tests at various gestation and postnatal age are shown in Tables 22.1 to 22.3[1, 16-18,24-29]. The proposed etiologies for the differences in the newborn hemostatic system relative to the adult system include; decreased synthesis of factors, enhanced clearance, general activation of the coagulation system at birth, with resultant consumption of factors, and synthesis of less active fetal forms of some proteins. The best known alteration in the neonatal hemostsis system involves the vitamin-K dependant factors. Coagulation factors II (prothrombin), VII, IX, and X and protein-C and protein-S undergo vitamin-K dependant post-translational γ-carboxylation of glutamic acid residues. These modified regions bind calcium and promote formation of coagulation factor complexes (e.g. the extrinsic and intrinsic tenase complex) on cell surface phospholipids, resulting in efficient localized clot formation. The levels of vitamin-K dependant proteins, factors IX, XII, prekalllikrein, and HMKW are low at birth and slowly reach adult levels by 6 months of age. The aPTT is generally not a useful test in the neonate because so many of the factors tested by the assay are physiologically low. Protein-C levels remain low until later in childhood[28]. Fibrinogen levels are normal and rise over the first week of life. Factors VII, V and XIII are normal at birth, thus allowing diagnosis of these factors in infancy. Antithrombin III and heparin cofactor II are also low' at birth. Several differences in fibrinolytic system exist in the newborn; plasminogen and α2-antiplasmin levels are low, whereas t-PA and PAI levels are twice the normal levels of adults. α2 macroglobulin, an inhibitor of many proteolytic enzymes, including thrombin and plasmin, has been reported in infants at twice the normal values for adults. The cumulative effect of these alterations leads to decrease in plasmin activity in the newborn. Other components of fibrinolysis, such as the naturally occurring activators and inhibitors, are usually present in amounts equivalent to the adult levels[1-6, 22]. Hence, both the coagulation and the fibrinolytic mechanisms are kept in dynamic equilibrium in the normal neonate[21]. This precarious balance can be upset in a wide variety of clinical conditions, which are discussed later in this chapter.

For an in-depth understanding of the biochemical and pathophysiological processes involved in blood coagulation, several monographs and review articles may be consulted[1-5, 8].

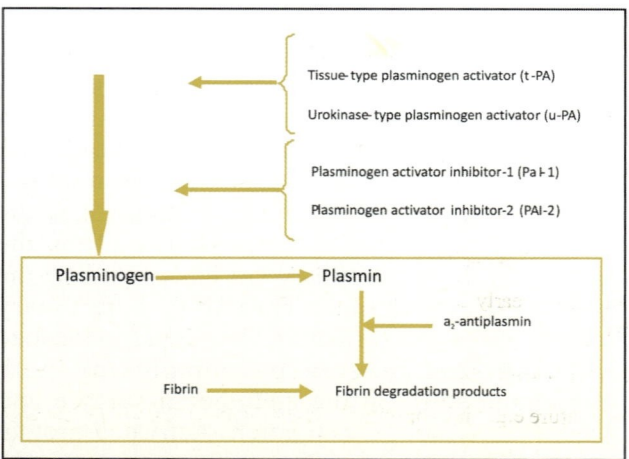

Figure 22.4 Fibrinogen activation cascade. The proenzyme, plasminogen is activated to the enzyme plasmin by tissue type plasminogen activator (t-PA) or urinary type plasminogen activator (u-PA). These two enzymes are inactivated after reaction with plasminogen activator inhibitor-1 (PAI-1) or plasminogen activator inhibitor-2 (PAI-2). Plasmin is capable of degrading fibrin clots to low-molecular weight fibrin degradation products. Plasmin may be inactivated by α_2 antiplasmin.

A PRACTICAL APPROACH TO THE BLEEDING NEONATE

In determining the cause of bleeding and its management in the newborn infant, a detailed history and physical examination along with a few screening laboratory tests provide valuable information.

History

The clues obtained from a few pointed questions asked to the parents can at times be more valuable than any laboratory test. It is important that a physician managing a bleeding neonate ask the following questions:

1. Is there a history of familial bleeding disorder such as hemophilia, von Willebrands disease, bruising, or bleeding in a previous sibling or any close relative?

2. Does the mother have lupus erythematosus, idiopathic thrombocytopenic purpura (past or present), excessive bruising, nose bleeds, preeclampsia, seizure disorder, cardiovascular disease?

3. Is there a history of herpes simplex or other maternal infection(s)?

4. Did the mother take drugs before or during delivery, such as aspirin, coumadin, anticonvulsants, rifampicin, isoniazid?

5. Was the infant's delivery complicated or precipitous for possible history of birth trauma?

6. Has vitamin K been given to the infant, and/or is the infant receiving breast milk or antibiotics?

Physical Examination

A rapid physical assessment of the bleeding newborn should be made to determine if the neonate has any evidence of systemic illness, e.g., sepsis, shock, hypoxia, that require immediate therapy while awaiting the laboratory tests. *Infants should be classified as either sick or well, as the differential diagnosis differs in these two easily separable clinical circumstances.* Commonly encountered diagnoses and the associated laboratory abnormalities in the sick and healthy groups of infants are listed in Table 22.4. If the overall impression is that the infant is sick as determined by the presence of severe asphyxia, acidosis, hypoxia, hypothermia, hypovolemia, hypoglycemia, seizures, prematurity with severe respiratory distress, hypotension or perinatal infections, the bleeding is likely to be a secondary phenomenon related to disseminated intravascular coagulation, peripheral platelet destruction, and/or liver dysfunction[3, 6, 30-34]. In these sick neonates, if one detects hepatosplenomegaly, it may suggest congenital or acquired infections, leukemia or erythroblastosis fetalis.

Table 22.4 An approach to the diagnosis of a bleeding neonate			
Laboratory Investigations			
Platelets	**PT**	**PTT**	**Possible diagnosis**
SICK NEONATES			
Decreased	Increased	Increased	Disseminated intravascular coagulation
Decreased	Normal	Normal	TORCH infections, early infections, (bacterial/fungal/viral), thrombotic-thrombocytopenia
Normal	Increased	Increased	Liver disease, heparinization
Normal	Normal	Normal	Altered vasculature e.g. "micropremie", severe hypoxia and/or acidosis
HEALTHY NEONATES			
Decreased	Normal	Normal	Immune thrombocytopenias, occult infection (fungal, CMV) or thrombosis, rarely bone marrow hypoplasia, leukemia
Normal	Increased	Increased	Vitamin-K deficiency
Normal	Normal	Increased	Hereditary clotting factor deficiencies
Normal	Normal	Normal	Swallowed materal blood, trauma, rarely qualitative platelet anomalies, Factor XIII deficiency, ulcer, hemangioma

Section 3

If congenital anomalies are detected along with thrombocytopenia, one should consider the diagnosis of thrombocytopenia with radial aplasia (TAR), Fanconi-pancytopenia, dyskeratosis congenita, osteopetrosis, trisomy 13 and 18, Chediak-Higashi, Wiskot-Aldrich and other syndromes[1, 5, 6, 8, 9, 35-38]. On the other hand, if the baby appears healthy, i.e., born at full term, vigorous, feeding well, not distressed and without evidence of systemic problems or physical anomalies, the etiology for the bleeding or the laboratory abnormality of the clotting studies is much more likely to be due to a primary bleeding disorder or a laboratory error. In healthy neonates, thrombocytopenia may also result from maternal drug ingestion, immune mediated, congenital, or due to a laboratory error or localized vascular lesion. If early diagnosis is not made in some of these infants, they may become sick. The physician may also obtain further clues from the nature and severity of the bleeding. Small scattered petechiae, ecchymoses (bruising), and bleeding from the gastrointestinal tract or central nervous system are commonly associated with thrombocytopenia[1, 2, 5, 6, 8, 14, 15, 35, 36]. In infants born with a nuchal cord or after a difficult delivery, petechiae may appear on the scalp, face or upper part of the trunk due to fragile vasculature[1, 5, 7, 15, 35].

Localized bleeding due to trauma, cephalhematoma, intramuscular hematoma secondary to vitamin K administration, umbilical stump hematoma, post circumcision bleeding, and hematoma or persistent oozing from skin puncture sites may be indicative of a specific coagulation factor deficiency, such as hemophilia or von Willebrand disease[1, 7, 18, 19, 39-44]. Presence of bright red blood in the vomitus or "tarry" stools are usually due to the newborn infant ingesting mother's blood and can be diagnosed by the Apt test[1, 13]. The principle of the Apt test is that the newborn infant's blood contains mainly fetal hemoglobin, which is resistant to denaturation with dilute alkali. Maternal blood, containing mainly hemoglobin A, is denatured and undergoes a color change to brownish-yellow. The procedure involves preparing a hemolysate by mixing 1 part of stool or vomitus with 5 parts of water, which is centrifuged to obtain pink supernatant. Five parts of this supernatant is mixed with 1 part of 1% (0.25 N) sodium hydroxide; the color is observed after 2 minutes. If the supernatant remains pink, it suggests infant's blood (Hb-F), whereas if it turns brownish-yellow it denotes swallowed mother's blood (Hb-A).

Generalized bleeding from skin, mucous membranes, venipuncture sites, gastrointestinal tract, the kidney or central nervous system can result from disseminated intravascular coagulation (DIC), platelet consumption, vitamin K deficiency, and severe liver disease[1-4, 6, 7, 33].

Laboratory Tests

In most neonates, the etiology of bleeding is clarified with three screening tests; platelet count, prothrombin time (PT), and partial thromboplastin time (PTT).[1, 65, 74-76] These routine tests are helpful when considered in the context of normal values for gestation and postnatal age (Tables 22.1 to 22.3).[12, 59] The platelet count in premature and full term newborn infants is the same as in adults, and ranges between 150,000 to 400,000/µl. Causes of laboratory errors in coagulation screening tests are listed in Table 22.5.

A diagnostic algorithm for a bleeding neonate is outlined in figure 22.5. The *platelet count* can be measured directly by phase microscopy or electronic cell counter, or manually by the conventional microscopic technique, or it can be quickly estimated by examining a well-prepared and stained peripheral smear. In order to estimate the platelet count in a peripheral smear, count the number of platelets per oil immersion field and multiply by 15,000 to 20,000. A count of 3 to 10 platelets per field would be considered adequate. In most laboratories, the manual method still remains a reliable method of platelet count and should be performed whenever the platelet count is below 50,000/ul[5, 7, 35] or platelet transfusion is contemplated. Use of electronic methods to count

Table 22.5 Causes of laboratory errors in coagulation screening tests	
Error	Cause
Platelet count falsely low	• Platelets adhere to heel after stick • Errors in dilution (manual technique) • Adherence to tube • Dilution with EDTA
PT and PTT falsely high	• Decreased plasma/citrate ratio (due to either too small a sample, or hematocrit > 65%) • Contamination with heparin from central line
PT and PTT falsely low	• Sample contaminated with tissue thromboplastin from difficult venipuncture

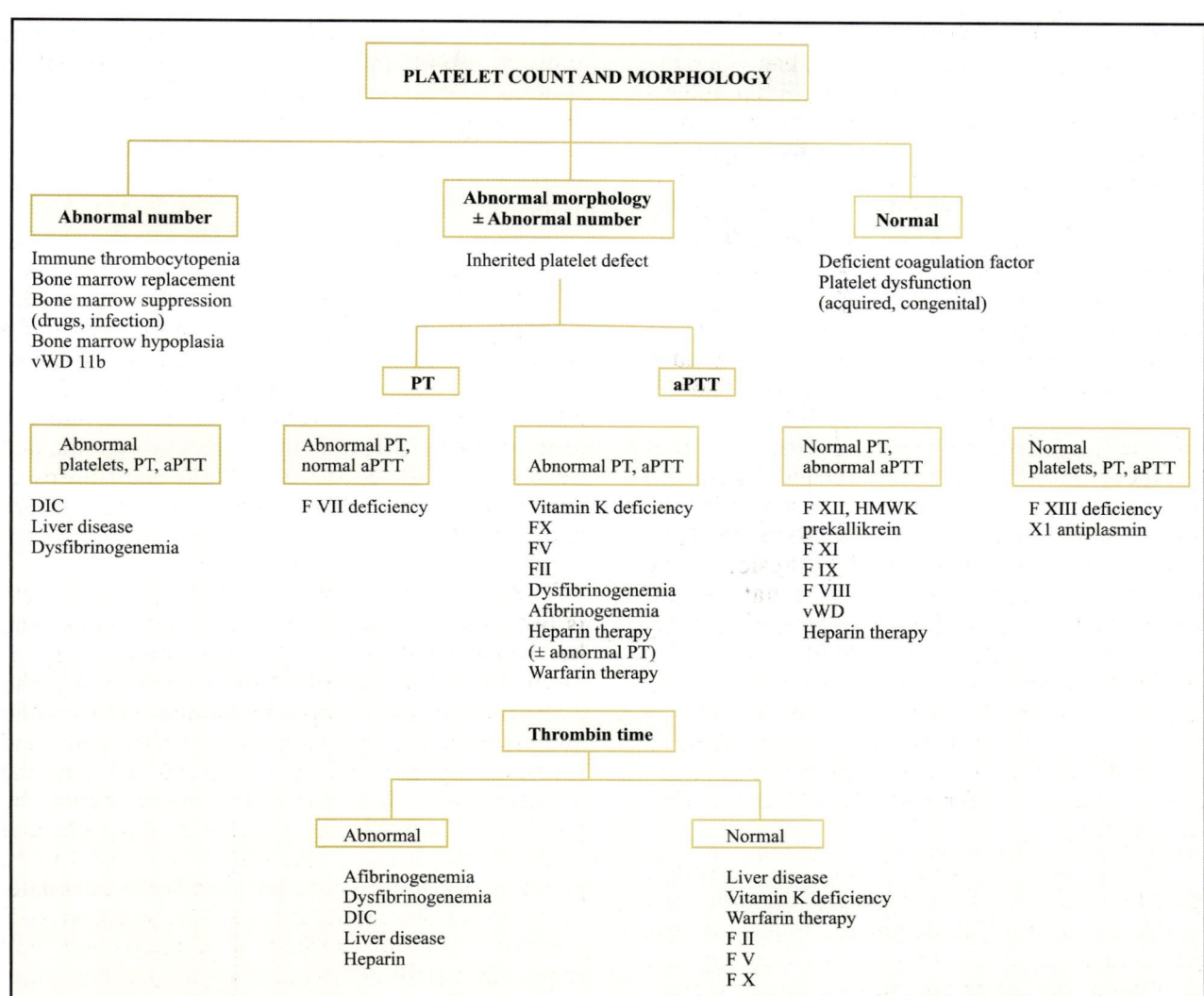

Figure 22.5 Diagnostic algorithm for a bleeding neonate. aPTT: activated partial thromboplastin time; DIC: disseminated intravascular coagulation; F: factor; plts: platelets; PT: prothrombin time; Rx: treatment; vWD: von Willebrand disease.
In an acquired or congenital coagulation factor deficiency state, a 50:50 mixture of patient plasma with pooled human plasma should yield normal results in a PT or a PTT assay. If these results are abnormal, investigation for a specific or nonspecific inhibitor of coagulation should be done.

platelets has been found to give better reproducibility, with a coefficient of variation of 4 percent as compared to 16 to 23 percent for the conventional microscopic techniques[5]. A major disadvantage of the automated platelet counters are their potential to over- or underestimate the actual number of platelets in certain clinical situations because they count particle size. Therefore, if the patient's platelet count falls outside this range, they are "not recognized" as platelets[5]. The count may be falsely lowered causing spurious thrombocytopenia by; (a) estimating it from blood obtained by difficult heel stick puncture, since the platelets adhere to the cut surface; (b) errors in dilution during the manual technique (normally 20 ul of blood is added to 1.98 ml of diluent); (c) presence of platelet autoaggulatinins giving rise to platelet clumping; (d) presence of giant platelets or megathrombocytes (with electronic platelet count); and (e) platelets adhering to the tube surface if not mixed immediately with EDTA, thus causing aggregation and a falsely low count called platelet satellitism (Table 22.5) [5-7, 45].

If the neonate has isolated thrombocytopenia, the mother's platelet count should be estimated[7, 8, 35, 46, 47-52]. She may have thrombocytopenia associated with preeclampsia or idiopathic thrombocytopenic purpura. Most infants who are not bleeding clinically and have platelet counts above 30,000/ μl do not require platelet transusion[7, 8, 35].

Rarely, the platelet count is normal. Platelet function, such as adhesion or aggregation (e.g.

salicylates, indomethacin therapy)[5, 8, 53-55] is altered and may be assessed clinically by measuring bleeding time (modified Ivy's method), and by examining a carefully prepared and stained peripheral blood smear[5, 8, 53, 55-57].

Prothrombin time (PT) and activated partial thromboplastin time (aPTT). These tests measure all soluble-clotting proteins, and therefore, are the most useful screening tests of blood coagulation. The *PT* is presumed to measure the *extrinsic coagulation pathway* and the aPTT, the *intrinsic pathway* (Figure 22.3a). They may be performed if the infant is bleeding or if the platelet count is low. The a*PTT* measures all factors except VII and XIII. *Activated PTT* is measured by most laboratories to standardize the procedure and thereby reduce errors. The aPTT may be abnormal when one or more of the factors is decreased by 20-40 percent of normal, and is, therefore, too sensitive a test for the preterm infant (Table 22.2). It is also influenced by markedly reduced quantities of contact factors (XI, XII, prekallikrein and high molecular weight kininogen) present in some of these babies. The normal values of platelets, PT, aPTT and other clotting factors at different gestational ages are summarized in Tables 22.1 and 22.2. Although it is important to remember that values may vary somewhat from one laboratory to another, a *PT greater than 17 seconds in a neonate at any gestational age and aPTT greater than 45 to 50 seconds in a term infant should be considered abnormal*[5, 29, 35]. In the preterm infant, the aPTT may not be useful because of the wide range of values, unless one has normal values for the neonate at varying gestational ages at the institution's laboratory. The PT and aPTT values may be falsely high if an insufficient blood sample is placed into the citrate tube or if the hematocrit is greater than 65 percent (Table 22.5). This occurs because of the disproportionately high citrate/plasma ratio and may be corrected by collecting the blood sample in the tube with half the citrate removed[5, 7, 8, 45]. Another source of error is contamination with heparin in the intravenous line, which will markedly elevate the aPTT and may cause a slight increase in the PT[1, 7, 58]. The reptilase test may be used to differentiate heparin effect on the sample from other coagulation disorders[45]. However, in general, specimens for blood coagulation tests should not be drawn from heparinized arterial catheters, even if they are initially flushed with a saline solution because an artifactually prolonged aPTT may still occur. A difficult, lengthy venipuncture, with associated tissue trauma and contamination of the needle with tissue thromboplastin, may also result in an unreliable PT and PTT, either due to small clots, fibrin strands or hemolysis with release of thromboplastic substances from red blood cells. If the PT, PTT, and platelets are truly abnormal, estimation of the fibrinogen level, fibrin split products (FSP) and D-dimers are performed. If the fibrinogen is decreased, along with the presence of FSP, a diagnosis of DIC is made[1-7, 33, 59].

In addition to controlling the bleeding in a sick neonate by replacing the appropriate clotting factors, therapy should be focused on the underlying disease(s) such as septicemia, herpes simplex, necrotizing enterocolitis, shock, hypovolemia, hypoxia or acidosis. *In managing a neonate who is bleeding, the physician's goal should be the well being of the infant rather than correcting the laboratory abnormality.* Blood products should be administered judiciously because of potentially serious side effects such as cytomegalovirus infection, hepatitis, acquired immune deficiency syndrome, malaria, hyperkalemia and hypervolemia occurring as a result of over-zealous transfusion therapy. Further therapeutic guidelines are provided in the discussion under specific bleeding disorders.

DIAGNOSIS AND MANAGEMENT OF COMMON NEONATAL BLEEDING DISORDERS

Disseminated Intravascular Coagulation (DIC), or Consumption of Platelets and/or Coagulation Factors

This is the most common and catastrophic cause of impaired hemostasis in a sick neonate, and may occur in up to 10 percent of sick infants admitted to a neonatal intensive care unit[1-7, 33].

Pathophysiology

Whereas normal hemostasis is a tightly regulated process, DIC involves diffuse inappropriate activation of clotting system throughout the vascular space. Bleeding primarily occurs due to depletion of clotting proteins and platelets. This process is exaggerated in neonates, particularly preterm infants, as a consequence of the limited capacity of their reticuloendothelial system to clear activated clotting factors from the circulation. Thrombosis with necrosis and/or organ dysfunction and microangiopathic hemolytic anemia may also occur. It has been proposed that the quality of coagulation factors consumed is dependent on the pathway by which DIC is initiated; with small vessel endothelial damage, or endotoxin release, intense platelet consumption occurs, while tissue factor release results in more marked fibrinogen consumption. The resultant alteration in the coagulation profile is dependent on substances consumed and the infant's capacity to synthesize more coagulation factors or platelets in response to their accelerated destruction.

Etiology

DIC is always a secondary event. Septicemia, including viremia is the most common cause of severe DIC in neonates. Other underlying causes include: obstetric complications, asphyxia, hypothermia, shock, respiratory distress syndrome or vascular lesions (Table 22.6) [1-7, 30, 33, 60-63]. Rarely, vascular malformations may be associated with DIC. The *Kasabach-Merritt syndrome* of giant hemangioma with thrombocytopenia and hypofibrinogenemia is associated with DIC and may include microangiopathic hemolytic anemia [64, 65]. The hemangiomas are not always obvious and may require radiographic imaging of the most common locations, i.e., brain, liver, spleen, and GI tract. The placenta may have chorangiomatous malformation leading to DIC. Rarely, massive hemolysis as seen in Rh incompatibility may trigger DIC.

Clinical Manifestations

There is a wide range of clinical severity associated with DIC. Although it is acute and fulminant in some infants with diffuse hemorrhage and ongoing consumption, other babies may have a milder picture with slight depression of clotting factor levels. The clinical manifestations of DIC are slight oozing from puncture sites to frank bleeding, either externally or from internal viscera, such as cerebral, pulmonary, gastrointestinal, or other organs. These patients often have melena,

shock, persistent acidosis, anemia (uncorrected by packed red cell transfusion), seizures or sclerema. Additional clinical findings may include blood oozing from body orifices, purpura, ecchymosis, and thrombosis of peripheral or central vessels with tissue ischemia, necrosis and gangrene. Therefore, a high index of suspicion of DIC is essential in these infants. Most infants appear extremely ill and are on assisted ventilation.

Diagnosis

The diagnosis of DIC is based on the characteristic laboratory findings in association with one or more of the etiological factors and clinical manifestations described earlier. Laboratory abnormalities include the presence of hemolytic anemia with irregularly contracted and fragmented erythrocytes detected in a peripheral blood smear, thrombocytopenia of variable degree, prolongation of PT and PTT, decrease in fibrinogen, elevated FSP or D-dimers. The levels of factor V and VIII are usually decreased. In some infants with infection, the vitamin K dependent factors (II, VII, IX and X) are reduced more than the labile factors (V, VIII), which are typically decreased in DIC [1]. The leukocytes frequently show toxic granulation, the white blood cell count is either decreased or increased with a shift to the left, suggesting septicemia and/or stress.

Treatment

Therapy must be primarily directed towards the underlying disease and coagulation abnormalities. If the condition that "triggered" DIC is brought under control, intravascular coagulation will usually cease. Therefore, appropriate antibiotics, correction of acidosis, electrolyte imbalance, hypotension, and adequate oxygenation

Table 22.6 Etiology of disseminated intravascular coagulation (DIC) in "sick" neonates		
Obstetric complications	**Neonatal infections**	**Miscellaneous**
• Placental abruption and vascular malformations	• Bacterial	• Extreme prematurity
• PIH: Chronic HTN	• Herpes	• Severe hemolysis
• Dead fetus multiple gestation	• Other viruses	• Hypoxia
• Fetal distress	• Congenital syphilis	• Shock
• Complicated breech extraction	• Candida albicans	• Giant hemangioma
• Amniotic fluid embolism		• Purpura fulminans
		(Protein-C or S, and antithrombin III deficiency)
		• Hepatitis

of tissues are mandatory. The decision to treat the abnormality with blood products must be based on the extent of clinical bleeding and laboratory abnormalities. Blood component replacement therapy should not be given in an otherwise stable infant with a positive guaiac test, slight skin bruising or a few petechiae. On the other hand, replacement transfusion therapy is indicated in an infant without obvious hemorrhage if the platelet count (done manually) is less than 10,000/µl or the PT is greater than 30 seconds[1-8, 35]. In premature infants with DIC, the PTT is often markedly prolonged because of contact factor depletion. In the diseases listed under Table 22.6, if frank bleeding or oozing occurs, or if intracranial or pulmonary hemorrhage is diagnosed, replacement therapy may be initiated along with treatment of the underlying disorder. Thus, judicious use of replacement therapy is essential to prevent the addition of fuel to the fire of intravascular coagulation. When treatment of the underlying disease and metabolic abnormalities may not be expected to result in prompt improvement, correction of the associated bleeding problem with either platelets, plasma, or cryoprecipitate is justified until the patient's clinical status is stabilized (Table 22.7). If the platelet count is less than 50,000/ul, one unit of platelets may be administered through a standard blood filter (microaggregate filters may trap platelets and therefore avoided.) One unit of platelet raises the platelet count by approximately 50,000/ul to 70,000/ul in a 3 kg term infant (one hour later). However, this may fall because of the consumptive process, consequently, platelet counts should be monitored along with other coagulation screening tests every 4 to 24 hours and transfusion repeated as indicated clinically. Fresh frozen plasma in a dose of 10 to 15 ml/kg is also given to correct the coagulation abnormality. Normally, platelets survive better at room temperature (22°C). However, the large volume of plasma (50 ml) required for storage of warm platelets may cause circulatory overload, particularly in the critically ill premature infant. This may be prevented by centrifuging the platelets and removing the excess plasma immediately before use. Usually platelet typing is not required and in an emergency, we suspend centrifuged platelets in AB-negative plasma. Another concern about using warm platelets in the newborn is the risk of bacterial contamination and its potential effects in immunocompromised recipients. As with all therapies, any decision to administer platelets to the newborn must balance the benefits and risks. If bleeding persists in patients with DIC after transfusion of plasma and platelets, one should consider transfusing cryoprecipitate. Cryoprecipitate contains large quantities of factors VII ahf, VIII vwf, XIII and fibrinogen. Normally one bag of cryoprecipitate contains 100 units of factor VIII (range 60-125 units) suspended in 10 to 15 ml plasma. The dose of cryoprecipitate is 0.5 u/kg (10 ml/kg). Therefore, one bag of cryoprecipitate will suffice (one unit of factor VIII/kg/dose will increase factor VIII activity by 2%). After correction of the coagulopathy, the patient should be monitored closely for bleeding, along with PT, PTT, and fibrinogen levels repeated in 4 to 6 hours to determine the continuation of DIC. In sick infants with DIC, replacement products are transfused as clinically indicated.

In DIC patients with fluid overload or congestive heart failure, exchange transfusion with fresh blood or reconstituted whole blood has been suggested in order to remove toxins, activated clotting factors, potentially harmful fibrin split

Product	Contents	Usual dose	Indications
FFP	All factors	10-20 mg/kg	DIC, liver disease protein-C deficiency
Exchange transfusion*	All factors	Double volume	Severe DIC, liver disease
Cryoprecipitate	Factors VIII, XIII,	1 bag + fibrinogen	DIC, liver disease, factor VIII, XIII deficiency, vW disease
Platelets**	Platelets	1-2 units/kg	Bleeding due to decrease in platelets
Vitamin K	–	1-2 mg	Suspected vitamin K deficiency
IV IgG	IgG	1-2 g/kg	NAIT, sepsis

Table 22.7 Products used for treatment of coagulation disorders

*Fresh whole blood; 1+ bag cryoprecipitate = 250 mg fibrinogen and 100 units of factor VIII
**Response variesNAIT: Neonatal alloimmune thrombocytopenia

products, and provide normal levels of clotting factors[66, 67]. Using the conventional push-pull technique may be hazardous in the immature infant due to the risk of intraventricular hemorrhage or necrotizing enterocolitis secondary to rapid changes in blood volume and thus cerebral venous or perfusion pressures. In a randomized controlled trial, infants receiving exchange transfusion did not have a better outcome when compared to those managed conservatively with treatment of the underlying disease or a third group receiving only judicious replacement transfusions[67]. Although in the past heparin therapy was widely used in DIC, its use is restricted to infants with vascular thrombosis. In view of the decrease in vitamin K-dependent factors in some patients with DIC, it may be prudent to administer 1 mg/kg of vitamin K to infants with DIC. Therapeutic caution with replacement therapy must be exercised to reach a desired end point of controlling major hemorrhage and not attempting to normalize laboratory tests, which is often not feasible[1, 6, 7, 33, 67]. In patients with shock, low antithrombin III levels may occur[68].

Hemorrhagic Disease of the Newborn (Vitamin K deficiency)

In 1894, Townsend described a series of 50 infants with self limiting bleeding that occurred mostly between the first and fifth day of life and that differed from classic hemophilia. As a medical student, Heinrich von Dam noted subcutaneous and intraperitoneal hemorrhages in chicks fed a fat-free diet and proposed that the bleeding was the result of a diet that was deficient in a fat soluble substance involved in coagulation, the *coagulation* vitamin, vitamin K. He went on to demonstrate that lowered plasma prothrombin levels correlated with occurrence of the deficiency-associated hemorrhagic disorder. Vitamin K was later shown to affect the functions of factors VII, IX, and X. Hemorrhagic disease of the newborn was formally defined by the AAP's Committee of Nutrition in 1961 as "a hemorrhagic disorder of the first days of life caused by a deficiency of vitamin K and characterized by a deficiency of prothrombin, proconvertin, and probably other factors".

Vitamin K is a fat soluble vitamin that is required for modifying coagulation protein II (prothrombin), VII, IX and X and anticoagulant proteins C and S. The vitamin is a membrane-bound component of a microsomal carboxylase system, which is proposed to couple carboxylation of coagulation zymogens with epooxidation of vitamin K. The post-translational γ-carboxylation of amino terminal glutamic acid residues form complexes with other hemostatic proteins, via calcium, on phospholipid surface. Localization of enzymes with their substrates and cofactors promote efficient reaction and forms localized blood clot rapidly. The vitamin K dependent carboxylation of the coagulation factors occurs in the rough endoplasmic reticulum of the hepatocyte. In the absence of vitamin K, synthesized prothrombin circulates in its noncarboxylated, functionally defective form[69, 70].

Three forms of vitamin K have been identified; vitamin K_1 (phytonadione), which is present in green leafy vegetables; vitamin K_2, which is synthesized by the gastrointestinal flora; and vitamin K_3 (menadione), a synthetic water soluble form, seldom used in neonates because of its association with hemolytic anemia. Placental transfer of vitamin K is poor and its levels are low in plasma and liver[70]. Breast milk is a poor source of vitamin K compared to cow's milk or infant formula supplemented with vitamin K[71-72]. The GI tract is sterile at birth, and its colonization with vitamin K-producing flora occurs after enteral feedings is instituted. Because lactation takes several days to be established, infants who are exclusively breast-fed or those who are not fed orally are at risk for vitamin K deficiency. Broad spectrum antibiotics can be associated with vitamin K deficiency if intestinal flora are eliminated. Until 1960s when vitamin K was not used prophylactically in all newborns, approximately 1 to 2 percent of breast fed infants developed cutaneous, mucosal or internal hemorrhage at 2 to 5 days of age due to vitamin K deficiency[69]. Vitamin K-dependent factors are deficient in most newborn infants because of the immaturity of the liver; therefore, routine use of 1 mg vitamin K parenterally soon after birth had been recommended. Hemorrhagic disease of the newborn had reemerged because vitamin K was not routinely administered in newborn infants[32, 72-75].

The vitamin K-dependent procoagulants, (factors II, VII, IX and X) are gestational age dependent (Tables 22.1 and 22.2), increasing with age; and in healthy neonates are about 30 to 60 percent of normal adult values[16, 17, 69]. The administration of vitamin K at birth prevents further depression of these factors. Normal adult values are usually reached by 6 weeks of age. Screening tests, such as the *PT*, *PTT* and thrombotest, reflecting the physiologic decrease in the vitamin K-dependent procoagulants are all prolonged at birth. In infancy, vitamin K-deficiency must be differentiated from normal physiologic decrease and from acquired and congenital coagulation disorders.

Section 3

Table 22.8 Differential diagnosis of neonatal thrombocytopenia

I. Primary fetal production/function defects

- TAR, Fanconi's anemia, trisomy 13 and 18
- Congenital amegakaryocytic thrombocytopenia
- Giant platelet syndrome: Bernard-Saulier, May-Hegglin and other leukocyte inclusions
- Thrombocytopenia, Robin sequence, agenesis of corpus callosum
- Parish-Trousseau with dysmegakaryopoietic thrombocytopenia, gaint platelets, gamma granules
- Renal disease: Alport syndrome

II. Thrombocytopenia secondary to increased platelet destruction

- DIC
- Infection (e.g. bacterial, viral, candida, NEC)
- Birth trauma, acidosis, hypoxia
- Thrombosis
- Malignancy (e.g., congenital leukemia)
- Giant hemagnioma (e.g., Kasabach-Merritt syndrome)

III. Thrombocytopenia: Mixed or Uncertain

- Rh hemolytic disease, non-immune hydrops, exchange transfusion
- Congenital infections
- Polycythemia
- Thrombotic thrombocytopenia, HUS
- Wiskott-Aldrich syndrome
- X-linked recessive thrombocytopenia
- Other hereditary causes

IV. Thrombocytopenia secondary to maternal factors

- Autoimmune neonatal thrombocytopenia
- Maternal autoimmune thrombocytopenia
- Pre-eclampsia, antiphospholipd syndrome
- Lupus, hyperthyroidism, diabetes mellitus
- Maternal medications

Neonatal thrombocytopenia associated with maternal immune thrombocytopenic purpura (ITP) or autoimmune thrombocytopenia

Neonatal thrombocytopenia resulting from maternal immune thrombocytopenia, also known as neonatal autoimmune thrombocytopenia, can occur in infants of mothers with immune thrombocytopenia due to ITP, lupus erythematosus, or other autoimmune disorders[35, 36, 46, 48, 50]. In neonates, the thrombocytopenia associated with maternal immune thrombocytopenia is generally milder than isoimmune thrombocytopenia. A large study of these patients revealed that the incidence of cord platelet counts less than 50,000/µl is only about 3%[1]. As a result, bleeding in these patients is usually not severe. Nevertheless, these infants should be followed closely, because platelet counts often fall in the days after birth. ITP is a distinct disorder in which antiplatelet antibody (primarily from spleen) are directed against both maternal and fetal platelets and must be differentiated from alloimmune thrombocytopenia and other causes (Table 22.8)[1, 35, 47-51, 89, 90]. Antiplatelet IgG antibodies from the mother are actively transported across the placenta to the fetus with resultant thrombocytopenia.

Maternal ITP is often diagnosed prior to delivery, although some mothers may have normal platelet count with megathrombocytes or "stress platelets". ITP in adults is often a chronic disease mediated by autoantibodies directed against cell surface glycoproteins of platelets (IIb/IIIa or Ib/IX). Although a low platelet count in the mother is suspicious of ITP, diagnosis is accomplished by a radiolabelled Coomb's test for detection of platelet associated IgG and C_3 complement. However, the severity of neonatal thrombocytopenia does not necessarily correlate with that of the mother. For example, mothers with a history of ITP and a persistent thrombocytopenia may give birth to infants with normal platelet counts, whereas mothers with ITP and normal platelet counts may give birth to infants with severe thrombocytopenia and hemorrhage. The overall mortality rate for infants born to ITP mothers is between 15 and 25 percent. The most common causes of mortality are stillbirth, prematurity, and hemorrhage.

Treatment of ITP during pregnancy is administered as per the guidelines published since 1996[50]. The main focus of *treatment of the mother with ITP* is to maintain her asymptomatic from hematological perspective rather than to achieve normal platelets[91]. Pregnant patients with ITP and platelet counts greater than 50,000/µl throughout gestation, as well as those with platelet counts of 30,000 to 50,000/µl, in the first or second trimester, do not routinely require treatment. Treatment in the form of glucocorticoids or intravenous immune globulin (IVIG) is indicated in patients with platelet counts less than 10,000/µl, and for those with platelet counts of 10,000 to 30,000/µl who are bleeding. For the symptomatic antenatal patient with ITP requiring treatment, corticosteroid therapy 1mg/kg per day results in an increase in platelet count in approximately three-fourth of patients within 2 weeks. Unfortunately, less than a third of these patients have sustained remission with prednisolone.

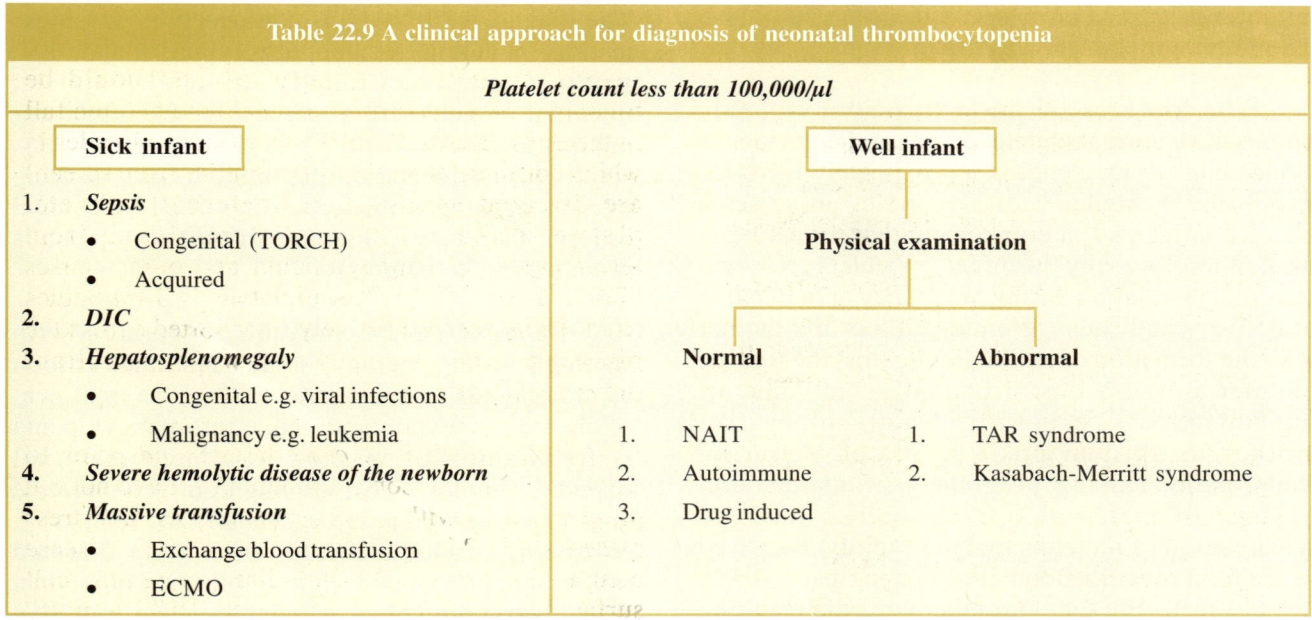

Table 22.9 A clinical approach for diagnosis of neonatal thrombocytopenia

Platelet count less than 100,000/µl		
Sick infant	**Well infant**	
1. *Sepsis*	**Physical examination**	
• Congenital (TORCH)		
• Acquired		
2. *DIC*	Normal	Abnormal
3. *Hepatosplenomegaly*		
• Congenital e.g. viral infections		
• Malignancy e.g. leukemia	1. NAIT	1. TAR syndrome
4. *Severe hemolytic disease of the newborn*	2. Autoimmune	2. Kasabach-Merritt syndrome
5. *Massive transfusion*	3. Drug induced	
• Exchange blood transfusion		
• ECMO		

Hence IVIG has been added to the therapeutic armamentarium to suppress the antiplatelet antibody. Often high doses (400 mg/kg per day for 5 days) of IVIG increase the platelet count to >50,000/µl in more than 80 percent of patients. An alternate regimen is to administer IVIG, 1gm/kg over 8 hours. This increases the platelet count in more than 50 percent of patients lasting for 2 to 3 weeks; for those patients in whom the platelet count does not increase, a second dose may be given on day 3. The main disadvantage of IVIG is that it is expensive and seldom produces a long-term remission. The value of fetal platelet count by fetal scalp sampling[1, 8] or percutaneous umbilical blood sampling (PUBS) has been questioned and discontinued[46, 48]. In a series of 165 pregnancies with ITP, 134 were delivered vaginally; 21 percent of whom had platelet counts <30,000/µl, but only one infant had non-fatal intracranial hemorrhage. Of the 31 infants delivered by cesarean section, 29 percent had platelet counts <30,000/µl, three of whom had severe intracranial hemorrhage. Thus it seems that the route of delivery for patients with ITP may not affect the incidence of intracranial hemorrhage. Therefore, the route of delivery in patients with ITP should be based on obstetrical indications alone. When glucocorticoid and IVIG therapy have failed, splenectomy is appropriate in the second trimester in women with platelet counts less than 10,000/µl who are bleeding. Platelet transfusion is indicated for women with counts less than 10,000/µl, before a planned cesarean section or for those who are bleeding and expected to deliver vaginally. In a recent retrospective study of 92 obstetric patients with ITP during 119 pregnancies over an 11 year period, platelet count lower than 150,000/µl was noted in 89% of mothers, and in 25% of neonates. Nine percent of these neonates had platelet counts less than 50,000/µl. Treatment for hemostatic impairment was necessary in 14% of neonates, two fetal deaths occurred, one due to hemorrhage.

The diagnosis in the neonate is made by a decrease in platelet count which may vary from slightly lower than normal to often as low as 5,000 to 10,000/µl, maternal history of ITP, and maternal thrombocytopenia (unless the mother is receiving corticosteroids or has previously had a splenectomy). Postnatal thrombocytopenia is found in 50 to 70 percent of neonates born to mothers with ITP[1, 5, 35, 48]. The thrombocytopenia is usually transient and is spontaneously corrected during the first week of life. They require close observation, but do not require platelet transfusion. Because of this transient thrombocytopenia, circumcision and other elective surgery should be deferred. The benefits of breast feeding should be weighed because small quantities of antiplatelet antibodies are present in breast milk and may prolong thrombocytopenia in these patients. For more severely affected infants, platelet transfusion is a stop-gap measure which can be used to limit the ongoing hemorrhage. Rarely, exchange transfusion has been used to remove antibodies and prevent recurrent thrombocytopenia. Corticosteroids (prednisone 2 mg/kg per day) and IVIG (1gm/kg per day for 1 to 3 days) have been used alone or in combination[1, 5, 9, 35, 90, 92, 93].

Alloimmune (Isoimmune) Neonatal Thrombocytopenic Purpura

The mothers of these thrombocytopenic infants have normal platelet counts and no evidence of bleeding. Its incidence is approximately 1 in 5000 live births or higher[1, 5, 35]. The infant possesses a platelet antigen of paternal origin that is lacking in the mother. Typically the infant's platelets cross into maternal circulation during pregnancy or at the time of delivery and cause immunization of the mother with the formation of antibodies against the foreign platelet antigen. Less frequently the cause of immunization is exposure of antigen-negative mother to antigen positive platelets during transfusion. During pregnancy, transplacental passage of maternal IgG antibodies leads to sensitization of platelets that are rapidly destroyed in the fetal reticuloendothelial system, particularly in the spleen with fetal thrombocytopenia resulting in-utero or at delivery. This mechanism is analogous to hemolytic disease of the newborn due to Rh-sensitization. The platelet specific antigen system most often involved in cases of neonatal alloimmune thrombocytopenia (NAIT) is PLA1.

The *diagnosis of NAIT* is suspected in a term neonate with thrombocytopenia and petechiae, bruising or rarely intracranial (occurring in 10 to 15% of cases) and other forms of bleeding, when other causes are excluded. Bussell and colleagues have estimated that one-fourth of the central nervous system hemorrhages associated with NAIT occur antenatally.[77] Early diagnosis and prevention of NAIT is therefore important. Unlike Rh-isoimmunization, the fetus may be affected in the first pregnancy. In subsequent pregnancies, approximately 75% of fetuses may be affected. Phenotyping of paternal platelets for both alleles of a diallelic antigen system may provide a clue that the current fetus must be affected. Currently most maternal protocols use PUBS early in gestation, preferably after 22 weeks (for technical reasons), with the thrombocytopenic fetuses treated with serial platelet transfusion. The problems with this treatment are; (a) The HPA-1 antibody has a much longer half life than the platelets themselves; and (b) HPA-1 antigen has been shown to be present on fetal platelets early in second trimester. Also weekly maternal transfusion with IVIG 1gm/kg with or without prednisolone has been used successfully in pregnancies at-risk for NAIT.[5,9,81] While optimal maternal therapy is being debated, several investigators have reported that all neonates born to mothers treated with IVIG had normal platelet counts.

The diagnosis of NAIT is confirmed by serologic testing, including immunophenotyping of maternal, paternal, and occasionally neonatal platelets; maternal or fetal serum can also be examined for antiplatelet antibody[1, 5, 35, 52]. Unfortunately, serologic evidence of alloantibodies are lacking in most of the possible cases identified by clinical criteria; therefore isoimmune thrombocytopenia is often a clinical diagnosis[1].

Because delays may be associated with serologic testing, therapy should be initiated as soon as the diagnosis is suspected[1, 5, 8, 35]. The treatment of choice for severe isoimmune thrombocytopenia is transfusion of washed irradiated maternal platelets (Figure 22.6); although antigen-negative donors may be used in subsequent affected siblings[1, 94]. No therapy is indicated for the mildly affected infants, but infants with signs of bleeding other than petechiae, or with platelet count less than 30,000/µl should receive specific therapy. Intravenous gamma globulin (1gm/kg for 2 days) or corticosteroids (methylprednisone 2mg/kg/day) or both can be used as temporary measures, although these interventions have limited benefit[1,5,35,48,90,95]. Corticosteroids are usually ineffective, although predelivery maternal therapy has been recommended. There is minimal or no response to platelet transfusion from a random donor (which is often used in clinical practice) because such platelets are likely to be PLA-1 positive and thus susceptible to antibody mediated destruction[1, 94, 96]. The donor platelets are ideally derived from the mother because they are certain to lack the target antigen. Most postpartum women can easily tolerate 1 to 2 unit platelet pheresis, as the plasma and red cells can be retransfused back to her. The platelets are gently washed several times to remove excess antibody, resuspended in AB-negative

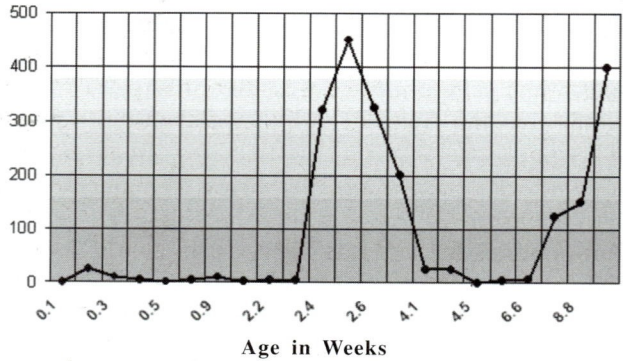

–•– **Platelets/mm³(x10⁻³)**

Figure 22.6 Treatment of isoimmune thrombocytopenia with washed, irradiated maternal platelets. (Adapted from Pearson HA et al. Isoimmune neonatal thrombocytopenic purpura: Clinical and therapeutic considerations. *Blood* 23:154,1964)

plasma, and thereafter slowly infused into the infant. Serial platelet counts are followed and the infant may require several transfusions in order to keep the platelet count above 30,000/µl or until clinically significant bleeding stops. If the life-span of transfused mother's platelets is extremely short, an alternative diagnosis, such as consumptive thrombocytopenia should be considered.

Platelets produced by neonates with isoimmune thrombocytopenia exhibit accelerated clearance for weeks until platelet antibody is removed from the circulation. Consequently, it is not unusual for additional transfusions with washed platelets to be required after the first few weeks. The likelihood is high that subsequent infants born to these mothers will be affected. Therefore, detailed counseling about the risk of recurrence should be provided to the family at the time of the first infant's diagnosis with neonatal alloimmune thrombocytopenia. It has been recommended that after the birth of an affected child with alloimmune thrombocytopenia, close relatives of the mother should be tested for the involved platelet antigen. In infants affected in the future, an antigen-negative donor should provide platelets.[7]

Congenital Deficiencies in the Coagulation Factors

Hemophilia

Prenatal diagnosis of hemophilia A or B is feasible. Intrauterine diagnosis of hemophilia A is confirmed in a male infant by measuring the ratio of factor VIII coagulant antigen to factor VIII-related antigen by immunological techniques, or by measuring the ratio of procoagulant factor VIII to factor VIII antigen in samples of pure fetal blood obtained by fetoscopy at approximately 20 weeks of gestation. Prenatal diagnosis of hemophilia B is made by an immunoradiometric assay for factor IX antigen in amniotic fluid between 16 to 20 weeks of gestation.

Hemophilia A (Factor VIII deficiency) and Hemophilia B (Factor IX deficiency) may present with bleeding symptoms in the newborn period. Because of sex-linked inheritance, male infants are affected. Affected cases can be diagnosed at birth because the lower limit of reference range for factor VIII (<50% or 0 - 0.05 U/ml) is similar to adult values. Severe (<1%) and moderate (1%- 5%) forms of hemophilia A and B cases can be confidently diagnosed in the newborn period.

However, infants with mild deficiency may be missed in neonatal period and require evaluation later if there is family history of bleeding because the factor IX levels fall within normal range of full term and premature infants. Delay in confirming the diagnosis is of no consequence; children with mild hemophilia B are not at-risk for spontaneous bleeding. These two disorders occur in about 1 per 5,000 male live births[1, 4, 97-99]. Approximately one-third to one-half of the infants develop bleeding during the neonatal period usually following trauma (e.g., circumcision, oozing from umbilicus or heel stick puncture). Rarely, intracranial hemorrhage in the form of subdural or subgalleal hematoma, subarachnoid or intraventricular hemorrhage may result from hemophilia[39, 41, 97-99]. Nevertheless, approximately one-third of severe hemophiliacs are not likely to have excessive bleeding following circumcision and it is presumed that bleeding may be prevented due to the liberation of tissue thromboplastin caused by the presence of circumcision clamp[39, 97-99]. The family history is usually negative in 50 percent of these cases. The infants otherwise appear normal. These are relatively healthy infants in whom the *PTT* may be prolonged, but the *PT* and platelet counts are always normal (Table 22.4). The diagnosis is confirmed by assaying factor VIII and IX in a specialized blood coagulation laboratory. Mild hemophilia B (factor IX deficiency) cannot always be differentiated from the normal physiologic reduction in factor IX during the newborn period; therefore, repeat assay at 3 to 4 months of age should be performed.

The therapy for hemophilia is outlined in Table 22.10. In emergency situation, fresh frozen plasma or cryoprecipitate may be administered[97-99]. Transfusion of these blood products in hemophiliacs is associated with potential risk of HIV infection and progression to AIDS,[100, 101] hence they have been recently treated with a virally safe factor VIII concentrate[102, 103]. Fibrin glue has been described as a useful treatment modality for circumcision in patients with bleeding diathesis and it is safer and cheaper than infusion of factor concentrate[39]. These patients and their families should be counseled and managed by a physician with knowledge and interest in this disease.

Management of bleeding involves infusion of factor VIII or IX to restore hemostasis. Factor IX concentrate should not be used in neonates other than those with severe deficiency because of the risk of undue thrombosis secondary to low antithrombin levels.

Section 3

Table 22.10 Treatment of hemophilia A and B		
Type of hemophilia	**Symptom**	**Treatment**
Hemophilia A (factor VIII deficiency)	Limited oral bleeding	Amicar 100 mg/kg PO q 6 hr
	Mild to moderate bleeding	Factor VIII 20 u/kg IV or DDAVP 0.3 ìg/ kg IV in patients known to have a satisfactory response
	Severe or life-threatening bleeding	Factor VIII 50 u/kg IV followed by repeated infusions of 20–25 u/kg IV q 12 hr
Hemophilia B (factor IX deficiency)	Limited oral bleeding	Amicar 100 mg/kg PO q 6 hr
	Mild to moderate bleeding	Factor IX 20 u/kg IV
	Severe or life-threatening bleeding	Factor IX 80 u/kg followed by 40 u/kg q 24 hr

Deficiency of factors II, V, VII, IX, X and fibrinogen are inherited as an autosomal dominant manner[1, 4, 104-106]. The homozygous form of the disorder may present with bleeding in the newborn period[23, 24, 27, 107]. Delayed bleeding from the umbilical stump is characteristic of homozygous factor XIII deficiency or of a severe qualitative or quantitative abnormality of fibrinogen. Laboratory findings in selected coagulation disorders are listed in Table 22.11. Screening coagulation tests (e.g., PT, PTT, thrombin time) are normal in patients with factor XIII deficiency, and the diagnosis should be confirmed by specific factor assay[1, 19, 23, 24, 27, 105, 106, 108]. Treatment of the coagulation factor deficiency involves infusion of stored plasma (except for factor V), fresh frozen plasma, or specific factor concentrates. Severe factor V deficiency can also present with intracranial hemorrhage in the newborn, hence a high index of suspicion should be maintained.

Bleeding is uncommon in neonates with von Willebrand disease (pseudohemophilia). The diagnosis of von Willebrand disease cannot be made with confidence in the newborn period because the levels of von Willebrand factor are elevated at birth masking the presence of most forms of von Willebrand disease[108].

THROMBOTIC DISORDERS

In the pediatric age group, arterial or venous thrombosis develops most often in the newborn period. Although thrombosis in neonates may occur frequently with vascular catheter placement, it may also occur spontaneously[1, 4, 22, 109, 110, 111-119]. Rarely, thromboembolism is associated with manifestations of bleeding or platelet and coagulation abnormality due to homozygous protein C or S deficiency or antithrombin III deficiency[12, 31, 60, 112, 116-121].

However, absence of thrombosis has been reported in subjects with heterozygous protein C deficiency[122].

Thrombosis Associated with Indwelling Catheters

Neonatal thromboembolism is associated with radial, brachial, temporal, pulmonary, and femoral arterial lines as well as central venous catheters inserted into the jugular and femoral and other veins. However, because of its widespread use, thromboembolism has been most often associated with placement of umbilical arterial catheters. End-hole catheters are less thrombogenic than side-hole catheters. Low umbilical arterial catheter position is associated with blanching and cyanosis of the extremities, but the incidence of radiographically proven thrombosis does not differ significantly whether the catheter tip is positioned high (between the seventh and eighth vertebrae) or low (at the third to fourth lumbar vertebrae). Often there are no clinical manifestations of thrombi, but serious morbidity, such as renal hypertension, intestinal necrosis, peripheral gangrene, paraplegia, cerebral infarct, and even death has been reported. In order to prevent catheter-associated thrombi, heparin infused intravenously in doses of 100-200 u/kg/day has been shown to improve catheter patency[1, 123, 124]. On the other hand, the possibility of bleeding associated with heparin, particularly in the premature infant is genuine due to technical difficulties in monitoring such patients. Because of the serious risk with umbilical venous catheters, such as pulmonary embolism and hepatic necrosis, its use in neonates has been reserved for extreme emergencies only, and should be removed as soon as percutaneous catheters can be placed[6, 7, 10, 12, 109].

					Table 22.11 Laboratory findings in selected coagulation defects

Factor	Bleeding time	PT	aPTT	Thrombin time	Comments
I (Afibrinogenemia)	A	A	A	A	Low fibrinogen level
Dysfibrinogenemia	N	A	±A	A	Fibrinogen activity lower than antigen levels
Heparin therapy	±N	N	A	A	Check factor level; PT, aPTT normalize with 50:50 mix
VII	N	A	N	N	Check factor level; PT corrects with 50:50 mix
IX	N	N	A	N	Check factor level; aPTT corrects with 50:50 mix
X	N	A	A	N	Check factor level; aPTT corrects with 50:50 mix
XI	N	N	A	N	Check factor level; aPTT corrects with 50:50 mix
XII, prekallikrein, HMW kininogen	N	N	A	N	Check factor levels; deficiencies do not cause clinical bleeding
XIII	N	N	N	N	Check factor level; check clot solubility
vWD	±A	N	±A	N	Check vWF antigen, factor VIII activity, RIPA (ristocetin-induced platelet aggregation), ristocetin cofactor, multimeric analysis
Inhibitor	N	±A	±A	N	Abnormality does not correct with 50:50 mix; check for lupus anticoagulant

A: abnormal; aPTT: activated partial thromboplastin time; HMW: high molecular weight; N: normal; PT: prothrombin time; vWD: von Willebrand disease; vWF: von Willebrand factor.

Section 3

Treatment of thrombosis is controversial, both because of absence of controlled clinical trials in neonates and because it is not possible to extrapolate from the adult literature. Consultation with a pediatric hematologist is recommended for any infant with thrombosis. Therapeutic options include supportive care, non specific measures (e.g. warming the involved or contralateral limb), anticoagulants, fibrinolytic agents, and surgical removal of the clot. Most infants with catheter related clots are clinically asymptomatic. In these infants, the thrombosis is rarely diagnosed and the patients receive supportive therapy, with good response. Patients who develop limb or organ dysfunction must be treated more aggressively. In other cases, anticoagulant or fibrinolytic therapy is used, but evaluation of the central nervous system for hemorrhage must precede treatment. The benefit of heparin therapy in the newborn with low antithrombin III (AT III) levels has been questioned, and enhancing the effects of heparin by concurrent infusion of AT III has been suggested. The guideline for heparin therapy in neonates is outlined in Table 22.12. Resistence to activated protein C may lead to thrombosis in some of these infants[125, 126]. Because of the difficulties in obtaining venous access and the need for frequent laboratory monitoring associated with heparin therapy, low molecular weight heparin (LMWH) have become accepted for treatment and prophylaxis of DVT in adults. LMWH has been reported in several studies in infants and children with documented safety and efficacy[127-129]. Table 22.13 outlines the current recommendations for LMWH, and the dosing is age and weight dependent. Infants younger than 2 months of age require higher doses than older children to maintain therapeutic anti-Xa level of 0.5 to 1.0 international units/ml. A large randomized, placebo control study is needed to compare the safety and efficacy of LMWH to the traditional unfractionated heparin (Table 22.12), and warfarin regimen (Table 22.14) for treatment of venous thrombosis in neonates and infants. Urokinase therapy has also been used, although it is often unsuccessful[130-134]. Protein C deficiency has been treated with protein C concentrate[142-144] in patients with renovascular hypertension due to aortic thrombus, nonsurgical therapy should be attempted prior to surgical removal of the clot[115, 155]. Warfarin therapy has also been used in children[136, 137]. Congental antithrombin III deficiency can be treated with antithrombin III concentrate[117, 125].

Table 22.12 Recommendations for unfractionated heparin therapy in neonates

Pretreatment laboratory testing: CBC with platelets, aPTT, PT, serum creatinine, ALT

Loading dose: 75 u/kg IV over 10 minutes

Maintenance dose: 28 u/kg/hr continuous infusion

Laboratory monitoring:

aPTT 4 hours after heparin loading dose is given (use table to adjust dosing), then daily

or

Daily anti-Xa level, unfractionated heparin–target range 0.35–0.6 anti-Xa units

or

Daily anti-factor lla level–target range 0.2–0.4 u/ml
Daily CBC with platelets

Unfractionated heparin dosing adjustments based on aPTT results				
aPTT (sec) (hr)	Bolus u/kg	Hold Infusion (min)	Percent change ininfusion rate	Repeat aPTT
<50	50	0	'!20	4
50-59	0	0	'!10	4
60-85	0	0	0	24
86-95	0	0	"!10	4
96-120	0	30	"!10	4
>120	0	60	"!15	4

Duration of therapy (see text):
10–14 days *or* 5–7 days; add warfarin or LMWH day 1 or 2 (extensive clot or PE: start warfarin on day 5 and treat with heparin for 14 days)

Precautions:

If platelet count drops < 150,000/µl, consider heparin-induced thrombocytopenia
Avoid IM injections and arterial punctures

Unfractionated heparin antidote: Protamine sulfate 10 mg/ml at a rate not to exceed 5 mg/min, maximum dose 50 mg		
Time elapsed since last heparin dose (min)	Protamine sulfate dose (mg/100 u heparin received) upto maximum 50 mg	aPTT after protamine (min)
<30	1	15
30-60	0.5-0.75	15
61-120	0.375-0.5	15
>120	0.25-0.375	15

ALT: alanine aminotransferase; aPTT: activated partial thromboplastin time; CBC: complete blood count; IM: intramuscular; IV: intravenous, LMWH: low-molecular-weight heparin; PE: pulmonary embolus; PT: prothrombin time. Adapted from the Protocol for Heparin Therapy, Hospital for Sick Children, Toronto, Canada, 1995.

Table 22.13 Recommendations for low molecular weight heparin (LMWH) therapy in neonates

Pretreatment laboratory testing:

    CBC with platelets, aPTT, PT with international normalized ratio

    ALT, AST, bilirubin total and direct, serum creatinine

Recommended therapeutic target range: 0.5–1.0 antifactor Xa u/ml

Therapeutic dosing

    Enoxaparirin

        <2 mo of age: 1.5 mg/kg q 12 hours

        >2 mo of age: 1.0 mg/kg q 12 hours

   Reviparin

        <2 mo of age: 150 u/kg q 12 hours

        >2 mo of age: 100 u/kg q 12 hours

Anti-Xa u/mL	Percent of prior dose	Repeat anti-Xa
<0.35	125	4 hours after next dose
0.35-0.49	110	4 hours after next dose
0.5-1.0	Same dose (100)	Next day
1.1-1.5	80	4 hours after dose
1.6-2.0	70	4 hours after dose
>2.0	Hold until anti–Xa < 0.5 u/ml, then 40	4 hours after dose

Laboratory monitoring

    Draw anti-Xa level 4 hours after dose given

    When anti-Xa level is 0.5–1.0 u/ml, repeat next day, then 1 week later and monthly after

Alt: alanine aminotransferase; AST: aspartate aminotransferase; aPTT: activated partial thromboplastin time; CBC: complete blood count; SQ: subcutaneous. Adapted from Lilleyman J et al (eds): Throboembolic Complications in Pediatric Hematology. 2nd ed. *New York, Churchill Livingstone,* 1999.

Renal Vein Thrombosis (RVT)

Approximately two-thirds to three-fourths of the reported cases are in the neonatal period. It may be unilateral or bilateral. The classic triad of hematuria, enlarged kidney(s) and thrombocytopenia is highly suggestive of RVT, but is not always present. The diagnosis is confirmed either by venography or ultrasonography[1-4]. Treatment comprises of adequate hydration, partial exchange transfusion for polycythemia and supportive measures (e.g., peritoneal dialysis). The role of heparin therapy and thrombolytic therapy awaits adequate future evlauation[121,125,126]. Nephrectomy during the acute phase of RVT has been abandoned.

Thrombosis Associated with Alteration in Blood Coagulation and Fibrinolysis[1-4, 122, 127, 138-144]

In keeping with Virchow's hypothesis, hypercoagulability and/or hypofibrinolysis would also predispose the newborn infant to thrombotic diseases. Both hereditary homozygous protein C deficiency and antithrombin III deficiency have lead to serious thromboembolic phenomenon including death in the newborn period. Plasma elimination of coagulation factors and inhibitors such as fibrinogen and antithrombin III are enhanced in neonates. Whether these findings are responsible for more rapid activation and consumption of these factors in the coagulation process is not yet known.

In the *management* of these patients, one should anticipate and prevent thromboembolism[1,7,9]. Prior to definitive therapy, the site and extent of thrombi should be delineated by contrast angiography and/or real-time 2-D ultrasound. Recommendations for treatment includes heparin as the drug of choice in mild to moderate vessel occlusion in doses of 5 to 10 u/kg/hr or less and supportive therapy[125, 126]. In severe disease, with critical impairment of blood flow, thrombolytic drugs, preferably urokinase may be used, even though

Table 22.14 Recommendations for warfarin therapy in neonates

Pretreatment laboratory testing

    CBC with platelets, aPTT, PT with international normalized ratio (INR)

    ALT, AST, bilirubin total and direct

Recommended target ranges for INR

    2.0"3.0, usual range 2.5"3.5, mechanical heart valves

Loading period

Lasts 3"5 days, or until a stable, therapeutic drug level is achieved

Begins 1"2 days after initiation of heparin therapy (for extensive DVT or pulmonary embolus, begin at day 5 of heparin therapy)

Dose on day 1: 0.2 mg/kg PO single daily dose, maximum 10 mg

    Fontan procedure patients: 0.1 mg/kg, maximum 5 mg

    Reduce loading dose if hepatic or renal dysfunction present or baseline INR > 1.2

    Monitor closely if potential for drug interactions exists

    Consider amount of vitamin K in diet and supplements

Warfarin dose adjustments during loading period*	
INR	**Percent of loading dose to be given**
1.1-13	100

Warfarin dose adjustments during maintenance period*	
INR	**Percent of previous dose to be given**
1.1-1.4	120
1.5-1.9	110
2.0-3.0	100
3.1-4.0	90
4.1-4.5	80
>4.5	Hold until INR < 4.5, then restart at 80

*Daily PO dose based on INR results.

Discontinue heparin 5 days after initiation of warfarin and when INR > 2.0 daily x 2.

Laboratory monitoring

    Daily INR until therapeutic level reached on 2 consecutive days

    INR weekly if stable; may require more frequent testing

Warfarin antidote

No bleeding; vitamin K_1

    Rapid reversal and anticipate warfarin treatment in future: 0.5-1 mg

    Rapid reversal and no future need for warfarin: 2 mg

Clinically significant bleeding: 2"5 mg vitamin K_1 IV over 10"20 min and fresh frozen plasma (20 u/kg) or factor IX concentrate containing other vitamin K"dependent factors (50 u/kg)

INR	Percent of loading dose to be given
1.1-13	100
1.4-3.0	50
3.1-4.0	25
>4.0	Hold until INR < 4.5, then restart at 50

*Daily PO dose based on INR results.Discontinue heparin 5 days after initiation of warfarin and when INR > 2.0 daily x 2.

DVT: deep vein thrombosis; IV: intravenous; SQ: subcutaneous. Adapted from the Protocol for Coumadin Therapy, Hospital for Sick Children, Toronto, Canada, 1995.

failure due to this therapy has been reported. Thrombolytic therapy with urokinase and recombinant tissue plasminogen (r-tPA) is listed in Table 22.15. The loading dose of urokinase is 4400 u/kg given intravenously over 10 minutes by constant infusion pump; maintenance therapy is initiated by a constant infusion of 4400 u/kg/hr, but should be adjusted until dissolution of the clot and/ or improved perfusion of the affected vessel is demonstrable[1, 130]. If impending gangrene is suspected, one may consider surgical removal of thrombi by a surgeon experienced in microvascular surgery[1, 7, 115].

When central venous catheters, e.g., Broviac are blocked, tPA may be used as outlined in Table 9.16. If umbilical venous or arterial catheters are blocked, they should be removed immediately.

SUMMARY AND CONCLUSIONS

Thrombocytopenia or alterations in coagulation factors occur frequently in the neonatal period. In some infants, this would manifest as either localized or generalized bleeding and/or thromboembolic phenomena. The physician taking care of such infants should quickly determine if the infant is well or sick, and undertake relevant history and physical examination as outlined previously. Three laboratory tests, *PT*, *aPTT* and platelet count are done to screen bleeding disorders encountered at this age.

Management of such patients comprises of anticipation and prevention of bleeding and/or thromboembolism in sick neonates. Whenever feasible, the physician must administer specific therapy for the underlying disorder that may be causing bleeding or thrombosis (e.g. septicemia, removal of vascular catheters, shock, hypoxia or

Table 22.16 Protocol for tPA use in blocked catheters
Instill tPA (2 mg/ml) into catheter; volume of tPA should be based on catheter type
Infant Broviac: 0.5 ml
Single-lumen Broviac: 1 ml
Double-lumen Broviac: 1.5 ml each lumen
Port-a-Cath: 2 ml
Allow the drug to dwell for 2 hours. At the end of 2 hours, the drug should be withdrawn.
This process may be repeated one additional time if needed.
tPA: tissue plasminogen activator.

Section 3

Table 22.15 Thrombolytic therapy						
Anti-coagulation	Loading dose	Continuous infusion	Pretreatment duration	Monitoring tests	Reversal tests	Agents
Urokinase	4400 u/kg	4400 u/kg/h	Up to 48 h or until clot lysis	CBC, platelets, PT, PTT, fibrinogen, FDP, cranial ultrasound	Fibrinogen, FDP, clot imaging*†	Fresh-frozen plasma, cryoprecipitate
Recombinant tissue Plasminogen activator (r-tPA)	0.5 mg/kg	0.04-0.5 mg/kg/h	48-72 h or until clot lysis If no response, consider concurrent plasminogen therapy	CBC, platelets, PT, PTT, fibrinogen, FDP, cranial ultrasound	Fibrinogen, FDP, clot imaging‡	Fresh-frozen plasma, cryoprecipitate

*Schmidt B, Andrew M: Report of Scientific and Standardization Subcommittee on Neonatal Hemostasis. Diagnosis and treatment of neonatal thrombosis. *Thromb Haemost* 67:381, 1992.

†Local treatment: Corrigan JJ: Neonatal thrombosis and the thrombolytic system: Pathophysiology and therapy. *Am J Pediatr Hematol Oncol* 10:83, 1988.

‡Dillon PW, *et al:* Recombinant tissue plasminogen activator for neonatal and pediatric vascular thrombolytic therapy.

CBC, complete blood count; FDP: fibrin degradation product; plts: platelets; PT: prothrombin time; PTT: partial thromboplastin time.

acidosis) along with prudent blood product replacement and other therapy to rapidly correct clinically significant bleeding. One should not be too eager to correct laboratory abnormalities in a patient without significant bleeding because of the dangers associated with transfusion of blood products. Informed consent must be obtained prior to administration of blood products unless the clinical condition is life-threatening.

REFERENCES

1.   Monagle P, Andrew M. Developmental hemostasis: Relevance to newborns and infants. In: Nathan and Oski's Hematology of Infancy and Childhood, 6th Edition Vol. 1; 2003, *Saunders Co., Philadelphia,* PA pp 121-168

2.   Nathan DG and Oski SH (Ed.). In: Hematology of Infancy and Childhood, *W.B. Saunders* Co. 1998; 5th edition, vol. 2, pp 1509-1717.

3.   Buchanan GR. Hemorrhagic diseases. In. Hematology of Infancy and Childhood, Nathan DG and Oski FA (eds). 3rd edition, *WB Saunders Co., Philadelphia* 1987; pp 104-127.

4.   Rosenberg RD. Physiology and diseases of coagulation: The fluid phase, In Hematology of Infancy and Childhood, Nathan DG and Oski FA (eds). 3rd ed, *WB Saunders Co., Philadelphia,* 1987; pp 1248.

5.   Stuart MJ, Kelton JG. The platelet: Quantitative and qualitative abnormalities. In: Hematology of Infancy and Childhood. Nathan DG and Oski FA (eds). 3rd ed, *WB Saunders Co, Philadelphia* 1987; pp 1343.

6.   Buchanan GR. Coagulation disorders in the neonate. *Pediatr Clin N Am* 1986; 333:203.

7.   Pramanik AK. Bleeding disorders in neonates. *Pediatr in Rev* 1992; 13:163.

8.   McMillan CW and Hilgartner S. Platelet and vascular disorders and coagulation disorders. In: Blood Diseases in Infancy and Childhood. Miller DP (ed), 3rd ed; *CV Mosby Co., St. Louis,* 1984; pp 784.

9.   Oski FA and Naiman JL (eds). Blood coagulation and its disorders in the newborn, and disorders of platelets. In: Hematologic Problems in the Newborn, 3rd ed. *WB Saunders Co., Philadelphia,* 1982; pp 137.

10. Schmidt B and Zipursky A. Thrombotic diseases in newborn infants. *Clin Perinatol* 1984; 11:461.

11. Schmidt B, Andrew M. Neonatal thrombotic disease: Prevention, diagnosis and therapy. *J Pediatr* 1988; 113:407.

12. Schmidt B, Andrew M. Neonatal thrombosis: Report of a prospective Canadian and international registry. *Pediatrics* 1995; 96:5:939-943.

13. Apt L, and Downey WS Jr., Melena neonatorum: The swallowed blood syndrome; A simple test for differentiation of adult and fetal hemoglobin in bloody stools. *J Pediatr* 1955; 47:6.

14. Aster RH. Gestational thrombocytopenia. A plea for conservative management. *N Engl J Med* 1990; 323:264-266.

15. Poley JR, Stickler GB. Petechiae in the newborn infant. *Am J Dis Child* 1961; 102:111.

16. M Andrew, B Paes, R Milner, *et al.* Development of the human coagulation system in the full-term infant. *Blood* 1987; 70:165-172.

17. Andrew M, Paes B, Milner R, *et al.* Development of the human coagulation system in the healthy premature infant. *Blood* 1988; 72:5:1651-1657.

18. Smith PS. Congenital coagulation protein deficiencies in the perinatal period. *Semin Perinatol* 1990; 14:384.

19. Barnard DR. Inherited bleeding disorders in the newborn infant. *Clin Perinatol* 1984; 11:309.

20. Lietman PS, McDonald MM, Hathaway WE. Anticoagulant therapy by continuous heparinization in newborn and older infants. *J Pediatr* 1982; 101:3:451-457.

21. Corrigan JJ Jr, Sleeth JJ, Jeter M, *et al.* Newborn's fibrinolytic mechanism: components and plasmin generation. *Am J Hematol* 1989; 32; 273-278.

22. Corrigan JJ Jr. Neonatal thrombosis and thrombolytic system: Pathophysiology and therapy. *Am J Pediatric Hematol Oncol* 1988; 10:83-91.

23. Cade JF, Hirsh J, and Martin M. Placental barrier to coagulation factors: Its relevance to the coagulation defect at birth and to hemorrhage in the newborn. *Brit Med J* 1969; 2:281.

24. Andrew M, Bhogal M, Karpatkin M, *et al.* Factors XI and XII and prekallikrein in sick and healthy premature infants. *N Engl J Med* 1981; 305:1130.

25. Forestier F, Daffos F, Galacteros F, *et al.* Hematological values of 163 normal fetuses between 18 and 30 weeks of gestation. *Pediatr Res* 1986; 20:342-346.

26. Bernard DR, Simmons MA. Physiologic coagulation studies in infants 24-31 week's gestation. *Pediatr Res* 1978; 12:466.

27. Barry A and Delage JM. Congenital deficiency of fibrin stabilizing factor. *N Engl J Med* 1965; 272:943.

28. Karpatkin M, Mannucci P, Bhogal M, *et al.* Low protein C in the neonatal period. *Br J Haematol* 1986; 62:137-142.

29. Male C, Johnston M, Sparling C, *et al.* The influence of developmental haemostasis on the laboratory diagnosis and management of haemostatic disorders during infancy and childhood. *Clin Lab Med* 1999; 19(1):39-69.

30. Chessels JM and Wigglesworth JS. Coagulation studies in severe birth asphyxia. *Arch Dis Child* 1971; 46:253.

31. Marlar RA, Neumann A. Neonatal purpura fulminans due to homozygous protein C or protein S deficiencies. *Semin Thromb Hemost* 1990; 16:299.

32. McNinch AW, Orme RLE, Tripp JH, *et al*. Hemorrhagic disease of the newborn returns. *Lancet* 1983; 1:1089.

33. Dube B, Bhargava V, Dube RK, *et al*. Disseminated intravascular coagulation in neonatal period. *Indian Pediatr* 1986; 23:925-931.

34. Boyd JF. Disseminated fibrin thromboembolism among neonates dying with 48 hours of birth. *Arch Dis Child* 1967; 42:401.

35. Andrew M and Kelton J. Neonatal thrombocytopenia. *Clin Perinatol* 1984; 11:359.

36. Mehta P, Vasa R, Neumann L, *et al*. Thrombocytopenia in the high-risk infant *J Pediatr* 1980; 97:791-794.

37. Ballmaier M, Schulze H, Cremer M, *et al*. Defective c-Mpl signaling in the syndrome of thrombocytopenia with absent radii. *Stem Cells* 1998; 16 Suppl 2:177-84.

38. Ballmaier M, Germeshausen M, Schulze H, *et al*. C-mpl mutations are the cause of congenital amegakaryocytic thrombocytopenia. *Blood* 2001; 97:1:139-146.

39. Kletzel M, Miller CH, Becton DL, *et al*. Post-delivery head bleeding in hemophiliac neonates. *Am J Dis Child* 1989; 143:1107.

40. Kulkarni R, Lusher JM. Intracranial and extracranial hemorrhages in newborns with hemophilia: A review of the literature. *J Pediatr Hematol Oncol* 1999; 21:4:289-295.

41. Michaud JL, Rivard GE, Chessex P. Intracranial hemorrhage in a newborn with hemophilia following elective cesarean section. *Am J Pediatr Hematol Oncol* 1991; 13:473.

42. Salooja N, Martin P, Khair K, *et al*. Severe factor V deficiency and neonatal intracranial hemorrhage: A case report. *Hemophilia* 2000; 6: 44-46.

43. Viola L, Chiaretti A, Lazzareschi I, *et al*. Intracranial hemorrhage in congenital factor II deficiency. *Pediatr Med Chir* 1995; 17:593-594.

44. Machin SJ, Winter MR, Davie SC, *et al*. Factor X deficiency in the neonatal period. *Arch Dis Child* 1980; 55:406-408.

45. Andrew M and Karpatkin M. A simple screening test for evaluating prolonged partial thromboplastin time in newborn infants. *J Pediatr* 1982; 101:610.

46. Cook RL, Miller RC, Katz VL, *et al*. Immune thrombocytopenic purpura in pregnancy: A reappraisal of management. *Obstet Gynecol* 1991; 78:578.

47. Stuart J, Breeze GR, Picken AM, *et al*. Capillary-blood coagulation profile in the newborn. *Lancet* 1973; pp 1467-1471.

48. Bussel J, Kaplan C, McFarland J. Recommendations for the evaluation and treatment of neonatal autoimmune and alloimmune thrombocytopenia. *Thromb Haemost* 1991; 65:631-634.

49. Chong BH. Diagnosis, treatment and pathophysiology of autoimmune thrombocytopenias. *Crit Rev Onc Hematol* 1995; 20:271.

50. George JN, Woolf SH, Raskob GE, *et al*. Idiopathic thrombocytopenic purpura: A Practice Guideline Developed by Explicit Methods for the American Society of Hematology. *Blood* 1996; 88:3-40.

51. Karpatkin M, Porges RF, Karpatkin S, *et al*. Platelet counts in infants of women with autoimmune thrombocytopenia: Effects of steroid administration to the mother. *N Engl J Med* 1981; 305:936.

52. Kaplan C. Immune thrombocytopenia in the fetus and the newborn: diagnosis and therapy. *Transfus Clin Biol* 2001; 8(3):311-314.

53. Stuart MJ, Gross SJ, Elrad H, *et al*. Effects of acetylsalicylic acid ingestion on maternal and neonatal hemostasis. *N Engl J Med* 1982; 307:909-912.

54. Gersony WM, Peckham GJ, Ellision RC, *et al*. Effects of indomethacin in premature infants with patent ductus arteriosus: Results of a national collaborative study. *J Pediatr* 1983; 102:895.

55. Corrazza MS, Davis RF, *et al*. Prolonged bleeding time in preterm infants receiving indomethacin for patent ductus arteriosus. *J Pediatr* 1984; 105:292.

56. Carcao, Blanchette, Dean, *et al*. The Platelet Function Analyzer (PFA-100®): A novel in-vitro system for evaluation of primary haemostasis in children. *Br J Haematol* 1998; 101:70-73.

57. Cariappa R, Wilhite T, Parvin, C, *et al*. Comparison of PFA-100 and bleeding time testing in pediatric patients with suspected hemorrhagic problems. *J Pediatr Hematol Oncol* 2003; 25:6:474-479.

58. Horgan MJ, Bartoletti A, Polansky S, *et al*. Effect of heparin infusates in umbilical arterial catheters on frequency of thrombotic complications. *J Pediatr* 1987; 111:5:774-778.

59. Johnson CA, Synder MS, Weaver RL, *et al*. Effects of fresh frozen plasma infusions on coagulation screening tests in neonates. *Arch Dis Child* 1982; 57:950.

60. Manco-Johnson MJ, Martar RA, Jacobson LJ, *et al*. Severe protein C deficiency in newborn infants. *J Pediatr* 1988; 113:2:359-363.

61. Zach TL, Cifuentes RF, Strom RL. Congenital mesoblastic nephroma, hemorrhagic shock, and disseminated intravascular coagulation in a newborn infant. *Am J Perinatol* 1991; 8:203-205.

62. Lynn JN, Pauly TH, Desai NS. Purpura fulminans in three cases of early-onset neonatal group B streptococcal meningitis. *J Perinatol* 1991; aa:44-146.

63. Adcock DM, Bronza J, Marlar RA. Proposed classification and pathologic mechanisms of purpura

fulminans and skin necrosis. *Semin Thromb Hemost* 1990; 16:333-340.

64. Hanna BD, Berstein M. Tranexamic acid in the treatment of Kasabach-Merritt syndrome in infants. *Amer J Pediatr Hematol and Oncol* 1989; 11:191-195.

65. Dreese MG, David M, Hume H, *et al*. Successful treatment of Kasabach-Merritt syndrome with prednisone and epsilon-aminocaproic acid. *Pediatr Hematol and Oncol* 1991; 8:329-334.

66. Gross S and Melhorn DK. Exchange transfusion with citrated whole blood for disseminated intravascular coagulation. *J Pediatr* 1971; 78:415.

67. Gross SJ, Filston HC, Anderson JC, *et al*. Controlled study of treatment of disseminated intravascular coagulation in the neonate. *J Pediatr* 1982; 100:445.

68. Schmidt BK, Muraji T, Zipursky A. Low antithrombin III in neonatal shock: DIC or non-specific protein depletion? *Eur J Pediatr* 1986; 145:500.

69. Lane PA and Hathaway WE. Vitamin K in infancy. *J Pediatr* 1985; 106:351.

70. Kotohara K, Endo F. Effect of vitamin K administration of a carboxy prothrombin (PIVKA-II) levels in newborns. *Lancet* 1985; 2:243.

71. Greer FR, Marshall S, *et al*. Vitamin K status of lactating mothers, human milk, and breast-feeding infants. *Pediatrics* 1991; 88:751.

72. American Academy of Pediatrics Committee on Fetus and Newborn: Controversies concerning vitamin K and the newborn. *Pediatrics* 2003; 112:1:191-192.

73. Malia RG, Preston FE, Mitchell VE, *et al*. Evidence against vitamin K deficiency in normal neonates. *Thromb Haemost* 1980; 44:159.

74. Shearer MJ, Rahim S, Barkhan P, *et al*. Plasma vitamin K in mothers and their newborn babies. *Lancet* 1982; 2:460.

75. Chaou WT, Chou ML, Eitzman DV. Intracranial hemorrhage and vitamin K deficiency in early infancy. *J Pediatr* 1984; 105:6:880-884.

76. Bleyer WA and Skinner AL. Fatal neonatal hemorrhage after maternal anticonvulsant therapy. *JAMA* 1976; 235:626.

77. Bonnar J. Warfarin anticoagulation and pregnancy. *Lancet* 1971; 1:862.

78. Blanchard RA, Furie BC. Subclinical vitamin K-deficiency in newborns and their mothers. *Blood* 1983; 62 (suppl.1):994.

79. Solves P, Altes A, Ginovart G, *et al*. Late hemorrhagic disease of the newborn as a cause of intracerebral bleeding. *Ann Hematol* 1997; 75:65-66.

80. Hathaway W, Isarangkura P, Mahasandana C, *et al*. Comparison of oral and parenteral vitamin K prophylaxis for prevention of late hemorrhagic disease of the newborn. *J Pediatr* 1991; 119:461-464.

81. Sutor A. Vitamin K deficiency bleeding in infants and children. *Semin Thromb Haemost* 1995; 21(3):317-329.

82. Anai T, Hirota Y, Yoshimatsu J, *et al*. Can prenatal vitamin K1 (phylloquinone) supplementation replace prophylaxis at birth? *Obstet Gynecol* 1993; 81:251.

83. Thorp JA, Parriott J, Ferrette-Smith D, *et al*. Antepartum vitamin K and phenobarbital for preventing intraventricular hemorrhage in the premature newborn: a randomized, double-blind, placebo-controlled trial. *Obstet Gynecol* 1994; 83(1):70-76.

84. Brousson MA, Klein MC. Controversies surrounding the administration of vitamin K to newborns: A review. *CMAJ* 1996; 154:307-315.

85. von Kries R, Hanawa Y. Neonatal vitamin K prophylaxis: Report of Scientific and Standardization Subcommittee on Perinatal Hemostasis. *Thromb Haemost* 1993; 69:293.

86. Chuansumrit A, Chantarojanasiri T, Isarangkura P, *et al*. Recombinant activated factor VII in children with acute bleeding resulting from liver failure and disseminated intravascular coagulation. *Blood Coagul Fibrinolysis* 2000; 11 Suppl 1: S101-105.

87. Chuansumrit A, Treepongkaruna S, Phuapradit P, *et al*. Combined fresh frozen plasma with recombinant factor VIIa in restoring hemostasis for invasive procedures in children with liver diseases. *Thromb Haemost* 2001; 85:748-749.

88. Albert T, Meng Y., Simms P, *et al*. Thrombopoietin in the thrombocytopenic term and preterm newborn. *Pediatrics* 2000; 105:6:1286-1291.

89. Samuels P, Bussel JB, Braitman LE, *et al*. Estimation of the risk of thrombocytopenia in the offspring of pregnant women with presumed immune thrombocytopenic purpura. *N Engl J Med* 1990; 323:229-235.

90. Roberts I, Murray N. Management of thrombocytopenia in neonates. *Br J Haematol* 1999; 105:4:864-870.

91. Salonvaara M, Riikonen P, Kekomäki R, *et al*. Clinically symptomatic central venous catheter-related deep venous thrombosis in newborns. *Acta Paediatr* 1999; 88:642-646.

92. Scott JR, Cruikshank DP, Kochenour NK, *et al*. Fetal platelet counts in the obstetric management of immunologic thrombocytopenic purpura. *Am J Obstet Gynecol* 1980; 136:495.

93. Karpatkin M. Corticosteroid therapy in thrombocytopenic infants of women with autoimmune thrombocytopenia. *J Pediatr* 1984; 105:623.

94. Adner MM, Fisch FR, Starobin SG, *et al*. Use of "compatible" platelet transfusions in treatment of congenital isoimmune thrombocytopenic purpura. *N Engl J Med* 1969; 280:244.

95. Kurtzberg J, Dunsmore K. IVIG therapy in neonatal isoimmune thrombocytopenic purpura and

alloimmunization thrombocytopenia.. In: *IVIG Therapy Today*, Ballow M (ed). *The Humana Press Inc., Totowa, NJ* 1992; pp 73.

96. McIntosh S, O'Brien RT, Schwartz AD, *et al*. Neonatal isoimmune purpura: Response to platelet infusions. *J Pediatr* 1973; 82:1020.

97. Baehner RL and Strauss HS. Hemophilia in the first year of life. *N Engl J Med* 1966; 275:524.

98. Lijung R, Petrini P, Nilsson IM. Diagnostic symptoms of severe and moderate hemophlia A and B. A survey of 140 cases. *Acta Pediatr Scand* 1990; 79:196-200.

99. Lusher JM, Warrier I: Hemophilia. *Pediatrics in Review* 1991; 12:9:275-281.

100. Schinaia N, Ghirardini A, Chiarotti F, *et al*. Progression to AIDS among Italian HIV-seropositive hemophiliacs. *AIDS* 1991; 5:385-391.

101. Williams AE, Sullivan MT. Transfusion-transmitted retrovirus infection. *Hematol Oncol Clin North Am* 1995; 9:1:115-136.

102. Evans JA, Pasi KJ, Williams MD, *et al*. Consistently normal CD4+ CD8+ levels in hemophilic boys only treated with a virally safe factor VIII concentrate (BPL 8Y). *Brit J Haematol* 1991; 79:457.

103. Williamson LM, Allain JP. Virally inactivated fresh frozen plasma. *Vox Sang* 1995; 69(3):159-165.

104. Ehrenforth S, Klarmann D, Zabel B, *et al*. Severe factor V deficiency presenting as subdural hematoma in the newborn. *Eur J Pediatr* 1998; 157:1032.

105. Kalla S, Menon NS. Neonatal congenital factor X deficiency. *Pediatr Hematol Oncol* 1991; 8:347-354.

106. Kitchens CS. Factor XI: A review of its biochemistry and deficiency. *Semin Thromb Haemost* 1991; 17:55.

107. Kashyap R, Saxena R, Chaudhry VP. Rare inherited coagulation disorders in India. *Hematologia* (Budap) 1996; 28:13-19.

108. Koster T, Andrew D, Briët E, *et al*. Role of clotting factor VIII in effect of von Willebrand factor on occurrence of deep-vein thrombosis. *Lancet* 1995; 345:152-155.

109. Bhettay E and Jacobs ME. Peripheral gangrene in the newborn. *Clin Pediatr* 1977; 16:573.

110. Bertina RM: Molecular risk factors for thrombosis: *Thromb Haemost* 1999; 82(2):601-609.

111. David M, Andrew M. Venous thromboembolic complications in children. *J Pediatr* 1993; 123:337.

112. Nowak-Gottl U, Dübbers A, Kececioglu D, *et al*. Factor V Leiden, protein C, and lipoprotein(a) in catheter-related thrombosis in childhood: A prospective study. *J Pediatr* 1997; 131:4:608-612.

113. Peters M, Ten Cate JW, Breederveld C, *et al*. Low antithrombin III levels in neonates with idiopathic respiratory distress syndrome: Poor prognosis. *Pediatr Res* 1984; 18:273.

114. Peters M, ten Cate JW, Koo LH, *et al*. Persistent antithrombin III deficiency: Risk factor for thromboembolic complications in neonates small-for-gestational age. *J Pediatr* 1984; 105:310.

115. Corrigan JJ Jr, Jeter M, Allen HD, *et al*. Aortic thrombosis in a neonate: Failure of urokinase thrombolytic therapy. *Am J Pediatr Hematol Oncol* 1982; 4:243.

116. Dahlback B, Carlsson M, and Svensson PJ. Familial thrombophilia due to a previously unrecognized mechanism characterized by poor anticoagulant response to activated protein C: Prediction of a cofactor to activated protein C. *Proc Natl Acad Sci USA* 1993; 90:1004-1008.

117. De Stefano V, *et al*. Antithrombin III in full-term and pre-term newborn infants: Three cases of neonatal diagnosis of AT III congenital defect. *Thromb Haemost* 1987; 57(3):329-331.

118. Rais-Bahrami K, Barry D, Naqvi M, *et al*. Thrombosis of the left heart in a newborn. *Clin Pediatr* 1992; 31:508.

119. Sills RH, Marlar RA, Montgomery RR, *et al*. Severe Homozygous protein C deficiency. *J Pediatr* 1984; 105:409.

120. Manco-Johnson MJ, Abshire TC, Jacobson LJ, *et al*. Severe neonatal protein C deficiency: Prevalence and thrombotic risk. *J Pediatr* 1991; 119:793.

121. Schmidt B, Andrew M. Report of Scientific and Standardization Subcommittee on Neonatal Hemostasis. Diagnosis and treatment of neonatal thrombosis. *Thrombosis and Haemostasis* 1992; 67(3):381-382.

122. Miletich J, Sherman L, Broze G. Absence of thrombosis in subjects with heterozygous protein C deficiency. *N Engl J Med* 1987; 317:16:991-996.

123. Hall RT, Rhodes PG, Turner EA, *et al*. Protamine sulfate titration for heparin activity in neonates with indwelling umbilical catheters. *J Pediatr* 1976; 88:467.

124. Marder VJ, Sherry S. Thrombolytic therapy: Current status. *N Engl J Med* 1988; 318:23:1512-1520 (part 1); and 1988; 318:24:1585-1595(part 2).

125. Shiozaki A, Arai T, *et al*. Congenital antithrombin III–deficient neonate treated with antithrombin III concentrates. *Thromb Res* 1993; 70:211.

126. Svensson PJ, Dahlback B. Resistance to activated protein C as a basis for venous thrombosis. *N Engl J Med* 1994; 330:517-522.

127. Massicotte P, Adams M, Marzinotto V, *et al*. Low molecular-weight heparin in pediatric patients with thrombotic disease: A dose finding study. *J Pediatr* 1996; 128:3:313-318.

128. Dix D, Andrew M, Marzinotto V, *et al*. The use of low molecular weight heparin in pediatric patients: A prospective cohort study [see comments]. *J Pediatr* 2000; 136:4:439-445.

129. Hirsh J, Levine MN. Low molecular weight heparin. *Blood* 1992; 79: 1-17.

130. Delaplane D, Scott JP, Silverman BL, *et al*. Urokinase therapy for a catheter-related right atrial thrombus. *J Pediatr* 1982; 100:149.

131. Dreyfus M, Magny JF, Bridey F, *et al*. Treatment of homozygous protein C deficiency and neonatal purpura fulminans with a purified protein C concentrate. *N Engl J Med* 1991: 325:1565.

132. Petrini P, Segnestam K, Ekelund H, *et al*. Homozygous protein C deficiency in two siblings. *Pediatr Hematol Oncol* 1990; 7(2):165-175.

133. Marlar RA, Montgomery RR, Broekmans AW. Diagnosis and treatment of homozygous protein C deficiency: Report of the working party on homozygous protein C deficiency of the subcommittee on protein C and protein S, international committee on thrombosis and haemostasis. *J Pediatr* 1989; 114:528.

134. Ettingshausen Ce, Veldmann A, Beeg T, *et al*. Replacement therapy with protein C concentrates in infants and adolescents with meningococcal sepsis and purpura fulminans. *Semin Thromb Hemost* 1999; 25:537-541.

135. Malin SW, Baumgart S. Nonsurgical management of obstructive aortic thrombosis complicated by renovascular hypertension in the neonatae *J Pediatr* 1985;106:630.

136. Andrew M, Marzinotto V, Brooker LA, *et al*. Oral anticoagulation therapy in pediatric patients: A prospective study. *Thromb Haemost* 1994; 71:265.

137. Streif W, Andrew M, Marzinotto V, *et al*. Analysis of warfarin therapy in pediatric patients: A prospective cohort study of 319 patients. *Blood* 1999; 94:3007-3014.

138. Hagstrom JN, Walter J, Bluebond-Langner R, *et al*. Prevalence of the factor V leiden mutation in children and neonates with thromboembolic disease. *J Pediatr* 1998; 133:6:777-781.

139. Mokrohisky ST, Levine RL, Blumhagen JD, *et al*. Low positioning of umbilical artery catheters increases associated complications in newborn infants. *N Engl J Med* 1978; 299:561

140. Zriek H, Bengur AR, Meliones JN, *et al*. Superior vena cava obstruction after extracorporeal membrane oxygenation. *J Pediatr* 1995; 127: 314.

141. Vailas GN, Brouillette RT, Scott JP, *et al*. Neonatal aortic thrombosis: Recent experience. *J Pediatr* 1986; 109(1):101-108.

142. Umbilical Artery Catheter Trial Study Group (Malloy M, Cutter G, Pramanik AK, *et al*). The relationship of intraventricular hemorrhage or death with the level of umbilical artery catheter placement: A multicenter randomized clinical trial. *Pediatrics* 1992; 90:881.

143. Spadone D, Clark F, *et al*. Heparin-induced thrombocytopenia in the newborn. *J Vasc Surg* 1992; 15:306.

144. Ambrus CM, Ambrus JL, Choi T, *et al*. The fibrinolysin system and its relationship to disease in the newborn. *Am J Pediatr Hematol Oncol* 1979; 1:251.

Section 3

Neonatal Seizures

Sourabh Dutta and GCM Pradeep

A seizure is clinically defined as a paroxysmal alteration in the neurologic function i.e. behavioral, motor or autonomic dysfunction. Seizures represent the most distinctive signal of neurologic disease in the newborn period. It is critical to recognize neonatal seizures, determine their etiology and treat them effectively. The exact incidence of seizures is difficult to delineate but it ranges from 0.5% in term babies to 20% in preterms.

PATHOPHYSIOLOGY

A seizure results when there is an excessive synchronous electrical discharge i.e. depolarization of neurons within the central nervous system. Although the fundamental mechanism of neonatal seizures is generally unknown, current data suggest that excessive depolarization may result due to following reasons[1].

(i)   Disturbance in energy production resulting in failure of sodium-potassium pump.

(ii) Relative excess of excitatory (glutamate) versus inhibitory neurotransmitters resulting in an excessive rate of depolarization.

(iii) Relative deficiency of the inhibitory (GABA) amino acids can result in an excessive rate of depolarization.

CLASSIFICATION

Four essential types of seizures can be recognized in neonates and within each type the seizures can be unifocal, multifocal or generalized. In many cases, more than one type of seizure occurs in a newborn baby over a period of time. The peculiar clinical characteristics of seizures in the newborn infant reflect the immature state of brain development. The relative underdeveloped organization of the cortex and undermyelination of axons usually underlies the disorganized convulsive activity and lack of orderly seizure propagation in the newborn period. For the same reason classic generalized "tonic-clonic" seizures are very rare in babies, in whom there is an additional problem of electro clinical dissociation.

Subtle seizures[2, 3]

Subtle seizures are the most common subtype, comprising about one-half of all seizures in term and premature newborns. Subtle seizures are rarely isolated and infants with subtle seizures will almost always have other seizure types as well. Subtle seizures include a broad spectrum of behavioral phenomena, occurring in isolation or in combination. Most common manifestations of subtle seizures in both term and preterm infants are ocular phenomenon. This includes tonic eye deviation, roving "nystagmoid" eye movements and sustained eye opening with apparent visual fixation. Oro-bucco-lingual phenomena includes chewing, sucking, or lip smacking movements and is often associated with a sudden increase in drooling. Various alternating limb movements have been described including pedaling, boxing, rowing, or swimming movements. Autonomic phenomenon, including sudden changes in skin color and capillary size, may occur alone or in combination with various motor manifestations. The frequency with which subtle clinical seizure phenomena are associated with concomitant EEG seizure activity is variable. Therefore, some caution should be used in attributing an epileptic origin to subtle clinical phenomena, particularly when these phenomena are the only manifestation of seizure in the infant.

Apnea can be a manifestation of a subtle seizure although most apneic episodes in preterm infants do not represent seizure activity. Such non-convulsive apnea is usually associated with bradycardia. Convulsive apnea, associated with EEG seizure activity, is more likely in term infants, particularly if the apnea is not accompanied by bradycardia but is associated with other subtle phenomena, such as eye opening, fixed staring, and deviation of eyes.

Clonic seizures

Clonic seizures are stereotypic and repetitive biphasic movements with a fast contraction phase and a slower relaxation phase. The rhythm of clonic seizure tends to be slower in the newborn period. Clonic seizures represent the seizure type associated most consistently with time-synchronised EEG seizure activity. Clonic seizure may be unifocal, multifocal, or generalized. Focal clonic seizure involves the face, upper or lower extremities on one side of the body, or axial structures on one side of the body. Multifocal clonic seizures involve several body parts often in migrating fashion (non-jacksonian manner). Generalized clonic seizures i.e. diffusely bilateral, symmetrical and synchronous movements are rarely if ever observed in the newborn.

Tonic seizures

Tonic seizures have a sustained episodes (seconds) of muscle contraction without repetitive feature. Tonic seizures may be generalized or focal. Latter are much more common than the former. Focal tonic seizures consist of sustained posturing of a limb or asymmetrical posturing of the trunk or neck. Generalized tonic seizures are characterized most commonly by tonic extension of both upper and lower extremities (mimicking "decerebrate" posturing) but also by tonic flexion of upper extremities with extension of lower extremities (mimicking "decorticate" posturing). Majority of these seizures are not usually associated with EEG discharges.

Myoclonic seizures

Myoclonic seizures are clinical episodes that as a group are not associated with time synchronised EEG discharges. Myoclonic movements are distinguished from clonic movements because of the more rapid speed of the myoclonic jerks and their predilection for flexor group of muscles. Three categories of myoclonic seizures are identified; focal, multifocal, and generalized. Myoclonic seizures are associated with diffuse and usually serious brain dysfunction and are likely to have poor long-term outcome.

Paroxysmal non-convulsive phenomena[4]

It may be difficult to distinguish some of the less discernible neonatal seizures from other paroxysmal episodes occurring in the newborn that are non-convulsive in origin. Jitteriness is a common benign neonatal movement disorder characterized by symmetrical tremors of the extremities, sparing the face. The movements are of equal rate and amplitude (clonic and myoclonic seizures have fast and slow components), occurring at a higher frequency than clonic movements (5-6 per second). Jitteriness is generally induced by an external stimulus and ceases with gentle restraint or passive flexion. It occurs in infants without neurological impairment and is not necessarily an abnormal feature. The most commonly identified causes are hypoxic-ischemic encephalopathy, hypoglycemia, hypocalcemia and narcotic withdrawal.

ETIOLOGY[4]

The common causes of neonatal seizures are listed in Table 23.1.

Table 23.1 Common causes of neonatal seizures
• **Hypoxia-ischemia ("asphyxia")**
• **CNS infection**   Meningitis, encephalitis, intrauterine infections
• **Intracranial hemorrhage**   Extradural, subdural, subarachnoid and periventricular hemorrhage (PVH)
• **Cerebral artery infarction**
• **Acute metabolic disturbances**   Hypoglycemia, hypocalcemia, hypomagnesemia, hyper- or hyponatremia (or rapidly changing sodium)
• **Inborn errors of metabolism**   Aminoaciduria, urea cycle defects, organic acidopathies, peroxisomal disorders, pyridoxine dependency
• **CNS malformations**   Cerebral dysgenesis, lissencephaly, and neuronal migration disorders, etc.
• **Maternal drug intoxication**   Cocaine, heroin, opium, methadone, etc.
• **Neonatal drug toxicity**   Theophylline, doxapram, aminofluoroquinolones
• **Benign neonatal seizures**   Benign familial neonatal convulsions (BFNC)   Benign idiopathic neonatal convulsions (BINC, "fifth day fits")   Benign neonatal sleep myoclonus
• **Hypertensive encephalopathy**
• **Neonatal epileptic syndromes**
• **Idiopathic**

Hypoxia-Ischemia

Hypoxic-ischemic (HIE) insults ("asphyxia") account for about 50% of all cases of neonatal seizures. Most asphyxiated infants with seizures have a moderate degree of encephalopathy presenting with subtle, focal, or multifocal fragmentary clonic seizures, usually within the first 24 hours[5]. Myoclonic and tonic seizures can occur in the most severe form of hypoxic-ischemic encephalopathy (HIE) and can be difficult to control pharmacologically. Other insults such as hypoglycemia, hypocalcemia, and subarachnoid hemorrhage may coexist and trigger postasphyxial seizures.

Central Nervous System Infection

Seizures may be the first manifestation of bacterial meningitis, underlining the importance of performing a lumbar puncture after a neonatal seizure. Additional investigations may be required if other CNS infections are suspected, such as herpes simplex encephalitis, and intrauterine infections.

Intracranial Hemorrhage

Subdural and subarachnoid hemorrhage can occur in term infants following birth trauma and may cause seizures independent of any associated asphyxial insult. In preterm infants severe intraventricular hemorrhage, with or without associated parenchymal venous infarction, may be followed within a few hours by generalised tonic seizures. Isolated germinal matrix hemorrhages are unlikely to produce seizures.

Cerebral Artery Infarction

In infants presenting with seizures, whose Apgar score was normal and subsequent investigations failed to reveal an infective or metabolic etiology, a high percentage of ischemic lesions were demonstrated by early magnetic resonance imaging before changes on cranial ultrasound scan became apparent.

Acute Metabolic Disturbances

Hypoglycemia

Hypoglycemia as an isolated cause of convulsions is seen in only 3% of cases, although it occurs frequently in infants with seizures because it coexists with other causes, such as hypoxia-ischemia, infection and inborn errors of metabolism etc[6]. The definition of hypoglycemia is also debated. The level constituting a risk for neurological impairment is variable, depending on the metabolic state of the infant. Nevertheless, when faced with a convulsing infant whose blood glucose is below 40 mg/dl most clinicians would advocate correction of the perceived hypoglycemia.

Hypocalcemia

Hypocalcemia presents typically either within the first 3 days of life or later in the neonatal period. Early-onset hypocalcemia occurs in infants of diabetic mothers, low birthweight infants, after exchange transfusion. Like hypoglycemia, it can also occur in association with other etiologies, particularly hypoxia-ischemia. Thus early-onset hypocalcemia is often associated with neonatal seizures but late onset hypocalcemic convulsions or tetany is now rare. The incidence of late-onset hypocalcemia has fallen due to introduction of low phosphate milk formulae and universal promotion of breast feeding.

Other Causes

Inborn errors of metabolism are a rare cause of neonatal seizures and should be considered when seizures are unresponsive to conventional treatment in neonates with a positive family history, onset of seizures with introduction of milk feeding, acidosis, or distinctive odor.

Pyridoxine dependency is a rare autosomal recessive defect in an enzyme involved in production of the inhibitory neurotransmitter GABA and presents with early-onset intractable seizures. The EEG may show generalised bursts of bilaterally synchronous high voltage 1-4 Hz activity with interspersed spikes, but the diagnosis is established by observing cessation of seizures within minutes of intravenous administration of 50-100 mg pyridoxine (normalisation of the EEG may be more gradual).

Benign familial neonatal convulsions (BFNC) represent a self-limiting (within 1-6 months) autosomal dominant syndrome presenting with clonic seizures on the second or third day of life. The infant has no abnormal neurological signs in the interictal period, investigations reveal no apparent cause, and subsequent development is usually normal[7]. It is related to mutations in the neuronal potassium channels KCNQ2 or KC NQ3[8].

Benign idiopathic neonatal convulsions (BINC or "fifth day fits") are multifocal clonic seizures, with a peak time of onset on the fifth day, and generally ceasing within 15 days. The cause is unknown, although low cerebrospinal fluid zinc concentrations have been described in some cases[9]. The term "fifth day fits" probably represents a meaningless diagnosis and should be avoided.

Benign neonatal sleep myoclonus consists of bilateral, synchronous myoclonic jerks occurring during quiet sleep. Onset is within the first week of life and resolves within two months. The EEG does not show any abnormal activity between or during these episodes. Neurological outcome is normal.

Two rare syndromes, early myoclonic encephalopathy (EME) and early infantile epileptic encephalopathy (EIEE)[10], characteristically present in the first weeks of life with severe recurrent seizures and are associated with inborn errors of metabolism (EME) and structural CNS abnormalities (EIEE). Both lead to severe subsequent neurodevelopmental impairment. During the neonatal period the seizures are fragmentary myoclonic and clonic in EME, and tonic in EIEE, both showing a burst-suppression EEG pattern.

DIAGNOSIS

The initial laboratory tests are directed against the two diseases that are especially dangerous but readily treated when recognized promptly; hypoglycemia and bacterial meningitis. Thus lumbar puncture and blood glucose (dextrostix) determination are performed urgently. In addition, blood should be drawn for determination of sodium, potassium, calcium, phosphorous and magnesium levels. Other metabolic determinations, radiological and imaging studies are guided by specific clinical features.

Imaging Studies

Cranial ultrasound scanning is readily available in most centers and is useful as a first line imaging investigation for exclusion of gross CNS pathology, CNS malformations, and periventricular hemorrhage. But it may fail to detect other forms of clinically important pathology, such as cerebral arterial infarction, subdural and subarachnoid hemorrhage. If the initial ultrasound examination is normal but the infant continues to have seizures or has abnormal interictal neurological signs, a computed tomogram or MRI examination should be carried out. Magnetic resonance imaging provides important information with respect to malformations. For symptomatic seizures due to HIE, abnormal T2, flair and diffusion weighted imaging can pinpoint regional injury and its severity.[11] Magnetic resonance spectroscopy can also predict severity and prognosis. An increased lactate to choline ratio and reduced N-acetyl-aspartate ratios is associated with higher disease severity.[12]

Electroencephalogram

EEG is usually obtained in the interictal period. Tracings obtained during the course of suspected seizures provide useful information regarding the presence of true epileptic phenomenon; however, there is evidence to suggest that some epileptic discharges may not be picked up by surface EEG. The importance and significance of EEG in the evaluation of neonatal seizures is given below:

(i) To help determine whether the infant with subtle clinical phenomena is experiencing an epileptic seizure.

(ii) To determine whether the paralyzed infant is experiencing convulsive phenomena.

(iii) To define the interictal background features, which may provide useful information to assess prognosis.

Delineation of seizure phenomenon by EEG requires awareness of the normal development of the EEG features in the neonate, availability of skilled technicians and experienced interpreters of the EEG tracings. Several general points regarding the electrical activity of the brain in the newborn should be recognized[13].

- Electrical seizures are not commonly accompanied by clinical seizure phenomena. This finding is particularly common in the most immature infants. A recent study showed that approximately 80% of EEG documented seizures are not accompanied by observable clinical seizures[14]. Occasionally electrical status epilepticus may also occur without clinical manifestations.

- Neonatal seizures tend to be brief, usually lasting less than 2 minutes.

- Neonatal electrical seizures tend to be focal and well localized, arising most commonly from temporal and central regions, less commonly from occipital regions, and least commonly from the frontal regions.

Full 20-lead EEG with concurrent video is the gold standard for monitoring and recording seizures in newborn babies. Since full 20-lead EEG is difficult to obtain on an emergency basis, amplitude integrated bed-side EEG (aEEG) is increasingly utilised. aEEG is obtained from a couple or limited number of leads and is displayed as a fast Fourier spectral transform. With aEEG, seizures are detected by acute alteration in spectral width and it has a relatively high specificity but low sensitivity[15]. Seizure activity that is brief, of low voltage or focal, is less likely to be detected on aEEG.

MANAGEMENT

The first step is to detect and treat the underlying cause of the seizures, paying special attention to associated acute metabolic disturbances, such as hypoglycemia and hypocalcemia. The second step is the assessment of the need to control the seizures, which involves balancing the benefits of stopping some or all of the seizures against any potential deleterious effects of anticonvulsant medications.

It is still not clear whether a neonate who has had seizures or is at risk for seizures (eg those with HIE) should undergo continuous EEG monitoring, and if electrographic seizures are detected, what should be done. Electrographic seizures have also been associated with brain injury. There is some consensus that short lasting and infrequent electrographic seizures need not be treated, but prolonged, frequent and persistent electrographic seizures should preferably be treated.

When neonatal seizures occur, a dextrostix should be obtained immediately. If there is hypoglycemia, 10% dextrose solution should be administered intravenously, followed by intravenous continuous glucose infusion (Table 23.2). When there are no metabolic abnormalities or seizures persist despite correction of metabolic abnormalities, anticonvulsants are administered in accordance with algorithm shown in Figure 23.1.

Anticonvulsants

If seizures persist and are recurrent, 20 mg/kg of phenobarbital should be administered intravenously, followed by additional 5 mg/kg boluses upto a maximum total dose of 40 mg/kg, preferably until all electrographic and clinical seizure activity is stopped. If respiratory depression is a concern, or in infants with hypoxic ischemic injury (who may not tolerate high-dose of phenobarbital), the infant should be given 20 mg/kg of intravenous phenytoin. Fosphenytoin, the salt ester of phenytoin is a preferred form of phenytoin. Fosphenytoin has major advantages for use in newborn babies, because it is an aqueous solution that is soluble in glucose-containing solutions, it can be administered more quickly than phenytoin, and it will not cause soft-tissue necrosis and injury that can occur with intravenous phenytoin, which is highly alkaline. If a neonate is in status epilepticus, lorazepam is the drug of choice. It has a rapid onset of action and a long half-life. The long half life of lorazepam is useful for sustained effect while diazepam is short acting because it is rapidly redistributed in the body fat. Lorazepam has a much smaller volume of distribution, accounting for its prolonged retention at high levels in the brain. The dosage should be 0.05 to 0.1 mg/kg.

Table 23.2 Acute management of neonatal seizures
• Stabilize vital functions by maintaining ABC
• Correct transient metabolic disturbances
o Hypoglycemia: 2 ml/kg of 10% dextrose IV bolus followed by 10% dextrose infusion at a rate of 8 mg/kg/min
o Hypocalcemia: 2 ml/kg of 10% calcium gluconate diluted with equal quantity of water IV slowly over 5-10 min
o Hypomagnesemia: When a suspected or known case of hypocalcemia does not respond to calcium therapy, a trial of magnesium therapy should be given. 50% magnesium sulphate 0.2 ml/kg IM every 12 hr till normal level is achieved
• Phenobarbitone 20 mg/kg IV loading dose. If necessary additional phenobarbitone 5 mg/kg IV every 5 min upto a maximum total dose of 40 mg/kg
• Phenytoin : 20 mg/kg IV (1mg/kg/min) in normal saline
• Lorazepam: 0.05-0.10 mg/kg IV

There has been recent interest in using lidocaine, a class Ia anti-arrhythmic agent, which is believed to suppress seizures through inhibition of sodium entry into neurons. A loading dose of 2 mg/kg, followed by infusion of 6 mg/kg/hour, is effective in treating neonatal seizures refractory to phenobarbitone. Prolonged infusion may result in accumulation of metabolites and may be responsible for recurrence of seizures on withdrawal. Clearance of lidocaine is reduced in preterm infants and monitoring of plasma concentration is advisable (therapeutic range 3-6 mg/l). *Lidocaine should not be used together with phenytoin because of risk of development of serious cardiac arrhythmias.*

Thiopental has been reported to be effective in the treatment of seizures in asphyxiated term newborns who do not respond to phenobarbitone. However, it is associated with a serious risk of development of hypotension. The adjunctive value of this mode of therapy remains to be established.

Paraldehyde has been shown to be a useful adjunct. It has a relatively short half life (12-24 hours); elimination is by hepatic metabolism and pulmonary transport and it is unaffected by altered renal function. Reported side effects include hepatic necrosis and pulmonary edema. A loading dose of 200-400 mg/kg can be given rectally or intravenously, followed by an infusion of 15-150 mg/kg/hour to achieve seizure control (0.3-3.0 ml/kg/hour of a 5% solution, made up in 5% dextrose). Glass syringes should be used for delivery of paraldehyde (because it reacts with plastic) and the solution should be protected from light.

Section 3

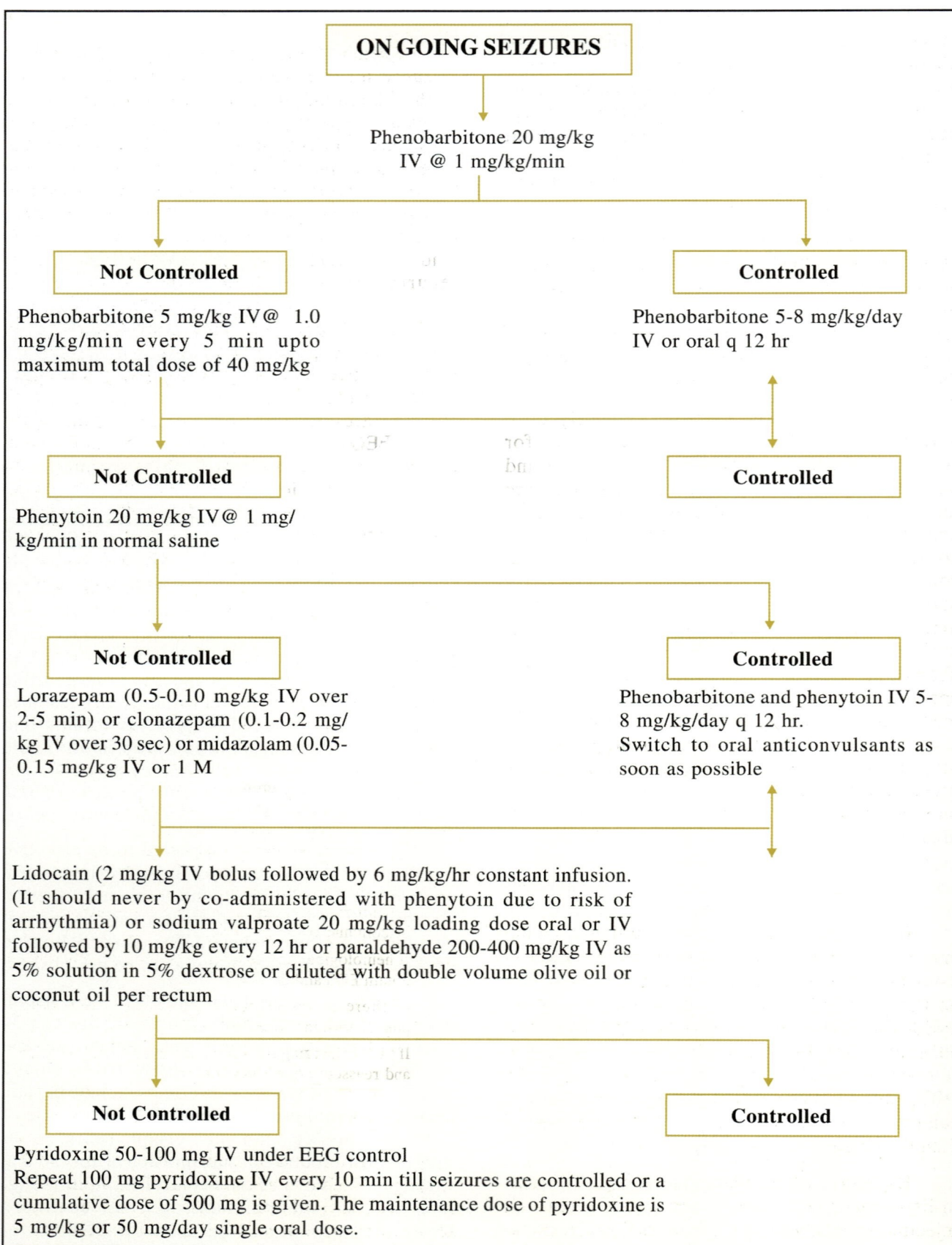

Figure 23.1 Algorithm for management of neonatal seizures

Sodium valproate has been used to treat intractable seizures, using an oral loading dose of 20 mg/kg, followed by 10 mg/kg 12 hourly. There is a wide variation in plasma clearance, necessitating monitoring of drug concentrations (therapeutic range 185-425 mMol/l). There are concerns about hepatotoxic effects of valproate because hyperammonemia is observed in all cases which may necessitate withdrawal of drug.

Carbamazepine has been reported to be effective as an initial agent in the treatment of neonatal seizures in a study of full term infants with birth asphyxia. All patients had a good clinical response. However, variability in blood levels suggests that more data are needed to determine the therapeutic utility of this agent.

The consensus is that the currently used antiepileptic drugs are not very effective for controlling neonatal seizures. Phenobarbital and phenytoin are equally efficacious but both are incompletely effective and either drug alone can control seizures in less than half of the EEG confirmed neonatal seizures[16]. There are also concerns that barbiturates and benzodiazepines may adversely affect brain development. Even brief systemic treatment with conventional antiepileptic drugs such as phenobarbitone, phenytoin, diazepam and valproate all increase apoptotic neuronal cell death in rodents[17]. However, newer antiepileptic agents such as topiramate and levetiracetam can be used as add-on drugs because they do not cause apoptosis. Both oral and IV preparations of levetiracetam are available while only oral formulation of topiramate is available at present.

Other Therapies[18]

Pyridoxine. Therapeutic trial with pyridoxine is reserved as a last resort. Intravenous preparation is not available in India and an IM preparation may be used instead (1 ml of neurobion has 50 mg pyridoxine and 1 ml each may be administered in either gluteal region or anterolateral aspect of thigh). Intravenous administration should be done in the NICU under EEG control as hypotension and apnea can occur. The maintenance dose of pyridoxine is 5 mg/kg single oral dose daily.

Exchange blood transfusion. It is indicated in life-threatening metabolic disorders, accidental injection of local anesthetic into fetal scalp, transplacental transfer of maternal drugs (chlorpropamide) and bilirubin encephalopathy.

Duration of Therapy

Optimal duration of therapy of infant with seizures in the newborn period relates principally to the likelihood of recurrence of seizures if the drugs are discontinued. The overall incidence of subsequent epilepsy in survivors has varied from 10% – 30% in different studies. Factors which determine the risk of development of subsequent epilepsy include status of neonatal neurological examination, cause of neonatal seizures and EEG findings. There is approximately 50% risk of recurrence of seizures if the neurological examination at discharge is abnormal. The risk of subsequent epilepsy after neonatal seizures secondary to perinatal asphyxia or hypoxic-ischemic encephalopathy is approximately 30%, while there is essentially no risk of recurrence with simple, late-onset hypocalcemia. Infants with normal EEG or "mild" depression have minimal risk of recurrence of seizures while infants with "marked" depression of electrographic activity on EEG have 40% risk of development of epilepsy. The duration of anticonvulsant therapy depends upon persistence of seizures or neurological signs and abnormalities on EEG and imaging studies (Table 23.3).

Table 23.3 Duration of anticonvulsant therapy
Neonatal period
• If seizures are controlled and neonatal neurological examination is normal, discontinue therapy before discharge

• If neurological examination is persistently abnormal
  o Identify etiology and obtain EEG
  o Continue phenobarbitone
  o Reevaluate after one month

One month after discharge
• If neurological examination has become normal discontinue phenobarbitone
• If neurological examination is persistently abnormal, obtain EEG and do imaging studies
• If there is no seizure activity on EEG, taper phenobarbitone over 4 weeks
• If EEG or imaging studies are abnormal, continue AEDs and reassess after 3 months

PROGNOSIS

The prognosis is determined primarily by etiology[19,20]. Due to advances in neonatal intensive care the survival has improved but long term adverse neuromotor outcome is as dismal as before[21]. The risk of mortality with prolonged neonatal seizures in term infants which was earlier

35% has now come down to 20%.[22] The prognosis following isolated hypocalcemia, subarachnoid hemorrhage or benign familial neonatal seizures is excellent. Early hypoglycemia, CNS infections, and hypoxia-ischemia have an intermediate prognosis (30-50% normal), while CNS malformations and inborn errors of metabolism are generally associated with a poor neurodevelopmental outcome.

Seizure characteristics which are associated with adverse outcome include generalised myoclonic or tonic seizures, intractable seizures requiring more than two antiepileptic drugs, and burst-suppression or persistent low voltage EEG states. A normal interictal EEG is associated with a good outcome. The presence of severe abnormalities in the background EEG pattern like burst suppression, prolonged (>20 sec) interburst interval, marked voltage suppression and electrocerebral silence are associated with poor outcome. Other clinical factors associated with poor outcome are persistent neurological abnormalities on clinical examination and very low birthweight. Only 25% of infants less than 31 weeks of gestation had a normal outcome following EEG confirmed seizures, compared with an abnormal 60% of term infants. Infants with an abnormal neuroradiologic study (CT/MRI) are likely to have a poor neuromotor outcome than those with normal study (36% vs 1%)[21]. The overall risk of development of recurrent seizures or epilepsy later in life among term babies is around 20%.

REFERENCES

1. Volpe JJ. Neonatal seizures. In: Neurology of the Newborn, 4th Ed. *Saunders Philadelphia,* pp 178-214.

2. WB Volpe JJ. Neonatal seizures. *Clin Perinatol* 1977; 4:43-63.

3. Volpe JJ. Neonatal seizures. *N Engl J Med* 1973; 289:413-416.

4. David E, Malcolm L. Neonatal seizures. *Arch Dis Child Fetal Neonatal Ed* 1998; 78:F70-F75.

5. Scher MS, Aso K, Beggarly ME, *et al.* Electrographic seizures in preterm and fullterm neonates: clinical correlates, associated brain lesion, and risk for neurologic sequelae. *Pediatrics* 1993; 91:128–134.

6. Calciolari G, Perlaman JM, Volpe JJ. Seizures in the neonatal intensive care unit of the 1980s: types, etiologies, timing. *Clin Pediatr (Phila)* 1988; 27: 119–23.

7. Pettit RE, Fenichel GM. Benign familial neonatal seizures. *Arch Neurol* 1980; 37:47–8.

8. Coppola G, Veggiotti P, Del Giudice EM, Bellini G, Longaretti F, Taglialatela M, Pascotto A. Mutational scanning of potassium, sodium and chloride ion channels in malignant migrating partial seizures in infancy. *Brain Dev* 2006;28:76-9

9. Goldberg HJ, Sheehy EM. Fifth day fits: an acute zinc deficiency syndrome? *Arch Dis Child* 1982; 57:633–535.

10. Ohtahara S, Ohtsuka Y, Yarnatogi Y, *et al.* The early infantile epileptic encephalopathy with burst suppression: developmental aspects. *Brain Dev* 1987; 9:371–6.

11. Grant PE, Yu D. Acute injury to the immature brain with hypoxia with or without hypoperfusion. *Radiol Clin North Amer* 2006: 44:63-77

12. Miller SP, Ramaswamy V, Michelson D, Barkovich AJ, Holshouser B, Wycliffe N, Glidden DV, Deming D, Partridge JC, Wu YW, Ashwal S, Ferriero DM. Patterns of brain injury in term neonatal encephalopathy. *J Pediatr.* 2005; 146:453-60

13. Clancy RR. Interictal sharp EEG transients in neonatal seizures. *J Child Neurol* 1989; 4:30-38.

14. Clancy RR. Prolonged electroencephalogram monitoring for seizures and their treatment. *Clin Perinatol* 2006; 33:649-65

15. de Vries LS, Toet MC. Amplitude integrated electroencephalography in the full-term newborn. *Clin Perinatol* 2006; 33:619-32.

16. Painter MJ, Scher MS, Stein AD, Armatti S, Wang Z, Gardiner JC, Paneth N, Minnigh B, Alvin J. Phenobarbital compared with phenytoin for the treatment of neonatal seizures. *N Engl J Med* 1999; 341:485-489.

17. Bittigau P, Sifringer M, Genz K, Reith E, Pospischil D, Govindarajalu S, Dzietko M, Pesditschek S, Mai I, Dikranian K, Olney JW, Ikonomidou C. Antiepileptic drugs and apoptotic neurodegeneration in the developing brain. *Proc Natl Acad Sci U S A.* 2002; 99:15089-94.

18. Upadhyay A, Aggarwal R, Deorari AK, Paul VK. Seizures in the newborn. *Indian J Pediatr* 2001; 68(10):967-972.

19. Bergman I, Painter MJ, Hirsh RP, *et al.* Outcome of neonates with convulsions treated in an intensive care unit. *Ann Neurol* 1983; 14:642-47.

20. Ledigo A, Clancy RR, Bermab PH. Neurologic outcome after electroencephalographically proven neonatal seizures. *Pediatrics* 1991; 88:583-596.

21. Tekgul H, Gauvreau K, Soul J, *et al.* The current etiologic profile and neurodevelopmental outcome of seizures in term newborn infants. *Pediatrics* 2006; 117:1270-1280.

22. Ronen GM, Buckley D, Penney S, Streiner DL. Long-term prognosis in children with neonatal seizures: a population-based study. *Neurology* 2007; 69:1816-1822.

Neonatal Sepsis

Vinod K Paul, Deepak Chawla and Meharban Singh

Neonatal sepsis or sepsis neonatorum refers to systemic infection of the newborn. It is characterized by a constellation of a non-specific symptomatology in association with bacteremia. The term "neonatal sepsis" used broadly in the clinical context encompasses diagnoses of septicemia, meningitis, pneumonia, arthritis, osteomyelitis and urinary tract infection in the newborn. This excludes local infections of the newborn infant such as omphalitis, pyoderma and conjunctivitis. Prompt recognition, appropriate parenteral antimicrobial therapy and judicious supportive care are the key determinants of positive outcome in this serious pediatric emergency. The ensuing discussion pertains primarily to neonatal infections due to aerobic bacteria, which account for an overwhelming majority of cases.

DEFINITION

Various definitions, both clinical and microbiological, have been used to describe neonatal sepsis. The microbiologic definition of neonatal sepsis encompasses isolation of the bacteria from the blood and/or CSF. Demonstration of the microbial pathogens is the gold standard for the diagnosis of sepsis. However, isolation of organism may not be feasible in all setups due to lack of culture studies and indiscriminate use of antibiotics. Hence, clinical definition of sepsis is acceptable for practical purposes. But there is no consensus on clinical definition of neonatal sepsis. A recent international consensus conference on pediatric sepsis has defined sepsis as SIRS (systemic inflammatory response syndrome) due to suspected or proven infection[1]. The diagnosis of SIRS is made if two of the following 4 criteria are met and at least one of the criteria is abnormal temperature or leukocyte count. This definition is applicable to full term neonates only.

1. Core temperature of >38.5°C or <36°C.
2. Unexplained heart rate of >180/min or <100/min for >30 min duration.

3. Mean respiratory rate >50/min (0-7days) or >40/min (8-28 days)/ requirement of mechanical ventilation for an acute illness not due to neuromuscular problem or due to general anesthesia.
4. Leukocyte count elevated or depressed for age or >10% immature neutrophils.

INCIDENCE

Neonatal infections are the single most common cause of neonatal mortality accounting for over one third of the 9 lakh newborn deaths each year in the country[2]. Sepsis is the commonest admitting diagnosis among neonates at referral facilities[3]. In the WHO Young Infant Study in five developing countries (viz. Bangladesh, Ghana, India, Pakistan and South Africa), severe infection (sepsis, meningitis and pneumonia) was the primary diagnosis in up to 44% of infants in 0-6 days age group and up to 70% of infants in the 7-59 days age group[4].

In 18-major hospitals in the country, the incidence of neonatal sepsis among intramural babies was 30 per 1000 live births as per the report of the National Neonatal Perinatal Database (NNPD)[5]. This contrasts with the reported incidence of 1 to 10 per 1000 live births in developed countries[6,7]. The incidence of bacterial meningitis in the west is 0.2 - 1.0 per 1000 live births[8]. In Indian NICUs, the incidence of meningitis was estimated as 3 per 1000 live births[5].

ETIOLOGY

Hospital-based Indian studies suggest that the predominant etiological agents of newborn sepsis are *Klebsiella pneumoniae, Staphylococcus aureus* and *Escherichia coli*. In the NNPD study, a total of 1248 organisms were grown from blood and CSF of neonates with sepsis in 18 centers in the country. *Klebsiella pneumoniae* was the commonest organism (32.5%), followed by *Staphylococcus aureus* (13%) and *Escherichia coli* (10.6%)[5]. In contrast *group B streptococci* (GBS), *E.coli* and *Streptococcus viridans* are leading pathogens in the west.

The etiology of neonatal sepsis from the community is not well understood. Perhaps the three commonest organisms are the same as in hospitals. However, *S.aureus* is probably more prevalent than *Gram-negative* organisms. At two Indian sites of the WHO Young Infant Study *S. aureus* was the most commonly isolated organism[9,10]. The other isolates included *Acinetobacter, E. coli* and *Klebsiella.*

Early-onset Versus Late-onset Neonatal Sepsis

Neonatal sepsis can be divided into two main groups depending on whether the onset of infection is in the first 48-72 hours of life or later. Early-onset septicemia is caused by organisms prevalent in the maternal genital tract, and often presents as perinatal hypoxia and respiratory distress (intrauterine pneumonia). Late-onset septicemia is of nosocomial or community acquired origin. Early-onset bacterial infections occur either due to ascending infection, with or without rupture of membranes, or during the passage of baby through the infected birth canal, or at the time of resuscitation in the labor room.

PREDISPOSING FACTORS

Host Factors

Newborn infants are immunodeficient even when they are born full-term (Table 24.1). Low birth weight neonates, both preterm as well as small-for-dates, are at an added disadvantage with regards to different components of immune system[11-13]. Infants with congenital malformations such as meningomyelocele and tracheoesophageal fistula are at increased risk to develop infection. Infants born to mothers with pre-eclampsia are more likely to have neutropenia and early-onset neonatal sepsis. Perinatal hypoxia appears to damage every organ of the baby including the im-mune system.

Breast feeding provides the single most effective protection to neonates against sepsis by providing hu-moral, cellular and other anti-infective factors[14].

Agent Factors

The agents causing neonatal sepsis has changed over decades in Western countries.

Table 24.1 Immune status of neonates compared to older children

Non-specific Factors

Skin
- Functionally immature against infection
- Presence of a surgical wound (i.e. umbilical stump)
- Frequent breaks in its integrity because of forceps, puncture marks, intravenous lines etc.

Gastrointestinal Tract
- Gastric acid secretion not well established
- Poor intestinal peristalsis
- Slower mucosal cell renewal times
- Lack of secretary IgA
- Poor biosynthesis of bile acids

Respiratory Tract
- Paucity of pulmonary alveolar macrophages
- Inefficient mucociliary clearance

Humoral Mediators

Immunoglobulins
- IgG (except IgG 2 sub-type) concentration is normal, while IgM, IgA, IgE concentrations are decreased.

Complement System
- Concentration of most components of classical as well as alternate pathway is diminished

Cellular Mediators

Lymphocytes
- Absolute number of lymphocytes is normal or increased
- Percentage of T-lymphocytes decreased, T-suppressor cells increased
- Large proportion of lymphocytes not identifiable by surface markers

Neutrophils
- Concentration is normal
- Chemotaxis and phagocytosis is poor
- Intracellular killing is normal

Other Mediators
- Reduced gamma interferon production
- Reduced fibronectin level

However, such change has not been documented in India in recent times. NNPD data of neonatal sepsis has shown that three bacterial organisms (*K. pneumoniae, S. aureus* and *E. coli*) have dominated as the main pathogenic agents for 2 decades. At the same time a significant change in antibiotic sensitivity has been seen over this period. Various causes that are associated with development of resistant strains include irrational use of antibiotics, easy availability of over the counter antibiotics, and use of broad spectrum antibiotics that promote selection of multi- drug resistant strains. Intrapartum use of antibiotics can also promote emergence of resistant bacteria.

The Environmental Factors

Maternal genital tract flora. Throughout pregnancy and until the rupture of membranes, the infant's environment is normally sterile. The human birth canal is colonized with a large number of aerobic and anerobic bacteria, mycoplasma, chlamydiae, fungi, yeasts and viruses. Rectal and urinary tract flora influence the genital tract colonization. The aerobic flora includes *E.coli, S. aureus, S. albus* and Klebsiella species.These organisms can get transmitted to the neonate and lead to early-onset sepsis. Maternal urinary tract infection also predisposes to early-onset sepsis in neonates.

Environmental flora. Neonates not only have enhanced vulnerability to infections, but also have an increased likelihood of getting infected from the immediate environment. This immediate environment can be either home (as in community acquired infection) or hospital. While exposure of VLBW neonates to nosocomial environment is an important issue in present day NICUs, community acquired infections in neonates still continues to be an important problem in developing countries. Poor hygienic conditions, dirty fomites and custom of giving a variety of prelacteal feeds lead to colonization of the vulnerable infants with pathogenic microbes.

Nosocomial infections of VLBW neonates is the leading cause of imorbidity and mortality in NICUs.The hands of the care-givers are a potent source of transmission of microbes unless due precautions are taken. Interventions such as needle sticks, venipunctures, long lines, infusions and sticking tapes breach the integrity of skin and increase the vulnerability of the baby to infection. In the nursery, high risk neonates are exposed to potential sources of pathogens such as incubators, cots, linen, suction and oxygen catheters, thermometers, endotracheal tubes, resuscitation equipment, ventilators etc. The congestion and overcrowding at home and in the nursery is associated with increased risk of infection. Lack of disposables (small-vein infusion sets, catheters, endotracheal tubes, syringes, needles etc), use of stock solution (heparinized saline for flushing and maintaining iv lines) and multi-dose drug vials are potent sources of infection[15]. Neonates requiring umbilical lines, intubation, ventilation, parenteral nutrition are at a particularly increased risk to develop infection. The type and density of nursery flora depends on the housekeeping routines, spectrum of antibiotics in use, colonization pattern of the personnel and type of neonatal admissions (intramural or extramural). Most neonatal units in India harbor Klebsiella, *E. coli, S. aureus, S. epidermidis* and *Pseudomonas aeruginosa* in their environment.

Presence of risk factors of early-onset sepsis may help in identification of at-risk neonates.[16,17] For example when *at least three* of the high risk factors outlined in 'Risk Score 2' are present, the baby is considered to have a very high probability of having early-onset sepsis and should be treated with appropriate antibiotics (Table 24.2).

CLINICAL FEATURES

The ability of a newborn baby to respond clinically to an infection or any other insult is limited to stereotyped responses. Hence, the presentation is often vague and non-specific. The illness may be silent in a very small baby who may suddenly die without having overt manifestations. A high index of suspicion is, therefore, mandatory to make an early diagnosis. Poor feeding, poor activity, poor cry, sluggish neonatal reflexes, hypothermia, excessive weight loss or inadequate weight gain, sick looking baby and abdominal distension are early features. Other manifestations include umbilical sepsis, regurgitation of feeds, vomiting or diarrhea. Respiratory distress (tachypnea with chest retractions or cyanosis) is common in early-onset septicemia. Apneic attacks, especially after the third or the fourth day, are suggestive of nosocomial septicemia. Exacerbation of jaundice with elevation of direct reacting bilirubin is occasionally a striking feature. Violaceous skin patches are seen in Pseudomonas and Klebsiella infections, salmon-colored maculopapular rash in listeriosis; and pustules, abscesses and exfoliative dermatitis (scalded skin syndrome) are common features of staphylococcal sepsis. Serious manifestations of sepsis include sclerema, bleeding due to DIC and a picture of necrotizing enterocolitis. Shock, respiratory failure and renal failure may supervene and herald death (Table 24.3).

Table 24.2. Examples of predictive 'risk scores' for early onset sepsis

Risk score 1		Risk score 2
Risk factor **Score**		1. Low birth weight or preterm
1. Prematurity 3		2. Febrile illness in the mother within 2 weeks prior to delivery
2. Birth asphyxia 2		3. Foul smelling and/or meconium stained amniotic fluid
3. Unclean vaginal examination 2		4. Prolonged rupture of membranes >24 hours
4. Foul smelling liquor 2		5. More than 3 vaginal examinations during labor
5. Maternal fever 2		6. Prolonged and difficult delivery with instrumentation
6. PROM >24 hr 1		7. Perinatal asphyxia (Apgar score <4 at 1 minute) or difficult resuscitation
7. Duration of labor > 24 hours 1		
Interpretation		*Interpretation*
0-3: Observe clinically		Presence of > 2 risk factors: Do sepsis screen
>4: Investigate		Foul smelling liquor or presence of three risk factors: Start antibiotics

---

Table 24.3 Cardinal manifestations of neonatal sepsis and meningitis

Neonatal sepsis/pneumonia

➤ General
- Lethargy, refusal to suck, poor cry, sluggish reflexes, sclerema
- Color change: Pallor, jaundice, cyanosis and mottling of skin
- Temperature fluctuations: Hypothermia or fever
- Excessive weight loss or poor weight gain

➤ Respiratory system: Tachypnea, grunting, chest retractions, apnea and gasping. Cough is usually absent.
➤ Circulatory system: Shock, prolonged capillary refill time
➤ Renal: oliguria and renal failure
➤ Abdominal: Abdominal distension, vomiting, diarrhea, hepatosplenomegaly, GI bleeding,
➤ Bones and joints: Abscess, swelling, pseudoparalysis and excessive crying
➤ Bleeding manifestations due to DIC

Neonatal meningitis

It is more common in late-onset septicemia. Setting of neonatal sepsis with presence of following additional manifestations point to meningitis:

➤ Fever
➤ Seizure(s)
➤ Bulging anterior fontanel
➤ Blank or staring look
➤ High pitched cry, excessive crying/irritability
➤ Neck retraction

Neonatal infections can readily disseminate to various body organs including meninges. Evidences of meningeal irritation are usually absent or minimal in newborn babies. In a baby with clinical profile and setting of septicemia, occurrence of fever, seizures, staring look, bulging anterior fontanel and high pitched or excessive crying should arouse the suspicion of meningitis. Inability to move a limb (pseudo-paralysis) or crying when baby is disturbed or picked up is suggestive of osteomyelitis/ arthritis. Local heat, swelling and redness also appear soon. Urinary tract infection does not produce specific manifestations. It is usually associated with unsatisfactory weight gain, vomiting and jaundice in a baby who does not look seriously sick.

Because of non-specific nature of signs and symptoms, differentiation of neonatal sepsis from other severe illnesses in neonates may be difficult at the time of presentation. Provisional diagnosis of serious bacterial infection warranting admission and further workup can be made if any of the following symptoms/signs is present: history of poor feeding, convulsions, movement only when stimulated, respiratory rate of 60 breaths per minute or more, severe chest indrawings, body temperature of 37·5°C or more or below 35·5°C.

INVESTIGATIVE WORK-UP

It is important that the supportive and antimicrobial therapy of a neonate with sepsis is instituted quickly. Hence, only a minimum number of essential investigations should be undertaken. A vast majority of neonates with sepsis present at facilities with no access to microbiologic and other investigations. It is quite appropriate in such a situation to manage these infants efficiently with a sense of urgency without investigations on the basis of clinical judgment.

Blood culture

Isolation of pathogens from blood confirms the diagnosis and guides antimicrobial therapy based on antibacterial susceptibility profile. It is essential to obtain blood specimen for culture through aseptic procedure (Table 24.4).

Table 24.4. Obtaining specimen for blood culture[18]

- Wash hands for 2 minutes and wear sterile gloves.

- Prepare a circular patch of skin over the venipuncture site about 5 cm in diameter by applying alcohol and allowing it to dry. Now apply povidone–iodine on the cleansed area starting in the centre and moving outward in concentric circles. Allow it to dry on the skin for at least one minute. Reapply alcohol and allow it to dry.

- Draw 1 ml of blood in a sterile syringe after venipuncture.

- Inject the blood into the culture bottle containing 10-20 ml of culture broth.

- Cleanse the site again with alcohol

The blood should be collected in an appropriate amount of culture medium. Maximal sensitivity has been reported when volume of blood sample is 10-20% of the culture media. It is preferable to take 1.0 ml of blood sample in 10-20 ml media bottles for reliable yield of pathogens. Blood specimens obtained from indwelling lines or from capillary prick are not appropriate for culture because they are likely to be contaminated. Blood culture positivity in clinically suspected neonates varies considerably in different centers. In advanced facilities, blood culture is positive in 80 percent of all cases of sepsis[19]. In the 18 center network of newborn units in India, 28.6 percent cases of clinical sepsis were reported to be culture positive[5]. In the WHO young Infant Study on Community-acquired sepsis in infants less than 2 months, bacteria were grown from 21-25% infants suspected of sepsis at the Indian sites[9,10].

The conventional blood culture methods provide the result in about 72 hours. It is possible to detect bacterial growth in 12 to 24 hours by improved microbiological techniques such as lysis centrifugation and instrument-based systems (such as BACTEC, BACTALERT etc.) because bacterial growth is continuously monitored in these systems.

CSF examination and culture

Routine lumbar puncture (LP) as a part of work-up of neonatal sepsis has been recommended because a significant proportion of cases of culture-positive septicemia are associated with meningitis[20].This policy has, however, been questioned more recently because the prevalence of meningitis is found to be much less (0-3.3%) in most studies[21-25]. Moreover, the LP is often dry, traumatic or inconclusive. It appears safe not to perform lumbar puncture in asymptomatic babies with only obstetric risk factors of early-onset sepsis[23]. *However, LP must be done in all neonates with clinical picture indicative of any form of late-onset sepsis even if signs of meningitis are absent.* Although the yield of meningitis will probably be less than 5 percent by this approach,this practice is worthwhile because there are serious implications in the management of such cases. Besides, in some cases CSF may yield a positive culture while the blood culture may be negative. In addition to culture, microscopy and Gram stain may provide useful information. It is important to remember that normal uninfected neonates have some white cells in the CSF (Table 24.5). Also, it is possible that the cells may be in the normal range, while CSF culture is positive or the organisms are seen on Gram's stain. The CSF protein and sugar levels are of a little help in most cases because of a wide range of normal values. In general, however, CSF microscopy/chemistry may be considered abnormal if there are more than 32 white cells (per mm^3) with 60 percent or more of polymorphs, and CSF to blood glucose ratio is less than 50 percent and protein is more than 150 mg/dl. Lumbar puncture can be performed even in sick infants provided the neck flexion is avoided and careful monitoring is done during the procedure. If the baby is critically sick and hemodynamically unstable, the procedure should be postponed till the condition improves.

Urine culture

In early-onset sepsis, urine cultures have a low yield and are not indicated. Although not well studied, it appears prudent to obtain urine culture in all suspected cases of late-onset sepsis as it may be the first marker of a urinary tract malformation. There is no point in sending the bag-samples of urine for culture, specimens obtained by suprapubic puncture alone are appropriate.

Table 24.5 Normal CSF findings in the neonate		
Test	Term mean (range)	Preterm mean (range)
1. Cells/cumm		
• WBCs	8 (0-32)	9 (0-29)
• Polymorphonuclear leukocytes	61%	57%
2. Protein (mg/dl)	90 (20-170)	115 (65-150)
3. Glucose (mg/dl)	52 (34-119)	50 (24-63)
4. CSF / blood glucose ratio (%)	51 (44-248)	75 (55-105)

Other microbiology tests

If there is any evidence of localized sepsis (viz. umbilical infection, pustules, abscess, conjunctivitis, cellulitis), smear and swab should be processed for Gram stain and culture.

Indirect Markers of Neonatal Infection

Though culture is the ideal method and gold standard for establishing the diagnosis, there are many pitfalls. It is time consuming and lacks sensitivity. This has led to use of various other indirect markers of infection in neonates. Because of the fulminant nature and high risk of mortality due to neonatal sepsis, there is a need for a rapid and reliable test with high sensitivity and adequate specificity. None of the following markers of neonatal sepsis are diagnostic *per se* but when a panel of screening tests (sepsis screen) is used, their sensitivity and specificity is enhanced.

White Blood Count

The total leukocyte count, neutrophil count, total immature neutrophils and ratio of immature or band cells to total neutrophils are the most helpful indirect markers of newborn sepsis (Table 24.6). They can be performed easily at the bed-side by the physician.

Total leukocyte count (TLC). There is a wide range of normal TLC, from 8,000 to 20,000 per cumm but high counts are uncommon. Neonatal sepsis is usually associated with leukopenia (TLC < 5000/cumm).

Neutrophil count. It is important to be familiar with the normal range of neutrophil count. Absolute neutrophil count (ANC) includes both immature and mature neutrophils. Neutrophil count is obtained by doing a differential leukocyte count on a stained smear or preferably by the automatic Coulter counter (after correction for nucleated red cells). Neutropenia is believed to be the best predictor of sepsis, while neutrophilia does not correlate well[6]. The normal curves generated by Manroe et al[26] and Mouzinho et al[32] (for very low birth weight neonates) are of immense help in classifying a given count as normal or abnormal. A count below the normal range is highly suggestive of sepsis. The lower limit of neutrophil count is 1800/cumm at birth, it rises to 7200/cumm by 12 hours, then declines to 1800/cumm after 72 hours and persists at that level. Among very low birth weight neonates, the lower limit of absolute neutrophil count is 500/cumm at birth, it rises to 2200/cumm at 18-20 hours, then declines to 1100/cumm at 60 hours and persists at that level[32]. Maternal hypertension, perinatal asphyxia and intraventricular hemorrhage can cause neutropenia and should be taken into account while interpreting a given result.

Immature to total neutrophil (I/T) ratio. Neonatal sepsis is a trigger for mobilization of immature neutrophils, essentially the band forms (or stab cells), from the storage pool to the peripheral blood. Manroe et al[26] have provided normal range of total immature neutrophils and I/T ratio at different ages. An I/T ratio of over 0.2 is a highly sensitive marker of neonatal sepsis[26](Table 24.6). It is obtained by examining the peripheral blood smear, counting the immature and mature neutrophils separately. A mature neutrophil has segmented nucleus and the segments are connected by characteristic thin filamentous strands. In contrast, the nucleus of a band cell is indented by more than one half of its breadth giving a uniform diameter (band-like configuration or a lobulated appearance) in which the isthmus between the lobules is broad enough to reveal two distinct margins with nuclear material between them[32]. Occasionally, metamyelocytes which are less mature

Table 24.6 Indirect markers for screening of neonatal sepsis[6,7, 19, 26-31]

	Test	Positive predictive value (%)	Negative predictive value (%)
	Individual components		
1.	White cells		
	• Total leukocyte count <5000/mm³	11-91	58-98
	• Neutropenia (less than Manroe* norms or <1750/mm³)	29-78	57-92
	• Immature to total neutrophil (I/T) ratio >0.2	27-71	65-98
2.	Platelet count (<150,000/mm³)	20-74	57-70
3.	C-reactive protein (CRP)	30-100	73-96
	Sepsis screens		
	(i) Philip and Hewitt 1980[29] TLC, CRP, I/T, mESR, haptoglobin (2 or more positive)	39	99
	(ii) Gerdes and Polin 1987[19] TLC, CRP, I/T, mESR (2 or more positive)	27	100
	(iii) Dollner et al 2001[31] (CRP, IL-6, or both)	28	99

*Manroe et al 1979[33]
TLC=Total leukocyte count; ANC=Absolute neutrophil count; 1/T=Immature to total neutrophil ratio; mESR=Micro-erythrocyte sedimentation rate; CRP = C- reactive protein

neutrophils than even the band cells, may also spill into the peripheral blood. The nucleus of a metamyelocyte shows only a marginal indentation (Figure 24.1). All bands and metamyelocytes are classified as immature neutrophils.

Other Markers

The neutrophils of neonates with sepsis have other abnormal features such as Dohle bodies (aggregates of rough endoplasmic reticulum which stain light

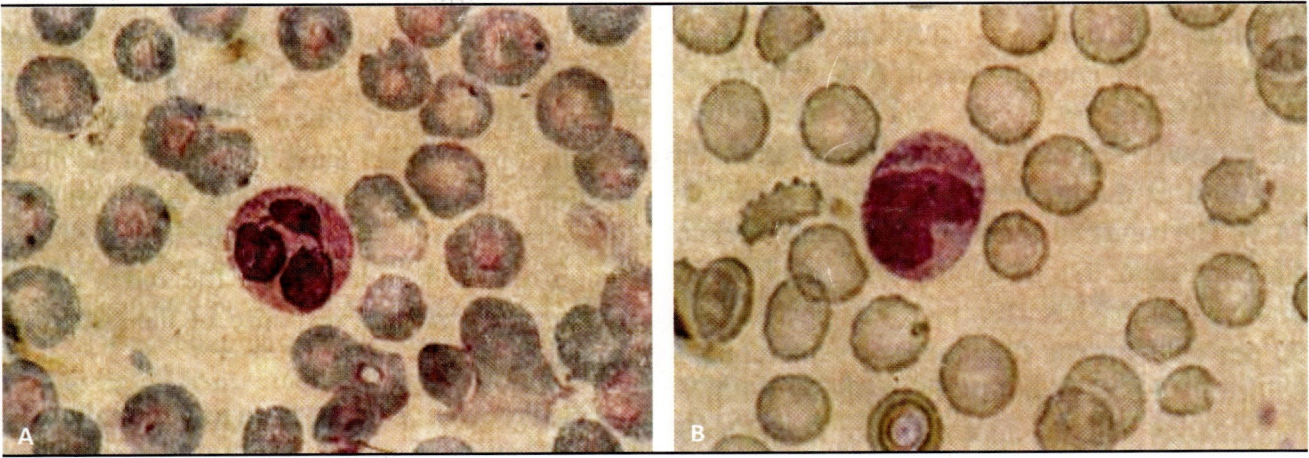

Figure 24.1a and b Morphological characteristics of mature and immature neutrophils in the peripheral blood smear. Both band neutrophils and metamyelocytes are immature neutrophils.

blue with Giemsa), toxic granulations (esosinophilic granules in the cytoplasm) and vacuolization. Detection of these findings requires some expertise and is of limited practical utility. Thrombocytopenia (<150,000/cumm) is another important indirect marker of sepsis in the newborn. However, thrombocytopenia is a late marker of sepsis and has low predictive value.

Acute Phase Reactants

C-reactive protein (CRP). CRP is an acute phase protein synthesized by the liver in response to an inflammatory stimulus within 6-8 hours. It serves as a sensitive marker of newborn sepsis. Normal levels of CRP are <1.6 mg/dl on day 1 and 2, and <1.0 mg/dl thereafter. A concentration above these levels indicates sepsis which is the commonest cause of inflammation in the newborn (Table 24.6). A positive rapid latex agglutination test on undiluted sample corresponds to a plasma CRP concentration of 0.8-1.0 mg/dl[6].The more accurate method is by using nephelometry. A serial decline in CRP indicates recovery from sepsis and may help in deciding the duration of antimicrobial therapy. CRP is also moderately elevated in the presence of meconium aspiration, birth asphyxia and shock.

Micro-erythrocyte sedimentation rate. Micro-ESR is obtained by collecting capillary blood in a standard pre-heparinized microhematocrit glass tube (75 mm length, internal diameter 1.1 mm, outer diameter 1.5 mm), placing it vertically and reading the fall in the red cell column after one hour. The normal value (mm 1st hour) is equal to the postnatal day of life plus 3 mm (thus, it is 5 on day 2 and 10 on day 7). Peak value is 15 mm 1st hour during the neonatal period[18]. High micro-ESR is a specific test but it has only moderate sensitivity (Table 24.6). The value is spuriously high in neonates with hemolysis and is low in babies with disseminated consumptive coagulopathy.

Procalcitonin. This is another acute phase reactant which may help in the diagnosis of sepsis. This is produced by monocytes in response to inflammation. The latent period is short about 4 hours and it peaks by 6-8 hours after the onset of infection. However, level of procalcitonin is affected by post-natal age necessitating careful interpretation especially in early-onset sepsis. An elevated level of procalcitonin has been shown to have a moderate sensitivity and specificity in both early and late-onset sepsis.

Cytokines. Interleukin-6 (IL-6), interleukin-8 (IL-8), tumor necrosis factor alpha (TNFa), interleukin IB (IL-IB) and interleukin 1receptor antagonist have been reported as early markers of neonatal sepsis[27,28]. Elevated IL-6 had a high sensitivity and negative predictive value of 89-91% for late-onset neonatal sepsis in one study[28]. IL-6 rise precedes the rise in CRP and, hence, it is a very early marker of sepsis. However, assays for estimation of cytokines are not feasible for clinical use at present.

Sepsis Screen

Newborn sepsis is potentially a life-threatening disease. Clinical symptomatology can be mild and non-specific, while definitive diagnosis based on culture is not available for at least 2 days. As a result, the clinician is often in a dilemma whether to give antimicrobial therapy or not. The indirect markers of sepsis discussed above provide practical help in this situation (Table 24.6). Because none of these tests alone have sufficient accuracy and reliability,[26,27]attempts have been made to assess their predictive utility in different combinations. These combinations are called as "sepsis screens". Table 24.6 lists a few of the reported studies on the value of sepsis screens.

Gerdes and Polin have underlined the significance of negative predictive value of repeat sepsis screen 12 to 24 hours after a suspected infant has yielded a negative screen[7]. If the second screen also turns out to be negative, the diagnosis of sepsis can be excluded with near certainty. Our experience also supports this observation.

On the basis of the contemporary literature and experience, we recommend a five-item sepsis screen consisting of TLC, absolute neutrophil count, immature to total neutrophil (I/T) ratio,micro-ESR and CRP by latex agglutination test (Table 24.7). However, the emphasis on accuracy of total and

Table 24.7 A practical "sepsis screen"*
1. Leukopenia (TLC <5000/mm³)
2. Neutropenia (as per Manroe/Mouzhino curves)
3. Immature to total neutrophil (I/T) ratio of >0.2
4. Micro-ESR of >15 mm 1st hour
5. C-reactive protein level >1mg/dl

* If two or more tests are positive, infant should be treated for the presumptive diagnosis of neonatal sepsis. If none or only one test is positive, screen should be repeated after 12 hours if clinical suspicion persists. If repeat screen is also negative, sepsis is unlikely.

differential count cannot be overstated. Subjective-bias and inter-observer variability should be minimized by training, supervision and quality control.

Laboratory Tests for Planning Therapy

Hematocrit should be checked and repeated periodically in all cases to detect anemia. Skiagram of chest (pneumonia) and abdomen (necrotizing enterocolitis/ileus) should be taken. Occult blood and reducing substance in stools is suggestive of necrotizing enterocolitis. Other investigations which help to plan management of newborn babies with sepsis include; arterial blood gases (to document respiratory failure/acidosis), blood sugar (to detect hypo- or hyperglycemia), serum bilirubin (both direct and indirect), blood urea/creatinine (to detect renal failure due to the disease or drugs), coagulation studies (bleeding diathesis or disseminated intravascular coagulation) and electrolytes (to detect dyselectrolytemia). Imaging studies like skiagram of bones/joints, ultrasound examination of abdomen, CT scan of brain etc. may be undertaken as indicated. Radionuclide bone and liver scan may be done if there is suspicion of osteomyelitis and pyemic liver abscesses.

TREATMENT

Therapy will be discussed under three headings, namely (a) antimicrobial treatment, (b) supportive care and treatment of complications, and (c) other therapeutic modalities.

Antimicrobial Treatment

Empiric therapy. The empiric therapy of neonatal sepsis is aimed at covering the major causative pathogens while awaiting reports of culture studies. Since the antimicrobial spectrum and susceptibility profile is different in different newborn care settings, it is not possible to have a universal recommendation of a single antibiotic regimen. Antibiotics are often used in neonates on the slightest suspicion of sepsis because of the grave and fulminant nature of neonatal sepsis. But unbridled overuse of antibiotics is associated with the serious risk of emergence of resistant strains of pathogens. Most newborn units in the country are already facing the problem of multi-drug resistant organisms such as *Klebsiella, E. coli, Enterobacter, Citrobacter* and *S. aureus*. Many strains have become resistant to even the third generation cephalosporins and amikacin, and the resistance to carbapenems looms large. The result is that our choice of antimicrobial therapy of sick neonates has become dangerously limited (Table 24.8). Rational use of antibiotics is the responsibility of every physician so that newer and potent anti-biotics are saved for the future generations of our infants.

Rational choice of antimicrobial agents for the treatment of neonatal sepsis is based on the following considerations:

(i) Sound knowledge of the microbial coverage of the available antimicrobials, their CSF penetration, safety, dosage and cost.

Table 24.8. Commonly isolated bacteria and their sensitivity				
Organism	Community and secondary level facilities	Tertiary hospitals		
	Likely sensitive	Likely sensitive	Intermediate	Likely resistant
Staphylococci	Penicillin, ampicillin, amoxycillin, co-trimoxazole, cloxacillin	Vancomycin, linezolid	Amikacin, cefoperazone, ciprofloxacin	Ampicillin, cloxacillin
Klebsiella	Gentamicin, amikacin, ciprofloxacin	Piperacillin, tazobactum, meropenem	Amikacin	Ampicillin, cefotaxime
E. coli	Gentamicin amikacin, ciprofloxacin	Amikacin, ciprofloxacin, piperacillin-tazobactum, meropenem	Gentamicin, cefotaxime	Ampicillin

(ii) Documentation of common pathogens causing neonatal infections in the concerned unit, region or community.

(iii) Antimicrobial susceptibility pattern of the prevalent pathogens.

(iv) Presence or absence of meningitis.

Each treating unit should adopt a suitable antibiotic policy on the basis of the above considerations. Based on changes in the spectrum of etiologic agents and the antibiotic sensitivity pattern, the choice of antibiotics must be periodically reviewed and modified. It is preferable to use a narrow spectrum antibiotic which is directed against the most likely pathogens.

Because the majority of the cases of newborn sepsis in our country are caused by *Klebsiella, S. aureus, and E. coli,* the initial regimen should provide coverage to these organisms. A combination of ampicillin and an aminoglycoside is the logical choice. A combination of oral co-trimoxazole and intramuscular gentamicin single daily dose IM has been found to be effective for ambulatory management of neonatal sepsis in the community[34].

In a hospital where majority of cases are coming from the community and antimicrobial resistance is not expected to be a problem, ampicillin plus gentamicin are again appropriate as initial antibiotics. However, if resistant strains are likely, as in the case of nosocomial pathogens of the nursery, the empiric choice could be ampicillin or cloxacillin in combination with amikacin. In some nurseries, the antibiotic susceptibility pattern is such that even this combination may be ineffective because of the multi-drug resistant strains of *Klebsiella or E. coli.* In this situation, a third generation cephalosporin (cefotaxime or ceftriaxone) is recommended in combination with amikacin (Table 24.9).

Nosocomial infections in many neonatal units in our country are caused by Gram-negative organisms, which have become resistant to the third generation cephalosporins. In such a situation, some neonatologists choose ciprofloxacin in combination with amikacin. Ciprofloxacin has a poor CSF penetration. Its use in neonates is not endorsed by experts in view of potential toxicity to the cartilage.

Table 24.9. Protocol for empirical therapy of neonatal sepsis and meningitis		
Examples	**Septicemia and pneumonia**	**Meningitis**
Situations where resistant strains are unlikely (*e.g. community-acquired pneumonia*)	Ampicillin *plus* gentamicin	Same as for septicemia/pneumonia *plus* cefotaxime
Situations where a few strains are likely to be resistant to common antibiotics (*e.g. nosocomial infections in intermediate care units that cater to stable preterm infants; also in units that adhere to rational antibiotic therapy and avoid indiscriminate use of broad-spectrum antibiotics*)	Ampicillin or cloxacillin *plus* amikacin	Same as for septicemia/pneumonia *plus* cefotaxime
Situations where most of the strains are likely to be resistant (*e.g. nosocomial infections in intensive care units that cater to high-risk, sick infants; also in units that use broad-spectrum antibiotics indiscriminately*)	Cefotaxime or piperacillin-tazobactam or ciprofloxacin plus amikacin. *Consider vancomycin if MRSA is suspected.*	Same as for septicemia/pneumonia (*but avoid ciprofloxacin*)
Special situations ° *No improvement / worsening of clinical condition despite 'appropriate' first-line antibiotic therapy*	Consider reserve antibiotics like cefoperazone-sulbactum, meropenem and aztreonam.	
° *Sudden outbreak of infections*	Based on the source of outbreak and the suspected/isolated organism (e.g. if due to MRSA, then use vancomycin)	

However, ciprofloxacin has been used in many nurseries in India without any reports of significant adverse effects. Nevertheless, ciprofloxacin should be reserved for situations where other options have been exhausted.

First- and second-generation cephalosporins (e.g. cefazolin, cefuroxime) are not commonly used for treatment of neonatal sepsis because of poor activity against some Gram-negative bacteria like Pseudomonas, poor CSF penetration and susceptibility to hydrolysis by beta-lactamase. Cefotaxime and ceftriaxone are third generation cephalosporins with similar antimicrobial coverage that includes most Gram-negative rods. Ceftazidime is particularly effective against Pseudomonas. They all have superb CSF penetration. These antibiotics have been an excellent choice for serious hospital-acquired neonatal septicemia, pneumonia and meningitis due to *Klebsiella pneumoniae, Escherichia coli, Enterobacter* species, *Acinetobacter* etc. Cefoperazone is another third generation cephalosporin, but it has poor CSF penetration. Cefepime is fourth-generation cephalosporin with activity against both Gram-positive and negative organisms including Pseudomonas. However, it is not active against MRSA. Extensive use of third- and fourth-generation cephalosporins can lead to emergence of resistance against even these beta-lactamase stable antibiotics. Therefore, routine use of wide-spectrum cephalosporins should be avoided.

Beta-lactam antibiotics combined with beta-lactamase inhibitors (e.g. piperacillin-tazobactam, ticarcillin-clavulanate and cefoperazone-sulbactam) are increasingly being used for treatment of neonatal infections. Advantages include bactericidal activity against many resistant organisms (including Pseudomonas but not MRSA).

Aminoglycosides like gentamicin, amikacin and tobramycin have good activity against Gram-negative bacteria. Extended dosage interval with preserved safety and efficacy makes gentamicin an attractive choice for treatment of sepsis. Amikacin is another widely used aminoglycoside because of lower susceptibility of development of resistance.

Aztreonam covers predominantly Gram-negative enteric bacilli. It has no activity against Gram-positive bacteria. Imipenem and meropenem have excellent activity against virtually all bacterial pathogens except MRSA and *Enterococcus faecium. However, imipenem has poor CSF*

penetration and should not be used for treatment of meningitis. Use of carbapenems must be restricted to only a rare situation of severe sepsis due to multi-drug resistant nosocomial organisms. Vancomycin and linezolid are effective against MRSA and should not be used unless MRSA has grown in bacterial culture or there is high probability of infection with resistant organisms.

Indications for Use of Empirical Antibiotics

Empirical antibiotic therapy is used in following clinical situations

1. In a symptomatic neonate where sepsis is a strong clinical possibility.
2. In a symptomatic neonate in whom sepsis screen is positive.
3. Asymptomatic neonate with ≥3 perinatal risk factors (Table 24.2).

Antibiotics should be modified based on clinical course and culture reports.

Duration of empiric antibiotic therapy

1. Empiric antibiotic therapy is continued till culture report is available after which the antibiotic is modified based on the sensitivity pattern.
2. If culture is negative but diagnosis of clinical sepsis is most likely and patient has shown clinical improvement, the same antibiotics should be continued for 7-10 days.
3. If culture is negative and patient is still asymptomatic, antibiotics can be stopped after 48-96 hours.

Culture Positive Sepsis

Antimicrobial therapy should be modified according to the culture and sensitivity report. When therapeutic response to initial antibiotics is excellent, they can be continued because of lack of correlation between *in-vivo* and *in-vitro* antibacterial sensitivity pattern. Table 24.8 lists the antibiotics of choice for various isolates. Neonatal sepsis due to *Pseudomonas aeruginosa* poses a difficult challenge. It is resistant to many antibiotics and hence piperacillin, piperacillin-tazobactam or ceftazidime should be considered if Pseudomonas sepsis is suspected. Penicillin resistant *S. aureus* can be treated with cloxacillin. Antimicrobials effective against MRSA (methicillin resistant *Staphylococcus aureus*) are ciprofloxacin,

Section 3

vancomycin and teicoplanin. Ampicillin is the drug of choice if listeriosis is suspected.

Neonatal Meningitis

The persistence of pathogens in the CSF correlates with increased risk of long-term complications. Also, it takes longer to eradicate Gram-negative enteric organisms from the CSF compared to Gram-positive cocci. Antibiotic penetration of blood brain barrier (BBB) for attaining minimal inhibitory concentration is an important consideration in selection of antibiotic. Intrathecal and intraventricular antibiotic therapy is not recommended in the management of meningitis as the prospective controlled trials conducted by the National Meningitis Cooperative Study Group have shown that these modes of treatment are of no additional therapeutic utility in neonatal meningitis[35, 36]. However, when ventriculitis is associated with septae and loculations, it is treated with bilateral intraventricular shunts.

First-generation cephalosporins, including cephaloridine and cefazolin do not diffuse across the blood-brain barrier. Cefuroxime is the only second generation cephalosporin with good CSF penetration but there is not enough data regarding its use in newborn babies. Cefotaxime, ceftriaxone, ceftazidime and piperacillin are not only highly effective against Gram-negative enteric organisms but also attain excellent CSF levels. These agents appear to be extremely effective in the management of neonatal meningitis. Data on ceftizoxime in this regard is inconclusive. Choramphenicol has superb penetration across all body cavities including the blood-brain barrier. However, there is a concern about its actual efficacy in the hospital-acquired infections due to resistant organisms. Aminoglycosides do cross inflamed meninges and achieve antibiotic concentration in the CSF above minimum inhibitory concentration. However, a penicillin or a third generation cephalosporin should be added to aminoglycosides for adequate therapy.

It is important to monitor cases of neonatal meningitis for complications such as hydrocephalus, ventriculitis and brain abscess. Ultrasound and CT head should be done. CSF examination repeated at 48-72 hours after starting treatment provides an excellent objective assessment of the progress of the baby. Infants whose CSF culture is still positive at this stage carry an adverse prognosis.

Table 24.10 Practical guidelines for management of a neonate with meningitis.

Treatment

- Select antibiotics with good CSF penetration.
- **Give correct dose**. For some antibiotics, the dose is higher for treatment of meningitis (refer to Table 24.11)
- Use intravenous route throughout the treatment
- Duration of therapy is at least 3 weeks or more
- Add anticonvulsant/mannitol, if required.

Monitoring/Investigations

- Monitor head circumference.
- Repeat CSF examination after 48 hours.
- If there is no improvement, conduct ultrasound examination of head for evidences of complications such as ventriculitis, ventriculomegaly and brain abscess. Perform CT as and when required.
- Follow-up neuromotor development.

Mode of Administration and Dosage of Antimicrobial agents

Table 24.11 gives details of the doses of antibiotics recommended in the neonates. It should be noted that for some antibiotics, the dose is higher in meningitis. Antibiotics must be administered intravenously at least during the initial phase of management and as long as intravenous fluids are being administered. Subsequently, except for the more fulminant infections, it is appropriate to give antibiotics intramuscularly. *In meningitis, arthritis and osteomyelitis, however, intravenous therapy must be ensured throughout the course of treatment.*

Duration of Therapy

Duration of therapy should be individualized. In general, antibiotics should be given for a period of 7-10 days in septicemia or pneumonia, 14 days in urinary tract infection and 21 days for meningitis. Longer periods of therapy may be required in poorly responding cases of meningitis. Surgical drainage, local rest and prolonged parenteral antibiotic therapy for 4-6 weeks is advocated for infants with osteomyelitis and arthritis.

Table 24.11 Dose (mg/kg per dose) and frequency of commonly used antimicrobial agents in neonates

Drug	Route	Birth weight < 2000 g		Birth weight >2000 g	
		0-7 d	>7 d	0-7 d	>7 d
Amikacin	iv, im	18 q 36 hr	15 q 24 hr	15 q 24hr	15 q 24 hr
Ampicillin					
Meningitis	iv	100 q 12 hr	100 q 8 hr	100 q 12 hr	100 q 8hr
Others	iv, im	50 q 12 hr	50 q 8 hr	50 q 12 hr	50 q 8 hr
Aztreonam	iv, im	30 q 12 hr	30 q 8 hr	30 q 8 hr	30 q 6 hr
Cefepime					
Meningitis	iv	30 q 8 hr	30 q 8 hr	30 q 8 hr	50 q 8 hr
Others	iv	30 q 12 hr	50 q 12 hr	30 q 12 hr	50 q 12 hr
Cefotaxime	iv, im	50 q 12 hr	50 q 8 hr	50 q 8 hr	50 q 8 hr
Ceftazidime	iv, im	50 q 12 hr	50 q 8 hr	50 q 8 hr	50 q 8 hr
Ceftriaxone					
Meningitis	iv, im	50 q 12 hr	50 q 12 hr	50 q 12 hr	50 q 12 hr
Others	iv, im	25 q 12 hr	25 q 12 hr	25 q 12 hr	25 q 12 hr
Cephalothin	iv	20 q 12 hr	20 q 8 hr	20 q 8 hr	20 q 6 hr
Cephazolin	iv, im	25 q 12hr	25 q 8 hr	25 q 12hr	25 q 8 hr
Chloramphenicol	iv, po	25 q 24 hr	25 q 24 hr	25 q 24 hr	25 q 12 hr
Ciprofloxacin	iv	5 q 12 hr	5 q 12 hr	5 q 12 hr	5 q 12 hr
	po	7.5 q 12 hr	7.5 q 12 hr	7.5 q 12 hr	7.5 q 12 hr
Clindamycin	iv, im, po	5 q 12 hr	5 q 8 hr	5 q 12 hr	5 q 8 hr
Cloxacillin					
Meningitis	iv	50 q 12 hr	50 q 8 hr	50 q 8 hr	50 q 6 hr
Others	iv, im	25 q 12 hr	25 q 8 hr	25 q 8 hr	25 q 6 hr
Erythromycin	po	10 q 8 hr	10 q 8 hr	10 q 8 hr	10 q 8 hr
Gentamicin	iv, im	4 q 36 hr	4 q 24 hr	4 q 24 hr	4 q 24 hr
Imipenem	iv, im	20 q 12 hr	20 q 12 hr	20 q 12 hr	20 q 8 hr
Meropenem					
Meningitis	iv	40 q 8 hr	40 q 8 hr	40 q 8 hr	40 q 8 hr
Others	iv	20 q 12 hr	20 q 12 hr	20 q 12 hr	20 q 12 hr
Metronidazole	iv, po	7.5 q 24 hr	7.5 q 12 hr	7.5 q 12 hr	7.5 q 12 hr
Mezlocillin	iv, im	75 q 12 hr	75 q 8 hr	75 q 12 hr	75 q 8 hr
Netilmicin	iv, im	4 q 36 hr	4 q 24 hr	4 q 24 hr	4 q 24 hr
Penicillin G					
Meningitis	iv	100,000 U q 12 hr	100,000 U q 8 hr	100,000 U q 8 hr	100,000 U q 6 hr
Others	iv, im	25000 U q 12 hr	25000 U q 8 hr	25000 U q 8 hr	25000 U q 6 hr
Piperacillin	iv, im	75 q 12 hr	75 q 8 hr	75 q 8 hr	75 q 6 hr
Piperacillin –tazobactum	iv, im	Calculate dose by piperacillin content as above			
Ticarcillin	iv, im	75 q 12 hr	75 q 8 hr	75 q 8 hr	75 q 6 hr
Ticarcillin –clavulanate	iv, im	Calculate dose by ticarcillin content as above			
Tobramycin	iv, im	4 q 36 hr	4 q 24 hr	4 q 24 hr	4 q 24 hr
Vancomycin	iv	15 q 12 hr	15 q 8 hr	15 q 12 hr	15 q 8 hr

Supportive Care and Treatment of Complications

Neonate should be nursed in a thermoneutral zone of ambient temperature (Table 24.12). If possible, servo-controlled incubator or open care system should be used. Intravenous fluids are started and enteral feeds are withheld in a sick baby for a couple of days. In case of documented hypoglycemia and when facilities to check blood sugar are not readily available, glucose (200 mg/kg or 2 ml/kg of 10% dextrose) should be given as a bolus. Blood glucose should be maintained between 60-100 mg/dl. Injection vitamin K 1 mg intravenously is given at admission and once a week till enteral feeds are re-established. Anemia is corrected with aliquots of packed cells. Metabolic acidosis and hypotension are managed by careful volume expansion (preferably with central venous pressure monitoring) and vasopressors. Normal saline or Ringer's lactate is used for volume expansion. Dopamine and dobutamine are commonly used vasopressors. Adrenaline (0.2 ug/kg/min constant infusion) has been used to combat shock when response to Ringer's lactate is unsatisfactory or ill sustained and other pressors like dopamine and dobutamine fail to maintain blood pressure. The dose of adrenaline can be tailored to patient's response[37]. Corticosteroids are indicated in gravely sick neonates with endotoxic shock, sclerema and adrenal insufficiency[38].

Hyperbilirubinemia should be managed with phototherapy and exchange blood transfusion. Oxygen and ventilatory therapy should be instituted in the event of respiratory failure as per the standard indications. Bleeding diathesis is managed by judicious administration of fresh blood, fresh frozen plasma, platelets and vitamin K. Efforts should be made to identify collection of pus in the body, and if present, it must be drained promptly. A high index of suspicion should be maintained to identify necrotizing enterocolitis (NEC) especially in preterm neonates. NEC is heralded by abdominal distension, gastrointestinal bleeding and cardio-vascular instability. In meningitis, seizures are treated with diazepam and phenobarbitone. In cases of severe manifestations of raised intracranial pressure, mannitol may be used.

Exchange blood transfusion. Exchange blood transfusion with fresh whole blood in critically sick neonates is a useful modality[39, 40]. It provides complement, granulocytes and antibodies; removes bacteria and toxins, corrects neutropenia and

---

Table 24.12 Outline of supportive treatment and monitoring of neonatal sepsis

Treatment

- Maintain body temperature: Provide warmth and prevent/treat hypothermia or hyperthermia.
- Establish intravenous line, use umbilical vein temporarily, if necessary .
- Infuse normal saline 10 ml/kg bolus, if capillary refill time is over 2 seconds; repeat if required.
- Initiate infusion of glucose (10%) with 0.18% saline. Give glucose bolus 200 mg/kg, if hypoglycemia is suspected or if blood sugar cannot be estimated.
- Administer appropriate antibiotic regimen in an adequate dosage.
- Use blood products judiciously as indicated.
- Consider anticonvulsants and mannitol in meningitis, if indicated.
- Treat shock using volume expansion and adrenaline or dopamine.
- Treat respiratory failure with oxygen and ventilation.
- Consider exchange blood transfusion in the presence of sclerema, rapid deterioration, hyperbilirubinemia and bleeding diathesis.

Monitoring/Investigations

- Vital signs: Temperature, respiratory rate, heart rate and blood pressure.
- Oxygen saturation, cyanosis, pallor, mottling.
- Capillary refill time, heart rate and peripheral pulses.
- Abdominal girth
- Body weight
- Urine output
- Blood pressure
- Central venous pressure, if in shock or CHF
- Icterus, bleeding, and sclerema
- IV site : Swelling, discoloration
- CNS : Fontanel, irritability, abnormal cry, seizures, tone, reflexes (Moro, suck, grasp), jitteriness, and neck stiffness

---

enhances neutrophilic function; improves the perfusion and corrects coagulation disturbances. It is advisable to perform exchange transfusion in sick infected babies in the presence of sclerema, disseminated intravascular coagulation, hyperbilirubinemia and rapid clinical deterioration. Since the candidate babies are often unstable, it is important to monitor them carefully during the procedure.

Other Therapeutic Modalities

Many other therapeutic modalities apart from antibiotics and supportive care have been tried in neonatal sepsis. Though initially they were promising, none of them later proved to be of use for routine practice. Currently, they are still experimental modalities and most of them have limited therapeutic utility.

Granulocyte transfusion. Neutropenia is a common finding during neonatal sepsis. Administration of viable granulocytes is thought to correct this abnormality. A few small studies using different methods of harvesting granulocytes and different transfusion protocols have documented conflicting and unconvincing results.[41]

Intravenous immunoglobulins (IVIG). The quantitative and qualitative deficiency of IgG among preterm neonates makes the proposition of immunoglobulin therapy very attractive. However, enough evidence is now available regarding futility of IVIG as an adjunct to treatment of sepsis or to prevent occurrence of sepsis in preterm babies.[42,43] Availability of specific monoclonal antibodes againt specific pathogens causing sepsis may hold promise.

G-CSF and GM-CSF. Limited capacity of neonates to mount an efficient granulocytic response to infection is in part due to the inadequacy of mononuclear cells to express granulocyte colony stimulating factor (G-CSF) and granulocyte macrophage colony stimulating factor (GM-CSF). With the availability of recombinant human G-CSF and GM-CSF, there is optimism about their role as an adjunctive therapy in neonatal sepsis. In septicemic animals GM-CSF induces neutrophilia and reduces mortality. It has been used in a dose of 10 ug/kg/d SC or slow IV for 7 days. However, a recent multi-center trial did not show any clinical benefit of GM-CSF in neonates with sepsis.[44] There is a concern about long term toxicity of GM-CSF therapy because it can enhance apoptosis of neutrophils and other cells through interleukin-1B-converting enzyme.

Other Experimental Therapies

Zinc, pentoxifylline, fibronectin, interferon and antilipid-A monoclonal antibodies are some of the other potential therapeutic modalities under investigation. At present these medications have no place in clinical practice.

MONITORING

Intensive care and monitoring is the key determinant of improved survival of neonates. The elements of monitoring in sepsis are not different from other life-threatening situations in newborn babies. The emergence of complications should be identified at the earliest in order to ensure timely intervention (Table 24.12). The periodicity of documenting the various parameters should be individualized.

PROGNOSIS

The outcome depends upon weight and maturity of the infant, type of etiologic agent, its antibiotic senstivity pattern; and adequacy of specific and supportive therapy. Associated congenital malformations like meningomyelocele, tracheoesophageal fistula and surgical procedure adversely affect the prognosis. The early-onset septicemia carries worse outcome than late-onset sepsis. Early and aggressive therapy is mandatory for better salvage. Complications such as endotoxic shock, sclerema, NEC, DIC etc. are associated with extremely high mortality. The reported mortality rates in neonatal sepsis in various studies from India ranges between 25-58 percent. Early diagnosis of infection, judicious and early use of specific antimicrobial therapy, close monitoring of vital signs and, above all, intensive supportive care with judicious use of fresh blood, FFP and immuno-therapy are associated with improved survival of neonates with sepsis.

REFERENCES

1. Goldstein B, Giroir B, Randolph A. International Consensus Conference on Pediatric Sepsis. Definitions for sepsis and organ dysfunction in pediatrics. *Pediatr Crit Care Med* 2005; 6(1):2-8.

2. Paul VK, Sachdev HPS, Mavalankar D, Ramachandran, P, Sankar J, Bhandari N, Sreenivas V, Sundararaman T, Govil D, Osrin D, Kirkwood B. Reproductive health, and child health and nutrition in India: meeting the challenge. *Lancet* 2011; 377(9762):332-349.

3. Paul VK, Ramani AV. Newborn care at peripheral health facilities. *Indian J Pediatr* 2000; 67:378-382.

4. The Young Infants Clinical Signs Study group. Clinical signs that predict severe illness in children under age 2 months: a multicentre study. *Lancet* 2008; 371(9607):135-145.

5. National Neonatology Forum: *National Neonatal Perinatal Database Report 2002-03.* Published by NNPD nodal center, All India Institute of Medical Sciences, New Delhi.

Section 3

6. Gerdes JS. Clinicopathologic approach to the diagnosis of neonatal sepsis. *Clin Perinatol* 1991; 18:361-381.

7. Gerdes JS, Polin R. Early diagnosis and treatment of neonatal sepsis. *Indian J Pediatr*1998; 65:63-78.

8. Klein JO, Marcey SM. Bacterial sepsis and meningitis. In: Infectious Disease in the Fetus and Newborn Infants. Remington JS, Klein JO (Eds.). *Philadelphia, WB Saunders,* 1995: p 835.

9. Deorari AK, Chellani H, Carlin JB, Greenwood P, Prasad MS, Satyavani A, Singh J, John R, Taneja DK, Paul P, Meenakshi M, Kapil A, Paul VK, Weber M. Clinico-epidemiological profile and predictors of severe illness in young infants (< 60 days) reporting to a hospital in North India. *Indian Pediatr* 2007;44(10):739-748.

10. Narang A, Kumar P, Narang R, Ray P, Carlin JB, Greenwood P, Muley P, Misra S, Weber M. Clinico-epidemiological profile and validation of symptoms and signs of severe illness in young infants (< 60 days) reporting to a district hospital. *Indian Pediatr* 2007;44(10):751-759.

11. Chandra RK. Influence of nutrition-immunity axis on perinatal infections. In: Neonatal infections: Nutritional and Immunologic Interactions. Ogra PL (ed). *Grune and Stratton Inc.* 1984; 229-246.

12. Edwards MS, Baker CJ. Bacterial infections. In: Neonatal Infections: Nutritional and Immunologic Interactions. Ogra PL (ed). *Grune and Stratton Inc., Orlando* 1984; pp 91-107.

13. Faden H, Rosales S. Infections in the compromised neonate. In: Neonatal Infections: Nutritional and Immunologic Interactions. Ogra PL (ed.) *Grune and Stratton Inc* 1984; pp 185-202.

14. Hylander MA, Strobino DM, Dhanireddy R. Human milk feedings and infections among very low birth weight infants. *Pediatrics* 1998; 102(3):E38.

15. Singh M, Paul VK, Deorari AK, Ray D, Murali MV, Sundaram KR. Strategies which reduced sepsis-related neonatal mortality. *Indian J Pediatr* 1988; 55:955-960.

16. Singh M, Narang A, Bhakoo ON. Predictive perinatal score in the diagnosis of neonatal sepsis. *J Trop Pediatr* 1994;40:365-368.

17. Sankar MJ, Agarwal R, Deorari AK, Paul VK. Sepsis in the newborn. *Indian J Pediatr* 2008;75:261-266.

18. Dutta R. Blood cultures. *Bull NNF* 1999; 13:43-46.

19. Gerdes JS, Polin RA. Sepsis screen in neonates with evaluation of plasma fibronectin. *Pediatr Infect Dis* 1987; 6:443-446.

20. Visser VE, Hall RT. Urine culture in the evaluation of suspected neonatal sepsis. *J Pediatr* 1979; 96:635-638.

21. Eldah M, Frenkel LD, Hiatt IM, Hegyi T. Evaluation of routine lumbar punctures in newborn infants with respiratory distress syndrome. *Pediatr Infec Dis J* 1987; 6:243-245.

22. Fielkow S. Reuter S, Gotoff SP. Carebrospinal fluid examination in symptom-free infants with risk factors for infection. *J Pediatr* 1991; 119: 971-243.

23. Kumar P, Sarkar S, Narang A. Role of routine lumbar puncture in neonatal sepsis. *J Pediatr Child* 1995; 31:8-10.

24. McIntyre P, Isaacs D. Lumbar puncture in suspected neonatal sepsis. *J Pediatr Child Health* 1995; 31:1-2.

25. Schwerenski J, McIntyre L, Bauer C. Lumbar puncture frequency and carebrospinal fluid analysis in the neonate. *Am J Dis Child* 1991; 145: 54-58.

26. Manroe DL, Weinberg AG, Rosenfeld ER, Brown R. The neonatal blood count in heath and disease I Reference values of neutrophilic cells. *J Pediatr* 1979; 95:89-98.

27. Doellner H, Arntzen KJ, HaereidPE, Aag S, Austgulen R. Interleukin-6 concentrations in neonates evaluated for sepsis. *J Pediatr* 1998; 132:295-299.

28. Misra PK, Kumar R, Malik GK, Mehra P, Awasthi S. Simple hematological tests for diagnosis of neonatal sepsis. *Indian Pediatr* 1989; 26:156-160.

29. Philip AGS, Hewitt JE. Early diagnosis of neonatal sepsis. *Pediatrics* 1980; 65:1036-1041.

30. Singh M, Narang A, Bhakoo ON. Evaluation of a sepsis screen in the diagnosis of neonatal sepsis. *Indian Pediatr* 1987; 24(1):39-43.

31. Døllner H, Vatten L, Austgulen R. Early diagnostic markers for neonatal sepsis: comparing C-reactive protein, interleukin-6, soluble tumour necrosis factor receptors and soluble adhesion molecules. *J Clin Epidemiol* 2001;54(12):1251-1257.

32. Mouzinho A, Rosenfeld CR, Sánchez PJ, Risser R. Revised reference ranges for circulating neutrophils in very-low-birth-weight neonates. *Pediatrics* 1994;94(1):76-82.

33. Williams WJ, Nelson DA. Examination of marrow. In: Hematology. Williams WT, Beutler El, Essler AJ, Lichtman MA (eds.). *McGraw Hill Co., New York,* 1991; p 28.

34. Bang AT, Bang RA, Baitule SB, Reddy MH, Deshmukh MD. Effect of home-based neonatal care and management of sepsis on neonatal mortality: field trial in rural India. *Lancet* 1999 Dec 4; 354(9194):1955-1961.

35. McCracken GH, Mize SG. A controlled study of intrathecal antibiotic therapy in Gram-negative enteric meningitis of infancy. *J Pediatr* 1976; 89:66-72.

36. McCracken GH, Mize SG, Threlkeld N. Intraventricular gentamicin therapy in Gram-negative bacillary meningitis of infancy. *Lancet*1980; 1:787-791.

37. Phillipos EZ, Barrington KJ, Robertson MA. Dopamine versus epinephrine for inotropic support in the neonate: A randomized blinded trial. *Pediatr Res* 1996; 39:238A.

Section 3

38. Singh M. Care of the Newborn. *Sagar Publications, New Delhi,* 7th ed, 2010, p. 223-230.

39. Mathur NB. Neonatal sepsis. *Indian Pediatr* 1996; 33:663-674.

40. Mathur NB, Subraniam BKM, Sharma VK, Puri RK. Exchange transfusion in neutropenic septicemic neonates: effects on granulocyte functions. *Acta Paediatr Scand* 1993; 82:939-993.

41. Pammi M, Brocklehurst P. Granulocyte transfusions for neonates with confirmed or suspected sepsis and neutropenia. *Cochrane Database of Systematic Reviews* 2011, Issue 10. Art. No.: CD003956. DOI: 10.1002/ 14651858. CD003956. pub 2.

42. Ohlsson A, Lacy J. Intravenous immunoglobulin for suspected or subsequently proven infection in neonates. *Cochrane Database of Systematic Reviews* 2010, Issue 3. Art. No.: C D001239. DOI: 10.1002/ 14651858.CD001239.pub3.

43. INIS Collaborative Group, Brocklehurst P, Farrell B, King A, Juszczak E, Darlow B, Haque K, Salt A, Stenson B, Tarnow-Mordi W. Treatment of neonatal sepsis with intravenous immune globulin. *N Engl J Med* 2011; 365(13):1201-1211.

44. Carr R, Brocklehurst P, Doré CJ, Modi N. Granulocyte-macrophage colony stimulating factor administered as prophylaxis for reduction of sepsis in extremely preterm, small-for-gestational age neonates (the PROGRAMS trial): a single-blind, multicentre, randomised controlled trial. *Lancet* 2009;373(9659): 226-233.

Section 3

Cardiac Emergencies in Newborn Babies

Anita Saxena and Rajnish Junjeja

INTRODUCTION

Cardiac emergencies in newborns are mostly secondary to congenital heart diseases (CHD). The prevalence of congenital heart disease is reported to be approximately 8 per 1000 live births.[1] Nearly half to one third of these infants are likely to die in the absence of immediate intervention[2]. It is likely that the prevalence is not much different in India, although data is not available. Considering a live birth rate of 20 million per year, India is likely to have 150,000 to 200,000 babies born with CHD every year. About 50,000 to 60,000 babies will have critical CHD requiring an early intervention for their survival.[3] Dealing with these patients is challenging for several reasons. Firstly, the symptoms of cardiovascular disease in newborns may be nonspecific, resembling those of more common disorders like neonatal sepsis, overwhelming pneumonia and RDS. Sometimes it may be difficult to differentiate a cardiac cause from the pulmonary cause when a newborn presents with cyanosis. Secondly, sudden deterioration can occur in a previously stable baby, not allowing enough time for transfer to a referral center with facilities for cardiac care.

Cardiac emergencies in neonates can arise secondary to congenital heart defects (ductus dependent lesions), cardiac arrhythmias or myocardial dysfunction. A more rational approach to the problem would be to classify the emergency according to the mode of clinical presentation. In this chapter, we describe the recognition and management of newborn babies presenting with;

1. Congestive heart failure/cardiogenic shock
2. Cyanosis
3. Rhythm disturbances

Fetal Circulation and Changes at Birth

In order to understand the influence of various congenital heart diseases in a newborn, knowledge of fetal circulation is essential. The basis of this understanding comes mostly from animal studies.

The placenta permits transport of oxygen from the mother to the fetus and carbon dioxide from fetus to mother. The least saturated blood from the upper part of the body returns through superior vena cava to the right atrium. It is joined by the coronary sinus return and is directed through the tricuspid valve to right ventricle and pulmonary artery. Most of this blood shunts through the ductus arteriosus into descending aorta, only a very small proportion goes into lungs. Thus lower part of the body gets deoxygenated blood some of which also flows through the umbilical arteries back to the placenta. Umbilical venous blood, which is highly oxygenated, reaches the inferior vena cava, partly directly through the hepatic circulation and partly through ductus venosus, bypassing the liver. The limbus of the foramen ovale helps to direct this blood into the left atrium. Left atrium also receives a small amount of oxygenated blood from pulmonary veins. Hence oxygenated blood reaches left atrium, left ventricle and ascending aorta. Thus aortic arch vessels, supplying the heart and the brain, receive fully oxygenated blood. A small amount of this blood passes through the isthmus to the descending aorta.

Fetal circulation is adjusted in such a manner that highly oxygenated blood reaches the heart and brain, and this is facilitated by three communications namely ductus venosus, patent foramen ovale and patent ductus arteriosus (Figure 25.1). Changes occur in fetal circulation within a few minutes after birth. The gas exchange function is transferred from placenta to the lungs, which expand at birth. Clamping of umbilical cord removes the low resistant circuit of the placenta, thereby increasing the systemic vascular resistance and decreasing the inferior vena caval return to the heart. With initiation of pulmonary ventilation, pulmonary vascular resistance falls and pulmonary blood flow increases by nearly ten times. By 24 hours, mean pressure in pulmonary artery decreases to half of systemic and then slowly falls further reaching adult levels in 2-6 weeks. The pulmonary venous return to left atrium increases, elevating the pressure in left atrium, which results in closure of the valve of fossa ovalis.

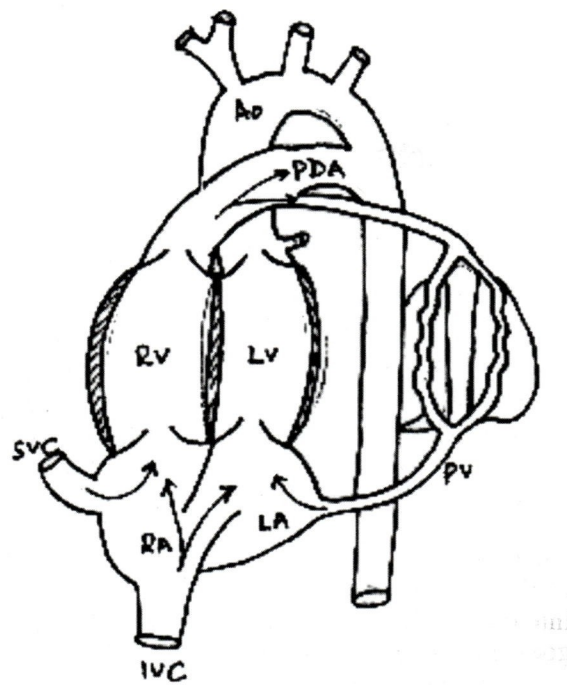

Figure 25.1 Showing fetal circulation. IVC and SVC are the inferior and superior cavas and RA, LA, RV and LV for the atria and ventricles, and PV for placental circulation

The ductus arteriosus starts shunting blood from aorta to pulmonary artery due to fall in pulmonary vascular resistance. It usually closes by the end of the first day mainly due to increase in oxygen tension. However, this closure is more functional rather than structural as ductus arteriosus is known to reopen with hypoxic episodes in the first week of life. The actual closure with ligament formation usually occurs by one to two months of age in majority of infants. In situations where pulmonary vascular resistance remains high, as in persistent fetal circulation, the foramen ovale may continue to shunt the blood right-to-left even after birth. In about 20 to 25 percent of normal adults, the foramen ovale remains open.

Due to the nature of fetal circulation, some of the complex congenital heart defects do not cause any problems during fetal life leading to normal fetal growth and development, e.g. transposition of great arteries, coarctation of aorta, ventricular septal defect, atrial septal defect, etc. In these cases, changes in fetal circulation after birth may make the newborn symptomatic, e.g. sudden deterioration occurring in a baby with transposition of great arteries or severe coarctation of aorta as ductus arteriosus closes. On the other hand, some other cardiac defects affect the heart growth during fetal life, e.g. in a case of mitral atresia, very little blood flows to left ventricle and aorta, making the left ventricle hypoplastic, there may be additional aortic isthmic hypoplasia or coarctation. In conditions like tricuspid and pulmonary atresia, the right ventricle is small, aorta is large and therefore associated coarctation of aorta is rare.

Congenital Heart Diseases in Neonates

Commonest cause of a cardiac emergency in newborns is congenital cardiac defect. Bedside diagnosis of a specific defect is often difficult, however broad generalizations can be made. The basic tools of cardiac evaluation used in children are less reliable in neonates due to circulatory changes that occur at birth. Some of the normal physical findings in a neonate include, fast heart rate of more than 100 to 150 beats per minute, varying degrees of acrocyanosis, mild arterial desaturation with PaO_2 of as low as 60 mmHg, single S_2 on first two days of life and pulmonary flow murmurs.

The types of CHD in neonates is different from that in older children and is given in Table 25.1. The commonest CHD in a neonate is a ventricular septal defect (VSD). The most lethal abnormality is hypoplastic left heart syndrome, majority of cases die by first year of life. Although

Table 25.1 Distribution of cardiac anomalies in neonates			
Lesion	Live births (% of all CHD)	Autopsy (% of all CHD)	Mortality by one year (% of all cases)
Ventricular septal defect	32	10	20
Patent ductus arteriosus	7	2	22
Coarctation of aorta	5	15	32
Tetralogy of Fallot	5	5	36
Complete transposition	5	15	62
Hypoplastic left heart syndrome	3	25	89
Pulmonary atresia with VSD	3	10	70
CHD: Congenital heart disease, VSD: Ventricular septal defect			

echocardiography remains the mainstay of diagnosing congenital cardiac defects with accuracy, a complete history and physical examination along with an X-ray chest and an ECG generally gives enough information for initial stabilization of these neonates in the emergency room. With advances in therapeutics including cardiac surgery, a corrective or definitive treatment is available for majority of infants with congenital heart disease.

CONGESTIVE HEART FAILURE

The causes of congestive heart failure according to the time of presentation are given in Table 25.2.

Table 25.2 Causes of heart failure in the neonate

A. Structural heart defects

At birth	❑ Hypoplastic left heart syndrome
	❑ Severe atrio-ventricular valve regurgitation e.g. tricuspid or mitral valve regurgitation
	❑ Large systemic arterio-venous fistula
Week 1	❑ Transposition of great arteries
	❑ Large patent ductus arteriosus in a preterm infant
	❑ Obstructive total anomalous pulmonary venous connection
Week 1-4	❑ Critical aortic or pulmonary stenosis
	❑ Preductal coarctation of aorta
	❑ Large ventricular septal defect, patent ductus arteriosus, atrioventricular septal defect
	❑ Anomalous origin of coronary artery from pulmonary artery
	❑ Cyanotic heart disease likes truncus arteriosus, single ventricle, tricuspid atresia, double outlet right ventricle

B. Myocardial diseases
- ❑ Myocarditis
- ❑ Transient myocardial ischemia with or without birth asphyxia
- ❑ Cardiomyopathy (seen in infants of diabetic mother)

C. Disturbances in heart rate
- ❑ Supraventricular tachycardia
- ❑ Atrial flutter
- ❑ Ventricular tachycardia
- ❑ Congenital complete heart block

D. Noncardiac causes
- ❑ Birth asphyxia
- ❑ Metabolic: hypoglycemia, hypocalcemia
- ❑ Severe anemia
- ❑ Neonatal sepsis
- ❑ Overtransfusion or overhydration

Clinical Picture

Symptoms such as fast breathing, rapid heart rate, feeding difficulties and excessive sweating are suggestive of congestive heart failure in a neonate. The weight gain is suboptimal. Tachypnea (respiratory rate of over 60/ min), tachycardia (heart rate of over 160 bpm), hepatomegaly and cardiomegaly are cardinal signs of heart failure. In addition there may be subcostal recessions, feeding difficulties and excessive sweating. Pedal edema, raised jugular venous pressure and basal crepitations over lung fields, features of congestive heart failure in older children and adults, are hardly ever seen in neonates and infants. In fact, presence of crepitation over lung fields may indicate associated respiratory infection. Bilateral rhonchi may be heard in advanced cases of heart failure. A loud third heart sound may be audible.

In advanced heart failure, the peripheral pulses become weak, perfusion is poor with mottled extremities and hypothermia. These babies may go into hypotension and shock if immediate help is not provided. Cardiogenic shock is more likely in neonates with left ventricular outflow tract obstruction like hypoplastic left heart, interrupted aortic arch, severe coarctation of aorta and critical aortic stenosis. Noncardiac causes of shock-like septicemia, meningitis etc. must be excluded.

Diagnosis of Specific Lesions

Diagnosing a specific lesion from the long list of causes of heart failure is not always possible at the bedside, but few clinical pointers may be helpful.

1. Bounding pulses with heart failure indicate presence of a patent ductus arteriosus, more so in preterm babies. High volume pulses are also noted in truncus arteriosus and arteriovenous malformations, which are less common causes of heart failure in neonates.

2. Weak or absent femoral pulses are seen in coarctation of aorta. It must be remembered that in the presence of a large patent ductus arteriosus in a newborn, the femoral pulses may be well felt. Coarctation usually manifests by the end of first week or later, hence one must palpate for femoral pulses at the time of discharge of the baby and at first follow up visit. The ECG in neonatal coarctation may show right axis deviation and right ventricular hypertrophy, instead of left ventricular hypertrophy, which is seen in older children.

3. An ejection systolic murmur heard at the base of the heart on day one of life suggests aortic or pulmonary stenosis.

4. Continuous murmur over the head in a newborn with heart failure, suggests arteriovenous malformation involving the vein of Galen (Figure 25.2). It should be suspected in a neonate with high output failure.

5. Mild cyanosis with a widely split second heart sound is suggestive of total anomalous pulmonary venous drainage. Other causes include Ebstein's anomaly and partial atrioventricular septal defect.

6. A systolic murmur due to atrioventricular valve regurgitation is a common finding in babies with a history of birth asphyxia. The murmur may be due to tricuspid regurgitation or due to papillary muscle dysfunction and mitral regurgitation. There may be ST-T wave changes in the ECG. These systolic murmurs are also heard in atrioventricular septal defect.

7. No significant murmur and muffled heart sounds suggest primary myocardial disease, myocarditis, or pericardial effusion.

8. A mid diastolic murmur at apex in a relatively older neonate with heart failure would suggest a large patent ductus or ventricular septal defect in an acyanotic baby and transposition of great arteries or persistent truncus arteriosus in a cyanotic neonate.

9. Some of these neonates have associated chromosomal anomalies. Specific syndromes are associated with specific heart defects, e.g. Down syndrome with atrioventricular septal defect and Noonan syndrome with pulmonary stenosis and hypertrophic cardiomyopathy.

Electrocardiography

An ECG shows right axis deviation and right ventricular dominance in a normal newborn. It should always be done, if a cardiac disorder is suspected. ECG also helps to diagnose arrhythmia in case the heart rate is either too slow (< 100 bpm) or too fast (> 160 bpm). Certain patterns may be diagnostic in the context of clinical picture.

1. Left axis deviation may point to atrioventricular septal defect, a muscular ventricular septal defect or tricuspid atresia as the the cause of underlying left-to-right shunt.

2. Short PR interval (< 0.08 sec), increased QRS voltages in a case of primary myocardial disease indicate underlying glycogen storage disorder like Pompe's disease (Figure 25.3).

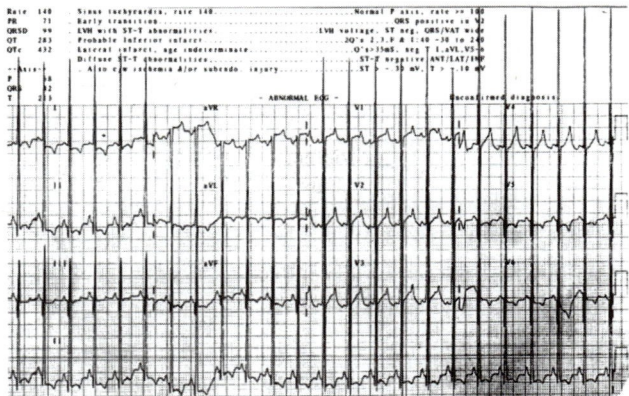

Figure 25.3 A 12 lead ECG from a child showing short PR interval and huge QRS voltages which is a classical finding in Pompe's disease.

3. Prominent q waves in lead I, aVL, V_4 to V_6 with or without ST-T wave changes is diagnostic of anomalous origin of left coronary artery from pulmonary artery (ALCAPA) in an infant with a picture of dilated cardiomyopathy (Figure 25.4).

4. Narrow QRS fixed rate tachycardia at a rate of 220-250 suggests supraventricular tachycardia as the cause of heart failure. The P waves are generally not discernible, but

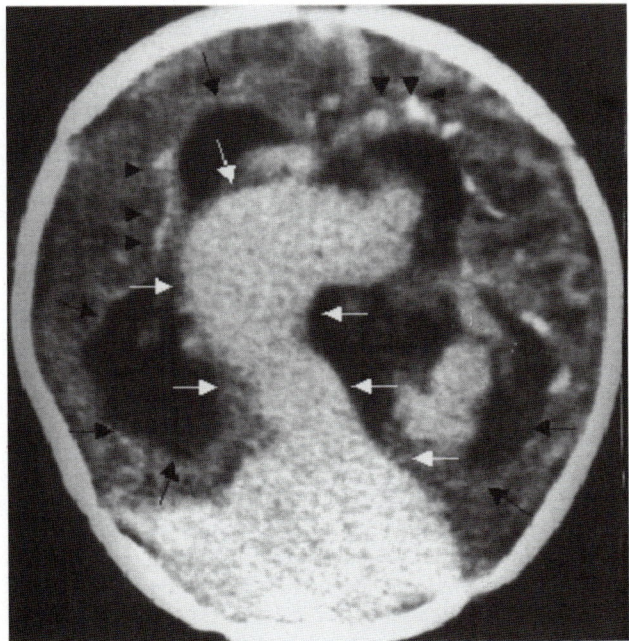

Figure 25.2 CT scan of the cranium showing vein of Galen malformation (white arrows), dilated lateral ventricles (black arrows), periventricular calcification (black arrowheads) and changes of encephalomalacia in both cerebral hemispheres. As a rule a CT scan in this setting should not be contrast enhanced. (reproduced from Indian Heart Journal, with permission).

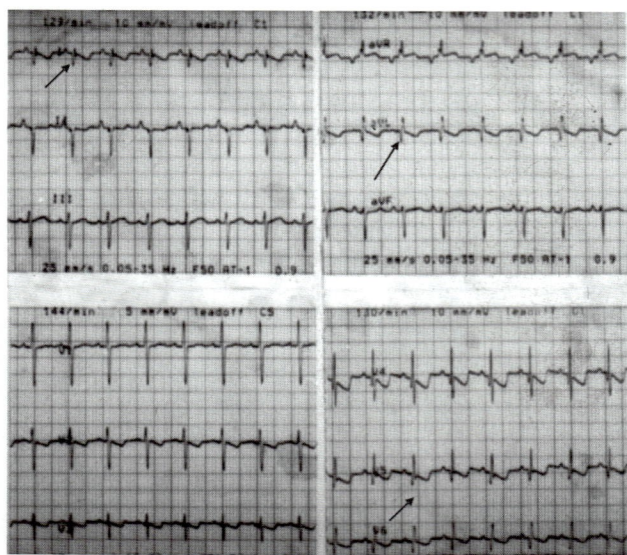

Figure 25.4 A 12 lead ECG in a child labeled as DCM q waves are clearly seen in lead I, aVL, V5 and V6 which is diagnostic of anomalous origin of left coronary artery from pulmonary artery (ALCAPA)

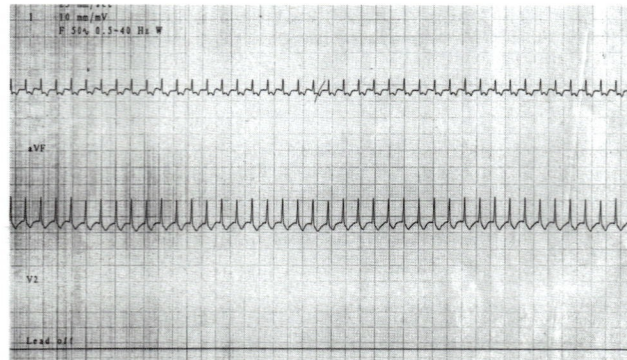

Figure 25.5 Narrow QRS tachycardia in a 2-day infant presenting with symptoms of lethargy and crying. Heart rate is around 250/min and no definite P waves are seen. Child most likely has an SVT, but it is imperative to take a 12 lead ECG or as many chest leads as feasible to be sure about the missing P waves. Recording a rhythm strip alone is incorrect practice

careful evaluation would suggest presence of notching on the ST–T waves which represents the P wave (Figure 25.5).

5.   A prolonged QT/QTc in an infant suggests hypocalcemia as a possible underlying cause of left ventricular dysfunction (Figure 25.6).

X-ray Chest

Although widely available, this important investigation is often omitted in the work up of a neonate with suspected cardiac disorder. An X-ray chest is a simple and an important investigation in categorizing a neonate to a specific group of congenital heart disease. The information about visceral situs, heart size, specific chamber enlargement, pulmonary blood flow, pulmonary and arterial venous hypertension, site of aortic arch and about pulmonary parenchyma is easily obtained from a chest radiograph.

A cardiothoracic ratio of more than 0.60 is indicative of cardiomegaly. A stomach bubble can localize the situs, normally present on the left side. In babies with situs inversion or situs ambiguous (where visceral situs is not clear with a central stomach bubble or midline liver) with a left sided heart, severe congenital heart defects are very common. Anatomy of right and left main bronchi, best seen in a penetrated film, is also helpful in recognition of situs. Enlargement of a specific chamber can also point towards a specific defect, e.g. cardiomegaly with right atrial enlargement points to atrial septal defect (if there is increased

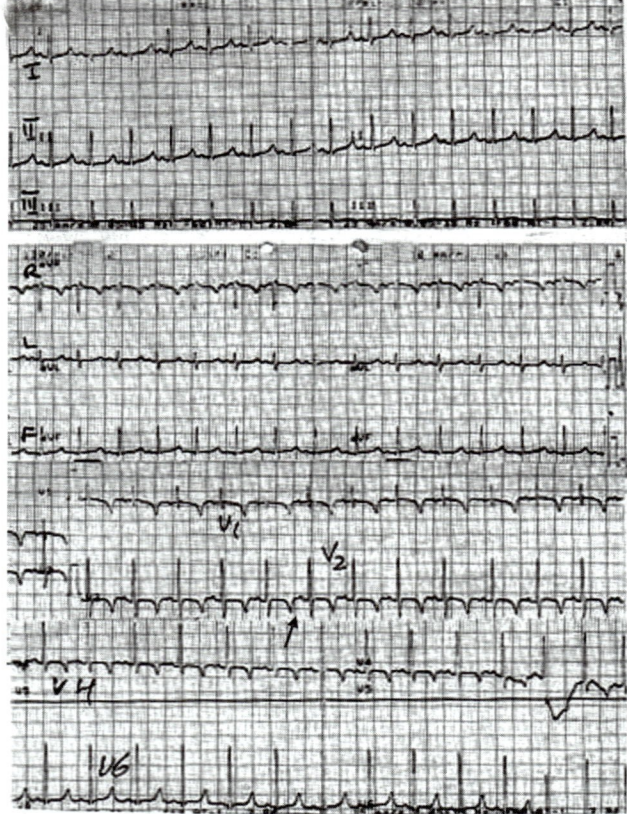

Figure 25.6 Infant with recurrent epileptic attacks and dilated cardiomyopathy. An ECG clearly reveals the long QT interval (arrow) suggesting hypocalcemia as the etiology of both

pulmonary blood flow) or tricuspid regurgitation. Left atrial enlargement goes in favor of ventricular septal defect, patent ductus arteriosus or left sided regurgitation.

An increased pulmonary blood flow, present in shunt lesions, is seen as more than five end-on vessels including both hila. Size of each vessel should be equal to or bigger than the size of accompanying bronchus (pulmonary plethora). The arteries are also increased in size and visible well beyond the periphery of the lung fields (Figure 25.7).

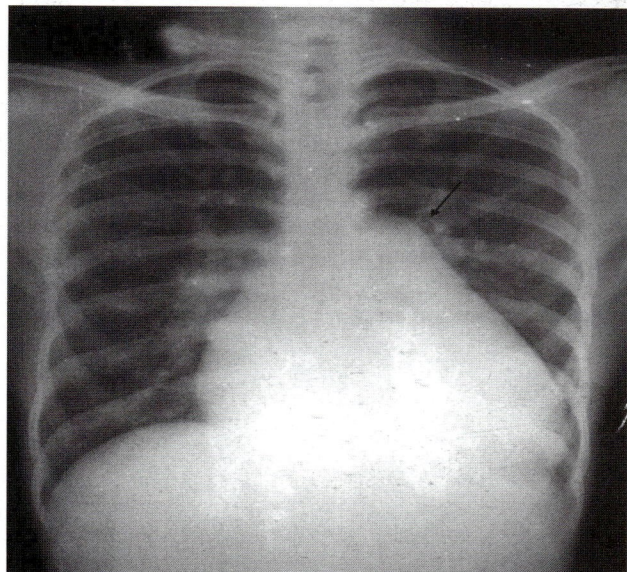

Figure 25.7 PA chest view of an infant with large left-to-right shunt. The cardiomegaly of LV type, RA enlargement, PA enlargement (arrow) and pulmonary plethora suggests large left-to-right shunt (probably additional atrial level shunt also)

Interpretation of chest X-rays should be systematic and must include assessment of rib cage and lungs. Most of the times an X-ray chest is not typical of any particular cardiac defect but provides important information for making a diagnosis. In a small proportion of cases, it can be diagnostic. These include ground glass appearance of lungs in obstructive total anomalous pulmonary venous drainage (Figure 25.8), a narrow pedicle and absence of thymus in a baby with transposition of great arteries (Figure 25.9). Presence of a pneumonic patch is not uncommon in these babies and may be the underlying precipitating factor for deterioration in the condition of the baby.

Echocardiography

Echocardiography should be performed as soon as the baby has been stabilized. The technique of using ultrasound to image the heart has been available for many years. With the advent of Doppler and color flow mapping, one is able to get complete anatomic and hemodynamic information non-invasively in a majority of cases. The technique is of special relevance in neonates with heart diseases as the imaging is excellent and the invasive

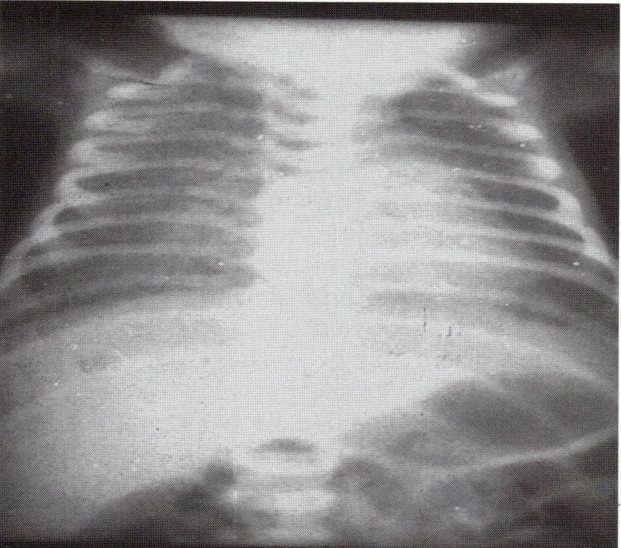

Figure 25.8 Classical ground glass appearance of the lung fields, no cardiomegaly and an enlarged liver, classical of an obstructed TAPVC

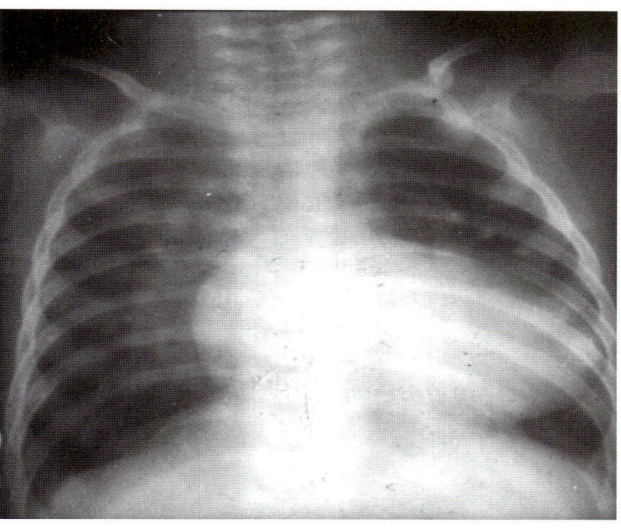

Figure 25.9 Chest skiagram showing classical egg on side appearance – the left ventricular side is the smaller side of the egg. The narrow pedicle is an integral part of the shape and is seen because of the absent thymus. Pulmonary blood flow is increased

tests like cardiac catheterization are associated with high-risk in these sick babies. The interpretation of echocardiographic findings is operator dependent to a large extent, and there is a wide scope for errors. Although screening echo may be done by the neonatologist, the details of CHD are best obtained by the trained personnel. It is not a substitute for an X-ray chest, as often practiced by several pediatricians/pediatric cardiologists.

The situs must be documented first by demonstrating the inferior vena cava, descending aorta and atrial appendage morphology. In rare cases of isomerism, situs identification may not be easy. The cardiac apex position should be defined next from a subcostal approach to check the cardiac postion e.g. levocardia, dextrocardia. The entry of at least three pulmonary veins can be shown by posterior tilt of the transducer. Subcostal view is also ideally suited for defining the interatrial septum and various types of atrial septal defects. However, subcostal view is often painful for the child with congestive heart failure and may wake up the neonate. Next, atrioventricular valves should be evaluated. There may be atresia of one valve with corresponding ventricle being hypoplastic. Atrioventricular canal defects (or endocardial cushion defects) can also be easily diagnosed by the presence of a common atrioventricular valve and primum atrial septal defect with or without a ventricular septal defect. The size, position and morphology of ventricles should be assessed as also the integrity of ventricular septum, best seen from the apex. Ventriculoarterial relationship is defined from the subcostal and parasternal regions. To differentiate pulmonary artery from aorta, its bifurcation should be identified. Aorta is identified by demonstrating the origin of coronary arteries from it. Occasionally, only one great artery is seen arising from both the ventricles as in persistent truncus arteriosus. The semilunar valves are evaluated for any thickening or stenosis. Finally, a suprasternal view must be obtained for defining the aortic arch, isthmus and entry of pulmonary veins into left atrium. The diagnosis of coarctation/arch interruption is possible from this view. Doppler evaluation of various valves and interatrial and interventricular septa must be combined with cross sectional imaging.

This segmental approach helps to prevent mistakes such as missing the diagnosis of transposition of great arteries (if bifurcation of posterior great vessel is not imaged, Figure 25.10) or total anomalous pulmonary venous connection (if the right-to-left flow across the atrial septal defect is not appreciated, Figures 25.11 and 25.12). Similarly failure to demonstrate origin of left coronary artery from pulmonary artery (in an infant with LV dysfunction) may result in labeling the infant as having dilated cardiomyopathy (Figure 25.13).

Treatment

Treatment of heart failure in newborns should focus on the treatment of the cause, precipitating factors (like anemia, infections, arrhythmias, etc), and treatment of the congested state.

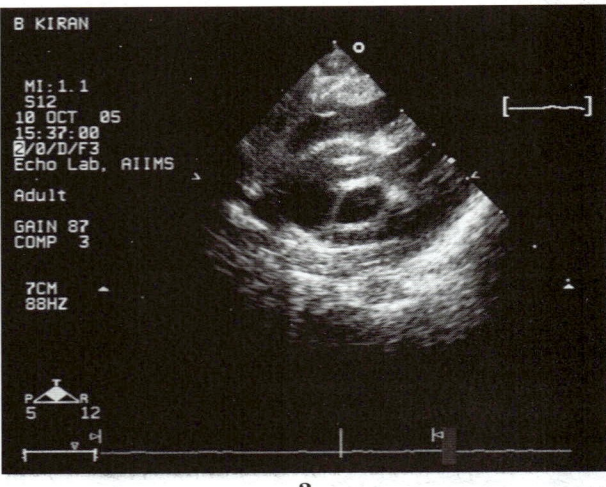

a

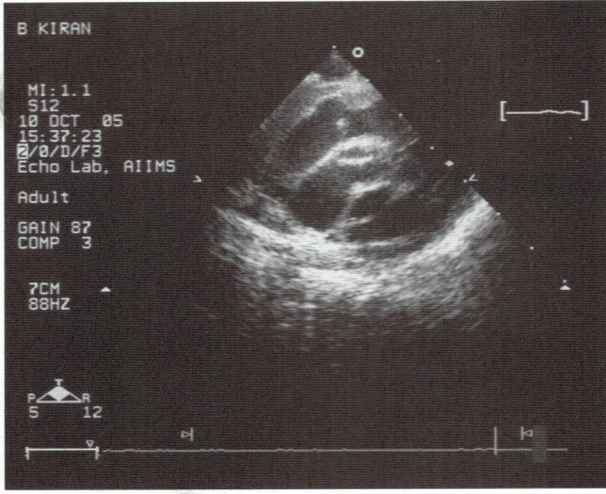

b

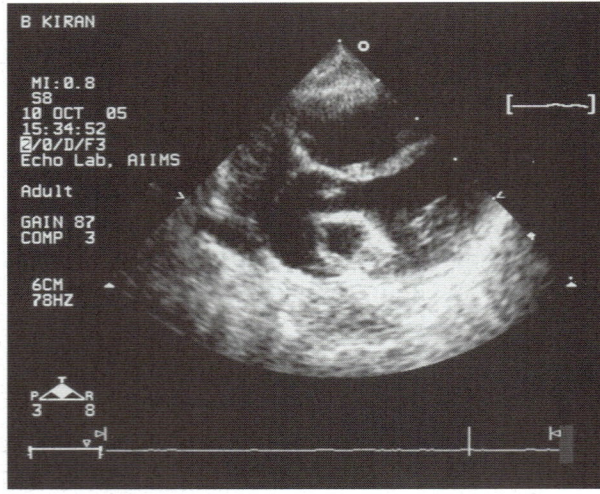

c

Figure 25.10 2-D echocardiogram in parasternal long axis view. It shows how easy it is to misdiagnose TGA as a normal heart. There is a vessel coming from LV and another from RV. Unless one looks at the bifurcation (10b) or focuses on the relationship of the vessels this may be diagnosed as abnormal heart

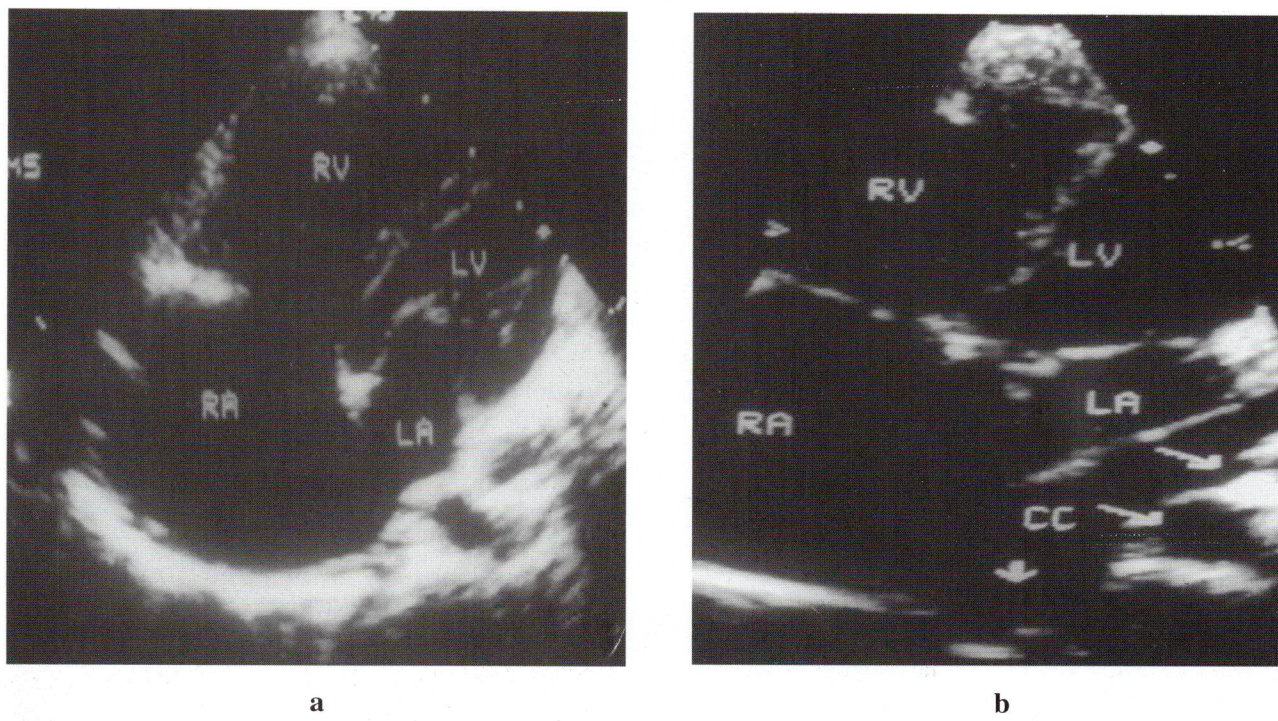

a   b

Figure 25.11 Apical 4 chamber views of a child with TAPVC. RA, RV dilatation is seen that may also be seen with an ASD. The pulmonary veins are seen at the usual place (arrow). It is only when a more posterior tilt is given or when the opening is sought does the common chamber become obvious (11b). Abbreviations are same as described before; CC is common chamber and PV is pulmonary vein

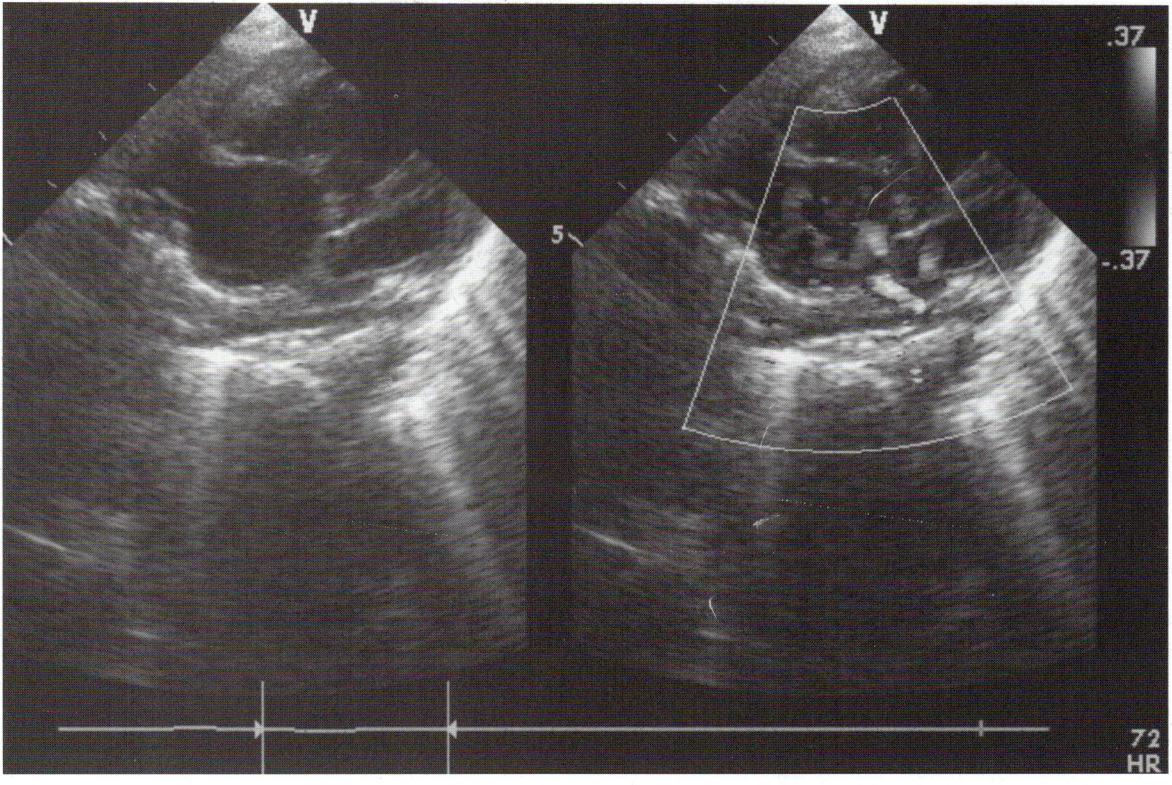

a   b

Figure 25.12 A TAPVC can be easily differentiated from an ASD by looking at the color Doppler that shows right-to-left flow (blue mosaic) instead of the usual left-to-right flow. Arrow in 12b shows the blue mosaic

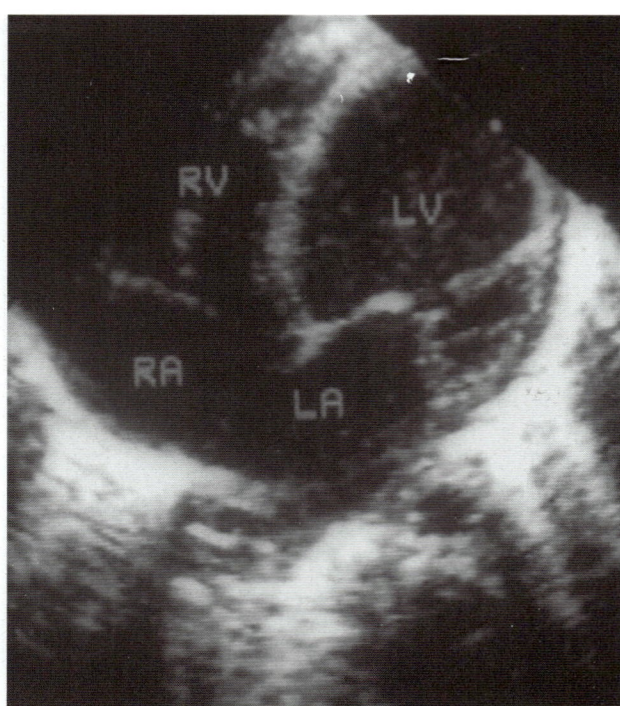

a

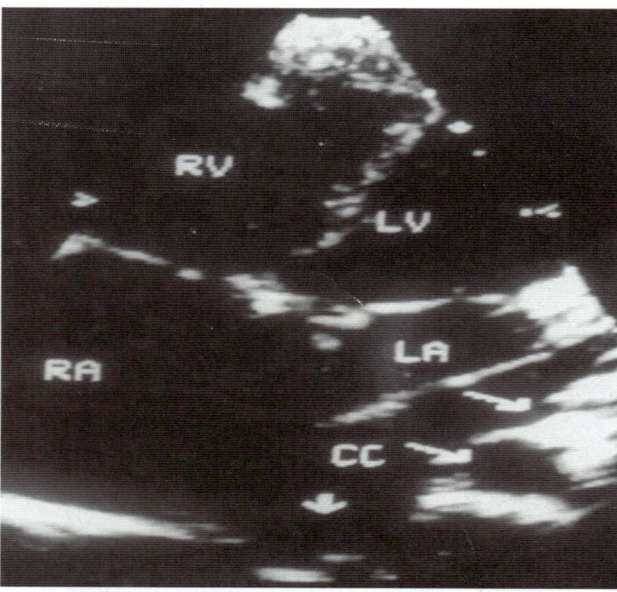

b

Figure 25.13 Apical 4 chamber views (a) and parasternal short axis view (b). Child labeled as dilated cardiomyopathy (DCM) because the coronary origin from the PA (arrow) was missed

General measures. These are directed towards improving cardiac performance, augmenting peripheral perfusion and decreasing systemic and pulmonary venous congestion. Umbilical vein catheterization is useful for infusion and medications. Sick neonates, especially those in cardiogenic shock, need to be intubated and mechanically ventilated.

1. **Maintenance of oxygenation.** The status of oxygenation should be monitored by blood gas determination in sick babies. Although estimation by pulse oximetry is readily available, it is subject to movement artifacts and is unreliable in infants with low cardiac output or poor skin perfusion. Infants with moderate to severe pulmonary edema may benefit from CPAP, but those with severe congestion resulting in persistent hypoxemia, hypercarbia and respiratory acidosis should receive IPPV with modest amount of PEEP. In lesions like hypoplastic left heart or severe coarctation, where ductus arteriosus is being kept open by infusion of prostaglandins, one should not try to achieve 100% oxygen saturation, as that would be achieved only by an over circulation of the pulmonary vascular bed. Also a high FiO_2 may decrease pulmonary vascular resistance and worsen pulmonary congestion, as oxygen is a potent pulmonary vasodilator. It may be necessary to ventilate these babies with room air to achieve the desired saturation of 75% – 80% and PaO_2 of 50-60 mm Hg that occurs with a pulmonary to systemic flow of nearly 1:1[4].

2. **Maintenance of adequate hydration and calorie intake.** Relatively stable newborns should be nursed orally with head end elevated. Small frequent oral feeds are better tolerated. If there is severe tachypnea, oral feeding should be withheld, as there is risk of aspiration. The fluid and caloric intake should be adequate as the requirement is increased during heart failure. Intravenous fluids are generally restricted to 65-80 ml/kg/day in newborns. It must be ensured that adequate calories are provided in restricted amount of fluids. Some sick neonates may have reduced intravascular volume at the time of admission to the emergency room. They should be given fluid boluses of 5 ml/kg normal saline every 20 to 30 minutes till they improve.[5]

3. **Maintenance of temperature and avoidance of hypoglycemia.** Hypothermia is a common problem in neonates and must be prevented. Similarly blood sugar should be closely monitored and corrected if there is hypoglycemia.

4. **Inotropic agents.** Digoxin is a commonly used inotropic agent and may be started orally

in stable neonates with heart failure. It is given in a loading dose of 20-40 mcg/kg and then maintained at 10 mcg/kg/day in two divided doses. Digoxin is a relatively safe drug in term neonates. Preterm babies and those with myocarditis are more sensitive to digoxin and therefore lower dose should be used in these babies. In sicker neonates, intravenous sympathomimetic amines are preferred. Dopamine and/or dobutamine are administered as continuous infusion in a dose of 5 – 20 mcg/kg/minute. Dobutamine may offer an advantage over dopamine as it has less arrhythmogenic potential and reduces afterload because of its vasodilatory effect.[5] In neonates with hypotension, dopamine may be used alone initially, dobutamine added later. Rarely infusion of milrinone is administered for its positive inotropic and after load reducing effects. Infusion of epinephrine is sometimes used for babies in cardiogenic shock.

5. **Diuretics.** Diuretic therapy plays an important role in management of heart failure by promoting diuresis and natriuresis. Furosemide is the most commonly used diuretic, it can be given orally or intravenously 2-4 mg/kg/day in two or three divided doses. The onset of action is within five minutes and peak effect is seen at 30 minutes. Serum electrolytes should be monitored on aggressive diuretic therapy. Supplementation of potassium is usually not required in neonates if the furosemide dose is $\leq$ 2 mg/kg.

6. **Vasodilators.** These drugs reduce the afterload and thus tend to augment the stroke volume without increasing the myocardial oxygen consumption. Vasodilators are contraindicated in neonates with heart failure secondary to obstructive lesions such as critical aortic, pulmonic or mitral stenosis. Commonly used vasodilators include angiotensin converting enzyme inhibitors (ACEI) and other drugs like hydralazine and nitrates. The doses and dominant site of action of various vasodilators is given in Table 25.3.

(a) *ACEI.* These drugs should be used cautiously as they may precipitate hypotension in the initial setting. Experience with ACEI is limited in neoantes and they are contraindicated in the presence of renal dysfunction. Of the various ACEI available, captopril is preferred as it has shorter duration of action. When using ACEI in neonates, renal function and urine output must be carefully monitored especially the first week of therapy.[6] One should start with a low dose of 0.1 mg/kg/day of captopril in three divided doses orally. ACEI are very helpful if tolerated, as there is excessive activation of renal angiotensin system in patients with congestive heart failure. Their role is proven in heart failure secondary to

Table 25.3 Doses and mode of administration of vasodilators

Agent	Site of action	Dose
Nitroglycerine	Venous	0.05-20 mcg/kg/min IV infusion
Iso-sorbide dinitrate	Venous	0.1 mg/kg q 6 hr PO (maximum dose 2 mg/kg/day)
Nitroprusside	Venous + Arterial	0.5-4.0 mcg/kg/min IV infusion
Hydralazine (Not available in India)	Arterial	0.5-1.0 mg/kg/IV q 6 hr, 1.7 mg/kg/day PO in 3-4 doses
Prazosin	Venous + Arterial	5-25 mcg/kg/dose PO q 6 hr
Nifedipine	Arterial	0.1-0.2mg/kg/dose q 6 hr PO
Captopril	Venous + Arterial	Neonate: 0.1-1.0 mg/kg/day PO Infants: 0.2-4.0 mg/kg/day in 3 div doses PO Children: 12.5 mg q 12 hr PO
Enalapril	Venous + Arterial	0.1-1.0 mg/kg/day in two divided doses PO
Losartan	Venous + Arterial	0.5 mg/kg/day once daily PO
Minoxidil	Arterial	0.2 mg/kg/day initial dose, increase slowly up to 1.0 mg/kg/day PO

IV: Intravenous, PO: Per oral

left-to-right shunts, myocardial dysfunction and atrioventricular valve regurgitation like mitral or aortic valve regurgitation.

(b) *Sodium nitroprusside.* It is a very potent vasodilator.[7] Hypotension is a common side effect and therefore intensive, preferably invasive monitoring of blood pressure is required during the infusion of this drug. When used for more than 48 hours, it can lead to thiocynate accumulation, agitation, twitchings and seizures.

7. Pharmacologic manipulation of ductus arteriosus. The patency of ductus arteriosus in newborns can be manipulated by certain drugs.

(a) *Prostaglandins.* These drugs are used for keeping the ductus open in conditions such as hypoplastic left heart, coarctation of aorta, critical aortic stenosis. Details of prostaglandin therapy are given later.

(b) *Indomethacin.* Indomethacin is used to close ductus arteriosus in preterm babies, the details are given in section on "PDA in preterm babies".

8. Specific measures. Most of the heart defects presenting, as emergencies in newborns require surgical treatment (Table 25.4). After initial stabilization, surgical correction is performed for defects like transposition of great arteries, coarctation of aorta, total anomalous pulmonary venous connection, persistent truncus arteriosus, large patent ductus arteriosus, large ventricular septal defect, complete atrioventricular septal defect etc. Lesions like single ventricle, multiple muscular ventricular septal defects, where complete correction is not possible, are initially palliated by performing banding of pulmonary arteries which reduces pulmonary artery pressure as well as pulmonary flow. Some of the cardiac defects can be managed by nonsurgical interventions in the catheterization laboratory as in valvular aortic stenosis.[8]

9. Treatment of arrhythmias. Arrhythmias occurring secondarily to metabolic factors rarely need management with antiarrhythmics unless life-threatening or associated with hemodynamic compromise. Sinus bradycardia is rarely significant enough to warrant any therapy. Atropine is useful for temporary relief while isoprenaline infusion can provide sustained benefit. Complete heart block and other forms of blocks are rarely seen in secondary forms; except due to digitalis toxicity and hyperkalemia. Tachyarrhythmias also need not be treated unless they are sustained. Isolated APC's or VPB's, couplets/triplets or bigeminy do not need any antiarrhythmics; but, the underlying cause like hypokalemia, digoxin toxicity, hypoxia and poor

Table 25.4 Timing of Surgery for Common Congenital Heart Disease in Neonates

Lesion	Type of surgery	Timing of surgery
Ventricular septal defect (a) Large, single (b) Multiple	Closure PA banding	< 6 months < 3-6 months
Large patent ductus arteriosus in full term baby	Ligation	< 3 months
Atrioventricular septal defect	Total repair	< 3-4 months
Severe coarctation of aorta	End-to-end anastomosis or subclavian flap repair	As soon as detected
Tetralogy of Fallot (a) Severe cyanosis (b) Mild cyanosis	Aortopulmonary shunt Total repair	As soon as detected 9 months – 1 year
Complete transposition of great arteries (a) with intact IVS (b) With VSD	Arterial switch operation Arterial switch operation	< 2-3 wks < 8-12 wks
Hypoplastic left heart	Norwood stage I	As soon as possible
Single ventricle with PAH	PA banding	< 8-12 wks

IVS: Intact ventricular septum, PA: Pulmonary artery PAH: Pulmonary arterial hypertension, VSD: Ventricular septal defect

myocardial function should be treated. Long QT syndrome associated with drugs and leading to early coupled VPB's warrants immediate withdrawal of the offending drug. In addition xylocaine and magnesium infusion may be needed especially if the QTc is > 500 msec and leading to early coupled VPB's. Torsades-de-pointes in this setting needs to be managed with above measures and isoprenaline/temporary pacing, as an after-depolarization following a long pause often triggers the arrhythmia. Maintaining a temporary pacing lead in a neonate/infant is obviously difficult and can be associated with complications like venous thrombosis, infection etc. Fortunately, Torsades is rarely seen in neonates in clinical practice.

10. **Other modalities**. Treatment of persistent pulmonary hypertension of the newborn is largely supportive. In severe cases high frequency ventilation and inhaled nitric oxide is used. Oral sildenafil has been successfully used by some workers; this approach is particularly useful in the settings where other treatment modalities are not available. [9] Similarly asphyxia-related myocardial damage and ischemia, are managed with infusion of inotropes. Most of these conditions have a good prognosis, provided the initial critical period is tided over effectively. There are several newer agents, the roles of which are still investigational, in adults and children. These include natriuretic peptides (e.g. nesiritide), calcium sensitizers (e.g. levosimendan), vasopressin antagonists (e.g. tolvaptan), renin inhibitors (e.g. aliskiren), endothelin antagonists (e.g. sitoxentan) etc.

Patent Ductus Arteriosus in Preterm Babies

With improvement in survival of premature babies, patent ductus arteriosus is being diagnosed with increasing frequency. The overall incidence of patent ductus arteriosus is 8/1000 in preterm infants, but it is very common in very low birth weight babies. Patent ductus arteriosus is present in 45% of infants weighing < 1750 gm and in 80% of those weighing < 1000 gm. Left-to-right shunting through a patent ductus can prolong dependency on ventilator and also lead to increased risk of developing bronchopulmonary dysplasia. Clinical diagnosis of patent ductus arteriosus can be made in the presence of hyperdynamic precordium, coupled with systolic murmur in second left upper intercostal space, bounding peripheral pulsations, sudden weight gain and increasing oxygen

requirements. A deterioration in the ventilatory status of a premature infant, recovering from respiratory distress syndrome, is often a strong indication of a significant left-to-right shunt through a patent ductus arteriosus. Increasing cardiomegaly may be another indication of patency of ductus. Echocardiography is very helpful to diagnose patent ductus arterious and to rule out other causes of deterioration like underlying pulmonary disease. It further helps in follow up of these babies as the partial or complete ductal closure can be documented after therapy.

Treatment includes restriction of fluids and administration of a diuretic like furosemide. Maintenance of adequate hematocrit and hemoglobin is very important as anemia further impairs cardiac function. Hematocrit should be maintained above 45. Caloric intake is often a major problem and intravenous hyperalimentation may be required. Indomethacin intravenously or through the nasogastric tube, given in a dose of 0.2 mg/kg/dose for 3 doses at 12 hourly intervals is safe and effective in closing the ductus in more than 70 percent of the cases. Babies weighing < 1000 gm have been shown to benefit from the use of prophylactic indomethacin therapy. Contra-indications include a raised BUN and / or creatinine, platelet count of < 80,000/ul, bleeding tendency, necrotising enterocolitis and hyperbilirubinemia. Ibuprofen has also been used with equivalent results and perhaps fewer side effects.[10] Patent ductus arteriosus in a term baby does not respond to indomethacin or ibuprofen. If patent ductus does not close with indomethacin therapy, surgical ligation is indicated. The ductus is clipped or ligated through a small lateral thoracotomy incision. Occasionally coils have been used to close ductus through transcatheter procedure.

CYANOSIS

It is usually easy to differentiate cyanosis due to a cardiac cause from a pulmonary cause. An elevated $paCO_2$ suggests primary lung or neurologic cause and a persistent low paO_2 favours the possibility of cyanosis due to a cardiac cause. However, in cases where the differentiation is difficult, a hyperoxia test is helpful. A paO_2 of more than 160 mm Hg upon inhalation of 100% oxygen for 5 to 10 minutes makes the cardiac cause of cyanosis unlikely, while a value of >200 mm Hg completely excludes it. Also, arterial saturation does not normalize with oxygen inhalation in infants with cyanotic cardiac defect, unlike those with primary lung pathology.

Section 3

Cyanosis should never be overlooked in a newborn, however mild it may be. The baby may be having a ductus dependent lesion, like pulmonary atresia and sudden deterioration will occur when ductus closes. A higher preductal paO_2 by 10 to 15 mm Hg as compared to postductal paO_2 is indicative of right-to-left shunt through patent ductus arteriosus as may be seen in persistent pulmonary arterial hypertension of the neonate, aortic atresia, hypoplastic left heart syndrome etc. Cyanosis is underestimated in the presence of anemia. Table 25.5 lists the various cardiac causes of central cyanosis in newborns, grouped under three headings.

I. **Cyanosis, murmur and absence of heart failure.** These babies are likely to have one of the cyanotic CHD lesions with reduced pulmonary blood flow, the classical example being tetralogy of Fallot (TOF). An ejection systolic murmur secondary to the obstruction to pulmonary outflow tract is usually audible. In cases with pulmonary atresia, there may be no murmur or a faint contnuous murmur in front or back due to the patent ductus arteriosus or collaterals. Some of these neonates present to the emergency room with deep cyanosis, hypoxemia and acidosis. Frank cyanotic spells are uncommon at this age. The clinical examination shows absence of heart failure. An X-ray chest typically shows a normal sized heart with oligemic, black looking lung fields. Further characterization into individual lesions may not be possible without the help of echocardiography, although tricuspid atresia is likely if the electrocardiogram shows left axis deviation, left ventricular hypertrophy and absence of right ventricular forces.

II. **Cyanosis, insignificant murmur and heart failure.** These features are typically seen in cyanotic lesions with increased pulmonary blood flow. These neonates present with clinical features of cyanosis and heart failure, as the pulmonary blood flow is increased. The baby has tachypnea, tachycardia, cardiomegaly and hepatomegaly in addition to mild cyanosis. Murmurs are soft, insignificant, and often diastolic due to increased flow across the mitral valve. The second heart sound is often single due to malposition of great arteries. Sometimes a split is appreciated with a loud P_2 component. In total anomalous pulmonary venous connection, the second heart sound is wide and fixed split. Presence of an early diastolic murmur favours truncus arteriosus. X-ray chest shows cardiomegaly

---

Table 25.5 Cyanotic heart diseases in the neonates

I. **Those associated with reduced pulmonary blood flow (have pulmonic stenosis)**

- ❑ Tetralogy of Fallot
- ❑ Tricuspid atresia
- ❑ Double outlet of right ventricle with pulmonary stenosis
- ❑ Transposition of great arteries with pulmonary stenosis
- ❑ Critical pulmonary valve stenosis or atresia
- ❑ Single ventricle with pulmonary stenosis
- ❑ Ebstein's anomaly

II. **Those associated with increased pulmonary blood flow (have pulmonary hypertension)**

- ❑ Transposition of great arteries
- ❑ Total anomalous pulmonary venous connection
- ❑ Persistent truncus arteriosus
- ❑ Double outlet of right ventricle
- ❑ Univentricular heart
- ❑ Atrioventricular septal defect

III. **Those associated with pulmonary venous congestion**

- ❑ Obstructed total anomalous pulmonary venous connection
- ❑ Hypoplastic left heart syndrome
- ❑ Pulmonary vein stenosis
- ❑ Cor triatriatum and mitral valve diseases

---

with increased lung markings due to pulmonary plethora. In some cases of transposition of great arteries, the X-ray chest may show a narrow pedicle, giving an "egg on side" appearance.

III. **Sick, cyanosed baby having respiratory distress, with insignificant murmurs.** This picture results from cyanotic CHD with pulmonary venous congestion. These neonates may develop hypotension and shock if not quickly supported. Tachypnea and tachycardia are prominent features, there may be hepatomegaly. Murmurs are usually absent. X-ray chest shows picture suggestive of pulmonary edema, at times difficult to differentiate from respiratory distress syndrome.

Treatment

General measures. These include correction of hypoxemia, acidosis, maintaining adequate hydration, avoidance of hypothermia and hypoglycemia etc. If heart failure is present, diuretics and inotropes are used.

Prostaglandin therapy. Prostagladin infusion is life saving in lesions which are dependent on the patency of arterial duct. Since its first description by Coceani and Wolfe in 1966, infusion of prostaglandin E_1 (PGE$_1$) has been extensively used in the practice of pediatric cardiology.[11] It helps in stabilizing the patient in the emergency room providing a grace period for definitive treatment.[12,13]

Indications. Prostaglandin E_1 infusion is indicated in three groups of lesions.

1. Congenital heart diseases with severe restriction to pulmonary blood flow e.g. pulmonary atresia, critical pulmonary stenosis (with or without a ventricular septal defect as in tetralogy of Fallot).

2. Congenital heart diseases with severe restriction to systemic blood flow e.g. hypoplastic left heart, severe coarctation of aorta, critical aortic stenosis, interrupted aortic arch etc.

3. Congenital heart diseases with inadequate mixing e.g. transposition of great arteries.

PGE$_1$ infusion is indicated in any sick neonate with hypoxemia and cyanosis even if the cardiac diagnosis is not clear and echocardiographic examination is pending. The only contraindication to its use is obstructed total anomalous pulmonary connection, wherein it may worsen or precipitate pulmonary edema.

Dosage. PGE$_1$ is given as a continuous infusion through an infusion pump. The initial dose is high, 0.05-0.1 mcg/kg/min, can be increased up to 0.4 mcg/kg/minute if there is no response. Once the desired effect is achieved (seen as either improvement in oxygen saturation or as improvement in systemic perfusion), the dose should be decreased gradually to 0.005-0.01mcg/kg/minute. The response is generally immediate and is much better when the drug is used in the first four days of life. Prostaglandin does not open the ductus that has closed anatomically and is therefore not likely to be useful in infants older than 4 to 6 weeks. Some workers have used intravenous atropine in a dose of 0.1 mg for keeping the ductus open while the prostaglandin infusion is being prepared.

Side effects. The major side effect is apnea which is seen in 12% of cases.[13,14] Apnea occurs more often in the cyanotic group and in babies weighing less than 2 kg. It is a dose related phenomenon. Facilities for assisted ventilation must be available when using PGE$_1$. Other common side effects include fever (14%) and flushing (10%).

Hypotension, bradycardia, irritability and increased rate of infection are less common side effects. Prostaglandin infusion should be used for as short a period as possible due to frequent side effects, some of which are serious. The newborn should be taken up for definitive treatment as early as possible because ductus arteriosus may become edematous and friable on long term PGE$_1$ therapy.

Specific Therapy

Lesions with reduced pulmonary blood flow. Severe hypoxia and desaturation in this group of patients is treated on the lines of cyanotic spell. The various measures recommended are given below.

1. Knee chest position. Parents should be asked to calm the child while pressing the knees against the chest.

2. Oxygen is administered, either using an oxygen hood or nasal prongs.

3. Morphine is very helpful, used in a dose of 0.1 to 0.2 mg/kg intravenously or subcutaneously.

4. Intravenous β-blockers like propranolol, atenolol or metaprolol, are given in a dose of 0.1 mg/kg.

5. Metabolic acidosis should be corrected by using sodium bicarbonate.

6. Proper hydration must be ensured with liberal infusion of intravenous fluids.

7. Anemia is an important precipitating cause especially in developing world and should be corrected by transfusing blood.

8. Infusion of PGE$_1$ for opening the ductus arteriosus.

9. In extremely severe cases, intubation and assisted ventilation may be required.

Severe cyanosis and hypoxemia are common indications for early surgical treatment. Once the baby is stabilized, further palliation is achieved by surgical creation of a systemic to pulmonary circuit shunt e.g. a modified Blalock Taussig shunt where a synthetic tube is interposed between subclavian artery and the ipsilateral branch of pulmonary artery. A complete correction or a definitive repair is done later. Pulmonary valve balloon dilatation has been performed in some cases where the pulmonary outflow obstruction is both valvular and infundibular.

Lesions with increased pulmonary blood flow. Transposition of great arteries is the most common cyanotic lesion in newborns, its incidence being 5-7% of all congenital heart diseases. In this condition the systemic and pulmonary circulation are in parallel and hence adequate mixing between the two circulations is essential for survival. This mixing often occurs through a patent foramen ovale or atrial septal defect and/or through a patent ductus. As the ductus and atrial communication start closing, severe hypoxia ensues. Creation of an interatrial communication by balloon atrial septostomy, performed under fluoroscopic or echocardiographic guidance, is life saving. It allows intercirculatory mixing with consequent improvement in arterial saturation and hypoxia. Presence of a ventricular septal defect may also help in mixing, but a further increase in pulmonary blood flow may result in pulmonary venous hypertension and pulmonary edema. Balloon atrial septostomy is helpful in this subgroup as it decompresses the left atrium, thereby relieving pulmonary venous congestion. Once stabilized, babies with transpostion of great arteries should undergo early surgery. An arterial switch operation is the ideal type of surgical procedure as it corrects both the anatomy and physiology. In this operation, aorta and pulmonary artery are transected and reanastomosed after switching, to the appropriate ventricles. Other lesions like total anomalous pulmonary venous connection, persistent truncus arteriosus are also corrected by surgical procedures. However, some of the lesions like single ventricle, are not correctable and require a pulmonary artery banding procedure initially.

Cyanosis with pulmonary venous congestion. An urgent surgical correction is the only treatment for obstructed total anomalous pulmonary venous connection, and the results are rewarding. Babies with hypoplastic left heart can be stabilized with PGE_1 infusion. But if the atrial communication is restrictive, balloon septostomy has to be done. Most parents opt for palliative care for babies born with hypoplastic left heart, as the long-term prognosis is not good.

CARDIAC ARRHYTHMIAS

The normal heart rate in newborn is fast, varying from 100 to 200 beats per minute. Sinus tachycardia is the commonest "tachyarrhythmia", that is often physiological, as seen in fever, crying, breast feeding or in response to hypovolemia, hypotension etc. Sinus bradycardia, when transient, may be seen during sleep, apnea, vomiting, electrolyte abnormalities but when persistent it is more often pathological as in severe acidosis, hypothermia, raised intracranial pressure or toxicity due to digoxin. Common arrhythmias that may

produce hemodynamic compromise or heart failure in a neonate are supraventricular tachycardia (SVT) and congenital complete heart block.

Supraventricular Tachycardia

It is the most common arrhythmia presenting to the emergency room.[15] In a neonate, SVT is usually caused by a reentrant circuit through a concealed or obvious accessory pathway, wherein a sinus rhythm ECG in the latter shows a short PR interval and a delta wave on the upstroke of QRS complex (Figure 25.14). Presence of underlying congenital heart defect is rare, although Ebstein's anomaly has a higher prevalence in the right sided and multiple pathways. Neonates show a persistent long RP tachycardia (PJRT) that is an AVRT using a slowly conducting concealed posteroseptal pathway with rates generally slower than a usual AVRT but leading to CHF due to its incessant behaviour (Figure 25.15). Ectopic atrial tachycardias can also lead to similar presentation and cause heart failure, more often in neonates than in older children. ECG shows a narrow QRS rhythm at a constant rate of 220-320 beats per minute and P waves are often not visible, though a careful scrutiny of the T wave would often show a sharp deflection occurring at the same point which is due to a P wave (Figure 25.16). In most SVT's the heart rate does not fluctuate with agitation and other autonomic influences thus differentiating it from sinus tachycardia. Initially the baby is irritable, lethargic and tachypneic with feeding difficulties. Eventually heart failure and sometimes, hypotension and shock set in if the arrhythmia continues.

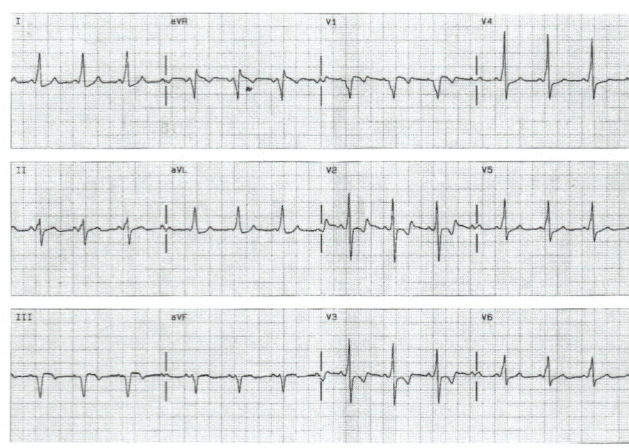

Figure 25.14 A 12 lead ECG from a child with preexcitation. The delta waves and short PR interval are apparent. The QS pattern in Lead VI suggests this to be septal pathway and the negative delta in III and aVF implies upward going initial forces. Thus this is a right posteroseptal pathway. This information helps in deciding about RF ablation therapy

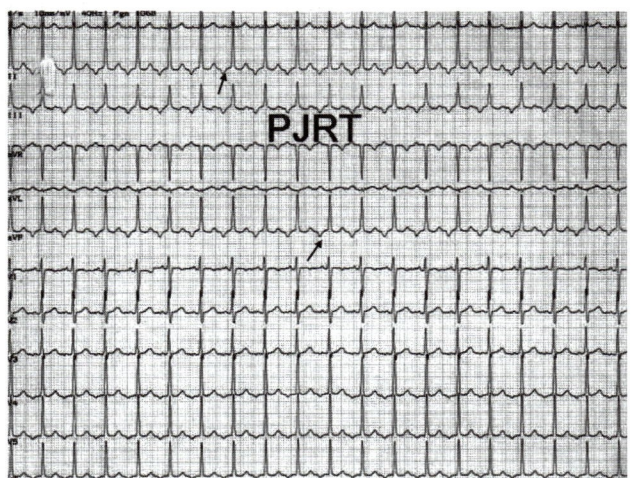

Figure 25.15 A 12-lead ECG from an infant with a narrow QRS tachycardia at the rate of 120/min. The arrow points to the inverted P waves in anterior leads as the pathway is typically a concealed posteroseptal one and hence the activation goes upwards in the atria. The RP (i.e., onset of R to next P) is longer then the PR interval that shows that the pathway conducts slowly. This is nearly diagnostic of a PJRT; can be seen in an ectopic atrial tachycardia

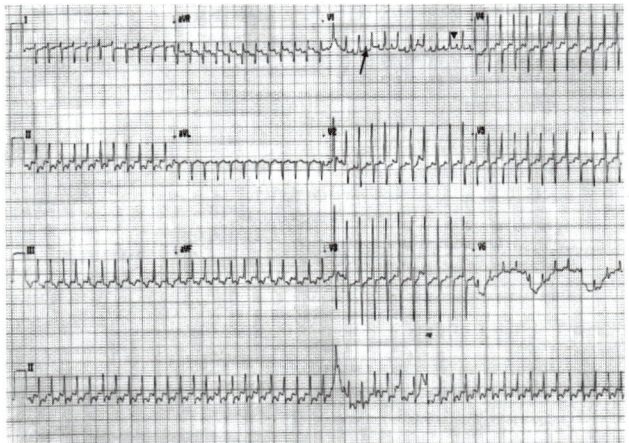

Figure 25.16 A 12-lead ECG of a neonate with atrial tachycardia at the rate of nearly 250/min. It is necessary in any tachycardia to hunt for the P waves and see their morphology and relation to R waves. The P waves are obvious only in lead V1 as the T wave cannot be so spiked and narrow. This ECG also emphasizes the need for a 12-lead ECG as no other lead shows the P so clearly. This tachycardia could be a reentrant tachycardia; use of adenosine would clarify the diagnosis

Treatment. In a hemodynamically unstable patient, synchronized cardioversion, in a dose of 0.5 – 1.0 Joules/kg body weight should be promptly used. If intravenous access is available, adenosine bolus of 0.2 to 0.3 mg/kg can be given. Adenosine is the drug of choice in neonates to break SVT.[16] It has a rapid onset of action, usually within 10 seconds. It should be given as a rapid intravenous

bolus as it has an extremely short half life (nine seconds). Since its half life is very short, it is ineffective when given slowly.[17] Its action is short lasting, so SVT may recur and it is usually ineffective in EAT and PJRT wherein the tachycardia resumes immediately. Lower doses are seldom successful through a peripheral line.

In a relatively stable baby with SVT, vagal maneuvers can be tried first. The most useful method is the application of crushed ice in a plastic bag to the baby's face for 10 seconds. Other vagal maneuvers are generally ineffective in neonates and eyeball massage is contraindicated. Digoxin is the other drug that has often been used for terminating an SVT in the past; however, intravenous digoxin is contraindicated in the presence of a manifest accessory pathway and given its low success rates is rarely used currently. In resistant cases, transesophageal atrial overdrive stimulation may be effective or one may have to resort to synchronized DC version. Intravenous verapamil or diltiazem, commonly used drugs to break SVT in adults, are contraindicated in infants due to the risk of hypotension and cardiogenic shock. Intravenous amiodarone may have to be resorted to in cases of EAT and PJRT that are unresponsive to usual measures. For chronic therapy, oral β blockers such as propranolol (1mg/kg/dose given three times a day that can be increased every 3-4 weeks depending on the heart rate and blood pressure) or digoxin are used. Infants may outgrow the arrhythmia in a large number of cases and the drug can be withdrawn after six months to one year.

Atrial Flutter

This is an uncommon arrhythmia in children with structurally normal heart, which is primarily limited to infants. It accounts for 30% of fetal tachycardias, 11-18% of neonatal tachyarrhythmias and occurs in < 10% in children beyond the first year of life. Incidence of underlying structural heart disease increases with the age at presentation and more than 90% of children who get the first episode after infancy have an abnormal heart. Presentation is varied with CHF in around 30%, hydrops in 20% and 50% are detected incidentally. The tachycardia can be made out typically by the flutter waves (Figure 25.17a and b), though rapid 1:1 or 2:1 conduction may mask the P waves and falsely confuse with an SVT. Ventricular rates can be very rapid reaching beyond 300/min and may lead to shock and death. Median ventricular rates in neonates are around 215 bpm with atrial rates of around 430 bpm. It is important to remember that typical atrial flutter is a macroreentrant arrhythmia

Section 3

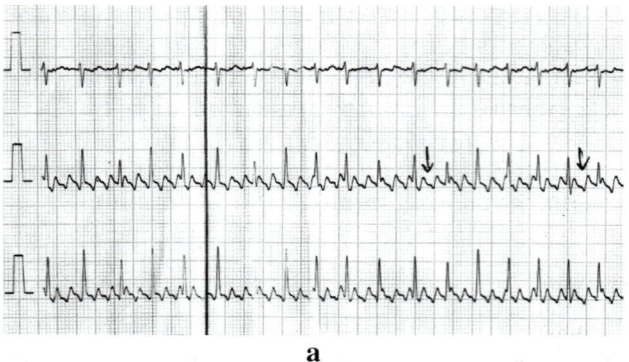

a

Figure 25.17a Atrial flutter in a neonate. The classic saw-tooth appearance of the baseline shows the flutter waves. The atrial rate is over 300/min (the PP interval occupies less than one big square). All the P waves are not transmitted to the ventricle and hence the ventricular rate is varying and is slower

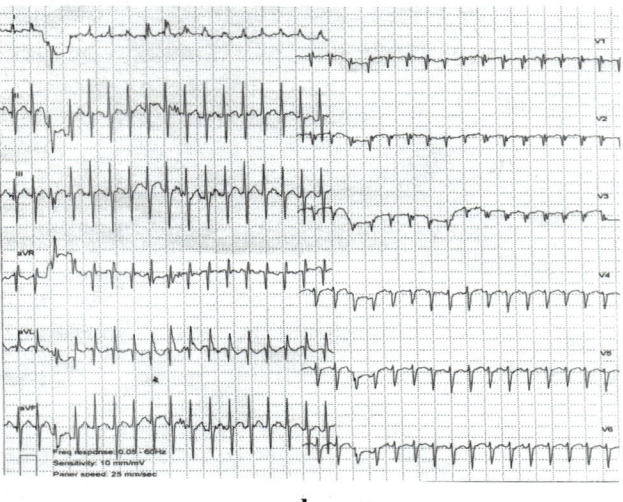

b

Figure 25.17b Show a flutter with a 1:1 conduction (different patient) with a ventricular rate of 280/min. This can be dangerous and needs immediate cardioversion. The flutter does not remain obvious at such a rate but can be unmasked by vagal maneuvers or iv adenosine

going around the right atrium. The diagnosis can be made easily by creating a transient AV block either by vagal maneuvers or giving adenosine IV, that unmasks the flutter waves transiently. Oral or intravenous digoxin leads to reversion in 25%, but a synchronized DC shock of 0.5-2 Joules/kg is more effective (success rates > 80%). Esophageal overdrive rarely works in neonates and infants. Oral digoxin is often prescribed prophylactically for 6 months, though there is no good evidence of its efficacy because tachycardia does not recur even without prophylactic therapy.

Ventricular Arrhythmias

Ventricular premature beats and ventricular tachycardia are rare, but the latter is a serious form

of arrhythmia in neonates. They often occur secondary to hypokalemia, asphyxia, hypomagnesemia, hypocalcemia and other electrolyte abnormalities. Occassionally ventricular arrhythmias may be associated with myocarditis, long QT syndrome and cardiac tumors. Treatment involves correction of underlying disorder or dyselectrolytemia. Antiarrhythmic drugs are rarely required. Hypomagnesemia is corrected by administration of magnesium sulphate in a dose of 50 mg/kg with a maximum of 2 gm over one hour. Hypokalemia should be corrected gradually to avoid hyperkalemia. Potassium is given in small dose of 0.25 mEq/kg, maximum of 10 mEq over 30 to 60 minutes, with repeat check for potassium levels prior to second dose. Hypocalcemia is corrected by administering either calcium chloride (0.1 to 0.2 ml/kg of 10% solution) or calcium gluconate (0.2 to 0.5 ml/kg of 10% solution)

Congenital Complete Heart Block

Complete heart block in a neonate may be associated with structural heart defects in 50% of cases. These lesions include corrected transposition of great arteries, atrioventricular septal defect, heterotaxy syndromes etc. In the rest 50%, there is no underlying heart defect, but often there is subclinical evidence of collagen vascular disease in the mother. The presentation is with bradycardia, the heart rates varying from 50-75 beats per minute (Figure 25.18). Some of the newborns develop heart failure due to the slow heart rate; in fact heart failure may start even in fetal life. These babies require insertion of an epicardial pacemaker soon after birth. The other indications for pacemaker are a very slow awake ventricular rate of < 55 beats per minute or < 30 bpm in sleep, broad QRS complex escape rhythm, prolonged QT/QTc interval or frequent ventricular ectopy. All such patients should undergo a detailed evaluation by a pediatric cardiologist, preferably a pediatric cardiac electrophysiologist, as soon as possible.

Transcatheter Therapeutic Cardiac Procedures

The concept of performing an interventional procedure in catheterization laboratory was first introduced by Dottes and Judkins in 1964, when they used a balloon catheter to dilate a peripheral vessel. Two years later, Rashkind performed the first intracardiac therapeutic procedure of "balloon atrial septostomy" in an infant with transposition of great arteries. A large number of reports appeared subsequently utilizing catheterization technique as therapeutic procedures in infants and children. The

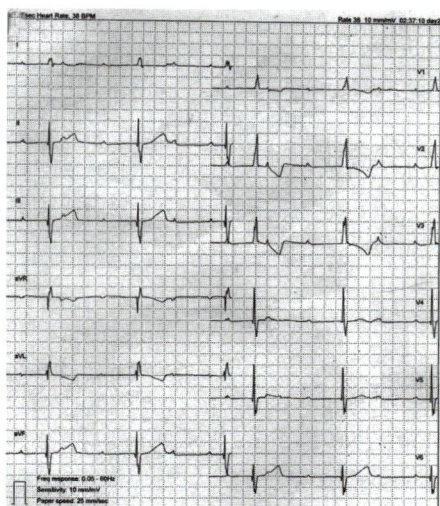

Figure 25.18 Congenital complete heart block in an infant. Note the complete lack of AV relationship and the slow regular ventricular rate (40/min). The QRS is relatively broad for the age of the child and the heart rate too slow. This is an indication for pacing

various interventional procedures that are performed in newborns and young infants can be grouped under following headings:

(i) Creation of defects eg balloon and blade septostomy

(ii) Balloon valvuloplasty for stenotic valves

(iii) Balloon angioplasty for stenotic vessels

(iv) Occlusion of unwanted vessels/collaterals or septal defects

(v) Others like radiofrequency perforation of atretic pulmonary valve, stenting of ductus arteriosus.

Interventional procedures in newborns are associated with higher complication rates as compared to older children and adults. It is, therefore, imperative that these procedures are performed in well-equipped centers and by experienced operators.

Balloon Atrial Septostomy

It is a life saving procedure for hypoxic, acidotic newborns with transposition of great arteries and inadequate mixing. The best results are obtained in neonates upto 4 weeks of age as the interatrial septum is thin and tears easily in the region of fossa ovalis. Conventionally this procedure is performed in the catheterization laboratory, but it can also be performed successfully under echocardiographic guidance at the bedside. The septostomy catheter is introduced through the umbilical or femoral vein and then advanced into left atrium through patent foramen ovale. The balloon at the tip of the catheter is inflated in left atrium and then pulled into the right atrium with a jerk, tearing the margins of fossa ovalis region. Creation of an atrial septal defect allows mixing, resulting in marked improvement of hypoxia. Complications are rare if the procedure is performed carefully, although cardiac perforation and avulsion of tricuspid valve may occur. Balloon atrial septostomy may also be used in infants with tricuspid atresia, mitral atresia, pulmonary atresia with intact ventricular septum and total anomalous pulmonary venous connection, if the atrial septal defect is restrictive.

Blade atrial septectomy. This procedure was first described by Park in 1975. In infants over 2-3 months of age, the interatrial septum becomes too tough to be torn by balloon septostomy. Blade atrial septostomy followed by balloon dilatation is performed for these cases. The indications are the same as for balloon septostomy.

Static balloon dilatation of atrial septum. It is an alternative to blade septostomy. This procedure appears to be safer than blade septostomy and entails dilatation of atrial septal defect by inflating a balloon across it.

Balloon Dilatation of Valves

Balloon valvuloplasty is useful for neonates with severe aortic or pulmonary valve stenosis. Inflation of balloon, introduced through a vein or artery, across a valve exerts a circumferential and linear wall stress splitting the fused commissures, thereby relieving the obstruction. It is important to use proper sized balloons to avoid cuspal tear and significant regurgitation of the valve. Echocardiography is useful in defining the severity of stenosis, function of the corresponding ventricle and for measuring valve annulus diameter for balloon sizing. The results of balloon dilatation are uniformly good for pulmonary stenosis, though the procedure may be technically challenging in those with right ventricular hypoplasia, right ventricular dysfunction and tricuspid regurgitation. Restenosis is rare. Pulmonary valve dilatation has sometimes been performed for neonates with tetralogy of Fallot when the right ventricular outflow obstruction is both infundibular and valvular. This procedure may obviate the need for an aortopulmonary shunt. In cases of aortic stenosis, balloon dilatation is a palliative procedure, majority of cases require one or more interventions including surgery, later in life. Complications are also more frequent than for pulmonary valve dilatation and include arrhythmias, bleeding, loss of femoral pulses, aortic regurgitation, etc.

Balloon Angioplasty for Coarctation of Aorta

The therapy of choice for coarctation of aorta in neonates is surgical relief of obstruction. In cases where the baby is very sick in spite of prostaglandin infusion (or has co-morbid conditions) one may have to resort to balloon dilatation. The immediate results are generally good but restenosis rates are very high, almost reaching 75% in the first year. Proper balloon sizing is important to avoid complications like dissection of aorta.

Occlusion of Patent Ductus Arteriosus

Transcatheter closure of ductus arteriosus is rarely performed in neonates, especially preterm babies. Surgical ligation is a simple and safe procedure for majority of such cases. Closure with coils has been performed in neonates and infants who pose higher risk for surgical ligation. The procedure is technically demanding and should be performed by skilled personnel. Complications include embolization of coils into pulmonary artery or aorta and obstruction of left pulmonary artery or aorta due to protrusion of coils in these structures.

Perforation of Atretic Pulmonary Valve

This procedure is performed in membranous pulmonary atresia with intact ventricular septum. Perforation of membrane with radiofrequency energy delivered through a wire is the safest and most successful method which has been used (Figure 25.19a and b). Once the valve has been perforated, balloon dilatation is performed to enlarge the opening. Complications include perforation of the right ventricular outflow region, dissection of pulmonary artery and cardiac tamponade. When successful, this procedure obviates the need for open heart surgery with its associated complications in a neonate.

Stenting of Ductus Arteriosus

Some of the congenital heart defects like pulmonary atresia and aortic atresia are ductus dependent. Infusion of prostaglandin helps to maintain ductal patency till definitive surgery is done. However, if immediate surgery is not contemplated for some reason, (e.g. unavailability of a donor for heart transplantation for a baby with hypoplastic left heart syndrome), long-term patency of the ductus is required. Stenting of the ductus is performed in such cases. Complications include

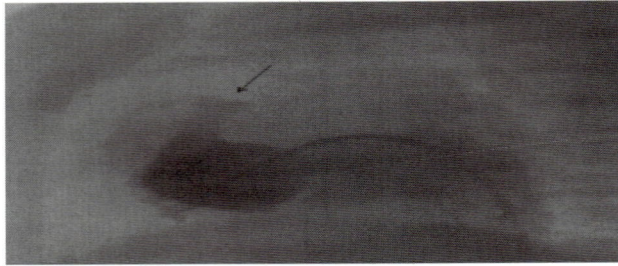

a

Figure 25.19a RV angiogram in lateral view showing the right ventricle (RV) and RV outlow. There is no contrast going into the PA a diagnostic feature of pulmonary atresia

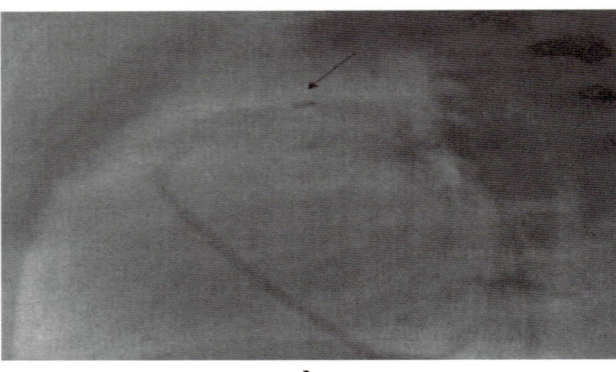

b

Figure 25.19b Radio opaque tip of Nykanen perforater wire (arrow) into the main pulmonary artery after RF perforation of the valve membrane, after which balloon dilatation is done. (Reproduced from Indian Heart Journal with permission)

stent thrombosis which can be prevented by aggressive anticoagulation therapy.

CONCLUSIONS

Successful management of neonatal cardiac emergencies requires an understanding of pathophysiology of common cardiac defects. The clinical picture is generally nonspecific and diagnosis of a specific lesion is often difficult. A possibility of a cardiac abnormality must be kept in mind in a neonate with pulmonary symptoms unresponsive to conventional therapy. General measures include maintenance of airway and adequate oxygenation, hydration and avoidance of hypoglycemia and hypothermia. If the baby is in shock, intravenous inotropes should be used. In cyanotic neonates who are sick and hypoxemic, an infusion of prostaglandin is indicated and could be life saving. An X-ray chest and ECG help to further identify the nature of cardiac problem. Echocardiographic examination is mandatory for making the specific diagnosis, which will help to institute the specific treatment. Transcatheter palliative procedures are life saving but they must be performed by skilled and experienced cardiologists because of high risk of complications in neonates.

REFERENCES

1. Fyler DC, Buckley LP, Hellenbrand WE, Cohn HE. Report of the New England Regional Infant Care Program. *Pediatrics* 1980; 65 (Suppl) : 375-461.

2. Hoffman JI, Kaplan S. The incidence of congenital heart disease. *J Amer Coll Cardiol* 2002; 39: 1890-900.

3. Saxena A. Congenital heart disease in India: a status report. *Indian J Pediatr* 2005; 72: 595-598.

4. Jobes DR, Nicolson SC, Steven JM, *et al.* Carbon dioxide prevents pulmonary over-circulation in hypoplastic left heart syndrome. *Ann Thorac Surg* 1992; 54: 150-51.

5. Schamberger MS. Cardiac emergencies in children. *Pediatr Ann* 1996; 25: 339-44.

6. Dutta S, Narang A. Enalapril induced acute renal failure in a newborn infant. *Pediatr Nephrol* 2003; 18: 570-572.

7. Benitz WE, Malachowski N, Cohen RS, Stevenson DK, Ariagno RL, Sunshine P. Use of sodium nitroprusside in neonates: efficacy and safety. *J Pediatr* 1985; 106: 102-110.

8. Allen H, Beekman R, Garson A, *et al.* Pediatric therapeutic cardiac catheterization: a statement for healthcare professionals from the Council on Cardiovascular Disease in the Young: American Heart Association. *Circulation* 1998; 97: 609-625.

9. Shah PS, Ohlsson A. Sildenafil for pulmonary hypertension in neonates. Cochrane Database of Systematic Reviews 2011, Issue 8.

10. McSeidner S, Chang LY, Waleh N, Ikegami M, Petershack J, Yoder B, Giavedoni L, Albertine KH, Dahl MJ, Wang ZM, Clyman RI. Ibuprofen-induced patent ductus arteriosus closure: physiologic, histologic, and biochemical effects on the premature lung. *Pediatrics* 2008;121: 945-956.

11. Coceani F, Wolfe LS. On the action of prostaglandin E_1 and prostaglandins from brain on the isolated rat stomach. *Canad J Physiol Pharmacol* 1966; 44: 933-950.

12. Freed MD, Hymann MA, Lewis AB, *et al.* Prostaglandin E_1 in infants with ductus dependent congenital heart disease. *Circulation* 1981; 64: 899-905.

13. Reddy SCB, Saxena A. Prostaglandin E_1: first stage palliation in neonates with congenital cardiac defects. *Indian J Pediatr* 1998; 65: 211-216.

14. Lewis AB, Freed MD, Hymann MA, *et al.* Side effects of therapy with prostaglandin E_1 in infants with critical heart disease. *Circulation* 1981; 64: 893-898.

15. Flynn P, Engle M, Ehlers K. Cardiac issues in the pediatric emergency room. *Pediatr Clin North Amer* 1992; 39: 955-986.

16. Losec J, Endom E, Dietrich A, *et al.* Adenosine and pediatric supraventricular tachycardia in the emergency department: multicenter study and review. *Ann Emerg Med* 1999; 33: 185-191.

17. Crosson J, Etheridge S, Milstein S, *et al.* Therapeutic and diagnostic utility of adenosin during tachycardia evaluation in children. *Amer J Cardiol* 1994; 74: 155-160.

Section 3

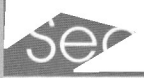
Emergencies in Children and Adolescents

26

Acute Gastroenteritis

Shinjini Bhatnagar, Mona K Chaturvedi and Meharban Singh

INTRODUCTION

Acute gastroenteritis is an inflammation of the stomach and the small intestine leading to acute onset of vomiting and diarrhea. Diarrhea is one of the commonest causes of death among under-5 children worldwide, following acute respiratory infection. Of the estimated 8.795 million global deaths in children younger than 5 years (U5) in 2008, diarrhea accounted for 15% of the total deaths[1]. In India, 13% of the 1.8 million U5 deaths are because of diarrhea accounting for more than 2,37,000 children a year. This represents almost one fifth of global child mortality due to diarrhea[1]. The estimated incidence of diarrhea in India is reported as 1.1 to 6 episodes in children aged 0 to 4 years[2]. The incidence and the risk of mortality from diarrheal diseases are greatest among children younger than 1 year of age, and thereafter rates decline incrementally. Infants aged 6 months to 11 months are at greatest risk possibly because of a shift from breast feeding to weaning[3]. Exclusive breast feeding protects against diarrhea because human milk is free from bacterial contamination and is replete with protective secretory IgA and other immunobiological agents[4].

The term diarrhea is often used interchangeably with acute gastroenteritis and it causes under nutrition or worsens milder forms of malnutrition because of increased and repeated loss of macro and micronutrients (vitamins and minerals) in stool, and increased catabolism due to infection[5,6]. Moreover, mothers often starve their children during the episode of diarrhea (due to the mistaken belief to provide rest to the gut) and sufficient emphasis on the need for continued feeding during diarrhea is not given by the health care providers. Malnutrition further increases the risk of diarrhea, its severity and mortality[7]. Other direct consequences of diarrhea include diminished growth and impaired cognitive development in resource-limited countries[8].

EPIDEMIOLOGY

An epidemiological definition of acute diarrhea is passage of at least three or more liquid or watery stools per day[9]. A recent change in the consistency or character of stools is a more important feature than the number of stools. Passage of frequent formed stools or pasty stools in breast-fed infants or passage of stools during or immediately after feeds due to initiation of gastrocolic reflex in young infants should not be mistaken with diarrhea. Frequent, loose greenish-yellow stools on day 3 or 4 of life is commonly referred to as transitional diarrhea which does not need any treatment.

The episode is termed as bloody diarrhea or dysentery when visible blood is present in the stool but does not include melena or presence of blood streaks on the surface of formed or hard stool. Episodes where blood is identified by microscopic examination or biochemical tests are not defined as bloody diarrhea[10]. The terms like bloody diarrhea, dysentery, bacillary dysentery and invasive diarrhea are often used interchangeably. Dysentery is defined as bloody diarrhea associated with fever, abdominal cramps, tenesmus and mucoid stools. However, in clinical practice all these accompanying features may not always be present. Dysentery caused by *Shigella* is called as bacillary dysentery and should be distinguished from amebic dysentery. Invasive diarrhea refers to diarrhea caused by bacteria like *Shigella*, some *Salmonella*, *E. coli* and *Campylobacter jejuni* that invade the bowel mucosa, causing inflammation and mucosal damage.

Most episodes of acute diarrhea terminate within 7 days and progressively smaller proportions persist beyond 14, 21 or 28 days. *When diarrheal symptoms persist for two or more weeks it is defined as persistent diarrhea.* The delineation of 14 or more days is arbitrary but is supported by data that case fatality rate increases to 13.9% for persistent episodes while it is similar in episodes lasting for 1-2 weeks duration[11]. A proportion of these episodes are termed as *"prolonged malnourishing diarrhea"* as they are associated with growth failure.

ETIOPATHOGENESIS

Etiologic spectrum varies during different seasons and in different geographic regions. In the developed countries, it is estimated that over 50 percent of acute diarrheas are caused by viruses including rotavirus, Norwalk-like virus and coronavirus. In developing countries bacterial enteropathogens are an important cause of acute diarrhea (Table 26.1). Isolation of *Escherichia coli* or other microorganisms from diarrheal stools does not imply an etiological role unless the organism is shown to be either toxigenic or invasive. Enterotoxigenic *E. coli* (ETEC) are responsible for 18-25% of all diarrheas in developing countries[12].

The enterotoxigenic organisms attach to the mucosa by means of fimbrial lectins and colonisation factors I and II produce heat labile (LT) and/or heat stable (ST) enterotoxins. The heat labile enteroxtoxins activate chloride hypersecretion and inhibition of sodium absorption by stimulating adenylcyclase on the membrane of mucosal cells. This results in the secretion of electrolyte-rich fluid into the small bowel and large voluminous diarrhea. The heat stable enterotoxin acts by activating guanylcyclase with increase in cyclic guanosine monophosphate (cyclic GMP). Certain serotypes of *E. coli* that cause epidemics of diarrhea in nurseries and sporadic infantile diarrhea are termed as enteropathogenic *Escherichia coli* (EPEC). They attach and efface the mucosal border, and are known to produce a shiga-like cytotoxin. EPEC may act by adhering to intestinal mucosal cells in a localised pattern and are also known as localized adherent *E. coli* (LAEC). The other serotypes are diffusely adherent (DAEC) or enteroaggregative *E. coli* (EAEC) which are identified by their characteristic diffuse or stacked brick adherence patterns on cell lines. Enteroinvasive *E. coli* invade the mucosa and enterohemorrhagic *E.coli* produce a cytotoxin. Hemorrhagic enterocolitis and hemolytic uremic syndrome have been reported with enterohemorrhagic *E. coli* 0157: H 7 infection.

Rotavirus is responsible for 20 to 25% of diarrheal episodes in children aged 6-24 months visiting treatment facilities and for 15% of cases in the same age group in the community. Most cases of diarrhea (98%) occurr during the first 2 years of life, peaking at 9-11 months of age. Incidence of rotavirus diarrhea-associated hospitalizations has been reported as high as 337 hospitalizations/100,000 children in under 5 years of age from urban slums in north India[13]. It causes patchy blunting of intestinal villi with reduction of mucosal disaccharidases which return to normal within 2-3 weeks. Shigellosis is endemic in most developing countries and is the most important cause of bloody diarrhea globally. It results in at least 80 million cases of bloody diarrhea and 700,000 deaths each year. Ninety-nine percent of infections caused by Shigella occur in developing countries, 70% cases

Table 26.1 Etiology of acute diarrhea among preschool children in Delhi (AIIMS data showing % isolates)		
Bacteria	**Patients (n=204)**	**Controls (n=98)**
Bacteria		
Escherichia coli		
Enterotoxigenic (ETEC)	23.02	7.14
Enteropathogenic (EPEC)	7.84	1.02
Shigella	2.94	--
Salmonella	2.45	--
Compylobacter jejuni	10.23	8.16
Yersinia enterocolitica	0.49	--
Viruses		
Rotavirus	20.58	2.04
Mixed		
Rota + ETEC	0.98	--
Rota + EPEC	0.98	--
Protozoa		
Giardia lamblia	3.92	1.02
Entamoeba histolytica	1.47	--
No pathogens	25.09	80.62

in U5, with 60% of deaths among children less than five years of age[14]. It invades and multiplies within colonic epithelial cells, causing cell death and mucosal ulcers. The virulence factors include a smooth lipopolysaccharide cell wall antigen and a Shiga toxin that is cytotoxic, neurotoxic, and perhaps also causes watery diarrhea. Shigella are subdivided into 4 serogroups; *S. flexneri* is the most common in developing countries while *S. sonnei* in developed countries. *S. sonnei* and *S. boydii* usually cause relatively mild illness in which diarrhea may be watery or bloody. *S. flexneri* is thechief cause of endemic shigellosis in developing countries. *S. dysenteriae type-1* also known as the Shiga bacillus (Sd1) causes epidemics of severe disease with high mortality. It produces a potent Shiga cytotoxin and develops resistance to antimicrobials more frequently than other species. Shigellosis is particularly severe in malnourished and formula fed infants. *Campylobacter jejuni* causes 5-15% of watery diarrhea in infants by invading the ileum and the large intestine. It is also known to produce a cytotoxin and a heat-labile enterotoxin.

Cholera manifests acutely with profuse watery diarrhea and vomiting that can rapidly lead to dehydration and shock. In the absence of treatment, case fatality is very high. World Health Organization has reported over 200,000 cholera cases with a case fatality rate of 2.7% from 52 developing countries[14]. In India the eastern regions have a high incidence with 1.6/1000/year cases being reported from Kolkata[15]. In endemic areas, cholera may account for 5-10% of hospitalized patients with diarrhea mostly in children under 5 years of age. Diarrhea is caused *by V. cholerae 01* (biotypes EL Tor and classical; and two serotypes Ogawa, Inaba) and 0139. It adheres to and multiplies on the small intestine mucosa where it produces an enterotoxin that results in secretory diarrhea. Salmonella is an uncommon cause of gastroenteritis in young children in most developing countries but can be responsible for 10% or more in urban children. Invasion of the ileal epithelium results in an exudative diarrhea and occasionally dysentery. Antibiotic resistant strains are found worldwide.

Giardia lamblia and *Entamoeba histolytica* are not a common cause of diarrhea in young children (<2%). Giardia lamblia infects the small bowel while *Entamoeba histolytica* invades the large intestine mucosa resulting in an inflammatory type of diarrhea. About 90% of *Entamoeba histolytica* infections are asymptomatic and are caused by non-pathogenic strains. In India, *Cryptosporidium parvum* may account for about 15% of childhood diarrhea. It attaches to the microvillous surface of enterocytes and cause fluid loss and malabsorption due to the resulting mucosal damage. It is common in immunosuppressed patients, particularly in those with acquired immune deficiency syndrome (AIDS) but is now being

Section 4

Table 26.2 Clinical features due to various etiologic agents	
Agent	**Features**
Rotavirus	Watery diarrhea, usually associated with vomiting and low-grade fever. Self-limiting with median duration being around 8 days.
ETEC	Watery, high purging diarrhea with or without fever.
Enteroinvasive pathogens (Shigella, Salmonella, EPEC)	Fever and watery diarrhea, or dysentery with fever, tenesmus, abdominal cramps and small mucoid bloody stools.
Vibrio cholerae	Acute onset high purging diarrhea with extreme prostration, severe dehydration and shock. Characteristic rice-water appearance of stools. There may be history of contact/epidemic.
Cryptosporidium	Acute onset high purging diarrhea, sometimes very large volume watery diarrhea.
Campylobacter jejuni	Watery diarrhea, in one-third blood and mucus appears in stools after a couple of days.
Giardia lamblia	Insidious onset with pale, large, semi-formed stools and abdominal distension, absence of dehydration.
Entamoeba histolytica	Insidious onset with marked tenesmus, little fecal matter which is mainly composed of blood and mucus, absence of toxemia and dehydration.
Candida albicans	Associated malnutrition, history of intake of broad spectrum antibiotics, oral thrush, perianal moniliasis.
Staphylococcal enterocolitis	History of eating infected food, affection of other family members, acute onset after 4-8 hours of ingestion of offending food, prompt recovery within 24 hours.

increasingly identified in immunocompetent children.

Diarrhea may also be associated with systemic infections (acute otitis media, pneumonia, urinary tract infection, septicemia, necrotizing enterocolitis) particularly in young infants and newborn babies.

CLINICAL FEATURES

The clinical picture is usually similar despite different etiological agents. It is characterized by acute onset of vomiting, loose or watery stools with or without fever (Table 26.2). The course of illness is generally self-limiting and usually lasts for 5 to 7 days. Abdominal cramps and tenesmus with blood and mucus in stools are characteristic of enteroinvasive pathogens. High purging rates exceeding 10 ml/kg per stool are sometimes seen with ETEC, *V. cholerae* and rotavirus diarrhea. Infection with Giardia or *Entamoeba histolytica* is an infrequent cause of acute diarrhea in children less than 5 years. *Cryptosporidium parvum* should be considered in cases with large volume diarrhea leading to dehydration. Chronic high volume diarrhea leading to malnutrition, extra intestinal manifestations and sometimes death are features of immunocompromised or severely malnourished children with cryptosporidiosis.

The child should be assessed for physical signs of dehydration, electrolyte disturbances, presence of extra intestinal infections e.g. septicemia, pneumonia, otitis media and nutritional status.

Fluid and Electrolyte Disturbances

The most serious and at times fatal consequences of acute gastroenteritis are the development of dehydration and electrolyte disturbances. There is loss of sodium, chloride, bicarbonate, and potassium in addition to water in the diarrheal stools. The loss of sodium is around 90 mEq/L in diarrhea due to *Vibrio cholerae* and upto 60 mEq/L in ETEC and rotavirus diarrhea[16]. Extreme lethargy, floppiness, poor or non acceptance of ORS may occur due to electrolyte disturbances as well as severe dehydration. Thus, in a child with some dehydration, change in the mental status should alert the clinician to the possibility of severe electrolyte disturbances.

Dehydration due to depletion of extra cellular fluid, unless the fluid losses are replenished by oral intake, is invariable. Children are more susceptible to develop dehydration due to the limited urinary concentration capacity of kidneys, their dependency upon adults to replenish their fluid losses and an exceedingly high daily turnover of water. The insensible water losses through skin and lungs are more in children due to the large surface area and rapid breathing rates. Excessive thirst and irritability are the earliest features of dehydration. Due to the relatively larger fraction of extra cellular fluid compartment in children, skin turgor is lost following dehydration. Severe dehydration is a life-threatening complication and is characterized by additional features of apathy, drowsiness, tachycardia, circulatory collapse, acidosis and severe oliguria or anuria.

Deep and rapid breathing indicates metabolic acidosis (defined by blood pH <7.1) and may be commonly seen in acute gastroenteritis. It occurs due to increased tissue catabolism and starvation, retention of H+ ions due to reduced glomerular filtration rate and anerobic tissue catabolism due to reduced perfusion of tissues. There is excessive loss of bicarbonates in the stools to buffer increased lactate production in the gut due to bacterial fermentation. Insufficient replacement of potassium losses during diarrhea can lead to potassium depletion and hypokalemia (serum K^+ <3.0 mEq/L) and can be an important cause of mortality especially in malnourished children. It can cause muscle weakness, paralytic ileus, abdominal distension, renal impairment, and cardiac arrhythmias. It is characterized by ST depression and T wave inversion on electrocardiogram.

Assessment of Severity of Dehydration

Several scoring systems have been designed to assess the severity of dehydration but have limited clinical utility. WHO recommends simple and practical assessment protocol that has been introduced through the Integrated Management of Neonatal and Childhood Illnesses (IMNCI) in the country. These criteria can be easily followed both in tertiary care hospitals and in remote peripheral health centers.

The hydration status should be assessed according to the IMNCI criteria, as given below, and classified as no, some or severe dehydration[17].

A young infant with **severe dehydration** has any two of the following signs i.e. lethargy or unconsciousness sunken eyes, or a skin pinch that goes back very slowly.

Two of the following signs: • Lethargic or unconscious • Sunken eyes* • Skin pinch goes back very slowly	Severe dehydration
* Ask the mother for presence of recent sunken eyes in her child whenever there is a doubt.	

Those with **some dehydration** have any combination of two of the following signs: restless/irritable, sunken eyes, skin pinch goes back slowly.

Two of the following signs:	
• Restless, irritable • Sunken eyes* • Skin pinch goes back slowly	Some dehydration

Those infants with diarrhea who do not have any signs to classify as severe or some dehydration are classified as **no dehydration.**

Not enough signs to classify as some or severe dehydration	No dehydration

* Ask the mother for presence of recent sunken eyes in her child whenever there is a doubt.

Evaluation of dehydration is difficult in both obese and malnourished children. In an obese child, the degree of dehydration may be under estimated because the skin turgor may be preserved despite loss of extracellular fluid. In marasmic children, the severity of dehydration may be overestimated (Box). The malnourished child may appear lethargic and have sunken eyes and a skin pinch that returns back very slowly. The skin turgor is lost due to a marked reduction in subcutaneous fat and connective tissue.

Dehydration is isotonic in nature in over two-thirds of patients. Hypotonic dehydration (serum $Na^+ < 130$ mEq/L) occurs in 15-20 percent of patients due to replacement of diarrheal losses by plain water. Hypertonic dehydration (serum $Na^+ > 150$ mEq/L) is a serious but less common problem in developing countries. It occurs due to greater loss of water without sodium due to excessive vomiting, low content of sodium in diarrheal stools, fever, sweating and rapid breathing. Reduced intake of plain water or ingestion of electrolyte-rich oral rehydration solution, commercial aerated drinks, or fruit juices are other important causes of hypernatremia[18]. In hypertonic dehydration extracellular fluid compartment is better preserved at the expense of intracellular dehydration and dysfunction. Skin turgor is preserved resulting in under estimation of the severity of dehydration. Skin feels dry, thick and doughy. Circulation and renal perfusion are maintained. These children are extremely thirsty which is out of proportion to other signs of dehydration. There may be associated acidosis, hyperglycemia and hypocalcemia. Woody tongue and doughy abdomen and brisk deep

Assessment of dehydration in severely malnourished children

It is best to assume that all severely malnourished infants and children with watery diarrhea have some dehydration. The basic format for assessment remains the same for severely malnourished children as for the well-nourished children; however, there are some signs that are not reliable:

o Mental state. They are usually apathetic when left alone or irritable when handled.

o Mouth, tongue and tears. They usually have a dry mouth and absent tears because of atrophied salivary and lacrimal glands.

o Skin turgor. Lack of supporting tissues and subcutaneous fat results in thin and loose skin. It may flatten or not flatten at all when pinched. Presence of edema may mask diminished turgor of the skin.

Signs that remain useful and reliable for assessing dehydration include history of excessive fluid loss through vomitings/or diarrhea, recent onset of sunken eyes, eagerness to drink (signs of some dehydration); prolonged capillary refill (>2 sec), weak or absent radial pulse and decreased or absent urine flow (signs of severe dehydration)

It is important to differentiate severe dehydration with shock and septic shock in a severely malnourished child

Septic shock should be considered if there are signs of severe dehydration in the absence of watery diarrhea. The hemodynamic status (increase in heart rate, prolonged capillary refill time) is out of proportion to diarrheal losses. Unexplained abdominal distension (normal potassium), coffee ground vomitus and dilated peripheral or skull veins are indicators of systemic infection. Isolated severe dehydration should be considered if there is rapid improvement on administration of intravenous fluids.

Adapted from the WHO manual on "Management of the child with a serious infection or severe malnutrition; Guidelines for care at the first-referral level in developing countries"

tendon reflexes may also be present. Irritability and seizures especially following rapid correction of hypernatremic dehydration carry a poor prognosis.

Associated Systemic Infections

Associated systemic infections like acute otitis media, pneumonia, urinary tract infection, and septicemia should be looked for, particularly in infants less than 2 months, and severely malnourished or immunocompromised children. Fever with toxemia and refusal to take feeds is suggestive of sepsis. These cases should preferably be admitted to the hospital and managed with systemic antibiotics.

Abdominal Distension

Abdominal distension seen with acute gastroenteritis is usually due to lactose intolerance, or paralytic ileus resulting from associated septicemia, necrotizing enterocolitis or hypokalemia. Sudden cessation of diarrhea with passage of currant-jelly stools and episodes of spasmodic crying with abdominal distension is diagnostic of acute intussusception. Excessive intake of aerated liquids, opium derivatives and gut sedatives may also lead to intestinal dysmotility and abdominal distension[19].

Convulsions

Generalized convulsions may occur following thrombosis of cerebral vessels due to hemoconcentration, rapid correction of hypernatremic dehydration, severe hyponatremia, hypocalcemia, hypomagnesemia, post-acidotic tetany or concomitant meningoencephalitis. Seizures occur in about one-fourth of children with shigellosis. Sagittal sinus thrombosis may rarely occur in severely dehydrated patients. It is usually characterized by signs of raised intracranial pressure, visible veins on the forehead, stupor and bulging anterior fontanel. Seizures and quadriparesis may occur. When thrombosis extends to the cortical veins, hemorrhagic infarction of the brain can be identified on CT scan. CSF pressure is usually elevated and it often contains red blood cells and elevated proteins.

Renal Shut Down

Oliguria of pre-renal onset due to reduced perfusion of kidneys and reduced glomerular filtration rate may occur but is reversible on rapid rehydration. Prolonged and severe circulatory collapse and shock may lead to acute tubular necrosis and should be differentiated from oliguria due to reduced perfusion of the kidneys for effective management (Table 26.3). Hemolytic uremic syndrome is a recognized complication of shigella dysentery and diarrhea due to enterohemorrhagic *E. coli* in children below 2 years of age. It is characterized by Coomb's negative microangiopathic hemolytic anemia, fragmented or burred erythrocytes, thrombocytopenia, leukocytosis, reticulocytosis, hematuria, proteinuria and marked azotemia. Hemoglobin concentration may be as low as 4g/dl. Bilateral renal vein thrombosis may mimic the clinical picture of hemolytic uremic syndrome and should be excluded.

Table 26.3 Differences between oliguria due to renal hypoperfusion and acute tubular necrosis

	Criteria	Pre-renal hypoperfusion	Acute tubular necrosis
1.	Reponse to rapid intravenous fluid therapy	Urinary flow is established	No effect with risk of pulmonary edema
2.	Urine specific gravity	>1.020	< 1.010
3.	Urinary osmolality	>500	< 300
4.	Urine/Plasma osmolality	>1.5	< 1.0
5.	Urine/Plasma creatinine	>40	< 20
6.	Urine/Plasma urea	>10	< 5
7.	Urine sodium (mEq/L)	< 20	> 40
8.	Blood urea/creatinine ratio	> 20	<20
9.	Renal failure index*	<1	>3
10.	Fractional excretion of sodium** (%)	<1	>3

$$ \text{* Renal failure index} = \frac{UNa\ (mEq/L)}{Ucr/Pcr} $$

$$ \text{** FeNa (\%)} = \frac{\text{Urine sodium} \times \text{serum creatinine}}{\text{serum sodium} \times \text{urine creatinine}} $$

INVESTIGATIONS

In most cases of acute diarrhea there is no role of laboratory investigations. Presence of more than 20 leukocytes per high power field is suggestive of invasive diarrhea but the fecal leukocyte count has poor specificity of around 50-60 percent. To identify cases for antibiotic therapy e.g. *Shigella* and *V. cholerae*, the presence of gross blood in stools and cholera-like clinical picture, respectively are more useful than culture. However, in bloody diarrhea determining antimicrobial sensitivity of isolates would help in the management. Documenting cholera on the basis of rice-water stools is of epidemiological importance. *E. coli* is often reported on stool cultures but most laboratories lack the ability to identify whether they are diarrheagenic or commensals. *Campylobacter jejuni* require special method for isolation. Nonavailability of facilities for microbiology or microscopy should not be the reasons for lack of effective or rational management.

Serum electrolyte estimation is not required for routine management of diarrhea with some dehydration. They should be monitored in patients with altered sensorium, marked irritability, extreme lethargy, seizures, abdominal distension or weak respirations. In malnourished children, infants under 2 months of age, seriously toxic patients with high fever or abdominal distension, blood culture should be taken to exclude septicemia. Monitoring BUN, glucose, acid-base parameters, urinary volume, specific gravity or osmolality would be useful in patients who develop severe dehydration or shock. Electrocardiogram is useful for urgent evaluation of tissue potassium status. There is no indication to test pH of stools or reducing substance in stools in children with acute diarrhea. *Lactose intolerance if present during acute diarrhea is transient and does not need any withdrawal of lactose feeds.*

MANAGEMENT

Most episodes of diarrhea are self-limited and the mainstay of management is correction of the existing fluid and electrolyte deficit depending on the signs of dehydration (rehydration therapy), replacement of ongoing losses due to continuing diarrhea to prevent recurrence of dehydration (prevention of dehydration) and provision of normal daily fluid requirements (maintenance therapy). The other important component of management is maintenance of optimal feeding during diarrhea to prevent malnutrition. Routine antimicrobial therapy is not required and is limited to episodes that have gross blood in stool, culture positive shigella infection, *Vibrio cholerae* with severe dehydration, diarrhea due to giardia or *E. histolytica* and associated non gastrointestinal systemic infection.

Indications for Referral to the Hospital

Most patients of acute diarrhea can be managed on an ambulatory basis but child should be admitted to the hospital in following situations.

- Gastroenteritis in infants below 2 months
- Persistent vomiting and high purge rate (almost every hour) with high risk of dehydration
- Severe dehydration, shock or poor urine output
- Severe abdominal pain, localized tenderness or mass
- Anemia, throubocytopenia, acute kidney injury due to hemolytic uremic syndrome
- Persistent diarrhea (> 2 weeks) with mal-nutrition
- Non-responding bloody diarrhea

Oral Rehydration Therapy

Oral rehydration therapy (ORT) is the most significant development in the management of diarrheal disease in children and is provided by administration of oral rehydration salt solution and other home based culturally acceptable fluids to prevent and treat dehydration during diarrhea. Importance of ORT must be emphasized to health care providers. One of the greatest advantages of ORT is that it can be brought to the patient's home and administered early at the onset of diarrhea.

Oral rehydration solution (ORS)

ORS consists of sodium chloride, sodium bicarbonate, potassium chloride, glucose and water and is based on the principle that optimal concentration of glucose effectively enhances the uptake and transport of sodium and water across the intestinal mucosa. For over three decades, UNICEF and WHO recommended a single formulation of glucose-based ORS (Table 26.4) irrespective of the cause or age group affected. It was effective even in young children with non-cholera diarrhea when used according to the recommended guidelines with ready access to plain water during oral rehydration. WHO-ORS was hailed as "potentially the most important medical advance of this century". It successfully rehydrated patients with diarrhea, and substantially reduced hospital case fatality rates, hospital admission rates and cost of treatment. However, it did not decrease duration of diarrhea or stool output.

Table 26.4 Composition of original ORS (mOsm/l)	
Content	**Osmolarity (mOsm/l)**
Glucose	111
Sodium	90
Chloride	80
Potassium	20
Citrate	10
Total osmolarity	**311**

Another main concern was the potential risk of hypernatremia with standard WHO-ORS in children with non-cholera diarrhea and the recognition that the standard WHO-ORS may provide too much sodium to edematous children. There were also reports of recurrent dehydration in young infants treated with standard WHO-ORS for replacement of ongoing stool losses that was promptly reversed when patients were kept nil orally and given intravenous fluids. The recurrent dehydration was attributed to high purging because of high glucose concentration in the ORS. All these concerns prompted formulation of low osmolar ORS with lower risk of complications than the standard WHO-ORS.

Improved oral rehydration salts solution

Meta-analysis of 7 double blind randomized controlled trials comparing amino-acid based ORS with standard WHO ORS found no clinical advantage over WHO-ORS in children with non-cholera diarrhea[20]. Rice-based and WHO-ORS solutions were found to be nearly equally effective for treating children with acute non-cholera diarrhea, when feeding was resumed promptly following initial rehydration[20]. These solutions were more efficacious in cholera but as they did not have any significant benefits in non-cholera diarrhea they were not introduced for treatment of dehydration in diarrhea in place of standard WHO-ORS.

Earlier laboratory experiments had shown that solutions with reduced osmolarity (sodium 60 mMol/l, glucose 80-120 mMol/l, osmolarity 240 mOsm/l) enhanced water and sodium absorption[21]. Several randomized clinical trials were done to evaluate reduced osmolarity ORS containing glucose, maltodextrin or sucrose (total osmolarity 210-268 mOsmol/l) and a sodium concentration ranging from 50 to 75 mEq/L[22]. These studies were conducted mainly in developing countries, included well-nourished and malnourished children aged 1 month to 5 years with acute diarrhea (duration <7 days) with dehydration. Four of the studies were done in India, two as part of large multi-center trials. Use

of reduced osmolarity ORS was associated with a 39% reduction in need for intravenous fluids, 19% reduction in stool output and 29% lower incidence of vomiting. The incidence of hyponatremia (serum sodium <130 mEq/L) at 24 hours evaluated in 3 clinical trials was greater among children given reduced osmolarity ORS but these differences were not significant and none of these children were symptomatic. The reduced osmolarity ORS was also found to be safe and effective for use in children with cholera. It was reported to be as effective as standard ORS in adults with cholera but was associated with asymptomatic hyponatremia[23].

The WHO meeting of experts after reviewing all the available data proposed that the reduced osmolarity ORS with 75 mEq/L of sodium and 75 mMol/l of glucose is effective both in adults and children with cholera[23]. Subsequently, Phase IV studies on more than 100,000 adults and children hospitalized with diarrhea (approximately 20% with cholera), reported no increased risk of symptomatic hyponatremia with low osmolarity ORS[24]. There were programmatic and logistic advantages of using a single solution globally for all causes of diarrhea at all ages. They also concluded that safety data in patients with cholera, while limited, are reassuring. Indian Academy of Pediatrics endorsed use of reduced osmolarity ORS as an acceptable oral rehydration solution for all age groups[25]. Reduced osmolarity ORS was introduced in the National Diarrheal Disease Control Program in the country in June 2004 and is now available commercially (Table 26.5).

Table 26.5 Composition of reduced osmolarity ORS	
Reduced osmolarity ORS	**grams/liter**
Glucose, anhydrous	13.5
Sodium chloride	2.6
Potassium chloride	1.5
Trisodium citrate	2.9
Total weight	**20.5**
Reduced osmolarity ORS	**mMol/liter**
Glucose, anhydrous	75
Sodium	75
Chloride	65
Potassium	20
Citrate	10
Total osmolarity	**245**

Treatment of Dehydration

Children with some dehydration or severe dehydration should be weighed without clothing, as an aid for estimating their fluid requirements. The fluid deficit can be estimated on the basis of severity of dehydration as shown in Table 26.6.

Table 26.6 Assessment of fluid deficit		
Assessment	Fluid deficit as % of body weight	Fluid deficit in ml/kg bodyweight
No signs of dehydration	<5%	<50 ml/kg
Some dehydration	5-10%	50-100 ml/kg
Severe dehydration	>10%	>100 ml/kg

Prevention of Dehydration (IMNCI Treatment Plan A)

ORS should be administered early during the course of diarrhea to prevent dehydration. If there is no dehydration, the child can be sent home after advising the normal daily fluid requirements and the replacement of ongoing losses to prevent dehydration. ORS should be recommended in amounts given in Table 26.7.

Table 26.7 ORS for prevention of dehydration		
Age	Amount of ORS to be given after each loose stool	Amount of total ORS in a day
Less than 24 months	50-100 ml	500 ml/day
2 to 10 years	100-200 ml	1000 ml/day
10 years or more	As much as wanted	2000 ml/day

Other fluids that can be given to prevent dehydration include fluids available at home, food based fluids and sugar-salt solution. Mothers should be educated to give safe plain water (preferably given with food), lemon water, soups with salt, butter milk (*lassi*) with salt and coconut water. Since many of these fluids lack a glucose precursor or salt or both they are likely to be effective only in the presence of continued feeding which provides starch and protein to promote absorption of luminal sodium. These fluids together with food provide oral rehydration therapy (ORT). Food based solutions like rice *kanji* or watery *dal* with salt can also be used for ORT. However, most food based solutions ferment within 6-8 hours of storage in tropical conditions. The need for cooking may reduce their actual use by mothers. There is also the risk that food-based solution may be confused with 'food'

by mothers, which has the potential danger that mothers will assume that concurrent feeding during diarrhea is not required. It should be noted that fluids (e.g. herbal teas, fruit juice, cola drinks and plain tea, etc) consumed in small amounts or glucose water without salt is not ORT and the latter may cause osmotic diarrhea.

Sugar salt solution is a mixture of sugar (sucrose) and salt (sodium chloride) that provides a final concentration of 4% sugar and 0.4% salt when properly prepared. It is prepared by taking two-finger pinch of table salt (0.8 g) and one heaped teaspoon (8 g) of sugar in a large cup or glass (200 ml) of water. It can be used as replacement for ORS but has several limitations. The lack of suitable utensils for measuring the ingredients and water, and the difficulty in educating mothers for its proper preparation and administration has often resulted in high sodium concentration (>120 mEq/L) solutions. These errors can be minimized by actually demonstrating to mothers how to measure ingredients and water in addition to verbal instructions.

The normal daily fluid intake of breast milk or formula feeds that the child was previously consuming and plain water should be continued.

Treatment of Some Dehydration (IMNCI Treatment Plan B)

Patients with some dehydration should be ideally treated in a health care facility. At least 75 ml/kg of ORS should be given during the first 4 hours with instructions to offer more if the child is keen to take. All ongoing stool losses (10-20 ml per kilogram body weight for each liquid stool) should be replaced with ORS. The mother should be shown how to mix ORS and instructed to give a teaspoonful every 1-2 minute for a child under 2 years and frequent sips from a cup for an older child. If the child vomits she should be asked to wait for 10 minutes and then give the solution more slowly; a spoonful every 2-3 minutes. Breast feeding should be encouraged and 100-200 ml extra water should be offered to non-breast fed infants less than 6 months. Approximate fluid estimates for deficit replacement are given in Table 26.8.

Signs of dehydration usually disappear within 4 hours. ORS should be continued, even after dehydration has been corrected, in volumes equal to diarrheal losses as maintenance fluids and to prevent dehydration. If the body weight is not known standard requirements may be followed as shown in Table 26.7. Plain water should be offered in between the ORS sips. Feeding should be

Section 4

Table 26.8 Guidelines for treating patients with some dehydration when body weight is not known

Age	Upto 4 months	4 months upto 12 months	12 months upto 2 years	2 years upto 5 years	5 years upto 14 years	14 years or older
Approximate weight in kg	<6 kg	6 -<10 kg	10 -<12 kg	12-<19 kg	20-<30 kg	≥30 kg
ORS in ml	200-400	400-700	700-900	900-1400	1400-2200	2200-4000
Approximate local measure (glass)	1-2	2-3	3-4	4-6	6-11	12-20

resumed soon after deficit replacement. If the child continues to have some dehydration after 4 hours, another 4 hours rehydration treatment with ORS solution should be repeated but feeding (milk, breast feeds and other foods) should be resumed immediately. When mother has to leave the clinic/center before completing the treatment, she should be advised how to prepare ORS solution and how much to give in order to finish the 4-hour treatment quota at home. Extra fluids and feeding should be continued and she should be told to return if any of the danger signs appear. ORS should not be continued once the diarrhea has stopped.

Severe dehydration (IMNCI Treatment Plan C)

Comatosed or lethargic children or those with severe dehydration, persistent vomiting or abdominal distension should be given intravenous rehydration. Children with severe dehydration or shock should be started on rapid IV infusion of Ringer's lactate with 5% dextrose. If Ringer's lactate is not available, normal saline solution (0.9% NaCl) in 5% dextrose should be given. The deficit amount of 100 ml/kg should be administered as shown in Table 26.9.

ORS (5 ml/kg/hr) should be started as soon as the child can take orally even while getting IV fluids. It is important to replace the ongoing stool

(10 ml/kg) and vomitus (2-5 ml/kg) losses with ORS or intravenous fluids. The child should be reassessed every 15-30 minutes until a strong radial pulse is present. If hydration status is not improving the IV fluids should be given more rapidly. Additional IV fluids (0.18% saline in 5% dextrose, calculated for age and weight) may be given for the next 8-24 hours for ongoing losses and maintenance requirements till oral intake improves. See Box for calculation and administration of fluids and electrolytes in a one year old infant with severe dehydration, acidosis and hypokalemia.

In situations where IV fluids cannot be given immediately, rehydration can be started with ORS using a NG tube at 20 ml/kg/hr (total of 120 ml/kg in 6 hours). The child should be reassessed every 1-2 hours and if found to have repeated vomiting or abdominal distension the fluids should be given more slowly. If the child shows improvement but still has signs of some dehydration after the full deficit correction for severe dehydration, ORS solution should be given for another 4 hours as for Plan B. Infants should be encouraged to breast feed.

If there are no signs of dehydration at the end of the rehydration period the child should be given appropriate amount of oral fluids (as for plan A) for ongoing stool and vomitus losses and for normal maintenance requirements. It is advisable to observe these children for at least 6 hours before discharge to confirm if the mother is able to maintain the child's hydration by giving ORS solution.

Fluid Therapy in a Severely Malnourished Child

Children with severe malnutrition are difficult to assess and manage. The recommended fluids and rates of administration are shown in Table 26.10 Children with severe malnutrition may have circulatory signs suggesting shock, but may have sepsis rather than hypovolemia. Whenever possible, avoid administration of intravenous fluids and use

Table 26.9 Intravenous fluid therapy in severe dehydration

Age	First give 30 ml/kg in	Then give 70 ml/kg in
< 12 months old	1 hour*	5 hours
Older children	30 minutes*	2 ½ hours

*Repeat bolus administration if the radial pulse is still very weak or not detectable or the patient has not passed urine.

Example. **Calculate the fluid and electrolyte requirements of one year old, 10 kg infant having severe dehydration (15%), acidosis and hypokalemia.**

Deficit fluid   15% dehydration
                         $150 \times 10 = 1500$ ml

Daily maintenance $120 \times 10 = 1200$ ml

Total requirements in 24 hours = 2700 ml
Administer one-half (1400 ml) of the above amount in first 8 hours and remainder in the next 16 hours.

First hour 30 ml/kg = 300 ml of Ringer's lactate solution (or 0.45% saline in 5% dextrose)
                    = 300/60 = 5 ml/minute
                    = 5×20 = 100 drops/minute

(Alternatively divide ml/hour by 3 to get drops/minute i.e. 300/3 = 100 drops/minute)

Next 7 hours give 1100 ml i.e. 157 ml/hour of Ringer's lactate = 157/3 i.e. 52 drops/min

Next 16 hours give 1300 ml i.e. 81 ml/hour of 0.18% saline in 5% dextrose = 81/3 i.e. 27 drops/minute

On-going losses Calculate fluid losses through vomiting and stools every 4-6 hours and replenish with N/2 dextrose-saline solution. For each diarrheal stool and vomiting provide additional fluids to the extent of 10 ml/kg and 2 ml/kg respectively. The commonest cause of persistence of dehydration is lack of adequate replacement of concurrent losses of fluids.

Moderate acidosis Administer 3 ml of 7.5% sodium bicarbonate/kg i.e. $3 \times 10 = 30$ ml
One-half i.e. 15 ml is given during first hour and the rest during next 7 hours

Give calcium gluconate 50 mg/kg following correction of acidosis to prevent post acidotic tetany

Hypokalemia   Potassium 4 mEq/kg = 40 mEq to be administered only when urine flow is established. Correct slowly over 24 hours. Do not exceed concentration of 40 mEq/L.

a nasogastric (NG) tube or oral fluids. Only if the child is lethargic or unconscious and cannot swallow a NG tube or is vomiting excessively, 15 ml/kg

Ringer's lactate or ½-strength normal saline with 5% glucose should be administered intravenously during 1 hour and child monitored carefully. If the child shows signs of improvement, another bolus of of IV 15 ml/kg should be repeated over I hour. The intravenous fluids should be discontinued if the pulse increases by 15 or the respiratory rate by 5/min. Subsequently the child can be managed on oral or nasogastric ORS. If the child fails to improve after the first 15 ml/kg IV, it should be assumed that the child has septic shock and should be managed accordingly (Figure 26.1).

If the child deteriorates during the IV rehydration (breathing increases by 5 breaths/min or pulse by 15 beats/min), stop the infusion because IV fluids can worsen the child's condition. Therefore, whenever possible, a dehydrated child with severe malnutrition but without shock should be rehydrated orally. ORS should be given orally or by nasogastric tube 5 ml/kg every 30 minutes for the first 2 hours and then 5-10 ml/kg/hour for the next 4-10 hours. Blood sugar should be monitored on a regular basis. After initial dehydration is corrected, 5-10 ml/kg of ORS should be continued for every loose stool. It is essential to initiate feeding during rehydration.

Hypertonic Dehydration

Continuation of breast feeding and offering plain water in between ORS is useful to prevent hypernatremia if the patient can drink orally. Convulsions are also less likely to occur when treatment is given with ORS rather than IV fluids. In children who cannot take orally or are in shock, circulatory adequacy should be restored with 20 ml/kg boluses of normal saline. The volumes of fluid to be given over the next 48 hours are decided by computing the clinically estimated fluid deficit and the maintenance requirement over next 48 hours. It is preferable to use N/5 saline for maintenance replacement. 10 ml of 10% calcium gluconate should be administered for every 500 ml. Ongoing losses should be replaced simultaneously preferably through a separate IV line.

Hypotonic Dehydration

ORS solution is safe and effective for treatment of hyponatremic dehydration. Intravenous fluids may be required in those patients who are unable to drink ORS because of altered sensorium or seizures. Symptomatic hyponatremia is corrected using 3% NaCl (0.5 mEq Na$^+$/ml). The goal is to achieve a serum sodium between 120–125 mEq/L. The required volume of 3% NaCl is calculated using

Section 4

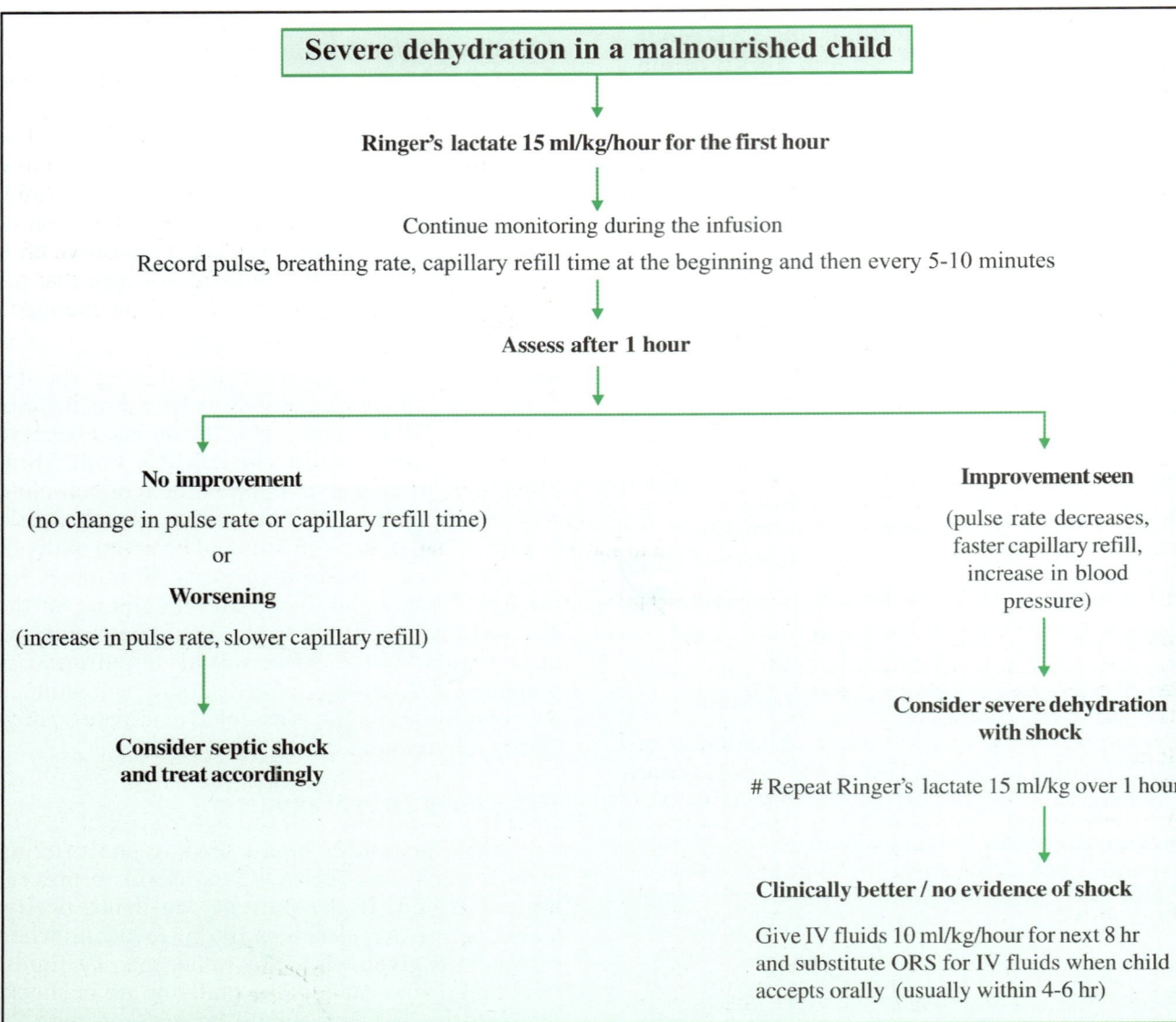

Figure 26.1 Fluid management in a malnourished child with severe dehydration

the formula 1.2 × body weight × (120 −Na$^+_{obs}$) ml. In those children who have serum sodium less than 120 mEq/L but are asymptomatic, normal saline can be infused slowly over 24 hours as maintenance fluids.

Hypokalemia

When the serum potassium is less than 2.0 mEq/L or less than 3.5 mEq/L with ECG changes or there is clinical evidence of paralytic ileus, 0.3

Table 26.10 Fluids and feeding in a severely malnourished child			

- Insert an IV line (and draw blood for emergency laboratory investigations).
- Weigh the child (or estimate the weight) to calculate the volume of fluids to be given.
- Give IV fluids 15 ml/kg over 1 hour. Use one of the following solutions :
  Half-normal saline with 5% glucose or Ringer's lactate with 5% glucose.
- Supplement zinc, vitamin A and correct potassium deficit.

Body weight (kg)	Volume of IV fluids over 1 hour (15 ml/kg)	Body weight (kg)	Volume of IV fluids over 1 hour (15 ml/kg)
4 kg	60 ml	12 kg	180 ml
6 kg	90 ml	14 kg	210 ml
8 kg	120 ml	16 kg	240 ml
10 kg	150 ml	18 kg	270 ml

- *Record the pulse and breathing rate at the start and every 5-10 minutes.*

If there are signs of improvement (pulse slows and capillary refill becomes faster) :
- Repeat IV bolus 15 ml/kg over 1 hour; then switch to oral or nasogastric rehydration with ORS, 5-10 ml/kg/hr up to 10 hours
- Initiate refeeding with starter F-75 (milk based diet providing 75 cal/100 ml)

If the child fails to improve after the first 15 ml/kg IV, assume the child has septic shock:
- Give maintenance IV fluids (4 ml/kg/hr).
- Initiate refeeding with starter F-75
- Start antibiotic treatment

If the child deteriorates during the IV rehydration (breathing increases by 5 breaths/min or pulse by 15 beats/min), stop the infusion because IV fluids can worsen the child's condition.

Whenever possible, a dehydrated child with severe malnutrition but without shock should be rehydrated orally. ORS should be given orally or by nasogastric tube 5 ml/kg every 30 minutes for the first 2 hours and then 5-10 ml/kg/hour for the next 4-10 hours. Blood sugars should be monitored continuously. After dehydration is corrected, 5-10 ml/kg of ORS should be continued for every loose stool. It is essential to initiate feeding early during rehydration.

mEq/kg/hour of potassium chloride should be given in the required volume of IV fluids. The infusion rate should be 1 mEq/kg/hour for arrhythmia or respiratory arrest. Maximum levels of potassium chloride in IV fluids should be limited to 40 mEq/I and 80 mEq/L (1.0 ml of 15% kcl provides 2.0 mEq K) in the peripheral or central veins respectively and given under cardiac monitoring. When serum potassium is between 2.0 mEq/L and 3.5 mEq/L, potassium deficits are corrected with ORS solution as given for rehydration therapy. Additional oral potassium at 4 mEq/kg/day till the serum potassium rises to greater than 3.5 mEq/L should be given. Foods rich in potassium, such as fruits (e.g. bananas) and intake of green coconut water should be encouraged during and after the episode of diarrhea.

Metabolic acidosis

Acidosis should be corrected with 7.5% sodium bicarbonate (calculated by the formula base deficit × weight in kg × 0.3) solution. When facilities for estimation of acid-base parameters are not available, 3-5 ml/kg sodium bicarbonate (7.5 %;1ml = 0.9 mEq) can be administered; one-half of the calculated amount diluted with an equal volume of distilled water should be administered slowly as a bolus followed by administration of the remaining amount during next 8 hours.

Zinc supplements

A number of trials in India and other low middle income countries have documented faster recovery and reduced severity of diarrhea following zinc supplementation during acute diarrhea[26,27,28,29]. Zinc deficiency is common in children living in such settings due to low intake of animal foods, high dietary phytate content, and overall inadequate diets[30]. This led to the WHO recommendation of supplemental zinc as syrup or tablets (10 mg/day elemental zinc for infants <6 months and 20 mg/day for children >6 months for 10 to 14 days) during acute diarrhea[31]. Addition of zinc to the case management strategy was evaluated in a cluster randomized study in six primary health centers in north India[32]. Prevalence and hospitalization for diarrhea decreased significantly in the villages that received low osmolarity ORS and zinc as compared to the control villages. It is important to note that the prescriptions for antibiotics by care providers and use of unwarranted injections were significantly less, and the ORS use rates significantly higher in the intervention villages. Additionally, zinc given during an episode of diarrhea reduced subsequent diarrheal morbidity. Similar benefits on reduction of antibiotic use during diarrhea were seen in a large multicenter study done across India, Brazil, Ethiopia, Egypt, and the Philippines[33]. Government of India included zinc in the national program for treatment of diarrhea in 2007. These recommendations have been endorsed by the Indian Academy of Pediatrics and the industry is being encouraged to prepare zinc formulations, which contain only zinc[24]. All salt preparations (sulfate, acetate or gluconate) of zinc can be used as the effects are not dependent upon the type of zinc salts[28,29]. Iron containing zinc formulations should not be used as it may interfere with zinc absorption. Zinc should not be mixed with ORS and should be administered separately during a diarrheal episode[34].

Therapeutic benefits of zinc administration during diarrhea are biologically plausible because of its effects on various components of the immune system and its direct gastrointestinal effects. Zinc has a critical role in metalloenzymes, polyribosomes, the cell membrane, cellular function, cellular growth and in the function of the immune system[35, 36]. Zinc is said to improve absorption of water and electrolytes by helping in early regeneration of intestinal mucosa and restoration of enteric enzymes[37]. Additionally zinc deficiency has been found to be widespread among children in developing countries, and occurs in most of Latin America, Africa, the Middle East and South Asia[38]. Intestinal zinc losses during repeated episodes of diarrhea aggravate pre-existing zinc deficiency[39].

Antimicrobial Therapy

The specific clinical indications for use of antimicrobial agents where they have been found to be useful are listed below:

(i)   Suspected cholera with severe dehydration

(ii) Bloody diarrhea (probably shigellosis)

(iii) Serious associated non-gastrointestinal infections e.g. pneumonia, septicemia, meningitis, urinary tract infection, acute otitis media, etc.

(iv) Severely malnourished or immune compromised children

(v)   Specific infections like giardia, amebiasis, cryptosporidium, *Clostridium difficile*, Salmonella in early infancy.

Cholera

The mainstay of treatment for cholera is rehydration with ORS (for some dehydration) or intravenous Ringer's lactate (for severe dehydration). Antimicrobials are used as adjuncts to ORT in children with cholera because they help to reduce the rate of stool output, minimize fluid requirements and decrease excretion of *Vibrio cholerae* in the stool. Antibiotics like tetracycline (12.5mg/kg four times a day for a period of 3 days), erythromycin (12.5 mg/kg given four times a day for 3 days), co-trimoxazole (trimethoprim 5 mg/kg or sulphamethoxazole 25 mg/kg twice a day for three days) and furazolidone (1.25 mg/kg four times a day for 3 days) have been used effectively in the past. Doxycycline (6 mg/kg single dose) is as effective as multiple doses of tetracycline in treatment of cholera[40,41]. The major concern is that resistance to these drugs has been reported. Studies in adults with *V. cholerae* 01 and 0139 have shown that single dose of 0.1g ciprofloxacin is effective in the treatment of cholera and is better than single dose of doxycycline in the eradication of the pathogens from the stool[42]. Norfloxacin 400 mg given twice a day for three days to adults has been reported to decrease the stool output, diarrheal duration and need for intravenous fluids[43]. There is preliminary evidence to suggest that fluoroquinolones can be safely used in children as an adjunct to oral rehydration therapy[44]. Extensive experience in the use of these drugs in children with typhoid, cystic fibrosis and dysentery has not shown any evidence of bone or joint toxicity, and impairment of linear growth[45-48].

Acute Dysentery

Prompt antimicrobial therapy in shigellosis decreases associated mortality, reduces malabsorption, hastens clinical recovery and increases elimination of *Shigella* from the stool. Absorbable, systemic antimicrobials are recommended as *Shigella* invades the intestinal mucosa and multiplies within the submucosa. Case-fatality among hospitalized patients with *Shigella dysenteriae type1* can be as high as 15% and may further increase if treatment is initiated with ineffective antimicrobials. The choice of antimicrobial should, if possible, be based on recent susceptibility data from *Shigella* strains isolated in the area. If information on local strains is not available, data from nearby areas or from recent regional epidemics should be used. In recent years, Shigella strains resistant to antimicrobials like ampicillin and co-trimoxazole have emerged and these are no longer recommended for treatment of shigellosis[49]. Over the last decade nalidixic acid (the drug of choice for the last several years) resistant *Shigella dysenteriae* type 1 have been reported from South and Middle-east Asia, Eastern and Southern Africa and in addition there has been a recent outbreak of nalidixic acid resistant *Shigella sonnei* from Israel[50-52]. WHO recommends ciprofloxacin, (15 mg/kg twice a day for 3 days) as the drug of choice for all patients with bloody diarrhea, irrespective of age[10]. Effective antimicrobial therapy should produce improvement within 48 hours by decreasing the blood in stools, the frequency of stools and fever. If no improvement is seen then antimicrobial resistance should be considered. Ofloxacin, ceftriaxone (50-100 mg/kg once a day intramuscular for 2-5 days), pivmecillinam (20 mg/kg four times a day for 5 days) and azithromycin (10-20 mg/kg or 1-1.5 g in adults once a day orally for 1-5 days) are effective for treatment of multi-resistant strains of *Shigella* in all age groups and are currently recommended as alternative antimicrobials[53-55]. It is recommended that these should only be used when local strains of *Shigella* are known to be resistant to ciprofloxacin. Ampicillin, chloramphenicol, co-trimoxazole, tetracycline, nitrofurans, aminoglycosides, first- and second-generation cephalosporins, amoxycillin and nalidixic acid are not effective against *Shigella*[10] (Figure 26.2).

Other uncommon causes of bloody diarrhea

Erythromycin is the drug of choice for *Campylobacter jejuni* but the treatment should be started early as most episodes recover by the time the laboratory diagnosis is made. Antimicrobial therapy in salmonella infection may prolong the carriage of the pathogens. Bloody diarrhea due to *Entamoeba histolytica* is uncommon in children. Amebiasis should be considered when two different antibiotics, usually effective for *Shigella* in the area, have been given sequentially without showing signs of clinical improvement, or trophozoites of *E. histolytica* with engulfed RBCs are identified in fresh stool samples in a reliable laboratory. Amebic dysentery should be treated with metronidazole in a dose of 10 mg/kg 3 times a day for 5-10 days. Specific treatment for protozoal diarrhea is detailed in Table 26.11.

Table 26.11 Antiprotozoal therapy	
Pathogen	**Drug, dose and duration**
Entamoeba histolytica (only if microscopic examination of fresh stool sample done in a reliable laboratory shows trophozoites of *E. histolytica* containing RBCs)	Metronidazole 10 mg/kg given three times a day for 5 - 10 days
Giardia lamblia (only if trophozoites are identified in stool or duodenal fluid)	1. Metronidazole 5 mg/kg is given 3 times in a day for 5 days 2. Tinidazole can be given in a single dose (50 mg/kg orally; upto a maximum of two doses). 3. Albendazole (10 mg/kg daily for 5 days) or mebendazole (200 mg thrice daily for 5 days) are equally effective and better tolerated than metronidazole[56]. 4. Recent evidence suggests that nitazoxanide (nitrothiazolyl-salicylamide derivative) is significantly better in achieving earlier recovery from diarrhea as compared to a placebo[57] but is similar in efficacy to metronidazole[58]. Presently limited evidence is available from randomized controlled trials to recommend routine treatment (100 mg twice daily for 3 days) with nitazoxanide for giardiasis.
Cryptosporidium parvum	Supportive therapy is the mainstay of treatment. Nitazoxanide (100 mg twice daily for 3 days) is presently the only FDA approved treatment available for children 1 to 11 years of age with normal immune function[59-61]. The role of nitazoxanide in treating cryptosporidiosis in immune compromised children is not clear. Parmomycin has been shown to have potential benefits but need further evaluation in immune compromised individuals.

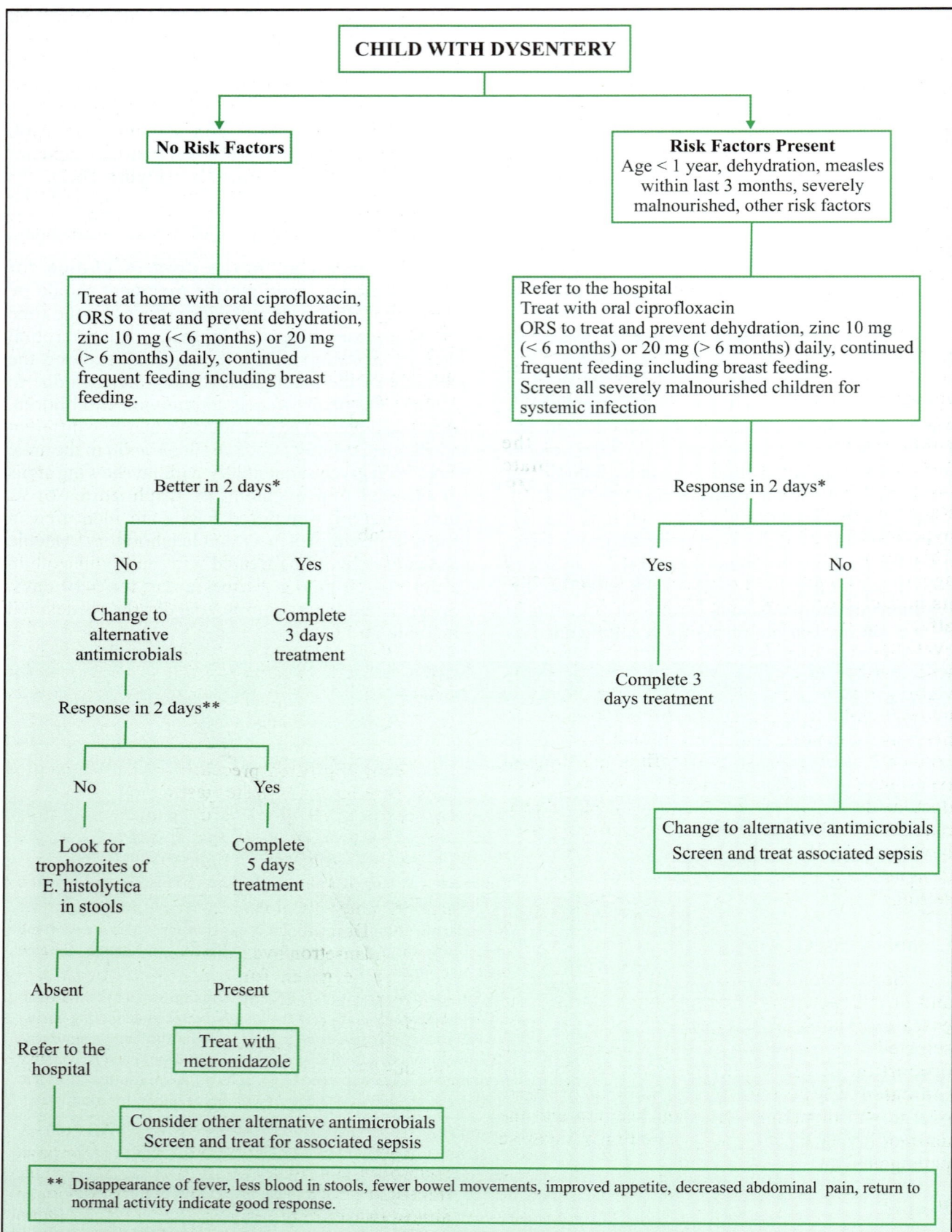

Figure 26.2 A suggested algorithm for treatment of dysentery

Section 4

Antidiarrheal Agents

Adsorbents (kaolin, pectin, activated charcoal, bismuth subcarbonate) are not indicated in the routine treatment of acute diarrhea. Motility suppressants (opiates, opiate-like compounds, tincture of opium, camphorated tincture of opium or paregoric, codeine, diphenoxylate with atropine, loperamide hydrochloride) decrease intestinal peristalsis and delay the elimination of the causative organisms. Their use particularly in infants is dangerous because of risk of causing paralytic ileus, respiratory depression, abdominal distension, bacterial overgrowth and toxic megacolon.

The antisecretory properties of the new synthetic enkephalinase inhibitor, racecadotril (acetorphan), are attributed to inactivation of endogenous enkephalins, secreted by myenteric and submucus plexus in the digestive tract. The enkephalins act as neurotransmitters in the gastrointestinal tract by activating δ-opiate receptors and thus reducing the level of cyclic AMP. Racecadotril has antisecretory action only when hypersecretion is present, not in the basal state[62]. This compound differs from μ-opiate receptor agonists like loperamide and diphenoxylate because its antisecretory mechanisms are independent of effects on intestinal motility. The drug has been evaluated in a small number of children and adults with diarrhea in randomized controlled trials with varying results. In a placebo-controlled study in under-3 children racecadotril (1.5 mg/kg/dose q 8 hr) was associated with 50% reduction in stool volume[63]. Nevertheless, the benefit of this drug for treatment of acute diarrhea has not been documented to an extent and in a manner that is required minimally to recommend its use. We need more evidence of its efficacy and safety from well-designed randomized controlled studies done in our settings[64].

Combination Therapy

Several combinations of antibacterial agents and of antibacterials with antidiarrheals offer no extra clinical benefit compared to a properly selected single antibacterial agent for the small proportion of diarrheal illness where they are indicated. Combination therapy can promote overgrowth of harmful resistant bacteria and the antimotility agents may delay excretion of invasive pathogens.

Probiotics

Possible therapeutic and preventive benefits of probiotics in childhood diarrhea have been evaluated over the last decade. The commonly studied strains have been *Lactobacillus rhamnosus GG, Lactobacillus reuteri, Lactobacillus casei, Lactobacillus acidophilus, Escherichia coli* strain Nissle 1917, *Bifidobacteria, Enterococci (Enterococcus faecium* SF68), and yeast – *Saccharomyces boulardii*. Systematic reviews have suggested some benefits with specific strains[65]. The evidence is primarily related to developed countries and shows modest effect for treatment of mild or moderate acute diarrhea, restricted to Rotavirus which is the cause of diarrhea in more than 75% of cases in studies from the west while it constitutes about 25% of diarrhea in hospitalized children and 15% in outpatient practice in India. However, it may not be possible to extrapolate the findings of these studies to our setting where the breast feeding rates are high and the microbial colonization of the gut is different. Also, stool output which is the objective parameter of improvement, has not been evaluated. Effects of one species cannot be extended to another species and treatment schedules are not well established or studied. As the efficacy of probiotics is dependent on the formulation and the host factors, it is desirable to conduct randomized controlled trials to assess their utility before they are recommended for routine use in diarrhea. The combination formulations containing prebiotics, probiotics and zinc are available in the market but need to be studied by randomized controlled trials.

Antiemetics

Vomiting often precedes or is associated in most children with acute gastroenteritis and may interfere with successful oral rehydration. Administration of small sips of ORS with a spoon (instead of gulps with a glass, cup or bottle) is usually well tolerated. Sips of ORS often relieve gastritis and control vomiting. Antiemetics are best avoided. Domperidone (0.2 mg/kg/dose every 4-6 hr) or ondansetron hydrochloride (2-4 mg/dose 4-6 hr) may be given for a couple of doses. The occurrence of small infrequent vomiting does not interfere with ORT but when vomiting is persistent and even sips of ORS are not retained, the child should be hospitalized for intravenous fluid therapy.

Dietary Management

There is no physiological basis to suggest that starvation provides rest to the gut and reduces intestinal peristalsis. Even during acute diarrhea, almost two-third of the normal absorptive capacity of the gut is preserved. Early feeding promotes rapid mucosal recovery and prevents or minimizes the deterioration of nutritional status that normally accompanies such illness. Breast feeding should be continued uninterrupted even during rehydration with ORS. Energy dense foods with the least bulk, which are easily available in the household should be offered in small quantities but frequently, at least once every 2-3 hours. Staple foods do not provide optimal calories per unit weight and these should be enriched with fat and oil or sugar. Some examples are rice dal gruel (*khichri*) with oil, rice with milk or curd and sugar, mashed banana with milk or curd, egg white, mashed potatoes with oil and lentil. Foods with high fiber content e.g. coarse fruits and vegetables should be avoided. *Cola drinks and fruit juices should not be given.* In non breast fed infants, undiluted cow or buffalo milk should be offered after correction of dehydration together with semisolid foods. Milk should not be diluted with water during any phase of acute diarrhea. In some cases with high purging diarrhea milk cereal mixtures e.g. porridge (*dalia*), sago, milk-rice-sugar mixtures (*kheer*), can be used. *Routine lactose free feeding is not required during acute diarrhea even when reducing substances are detected in the stools.* Lactose malabsorption or clinical lactose intolerance requiring dietary modification is rare in acute diarrhea. Such cases usually respond to milk cereal mixtures. During recovery, an intake of at least 25% more than basal calories should be attempted with nutrient-dense foods; it should continue until the child reaches pre-illness weight and ideally until the child achieves normal nutritional status, as measured by expected weight-for-height or weight-for-age. This might take several weeks or months, depending on the degree of deficit. Feeding in severely malnourished children needs special attention (Box).

PREVENTION

Acute diarrheal disease is preventable by ensuring adequate nutrition and health education. Exclusive breast feeding (not even water should be given in hot summer months) should be encouraged for initial six months till weaning foods are introduced. Breast feeding should be continued as long as possible. Adequate nutrition should be maintained by ensuring satisfactory intake of home-made weaning foods, intake of zinc and other micronutrients. In formula-fed babies, the bottle and nipple should be properly sterilized by boiling for at least 15 minutes. Top-fed babies should preferably be fed with the help of cup and spoon or *paladey* because they can be readily cleaned. Pacifiers or dummy nipples are potential sources of infection and should be avoided. Environmental sanitation,

---

Feeding of severely malnourished children with diarrhea

Feeding should be initiated as early as possible if there is no vomiting and if the child is alert and drinking, the diet should be started immediately even before the rehydration is complete.

Feeding during the initial phase when the child is sick and dehydrated

- The initial feeds should have at least 75 calories/100 g and should be offered at 80-100 kcal/kg/day, 130 ml/kg/day (100 ml/kg/d if the child has severe edema) and 1.0-1.5 g protein/kg/day
- Small feeds of low lactose and low osmolarity should be given to avoid overloading the intestine, liver and kidney.
- Feeding should be frequent (every 2 hours) and continued throughout day and night for at least 3-hourly feeds.
- The feed volume should be gradually increased.
- Feeds should be given orally with cup and spoon and the amount left may be fed using NG tube (NG feeding may be given till 3/4th of all feeds are accepted orally or two consecutive feeds are accepted orally)
- *Ad-libitum* breast feeding should be encouraged

Feeding during the rehabilitation (catch-up) phase

- Higher intakes should be encouraged. The frequency of feeds should be gradually decreased (6 feeds /day) and the volume offered at each feed increased.
- The energy density and proteins should be increased to 100 kcal/100 g and 2.5-3.0 g/100 g respectively.
- The calories offered should be increased to 150-220 kcal/kg/d and proteins to 4 g/kg/d over the next few days.
- Breast feeding should be continued *ad-libitum*.

---

personal hygiene, clean potable water supply, and proper drainage facilities are essential. The foods should be kept covered and adequately protected against dust and flies. Infants are known to put their hands and toys frequently into their mouth especially during teething. Their hands and toys should be kept free from contamination by frequent cleaning.

Health education regarding personal hygiene and avoidance of fecal contamination must be imparted and popularized through available mass media. The health workers should teach, encourage and set a good example to influence community members to adopt these preventive practices.

The multiplicity of enteropathogens has discouraged attempts to produce effective vaccines for acute diarrheal disorders. There is a need for oral vaccines to provide protection against rotaviruses, *Escherichia coli* and *Shigella*. Currently, two vaccines against rotavirus have been approved, a live oral vaccine (RotaTeq™) made by Merck, and GSK's Rotarix™ for use in children. Field trials for rotavirus vaccine using Indian strains are currently under way in India[66, 67]. In vaccine development novel delivery systems are being studied including oral[68] and transcutaneous administration of antigens. While vaccines will help reduce pathogen specific diarrhea, improvements in personal hygiene and environmental sanitation are more crucial before overall rates of diarrhea can be reduced in the vulnerable populations.

CONCLUSIONS

In conclusion, ORS remains the mainstay of therapy during acute diarrhea and zinc given as an adjunct to ORS has an additional benefit to reduce the stool volume and diarrheal duration. Probiotics and antisecretory drugs are not recommended. Antimicrobials should be restricted to bloody diarrhea, culture positive Shigella, cholera with severe dehydration, associated non-gastrointestinal infections, severely malnourished and immune compromised children.

However, despite the well known benefits of WHO ORS, the National Health Family Survey-3 suggests that only 33% mothers administer ORS as a part of treatment of diarrhea to their children. Also the WHO-UNICEF Joint Statement, Clinical Management of Acute Diarrhea suggests prescriptions of zinc for treatment of acute diarrhea are currently restricted to only 1% children globally. To improve case management of acute diarrhea, it is necessary to continue professional development programs targeting the practitioners of all systems of medicine. Additionally, we must reinstate the commitment to rational management of diarrhea, a disease that continues to affect millions of children in the developing world.

REFERENCES

1. Black RE, Cousens S, Johnson HL, *et al.* Child Health Epidemiology Reference Group of WHO and UNICEF: Global, regional, and national causes of child mortality in 2008: a systematic analysis. *Lancet* 2010, June 5, 375 (9730):1969-87 Epub 2010 May 11.

2. Kosek M., Bern C., Guerrant R. The Global Burden of Diarrheal Disease, As Estimated from Studies Published Between 1992 and 2000. *Bull World Hlth Organ* 2003; 81:197–204.

3. National Family Health Survey (NFHS-3) India, 2006-2007.

4. Quigley MA, Kelly YJ, Sacker A. Breastfeeding and hospitalization for diarrheal and respiratory infections in the United Kingdom Millennium Cohort Study. *Pediatrics* 2007 Apr;119(4):e837-42.

5. Castillo-Duran C, Vial P, Uauy R. Trace mineral balance during acute diarrhea in infants. *J Pediatr* 1988; 113(3):452-7.

6. Stephensen CB, Alvarez JO, Kohatsu J, Hardmeier R, Kennedy JI Jr, Gammon RB Jr. Vitamin A is excreted in the urine during acute infection. *Am J Clin Nutr* 1994; 60(3):388.

7. Caulfield LE, de Onis M, Blossner M, Black RE. Undernutrition as an underlying cause of child deaths associated with diarrhea, pneumonia, malaria, and measles. *Am J Clin Nutr* 2004; 80(1):193-8.

8. World Gastroenterology Organisation practice Guidelines: Acute diarrhea March 2008.

9. S. K. Mittal, Vyom Aggarwal and KK Kalra. Chronic diarrhea in children of tropics *Indian J Pediatr*, Volume 61, Number 6, 635-642, DOI: 10.1007/BF02751970.

10. Guidelines for the control of shigellosis, including epidemics due to *Shigella dysenteriae type 1*. WHO 2005.

11. Bhan MK, Arora NK, Ghai OP, Ramachandran K, Khoshoo V, Bhandari N. Major factors in diarrhea related mortality among rural children. *Indian J Med Res* 1986; 83:9-12.

12. Firdausi Qadri, Ann-Mari Svennerholm, A.S.G. Faruque, R. Bradley Sack.Enterotoxigenic *Escherichia coli* in developing countries: Epidemiology, microbiology, clinical features, treatment, and prevention; *Clin Microbiol Rev* 2005 July; 18(3): 465–483.

13. Bahl R, Ray P, Subodh S, Shambharkar P, Saxena M, Parashar U, Gentsch J, Glass R, Bhan MK. Incidence of severe rotavirus diarrhea in New Delhi, India, and G and P types of the infecting rotavirus strains. Delhi Rotavirus Study Group *J Infect Dis* 2005 Sep 1;192 Suppl 1:S114-S119.

14. WHO. Cholera 2006. *Weekly Epidemiological Record* 2007; 82:273–84.

15. Jacqueline L. Deen, Lorenz von Seidlein, Dipika Sur, MagdarinaAgtini, Marcelino E. S. Lucas, Anna Lena Lopez, Deok Ryun Kim, Mohammad Ali, John D. Clemens. The high burden of cholera in children: Comparison of incidence from endemic areas in Asia

and Africa *PLoS Negl Trop Dis* 2008 February; 2(2): e173 doi: 10.1371/journal. pntd. 0000173.

16. Molla AM, Rahman M, Sarkar SA, *et al.* Stool electrolyte content and purging rates in diarrhea caused by rotavirus, enterotoxigentic*E.coli*and *V. Cholerae* in children. *Trop Pediatr* 1981; 98:835.

17. World Health Organization, Division of Child Health and Development. Integrated Management of Childhood Illness. Geneva: *World Health Organization;* 2009.

18. Walker SH, Gahol VP, Quintero BA. Sodium and water content of feedings for use in infants with diarrhea. *Clin Pediatr* 1989; 20:199.

19. Hamdi IA, Dodge JA. Toddler diarrhea: Observations on the effects of aspirin and loperamide. *J Pediatr Gastroenter Nutr* 1985; 4:362.

20. Bhan MK, Mahalanabis D, Fontaine O, Pierce NF. Clinical trials of improved oral rehydration salt formulations: a review. *Bull World Health Organ* 1994; 72(6):945-55.

21. Farthing MJ. Studies of oral rehydration solutions in animal models. *Clin Ther* 1990; 12 Suppl A:51-62.

22. Hahn SK, Kim YJ, Garner P. Reduced osmolarity oral rehydration solution for treating dehydration due to diarrhea in children: systematic review. *BMJ* 2001; 323:81-5.

23. Reduced osmolarity oral rehydration salts (ORS) formulation. A report from a meeting of experts jointly organized by UNICEF and WHO. UNICEF House, New York, USA, 18 July, 2001. WHO/FCH/CAH/ 0.1.22.

24. Alam NH, Yunus M, Faruque ASG, Gyr N, Sattar S, Parvin S, *et al.* Symptomatic hyponatremia during treatment of dehydrating diarrheal disease with reduced osmolarity oral rehydration solution. *JAMA* 2006; 296: 567-573.

25. Bhatnagar S, Lodha R, Choudhury P, *et al.* IAP Guidelines 2006 on Management of Acute Diarrhea. *Indian Pediatrics* Vol 44-May 17, 2007.

26. Bhutta ZA, Bird SM, Black RE, Brown KH, Gardner JM, Hidayat A, *et al.* Therapeutic effects of oral zinc in acute and persistent diarrhea in children in developing countries: pooled analysis of randomized controlled trials. *Am J Clin Nutr* 2000; 72: 1516-1522.

27. Bhatnagar S, Bahl R, Sharma PK, Kumar GT, Saxena SK, Bhan MK. Zinc with oral rehydration therapy reduces stool output and duration of diarrhea in hospitalized children: a randomized controlled trial. *J Pediatr Gastroenterol Nutr* 2004; 38: 34-40.

28. Lazzerini M, Ronfani. Oral zinc for treating diarrhea in children. Cochrane Database of systematic Reviews 2008, Issue 3. DOI: 10.1002/14651858.

29. Lukacik M, Ronald L. A meta-analysis of the effects of oral zinc in treatment of acute and persistent diarrhea. *Pediatrics* 2008;121;326.

30. Walsh CT, Sandstead HH, Prasad AS, Newberne PM, Fraker PJ. Zinc: health effects and research priorities for the 1990s. *Environ Health Perspect* 1994; 102 Suppl 2: 5-46.

31. Fontaine O. Effect of zinc supplementation on clinical course of acute diarrhea. *J Health Popul Nutr* 2001; 19: 339-346.

32. Bhandari N, Mazumder S, Taneja S, Dube B, Agarwal RC, Mahalanabis D, *et al.* Effectiveness of zinc supplementation plus oral rehydration salts compared with oral rehydration salts alone as a treatment for acute diarrhea in a primary care setting: a cluster randomized trial. *Pediatrics* 2008; 121: e1279-1285.

33. Awasthi S. Zinc supplementation in acute diarrhea is acceptable, does not interfere with oral rehydration, and reduces the use of other medications: a randomized trial in five countries. *J Pediatr Gastroenterol Nutr* 2006; 42: 300-305.

34. Wadhwa N, Natchu M, et al. ORS containing Zinc does not reduce diarrhea or stool volume of acute diarrhea in Hospitalized children. *J Pediatr Gastroenterol Nut* August 2011; vol 53; Issue 2:161-167.

35. Bettger WJ, O'Dell BL. A critical physiological role of zinc in the structure and function of biomembranes. *Life Sci* 1981; 28:1425-38.

36. Shankar AH, Prasad AS. Zinc and immune function: the biological basis of altered resistance to infection. *Am J Clin Nutr* 1998; 68 (suppl.2): 447S-463S.

37. Wapnir R. Zinc deficiency, malnutrition and the gastrointestinal tract. *J Nutr* 2000; 130 (5S Suppl): 1388-92.

38. World Health Organization. Complementary feeding of young children in developing countries: a review of current scientific knowledge. *Document WHO/NUT/ 98.1. Geneva: World Health Organization;* 1998.

39. Ruz M, Solomons NW. Fecal zinc of endogenous zinc during oral rehydration therapy for acute diarrhea. *J Trace Elem Exp Med* 1995; 7:89-100.

40. WHO Global Taskforce on Cholera Control 2010.WHO CDS CSR NCS 2003. 7.

41. Facility based Integrated Management of Neonatal and Childhood Illness, WHO/UNICEF, Ministry of Health and Family Welfare, Govt. of India, 2009.

42. Khan WA, Bennish ML, Seas C, Khan EH, Ronan A, Dhar U, Busch W, Salam MA. Randomised controlled comparison of single-dose ciprofloxacin and doxycycline for cholera caused by *Vibrio cholerae* 01 or 0139. *Lancet* 1996; 348(9023):296-300.

43. Dutta D, Bhattacharya SK, Bhattacharya MK, Deb A, Deb M, Manna B, Moitra A, Mukhopadhyay AK, Nair GB. Efficacy of norfloxacin and doxycycline for treatment of *vibrio cholerae* 0139 infection. *J Antimicrob Chemother* 1996; 37(3):575-81.

Section 4

44. Moolasart P, Eampokalap B, Supaswadikul S. Comparison of the efficacy of tetracycline and norfloxacin in the treatment of acute severe diarrhea. *Southeast Asian J Trop Med Public Health* 1998; 29(1):108-11.

45. Schaad UB, abdus Salam M, Aujard Y, Dagan R, Green SD, Peltola H, *et al*. Use of fluoroquinolones in pediatrics: consensus report of an International Society of Chemotherapy Commission. *Pediatr Infect Dis J* 1995; 14(1):1-9.

46. Pradhan KM, Arora NK, Jena A, Susheela AK, Bhan MK. Safety of ciprofloxacin therapy in children: magnetic resonance images, body fluid levels of fluoride and linear growth. *Acta Paediatr* 1995; 84(5):555-60.

47. Bethell DB, Hien TT, Phi LT, Day NP, Vinh H, Duong NM, *et al*. Effects on growth of single short courses of fluoroquinolones. *Arch Dis Child* 1996; 74(1):44-46.

48. Doherty CP, Saha SK, Cutting WA. Typhoid fever, ciprofloxacin and growth in young children. *Ann Trop Paediatr* 2000; 20(4): 297-303.

49. Dutta S, Rajendran K, Roy S, Chatterjee A, Dutta P, Nair GB, Bhattacharya SK, Yoshida SI. Shifting serotypes, plasmid profile analysis and antimicrobial resistance pattern of shigella strains isolated from Kolkata, India during 1995-2000. *Epidemiol Infect* 2002; 129(2):235-43.

50. Anh NT, Cam PD, Dalsgaard A. Antimicrobial resistance of Shigella species isolated from diarrheal patients between 1989 and 1998 in Vietnam. *Southeast Asian J Trop Med Public Health* 2001; 32(4):856-62.

51. Iwalokun BA, Gbenle GO, Smith SI, Ogunledun A, Akinsinde KA, Omonigbehin EA. Epidemiology of shigellosis in Lagos, Nigeria: trends in antimicrobial resistance. *J Health Popul Nutr* 2001; 19(3):183-90.

52. Ashkenazi S, May-Zahav M, Sulkes J, Zilberberg R, Samra Z. Increasing antimicrobial resistance of Shigella isolates in Israel during the period 1984 to 1992. *Antimicrob Agents Chemother* 1995; 39(4):819-23.

53. Vinh H, Wain J, Chinh MT, Tam CT, Trang PT, Nga D, Echeverria P, Diep TS, White NJ, Parry CM. Treatment of bacillary dysentery in Vietnamese children: two doses of ofloxacin versus 5-days nalidixic acid. *Trans R Soc Trop Med Hyg* 2000; 94(3):323-326.

54. Salam MA, Dhar U, Khan WA, Bennish ML. Randomised comparison of ciprofloxacin suspension and pivmecillinam for childhood shigellosis. *Lancet* 1998; 352(9127):522-527.

55. Leibovitz E, Janco J, Piglansky L, Press J, Yagupsky P, Reinhart H, Yaniv I, Dagan R. Oral ciprofloxacin vs. intramuscular ceftriaxone as empiric treatment of acute invasive diarrhea in children. *Pediatr Infect Dis J* 2000; 19(11):1060-1067.

56. Misra PK, Kumar A, Agarwal V, Jagota SC. A comparative clinical trial of albendazole versus metronidazole in children with giardiasis. *Indian Pediatr* 1995; 32(7):779-782.

57. Rossignol JF, Ayoub A, Ayers MS. Treatment of diarrhea caused by *Giardia intestinalis* and *Entamoeba histolytica* or *E. dispar*: a randomized, double-blind, placebo-controlled study of nitazoxanide. *J Infect Dis* 2001; 184(3):381-384.

58. Ortiz JJ, Ayoub A, Gargala G, Chegne NL, Favennec L. Randomized clinical study of nitazoxanide compared to metronidazole in the treatment of symptomatic giardiasis in children from Northern Peru. *Aliment Pharmacol Ther* 2001; 15(9):1409-1415.

59. Rossignol JF, Ayoub A, Ayers MS. Treatment of diarrhea caused by *Cryptosporidium parvum*: a prospective randomized, double-blind, placebo-controlled study of nitazoxanide. *J Infect Dis* 2001; 184:103-106.

60. Rossignol JF, Hidalgo H, Feregrino M, Higuera F, Gomez WH, Romero JL, Padierna J, Geyne A, Ayers MS. A double-blind placebo-controlled study of nitazoxanide in the treatment of cryptosporidial diarrhea in AIDS patients in Mexico. *Trans R Soc Trop Med Hyg* 1998; 92(6):663-666.

61. Jean-François A. Rossignol, Ayman Ayoub and Marc S. Ayers. Treatment of diarrhea caused by *Cryptosporidium parvum:* A prospective randomized, double-blind, placebo-controlled study of nitazoxanide. *Infect Dis* Vol. 184, No. 1 (Jul. 1, 2001), 103-106.

62. Primi MP, Bueno L, Baumer P, *et al*. Racecodatril demonstrates intestinal anitsecretary activity *in vivo*. *Aliment Pharmacol Ther* 1999; 13-Suppl 6:3-7.

63. Salazar-Lindo E, Santisteban-Ponce J, Chea-woo E, Gutierrez M. Racecodatril in the treatment of acute watery diarrhea in children. *N Engl J Med* 2000; 343: 463-467.

64. Bhan MK, Bhatnagar S. Racecadotril- Is there enough evidence to recommend it for treatment of acute diarrhea? *Indian Pediatr* 2004; 41(12):1203-1204.

65. Allen SJ, Martinez EG, Gregorio GV, Dans LF. Probiotics for treating acute infectious diarrhea. Cochrane Database of Systematic Reviews 2010, Issue 11. Art. No.: CD003048. DOI: 10.1002/14651858. CD003048.pub3

66. A Phase III Clinical Trial to Evaluate the Protective Efficacy of Three Doses of Oral Rotavirus Vaccine (ORV) 116E (ROTAVAC) *clinicaltrials.gov/ct2/show/ NCT01305109*.

67. Glass RI, Bhan MK, Ray P, Bahl R, Parashar UD, Greenberg H, Rao CD, Bhandari N, Maldonado Yvonne, Ward RL, Bernstein DI, Gentsch JR (2005) Development of candidate rotavirus vaccines derived from neonatal strains in India. *J Infect Dis* 192 (S1): S30-S35. ISSN 0022-18.

68. Sack D. Shimko J. Randomized double blind, safety and efficacy of a killed oral vaccine for enterotoxigenic E. coli diarrhea of travelers to Guatemala and Mexico. *Vaccine* 2007; 25 (22): 4392-4400.

Section 4

27

Serious Bacterial Infections

Gouri Rao Passi

When the harmony between man and the complex microenvironment of millions of microorganisms is broken, infection results. Serious bacterial infections like septicemia and meningitis occur when there is a major disruption of this environment (such as in an ICU setting where broad spectrum antibiotics and invasive venous catheters are used); or the organism is particularly aggressive (such as meningococcus); or the host immune response is seriously impaired (children on chemotherapy, children with burns, preterm neonates or children with HIV or sickle cell anemia). In the last decade, we have learnt many new things about how bacteria initiate damage and how the human body responds to this attack. This has helped us improve the way we manage patients with severe bacterial infections and improve survival.

SEPTICEMIA

Definitions and Terminology

Sepsis has a wide spectrum of manifestations. When there is mere bacterial invasion it is called bacteremia and when the body recognizes the invasion and mounts an inflammatory response it is called SIRS (systemic inflammatory response syndrome). When the inflammatory response is excessive or the body is overwhelmed by the

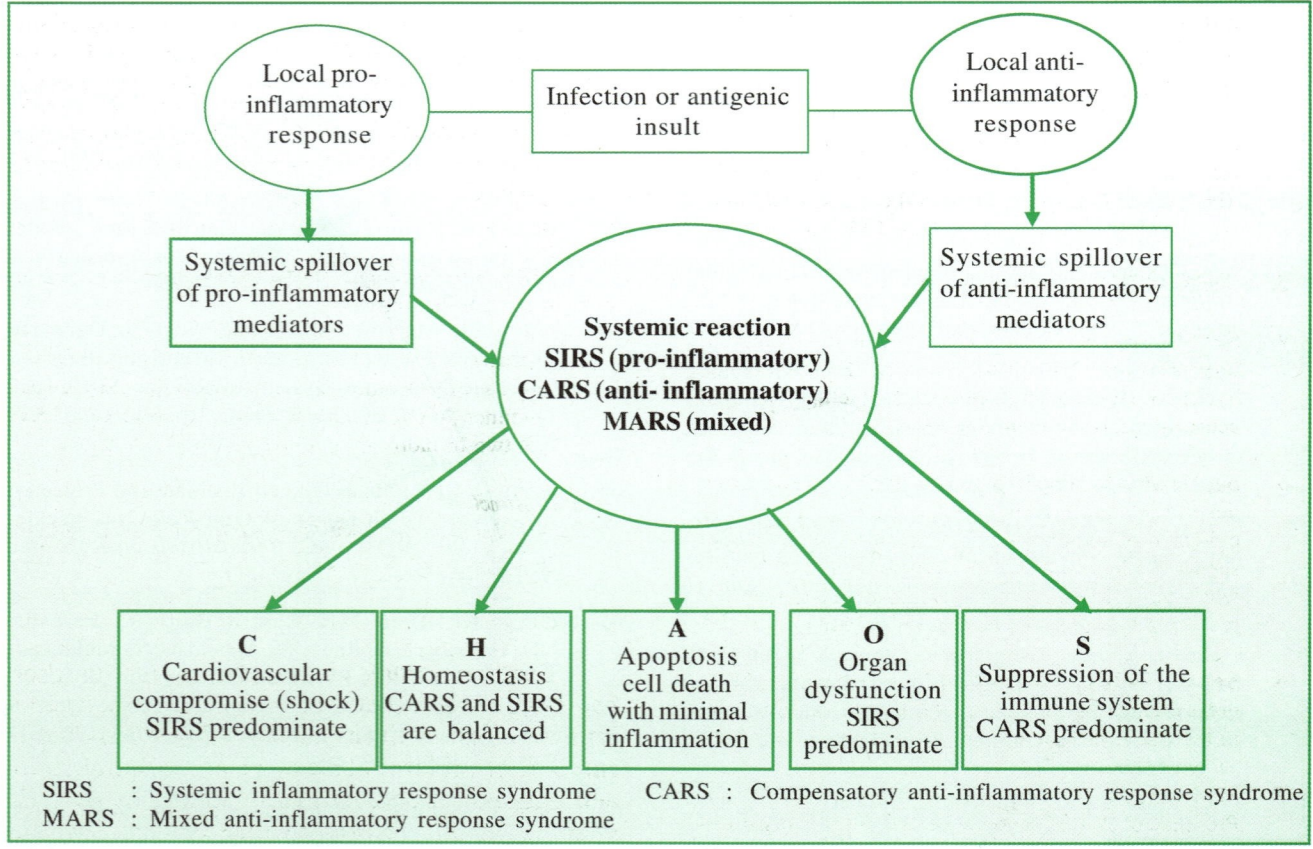

Figure 27.1 Interaction between systemic pro-inflammatory and anti-inflammatory responses following serious bacterial infection leading to life-threatening consequences and "CHAOS". Adapted from Bone RC *et al. Chest* 1997; 112:235-43.

bacterial invasion, initially there is organ hypoperfusion followed by organ dysfunction. As the clinical status worsens, refractory hypotension sets in, followed by multi-organ failure (Figure 27.1).

The American College of Chest Physicians/ Society of Critical Care Medicine (ACCP/SCCM) has put forth a consensus definition that differentiates the various stages of sepsis[1-2] (Tables 27.1 to 27.4). The definitions for sepsis and organ dysfunction have recently been modified for pediatric age group. The key differences are that temperature and leukocyte abnormalities have been given more weightage than tachycardia and tachypnea. Bradycardia may be a sign of SIRS in the newborn age group but not in older children. If overwrapping is suspected, baby should be unbundled and temperature recorded after 15-30 minutes.

Table 27.1 Terminology of sepsis and its sequelae

1. **Bacteremia.** Positive blood culture with viable bacteria in the blood.

2. **Systemic inflammatory response syndrome (SIRS).** Severe clinical insult leading to a systemic inflammatory response manifested by two or more of the following features:

    (i) Temperature >100.5°F (>38°C) or < 96.0°F (<36°C)

    (ii) Heart rate >2 SD above normal for age

    (iii) Respiratory rate >2SD above normal for age

    (iv) Peripheral white blood cell count < 4000/mm³, $\geq$12000/mm³, or more than 10% band cells

3. **Sepsis.** SIRS due to an infection

4. **Severe sepsis.** Sepsis plus organ dysfunction, hypoperfusion or hypotension. Evidences of hypoperfusion may include oliguria, lactic acidosis or acute alteration in mental state.

5. **Septic shock.** Sepsis associated with hypotension despite adequate fluid resuscitation in addition to evidence of hypoperfusion as defined under severe sepsis. Patient may not be hypotensive at the time when perfusion abnormalities are noted if they are receiving vasopressors or inotropic agents.

6. **Sepsis induced hypotension.** Systolic blood pressure measurement >2 SD below the mean for age in the absence of other causes of hypotension.

7. **Multiorgan dysfunction syndrome (MODS).** Presence of altered function of two or more organs in an acutely ill patient so that homeostasis cannot be maintained without intervention.

Table 27.2 Definitions for sepsis based on international pediatric sepsis consensus conference

SIRS

Presence of atleast 2 of the 4 criteria of which one must be either (1) or (2).

1. Core temperature of more than 101°F (38.5°C) or less than 96°F (< 36°C)

2. Leukocyte count elevated or depressed for age (not secondary to chemotherapy), or > 10% immature neutrophils.

3. Tachycardia >2 SD above normal for age (Refer to Table 27.3) in the absence of medications, painful stimulus or otherwise persistent unexplained elevation for 0.5 to 4 hours OR for children <1 year; bradycardia <10th percentile for age in the absence of external vagal stimulus, ß blockers, congenital heart disease or otherwise unexplained for 0.5 hour period.

4. Mean respiratory rate >2 SD above normal for age or mechanical ventilation for acute process not related to underlying neuromuscular disease or general anesthesia (Refer to Table 27.3).

Infection

A suspected or proven infection (by positive culture, tissue stain, or polymerase chain reaction test) caused by any pathogen.
OR
A clinical syndrome associated with a high probability of infection as evidenced by positive findings on clinical examamination, imaging, laboratory tests i.e. white blood cells in a normally sterile body fluid, perforated viscus, chest radiograph suggestive of pneumonia, petechial or purpuric rash or purpura fulminans.

Sepsis

SIRS in the presence of or as a result of suspected or proven infection.

Severe sepsis

Sepsis plus evidences of cardiovascular organ dysfunction OR acute respiratory distress syndrome OR two or more organ dysfunction (Table 27.4).

Septic shock

Sepsis and cardiovascular organ dysfunction as defined in Table 27.4.

Epidemiology

Septicemia most commonly occurs in newborn babies especially preterms, hospital settings and in immunocompromised patients. Due to increased survival of preterm babies, greater hospitalization and aggressive chemotherapy strategies over the years, it is not surprising that the incidence of septicemia is increasing. There is limited information regarding the demography of sepsis from India.

Age group	Heart rate (beats/min) Tachycardia	Heart rate (beats/min) Bradycardia	Respiratory rate (breaths /min)	Leukocyte count /mm³	Systolic BP (mm Hg)
0 –7 d	>180	<100	>50	>34,000	<65
7d – 1 mo	>180	<100	>40	>19,500 or <5000	<75
1 mo – 1 yr	>180	<90	>34	>17,500 or <5000	<100
2 – 5 yr	>140	NA	>22	>15,500 or <6000	<94
6 – 12 yr	>130	NA	>18	>13,500 or <4500	<105
13 – 18 yr	>110	NA	>14	>11,000 or <4500	<117

Table 27.3 Age specific vital signs and laboratory variables (5th – 95th centile)

NA: Not applicable

Table 27.4 Criteria for organ dysfunction

Cardiovascular

Despite administration of isotonic intravenous fluid bolus of ≥ 40 ml/kg in one hour

1. BP <5th centile for age
   OR
2. Need for vasoactive drugs to maintain BP in normal range (dopamine >5 ug/kg/min or dobutamine, epinephrine or norepinephrine at any dose)
   OR
3. Two of the following criteria:
   (a) Unexplained metabolic acidosis; base deficit >-5 mEq/L
   (b) Increased arterial lactate of >twice upper limit
   (c) Oliguria <0.5 ml/kg/hour
   (d) Prolonged capillary refill >3 sec
   (e) Core to periphery temperature gap of >3°C

Respiratory

1. PaO_2/FiO_2 <300 in the absence of cyanotic heart disease or preexisting lung disease
   OR
2. $PaCO_2$ >65 mmHg or >20 mmHg above base line
   OR
3. Proven need for >50% FiO_2 to maintain arterial oxygen saturation of >92%
   OR
4. Need for non-elective invasive or non-invasive ventilation

Neurologic

1. Glasgow coma score <11
2. Acute decrease in Glasgow coma score by >3 points from abnormal baseline.

Hematologic

1. Platelet count <80,000 per mm³ or decrease by >50% in last 3 days
2. International normalized prothrombin ratio >2

Renal

1. Serum creatinine >2 SD for age or 2 fold increase in baseline creatinine

Hepatic

1. Total bilirubin >4 mg/dl (not applicable for newborns)
2. ALT 2 times upper limit of normal

American data is based on a very comprehensive study of the epidemiology of sepsis in the USA from 1979 to 2000. In this period there was an increase in the incidence of sepsis from 82.7/ 100, 000 population to 240.4/ 100,000 population. However, the mortality in hospitalized children has fallen from 27.8% to 17.9% during this period. Another key finding of this study has been an increase in Gram-positive organisms and fungal sepsis over the last two decades[3, 4].

According to PICU data, nosocomial infections are twice as common as community-acquired septicemias. Central lines, invasive procedures, endotracheal intubation and catheterization have all predisposed the PICU patients to develop bacteremias and sepsis. Patients with splenic dysfunction such as sickle cell anemia or post splenectomy patients are at increased risk for infection with capsulated organisms. Patients on chemotherapy such as children with leukemia, immunocompromised children e.g. with AIDS or patients in PICU are at an increased risk for development of infection with *Pseudomonas aeruginosa* and *S. aureus*.

Etiological Agents

Blood cultures are positive for bacteria or fungi in 20-40% cases of severe sepsis and 40-70% patients in septic shock. In American data from a PICU setting, 62% of blood cultures grew Gram-positive organisms, 31% Gram-negative organisms and 5.6% fungi[4]. The nature of pathogens varies depending upon the age of the patient and immunological status of the host.

Early-onset neonatal sepsis. *Streptococcus agalactiae (Group B Streptococcus), Escherichia coli, Haemophilus influenzae,* and *Listeria monocytogenes* are the most frequently encountered organisms.

Late-onset neonatal sepsis. *Coagulase-negative Staphylococcus, Staphylococcus aureus, E. coli, Klebsiella species, Pseudomonas aeruginosa, Enterobacter species, Candida species, S. agalactiae, Serratia species, Acinetobacter species,* and various anerobes are the most commonly involved organisms.

Sepsis in infancy. *H. influenzae* type b (*Hib*), *S pneumoniae, N meningitidis,* and *Salmonella* species are the most frequent pathogens causing sepsis among infants worldwide. Even in India, Hib has been shown to be a significant burden[5]. *Streptococcus pneumoniae* and *Neisseria meningitidis* predominate in the United States and the developed world because Hib conjugate vaccination has effectively eliminated the disease caused by that organism.

Sepsis in childhood. The aforementioned pathogens also cause SIRS in childhood, although the presence of encapsulated organisms generally becomes less frequent as the child's immune response to polysaccharide antigens improves with age.

Pathophysiology

The pathophysiology of septicemia is variable depending on the infecting organism, host immune status and other iatrogenic interventions such as endotracheal intubation, long lines, indwelling catheters etc. In sepsis, bacteremia is followed by a complex immune response to bacterial antigens. The inflammatory response includes activation of various immunological markers including the complement, cytokine cascades, arachidonic acid metabolites, cell-mediated immunity, the clotting cascade, and humoral immune mechanisms. This generalized pro-inflammatory state is called SIRS, systemic inflammatory response syndrome. The biological effects of the various cytokines (TNF alpha, IL-1, IL-6, etc.) include fever, shock, myocardial suppression, capillary leak, coagulation and metabolic abnormalities[6]. Depression of myocardial function results in reduced ejection fraction and poor ventricular response to fluid challenge. Activation of the coagulation pathway results in disseminated intravascular coagulation. Almost all patients with septic shock have coagulation abnormalities. Initial activation of the coagulation pathway is followed by dysregulation with suppression of the antifibrinolytic systems.

In severe sepsis there may be excessive neutrophil activation and prolonged survival. These neutrophils induce endothelial dysfunction, release cytotoxic molecules and lead to inflammatory host organ injury. Further there is accelerated apoptosis of lymphocytes resulting in lymphocyte depletion.

Early uncomplicated sepsis is characterized by high circulating catecholamine levels whereas septic shock is associated with depletion of endogenous catecholamine stores and possible catecholamine resistance.

TNF-α, IL-1 and NO are associated with myocyte dysfunction and may explain the early myocardial depression seen in sepsis[7]. Activation of neutrophils, release of free radicals, leukocyte aggregation and endothelial damage of the pulmonary microvasculature result in ARDS (acute respiratory distress syndrome).

Section 4

Glycolysis, gluconeogenesis and a relative insulin resistance are common. There is initial hyperglycemia and later hypoglycemia when glycogen stores are depleted. Lactic acidosis due to cellular hypoxia results as organ hypoperfusion sets in. Transient hypoparathyroidism and increased levels of procalcitonin are associated with hypocalcemia in both adults and children with sepsis.

Identifying febrile children at-risk for a serious illness

NICE (National Institute for Clinical Excellence) of the UK has laid down some guidelines to identify children with fever who may have serious illness[8, 9] (Table 27.5).

History and physical examination will often clarify whether the initial focus of infection is the respiratory tract, skin, gastrointestinal tract, bones and joints, central nervous system or urinary tract. The commonest initial focus of infection is the respiratory tract, followed by the abdominopelvic region and the urinary tract. In more than 15% cases the site of primary infection is unknown[10]. Even when there is no focus, 25% of healthy babies between 3 and 36 months with a fever of more than 105.8°F (41°C) will have bacteremia. An excessively irritable baby who cannot be consoled despite optimal care and comfort is a highly suggestive of serious infection. Chills, nausea and vomiting are also suggestive of bacteremia. Presence of petechiae in a febrile child is an ominous sign. When bacteremia progresses to a generalized pro-inflammatory state of SIRS, tachycardia, and tachypnea become evident. Tachypnea disproportionate to fever or respiratory involvement occurs because of stimulation of the medullary centers for respiration and is an early sign of serious infection.

As sepsis progresses evidences of hypoperfusion and organ dysfunction set in. Alterations in mental status and oliguria are the earliest markers of hypoperfusion of brain and kidneys. When the extremities are cold and clammy and blood pressure has started dropping, septic shock is well established and the prognosis is grim.

It is difficult to make an etiological diagnosis of sepsis on clinical grounds but certain features may provide clues. Preceding history of skin infection, empyema, indwelling vascular catheter, tampon use in adolescent girls are useful clues for the diagnosis of staphylococcal infection. Petechiae are often seen with *N. meningitidis* infections while ecthyma gangrenosum and purpura fulminans are suggestive of pseudomonal infections. Generalized erythroderma in a septic patient suggests *Staphylococcus aureus* or *Streptococcus pyogenes* as possible pathogens. A history of diarrhea is suggestive of Gram-negative infection due to salmonella species.

Differential Diagnosis

A large number of non-bacterial and non-infective conditions should be considered in the differential diagnosis:

Table 27.5 Risk assessment of febrile children			
Parameter	Low risk	Intermediate risk	High risk
Awareness	awake, alert and responsive	Responds to prolonged stimulation	Unable to arouse and if aroused does not stay awake
Cry	Normal	Feeble	Weak or high-pitched or inconsolable crying
Feeding in infants	Satisfactory	Poor	Unable to feed
Evidence of dehydration	Nil	Mild to moderate	Poor tissue perfusion with hypotension
Anterior fontanel	Normal	Normal or depressed	Bulging or non-pulsatile
Vital signs	Normal	some alteration	Severe alterations

Source: Adapted from Feverish Illness in Children: Assessment and initial management in children younger than 5 years. NICE Clinical Guidelines, No. 47. National Collaborating Centre for Women's and Children's Health (UK). London (UK): *RCOG Press;* May 2007.

1. Non bacterial infections
   (a) Viral infection: dengue hemorrhagic fever, enteroviral, adenoviral infections, etc.
   (b) Fungal sepsis: Candida sepsis in preterm or immunocompromised children
   (c) Protozoal infections: malaria

2. Metabolic and endocrine abnormalities
   Inborn errors of metabolism, hypoglycemia, Reye's syndrome, electrolyte disturbances, adrenal insufficiency, diabetic ketoacidosis etc.

3. Surgical catastrophes
   Appendicitis, intussusception, volvulus, perforation, peritonitis etc.

4. Hematological disorders
   (a) Malignancies: leukemia, lymphoma etc.
   (b) Aplastic anemia
   (c) Sickle cell crisis

5. Autoimmune disorders
   Kawasaki disease, juvenile rheumatoid arthritis, systemic lupus erythematosus

6. Miscellaneous conditions
   Hemolytic uremic syndrome, thrombotic thrombocytopenic purpura, erythema multiforme, intoxications, etc.

Complications

Sepsis may be followed by failure of various body organs which often follow a particular pattern of sequence. Lung dysfunction including ARDS often occurs early in the course of sepsis and persists with a mean duration of 9 days. Shock and oliguria may occur early but either resolves rapidly or proves fatal. CNS dysfunction has a delayed onset usually after 24–48 hours but resolves within 4-5 days. Fortunately, majority of organ failures resolve within one month among the survivors of sepsis[10].

1. **Cardiopulmonary complications.** The increased pulmonary capillary permeability leads to exudation of alveolar fluid, decreased pulmonary compliance and reduced arterial oxygen concentration. Diffuse pulmonary infiltrates, reduced pulmonary compliance with refractory hypoxemia signal the development of ARDS. Septic shock is usually due to severe decrease in systemic vascular resistance. Initially cardiac output is normal or increased. Myocardial depression usually sets in later and worsens the hypotension.

2. **Renal complications.** Acute tubular necrosis is often due to hypotension and reduced renal perfusion. Capillary injury and damage by drugs may aggravate renal dysfunction.

3. **Coagulation abnormalities.** Thrombocytopenia occurs in 10-30% cases due to combination of various factors. When DIC sets in due to diffuse endothelial injury and consumption of platelets, there are wide spread bleeding manifestations.

4. **Neurological complications.** Alteration in sensorium may herald hypoperfusion to the brain. A generalized "critical illness" polyneuropathy may delay extubation from the ventilator.

Laboratory Evaluation

A leukocyte count of more than 15,000/mm³ or less than 5000/ mm³ has a high predictive value for bacteremia. Other useful screening tests for serious bacterial infections include an erythrocyte sedimentation rate of >30 mm/hr or an elevated CRP and procalcitonin. A meta-analysis to evaluate the accuracy of procalcitonin found that it has higher sensitivity (88% vs 75%) and specificity (81% vs 67%) than CRP in differentiating bacterial from non-infective causes of inflammation[11]. A careful examination of the peripheral blood smear may show an elevation of band cells, toxic granules, thrombocytopenia and fragmented RBC's. Howell-Jolly bodies on the smear would indicate splenic dysfunction, which predisposes the child to severe sepsis.

An elevated serum lactate level indicates tissue hypoperfusion and serial reduction of lactate levels with therapy has been associated with good outcome in serious bacterial infections. Metabolic parameters, which need monitoring and correction, include blood sugar, serum sodium, potassium and calcium levels and arterial blood gases. Disseminated intravascular coagulation (DIC) is suspected when there is thrombocytopenia, prolonged prothrombin and partial thromboplastin times, reduced serum fibrinogen levels and elevated fibrin split products and D-dimers.

Isolating the causative organisms from blood and when appropriate the CSF, urine, and other body fluids is crucial to fine tune the choice of antibiotics. To evaluate organ dysfunction serum creatinine, transaminases, and skiagram of chest should be taken. The presence of bilateral fluffy shadows in the chest are suggestive of ARDS. A urine to serum osmolality ratio of more than 1.5, and urine osmolality of more than 400 mOsm/kg rule out the presence of serious renal dysfunction.

Management

The appropriate management of severe bacterial infections is based on following principles:

1. Rapid cardiopulmonary assessment and clinical evaluation
2. Choice of appropriate antibiotics
3. Optimal supportive therapy
4. Surgical drainage of pus collection or septic focus

Rapid cardiopulmonary assessment and clinical evaluation

1. Mental status: Restlessness, agitation, lethargy, and decreased responsiveness are red flags for severe infection
2. Check airway patency and stability
3. Breathing: Check for respiratory distress, air entry, crepitations and rales (early ARDS).
4. Circulation: Assess heart rate (tachycardia is an early sign), blood pressure (diastolic pressure falls early with wide pulse pressure and systolic pressure falls later causing narrow pulse pressure), CRT > 3 sec is abnormal, hepatomegaly and raised JVP signal myocardial dysfunction.
5. Urine output in the last 6 hours must be assessed.

Antibiotic therapy

The principles of antibiotic therapy in severe sepsis are listed below:

1. Empiric antibiotic regimens should provide 100% coverage of the likely pathogens for the suspected source of infection

2. Intravenous broad spectrum antibiotics should be administered immediately (preferably <30 min) following the clinical diagnosis of septic shock.
3. The doses of antibiotics should be at the higher end of the range in all patients with life-threatening illness.
4. Multidrug antimicrobial therapy is preferred for initial empiric therapy of septic shock
5. Empiric therapy should be adjusted to a narrower regimen if plausible pathogen is identified or when patient stabilizes (ie shock resolves)
6. Wherever possible early source control should be implemented i.e. drainage of abscess, empyema and removal of implanted devices.

In a stable child when bacteremia is suspected (a febrile child 3 –36 months old with a fever > 39°C and leukocyte count of >15,000/mm^3), a blood culture should be taken and child started on oral amoxicillin or amoxycilin-clavulanic acid combination or parenternal ceftriaxone. A close watch should be kept on the vital signs and feeding behaviour.

In a toxic, sick looking child with or without impending shock, the child must be admitted to the hospital and started on parenteral antibiotics (Table 27.6). When there is no focus of infection or specific features, in a young child we need to cover *S. pneumoniae, S. aureus, S. pyogenes, N.meningitidis* and *H.influenzae type b*. A combination of ceftriaxone or cefotaxime with cloxacillin or vancomycin will provide an adequate coverage.

When staphylococcus is strongly suspected on the basis of bilateral fluffy pulmonary lesions or pneumatoceles, empyema, arthritis or presence of long lines, cloxacillin or vancomycin with an aminoglycoside is recommended. Because cloxacillin may be more effective than vancomycin

Table 27.6 Empirical antibiotic regimens for septic shock in infants and children	
Clinical background	**Antibiotics**
❑ Normal child or skin findings suggestive of meningococcemia or preceding skin trauma or varicella	Cefot/Ceftr + Vanco
❑ Urinary tract infection	Cefot/ Ceftr + AG
❑ Intra-abdominal or pelvic site	Clinda + AG + Amp/Pip or Pip-tazo
❑ Immunocompromised child i.e. malignancy, immunodeficiency state, neutropenia and central line	Vanco+ AG + CTZ/Pip-tazo/Tic-clav
❑ Asplenia and splenic dysfunction	Vanco + Ceftr/ Cefot

(Cefot = cefotaxime, Ceftr = ceftriaxone, Vanco = vancomycin, Clinda = clindamycin, AG = aminoglycoside, Pip = piperacillin, Tazo = tazobactum, CTZ = ceftazidime, Tic-clav = ticarcillin-clavulanic acid)

Section 4

in community acquired MRSA, some authorities recommend using a combination of cloxacillin, vancomycin and aminoglycoside empirically in life-threatening infections.

Infections with a gastrointestinal or genitourinary focus need a cover for Gram-negative infections (ceftriaxone or cefotaxime) and anerobes (metronidazole or clindamycin or ticarcillin-clavulanate or piperacillin-tazobactam) with or without an aminoglycoside.

When organisms producing extended spectrum B lactamases such as Klebsiella or Enterobacter are isolated, treatment failures with 3rd generation cephalosporins such as ceftriaxone are common despite in-vitro sensitivities. Carbapenems (imipenem-cilastin or meropenem) or piperacillin with tazobactum and aminoglycosides are the drugs of choice in this situation. Immunocompromised hosts need an antibiotic cover for *Pseudomonas aeruginosa* and *S. aureus* (ceftazidime, cefepime, cefpirome, aminoglycoside and vancomycin) and candida[13].

Antibiotic resistance has become a major problem in critically sick children. Methicillin resistant *S. aureus* (MRSA) can be treated with vancomycin, while vancomycin-resistant enterococci (VRE) may need newer compounds such as quinpristin-dalfopristin, linezolid and daptomycin. Plasmid mediated beta lactamases which mediate resistance to ampicillin, piperacillin and other cephalosporins can be treated with beta lactams/beta lactamase inhibitor combinations and carbapenems. Metallo-beta-lactamases (eg NMD mutation) that make Gram negatives resistant to even carbapenems are increasingly being reported. Marginal agents like colistin may have to be used for pan resistant organisms[14].

Supportive Therapy

(a) Maintenance of perfusion of vital organs and tissues. The critical factor for the development of SIRS is believed to be hypo-perfusion of tissues. Intravascular volume depletion, peripheral vasodilation, myocardial depression and increased metabolic rate lead to global tissue hypoxia. This initiates the cascade of cytokine release and the generalized pro-inflammatory response which progresses inexorably towards multi-organ dysfunction if management is delayed. *"Early goal directed therapy"* when initiated well in time has shown to improve overall survival of patients with severe sepsis[15]. The sequence of events can be prevented and effectively managed by supporting cardiac preload, afterload and contractility along with effective oxygenation in the lungs. The protocol for aggressive management is outlined below:

1. **Step 1: 0-5 min**
    1. Recognize depressed mental status and decreased perfusion
    2. Begin high flow oxygen (venturi or non rebreathing mask may be used)
    3. Establish intravenous or intraosseous access.
    4. Intubate and ventilate if airway is unstable, if there is inadequate oxygenation or ventilation, hypotension on arrival, convulsive seizures non responsive to 2 doses of benzodiazepines, persistent GCS <8 and signs of raised ICT.

2. **Step II: 5-40 minutes**
    (ii) Bolus of 10 ml/kg crystalloid (Normal saline or Ringer's lactate) q 30 min till CVP reaches 8-12 mmHg or blood pressure and capillary refill are restored. If there is no improvement following administration of 60 ml/kg of crystalloid, myocardial dysfunction should be considered. Rapid infusion of fluid may be given using infusion pumps or the push pull method using a 3-way stop-cock or gravity.

    (iii) Start IV antibiotics.

    (iv) Establish second intravenous access.

    (v) Correct hypocalcemia and hypo- and hyperglycemia. A tight control of blood sugars to maintain them between 80–120 mg/dl with insulin therapy has been shown to reduce the mortality in sepsis irrespective of previous history of diabetes. Hyperglycemia is known to reduce the phagocytic effect of neutrophils and insulin *per se* reduces apoptotic cell death due to several mechanisms[16]. However, the effect of tight control of sugar on survival is still unclear and hence the Critical Care Chapter of the IAP recommends the use of insulin only if there is "significant glucosuria and polyuria leading to difficulty in fluid management".

3. **Step III: 40-60 minutes**
    (i) Recognize fluid refractory shock: Administer vasopressors (dopamine usually at least 10 ug/kg/min with or without dobutamine) to maintain mean arterial pressures within normal range (keep mean BP >40 mmHg between

1- 4 mo, >45 mmHg 5 mo- 4 yr, >50 mmHg 6-7 yr, >55 mmHg >8 yr).

(ii)   Establish central venous line.

(iii)   Reasses need for ventilation. *Elective ventilation* reduces the work of breathing which accounts for 15–30% of oxygen consumption. When used early in children with septic shock, it improves oxygenation by providing PEEP and correcting metabolic acidosis.

4.   Step IV: Beyond 60 minutes

(i)   Recognize dopamine resistant shock

(ii)   Monitor CVP, ECHO, MAP

(iii)   Reverse cold shock resistant to dopamine (low or normal BP) with epinephrine (0.05–0.3 ug/kg/min. maximum 1ug/kg/min) via central line

(iv)   Reverse warm shock resistant to dopamine (wide pulse pressure with low to low normal blood pressure) with norepinephrine (0.05–1 ug/kg/min).

(v)   Intravenous hydrocortisone 50 mg/m^2 every 6 hourly for catecholamine resistant shock or suspected or proven adrenal insufficiency is recommended by the Critical Care Chapter of the IAP. Several studies have failed to document improved outcome with high doses of corticosteroids. They may in fact increase the case fatality rate by increasing the incidence of secondary infection[17]. However, there is some evidence that low or "physiological doses" of steroids, especially if adrenal insufficiency has been documented, improves outcome. A random cortisol level below 20 ug/dl or a failure of cortisol to increase by at least 9 ug/dl after ACTH may indicate relative adrenal insufficiency. These studies have used hydrocortisone in a dose of 25-50 mg followed by an infusion at a rate of 0.18 mg/kg/hr and shown beneficial effects[18].

(vi)   When vasopressors are ineffective, consider phosphodiesterase inhibitors (milrinone 50 – 75 ug/kg loading dose over 15 minutes followed by 0.25-0.75 ug/kg/min) improve myocardial contractility, facilitate diastolic relaxation and decrease systemic venous resistance (SVR).

(vii)   In warm shock resistant to nor epinephrine low-dose vasopressin (0.3-2 milliunits/kg/min or 0.01 -0.12 units/kg/hour) may restore SVR.

(viii)   Continuous monitoring of central venous saturation (ScvO$_2$) with computerized spectrophotometer. If PCV is <30 and ScvO$_2$ <70%, packed cells are transfused and if PCV is >30 and ScvO$_2$ <70%, dobutamine is likely to be more useful.

(b)   *Blood transfusions* are often required to maintain the hemoglobin between 8 –10 g/dl. DIC should be treated by administration of fresh frozen plasma, cryoprecipitate and platelets.

(c)   *Nutrition.* Protein calorie requirements in sepsis are high. Prolonged malnutrition is deleterious because it adversely effects the immunological status. There are many advantages of enteral feeding over parenteral nutrition. However, enteral feeds may be withheld for a day or two till patient is hemodynamically stable.

(d)   *Drotrecogin alfa.* Human recombinant activated Protein C when used within 24 hours of onset of organ dysfunction in sepsis is shown to reduce the relative risk of death by 19.4% in adults[19]. It is given as a continuous infusion at 24 ug/hr. The major limitation is cost and risk of serious bleeding in 3.5% of cases. Its use is contraindicated in patients with platelet counts <30,000/mm^3 or an INR >3. Trials in children are currently underway[20].

(e)   *Double volume exchange* blood transfusion has been used in neonatal sepsis with good outcomes. It is technically more difficult in older children wherein its efficacy has not been studied.

(f)   Deep vein thrombosis prophylaxis is recommended for post pubertal children with severe sepsis.

(g)   Veno-venous hemofiltration may be useful in children with anuria and oliguria with symptomatic volume overload.

(h)   *Veno-arterial ECMO* provides respiratory and cardiac support, while veno-venous ECMO gives respiratory support and a ventricular assist device can be used for cardiac support. It has been shown to improve outcome in children with refractory septic shock with multi-organ dysfunction receiving multiple vasopressors[18].

(i)   *Intravenous immunoglobulins (IVIG).* Though some pediatric studies have supported the use of IVIG, large clinical trials and consensus guidelines do not recommend its widespread use[21]

(j) Numerous other trials of agents that block the inflammatory cascade such as tumour necrosis factor antagonists, monoclonal anti-endotoxin antibodies, interleukin-1 receptor antagonists have failed to reduce mortality in severe sepsis[6].

Surgical drainage of septic focus or pus collection

Any significant pus collection like an empyema or a large abscess must be drained. If the initial focus is an intestinal perforation such as appendicitis, the abdomen must be explored. MRI studies are useful to outline fluid and pus collection in visceral cavities. In patients with disseminated staphylococcal disease, daily thorough clinical examination to look for fresh collection of pus and its drainage is the key to good outcome.

Outcome

It depends on the nature and virulence of infecting organisms, duration of infection, immune status of the patient, adequacy of treatment and the number of the dysfunctional organs. The average risk of death increases by 15–20% with every additional organ involved. When on an average two organs fail in a patient with severe sepsis, the associated mortality is around 30-40% [10].

Prevention

Most episodes of severe sepsis and septic shock are nosocomial. Nosocomial infections should be prevented by strict hand washing, early use of enteral nutrition, reduction of invasive procedures and indwelling catheters. Monitoring antibiotic resistance patterns and rational use of antibiotics will prevent the proliferation of multidrug resistant organisms.

POST NEONATAL MENINGITIS

Definition

Bacterial meningitis is defined as inflammation of the meninges secondary to bacterial infection.

Epidemiology

Bacterial meningitis was uniformly fatal before the discovery and use of antibiotics. The commonest age group for meningitis is between 6 and 12 months. Ninety percent of meningitis occurs below 5 years of age. In the United States the incidence of meningitis in the 1970's was 5.4-7.3 per 100,000 population. Since the introduction of *Haemophilus influenzae type b* (Hib) vaccine, meningitis due to Hib has dramatically reduced in the last decade in the USA. In the last few years incidence of pneumococcal meningitis in children has also gone down because of compulsory pneumococcal vaccination in the USA.

Etiology

In the post neonatal period the commonest organisms causing meningitis include *Hib, S. pnemoniae* and *N. meningitidis*. However, the epidemiology of these infections have been greatly modified in the last decade in the USA because of compulsory vaccination against *Hib* and Pneumococcus. The American Academy of Pediatrics introduced vaccination against *Hib* in 1991 and by 1997 there was a 99% reduction in meningitis due to *Hib* in the USA[16]. Risk factors for pneumococcal meningitis include sickle cell disease, underlying systemic disease and lack of breast feeding. Meningitis due to *Neisseria meningitides* sometimes occur in epidemics and complement deficiencies predispose to development of these infections. *Staphylococcus epidermidis* is often the culprit in CSF shunt infections or after neurosurgical procedures. Other risk factors for bacterial meningitis include immunocompromised state, HIV infection, asplenia, terminal complement deficiencies, immunoglobulin deficiencies, penetrating head injuries and CSF leaks. Patients with cochlear implants have a more than 30 fold increased incidence of pneumococcal meningitis[22]

Pathogenesis

The stages in the pathogenesis of meningitis are characterized by; (i) respiratory tract colonization or infection, (ii) bacteremia, (iii) seeding of the meninges and (iv) inflammation of the meninges and brain. Occasionally the meninges are seeded from contiguous foci such as mastoid, fracture through the paranasal sinus or infected dermal sinus. Head injury disturbs blood brain barrier and may precede development of meningitis. The lack of complement and opsonic proteins results in unimpaired proliferation of bacteria in the CSF. Bacterial products such as Gram-negative lipopolysaccharide or Gram-positive peptidoglycan stimulate production of cytokines such as IL-2 and TNF. The resultant inflammatory cascade causes an increase in intracranial tension, vasculitis and sometimes development of a subdural collection of albumin rich fluid. Thrombosis of the small cortical veins resulting in cerebral necrosis and of the major venous sinuses may occur. Inappropriate secretion

Section 4

of antidiuretic hormone may cause hyponatremia. Hypoglycorrhachia occurs due to abnormal glucose transport across the choroid plexus and increased glucose utilization by host tissues and bacteria.

Clinical Features

A child with pyogenic meningitis classically presents with fever, confusion, headache, vomiting, neck rigidity and photophobia. Kernig's sign is elicited by flexing the thigh on the abdomen to 90°, which is followed by inability to extend the knee beyond 135°. In Brudzunski's sign, when the neck is flexed the thighs and knees flex towards the abdomen. In infancy, classical neck rigidity may not be seen in 30% cases. Neck rigidity is also absent in the comatose and severely malnourished child or a child with diffuse neurological impairment. Irritability, restlessness and poor feeding are non-specific features of meningitis in infants. Raised intracranial tension is invariable and presents with headache in the older child and bulging anterior fontanel and open sutures in infants. Papilledema is uncommon in acute meningitis. Its presence may suggest sub-dural collection, venous thrombosis or brain abscess. The presence of focal neurological deficit implies cortical necrosis, occlusive vasculitis or thrombosis of cortical veins and is a marker of long-term poor prognosis and residual deficits. Focal deficits include III, IV, VI, VII, and VIII cranial nerve deficit, hemiparesis, quadriparesis, ataxia and torticollis. Overall 30% of children with pyogenic meningitis have seizures. Seizures occurring beyond 4 days and those that are focal and persistent are more commonly associated with long-term sequelae while seizures during first 4 days are usually benign.

Subdural collections are seen in 43% of *Hib* meningitis, 30% with pneumococcal meningitis and 22% with meningococcal meningitis. They present as increasing head size, bulging anterior fontanel, persistent vomitings reappearance of fever and abnormal transillumination of the skull.

Shock, petechiae, pupura, arthritis and DIC occur most commonly with meningococcal meningitis but have been recorded with pneumococcal and *Hib* meningitis too.

Differential Diagnosis

1. Non bacterial CNS infections
    (a) Viral meningoencephalitis
    (b) Tubercular meningitis
    (c) Cerebral malaria, toxoplasmosis, cysticercosis
    (d) Fungal meningitis e.g. Cryptococcal

    (e) Focal bacterial CNS infections e.g. brain abscess or subdural empyema
2. Cerebrovascular accidents
    (a) Subarachnoid hemorrhage
    (b) Intracerebral bleed
    (c) Embolus
3. Chemical meningitis due to drugs, radiocontrast material or anesthetic agents.
4. Meningismus due to non-CNS systemic infections.
5. Tetanus, strychnine poisoning, over dose of anti-emetic drugs.

Diagnosis

The diagnosis of meningitis is based on CSF findings. A lumbar puncture must be done as soon as possible. A lumbar puncture may be deferred if there is papilledema, focal neurological deficit, and suggestion of intracranial space occupying lesion, cerebellar herniation, hydrocephalus or trauma.

Beyond 3 months of age a normal CSF has <6 WBC's/HPF and even a single polymorph is considered abnormal. In case of a traumatic CSF the total number of RBCs and WBCs may be counted. The normal ratio is generally considered to be 1 WBC per 1000 RBCs. Deviation from this ratio could suggest meningitis. Generally the WBC count in pyogenic meningitis is in thousands with 80 – 95% being neutrophils. A CSF to serum glucose ratio of <0.4 is said to be 80% sensitive and 98% specific for the diagnosis of pyogenic meningitis in children >2 months of age[24].

A Gram stain of the CSF identifies the organisms in 60-80% cases. The yield is reduced by 20% by prior treatment with antibiotics. Rapid antigen detection methods like latex agglutination; countercurrent immunoelectrophoresis and coagglutination have 70 –100% sensitivity in picking up causative organisms. It may be useful in patients who have received prior antibiotic treatment but its routine use is not recommended by the Practice Guidelines Committeee for bacterial meningitis since it does not seem to affect treatment decisions. The limulus lysate assay picks up endotoxin in CSF and may be useful in Gram-negative meningitis but is not routinely recommended. The broad based PCR, which uses a wide range of primers, has a sensitivity of 100% and specificity of 98.2% and is useful to exclude a diagnosis of meningitis. Further refinements of technique will increase its utility in day-to-day clinical practice.

Differentiating between viral and bacterial meningitis has always been tricky. A CSF glucose less than 34 mg/dl, CSF to blood glucose ratio of <0.23, a CSF protein of >220 mg/dl, a CSF leukocyte count of >2000/mm³, a CSF neutrophil count >1180/mm³ have been shown to predict bacterial meningitis in over 99 percent cases. A CSF lactate of >4.2 mmol/l, an elevated serum CRP, and serum procalcitonin levels have high predictivity for the diagnosis of bacterial meningitis.

Treatment

Treatment of meningitis consists of administration of appropriate antimicrobials and supportive therapy.

1. Antibiotics

Antibiotic therapy should be started as early as possible and preferably through intravenous route. Empirical antibiotics must be started without waiting for confirmation of etiologic organisms (Table 27.7). Use appropriately high doses well above those used in other indications and ensure adequate length of therapy[24] (Table 27.8). While the intravenous route is the best route to use, intraosseous route has occasionally been used with cefotaxime with good results. When patient has been stabilized after initial IV chloramphenicol for several days, oral chloramphenicol can be used subsequently.

The usual organisms that should be covered in post neonatal meningitis include *Hib*, *pneumococcus* and *meningococcus*. Ceftriaxone or cefotaxime provide good cover except when penicillin resistant pneumococcus or staphylococcus is isolated (Table 27.9). Vancomycin is a good choice for resistant pneumococcus but rifampicin should be added if the level of resistance is high. If a patient is allergic to vancomycin, teicoplanin is a useful alternative as it has wide coverage and good CNS penetration. A lumbar puncture is generally not repeated except in neonatal meningitis or if there is lack of clinical improvement in 48 hours.

2. Adjunctive therapy

(a) *Fluids and electrolytes.* As far as possible give full maintenance isotonic fluids to patients with meningitis. Maintaining good cerebral perfusion reduces ischemia and improves long-term outcome. Fluid restriction is indicated if there is syndrome of inappropriate ADH secretion (SIADH).

(b) *Anticonvulsants.* The commonest anticonvulsant used is phenytoin but occasionally phenobarbitone and midazolam infusion is required if seizures are uncontrolled. Anticonvulsants are tapered off within few days or weeks after discharge.

(c) *Antiedema measures* include raising the head end of the patient, IV mannitol, steroids and careful hyperventilation.

Table 27.8 Duration of antimicrobial therapy for bacterial meningitis based on isolated pathogens

Microorganism	Duration of therapy (days)
Neisseria meningitidis	7
Haemophilus influenzae	7
Streptococcus pneumoniae	10-14
Streptococcus agalactiae	14-21
Aerobic Gram-negative bacilli	21
Listeria monocytogenes	>21

Table 27.7 Recommendations for empirical antimicrobial therapy for purulent meningitis based on patient's age and specific predisposing conditions

Predisposing factors	Common bacterial pathogens	Antibiotics
Age		
• 1-23 months	S. Pneumoniae, N. meningitides	Vanco + Cefot/Ceftr
• >2 years	N. meningitidis, S. pneumoniae, Hib	Vanco + Cefot/Ceftr
Head trauma		
• Basilar skull fracture	S. pnemoniae, Hib, Gr A β-hemolytic streptococci	Vanco + Cefot/Ceftr
• Penetrating trauma and post neurosurgery CSF shunt	S. aureus, S. epidermidis P. aeruginosa	Vanco+ Cefepime, Vanco+Ceftaz, Vanco+Mero
Impaired cellular immunity	L. monocytogenes, Gram-negative bacilli, S. pneumoniae	Vanco+ceftazidime+ampicillin

Cefot = cefotaxime, AG = aminoglycoside, Vanco = vancomycin, Ceftr = ceftriaxone, Ceftaz = ceftazidime, Mero = meropenem

Section 4

Table 27.9 Recommendations for use of antibiotics based on organisms isolated and their susceptibility to antibiotics

Microorganisms and susceptibility	Standard therapy	Alternative antibiotics
S. pneumoniae Penicillin MIC		
<0.1ugm/mL	Pen G, Amp	Cefot/Ceftr/Chloro
0.1 – 1.0 ugm/mL	Cefot/Ceftr	Cefepime, Mero
>2.0 ugm/mL	Vanco + Cefot/Ceftr	Fluoroquinolone/Moxiflox
N. meningitidis Penicillin MIC		
<0.1 ugm/mL	Pen G/Amp	Cefot/Ceftr/Chloro
0.1 – 1 ugm/mL	Cefot/Ceftr	Chloro/Fluoroquinolone/Mero
Listeria monocytogenes	Amp/ Pen G	Trim-sulph, Mero
Group B streptococcus	Amp/Pen G	Cefot/Ceftr
E. coli, Enterobacteriaciae	Cefot/Ceftr	Aztreonam, Fluoroquinolone, Mero, Trim-sulph, Amp
P. aeruginosa	Cefepime/ Ceftaz	Aztreonam, Mero, Cipro
Hib	Amp	Cefot/Ceftr, Cefipime,Chloro, Fluoroquinolone
S. aureus	Cloxacillin	Vanco, Mero, Trim-sulph, Linezolid
S. epidermidis	Vanco	Linezolid
Enterococcus		
Amp sensitive	Amp + Genta	
Amp resistant	Vanco + Genta	
Amp + Vanco resistant	Linezolid	

Pen G = penicillin G, Amp = ampicillin, Cefot = cefotaxime, Ceftr = ceftriaxone, Chloro =chloramphenicol, Mero = meropenem, Trim-sulph = trimethoprim– sulphamethoxazole, Ceftaz = ceftazidime, Vanco = vancomycin, Genta = gentamicin, Cipro = ciprofloxacin

(d) *Corticosteroids.* Dexamethasone in a dose of 0.15 mg/kg/dose 6 hourly when given with antibiotics for the first 4 days has been shown to improve outcome and reduce the incidence of hearing deficit in *Hib* meningitis[25]. Its therapeutic utility in pneumococcal meningitis is unclear. It may reduce CSF levels of vancomycin by reducing the meningeal inflammation. Its first dose must be given 10-20 minutes prior to the first dose of antibiotic.

(e) *Shunt infection.* Removal of the shunt with some form of external drainage is the best way to treat shunt infections. In coagulase negative staphylococcus, if after 3-7 days of antibiotics, the CSF is normal, shunt may be replaced. In meningitis due to *S. aureus* 7 days and Gram-negative organisms 10-14 days of therapy must be given before shunt replacement. In persistent ventriculitis, intraventricular antibiotics have been used[26].

(f) *Treating contacts.* Prophylaxis is given to contacts in following situations (Table 27.10).

- *Hib* meningitis. To all household contacts when there are children <4 years in the house; all staff and children in a day care center where 2 or more children developed infection.

- *N. meningitidis meningitis.* To all household or nursery school contacts, medical personnel with close contact with oral secretions.

Complications

Sub-dural effusion occurs in 10-30% cases of meningitis but is asymptomatic in majority of patients. Symptoms include bulging anterior fontanel, sutural diastasis, focal and persistent seizures, persistent fever, vomitings or neurological deterioration after 72 hours of antibiotics. If there

Table 27.10 Guidelines for chemoprophylaxis		
Drug	**Age of contacts**	**Dosage**
H. Influenzae		
Rifampicin	<1 month 1month to 12 years	10 mg/kg daily for 4 days 20 mg/kg daily for 4 days
Meningococcal disease		
Rifampicin	<1 month 1 month to 12 years	5 mg/kg BD for 2 days 10 mg/kg BD for 2 days
Ceftriaxone	<12 years >12 years	125 mg IM single dose 250 mg IM single dose
Ciprofloxacin	–	20 mg/kg single dose PO

is evidence of raised intracranial tension or depression of sensorium it may require tapping. Some neurosurgeons follow a technique of repeated tappings of not more than 30 ml of CSF per day for upto 2 weeks. If this fails, closed extra-dural drainage may be tried till sub-dural protein reduces, followed by a sub-dural peritoneal shunt.

Ventriculitis is common in neonatal meningitis and occurs in upto 92% of fatal cases but it is rare in older children. If there is additional obstruction at aqueduct of Sylvius it behaves like a bag of pus and child deteriorates rapidly. It is treated with large doses of antibiotics for a prolonged period. Intraventricular antibiotics with an external ventriculostomy or shunt reservoir may be required if the infection is difficult to eradicate. The empiric doses of intraventricular antibiotics are shown in Table 27.11. Additional doses can be determined by calculating the "inhibitory quotient". Prior to the next dose, a sample of CSF is withdrawn and trough level of antibiotic is determined. The trough level is divided by the MIC of the drug for the isolated organism; it must exceed 10-20 for consistent CSF sterilization.

Prevention

Effective vaccines are available to prevent pyogenic meningitis due to three common pathogens i.e. Hib, meningococci and pneumococci (Table 27.12).

Prognosis

Prognosis of pyogenic meningitis has improved with early diagnosis and antibiotic therapy. The case fatality rate varies between 1-8%. Severe neurodevelopment sequelae may occur in 10-20% cases while subtle neurobehavioural deficits are seen in 50% of survivors. Audiometric evaluation

Table 27.11 Recommended doses of antimicrobials by intraventricular route	
Antimicrobial agents	**Daily intraventricular dose (mg)**
Vancomycin	5 – 20
Gentamicin	1-8
Tobramycin	5 – 20
Amikacin	5 –50
Polymyxin B	5
Colistin	10
Quinupristin/dalfopristin	2-5
Teicoplanin	5-40

of hearing is mandatory in all survivors because deafness may occur in 10-30% cases after recovery.

TOXIC SHOCK SYNDROME

Definition

Toxic shock syndrome (TSS) is an acute multi-system disease with high grade fever, hypotension, diffuse erythematous skin rash, renal failure, mucosal erythema, vomitings, diarrhea and non-focal neurological abnormalities[27].

Etiology

It is caused by TSS-1 producing strains of *S. aureus* and occasionally by *Group A Streptococcus*. The exotoxin directly or via various cytokines including tumor necrosis factor and interleukin-1 cause a generalized inflammatory response.

Epidemiology

This syndrome was initially described in menstruating women who were using tampons.

Table 27.12 Vaccinations against meningitis

Vaccine	Dose	Age of administration	Indications
H influenzae type B (HiB)	0.5 ml im	6,10,14 weeks, booster 15-18 months	Routine
Pneumococcal conjugate vaccine (PCV-13)	0.5 ml im	2,4,6 month, booster 15 months	Routine in USA
Pneumococcal polyvalent polysaccharide vaccine (PPV)	0.5 ml im or sc	>2 years single dose	Sickle cell disease, asplenia, nephrotic syndrome, CRF*, HIV, chronic cardiopulmonary disease, CSF leaks
Meningococcal polysaccharide quadrivalent A,C, Y, W-135	0.5 ml im or sc	>2 years single dose followed by boosters every 2-3 years	Meningococcal outbreaks for health personnel and close contacts, Haj pilgrims, asplenia, complement deficiencies

* CRF: Chronic renal failure

Over the years, the use of hyperabsorbent tampons has slowly declined, followed by sharp decline in the incidence of TSS. Currently TSS is usually associated with burns, nasal packing, wound infections and osteomyelitis.

Pathogenesis

S. aureus mediated TSS develops when toxins such as TSS-toxin1 (75%), enterotoxin-B (23%) or enterotoxin-C (2%) are released into the circulation. These are superantigens which stimulate a massive non-specific T cell inflammatory response but specific antigen recognition does not occur. The conventional antigens activate only about 0.01% to 0.1% of the T-cell population, whereas, the superantigens activate 5-30% of the entire T-cell population. The net effect is massive production of cytokines that are capable of mediating shock and tissue injury. As part of this T cell response, interferon–gamma is also produced, which subsequently inhibits polyclonal immunoglobulin production. This failure to develop antibodies may explain why some patients are predisposed to relapse after a first episode of TSS. Subsequently generalized capillary permeability and multi-organ dysfunction sets in. Hyperabsorbent tampons in menstruating women which were commonly associated with TSS, increase partial pressure of oxygen in the vagina, provide surfactants and bind magnesium, all of which increase the production of toxins. The clinical picture of streptococcal TSS is slightly different from staphylococcal TSS and is mediated by streptococcal pyrogenic exotoxin A and B.

Clinical features

The illness starts abruptly with fever, chills, vomitings, profuse watery diarrhea and generalized erythroderma and myalgias. Fever and generalized erythroderma are universally present while diarrhea, vomitings and myalgias are present in >90% cases. Headache, sore throat and conjunctival hyperemia is seen in over 50% of cases. Because of the loss of peripheral vascular resistance there is hypotension with multi-organ dysfunction. Alteration in sensorium, oliguria, hepatic dysfunction and DIC sets in subsequently. After a week or so, generalized desquamation occurs.

The following criteria are useful for clinical diagnosis of TSS:

- Body temperature higher than 38.9°C.
- Systolic blood pressure lower than 90 mm Hg.
- Skin rash with subsequent desquamation, especially on the palms and soles.
- Involvement of 3 or more of the following organ systems:
  o Gastrointestinal tract: Vomitings and profuse diarrhea
  o Mucous membranes (vagina, conjunctivae, pharynx): Marked hyperemia
  o Muscles: Severe myalgia or greater than 5-fold increase in creatine kinase levels
  o Central nervous system: Disorientation without focal neurologic signs
  o Renal system: BUN or creatinine levels at least twice the upper reference range limit or pyuria in the absence of urinary tract infection

o Hepatic system: Bilirubin, serum aspartate aminotransferase (AST), or serum alanine aminotransferase (ALT) levels at least twice the upper reference range limit

o Blood: Thrombocytopenia (platelet count <100,000/mm^3)

The serologic tests for Rocky Mountain spotted fever, leptospirosis, and measles should be negative. Streptococcal TSS differs from staphylococcal TSS because invasive disease is commoner and blood culture may be positive in 60% cases of streptococcal TSS. Erythroderma and GI symptoms like vomitings and diarrhea are less common and mortality (33%) is 10 times that of staphylococcal TSS (3.3%).

Investigations

Leukocytosis is uncommon but neutrophils account for >90% of total leukocytes. Anemia and thrombocytopenia along with prolonged prothrombin and partial thromboplastin time are common early markers of the disease. Evidences of multiorgan dysfunction with elevated SGPT, creatinine, CPK and low albumin are common. Profoundly low serum calcium reflect low albumin and elevated calcitonin-like substance. Sterile pyuria and CSF pleocytosis indicate generalized involvement of mucosal membranes.

Treatment

1. *Locate and drain the infected site.* Even a small undrained focus of infection can have serious consequences due to the continued production of toxin. If the condition occurs post-operatively, the surgical site must be presumed to be the culprit no matter how benign it looks

2. *Antimicrobial therapy.* Start with anti-staphylococcal antibiotics intravenously in maximal doses. Additionally clindamycin is used because of its unique property of inhibiting toxin production. Once the child is stable, oral antibiotics are continued to complete 10–14 days course. For community-acquired TSS, β-lactamase resistant penicillin such as cloxacillin with clindamycin is a good choice while for hospital-acquired TSS, vancomycin with clindamycin are more appropriate.

3. *Fluid replacement.* Aggressive fluid replacement with crystalloids and colloids with close monitoring of central venous pressure and other vitals as discussed in the management of septic shock are essential in the initial management of these patients.

4. *Intravenous immunoglobulins.* A single dose of 400 mg/kg of intravenous immunoglobulins over several hours has shown remarkable reduction of mortality in animal studies and anecdotal case reports[28].

5. *Corticosteroids.* Short courses of methyl prednisolone and dexamethasone early in the course of illness has reduced fever and severity of illness but not made a dent on overall mortality.

6. In recent years, research is continuing to develop either monoclonal antibodies against TSST-1 or other peptides to block the ability of bacterial toxins to activate T cells, therefore blocking the toxicity cascade.

Outcome

Death occurs in 3.3% cases of staphylococcal TSS and 30% of patients with streptococcal TSS. It is usually early in the course of illness and due to fatal arrhythmia, refractory respiratory failure or bleeding. Recurrences are also known and prophylaxis has been used in menstrual TSS with rifampicin or clindamycin during menses. Long term sequelae like lack of concentration, and chronic fatigue syndrome have been reported.

PYOGENIC LIVER ABSCESSES

Pyogenic liver abcesses are uncommon due to the rich vascular supply, unique architecture and active reticuloendothelial system of the liver. In children the commonest mode of infection is hematogenous spread of bacteria to the liver whereas biliary tract disease like cholangitis, pancreatitis and penetrating duodenal ulcers are the chief causes of liver abscess in adults. In neonates, umbilical catheterization, omphalitis, and necrotizing enterocolitis result in infection via the portal system. Intra-abdominal infections like appendicitis, ulcerative colitis and peri-rectal abscesses also result in portal venous bacteremia and subsequent liver abscess. Other predisposing causes include chronic granulomatous disease, penetrating trauma, liver infarcts and immunocompromised states like leukemia. The commonest organism in children is *S. aureus* followed by Gram-negative organisms. Anerobic organisms are also common and mixed infections are seen in almost half the cases.

Clinical features are subtle and often missed unless carefully examined by an astute physician.

Section 4

Non-specific complaints like fever, vomitings, malaise may go unnoticed for weeks before the diagnosis is made. Hepatomegaly occurs in 40-80% cases and intercostal tenderness should be carefully elicited in all patients. Jaundice, abdominal distension and pleural involvement are less common.

Anemia and leukocytosis are non-specific findings. The first investigation that usually alerts a clinician is an elevated right hemi-diaphragm on skiagram of chest. Mild elevation of transaminases with significant elevation of alkaline phosphatase with a rapidly enlarging tender hepatomegaly must make one suspect a liver abscess. Ultrasonography is useful first line investigation to confirm the diagnosis. A CT scan may be needed for the diagnosis of very small abscesses (upto 1 cm in diameter) and is useful to clearly define their extent. MRI has no added benefit. Blood culture is usually sterile except in patients with multiple abscesses.

Surgical drainage is the key to successful treatment. Percutaneous drainage via CT or ultrasound guidance has also been described but may not be successful in multiloculated or multiple abscesses. The choice of antibiotics should be based on the isolation of pathogens and their antibacterial sensitivity pattern. Initial empiric therapy may include cloxacillin with an aminoglycoside and an anerobic cover such as clindamycin, metronidazole or chloramphenicol. At least 2-4 week therapy is essential and end point is determined by radiological findings and clinical recovery.

PELVIC ABSCESS

These are uncommon in children but usually occur as a complication of appendicular or other intestinal perforations. Rarely inflammatory bowel disease or pelvic inflammatory disease in adolescents may be the predisposing condition. They present as prolonged unexplained fever with vague abdominal pain. Rectal examination may reveal a boggy tender mass. Ultrasound localizes the lesion and CT may be required for more accurate delineation. Organisms isolated are usually Gram-negative or anerobic. Surgical drainage and in recent years ultrasound guided percutaneous drainage is the key to effective treatment. Antibiotics such as clindamycin with an aminoglycoside are most appropriate.

REFERENCES

1. Muckart DJ, Bhagwanjee S. American College of Chest Physicians/Society of Critical Care Medicine Consensus Conference. Definitions of the systemic inflammatory response syndrome and allied disorders in relation to critically injured patients. *Crit Care Med* 1997; 25: 1789-1795.

2. Goldstein B, Giroir B, Randolph A, and the members of the International Consensus Conference on Pediatric Sepsis. International Pediatric Sepsis Consensus Conference: Definitions for sepsis and organ dysfunction in pediatrics. *Pediatric Crit Care Med* 2005; 6:2-8.

3. Martin GS, Mannino DM, Eaton S, Moss Marc. The epidemiology of sepsis in the United States from 1979 through 2000. *N Engl J Med* 2003; 348:1546-1554.

4. Gray J, Gossain S and Morris K. Three-year survey of bacteremias and fungemia in a pediatric intensive care unit. *Pediatr Infect Dis J* 2001; 20:416-421.

5. Invasive Bacterial Infections Surveillance (IBIS) Group of the International Clinical Epidemiology Network. Are Haemophilus influenzae infections a significant problem in India? A prospective study and review. *Clin Infect Dis* 2002; 34: 949-957.

6. Hotchkiss RS, Karl IE. The pathophysiology and treatment of sepsis. *N Engl J Med* 2003; 348:138-150.

7. Nduka OO. Parrilo JE. The pathophysiology of septic shock. *Crit Care Clin* 2009; 25: 677-702.

8. Feverish Illness in Children: Assessment and Initial Management in Children Younger than 5 Years. NICE Clinical Guidelines, No. 47. National Collaborating Centre for Women's and Children's Health (UK).London (UK): *RCOG Press;* 2007 May.

9. Vincent J-L, Martinez EO, Silva E. Evolving concepts in sepsis definitions. Sepsis. *Crit Care Clin* 2009; 25: 665-675

10. Wheeler AP, Bernard GR. Treating patients with severe sepsis. *N Engl J Med* 1999; 340: 207-214

11. Simon L, Gauvin F, Amre DK, Saint-Louis P, and Lacroix J. Serum procalcitonin and C-reactive protein levels as markers of bacterial infection: A systematic review and meta-analysis. *Clinical Infect Dis* 2004; 39:206–217

12. Hatherill M, Tibby SM, Turner C, Ratnavel N and Murdoch IA. Procalcitonin and cytokine levels: Relationship to organ failure and mortality in pediatric septic shock. *Critical Care Med* 2000; 28:2591-2594.

13. Kaplan S. Bacteremia and septic shock. In: Textbook of Pediatric Infectious Diseases. Feigin RD, Cherry JD, Demmler GJ, Kaplan SL (Eds), 5th edition, *Philadelphia, Saunders* 2004; pp. 810-824.

14. Kumar A. Optimizing antimicrobial therapy in sepsis and septic shock. *Crit Care Clin* 2009; 25:733-751.

Section 4

15. Rivers E, Nguyen B, Havstad S, *et al*. Early goal-directed therapy in the treatment of severe sepsis and septic shock. *N Engl J Med* 2001; 345:1368-1377.

16. Van den Bergh G, Wouters P, Weekers F, *et al*. Intensive insulin therapy in critically ill patients. *N Engl J Med* 2001; 345:1359-1367.

17. Cronin L, Cook DJ, Carlet J, *et al*. Corticosteroid treatment for sepsis: a critical appraisal and meta-analysis of the literature. *Crit Care Med* 1995; 23: 1430-1439.

18. Annane D. Corticosteroids for septic shock. *Crit Care Med* 2001; 29 :(suppl), S117-S120.

19. Bernard GR, Vincent JL, Laterre PF, *et al*. Efficacy and safety of recombinant human activated protein C for severe sepsis. *N Engl J Med* 2001; 344:699-709.

20. Butt W. Septic shock. *Pediatric Clin N Amer* 2001; 48:601-605.

21. Werdan K, Pilz G, Bujdoso O, Fraunberger P, Neeser G, Schmieder RE, *et al*. Score-based immunoglobulin G therapy of patients with sepsis: The SBITS study. *Crit Care Med* 2007; 35:2693-2701.

22. Reefhuis J, Honein MA, Whitney CG, et al. Risk of bacterial meningitis in patients with cochlear implants. *N Engl J Med* 2003; 349:435-445.

23. Centre for Disease Control and Prevention: Progress towards eliminating *Haemophilus influenzae type b* disease among infants and children, United States. 1987-1997. *MMWR* 1998; 47:993-998.

24. Tunkel AR, Hartman BJ, Kaplan SL, Kaufman BA, Roos KL, Scheld M, *et al*. Practice guidelines for the management of bacterial meningitis. *Clin Infect Dis* 2004; 39:1267-1284.

25. McIntyre PB, Berkley CS, King SM, *et al*. Dexamethasone as adjunctive therapy in bacterial meningitis: a meta-analysis of randomized clinical trials since 1988. *JAMA* 1997; 278:925-931.

26. Tunkel AR, Kaufman BA. Cerebrospinal fluid shunt infections. *In*: Principles and Practice of Infectious Diseases. Mandel GL, Bennet JE, Dolin R, (eds). *Philadelphia: Elsevier Science,* 6th ed. 2004: pp. 1126-1132.

27. Chesney PJ, Davis JP. Toxic shock syndrome. In: Textbook of Pediatric Infectious Diseases Vol 1, Feigin RD, Cherry JD, Demmler GJ, Kaplan SL (Eds). *Saunders, Philadelphia.* 5th ed. 2004; pp. 836-859.

28. Barry W, Hudgins L, Donta ST, *et al*. Intravenous immunoglobulin therapy for toxic shock syndrome. *JAMA* 1992; 267:315-317.

Section 4

28

Cerebral and other Forms of Severe Malaria

Yogesh Jain, Anju Kataria and Meharban Singh

Falciparum malaria is the most common serious parasitic disease of human beings, accounting for one million deaths every year. In India, about 8 lakh cases of falciparum malaria and about 1000 deaths were reported in 2010[1]. The estimated magnitude shown in a recent study that pegs the number of deaths by over 200 times has been questioned by some, this study seriously questions routine data collection and every one agrees that there is gross under-reporting[2]. Malaria may be caused by any of the five plasmodium species, only infections due to *P. falciparum* can present with severe symptoms and rapid progression, which if untreated can lead to death. Recently, severe disease has been reported to occur with *P vivax* as well. The disease is severe with multi-organ involvement especially in the non-immune individual. It is a disease of the poor and those who have poor access to health care services, and are denied good quality health services. Most cases of falciparum malaria occur in the poorer and tribal dominated central Indian states (Figure 28.1) of Orissa, Chhattisgarh, MP, Jharkhand and the North East states[3]. Not surprisingly, although only 8% of the country's people are adivasis (tribals), more than 50% of the cases and deaths due to falciparum malaria occur among them[4] (Figure 28.2).

While the disease is caused by plasmodium that is transmitted by the vector Anopheles, the extent and severity of the disease is determined by the host. Overall, falciparum malaria has a mortality of 0.1% in the healthy immune population. However, if diagnosis is delayed, then as many as 30% of episodes with falciparum malaria are likely to become severe. And once the illness is characterized as 'severe' the therapeutic options are scarce and risk of mortality is high anywhere in the world and is at least 15 to 20%. Outbreaks of falciparum malaria are almost always man made and occur most where there is breakdown of public health facilities. It is important that pediatricians should be aware of this fact because they would often be called upon to deal with a sick child with severe malaria in the setting of an outbreak or epidemic, when the demands on their clinical expertise would need to be supplemented with a sound use of the primary health care approach.

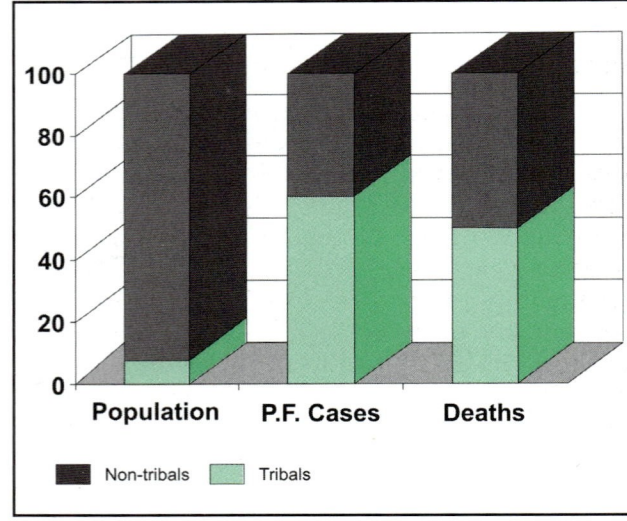

Figure 28.2 Falciparum malaria in tribals and non-tribals

The rising proportion of cases due to *P. falciparum* (almost 50%) and increasing resistance to chloroquine (Figure 28.3) and frequent administration of sulphadoxime-pyremethamine therapy in India has made the situation worse[4],[5].

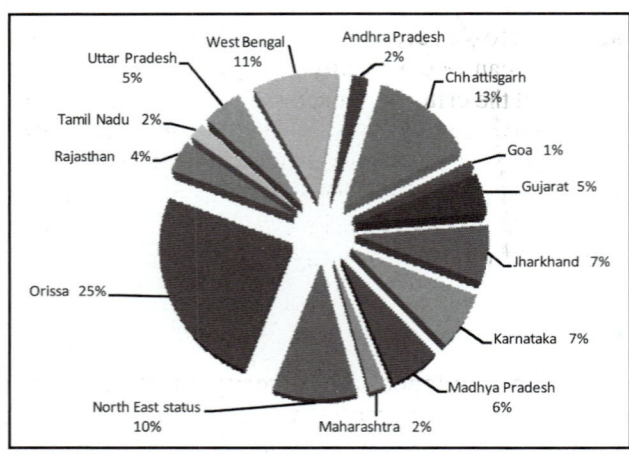

Figure 28.1 Contribution of different states to malaria in India

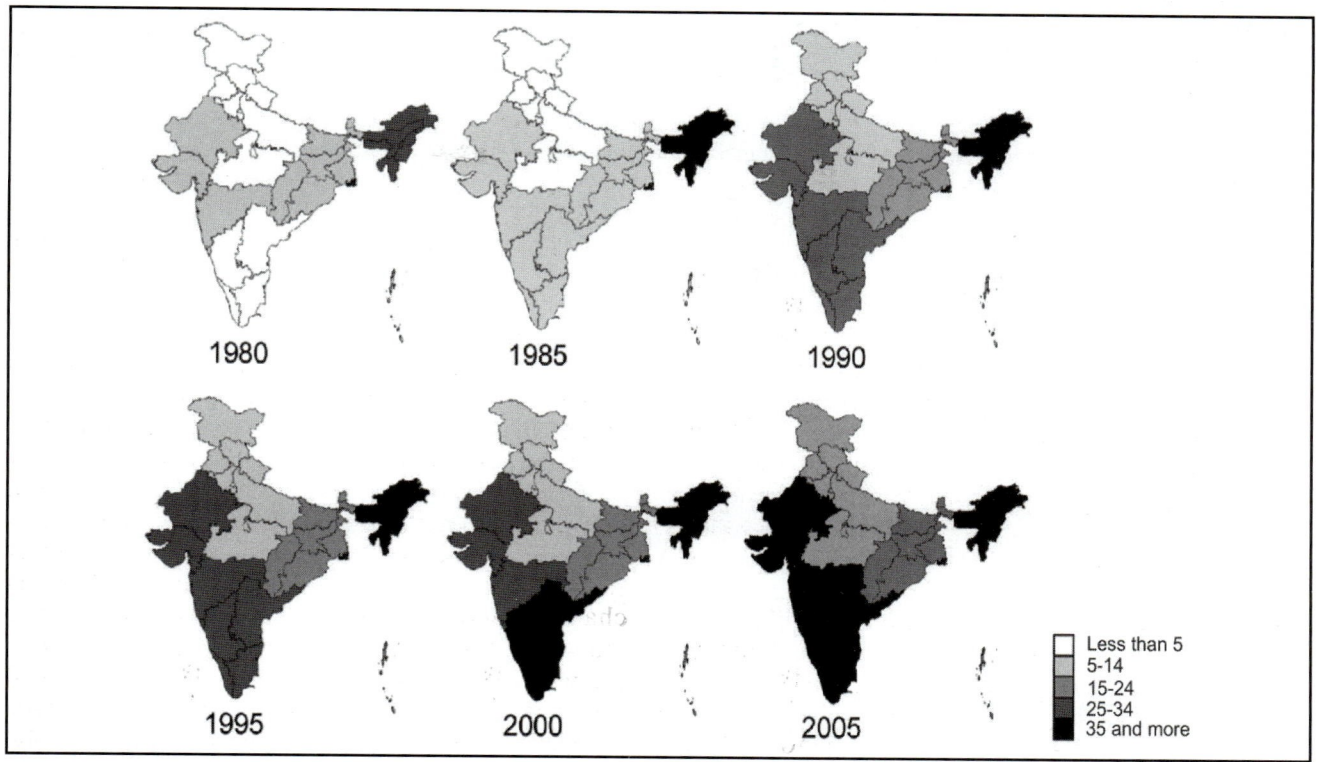

Figure 28.3 The increasing trend of resistance to chloroquine in falciparum malaria in the country. A 25% cut off for resistance merits a change in the first line drug against the disease.

The World Health Organization (WHO) has proposed the term 'Severe Malaria' to identify those symptomatic malaria infections which can lead to death if not treated appropriately. It is defined as presence of asexual forms of *P. falciparum* in the peripheral blood along with one or more of the signs[6, 7] (major or minor) listed in Table 28.1

Pediatricians, however, should not unduly worry about definitions or semantics. The clinical suspicion of severe malaria, even if it does not fit into the aforementioned criteria or there is lack of parasitological confirmation, merits immediate treatment because there is a highly significant relationship between delay in starting chemotherapy and mortality in severe malaria. The clinical features of severe malaria in children depends on the level of endemicity in an area. In areas with high level of transmission; holoendemic (>75 percent) and hyperendemic (50-75 percent) spleen rates, it presents most frequently as severe anemia in children below 5 years[8]. In areas with less intense transmission, the age range affected by severe malaria extends upto 10 years, and cerebral malaria becomes a more prominent manifestation. In areas with low transmission (non-immune individual), cerebral malaria is an important manifestation at all ages and the disease is unlikely to occur in small children. However, this clear demarcation of presentation is not always persent. In the year 2010, when several central Indian states saw a major epidemic of falciparum malaria, the authors found that over 70% of all patients with severe malaria and 79% of all those who died, were children in Bilaspur district in Chhattisgarh, which is an area known for its unstable pattern of malaria transmission[9].

In general, convulsions, severe anemia, hypoglycemia and lactic acidosis with hypotension are common presenting features of severe malaria in children while jaundice, pulmonary edema and acute renal failure are more commonly seen in adults. However, cerebral malaria, shock and acidosis can occur at any age. In 2000, the WHO modified the criteria[7] for severe malaria by including the previous two minor criteria of heavy parasitemia (more than 5% parasitized RBCs) and jaundice as major manifestations. However, some subsequent series on severe malaria did not find these two criteria of much discerning value[10].

EPIDEMIOLOGY

The incidence and severity of *Plasmodium falciparum* has increased in the last few years in India and South East Asia, partly because of increasing incidence of multi-drug resistance of the

Section 4

Table 28.1 Manifestations of severe malaria[7]

MAJOR CRITERIA

1.	Cerebral malaria/ unarousable coma not attributable to any other cause	Failure to localize or respond appropriately to noxious stimuli (Glasgow coma score $\leq$ 8). Coma should persist for >30 min after a seizure to differentiate it from transient postictal state.
2.	Severe normocytic normochromic anemia	Hematocrit <15%, or hemoglobin < 5 g/dl.
3.	Renal failure	Urine output < 0.5 ml/kg/hr with no improvement on rehydration and serum creatinine > 3 mg/dl.
4.	Pulmonary edema	Acute respiratory distress syndrome
5.	Hypoglycemia	Whole blood glucose < 40 mg/dl
6.	Hypotension/shock	Systolic BP < 50 mm of Hg in children aged 1-5 years, < 80 mm Hg in adults, with cold and clammy extremities (core-skin temperature difference of > 2° C).
7.	Bleeding/DIC	Spontaneous bleeding and hemorrhages from gums, nose, GIT or evidences of DIC.
8.	Convulsions	More than two generalized convulsions in 24 hr despite cooling
9.	Acidemia/acidosis	Arterial pH < 7.25, plasma HCO_3 < 15 mMol/1, or venous lactate > 6 mMol/l.
10.	Macroscopic hemoglobinuria	
11.	Post mortem diagnosis of malaria on needle biopsy of brain	

MINOR CRITERIA

1. Impaired consciousness: Less severe alteration of sensorium should also be considered as an important correlate of cerebral malaria.
2. Extreme weakness. Profound weakness so that the patient cannot sit or walk, with no obvious neurological explanation.
3. Hyperparasitemia (parasite count >250,000/μl or >5% RBCs are parasitized)
4. Jaundice detected clinically or serum bilirubin >3 mg/dl
5. Hyperpyrexia (rectal temperature of >40° C)

parasite and partly due to resistance of the vector to insecticides. Unsatisfactory malaria control strategies has also contributed to the current dismal situation. It is estimated that over 50 percent of all cases of malaria in the country are due to *P. falciparum* infections. Multi-drug resistant *P. falciparum* malaria is widely prevalent in India with highest incidence in North-Eastern States (Assam, Arunachal Pradesh, Meghalaya, Nagaland, Mizoram), Orissa and tribal populations settled in the forests. Figure 28.3 gives a pictorial description of the areas where chloroquine resistance in Falciparum malaria has been reported to be more than 10%. This widespread prevalence of resistance has prompted the Nation Vector Borne Disease Control Programme (NVBDCP) to change the drug policy for falciparum malaria drastically in 2008 to make Artesunate Combination Therapy (ACT) as the standard of care[11].

CLINICAL SYNDROMES OF SEVERE MALARIA

Severe malaria is caused by *P. falciparum* infection which can present with dysfunction of any one or multiple organ systems of the body. As many as 30% of episodes of falciparum malaria may become severe if diagnosis and treatment is delayed. Rarely, sporadic cases of *P. vivax* may cause severe disease in humans including pulmonary edema, renal failure, hemoglobinuria and altered sensorium[12].

There are no clinical features that reliably distinguish severe malaria from other severe infections in children[13]. Therefore, it is wise to consider severe malaria as a differential diagnosis in any sick child who presents with fever. However, the most important manifestations of severe *P. falciparum* infection in children are cerebral malaria, severe anemia and respiratory distress.

Fever with acute encephalopathy. Although 'cerebral malaria' implies a distinct disease entity, the clinical syndrome is highly variable, with most cases having one of the following symptoms such as (i) coma associated with other severe systemic derangements such as severe anemia, metabolic acidosis, respiratory distress or shock; (ii) coma with protracted or multiple seizures, where unconsciousness might be caused by a long (>1 hr) post-ictal state or by subclinical or subtle seizure activity, characterised by conjugate eye deviation, nystagmus, salivation, and hypoventilation[14] and (iii) a pure neurological syndrome of coma and abnormal motor posturing, which might be complicated by raised intracranial pressure and recurrent seizures[15]. In fact, sudden hypoventilation and apnea due to respiratory centre depression is not uncommon, and should be anticipated and managed with early ventilator support when necessary[10,16].

Convulsions are common both before and after the onset of coma. They are significantly associated with increased morbidity and sequelae. They may present in very subtle ways; important signs include intermittent nystagmus, salivation, minor twitchings of a single digit or a corner of the mouth and an irregular breathing pattern. In some children, extreme opisthotonos is seen. In children with profound coma, corneal reflexes and "doll's eye" movements may be abnormal.

On examination, the child is usually febrile and unarousable. Signs of meningeal irritation are absent but occasionally there may be some passive resistance to neck flexion. The features are those of symmetrical encephalopathy and focal signs are unusual. There is no gaze paresis and other cranial nerves are usually normal. There may be forced jaw closure with repetitive spontaneous teeth grinding (bruxism) and the pout reflex may be present. The tone may be normal, increased or decreased. Episodes of increased muscle tone with decorticate and decerebrate posturing may occur. The deep tendon reflexes may be brisk or depressed; plantars are extensors in half the patients.

The pupils are usually mid sized and often react to light. Fundus examination is useful for detecting retinopathy. Malarial retinopathy consists of a group of retinal abnormalities that are unique to severe malaria and common in children with cerebral malaria. Retinal hemorrhages may be seen in 15 percent of the cases. A large, prospective autopsy study of children who died from cerebral malaria in Malawi showed that malarial retinopathy was better than any other clinical or laboratory feature for distinguishing malarial from nonmalarial coma[17].

The CSF is usually unremarkable. CSF pressure is often raised and there may be up to 10 cells/ml (rarely upto 50), most of them being lymphocytes. The protein is elevated upto 200 mg/dl and the glucose is slightly low relative to blood glucose level. The CSF lactate is raised proportionate to the severity of disease process.

Fever with severe anemia. If there is associated splenomegaly or hemoglobinuria ('black water fever') it strongly supports the possibility of malaria. Anemia is more likely to occur with high parasitic load. Mortality of children with asymptomatic severe malarial anemia is low (around 1%), but rises to more than 30% when anemia is complicated by severe respiratory distress and metabolic acidosis[13].

Fever with jaundice. The jaundice results from hemolysis or associated viral hepatitis and is chiefly unconjugated. Jaundice is more common in patients who develop renal dysfunction. As mentioned above, jaundice is usually a minor manifestation, though recently it has been included as a major criteria.

Fever with acute renal failure may occur due to acute tubular necrosis, hemoglobinuria and administration of NSAIDs. However, this is rather uncommon in children.

Fever with bleeding. Gastrointestinal hemorrhage is common, especially in cerebral malaria due to consumption of platelets in the brain or development of disseminated intravascular coagulation.

Fever with diarrhea and/ or hypovolemic shock. It is called Algid malaria and is often associated with Gram-negative sepsis. Shock is not a common feature of uncomplicated cerebral malaria and should alert the pediatrician for concomitant presence of septicemia.

Fever with cough and respiratory distress. Respiratory distress (deep breathing, or Kussmaul's respiration) is a common clinical manifestation of severe disease and is a sign of metabolic acidosis[18], and has emerged as a powerful independent predictor of fatal outcome in falciparum malaria[19]. It can be misinterpreted as cardiac failure and circulatory overload, especially if associated with severe tachycardia. In children, this manifestation may be commonly associated with severe dehydration and acidosis.

Hypoglycemia (blood glucose concentration < 2.2 mMol/l or < 40 mg/dl) is associated with a poor outcome in children with malaria

While any of the above manifestations may occur independently, a combination of two or more of the above criteria is far more common. For example, a common presentation seen in children is that of severe anemia, acidosis and shock, with/ without features of cerebral malaria. Since severe malaria is a multisystem, multi-organ disease, children frequently present with more than one of the classic clinical phenotypes i.e. cerebral malaria, respiratory distress, severe malarial anemia, hypoglycemia. A typical case scenario is shown in the Box.

A typical case scenario in a young child

Kiran baiga, 2 years old, weighing 8 kg presents with a 3 days history of fever, pallor, and rapid breathing; history of 3 seizures on the way to the hospital, now drowsy and unable to feed. On examination, the child had rectal temperature 39.6°C; pale yellow palms; breathing rate 60/min, deep breathing with subcostal recessions (respiratory distress); pulse 160/min; blood pressure 76/50 mm Hg; capillary refill time 4 sec; Blantyre coma score 2; hepatomegaly 1 cm below costal margin. Investigations revealed haemoglobin 1.8 g/dl; thick smear P. falciparum asexual forms 180,000 per ml; blood glucose 36 mg/dl; creatinine 0.7 mg/dl.

Questions: What should be the sequence of management? Should we ventilate him? Should we give blood or a colloid in the first go (meaning thereby that we give blood transfusion as an emergency measure)? or should we hydrate him first as a response to the deep breathing and acidosis because he had not taken orally for over 12 hours?

In endemic areas, it is also not uncommon to have multiple infections in the same child e.g. malaria with enteric fever or other acute infections like viral hepatitis or sepsis. Therefore, malaria should still be considered as a possibility even if there is evidence of some other infection and the child is not improving.

PATHOPHYSIOLOGY

Cytokines and tumor necrosis factor are implicated as a cause of fever, lethargy and anorexia. They are not directly responsible for either cerebral symptoms or the organ failure which are so common in severe malaria. High plasma concentrations of TNF-α in patients with cerebral malaria also correlate with disease severity including hypoglycemia, hyperparasitemia and death[20]. Cytokines are known to release nitric oxide which is neurotoxic leading to coma. Erythrocytes infected with mature *P. falciparum* demonstrate cytoadherence to specific receptors at the venular microvasculature and thus disappear from circulation (sequestration). The high molecular transmembrane protein *P. falciparum* erythrocyte membrane protein 1 (PfEMP-1) is the most important ligand for cytoadherence[21]. The sequestration in vital organs causes tissue hypoperfusion. Besides, these infected erythrocytes tend to adhere to each other (rossetting) and further compromise tissue perfusion[22]. Rossetting is a central mechanism in cerebral malaria while cytoadherence is associated with other organ system dysfunction. Cytoadherence of erythrocytes in the microcirculation is aggravated by accumulation of platelets which form a sticky bridge between infected erythrocytes and the endothelium. Further, lack of deformability or rigidity of the infected erythrocytes compounds the problem of hypoperfusion leading to sluggish microcirculation. Reduced blood flow in the microcirculation of vital organs leads to hypoxia, anerobic metabolism and lactic acidosis which is a strong predictor of poor outcome. Severe malaria has features in common with severe sepsis syndrome. The pathophysiology of both disorders might reflect a cytokine-driven systemic inflammatory response[23].

It has now been clearly shown that cerebral edema is not a common feature of cerebral malaria. However, raised intracranial pressure may be seen in as many as 80 percent of children, but the rise in pressure is much less than in pyogenic meningitis[24]. The rise in intracranial pressure is due to increased cerebral blood volume which in turn is consequent to the body's attempt to increase cerebral perfusion which is adversely affected by the sequestered biomass of infected erythrocytes.

DIAGNOSIS

Severe malaria can be confused with many other febrile illnesses in children. Therefore, a rapid and accurate diagnosis of malaria is mandatory for prompt and effective management. It is also important to quantify the degree of parasitemia because it has therapeutic and prognostic significance. As already mentioned, parasitemia of 5 percent or more RBCs along with other clinical manifestations signifies severe malaria.

Though there are many new investigative modalities, parasite examination on thick and thin blood smears by a competent microscopist is still the most cost-effective, simple and highly sensitive method. A thick smear can pick upto 4-10 parasites per μl while a thin smear can pick up to 100 parasites per μl. It is highly unlikely that a child has evidence of severe malaria with parasite counts lower than the thresholds mentioned above. Smear examination not only helps in the diagnosis, but it is useful to monitor response to antimalarial drugs. However, blood smears may be negative in children with severe malaria, particularly if the staining techniques are faulty or the skills of the microscopist are inadequate. It may take upto 30 minutes for a proper examination of a single smear to be sure that there are no malarial parasites. Thick smears are useful for screening while thin smears are mandatory for study of the morphological characteristics of the parasite for specific diagnosis. If a blood smear is negative, it should be repeated every 6 hours for 24 hours.

The tests such as fluorochrome staining of the parasites in the whole blood called as quantitative buffy coat (QBC) technique[25] have the advantage of being rapid (taking only 10 minutes) and have a sensitivity of 94 percent and specificity of 92 percent. They, however, require a fluorescent microscope and an experienced technician.

Tests based on detecting malarial antigens in blood by ELISA technique such as histidine rich protein 2 of *P. falciparum* antigens (PfHRP2 and pLDH) can be rapidly performed as a dipstick test. A host of kits have flooded the market over the last few years. Many of them are specific for *P. falciparum*, while others are for non specific plasmodium antigen. Even the NVBDCP is also actively encouraging its use in malaria diagnostics as it obviates the need for microscopy, and also offers the results in minutes. It recommends that all peripheral health workers use these kits to diagnose falciparum malaria and institute treatment promptly.

However, one should exercise caution in its use. The kits are heat labile, and don't tolerate temperatures of over 30°C when the sensitivity and specificity of falciparum specific kits decline rapidly. Second, they don't tell us the parasite density. Third, they remain positive for several weeks after the recovery of patient and may not be appropriate for the diagnosis of recrudescences. They have a sensitivity and specificity of 94 percent and 95 percent respectively.

DNA probes have been developed for the diagnosis but they are time consuming, expensive and have low sensitivity. However, sensitivity of PCR assay is very high which can detect even one parasite per ml of blood.

In conclusion, malaria microscopy remains the modality of choice for diagnosis in most centres, as it has the highest sensitivity, allows identification of species and assessment of parasite density. Where such services are not available, rapid diagnostic kits offer a second option, with all its limitations as outlined above.

Other investigations that help in assessing the severity and aid management include a complete blood count (CBC), blood glucose, serum electrolytes, liver function tests including prothrombin time, blood urea, serum creatinine, blood gases and acid base parameters. Anemia is usually severe and often normocytic normochromic on peripheral blood smear. Anemia may increase in severity even after treatment and improvement and therefore hemoglobin must also be checked 24 hours after hospitalization.

A chest skiagram must be obtained in the event of respiratory distress and blood culture should be taken if coexistent Gram-negative septicemia is suspected. A CSF examination is mandatory to rule out other causes of febrile encephalopathy.

However, in most low resource settings where severe malaria is likely to be managed, the bare minimum requirements of investigations include hemoglobin, blood glucose, serum creatinine, parasite counts and at times a CSF examination. Blood glucose should be monitored every 4 hr and hemoglobin and parasite count every 12–24 hr, with additional measurements prompted by any deterioration in the level of consciousness.

A CT scan of the head should be done in those children who have repeated convulsions and altered sensorium to rule out any intracranial space occupying lesion, viral encephalitis, brain abscess, infarction or hemorrhage.

MANAGEMENT

Majority of deaths in malaria occur at home or on the way to the hospital. In remote areas, it may take several hours for the patient to reach a health facility. Since early parenteral treatment is a crucial determinant of outcome, rectal administration of artesunate at home by a peripheral health worker can be life saving[26,27]. Unfortunately rectal formulation is still not available in India. Even when children reach the hospital, more than 50% of deaths from severe childhood illnesses, including malaria, occur within 24 hr of hospital admission[28].

All children with severe malaria should ideally be managed in an intensive care unit. They need early and effective anti-malarial therapy, excellent supportive management and nursing care.

Antimalarial Therapy

Severe malaria must to be treated promptly with parenteral anti-malarials. There is no role of oral anti-malarials as the primary treatment modality of patients with severe malaria. When clinical suspicion of cerebral malaria is strong i.e. acute onset febrile encephalopathy with severe anemia, splenomegaly and hypoglycemia, antimalarial therapy may be started even when initial blood smear is reported as negative for malarial parasites.

Choice of Antimalarial Drugs

In view of the wide spread prevalence of chloroquine resistance of the parasite in Asia, its use is no longer recommended for treatment of severe malaria. In places where chloroquine resistance is prevalent or its status is not known, artemesinin compounds are the drug of choice. Among the artemisinin compounds; artesunate and artemether are effective in both chloroquine and quinine resistant cases of malaria. They are more convenient to use and are credited to have a more rapid schizonticidal effect. They act at all stages of the life cycle of the parasite unlike quinine which acts only on the middle third of the life cycle of the malarial parasite. The large multicentric, multinational randomized trial of 1461 primarily adult patients in Southeast Asia has clearly established the superiority of intravenous artersunate over quinine in the treatment of severe malaria. Mortality was 35% lower in the artesunate treated patients with reduced risk of hypoglycemia compared to quinine[29]. However, their use is limited by their availability and risk of disease recrudescence if used alone, and thus its use is always combined with another antimalarial drug.

This combination of an artemisinin compound with another drug (called ACTs) is achieved by using a drug with short half life such as artemesinin compounds and a long acting drug like sulphadoxine- pyrimethamine (S-P). Artemisinin and its derivatives achieve the highest parasite killing rates and target asexual and sexual stages of parasite development in the blood with two important therapeutic consequences; prevention of clinical deterioration and interruption of transmission[30]. Combination of an artemisinin derivative with a long acting antimalarial drug reduces treatment duration from 7 days to 3 days and prevents recrudescence of the illness.The main ACTs are artesunate combined with either sulphadoxine-pyrimethamine or amodiaquine, artemether combined with lumefantrine, and dihydroartemisinin with piperaquine.

However, caution should be exercised in the manufacture, sale and use of artemesinin compounds, whether as oral medicines or parenteral formulations, since its overuse or use as monotherapy or irrational use can lead to rapid development of resistance, and we might lose the last weapon in our antimalarial armamentarium. The use of monoartesunate compounds should be strictly prohibited.

In India, reports of quinine resistance are extremely uncommon. Thus, quinine may offer an alternative in case artemesinin is not available. It is a rather safe drug if administered according to standard guidelines. There is a need to attain therapeutic levels of quinine as soon as possible for adequate antimalarial activity. Moreover, the levels of glycoproteins to which the quinine is partially bound, are raised during the acute phase of the malarial illness[31]. A loading dose will help in reaching the necessary concentration of unbound quinine. However, if the child has received oral quinine or mefloquine in the past two days, the loading dose should be avoided.

Quinine is a safe drug if used correctly. There is little or no hypoglycemia if the infusion is given slowly over four hours. It may cause orthostatic hypotension at times. If the infusion is slow, it is usually safe, although ventricular arrhythmias and hypotension are known to occur with quinine poisoning. Intramuscular injections of quinine are painful, but not dangerous. The dose of quinine should be reduced to one-half or one-third if the patient remains seriously ill for 48 hours or develops acute renal failure. The drug should be made oral as soon as feasible. The total duration of therapy should be 7 days.

Adverse effects due to quinine (cinchonism) include tinnitus, high tone deafness, nausea, malaise and blurring of vision. Blood glucose should be monitored every 3 hours due to risk of hypoglycemia because quinine is known to increase pancreatic insulin secretion.

Treatment schedule. Once the diagnosis is made and the decision to use an antimalarial is taken, one must weigh the child. Always calculate doses as mg/kg of body weight. If artemisinin derivatives are used, parenteral therapy should be switched over to oral artesunate 1 mg/kg/day for a total duration of 5-7 days. The dosage schedule for various antimalarial drugs for life-threatening malaria are given in Table 28.2. Therapy should be continued for 7 days (both parenteral + oral) along with doxycycline (4 mg/kg/day for 7 days) except in small children and pregnant women. Mefloquine is not recommended as maintenance antimalarial drug

Table 28.2 Drugs and their dosages for the management of severe malaria

Drugs	Preparation	Dose	Route	Method of administration	Duration
1. Quinine	Quinine dihydrochloride (cinkona 300 mg/ml, tabs of quinine sulphate 100 mg, 300 mg, 600 mg) Quinine dihydro-chloride 12 mg is equivalent to 10 mg base	20 mg/kg of salt (loading) and then 10 mg/kg/dose q 8 hr	IV/IM Oral	Dilute in 10 ml/kg of 5% dextrose or normal saline and infuse over 4 hrs (both loading and maintenance doses). Start oral therapy as soon as patient is able to take	7 days
2. Artesunate	Falcigo®/Arnate® 60 mg/ml; falcigo tab 50 mg, 100 mg, 200 mg as ACT	2.4 mg/kg followed by 1.2 mg/kg after 12 and 24 hours and then daily till patient is able to take orally. 4 mg/kg/day	IM/IV Oral once a day	Doxycycline 4 mg/kg/day for 7 days except in under-five children and pregnant women or single dose of 25 mg/1.25 mg sulfadoxine-pyremethamine	5-7 days
3. Artemether*	Paluther® 80 mg/ml	3.2 mg/kg (loading) 1.6 mg/kg after 12 hr and then 1.6 mg/kg daily	IM	- do -	5 days

* Artemether is an oil-based formulation, which releases drug slowly and erratically.

because of its association with post-malaria neurological syndrome[25].

There is no risk of relapse in patients with falciparum malaria but a single dose of primaquine 0.75mg/kg oral may be given to destroy gametocytes and prevent the spread of disease. Primaquine is contraindicated in G6PD deficient individuals, children below 1 year and pregnant women. There is still a need to administer primaquine following therapy with artemisinins because they do not have gametocidal effect. Antimalarial chemotherapy of chloroquine resistant severe malaria is summarized in the Box.

Supportive Therapy

Meticulous nursing care and strict maintenance of input output chart, blood sugar and electrolytes are important aspects of supportive management. Hyperpyrexia should be controlled by giving an antipyretic like paracetamol (15 mg/kg/dose q 4-6 hr), and use of tepid water sponging and fanning. Hydration should be maintained as children are often fluid depleted because of poor intake, vomiting, fever or stool losses. In a critically sick child, if possible, a central venous line or Swan-Ganz catheter should be inserted to guide fluid therapy.

The level of sensorium should be assessed by using the simple Blantyre score[32] (Table 28.3). The comatosed child should be nursed in lateral decubitus taking due care of airways, breathing, circulation, eye care, urethral catheter etc. It is strongly recommended to insert a nasogastric tube and suck out the stomach contents to minimize the risk of aspiration pneumonia. Aspiration pneumonia is a common and potentially fatal complication that must be prevented and promptly managed if it occurs. The child should be turned every 2 hours and particular attention be paid to pressure points. Do not allow the child to lie in a wet bed.

Mechanical ventilation is indicated in critically sick children with intercurrent pneumonia, pulmonary edema and ARDS. If it is decided to ventilate, the process of intubation and starting assisted ventilation should be very swift because even transient hypercapnia can further increase the already increased intracranial pressure of a parasite sequestered brain of a child.

Hypoglycemia is observed in 20%-35% of children with severe malaria at the time of presentation to the hospital. It seems that it is related to the severity of infection, rather than the side effects of any drug. Hypoglycemia is particularly common in children under 3 years and in those with

Section 4

Antimalarial chemotherapy of severe falciparum malaria and chloroquine-resistant malaria or when sensitivity is not known

Quinine: 20 mg dihydrochloride salt/kg (loading dose) diluted in a concentration of 1 mg/ml of normal saline or 5% dextrose is given as IV infusion over 4 hours; then 12 hours after the start of the loading dose, give a maintenance dose of quinine, 10 mg salt/kg, over 4 hours. This maintenance dose should be repeated every 8 hours, calculated from the beginning of the previous infusion, until the patient can swallow, then quinine sulfate tablets, 10 mg salt/kg, 8-hourly to complete a 7-day course of treatment and a single dose of 25 mg /kg sulfadoxine and 1.25 mg/kg pyrimethamine on day 1.

If IV infusion is not possible, quinine can be given IM . (If for some reason quinine cannot be administered by infusion, quinine dihydrochloride can be given in the same dosages by IM injection in the anterior thigh but not in the buttock. The dose of quinine should be divided between two sites – half the dose in each anterior thigh. If possible, for IM use, quinine should be diluted in normal saline to a concentration of 60–100 mg salt/ml and add xylocaine 0.5 ml of 2% solution to reduce local pain.

In areas where a 7-day course of quinine is not curative , add an oral course doxycycline 3 mg/kg once daily, for 3–7 days, as soon as the older child can swallow (Avoid in children under 8 years and pregnant women); If there is no clinical improvement after 48 hours of parenteral therapy, the maintenance dose of quinine should be reduced by one-third to one-half (i.e. 5–7 mg quinine dihydrochloride/kg 8-hourly).

Total daily doses of IV quinine in those patients who are not improving after 48 hours of parenteral therapy are as follows:

Day 1: 20 mg salt/kg of body weight

Day 2 and subsequent days: 10–14 mg salt/kg of body weight

It is unusual to continue IV infusions of quinine for more than 4–5 days. If it is more convenient, quinine may be given by continuous infusion (Infusion rates should not exceed 5 mg salt/kg of body weight per hour.) A loading dose of quinine should not be used if the patient has received quinine or mefloquine within the preceding 12 hours.

OR

Artesunate: 2.4 mg/kg (loading dose) IV, followed by 1.2 mg/kg at 12 and 24 hours, then 1.2 mg/kg daily for 6 days. If the patient is able to swallow, the child can be shifted to ACT which is given orally.

OR

Artemether: 3.2 mg/kg (loading dose) IM, followed by 1.6 mg/kg daily for 6 days. If the patient is able to swallow, the child can be shifted to ACT which is given orally

Artesunate suppositories: 200 mg intrarectally at 0, 12, 24, 36, 48 and 60 hours may prove to be highly effective and is on trial. A loading dose of 4 mg/kg intrarectally, followed by 2 mg/kg at 4, 12, 48 and 72 hours has been used in Vietnam. This treatment should be followed by an oral antimalarial drug.

N.B. If parenteral administration is not possible, and if artemisinin or artesunate suppositories are available, they may be given.

---

convulsions or hyperparasitemia or in profound coma. Although the threshold for treatment of hypoglycemia is blood glucose concentration less than 40 mg/dl, recent data suggest that use of a higher treatment threshold (around 72 mg/dl) might be more appropriate[33]. An interesting study which compared sick children with malarial and non malarial infections found an identical prevalence of hypoglycemia in both the groups[34]. It does not occur due to administration of quinine if it is infused slowly. Whatever be the cause, hypoglycemia is an important risk factor for morbidity and mortality in falciparum malaria[35]. Blood sugar should be monitored in all children with severe malarial infections. During treatment, blood sugar should be monitored every 4-6 hours till recovery of consciousness or till 48 hours.

If hypoglycemia occurs, give intravenous 50% dextrose in a dose of 1.0 ml/kg of body weight (0.5 g/kg) diluted in approximately the same volume of IV fluid slowly over several minutes or give 5 ml/kg of 10% dextrose bolus intravenously followed by a continuous infusion to maintain blood glucose levels. One should remember that hypoglycemia

Table 28.3 Blantyre coma scale for children

The "Blantyre coma scale" is a modified Glasgow coma scale (1974) and is designed to assess coma in children with malaria who have not learned to speak

	Score
Best motor response	
Localizes painful stimulus	2
Withdraws limb from painful stimulus	1
Best verbal response	
Appropriate cry with pain	2
Moans or inappropriate cry	1
No response	0
Eye movements	
Watches or directed (e.g. follows mother's face)	1
Fails to watch or follow is not direct	0
Nonspecific or absent response	0

The minimum Blantyre coma score is 0 which indicates poor outcome. The maximum score of 5 indicates good outcome. The score under 5 is considered as abnormal.

can occur even if the patient is on IV fluids. If it is not possible to give IV drugs or fluids, one can give 1 ml/kg of body weight of 50% dextrose or of any other sugar-based solution through a nasogastric tube.

If seizures occur, intravenous or intrarectal benzodiazepines, or intramuscular paraldehyde may be given. There is no role for prophylactic phenobarbital. In a large, randomised, controlled study in unventilated Kenyan children aged 9 months to 13 years with cerebral malaria, a single intramuscular dose of phenobarbital 20 mg/kg on admission was associated with substantially decreased frequency of seizures but increased mortality, possibly from respiratory depression[36.] Whether a lower dose of phenobarbital could reduce frequency of seizures without a concomitant rise in mortality remains to be seen. If seizures recur, phenytoin 15 mg/kg body weight may be given intravenously as a loading dose followed by 4-8 mg/kg daily till the day of discharge. However, hypoglycemia must always be ruled out and treated in children with malaria and seizures.

Children with cerebral malaria may continue to have altered sensorium even after correction of hypoglycemia and seizure control. As mentioned above, the raised intracranial pressure (ICP) seen in some children is not due to cerebral edema, hence steroids have no role. Meta-analysis of steroid therapy is cerebral malaria has shown greater risk of complications like GI bleeding and seizures, and delayed recovery of consciousness[37]. If there is evidence of raised ICP, osmotic diuretics may be used, though its role is controversial. Evidence from randomised trials does not support the use of single-dose mannitol as an adjunctive treatment[38]. Hemoconcentration due to diuresis may further slow the cerebral circulation and aggravate sludging.

As mentioned above, mortality of children with severe malarial anemia rises to 30–40% for children in whom anemia is complicated by severe respiratory distress and metabolic acidosis. Rapid blood transfusion can be life saving, The optimum volume and speed of transfusion are unknown[15, 39]. The sicker the child the more rapidly the transfusion needs to be given. If the hematocrit is less than 15% or the haemoglobin concentration is less than 5 g/dl in a child with signs of metabolic acidosis, give screened whole blood, 10 ml/kg of body weight over 30 minutes and a further 10 ml/kg of body weight over 1–2 hours[32]. A diuretic is usually not indicated as most of these children are hypovolemic. During convalescence supplements of folic acid should be given.

Acute renal failure is unusual in children with severe malaria. If it occurs, the maintenance dose of quinine is reduced to one-half or one-third. Peritoneal dialysis is indicated in case of persistent oliguria and rising creatinine levels. If available, hemodialysis is a better option. Indwelling urinary catheter should be removed as soon as it is no longer necessary.

Hemoglobinuria may occur and is, usually associated with high degree of parasitemia. In most cases it is not accompanied by renal failure and the normal doses of antimalarials including quinine can be continued. Blood transfusion may be required when it leads to severe anemia.

Gram-negative septicemia is a common superinfection in children with severe falciparum malaria. 127 (6%) of 2048 children admitted to hospital in Kenya and Mozambique with severe falciparum malaria had concurrent positive blood cultures (an underestimate of bacteremia), and case fatality increased in parasitemic children with invasive bacterial infection[40,41]. The indications for empiric antibiotic therapy include (i) fever that persists 48 hours after starting antimalarials, (ii) presence of shock or respiratory distress, (iii) those who are younger than one year and (iv) those with severe anemia.[42] Malaria and bacterial co-infection mainly occur with multidrug-resistant Gram-negative bacteria, particularly non-typhoidal salmonellae and the best choice of antibiotic would therefore be either a quinolone or third generation cephalosporin[43].

Section 4

While lethal hemorrhage is unusual in severe malaria, clinically significant bleeding, usually in the form of gastrointestinal hemorrhage may be seen in upto 10 percent of children. It may result due to thrombocytopenia or disseminated intravascular coagulation. The use of drugs that increase the risk of gastrointestinal bleeding such as aspirin and corticosteroids should be avoided. Supportive therapy with ranitidine, blood components and vitamin K is sometimes necessary; most patients, however, improve rapidly with antimalarial therapy.

Role of Exchange Blood Transfusion

Small isolated studies have documented therapeutic utility of exchange blood transfusion in children with life-threatening malaria but no randomized controlled trials exist. However, there is little, if any justification for doing this after the availability of artemesinin compounds since they bring the down the malarial counts very fast. More over, this procedure is not feasible in most endemic malaria situations and in older children. Exchange transfusion is no longer recommended for asymptomatic heavy parasitemia, whatever be the severity.

Common Errors in the Diagnosis and Management of Malaria

Although severe malaria is a common illness and most institutions provide effective therapy for it, errors in diagnosis and management of severe malaria are rather common, which contribute to adverse outcome. Many of these are avoidable, and must be remembered. The most frequent errors are listed below.

Errors in diagnosis

1. Failure to think of malaria in a patient with either typical or atypical illness.
2. Failure to elicit a history of exposure (travel history) to an area of high transmission.
3. Misjudgement of severity, especially in those who are conscious and yet sick or toxic.
4. Failure to do a thick blood film as a diagnostic test, and only relying on a thin smear.
5. Failure to identify *P. falciparum* in a dual infection with *P. vivax* (the latter may be more obvious).
6. Missed hypoglycemia either because there is no glucometer or not considering it as a problem among those who are conscious but sick.

7. Failure to diagnose other associated infections (bacterial, viral including HIV, etc.).
8. Failure to recognize respiratory distress (metabolic acidosis, ARDS).
9. Failure to carry out an ophthalmoscopic examination for the presence of papilledema, and retinal hemorrhages.

Errors in management

1. Inadequate nursing care , not keeping the patient on the side, not putting an NG tube in an unconscious patient.
2. Delay in starting antimalarial therapy, waiting for a positive report before giving the first dose of parenteral antimalarlals.
3. Use of inappropriate therapy i.e. chloroquine in areas of resistance and unjustified withholding of an antimalarial drug
4. Inappropriate dosage and route of administration of antimalarials like (i) inappropriate route of administration, (ii) unjustified cessation of treatment, (iii) failure to prevent cumulative toxic effects of antimalarial drugs.
5. Failure to switch patients from parenteral to oral therapy as soon as they can take oral medication.
6. Unnecessary continuation of chemotherapy beyond the recommended duration of treatment and failure to review antimalarial treatment in a patient whose condition is deteriorating.
7. Errors of fluid and electrolyte replacement due to failure to control the rate of intravenous infusion.
8. Failure to identify or treat metabolic acidosis.
9. Unduly delayed endotracheal intubation and ventilation where this is indicated.
10. Failure to control convulsions.
11. Failure to recognize and treat severe anemia.
12. Failure to give antibiotics for possible pyogenic meningitis if the decision is made to delay lumbar puncture.

PROGNOSIS

Mortality rates in severe malaria are still as high as 15 to 30% even if optimal and early treatment is instituted. Parasite density, hypoglycemia, lactic acidosis, severe anemia, multi-organ dysfunction, deep coma at admission and persistent seizures are recognized poor prognostic correlates. Although most children with cerebral malaria regain consciousness within 48 hours and seem to make a full neurological recovery, around 10 percent of children with cerebral malaria may have persistent neurological deficit in the form of protracted coma, cerebellar ataxia, hemiparesis, speech disorders, cortical blindness, behavioural disturbances, hypotonia or generalized spasticity and cranial nerve palsies[44]. As many as 50 percent of these recover completely within 6 months, while the rest may have variable degree of neurological deficits.

PREVENTION

Children with severe malaria and their families are perhaps the most receptive people to accept the advice for prevention. Use of a insecticide treated bednet at night and use of repellants at dusk time as personal protection measures should be recommended. Primaquine for gametocidal effect is advised for all children who are more than one year old. Often falciparum malaria attacks several family members almost at the same time. One must specifically ask about others in the family, so that they are investigated and treated in a timely fashion.

REFERENCES

1   http://www.nvbdcp.gov.in/Doc/Malaria-situation-april11.pdf, accessed on June 10, 2011

2.   Dhingra N, Jha P, Sharma VP, *et al.* for the Million Death Study Collaborators. Adult and child malaria mortality in India: a nationally representative mortality survey. *Lancet* 2010 Nov 20;376(9754):1768-74.

3.   A Profile of National Institute of Malaria Research. Estimation of True Malaria Burden in India. pp 91-99. Available at http://www.mrcindia.org/MRC_profile/profile2/Estimation of true malaria burden in India.pdf

4.   Kumar A, Valecha N, Jain T,. Dash AP. Burden of malaria in India: Retrospective and prospective view. *Amer J Trop Med Hyg* 77(Suppl 6), 2007, 77 (Suppl 6): 69–78.

5.   Singhal T. Management of severe malaria. *Indian J Pediatr* 2004; 71:81-88.

6.   World Health Organization. Division of Control of Tropical Diseases: Severe and complicated Malaria. *Trans R Soc Trop Med Hyg* 1990; 84 (suppl 2):1-65.

7.   World Health Organization. Severe falciparum malaria. *Trans R Soc Trop Med Hyg* 2000;94:1–90.

8.   Dondorp AM. Pathophysiology, clinical presentation and treatment of cerebral malaria. *Neurolgy Asia* 2005; 10:67-77.

9.   Jain Y, Kataria A, Kataria R, Jain R, D'Souza R. Stoop to conquer: an analysis of the epidemic of falciparum malaria in Chhattisgarh. Presentation made to the Department of Health, Government Of Chhattisgarh, Raipur, May 2, 2011.

10. Bruneel F, Hocqueloux L, Alberti C, Wolff M, Chevret S, Be´dos J-P, Durand R, Le Bras J, Re´gnier B, Vachon F. The clinical spectrum of severe imported falciparum malaria in the intensive care unit: report of 188 cases in adults. *Amer J Respir Crit Care Med* 2003;167: 684–689.

11. Drug Policy for Malaria, National Project Implementation Plan for National Vector Borne Disease Control Project (2008-2013), June 2008, pp 33-38.

12. Kocher DK, Saxena V, Singh N, *et al.* Plasmodium vivax malaria. *Emerg Infect Dis* 2005; 11:132-134.

13. Marsh K, Forster D, Waruiru C, *et al.* Indicators of lifethreatening malaria in African children. *N Engl J Med* 1995; 332: 1399–1404.

14. Crawley J, Smith S, Muthinji P, Marsh K, Kirkham F. Electroencephalographic and clinical features of cerebral malaria. *Arch Dis Child* 2001; 84: 247–53.

15. Idro R, Otieno G, White S, *et al.* Decorticate, decerebrate and opisthotonic posturing and seizures in Kenyan children with cerebral malaria. *Malar J* 2005; 4: 57.

16. White NJ. The management of severe falciparum malaria. *Am J Respir Crit Care Med* 2003 : 167; 673–677.

17. Beare NA, Taylor TE, Harding SP, Lewallen S, Molyneux ME. Malarial retinopathy: a newly established diagnostic sign in severe malaria. *Am J Trop Med Hyg* 2006; 75: 790–97.

18. English M, Waruiru C, Marsh K. Transfusion for respiratory distress in life-threatening childhood malaria. *Am J Trop Med Hyg* 1996; 55: 525–30.

19. Schellenberg D, Menendez C, Kahigwa E, *et al.* African children. with malaria in an area of intense *Plasmodium falciparum* transmission: features on admission to the hospital and risk factors for death. *Am J Trop Med Hyg* 1999; 61: 431–38.

20. Grau GE, Taylor TE, Molyneux ME, Wirima JJ, *et al.* Tumor necrosis factor and disease severity with flaciparum malaria. *N Engl J Med* 1989; 320:1586-1591.

21. Magowan C, Wollish W, Anderson L, Lecch J. Cytoadherence by *Plasmodium falciparum* infected erythrocytes is correlated with expression of a family of variable proteins on infected erythrocytes. *J Exp Med* 1988; 168:1307-1320.

22. Handunnetti SM, David PH, Perera KLRL and Mendis KN. Uninfected erythrocytes form 'rosettes' around *Plasmodium falciparum* infected erythrocytes. *Am J Trop Med Hyg* 1989; 40:115-118.

23. Clark IA, Budd AC, Alleva LM, Cowden WB. Human malarial disease: a consequence of inflammatory cytokine release. *Malar J* 2006; 5: 85.

Section 4

24. Waller D, Crawley J. Nosten F, *et al.* Intracranial pressure in childhood cerebral malaria. *Trans R Soc Trop Med Hyg* 1991; 85:362-264.

25. Spielman A, Perrone JB. Teklehaimanot. A, *et al.* Malaria diagnosis by direct observation centrifuged samples of blood. *Am J Trop Med Hyg* 1988; 39:337-342.

26. Jane Crawley, Cindy Chu, George Mtove, François Nosten. Malaria in children *Lancet* 2010; 375: 1468–1481.

27. Gomes MF, Faiz MA, Gyapong JO, *et al.* for the Study of 13 Research Group. Pre-referral rectal artesunate to prevent death and disability in severe malaria: a placebo-controlled trial. *Lancet* 2009; 373: 557–566.

28. Molyneux EM, Maitland K. Intravenous fluids—getting the balance right. *N Engl J Med* 2005; 353: 941–944.

29. The South East Asian Quinine Artesunate Malaria Trial (Seaquamat) Group. Artesunate versus quinine for treatment of severe falciparum malaria: a randomized trial. *Lancet* 2005; 336:717-725.

30. Sinclair D, Zani B, Donegan S, Olliaro P, Garner P. Artemisinin based combination therapy for treating uncomplicated malaria.Cochrane Database Syst Rev 2009; 3: CD007483.

31. Mansor SM. Molyneux ME, Taylor TE, *et al.* Effect of plasmodium falciparum malaria infection as the plasma concentration of alpha acid glycoprotein and the binding of quinine in Malawian children. *Br J Clin Pharmacol* 1991; 32:317-325.

32. Management of Severe Malaria: A Practical Handbook, *WHO, Geneva* 2000.

33. Achoki R, Opiyo N, English M. Mini-review: management of hypoglycemia in children aged 0–59 months. *J Trop Pediatr* 2009; published online Nov 23. DOI:10.1093/tropej/fmp109.

34. White NJ, Miller KD, Marsh K, *et al.* Hypoglycemia in African children with severe malaria. *Lancet* 1987; I: 708-711.

35. Taylor TE, Molyneaux ME, Wirima JJ, *et al.* Blood glucose levels in Malawian children before and during the administration of intravenous quinine in severe falciparum malaria. *N Engl J Med* 1988; 319:1040-1047.

36. Crawley J, Waruiru C, Mithwani S, *et al.* Effect of phenobarbital on seizure frequency and mortality in childhood cerebral malaria: a randomised, controlled intervention study. *Lancet* 2000; 355: 701–706.

37. Prasad K, Garner P. Steroids for treating cerebral malaria. *The Cochrane Database of Systematic Reviews.* 1999; Issue 3, Art No. CD 000972 D01:10.1002/14651858. CD000972.

38. Namutangula B, Ndeezi G, Byarugaba JS, Tumwine JK. Mannitol as adjunct therapy for childhood cerebral malaria in Uganda: a randomized clinical trial. *Malar J* 2007; 6: 138.

39. Maitland K, Pamba A, Newton CR, Levin M. Response to volume resuscitation in children with severe malaria. *Pediatr Crit Care Med* 2003; 4: 426–431.

40. Bassat Q, Guinovart C, Sigauque B, *et al.* Severe malaria and concomitant bacteremia in children admitted to a rural Mozambican hospital. *Trop Med Int Health* 2009; 14: 1011–1019.

41. Berkley JA, Bejon P, Mwangi T, *et al.* HIV infection, malnutrition, and invasive bacterial infection among children with severe malaria. *Clin Infect Dis* 2009; 49: 336–343.

42. Bronzan RN, Taylor TE, Mwenechanya J, *et al.* Bacteremia in Malawian children with severe malaria: prevalence, etiology, HIV coinfection, and outcome. *J Infect Dis* 2007; 195: 895–904.

43. Graham SM, English M. Non-typhoidal salmonellae: a management challenge for children with community-acquired invasive disease in tropical African countries. *Lancet* 2009; 373: 267–269.

44. Brewster DR, Kwiatkowski D, White NJ. Neurological sequelae of cerebral malaria in children. *Lancet* 1990; 336:1039-1043.

29

Dengue Fever and Severe Dengue Infection

SK Kabra, Rakesh Lodha and Tanu Singhal

INTRODUCTION

Dengue fever is caused by infection due to any one of the four serotypes of dengue viruses (Den 1, 2, 3 & 4). Dengue virus (DV) is a single-stranded RNA virus that belongs to the *flavivirus* genus of the Flaviviridae family. Infection is transmitted by female Aedes mosquitoes (*Aedes aegypti, Aedes albopictus*). In the past, dengue infections were classified by the WHO on the basis of severity as dengue fever, dengue hemorrhagic fever (DHF) and dengue shock syndrome (DSS). The accuracy of these terms in classifying dengue infections in endemic areas such as India and Thailand has recently been questioned. Hence, it may be more appropriate to refer to DHF and DSS as severe dengue infections[1, 2].

Dengue infections have become endemic in most of the South-East Asian countries including India. In the recent past several minor or major outbreaks have been reported from various parts of India[3]. Documented concurrent infections with all serotypes in Delhi indicates that this metropolitan city is now truly hyperendemic for dengue infection[4]. It has been observed that a large number of asymptomatic dengue infections precede and accompany severe dengue epidemics. It is estimated that during outbreaks, about 150-200 mild to silent infections occur in the community for each case of severe dengue infection[5]. Therefore, only a minority of individuals (3%) infected with DV develop severe dengue fever.

In the last 50 years, incidence of dengue fever has increased 30-fold with increasing geographic expansion to new countries and, in the present decade, from urban to rural settings. An estimated 50 million dengue infections occur annually and approximately 2.5 billion people live in dengue endemic countries[6].

PATHOGENESIS

Despite our growing understanding of various facets of the infection, its pathogenesis still remains unclear, with the possibility of several mechanisms being involved simultaneously. The virus is taken up by dendritic cells, and after antigen processing, presents it to T cells, leading to immune activation and release of a cascade of cytokines that are believed to mediate the systemic effects of plasma leakage and circulatory insufficiency. Thrombocytopenia develops due to the presence of cross-reacting antibodies to platelets and is responsible for the bleeding diathesis. The phenomenon of *'original antigenic sin'* may explain the increased severity of illness during secondary infections, due to the presence of antibodies to the previously infecting serotype. This leads to immune enhancement followed by development of severe dengue disease. In addition, there is evidence for increased apoptosis and endothelial cell dysfunction, which may also contribute to its pathogenesis. Dengue virus infection in infants may cause increased morbidity due to the presence of pre-existing maternal antibodies in endemic areas[7]. An alternative explanation for severe dengue suggests that certain strains of the dengue virus (South-East Asian) may be inherently capable of supporting severe antibody-enhanced infection than the virus in other geographic areas[8].

The major pathophysiologic changes that determine the severity of disease and differentiate it from dengue infection are plasma leakage into third space and abnormal hemostasis leading to rising hematocrit values and moderate to marked thrombocytopenia along with varying degree of bleeding manifestations[9]. The cause of abnormal leakage of plasma, which is a characteristic feature of severe dengue infection, is not known. However, rapid recovery without residual abnormality in vessels suggests that it is the result of release and interaction of biological mediators which are capable of producing severe illness with minimal structural injury[7].

CLINICAL MANIFESTATIONS

Dengue infection has a broad range of clinical manifestations and often with unpredictable clinical evolution and outcome. Incubation period varies between 4-10 days. Most infections are subclinical. Infants and young children may present with an undifferentiated febrile illness. The classic presentation of dengue fever is usually seen in older children, adolescents and adults and can be described under three phases; febrile, critical and recovery phases[6].

1. *Febrile phase.* It is characterized by sudden onset of high-grade fever that may last for 2–7 days. There may be facial flushing, skin erythema (scarlitiniform or maculopapular skin rash), generalized body aches, myalgias, arthralgias, headache, pain in eyes, back ache, anorexia, nausea and vomiting. Occasionally child may have sore throat, injected pharynx and conjunctival injection. Relative bradycardia and electrocardiographic changes may be seen in older children and adults. A positive tourniquet test may be seen in some patients. Minor hemorrhagic manifestations; petechiae and mucosal bleeding (e.g. nose and gums) may be seen in some patients. Liver may be enlarged and tender after 2-5 days and indicates risk for development of severe illness. There is progressive decrease in total white cell count and platelet count,

2. *Critical phase.* This phase is seen between 3-7 days of onset of fever when defervescence sets in. Child may develop bleeding manifestations and shock with fall in platelet count and increase in packed cell volume (PCV). During defervescence of fever, the patient develops features of capillary leakage in the form of puffiness, edema, ascites and pleural effusion especially on the right side. The profound leakage of plasma from capillaries may lead to hypovolemia resulting in shock-related symptoms in the form of restlessness, cold and clammy extremities, rapid thready pulse, low blood pressure with narrow pulse pressure (< 20 mm Hg), poor tissue perfusion (delayed capillary refill) and oliguria. Some children may develop organ dysfunction such as severe hepatitis, encephalitis or myocarditis and/or severe bleeding without any obvious plasma leakage or shock.

3. *Recovery phase.* After 24-48 hour of critical phase, a gradual reabsorption of extravasated fluid takes place in 48-72 hours. General well-being improves, appetite returns, gastro-intestinal symptoms abate, haemodynamic status stabilizes and diuresis ensues. Some patients may have a skin rash suggestive of *"isles of white in the sea of red"*. During recovery patents may demonstrate desquamation with marked itching of extremities, palms and soles. Due to reabsorption of extravasated plasma back into vascular compartment some children may develop respiratory distress due to pulmonary edema during recovery. PCV stabilizes or may become lower due to the dilution. Total leukocyte count returns back to normal after defervescence but rise in platelet count is slow. The following clinical and laboratory features may suggest presence of severe dengue infection.

Clinical criteria. Acute onset of high-grade fever, hemorrhagic manifestations (at least a positive tourniquet test), tender hepatomegaly, effusion in body cavities and or shock.

Laboratory criteria. Thrombocytopenia (1,00,000 cells per cubic mm or less or less than 1-2 platelets per oil immersion field), and rising hematocrit.

DIFFERENTIAL DIAGNOSIS

During an epidemic, diagnosis of dengue fever is easy. Differential diagnosis for dengue infection include influenza, malaria, enteric fever, leptospirosis and less commonly meningococcemia and rickettsial infections. Malaria, leptospirosis, flu and enteric fever may also be coinfected with dengue[10]. Several other viruses known to cause severe hemorrhagic fever like Ebola viruses and Marburg viruses have not been reported from India as yet. Two other hemorrhagic fever viruses Hanta virus and Crimean Congo hemorrhagic virus have been reported recently in India[11, 12]. Wide spread chikungunya virus infections have occurred in various parts of India and South-East Asia. Its clinical manifestations are similar to dengue. However, fever is of shorter duration, thrombocytopenia and bleeding manifestations are less common. Other clinical features that are more common in chikungunya include skin eruptions, mucosal lesions, polyarthralgia and encephalopathy[13]. Since dengue as well as chikungunya infections are endemic in most parts of India, both infections may occur together[14].

LABORATORY INVESTIGATIONS

During the course of illness, children with severe dengue infection show gradual increase in packed cell volume (PCV), decrease in platelet and leukocyte count with increase in lymphocyte population. Rising hematocrit or a single hematocrit value of more than 40% or retrospectively when peak hematocrit is more than 20% of the hematocrit at the time of recovery are suggestive of hemoconcentration due to wide spread capillary leakage. A low WBC count in a child with febrile illness during the endemic season is a pointer towards possible dengue infection. However, malaria and typhoid/paratyphoid may also present with low WBC count though the leukopenia tends to be more severe in dengue. The peripheral smear may show transformed lymphocytes[15, 16]. In severe illness with shock there may be evidences of disseminated intravascular coagulation (DIC).

Serum chemistry may show decrease in total protein and albumin, which is more marked in patients with shock[17]. Levels of transaminases are usually raised. A higher increase in SGOT than SGPT suggests the possibility of dengue infection rather than other viral infection[18]. In severe cases there may be hyponatremia, and acidosis along with increase in blood urea nitrogen and creatinine[19].

Skiagram of the chest or ultrasound examination may show varying degrees of pleural effusion, commonly on the right side and occasionally bilateral[20]. Ultrasonography of abdomen may show ascites and enlarged gall bladder due to wall edema[21]. Abnormal electrocardiogram and myocardial dysfunction on echocardiogram has also been reported[22, 23]. The mechanism of decreased cardiac output during toxic stage of DHF is complex. Decreased preload is accompanied by decreased left ventricular performance, and possibly a subnormal heart rate response in some patients[24]. Activation of complement system leads to profound depression of C_3 and C_5 levels.

Confirmation of diagnosis of dengue may be established by direct methods of isolation of virus by culture, genome detection by PCR and NS1 antigen detection[25]. Virus isolation or PCR requires the sample to be obtained within the first 5 days of fever, is technically demanding, not universally available, expensive and hence of limited practical use. NS1 antigen is a highly conserved glycoprotein of dengue virus and secreted during the initial phase of illness. It disappears as the antibodies appear and its level declines as illness advances and in secondary dengue infections. The specificity of NS1 antigen is nearly 100% and sensitivity in the first

four days of illness is 90% in primary dengue and 70% in secondary dengue infection[26].

Indirect methods for diagnosis of dengue infection based on antibody determination need careful interpretation[27]. Following primary dengue infection, 80% of patients will have detectable IgM antibodies by day 5 and 99% by day 10. IgM antibodies peak by day 14 and are undetectable by two to three months. Dengue-specific IgG antibodies rise later, peak to levels which are lower than IgM, decline slowly and remain detectable at low levels for life. Following secondary dengue infection, there is a rapid IgG response in the first 2-3 days, peaking to levels much higher than primary dengue infection. In secondary dengue infection, the IgM antibodies rise later, are blunted and may be absent in some patients. *Therefore, diagnosis of primary dengue infection is based on elevation of dengue-specific IgM and that of secondary dengue infection by early and rapid elevation of dengue-specific IgG antibodies.* Since, diagnosis of secondary dengue is of clinical importance, commercial kits which are able to differentiate the IgG response of secondary dengue from primary or past dengue infection should be used. Rapid tests do not usually fulfill this requirement. The drawbacks of serologic diagnosis include false negativity in early illness, cross reactivity with other flavivirus infections such as Japanese encephalitis, marked variability between kits and different cut offs in different endemic areas. The role of serology is hence limited to provide a retrospective diagnosis and is of no use in management of the patient.

> *Early and rapid elevation of dengue-specific IgG antibodies is a reliable marker of secondary infection with dengue virus and is associated with an increased risk of severe dengue infection.*

The cornerstone for diagnosis and patient management still remains rigorous serial clinical and blood count monitoring. However, if serologic diagnosis of dengue is attempted, the best sensitivity is achieved with estimation of NS1 antigen, dengue-specific IgM and IgG all together in a single sample at the time of presentation[28].

MANAGEMENT

Patients with dengue infection can be classified as asymptomatic or may have symptomatic undifferentiated fever, dengue without warning signs, dengue with warning signs and severe dengue infection.

(i) **Undifferentiated fever**. These patients have non specific symptoms and are diagnosed during an epidemic. They are treated with supportive measures like administration of paracetamol, nursing in a cool room, intake of plenty of fluids and regular monitoring for development of any complications.

(ii) **Dengue infection without warning signs**. Patients with fever, bodyaches, rashes or minor bleeding may be treated symptomatically. Fever and bodyaches are best treated with paracetamol.

> *During an epidemic of dengue fever, every febrile episode should preferably be treated with paracetamol. NSAIDs and aspirin should be avoided due to potential risk of aggravating bleeding manifestations.*

Salicylates and other non-steroidal anti-inflammatory drugs (NSAIDs) should be avoided as these may predispose the child to develop mucosal bleeds. Child should be encouraged to drink plenty of fluids. There is no specific antiviral therapy. In an epidemic setting all patients need regular monitoring by a primary care physician for early detection of severe disease. The primary care physician/health care worker should monitor the patient for warning signs along with hematocrit and platelet counts. Any patient who develops warning signs as listed below should be admitted to a hospital.

(iii) **Dengue with warning signs**. Children with suspected dengue infection who have any of the following features should be admitted to the hospital.

- Abdominal pain or tenderness
- Persistent vomiting
- Fluid accumulation in pleural cavity, abdomen or subcutaneous tissues
- Mucosal bleeds
- Lethargy, restlessness or irritability
- Liver enlargment >2 cm
- Progressive increase in HCT with concurrent decrease in platelet count.

These patients should be admitted in the hospital and given intravenous fluids. Crystalloids are the preferred fluids. A study comparing different fluid regimes suggested some benefits of colloids in children presenting with lower pulse pressures[29]. Further large-scale studies, stratified for pulse pressure, are required before making a general recommendation. The management of severe dengue infection demands high levels of expertise and skills for administration of fluids and electrolytes to correct hypovolemia due to leakage of serum from capillaries into the extravascular compartment. In the hospital, all children should be given Ringer's lactate or normal saline infusion at a rate of 7 ml/kg over one hour. After one hour, if PCV has decreased and vital parameters are improving, fluid infusion rate should be decreased to 5 ml/kg over next hour and to 3 ml/kg/hour for subsequent 24-48 hours with frequent monitoring of PCV and vital parameters. When the patient is stable as indicated by normal blood pressure, good oral intake and urine output, the child can be discharged.

If after one hour PCV is rising and vital parameters do not show improvement, fluid infusion rate is increased to 10 ml/kg over next hour. In case of no further improvement, fluid infusion rate is further increased to 15 ml/kg over next hour (3rd hour). If no improvement is observed either in vital parameters or PCV at the end of 3 hours; colloids or plasma infusion in doses of 10 ml/kg is administered (Figure 29.1). Once the PCV and vital parameters are stable the infusion rate is gradually reduced and discontinued over 24–48 hours.

(iv) **Severe dengue**. Children presenting or developing any of the following complications are diagnosed to have severe dengue infection.

- Severe plasma leakage leading to
  - Shock, delayed capillary refill or oliguria
  - Fluid accumulation in serosal cavities with respiratory distress
- Severe bleeding manifestations
- Severe organ involvement
  - Liver: Hepatomegaly, liver failure, AST or ALT $\geq$1000 units
  - CNS: Impaired consciousness
  - Heart: Myocardial dysfunction

Children classified as severe dengue should be hospitalized (preferably in PICU) and treated aggressively with supportive care. Normal saline or lactated Ringer's solution; 10-20 ml/kg is infused over one hour or given as a bolus if blood pressure is unrecordable (DSS IV). Normal saline is better and preferred solution because Ringer's lactate is hypotonic. In critically sick children it is preferable to establish two IV lines, one for administration of normal saline and other for infusing 5% dextrose

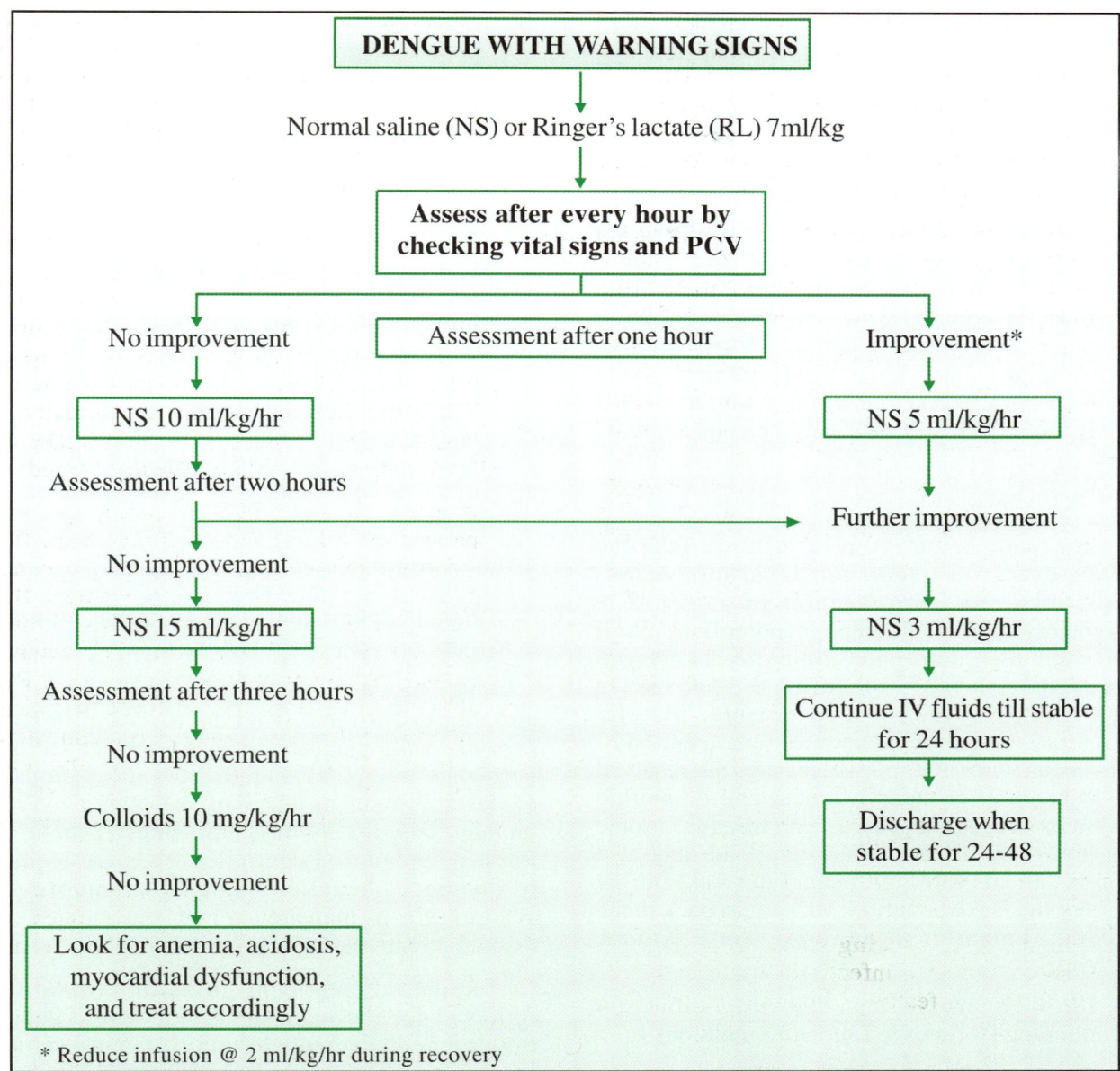

Figure 29.1 Protocol for intravenous fluid therapy

and potassium. If there is no improvement in vital parameters and PCV is rising; colloids 10 ml/kg is infused rapidly. Alternatively if PCV is falling without any improvement in vital parameters; blood transfusion should be given with the presumption that lack of improvement is due to occult blood loss (Figure 29.2). Once improvement starts the infusion rate of fluids is gradually decreased. In addition to fluid management, oxygen should be administered to all patients with shock.

The child should be closely monitored for various complications which should be identified early and managed effectively.

Bleeding manifestations

For uncontrolled bleeding in severe dengue infection, the role of plasma or platelet infusion remains unclear[30, 31]. Platelet counts are unreliable to predict bleeding. In a small study in which children with severe thrombocytopenia were included, platelet infusion did not alter the outcome of patients[32].

(a) *Petechial spots or mild mucosal bleed but hemodynamically stable.* These patients needs supportive care including bed rest, maintenance of hydration and monitoring. Avoid IM injections. There is no role of prophylactic platelet rich plasma (PRP) infusions even with severe thrombocytopenia. Avoid any procedures predisposing to mucosal trauma. If indicated insert NG tube with great care.

(b) *Severe bleeding, hemodynamic instability and excessive mucosal bleeds.* These patients should be treated with blood transfusion and monitoring. There is little evidence to support the practice of transfusing platelet concentrates and/or fresh-frozen plasma for severe bleeding. When massive bleeding cannot be managed with fresh whole blood/fresh-packed cells and possibility of DIC is there, FFP and PRP may be considered.

Fluid overload[6]

The causes of fluid overload in dengue infection include excessive and/or too rapid intravenous fluids; incorrect use of hypotonic rather than isotonic crystalloid solutions; inappropriate use of large volumes of intravenous fluids in patients with unrecognized severe bleeding; inappropriate transfusion of fresh-frozen plasma, platelet concentrates and cryoprecipitates; continuation of intravenous fluids after plasma leakage has resolved (24-48 hours after defervescence) and co-morbid conditions such as congenital heart disease, chronic lung and renal disease. Fluid overload may also occur in patients with significant fluid leak. During recovery the leaked out fluid will return back to the vascular compartment and may cause volume overload.

Fluid overload can be prevented by discontinuing IV fluids in following situations.

- Cessation of signs of plasma leakage as suggested by stable blood pressure, pulse volume and peripheral perfusion; and decrease in hematocrit in the presence of a good pulse volume.
- Afebrile for more than 24–48 days (without the use of antipyretics).
- Resolving bowel/abdominal symptoms.
- Improving urine output.

(i) *Fluid overload with stable hemodynamic status and the patient is out of the critical phase (more than 24-48 hours of defervescence).* In such patients stop intravenous fluids but continue close monitoring. If necessary, give oral or intravenous furosemide 0.1–0.5 mg/kg/dose once or twice daily, or a continuous infusion of furosemide 0.1 mg/kg/hour. Monitor serum potassium and correct any hypokalemia.

(ii) *Fluid overload with stable hemodynamic status but patient is still in a critical phase.* Reduce the intravenous fluids gradually. Avoid diuretics during the plasma leakage phase because they may lead to intravascular volume depletion. Patients who remain in shock with low or normal hematocrit levels but show signs of fluid overload may have occult hemorrhage. Further infusion of large volumes of intravenous fluids alone will lead to a poor outcome. Careful fresh whole blood transfusion should be given as soon as possible. If the patient remains in shock and the hematocrit is elevated, repeated small boluses of a colloid solution may be administered.

Other supportive measures

Renal replacement therapy. Renal failure is best managed with veno-venous hemodialysis.

Vasopressor and inotropic therapies. They are indicated if there is no improvement in blood pressure with adequate fluid replacement despite normal or raised CVP. In refractory shock, infusion of desmopressin in doses of 0.3 mg/kg over 30 minutes daily for 3-4 days have shown benefit[33, 34]. Further randomized controlled trials are required to document beneficial role of desmopressin/ vasopressin in management of shock in severe dengue infections.

Standard treatment guidelines should be followed for the management of severe hepatic involvement, encephalopathy or encephalitis, cardiac conduction abnormalities and fluid and electrolyte abnormalities.

There is no therapeutic utility of corticosteroids[35]. Broad spectrum antibiotics are indicated for treatment of superadded bacterial infection. Blood transfusion (20 ml/kg) is indicated when shock persists despite declining hematocrit values (which are indicative of adequate fluid replacement) due to overt or internal hemorrhage. There is no role of intravenous immunoglobulins or recombinant activated Factor VII[6].

All children with hypotension should receive oxygen inhalation by nasal cannula/ face mask or oxygen hood. A small study on 37 children in severe dengue with respiratory failure demonstrated significant benefit of nasal CPAP over oxygen by nasal cannula[36].

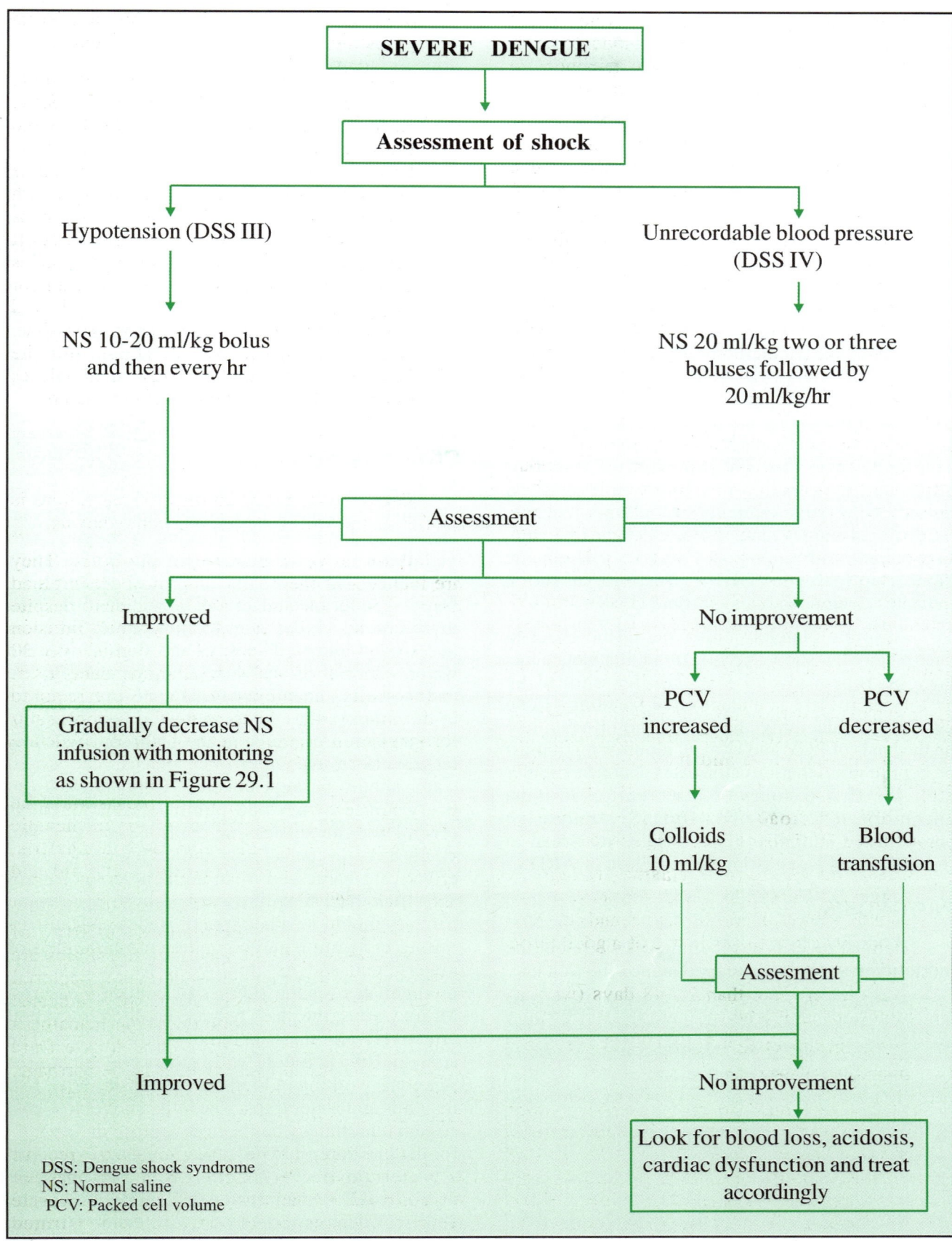

Figure 29.2 Treatment algorithm for severe dengue infection

MONITORING

In view of the dramatic course of severe dengue, monitoring of the patient is crucial in the first few hours of illness. Heart rate, respiratory rate, blood pressure and pulse pressure should be monitored every 30 minutes till the patient is stable, thereafter monitoring should be continued every 2-4 hours as long as the child is in the hospital. In critically ill children, central venous pressure and accurate urine output with an indwelling urinary catheter should be monitored. However, difficulties encountered in monitoring CVP in critically sick children is a limiting factor for its routine use. The laboratory monitoring includes PCV measurement by microhematocrit method every one hour for first 4 hours or till it shows a stable result. In monitoring hematocrit, one should bear in mind the possible effect of pre-existing anemia, severe hemorrhage and early volume replacement therapy. Presence of pleural effusion on skiagram of chest or ultrasound examination or hypoalbuminemia can provide supportive evidences of plasma leakage, the distinguishing feature of severe dengue infection. In a patient with provisional diagnosis of dengue hemorrhagic fever (DHF), presence of shock indicates dengue shock syndrome (DSS).

Absolute platelet counts should be checked once a day till it shows a rising trend. Platelet counts may be repeated and DIC studies should be performed if there is uncontrolled bleeding (Table 29.1). While deciding about the fluid infusion rate on the basis of PCV and clinical monitoring, it must be kept in mind that infusion rates decrease rapidly after the first 6 hours of intervention in most uncomplicated cases of DHF/DSS[37]. Excessive unmonitored administration of fluids may lead to fluid overload, congestive heart failure or ARDS.

PROGNOSIS

Dengue fever is a self-limited disease but the mortality in severe secondary dengue infection may be as high as 40–50 percent if left untreated. Early recognition of illness, careful monitoring and appropriate fluid therapy alone has resulted in reduction of case fatality rate to 1-5 percent[38]. There are several other causes of viral hemorrhagic fever that have worst outcome. Early recognition of shock is of paramount importance as the outcome of a patient with DSS depends on the duration of shock. If shock is identified when pulse pressure starts getting narrow and intravenous fluids are administered at this stage, the outcome is excellent. Recovery is fast and majority of patients recover completely in 24-48 hours without any residual sequelae. The prognosis is grave in patients with prolonged shock and when blood pressure is not recordable. Other adverse correlates of outcome include encephalopathy, DIC, myocardial dysfunction and ARDS.

PREVENTION

Preventive measures are directed towards elimination of adult mosquitoes and their larvae. During epidemics aerial spraying or fogging with malathion is recommended for control of adult mosquitoes. However, larval control measures by source reduction and use of larvicides are even more crucial. *Aedes aegypti* mosquitoes breed in and around human dwellings and flourish in fresh water. Special drives should be launched during and soon after the rainy season to interrupt breeding cycle of mosquitoes. There should be no opportunity for stagnation of water in the bathroom, kitchen, terrace, lawn and other open places. The stored water should be kept covered. Cooperation from every house owner and public establishment is crucial for the success of control program. The youth force in the schools and colleges should be effectively harnessed to strengthen vector control activities. The hospital wards admitting dengue patients should be made free of Aedes mosquitoes. Strong motivation and commitment on the part of government and its employees are fundamental prerequisites for the success of control measures. Mesocyclops, the shell fish are credited to eat and effectively eliminate larvae of *Aedes aegypti*. The strategy has been used with success by Australian scientists working in Vietnam by growing shell fish in ponds and water traps. Recently a novel low cost sustainable strategy has been developed in Australia for dengue control by infecting *Aedes aegypti* with a bacterium *Wolbachia pipientis*. The presence of *Wolbachia* in the infected mosquitoes blocks the ability of dengue virus to grow in them. When an infected male mosquito mates with an uninfected female, all her eggs die. And when an infected,

---

Table 29.1 Monitoring of critically sick children with severe dengue infection

- Vital signs every 30 min till stable
- Hematocrit every one hr for first 4-6 hr, then every 4 hr for 24 hours. Monitor 12 hourly during recovery.
- Fluid balance sheet: Type of fluid, amount, rate etc.
- Accurate urine output
- Platelet count, serum electrolytes, blood gases and acid base parameters every 12-24 hr.
- DIC profile, liver and renal function tests as and when indicated.
- Weight every 12 hr

female mosquito mates with an uninfected male, the eggs do hatch normally but all the eggs carry *Wolbachia*. When this process continues over a period of time, all the species of *Aedes aegyptiae* are likely to get infected with *Wolbachia* and these mosquitoes become incapable of transmitting dengue infection. A live attenuated quadruple vaccine is undergoing clinical trials but there are concerns whether vaccine may predispose to development of DHF in some cases. Education of parents for rational management of febrile children with adequate fluids and early recognition of danger signs of DHF or evidence of shock would go a long way to improve their survival.

REFERENCES

1. Srikiatkhachorn A, Gibbons RV, Green S, *et al.* Dengue hemorrhagic fever: the sensitivity and specificity of the World Health Organization definition for identification of severe cases of dengue in Thailand,1994-2005. *Clin Infect Dis* 2010; 50: 1135-1143.

2. Gupta P, Khare V, Tripathi S, *et al.* Assessment of World Health Organization definition of dengue hemorrhagic fever in north India. *J Infect Dev Countr* 2010 Mar 29; 4(3):150-155.

3. Chaturvedi UC, Nagar R. Dengue and dengue haemorrhagic fever: Indian perspective. *J Biosci* 2008; 33: 429-441.

4. Bharaj P, Chahar HS, Pandey A, Diddi K, Dar L, Guleria R, Kabra SK, Broor S. Concurrent infections by all four dengue virus serotypes during an outbreak of dengue in 2006 in Delhi, India. *Virology J* 2008, 5:1.

5. Anonymous. Clinical diagnosis. In: Dengue haemorrhagic fever, Diagnosis, Treatment, Prevention and Control; 2nd edition, *Geneva, World Health Organization* 1997; pp 12-23.

6. Anonymous. Dengue Guidelines for Diagnosis, Treatment, Prevention and Control. A joint publication of the World Health Organization (WHO) and the Special Programme for Research and Training in Tropical Diseases (TDR), 2009.

7. Guglani L, Kabra SK. T-cell immunopathogenesis of dengue virus infection. *Dengue Bulletin* 2005; 29: pp. 58-69.

8. Halstead SB. Dengue hemorrhagic fever. In: Hand book of Viral and Rickettsial Haemorrhagic Fevers. Gear JHS (Ed). *Boca Raton, Florida CRC Press* 1988, pp. 85-94.

9. Navarro-Sanchez E, Despres P, Cedillo-Barron L. Innate immune response to dengue virus. *Arch Med Res* 2005; 36:425-435.

10. Karande S, Gandhi D, Kulkarni M, Bharadwaj R, *et al.* Concurrent outbreak of leptospirosis and dengue in Mumbai, India. *J Trop Pediatr* 2005; 51:174-181.

11. Chandy S, Abraham S, Sridharan G. Hantaviruses: an emerging public health threat in India? A review. *J Biosci* 2008 Nov; 33(4):495-504.

12. WHO. First documented case of human Crimean-Congo Haemorrhagic Fever (CCHF) in India. Accessed on 14/7/2011. Available at URL http://www.searo.who.int/en/Section10/Section369/Section2504_15923.htm

13. Sebastian MR, Lodha R, Kabra SK. Chikungunya infection in children. *Indian J Pediatr* 2009; 76: 185-189.

14. Chahar HS, Bharaj P, Dar L, Guleria R, Kabra SK, Broor S. Co-infections with chikungunya virus and dengue virus in Delhi, India. *Emerg Infect Dis* 2009; 15: 1077-1080.

15. Suvatte V, Longsaman M. Diagnostic value of buffy coat preparation in dengue hemorrhagic fever. *South East Asian J Trop Med Pub Health* 1979; 10:7-12.

16. Nimmannitya. Clinical manifestations of dengue/dengue hemorrhagic fever. In: Monograph on Dengue/Dengue Hemorrhagic Fever, *New Delhi. WHO regional publication SEARO* 22, 1993, pp 48-54.

17. Sumarmo HW, Jahja E, Guber DJ, Subaryono W, Soremsem K. Clinical observations on virologically confirmed fatal dengue infection in Jakarta. *Bull WHO* 1983; 61: 693-701.

18. Nguyen TL, Nguyen TH, Tieu NT. The impact of dengue hemorrhagic fever on liver function. *Res Virol* 1997; 148: 273-277.

19. Pongphanich B, Kumponpant S. Studies of dengue hemorrhagic fever, hemodynamic studies of clinical shock associated with dengue hemorrhagic fever. *J Pediatr* 1973; 83: 1073-1077.

20. Kabra SK, Verma IC, Arora NK, Jain Y, Kalra V. Dengue hemorrhagic fever in children in Delhi. *Bull WHO* 1992; 70:105-108.

21. Setiawan MW, Samsi TK, Pool TN, Sugianto D, Wulur H. Gall bladder wall thickening in dengue hemorrhagic fever: an ultrasonographic study. *J Clin Ultrasound* 1995; 23:357-362.

22. Wong HB, Tan G, Cardiac involvement in haemorrhagic fever. *J Singapore Pediatr Soc* 1967; 9:28-35.

23. Kabra SK, Juneja R, Madhulika, *et al.* Myocardial dysfunction in children with dengue hemorrhagic fever. *Natl Med J India* 1998,11; 59-61

24. Khongphatthanayothin A, Suesaowalak M, Muangmingsook S, Bhattarakosol P, Pancharoen C. Hemodynamic profiles of patients with dengue hemorrhagic fever during toxic stage: an echocardiographic study. *Intensive Care Med* 2003; 29: 570-574.

25. Shu PY, Huang JH. Current advances in dengue diagnosis. *Clin Diag Lab Immunol* 2004, 11: 642–650.

26. Datta S, Wattal C. Dengue NS 1 antigen. A useful tool for early diagnosis of dengue virus infection. *Indian J Med Microbiol* 2010; 28: 107-110.

Section 4

27. Anonymous. Laboratory diagnosis. In: Dengue Haemorrhagic Fever: diagnosis, treatment, prevention and control, 2nd edition. *Geneva, World Health Organisation* 1997; pp 34-47.

28. Mui Wang SM, Sekaran SD. Evaluation of a commercial SD dengue virus NS1 antigen capture enzyme-linked immunosorbent assay for early diagnosis of dengue virus infection. *J Clin Microbiol* 2010; 48: 2793-97.

29. Ngo NT, Cao XT, Kneen R, et al. Acute management of dengue shock syndrome: a randomized double-blind comparison of 4 intravenous fluid regimens in the first hour. *Clin Infect Dis* 2001; 32:204-213.

30. Lum LC, Goh AY, Chan PW, El-Amin AL, Lam SK. Risk factors for hemorrhage in severe dengue infections. *J Pediatr* 2002; 140:629-631.

31. Chuansumrit A, Phimolthares V, Tardtong P, Tapaneya-Olarn C, Tapaneya-Olarn W, Kowsathit P, Chantarojsiri T. Transfusion requirements in patients with dengue hemorrhagic fever. *Southeast Asian J Trop Med Public Health* 2000; 31:10-14.

32. Kabra SK, Jain Y, Madhulika, *et al*. Role of platelet transfusion in dengue hemorrhagic fever. *Indian Pediatr* 1998; 35: 452-454.

33. Vasudevan A, Lodha R, Kabra SK. Vasopressin infusion in children with catecholamine-resistant septic shock. *Acta Paediatr* 2005; 93: 380- 383.

34. Pea L, Roda L, Moll F. Desmopressin treatment for a case of dengue hemorrhagic fever/dengue shock syndrome. *Clin Infect Di*s 2001; 33:1611-1612.

35. Tassniyom S, Vaanawathan S, Chirawatkal V, Rojanasuphot S. Failure of high dose methyl prednisolone in established dengue shock syndrome: A placebo controlled double blind study. *Pediatrics* 1993; 92; 111-115.

36. Cam BV, Tuan DT, Fonsmark L, Poulsen A, Tien NM, Tuan HM, Heegaard ED. Randomized comparison of oxygen mask treatment vs. nasal continuous positive airway pressure in dengue shock syndrome with acute respiratory failure. *J Trop Pediatr* 2002; 48:335-339.

37. Kabra SK, Jain Y, Pandey RM, *et al*. Dengue hemorrhagic fever in children in the 1996 Delhi epidemic. *Trans Royal Society Trop Med Hygiene* 1999; 93:1-5

38. Halstead SB. Global epidemiology of dengue; health system in disarray. *Trop Med* 1993; 137-146.

Acute Severe Asthma

GR Sethi and Vineet Sehgal

Acute exacerbations of asthma are acute episodes of progressively worsening shortness of breath, cough, wheezing, chest tightness or a combination of these symptoms. An acute severe exacerbation of asthma that does not respond to conventional therapy is called status asthmaticus.

Acute severe attack of asthma is an important cause of morbidity, school absenteeism and frequent visits to the clinic or hospital. There is enough data globally to prove that the prevalence and severity of asthma is increasing[1-4]. There has been an increase in mortality as well, particularly in younger age groups[5-8]. This chapter deals with management of acute severe asthma. A stepwise approach is necessary for appropriate management. The steps in management are:

1. Assessment of severity and identification of life threatening attack.
2. Initiation of therapy
3. Assessment of response to initial therapy
4. Modification of or additions to therapy and referral.

Step 1. INITIAL ASSESSMENT OF SEVERITY

Identification of Life-threatening Attack

Initial assessment is necessary to rapidly determine the degree of airway obstruction and hypoxia. One can immediately identify severe or life- threatening patients and give them vigorous therapy even before undertaking a detailed assessment (Tables 30.1 and 30.2).

Table 30.1 Estimation of severity of acute exacerbation of asthma			
Symptom/sign	**Mild**	**Moderate**	**Severe**
• Respiratory rate	Normal	Increased	Increased or gasping
• Alertness	Normal	Normal	May be restless or drowsy
• Dyspnea	Absent or mild, speaks in complete sentences	Moderate; speaks in phrases or partial sentences	Severe; speaks only in single words or short phrases
• Pulses paradoxus	<10 mm Hg	10-20 mg Hg	20-40 mm Hg
• Accessory muscle use	No or mild intercostal retractions	Moderate intercostal retractions with tracheosternal retractions, use of sternocleido-mastoid muscles	Severe intercostal and tracheosternal retractions with nasal flaring
• Color	Pink	Pale	Ashen grey or cyanotic
• Auscultation	End expiratory wheeze only	Wheeze during entire expiration and inspiration	Breath sounds becoming almost inaudible
• Oxygen saturation	>95%	90-95%	<90%
• $paCO_2$	<35 mm Hg	35-40 mg Hg	>40 mm Hg
• PEFR	70-90% of predicted or personal best	50-70% of predicted or personal best	< 50% of predicted or personal best

PEFR: Peak expiratory flow rate.

Table 30.2 Assessment of severity of acute attack of asthma		
Life-threatening asthma	Any one of the following in a child with severe asthma:	
	Clinical signs	**Measurements**
	• Silent chest • Cyanosis • Poor respiratory effort • Hypotension • Exhaustion • Confusion	• SpO$_2$ <92% • PEFR <33% best or predicted

Acute severe asthma	• Can't complete sentences in one breath or too breathless to talk or feed
	• SpO$_2$ <92%
	• PEFR 33-50% best or predicted
	• Pulse >140 in children aged 2-5 years
	             >125 in children aged > 5 years
	• Respiration > 40 breaths/min aged 2-5 years
	              > 30 breaths/min aged 7-5 years	

Moderate asthma exacerbation	• Able to talk in sentences
	• SpO$_2$ ≥ 92%
	• PEFR ≥ 50% best or predicted
	• Heart rate ≤ 140/min in children aged 2-5 years
	              ≤ 125/min in children > 5 years
	• Respiratory rate ≤ 40/min in children aged 2-5 years`
	                ≤ 30/min in children > years	

Based on British Guidelines on Management of Asthma 2009		

The features of a life-threatening attack of asthma are as follows:

(i) Cyanosis, silent chest or feeble respiratory efforts.
(ii) Fatigue or exhaustion.
(iii) Agitation or reduced level of consciousness.

Any child with features suggestive of a life-threatening attack should ideally be treated in a hospital where intensive care facilities are available. However, the child should receive oxygen, bronchodilator and a dose of steroids before making arrangements for transfer to a tertiary level health facility. Oxygen and inhalation therapy (MDI with a spacer) should be care continued while the child is being transferred.

Detailed Clinical Assessment

A detailed clinical assessment is done on the basis of history, physical examination and objective measurement of degree of airway obstruction and hypoxia.

History

Once an appropriate level of management has been instituted in a sick child, a detailed history should be taken with emphasis on certain points. It is necessary to know the duration of worsening and any specific allergen or irritant which could have triggered the attack, any history of previous hospitalizations, frequent emergency visits, chronic corticosteroid use or recent withdrawal from systemic steroids and history of previous admissions to an intensive care unit or intubation. These factors, if present, indicate an increased risk of the attack becoming very severe and such children should be intensively monitored.

Physical examination

The initial examination should rapidly determine the severity of airflow obstruction, degree of hypoxia, and identify complications. Categorization of an acute exacerbation of asthma into mild, moderate or severe can be done based on physical examination and objective parameters as shown in Table 30.1. In any child with severe degree of respiratory distress; presence of alteration of sensorium, confusion, and cyanosis will suggest respiratory failure. Examination should be repeated after each step of treatment to assess the response.

Objective assessment

Many patients may not perceive any distress even when they have moderate degree of airway obstruction. More importantly, even when symptoms and physical signs are minimal, the patient may have considerable level of airflow obstruction. An objective measurement of lung function thus becomes necessary. The two methods of objective measurement of lung function that can be used are (i) measurement of air flow obstruction by peak expiratory flow rate (PEFR) or forced expiratory volume in the first second (FEV1) and (ii) arterial blood gas analysis (ABG) or pulse oximetry.

PEFR can be measured using a simple peak flow meter. A child is made to use the peak flow meter in a standing position, three times and the best of the three values is taken as the child's PEFR during the acute attack (Figure 30.1). This is compared with the child's personal best or predicted PEFR. Figure 30.2 depicts a simple nomogram to predict PEFR of children between 5-18 years of age.

In children who are very young (< 5 years) or those who are very sick, arterial blood gas analysis or pulse oximetry should be used to assess the response to therapy and take a decision to transfer the child to intensive care unit.

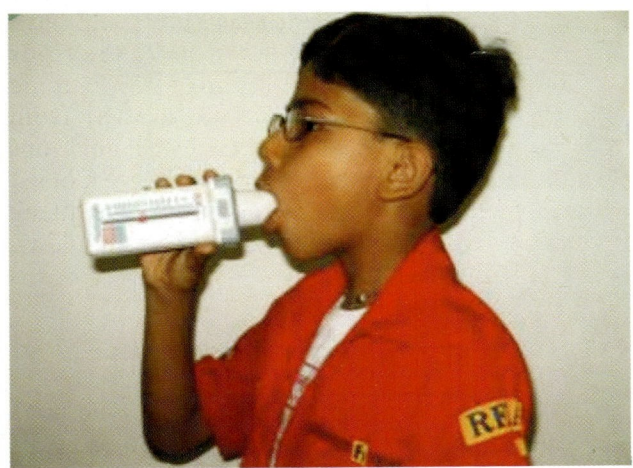

Figure 30.1 Method for recording PEFR with a mini-Wright peak flow meter

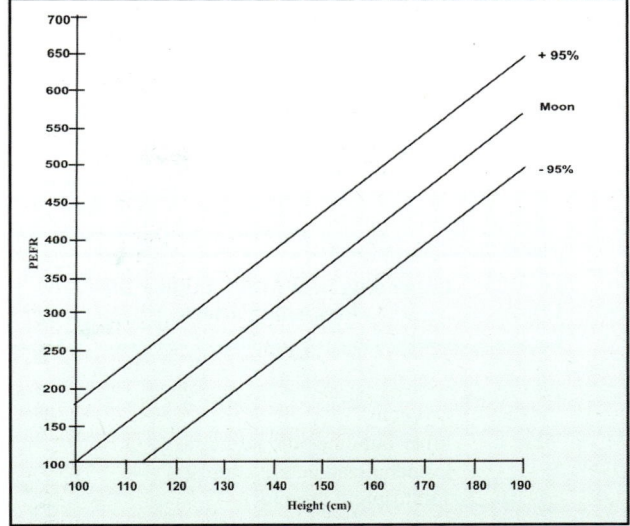

Figure 30.2 Nomogram of PEFR in children between 5-18 yrs of age in relation to height

Chest radiograph and other laboratory studies

Laboratory studies are generally not indicated in most cases of acute attack of bronchial asthma. However, if the child is unusually ill or there is a possibility of an infection, blood samples can be taken for (i) white blood cell count for detecting polymorphonuclear leukocytosis and elevation of band cells which suggests bacterial infection, (ii) serum electrolytes since both beta-2 agonists and corticosteroids may cause hypokalemia and (iii) serum theophylline levels (if facilities are available). If the child is already on theophylline, these levels may be necessary before institution of further systemic drug therapy as it has a very low safety margin.

A chest radiograph is indicated when the diagnosis of bronchial asthma is doubtful, there is poor response to treatment or there is a suspicion of a foreign body. It is also useful in a child with persistent unilateral chest signs or any other findings suggestive of lobar collapse, consolidation or complications due to air leaks.

Step 2. INITIATION OF THERAPY

Principles of Therapy

- The goal of therapy is to rapidly reverse the acute air-flow obstruction with consequent relief of respiratory distress. This is achieved by repeated use of inhaled beta-2 agonists (Figure 30.3).

- Hypoxia is treated by proper oxygenation of all acutely sick children.

Section 4

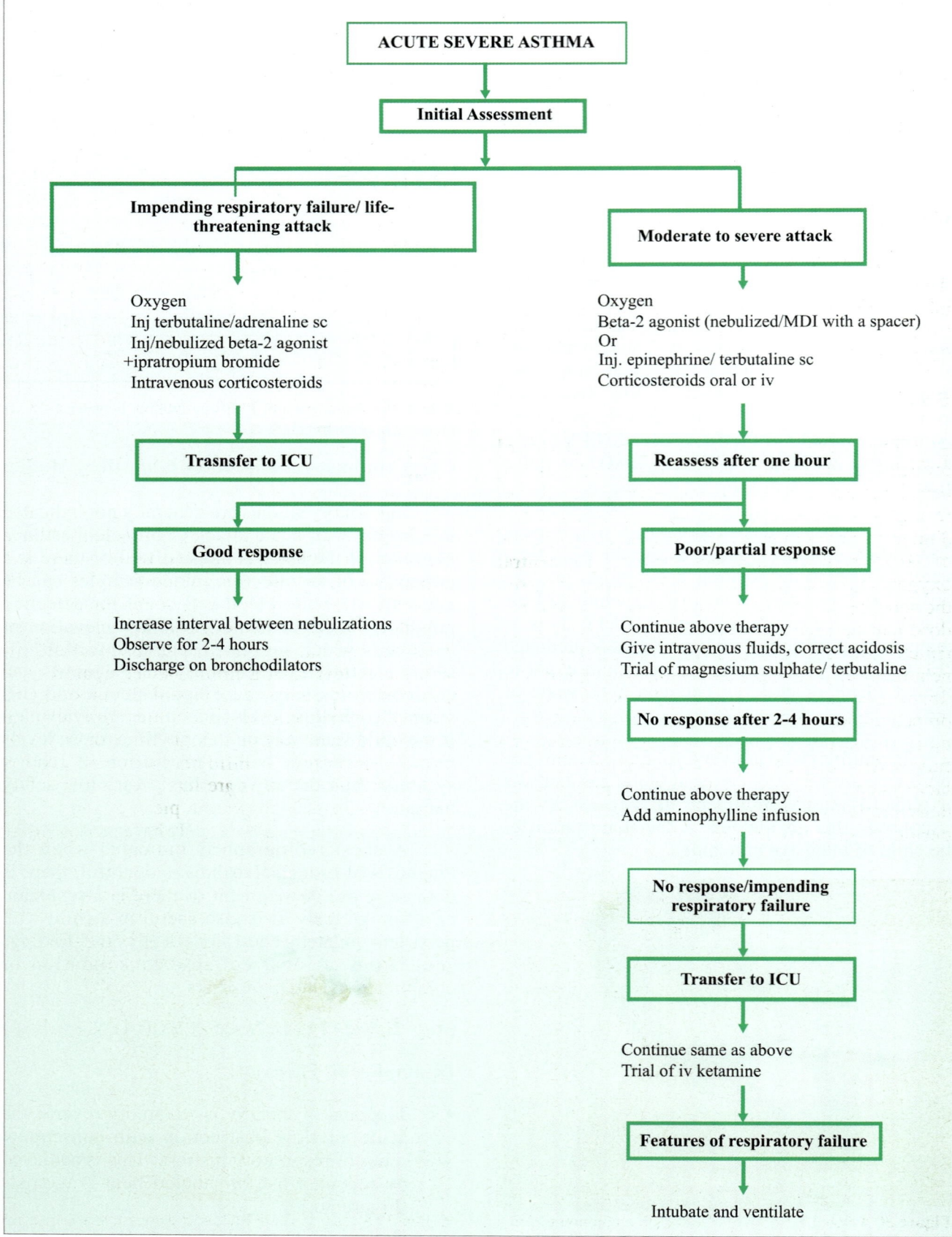

Figure 30.3 Algorithm for management of acute severe asthma

- Corticosteroids are added early in an acute attack if the response to inhaled bronchodilators is not satisfactory.

- Repeated clinical and objective assessment is done to evaluate the response to above measures, other drugs are added if necessary and patient is closely watched to detect impending respiratory failure at the earliest.

Oxygen

All patients of acute severe asthma have some degree of hypoxia. Oxygen at the rate of 3-6 liters/minute should be started. The flow should be enough to maintain arterial oxygen saturation (SaO_2) above 92 percent.

Beta-2 agonists

The currently recommended standard bronchodilator therapy is repeated inhalations of beta-2 agonist aerosol. Salbutamol nebulizer solution (5 mg/ml) in a dose of 0.1-0.15 mg/kg diluted in 3 ml of normal saline is administered over a period of 10-15 minutes. It is preferable to use central oxygen supply at the rate of 6-7 liters/ min to run the nebulizer, at least initially, to avoid hypoxia. The dose can be repeated every 20 minutes for three times and the child reassessed after each nebulization. The rationale behind giving repeated doses of inhaled bronchodilators is that the bronchodilatation that follows the initial dose allows more distal deposition of drug particles during further dosing. This results in dilatation of smaller airways and the short dosing interval prevents any deterioration of clinical status in the intervening period (Figure 30.4)[9]. Recent studies, however, suggest that continuous nebulization (CN) may be more effective than intermittent nebulization[10-13]. This method of therapy can continue for a prolonged period without having to set up nebulization at regular intervals.

Also patients are more likely to get acclimatized to continuous nebulization and therefore maintain a more constant breathing pattern. This would result in subsequent reduction of inspiratory flow and more peripheral deposition of inhaled bronchodilator aerosol[13]. Recommended doses are 0.1-0.5 mg/kg/hr via a delivery system comprising preferably of a constant infusion pump and central oxygen supply. Higher doses of 3.4± 2.2 mg/kg/hr have been used in ventilated patients[12, 14]. This set up is difficult to maintain, since it requires power and oxygen supply for a prolonged period. However, the superior efficacy of continuous nebulization over intermittent nebulisation has not yet been unequivocally proven. Table 30.3 summarizes various drugs, their doses and mode of administration.

Alternatively, metered dose inhaler (MDI) can be used with a spacer device to give repeated inhalations of beta-2 agonist (Figure 30.5). It is considered equivalent[15] or better[16] than nebulizer driven by compressed air. It does not cause oxygen desaturation unlike the former. The duration of therapy is less than a minute as compared to 15 minutes with a nebulizer. Use of MDI reduces the cost of therapy, is easily performed, and does not require power supply. MDI + spacer is the preferred option in mild to moderate asthma. Children aged <3 years are likely to require a face mask connected to the mouth piece of a spacer for successful drug delivery. Inhalers should be

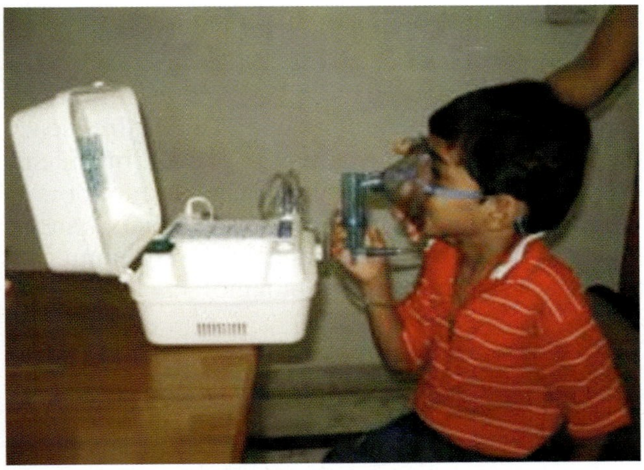

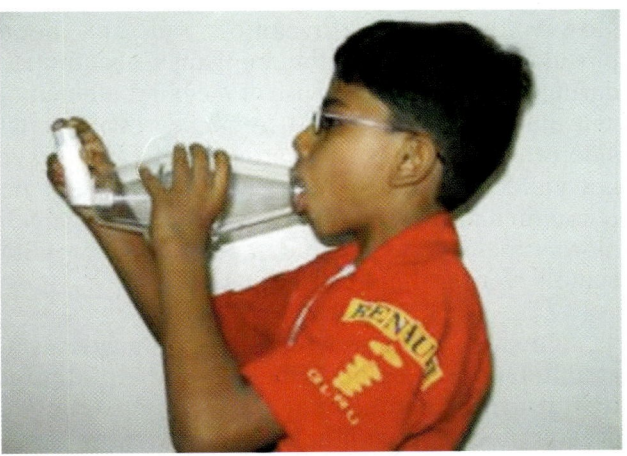

Figure 30.4 Nebulization with the help of a compressor. In a life-threatening situation, oxygen should be used at a flow rate of 6-7 liters/min

Figure 30.5 Method to use MDI with a commercially available spacer

actuated into the spacer in individual puffs and inhaled immediately by tidal breathing (for five breaths). Frequent doses of beta-2 agonists are safe for the treatment of acute asthma, although children with mild symptoms benefit from lower doses. Single puff given one at a time, followed by 5 tidal breaths, every 1-2 minutes can be used for upto 10 times[17]. One can use a commercially available spacer device with a valve and mask in children below 5 years (Figure 30.6).

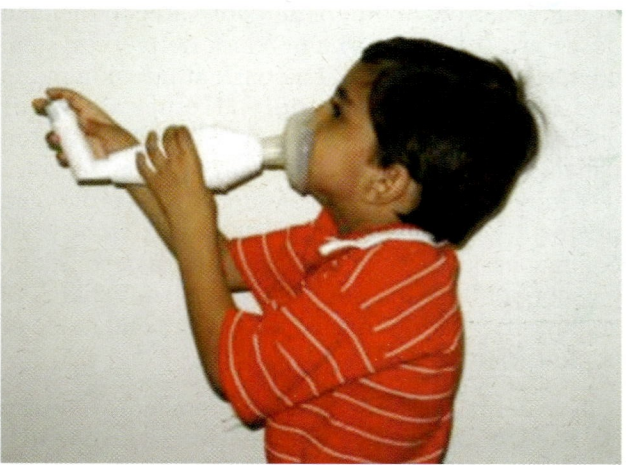

Figure 30.6 Method for using MDI with a spacer and mask in a 3-year-old child

Recently, some attention has turned to levo salbutamol, the pure or homochiral formulation of (R)–salbutamol. Conventional, or racemic salbutamol is a 50/50 mixture of (R)-salbutamol and (S)-salbutamol. (S) salbutamol, previously thought to be an inert compound, may exaggerate airway hyperesponsiveness[18] and also may have a proinflammatory effect[19]

As (S)-salbutamol is metabolized much more slowly than (R)-salbutamol[20], it has been postulated[21] that (S)-salbutamol may accumulate during frequent, repeated use of racemic salbutamol and thus lead to increased frequency of potential side effects. Studies comparing the two[21, 22] have not yielded any definite results, so presently no recommendation regarding the use of the much more expensive (R) salbutamol in children with acute severe asthma can be made.

In some children with severe bronchospasm, an initial dose of epinephrine may be helpful prior to initiating inhalational treatment[23]. Oxygen desaturation seen with nebulisation therapy is not seen with this form of therapy. On the contrary transient increase in paO$_2$ has been noticed by some workers[25, 26]. Injectable terbutaline may also be used

in place of epinephrine. Use of epinephrine is limited by its shorter duration of action, cardiac side effects and it cannot be repeated more than 2-3 times. Terbutaline has a longer duration of action and a repeat dose may not be required for 2-6 hours. Long acting beta-2 agonists, such as salmetrol, is contraindicated in children with status asthamaticus due to increased risk of mortality[27].

Anticholinergics

Some studies have shown that concomitant use of inhaled anticholinergics and a selective beta- 2 agonist produces significantly greater improvement in lung function than beta-2 agonists alone[28, 29]. Only ipratropium bromide is used in view of its negligible side effects[29]. Transient anisocoria and angle closure glaucoma have been noticed in adults[30, 31]. As it has few systemic adverse effects, its use is advocated for patients with life-threatening features or those who do not respond to initial high dose inhaled beta-2 agonists[32, 33]. Since ipratropium bromide is an acetylcholine antagonist while salbutamol is a beta-2 agonist, both acting at different sites in the lung and via different pharmacologic mechanisms, provides the basis for using these drugs together for their additive effect. There are, however, some studies which have shown no benefit of using anticholinergic drugs[35, 36]. In a recent meta-analysis of 13 studies, adding multiple doses of anticholinergic to beta-2 agonist was found to be safe and improved lung functions to avoid hospital admission in one of 12 such treated patients Repeated doses of ipratropium bromide should be given early to treat children who are poorly responsive to β2-agonists[36].

An optimal dose of 250 ug ipratropium bromide contained in 1. 0 ml of the respirator solution, may be mixed with salbutamol solution and both given together at an interval of 20 minutes with the nebulizer[37]. It may also be given alternating with the dose of nebulised salbutamol. Dosing frequency may be reduced as the patient improves. In patients who suffer from tachycardia or marked tremors in response to standard dose of beta-2 agonists and in younger age group (3-30 months) ipratropium may be more effective than salbutamol[38,].

Corticosteroids

Since inflammation is an important component of airway obstruction in an acute attack of asthma, there is no doubt that the use of steroids in an acute exacerbation is useful in resolving the obstruction[39,40]. But it is somewhat difficult to decide

Table 30.3 Drug dosages in children with acute attack of bronchial asthma

Drug	Available form	Dosage
Inhaled beta-2 agonists		
Salbutamol		
Metered dose inhaler with a spacer	100 ug/puff	2 inhalations every 5 min for a total of 10-20 puffs, with monitoring of PEFR or FEV1 to document response
Nebulizer solution	0.5% (5 mg/ml)	0.1-0.15 mg/kg/dose upto 5 mg every 20 min for 1-2 hr (minimum dose 1.25 mg/dose) or 0.1-0.5 mg/kg/hr by continuous nebulization (maximum 15 mg/hour) or 3.4 ± 2.2 mg/kg/hr in ventilated patients.
Terbutaline		
Metered dose inhaler	200 ug/puff	2 inhalations every 5 min for a total of 10-20 puffs. <20 kg: 2.5 mg >20 kg: 5 mg
Nebuliser solution	10 mg/ml	
Systemic beta-2 agonists		
Epinephrine hcl	1:1000 sol (1 mg/ml)	0.01 mg/kg upto 0.3 mg subcutaneously every 20 min for 3 doses
Terbutaline	0.05% (0.5 mg/ml) solution for injection in 0.9% saline	0.005 mg/kg upto 0.3 mg sc every 2-6 hours as needed. Intravenous bolus of 10 ug/kg over 30 minutes followed by IV infusion at the rate of 0.1 ug/kg/min. Increase as necessary by 0.1 ug/kg/min every 30 min. Maximum dose 4 ug/kg/min.
Inhaled anticholinergics		
Ipratropium bromide		
Nebulizer solution	250 ug/ml	1 ml diluted in 3 ml normal saline every 20 minutes for 1-2 hours. This may be mixed with salbutamol nebulizer solution or alternated with salbutamol.
Metered dose inhaler	20 µg/puff	2 inhalation every 5 min for a total of 10-20 puffs
Aminophylline	80% anhydrous theophylline (250 mg/10 ml inj.)	Give a loading dose of 5-6 mg/kg and maintain at 0.9 mg/kg/hr. If patient is already receiving theophylline, avoid bolus dose.
Prednisolone	5 mg, 10 mg, 20 mg tabs	1-2 mg/kg/dose every 6 hr for 24 hr, then 1-2 mg/kg/day in divided doses every 8-12 hr for 5-7 days.
Hydrocortisone	50 mg/ml inj.	10 mg/kg IV bolus followed by 2.5-5.0 mg/kg q 6 hr
Methylprednisolone	40 mg/ml inj.	4 mg/kg IV single dose
Magnesium sulphate	50% soln. for inj. (500 mg/ml)	30-70 mg/kg in 30 ml N/5 saline iv infusion over 30 minutes.

Section 4

precisely when steroids should be administered. It has been proved both in adults and children[41, 42,43] that steroids given for a short duration of 3-7 days, improve the resolution and reduce the chances of an early relapse. The beneficial effects of corticosteroids on airway mechanism in status asthamaticus usually becomes evident between 6 to 12 hours after the first dose[44].

It is evident that the timing of initiation of steroid therapy plays an important role in the subsequent outcome of the attack. Studies have shown that the efficacy of steroid therapy is maximal when they are started soon after the patient presents in the emergency room[45, 46]. In contrast, benefits were minimal when steroids were initiated 24-48 hours after observation[48, 49]. A single dose of intramuscular methyl-prednisolone in a dose of 4 mg/kg, when given as an early adjunct to the beta-2 adrenergic therapy has been reported to reduce the hospitalization rates[50]. Oral steroids work as quickly and effectively as systemic steroids.In following situations, steroids can be started at the outset:

(i)   A child with a very severe attack of asthma.
(ii)   Previous history of life-threatening attack or severe attacks not responding to broncho-dilators.
(iii)   If the child is on oral steroids or high doses of inhaled steroids for prophylaxis. An oral dose of 1-2 mg/kg of prednisolone may be as effective as an equivalent dose of hydro-cortisone given intravenously, because the time for onset of action is the same. The total duration of therapy may be 3-7 days depending upon the response. Tapering doses are not required unless duration of oral/systemic steroids has been more than 14 days. However, children who have already been on long term oral steroids would require a longer course with tapering of doses over 5-10 days.

Role of Inhaled Steroids

A number of studies have been carried out to assess the efficacy of inhaled steroids in acute exacerbation of asthma. Inhaled dexamethasone was the first to be compared with oral prednisolone in management of acute severe asthma. This study suggested that inhaled steroids were quicker acting than oral[51]. This was followed by number of studies comparing budesonide with oral prednisolone[52, 53]. These also suggested that inhaled steroids were effective in acute severe attack. However, there were doubts whether high doses of inhaled steroids could lead to systemic effects after local absorption from the airways. A controlled trial of high dose of fluticasone, another inhaled steroid which is sparingly absorbed, did not find inhaled steroids to be effective, instead there were few patients in the study group who showed worsening of lung functions[54]. A recent meta-analysis of controlled trials with inhaled steroids suggested that there is no clear evidence at present that inhaled steroids are better than systemic steroids[55]. There is insufficient evidence to support the use of inhaled steroids as alternative or additional treatment to oral or intravenous steroids for acute asthma.

Step 3. ASSESSMENT OF RESPONSE TO INITIAL THERAPY

The patient must be closely watched for any signs of improvement or deterioration during therapy. The patient should be assessed after initial therapy of 2-3 doses of bronchodilator aerosols along with oxygen over a period of one hour. The plan for further management will depend on whether the response to initial therapy has been good, partial or poor.

Good response

The subject with good response to initial therapy will become free of wheeze and without any breathlessness. Heart rate and respiratory rate will decrease. Auscultation of chest will show minimal or no rhonchi and PEFR or FEV1 will improve to more than 70 % of the predicted or personal best. Such a child can be observed in the emergency room for 2-4 hours and if remains stable, can be discharged on bronchodilators (inhaled or oral) for a period of 5-7 days. The parents should be advised to come for follow-up and all other necessary instructions should be given for prophylaxis.

Partial response

A child may show some response after bronchodilators but may still have breathlessness and wheezing. Physical examination will reveal persistence of rhonchi. Heart rate and respiratory rate will be above the physiologic levels. Pulsus paradoxus of 10-15 mmHg and oxygen saturation of 91-95% may be observed. PEFR will be between 40% to 70% of the predicted normal. Treatment of a child with partial response is discussed later.

Poor response

If there is no subjective or objective improvement after initial therapy, it indicates a poor response. This child will continue to have severe respiratory distress and wheeze. Physical examination will reveal severe airway obstruction as indicated by significant pulsus paradoxus (≥ 15 mmHg), use of accessory muscles and extensive rhonchi. Oxygen saturation of $\leq 90\%$ and PEFR < 40% of predicted normal may be observed. Therapeutic efficacy of inhaled bronchodilators depends upon the proper maintenance and correct technique of administration of beta-2 agonists and other medications with a nebuliser and metered dose inhaler (Tables 30.4 and 30.5).

Step 4. MODIFICATION OF THERAPY FOR PATIENTS WITH PARTIAL AND POOR RESPONSE TO INTIAL THERAPY

Continue Oxygen and bronchodilator therapy

If the response to the initial therapy is not good, oxygen and beta-2 agonist inhalation should be

Table 30.4 Correct use of a nebulizer

1. It is preferable to use central oxygen supply source or oxygen from a cylinder at a rate of 6-8 liters/min to nebulise the drug during an acute attack. However, if oxygen is not available, compressed air can be used. Face mask or mouth device is used depending upon the age and cooperation of the child.

2. The drug volume should be at least 3 ml. If residual volume (volume after nebulisation is over) is more than 1 ml, a larger amount of drug volume should be prepared. Three doses of the drug should be nebulised after every 20 minutes during first hour of therapy.

3. Patient should be instructed to inhale from his mouth. Although it may be difficult to control breathing pattern during an acute attack but deep and slow breathing is advocated.

4. Drug should be nebulised over a period of 8-10 minutes. If the procedure is taking longer than 10 minutes either chamber is malfunctioning or supply of compressed air/oxygen is defective.

5. A good mist formation suggests that the procedure of nebulization is satisfactory.

Cleaning the Nebulizer

It is preferable to use either disposable or separate nebuliser chamber for each patient. However, if that is not possible, cleaning the nebuliser and tubings thoroughly in-between patients is mandatory. A light detergent can be used followed by plain water to wash the equipment. 1% vinegar solution can be used for overnight immersion to disinfect the nebulizer and tubings. After sterilization and before next use, the nebuliser should be run dry for a few minutes.

Table 30.5 Correct use of MDI with a spacer

1. MDI alone is not advocated in children because of poor hand–lung coordination. A spacer device preferably with a mask is a must while using MDI in children.

2. Drug is held in suspension after actuation for a period of at least 10 seconds in the holding chamber.

3. A slow deep breathing through mouth is advised after actuation of MDI and provides better delivery of drug in the lungs.

4. Breath holding after a deep slow breath is not advocated, particularly during an acute attack because it may be very uncomfortable or impossible. Continuous slow and deep breathing is recommended.

5. Two puffs should be used every 5 minutes during first hour of therapy. In between puffs child should receive oxygen therapy.

6. While using a commercially available spacer, it must be ensured that the patient is able to operate the valve with each inspiration. The click of the valve should be audible with each breath.

7. A smaller volume (250 ml) spacer for younger children and a large volume (750 ml) spacer for older children is preferable. However, a large volume spacer can be used for all age groups.

8. Indigenously fabricated spacer is as good as a commercial device in treating an acute attack. Absence of valve in fact makes it easier to use in younger and sicker children.

9. MDI with a spacer is as good as a nebuliser. However, 4-6 doses of MDI are equivalent to one dose administered through a nebuliser.

10. The spacer should be washed with a detergent every week and air dried.

continued. The frequency of inhalation should be decided depending upon the severity of respiratory distress. Children who do not have severe respiratory distress and have shown partial response may only require inhalations 2-4 hourly while children with severe distress should be given more frequent inhalations. Inhalation therapy as frequently as every 20 min, or even continuously, can be given without side effects for the next two hours and child reassessed. If ipratropium is not used at the onset, it is added at the end of first hour as described earlier. MDI with a spacer can also be used frequently as an effective alternative device.

Intravenous fluids and correction of acidosis

Children admitted with an acute severe attack of asthma often have mild to moderate dehydration. Dehydration may produce more viscous mucus, leading to bronchiolar plugging.[56] Humidification of inspired air and correction of dehydration, therefore, are always indicated. However, at the same time, inappropriate antidiuretic hormone secretion has been reported in some cases of bronchial asthma. Hence fluid therapy should be individualized to keep the child in normal hydration.

Hypokalemia has been reported with frequent beta adrenergic and corticosteroid therapy.[57] It should be corrected when present. Metabolic acidosis that occurs during an acute attack may decrease the responsiveness of bronchi to bronchodilators. It has been recommended that if pH is less than 7. 3 or base deficit is greater than 5 mEq, intravenous correction with sodium bicarbonate is indicated, initially using half the calculated dose and then repeating the ABG.

Section 4

Monitoring

If the child is very sick and is deteriorating, he may require continuous monitoring. Repeated clinical assessments are necessary, at least at hourly intervals, in less sick children. In critically sick children, PEFR or FEV1, wherever possible, and ABG should be assessed for an objective evaluation.

If the patient has improved on continuation of the above therapy for about two hours, he can be observed for 2-3 hours and then discharged with proper advice. In case there is no improvement, treatment is intensified with addition of other drugs and the child is transferred to a place where intensive care facilities are available.

Addition of other or second line drug

Children with continuing severe asthma inspite of frequent nebulised β2-agonists, ipratropium bromide plus oral steroids, and those with life threatening features, need urgent review for transfer to a high dependency unit or pediatric intensive care unit (PICU) to receive second line intravenous therapies. The options available are β-2 agonists (salbutamol/ terbutaline), aminophylline and magnesium sulphate.

Role of aminophylline

The role of aminophylline in an acute attack of bronchial asthma is still controversial. There is no doubt that methylxanthines have bronchodilator activity but it is uncertain whether this adds to the bronchodilator effect achieved by beta-2 agonists and corticosteroids. In a meta-analysis of 13 controlled trials of intravenous aminophylline in acute asthma, no benefit of routine addition of aminophylline to inhaled beta-2 adrenergic agents and corticosteroids was documented. It has been proved in adult studies that aminophylline does not have additional bronchodilator effect[58, 59]. In addition methylxanthines have a very low margin of safety and side effects can be numerous and serious.

However, in a recent double blind placebo-controlled trial on hospitalized children, a clear benefit of aminophylline was demonstrated[61]. Two recent prospective randomized controlled trials in children have shown clear benefit of intravenous aminophylline in preventing respiratory failure in severe acute attack of asthma[62, 63]. Aminophylline is not recommended in children with mild to moderate acute asthma. Its use is recommended in a HDU or PICU setting for children with severe or life-threatening bronchospasm unresponsive to maximal doses of bronchodilators plus steroids. It is believed that aminophylline may act by mechanisms other than bronchodilation as well, such as stimulation of the respiratory drive, reduction in respiratory muscle fatiguability and enhancement of mucociliary clearance[63]. Moreover, aminophylline infusion is equally efficacious and more cost effective compared to terbutaline infusion[64].

A bolus dose depending upon previous treatment with methylxanthines is given followed by infusion of maintenance dose. The dose of theophylline is reduced in fever by 50%, and by 25-30% when concomitantly used with drugs like erythromycin, aminoquinolones, cimetidine and related drugs[58]. The dose may have to be increased in children getting drugs like rifampicin, phenytoin and phenobarbitone. If facilities are available drug levels should be monitored to ensure its safety and efficacy. As soon as the patient shows response, aminophylline infusion may be substituted by injectable deriphylline (6 hourly bolus) or even oral theophylline if patient is able to take orally.

Intravenous terbutaline

In children with low inspiratory rates where nebulization of beta-2 agonists have failed, intravenous terbutaline infusion, has been tried.[65,66] Therapy is started with an initial bolus of 10 ug/kg over 30 minutes, followed by an infusion at the rate of 0.1ug/kg/min which may be increased by 0.1ug/kg/min every 30 minutes, upto a maximum of 4 ug/kg/min or until there is a fall in $paCO_2$, with clinical improvement[67]. Dose of terbutaline should be reduced by half, if theophylline is used concomitantly[68]. Significant adverse effects noted with intravenous terbutaline include tachycardia, arrhythmias, hypertension, myocardial ischemia, hyperglycemia, hypokalemia, rhabdomyolysis, lactic acidosis and hypophosphatemia[67,69].

Magnesium sulphate

Some patients with acute severe asthma, treated with intensive initial nebulization therapy with beta-2 agonists and corticosteroids may not show improvement and progress to respiratory failure. One drug which may be worth trying in these refractory patients, to avert mechanical ventilation, is magnesium sulphate. Although there are very few controlled trials in children using this drug, a recent double blind placebo-controlled trial suggests that early institution of intravenous magnesium sulphate along with conventional therapy may result in early relief of airflow obstruction[70].

It acts by counteracting calcium mediated smooth muscle contractions, through its effects on calcium homeostasis,[71] inhibition of acetylcholine release[72] at the neuromuscular junction, inhibition of histamine release,[73] direct inhibition of smooth muscle contraction and sedation[74]. The recommended dose for infusion is 30-70 mg/kg over 20-30 minutes[75]. It is available as a 50% solution, 0.2 ml/kg of which can be given as an infusion in 30 ml N/5 normal saline in 5% dextrose over 30 minutes[76]. Serum levels greater than 4 mg/dl are necessary for bronchodilation. Onset of action occurs within a few minutes of iv infusion and lasts for 2 hours[77, 78]. Side effects include transient sensation of facial warmth, flushing, malaise and hypotension. At serum levels greater than 12.5 mg/dl side effects like areflexia, respiratory depression and arrythmia may be noted, but this is likely to happen when magnesium sulphate is administratered in a dose greater than 150 mg/kg[76-78]. Two recent meta-analyses [79, 80] of controlled trials on efficacy of magnesium sulphate in acute severe asthma suggests that it is safe and beneficial when conventional therapy with beta-2 agonist and steroids has failed. One of the studies [79] suggests that practice guidelines need to be changed to reflect these observations. Intravenous magnesium sulphate is a safe treatment for acute asthma although its place in management is not yet established. The current evidence recommendation favors use of magnesium sulfate over iv terbutaline in a patient who has failed to respond to initial therapy.

Role of antibiotics

Respiratory tract infections that trigger exacerbations of asthma are usually viral. Bacteria and mycoplasma may be infrequently associated. Role of antibiotics, hence, is limited to; (i) patients who are running high grade fever, look sick, and toxic; (ii) there is polymorphonuclear leukocytosis, (iii) sputum is purulent with presence of polymorphs and not eosinophils and (iv) chest radiograph shows consolidation or patchy opacities. In all other cases, even when steroids are used, there is no need to administer antibiotics.

Role of antihistaminics, mucolytics, cough syrups and sedatives

There is no evidence that addition of antihistamines, mucolytics or cough syrups are in any way helpful to the patient with acute asthma. Antihistaminics may make the bronchial secretions more viscid and difficult to expectorate. Sedation may be harmful in patients who are anxious and irritable because of hypoxia, and should be avoided. Instead measures to treat hypoxia should be made more effective. Occasionally younger infants may cry excessively due to reasons other than hypoxia, like hunger and unknown surroundings. This may increase the oxygen demand and also make management more difficult. The best way is to treat these children in the lap of mother. Rarely, sedation may be required and triclofos is a safe drug for this purpose.

Step 5. INTENSIVE CARE MANAGEMENT

Indications for Transfer to an Intensive Care Unit

The patient is observed on aforementioned therapy for next few hours and is monitored frequently. The decision to transfer to Intensive Care Unit (ICU) will depend upon the status of the child at the time of presentation and response to therapy. Any child with signs of life-threatening attack, should be immediately transferred to the ICU. If the child has been receiving therapy and has shown poor response after being observed for a few hours or develops clinical signs of impending respiratory failure like persistent hypoxemia, exhaustion or change in the level of sensorium, he should be immediately transferred to ICU. Continuous monitoring with the help of pulse oximetry or repeated ABG analyses are mandatory since most of these patients may not be in a position to perform PEFR.

Continuation of Therapy in PICU

The focus of care continues to be close observation and delivery of frequent nebulized beta-2 agonists, combined with corticosteroids and possibly aminophylline. As mentioned earlier, a trial of intravenous terbutaline and magnesium sulphate is desirable in a child who has not responded to above therapy due to low inspiratory flow rates.

Intubation and Controlled Ventilation

Despite maximal pharmacologic therapy, some children do not respond favourably and require intubation and mechanical ventilation. The decision to ventilate is usually reserved as a last option.

Indications for Mechanical Ventilation

1. Failure of maximal pharmacologic therapy.

2. Cyanosis and hypoxemia (paO_2 less than 60 mmHg).
3. $paCO_2$ greater than 50 mmHg and rising by more than 5 mmHg/hr.
4. Minimal chest movements.
5. Minimal air exchange.
6. Severe chest retractions.
7. Deterioration in mental status, lethargy or agitation.
8. Recumbent and diaphoretic patient.
9. Pneumothorax or pneumomediastinum.
10. Respiratory or cardiac arrest.

ABG values alone are not indicative of the need for mechanical ventilation and should be interpreted in context of the clinical picture. Frequently, more than one of these indications is present before the decision to ventilate is made. However, it must be stressed that inspite of being aware of the morbidity that ventilation entails, it is better to intubate a child electively rather than to wait for cardiorespiratory arrest to occur.

The patient should be stabilised using 100 percent oxygen administered with a bag and mask. Oral and airway secretions should be cleared and stomach decompressed using nasogastric tube, to diminish risk of aspiration. Pre-medication with intravenous atropine and topical anesthesia to hypopharynx and larynx, helps to decrease bronchospasm and laryngospasm, which may be produced as a result of upper airway manipulation. An ideal sedative that may be used for intubation is intravenous ketamine in a dose of 1-3 mg/kg[81,82]. The largest recommended endotracheal tube should be used. Muscle relaxation eliminates ventilator-patient asynchrony and improves chest wall compliance. It reduces $paCO_2$ for any given level of minute ventilation. Additionally, this gives the patient with respiratory muscle fatigue, a period of desperately needed physical rest. Vecuronium bromide, with an intermediate duration of action and without any cardiovascular or autonomic side effects, in a dose of 0.2-0.3 mg/kg may be used. Succinylcholine may be used too, but it has a short duration of action. A volume cycled ventilator is recommended with low respiratory rate (8-12 per min) and long expiratory time (I:E ratio of 1:4 or 1:3) to prevent hyperinflation. Airway obstruction in itself causes intrinsic PEEP, therefore end expiratory pressure (PEEP) should be minimal. Tidal volume of 10-12 ml/kg and peak airway pressure less than 40-50 cm of water should be maintained. High inspiratory flow rates should be kept to improve gas exchange. This can usually be achieved with heavy sedation or use of muscle relaxants.

Throughout ventilation, beta-2 agonists are nebulized into the inspiratory circuit of ventilator.

In the ventilated patients, therapeutic bronchoscopy with lavage after administration of saline, sodium bicarbonate and acetylcysteine[83] has been used in very ill patients with persistent mucus plugging, to prevent atelectasis and nosocomial pneumonia.

Role of leukotriene receptor antagonists

Initiating oral montelukast in primary care settings, early after the onset of acute asthma symptoms, can result in decreased asthma symptoms and reduced need for subsequent healthcare attendances in those with mild exacerbations[84]. There is no clear evidence to support the use of leukotriene receptor antagonists for moderate to severe acute asthma.

Role of droperidol

Dyspnea promotes anxiety, which may impair ventilation and interfere with efficacy of aerosol therapy. Therefore, in pediatric ICU set up, one may use safe sedatives with bronchodilator properties. Droperidol which has both of these properties may be used in asthmatics on assisted ventilation. It antagonises bronchoconstriction mediated by alpha-adrenergic receptors in peripheral airways. Recommended dose is 0.22 mg/kg and its main side effect is hypotension[85].

Role of ketamine

This drug is a disassociative anesthetic with excellent sedative and analgesic properties. It relaxes smooth muscle directly, increases chest wall compliance and also decreases bronchospasm in ventilated asthmatic children. It is given in a loading dose 0.5-1.0 mg/kg, followed by an infusion at 1.0-2.5 mg/kg/hr in ventilated children[81]. The common side effects include arrythmias, increased secretions and laryngospasm. It has been used in sub-anesthetic doses in non-ventilated adults in ICU set up in a bolus dose of 0.75 mg/kg over 10 minutes, followed by an infusion at a rate of 0.15 mg/kg/hr[82]. Thus intravenous ketamine is useful to relieve acute intractable bronchospasm, provided expert anesthetic help is available at hand.

Heliox

Helium-oxygen mixture has been used to reduce air viscosity and treat upper airway obstruction. Though there are no published controlled trials, some workers have reported a return of normal blood gases following this treatment, in patients with alveolar hypoventilation due to severe acute asthma[87,88]. The use of heliox, (helium/oxygen mixture in a ratio of 80:20 or 70:30), either as a driving gas for nebulisers, as a breathing gas, or for artificial ventilation in adults with acute asthma is not supported on the basis of present evidence. Heliox is not recommended for use in acute asthma outside a clinical trial setting.

Inhaled anesthetic agents

Patients who fail to improve with mechanical ventilation, with beta-2 agonists continuously delivered through ventilator tubing, a trial of inhaled anesthetic gases may be given. Use of halothane 1.0-1.5%,[89, 90] isoflurane 1%[91] and ether have been shown to produce significant improvement within one hour. Inhalation may be discontinued within 12 hours, though some patients require extended therapy. The exact mechanism of action of anesthetic agents is unclear. They may relax airway smooth muscle directly[92], inhibit the release of bronchoactive mediators, or inhibit vagal induced bronchospasm. It is suggested that halothane has an action similar to beta-2 agonists[93]. Administration of anesthetic agents can be done by fitting a standard ventilator with an anesthetic gas vaporiser.

The resolution of bronchospasm in ventilated asthmatic patient will become evident when $paCO_2$ values fall, while the same or lower peak airway pressure is being used. Once the $paCO_2$ is less than 45 mm Hg, the peak airway pressure is less than 35 cm water and there is mild or no bronchospasm on auscultation, the muscle paralysis can be stopped. As soon as respiratory muscle function returns to normal, the patient can be placed on spontaneous ventilation. If the child can maintain a $paCO_2$ of less than 45 mm Hg without assisted ventilation, extubation may be safely done.

Management During Recovery Phase

During the recovery phase of acute asthma, the frequency of inhalation should be reduced gradually, and oral drugs should be instituted in place of intravenous medications. The patient can be discharged once symptoms have cleared and lung functions stabilized (PEFR >75% predicted). Bronchodilator therapy consists of oral or inhaled beta-2 agonist depending upon the age of the child and affordability, and a long acting theophylline. The instructions to the parents and the child regarding the importance of correct timing of the drugs and proper inhalation techniques are of utmost importance. The child should be called for follow-up to detect any early relapse and observe the medication techniques. The parents must be told to monitor the child's symptoms and wherever possible, objective measurements like PEFR should be recorded to detect any worsening.

PREVENTION OF FUTURE ATTACKS

The following guidelines must be kept in mind to prevent future exacerbations of asthma[94].

1. Parents should be given proper education regarding home management of asthma. They should be provided with written instructions regarding the administration of drugs during acute asthma episode, and taught how to recognize deteriorating control, both clinically and by measurement of PEFR in older children.

2. Children should be supervised regularly and parents should know when and where to seek medical help.

3. A proper prophylactic therapy should be planned depending upon the age and affordability. A child who has suffered from a very severe attack will generally require inhaled steroids.

4. Simple methods of delivery like MDI with spacer and rotacap inhalers should be made available to as many patients as possible.

5. Hospitals should follow written protocols giving clear guidelines for management of acute as well as chronic asthma.

6. Avoidance of house-hold allergens like carpet dust, house mites, cockroaches, pet animals, synthetic edible colors and food preservatives (soft drinks, chiclets, gems, sauce, canned foods, tetrapack drinks, etc.) may reduce the frequency and severity of exacerbations. There is some evidence that negative ion generators may be useful to purify the air in the dwellings but they are expensive.

7. Children with asthma should avoid smoky, stuffy, overcrowded and polluted places. The use of insect sprays, strong perfumes, *agarbati* and mosquito repellents should preferably be avoided.

Section 4

8. The physical activity should be limited to the tolerance level of the child. Breathing exercises and yoga are useful to improve the vital capacity of the lungs.

9. Skin testing is unreliable for identification of allergens in children and is not routinely undertaken.

10. The resistance of the body against allergy and infections can be enhanced by taking antihistaminic, calcium and micronutrients like vitamin A, vitamin C, zinc and selenium.

REFERENCES

1. Burr ML, Butland BK, King S, Vaughan WE. Changes in asthma prevalence: Two surveys 15 years apart. *Arch Dis Child* 1989; 64:1452-1456.

2. Evans R, Mullally DI, Wilson RW, Gergan PI, Rosenberg HM, Grauman JS, *et al*. National trends in the morbidity and mortality of asthma in the US. Prevalence, hospitalization and deaths from asthma over past two decades: 1965-1984. *Chest* 1987; 91:(suppl6) S65-S74.

3. Portnoy J, Jones E. Pediatric asthma emergencies. *J Asthma* 2003; 40: 537-545.

4. Sly RM. Changing prevelance of allergic rhinitis and asthma. *Ann Allergy Asthma Immunol* 1999; 82:232-248.

5. Burney PGJ. Asthma mortality in England and Wales: Evidence for a further increase, 1974-84; *Lancet* 1986; 2:323-326.

6. Mao Y, Scmencin R, Morrison H, Mcac Williams L, Davies J, Wigle D. Increased rates of illness and death from asthma in Canada. *Canada Med Assoc J* 1987; 137:620-624.

7. So SY, Ng MMT, Ip MSM, Lam WK. Rising asthma mortality in young males in Hong Kong. 1976-85. *Respir Med* 1990; 84:457-461.

8. Weiss KB, Wagenar DK. Changing patterns of asthma mortality. Identifying target population at risk. *JAMA* 1990; 264:1683-1687.

9. Robertson CF, Smith F, Beck R, Levison H. Response to frequent low doses of nebulized salbutamol in acute asthma. *J Pediatr* 1985; 106:672-674.

10. Calcone A, Wolkove N, Stem E. Continuous nebulization of albuterol in acute asthma. *Chest* 1990; 97:693-697.

11. Moler FW, Hurwitz ME, Custer JR. Improvement in clinical asthma score and paCO$_2$ in children with severe asthma treated with continuously nebulized terbutaline. *J Allergy Clin Immunol* 1988; 81:1101-1109.

12. Papo MC, Frank J, Thompson AE. A prospective, randomized study of continuous versus intermittent nebulized albuterol for severe status asthmaticus in children. *Crit Care Med* 1993; 21:1479-1486.

13. Ryan G, Dolovier MB, Eng P, Obminski G, Cockroft DW, Juniper E. Standardization of inhalation provocation tests, influence of nebulizer output, particle size and method of inhalation. *J Allergy Clin Immunol* 1981; 67:156-161.

14. Katz RW, Kelly W, Crowley MR. Safety of continuous nebulized albuterol for bronchospasm in infants and children. *Pediatrics* 1993; 92:666-669.

15. Yung-Zen Lin, Kue-Hsiung Hsich. Metered dose inhaler and nebulizer in acute asthma. *Arch Dis Child* 1995; 72:214-218.

16. Batra V, Sethi GR, Sachdev HPS. Comparative efficacy of jet nebulizer and metered dose inhaler with spacer device in the treatment of acute asthma. *Indian Pediatr* 1997; 34:497-503.

17. Powell CV, Maskell GR, Marks MK, South M, Robertson CF. Successful implementation of spacer treatment guidelines for acute asthma. *Arch Dis Child* 2001; 84(2): 142-146.

18. Johansson F, Rydberg I, Aberg G, *et al*. Effects of albuterol enantiomers on *in-vitro* bronchial reactivity. *Clin Rev Allergy Immunol* 1996; 14:57-64.

19. Volchek GM, Bleich Gj, Kita II. Pro and anti-inflammatory effects of â-adrenegic agonists on eosinophil response to IL-5 [abstract]. *J Allergy Clin Immunol* 1998; 101:S35.

20. Walle T, Eaton EA, Walle UK, *et al*. Stereoselective metabolism of RS-albuterol in humans. *Clin Rev Allergy Immunol* 1996; 14:101-113.

21. Nelson IIS, Bensch G, Pleskow WW, *et al*. Improved bronchodilation with levalbuterol compared with racemic albuterol in patients with asthma. *J allergy Clin Immunol* 1998; 102(6 pt 1):943-952.

22. Gawechik SM, Saccar CL, Noonan M, *et al*. The safety and the efficacy of nebulized levalbuterol compared with racemic albuterol and placebo in the treatment of asthma in pediatric patients. *J Allergy Clin Immunol* 1999; 103:615-621.

23. Stempel DA, Redding GJ. Management of acute asthma. *Pediatr Clin North Am* 1992; 39:1311-1325.

24. Kartzky MS. Acute asthma. The use of subcutaneous epinephrine in therapy. *Ann Allergy* 1980; 44:12-14.

25. Peirson WG, Bierman CW, Stamm SL. Double-blind trial of aminophylline in status asthmaticus. *Pediatrics* 1971; 48:642-646.

26. Greenough A, Yuksel B, Everett L. Inhaled ipratropium bromide and terbutaline in asthmatic children. *Respir Med* 1993; 87:111-114.

27. Servent (Salmetrol xinaforte) aerosol (package insert) Research Triangle Park, NC : *Glaxo Wellcome*, 1994.

28. Reisman J, Galdes-Sebalt M, Kazim F. Frequent administration by inhalation of salbutamol and ipratropium bromide in the initial management of severe asthma in children. *J Allergy Clin Immunol* 1988; 81:16-20.

Section 4

29. British Thoracic Society guidelines for management of acute asthma. *Thorax* 2003; 58(Suppl I):132-150.

30. Jannum DR, Mickel SF. Anisocoria and aerosolized anticholinergics. *Chest* 1986; 90:148-149.

31. Shah P, Dhurjon L, Metcalfe T, Gibson J. Acute angle closure glaucoma associated with nebulized ipratropium bromide and salbutamol. *Brit Med J* 1992; 304:40-41.

32. Sly RM. New guidelines for diagnosis and management of asthma. *Ann Allergy Asthma Immunol* 1997; 78:27-37.

33. The British Guidelines on Asthma Management: 1995 review and position statement. *Thorax* 1997; 52(Suppl 1):51-52.

34. Partridge M, Saunders K. Site of action of ipratropium bromide and clinical and physiological determinants of response in patients with asthma. *Thorax* 1981; 36:530-533.

35. Storr 1. Lenney W. Nebulized ipratropium and salbutamol in asthma. *Am J Dis Child* 1986; 61:602-603.

36. Plotnick LH, Duarme FM. Combined inhaled anticholinergics and beta-2 agonist for initial treatment of acute asthma in children. *The Cochrane Library*-2001, Issue-2.

37. Milner AD, Henry RL. Acute airways obstruction in children under five. *Thorax* 1982; 37:641-645.

38. Stokes GM, Milner AD, Hodges IGC, Henry RL. Nebulized ipratropium bromide in wheezy infants and children. *Eur J Respir Dis* 1983; 64 (SuppI 128): 494-498.

39. Fanta CH, Rossing TH, McFadden ER. Glucocorticoids in acute asthma: A critical controlled trial. *Am J Med* 1983; 74:845-851.

40. Ratto D, Alfaro C, Spisey J, Giovsky MM, Sharma OP. Are intravenous steroids required in status asthmaticus? *JAMA* 1988; 260:527-529.

41. Chapman KR, Vercheek PR, White JG, Rebuck AS. Effect of a short course of prednisolone in prevention of early relapse after the emergency room treatment of acute asthma. *N Engl J Med* 1991; 324:788-794.

42. Shapiro GG. Double blind evaluation of methyl prednisolone versus placebo for acute asthma episodes. *Pediatrics* 1983; 71:510-514.

43. Fiel SB, Schwartz MA, Glanz K, *et al*. Efficacy of short term corticosteroid therapy in outpatient treatment of acute bronchial asthma. *Am J Med* 1983; 75:259-262.

44. Fanta CII, Rossing TII, Mc Fadden ER. Glucocorticoid in acute asthma: a critical controlled trial. *Am J Med* 1983; 74:845-851.

45. Harris JB, Weinberger MM, Nassif E, *et al*. Early intervention with short course of prednisone to prevent progression of asthma in ambulatory patients incompletely responsive to bronchodilators. *J Pediatr* 1987; 110:627-633.

46. Littenberg B, Gluck EH. A controlled trial of methyl prednisolone in the emergency treatment of acute asthma. *N Engl J Med* 1986; 314:150-152.

47. Pierson WE, Bierman W, Kelly VC. A double blind trial of corticosteroid therapy in status asthmaticus. *Pediatrics* 1983; 71:510-514.

48. Kattan M, Gurwitz D, Levison H. Corticosteroids in status asthmaticus. *J Pediatr* 1980; 96:596-599.

49. Webb MSC, Henry RL, Milner AD. Oral corticosteroids for wheezing attacks under 18 months. *Arch Dis Child* 1986; 61:15-19.

50. Tal A, Levy N, Bearman JE. Methyl prednisolone therapy for acute asthma in infants and toddlers: A controlled trial. *Pediatrics* 1990; 86:350-356.

51. Scarfone RJ, Loiselle JM, Wiley JP, Deeker JM, Henretig M, Joffe MD. Nebulized dexamethasone versus oral prednisone in the emergency treatment of asthmatic children. *Ann Emerg Med* 1995; 26: 480-486.

52. Arth N, Prapam Y, Suchai C, Jacob B, Class GD, Olof S, *et al*. High dose of inhaled budesonide may substitute for an oral therapy after an acute asthma. *Acta Paediatr Scand* 1999, 88:835-840.

53. Devidyal, Singhi S, Kumar L, Jayshree M. Efficacy of nebulized budesonide compared to oral prednisolone in acute asthma. *Acta Paediatr Scand* 1999; 88:835-840.

54. Schuh S, Reisman I, Alsheri M, Dupuis A, Corey M, Arsenault R, *et al*. A comparison of inhaled fluticasone and oral prednisolone for children with severe acute asthma. *N Eng J Med* 2000; 343:689-694.

55. Edmonds ML, Camargo CA, Pollock CY, Rowe BH. Early use of inhaled corticosteroids in the emergency department treatment of acute asthma. Cochrane Review, *The Cochrane Library*, Issue 2, 2001.

56. Chopra SR, Taplia GV, Simmons DH, *et al*. Effects of hydration and physical therapy on tracheal transport velocity. *Am Rev Respir Dis* 1977; 115:1009-1014.

57. Haalboon JRE, Denstra M, Stuyvenberg A. Hypokalemia induced by inhalation of fenoterol. *Lancet* 1985; 1:1125-1127.

58. Littenberg B. Aminophylline treatment in severe acute asthma: a meta-analysis. *JAMA* 1988; 259:1678-1684.

59. Self TH, Abou-Shala N, Burns R, *et al*. Inhaled albuterol and oral prednisolone in hospitalized adult asthma: Does theophylline add any benefit? *Am Rev Respir Dis* 1990; 98(6):1317-1321.

60. Pierson WE, Bierman W, Kelly VC. A double blind trial of corticosteroid therapy in status asthmaticus. *Pediatrics* 1983; 71:510-514.

61. Ream RS, Loftis LL, Albers GM, Backer BA, Lynch RE, Mink RB. Efficacy of intravenous theophylline in children with severe status asthmaticus. *Chest* 2001; 119: 480-488.

Section 4

62. Yung M, South M. Randomized controlled trial of aminophylline for severe acute asthma. *Arch Dis Child* 1998; 79:405-410.

63. Jenne JW. Theophylline use in asthma. *Clin Chest Med* 1984; 5:645-658.

64. Wheeler DS, Jacobs BR, Kenreigh CA. Theophylline versus terbutaline in treating critically ill children with status asthamaticus: a prospective RCT. *Pediatr Crit Care Med* 2005; 6(2):142-147.

65. Hill JH. Acute severe asthma. In : A Practical Guide to Pediatric Intensive Care, Blummer JL (Ed) 3rd edn. *St.Louis, Mosby Year-Book*, 1990.

66. Williams SJ, Winner SJ, Clark TJH. Comparison of inhaled and intravenous terbutaline in acute severe asthma. *Thorax* 1981; 36:629-631.

67. Dietrich KA, Conrad SA, Romero MD. Creatinine kinase isoenzymes in pediatric status asthmaticus treated with intravenous terbutaline. *Crit Care Med* 1991; 19 (Suppl):539.

68. Fuglsang G, Pedersen S, Borgstrom L. Dose response relationship of intravenously administered terbutaline in children with asthma. *J Pediatr* 1989; 114:315-320.

69. De Nicola KL, Monem GF, Gayle MO, Kissoon N. Treatment of critical status asthmaticus in children. *Pediatr Clin N Am* 1994; 41:1293-1323.

70. Pullela RD, Kumar L, Singhi SC, Prasad R, Singh M. Intravenous magnesium sulphate in acute severe asthma not responding to conventional therapy. *Indian Pediatr* 1997; 34:389-397.

71. Leff A. Pathophysiology of asthmatic bronchoconstriction. *Chest* 1982; 92 (suppl):135-145.

72. Delcastillo J, Engback L. The nature of neuromuscular block produced by magnesium. *J Physiol* 1954; 124:370-384.

73. Bois P. Effect of magnesium deficiency on mast cells and urinary histamine in rats. *Brit J Experiment Pathology* 1963; 44:151-155.

74. Altera BM, Altera BT, Carella A. Magnesium deficiency induced spasm of umbilical vessels: Relation to pre-eclampsia, hypertension, growth retardation. *Science* 1983; 221:376-378.

75. Okayama H, Okayama M, Aikawa T, et al. Treatment of status asthmaticus with intravenous magnesium sulphate. *J Asthma* 1991; 28:11-15.

76. Mudge GH, Wriner IM. Water, salt and ions. In: Textbook of the Pharmacologic Basis of Therapeutics. Goodman LS, Gilman AG (Eds): *New York, Macmillan*, 1996; p704.

77. Noppen N, Vanmaele L, Impens N, Wouter S. Bronchodilating effect of intravenous magensium sulphate in acute severe bronchial asthma. *Chest* 1990; 97:373-376.

78. Okayama H, Aikawa T, Okayama M, Sasaki H, Mue S, Takishima T. Bronchodilating effect of intravenous magnesium sulphate in acute severe asthma. *JAMA* 1987; 257:1076-1078.

79. Rowe BH, Jennifer AB, Bourdon C, Bota GW, Camargo CA. Intravenous magnesium sulfate for acute asthma in the emergency department. A systemic review of the literature. *Ann Emerg Med* 2000; 36:181-190.

80. Alter HJ, Koepsell TD, Hilty WM. Intravenous magnesium sulfate as an adjunct in acute bronchospasm: A meta-analysis. *Ann Emerg Med* 2000; 36:191-197.

81. Rock MJ, Reyes De La Rocha S, Hommedieu C, Truemper E. Use of ketamine in asthmatic children to treat respiratory failure refractory to conventional therapy. *Crit Care Med* 1986; 14:514-516.

82. Sarma VI. Use of ketamine in acute severe asthma. *Acta Anaesthiol Scand* 1992; 36:106-107.

83. Luksza AR, Smith P, Coakley J, et at. Acute severe asthma treated by mechanical ventilation: 10 years experience from a district general hospital. *Thorax* 1985; 41:459-463.

84. Harmanci K, Bakirtas A, Turktas I, Degim T. Oral monteleukast treatment of preschool aged children with acute asthma. *Ann allergy, asthma immunol* 2006; 96(5):731-735

85. Prezant DJ, Aldrich TK. Intravenous droperidol for the treatment of status asthmaticus. *Crit Care Med* 1988; 16:96-98.

86. Bierman MI, Brown M, Muren O, et al. Prolonged isoflurane anesthesia in status asthmaticus. *Crit Care Med* 1986; 14: 832-833.

87. Martin-Barbaz F, Bamoud D, Carpentier F. Use of helium and oxygen mixtures in status asthmaticus. *Rev Pneumol Clin* 1987; 43:186-188.

88. Radrigo GJ, Radrigo C, Pollock CV, Rowe B. Use of Helium oxygen mixture in the treatment of acute asthma: a systematic review. *Chest* 2003; 123(3):891-896.

89. O'Rourke PP, Crone RK. Halothane in status asthmaticus. *Crit Care Med* 1982; 10:341-343.

90. Rosseel P, Lawers LF, Bante L. Halothane treatment in life-threatening asthma. *Intensive Care Medicine* 1985; 11:241-246.

91. Johaston RG, Noseworthy TW, Friesen EG, et al. Isoflurane therapy for status asthmaticus in children and adults. *Chest* 1990; 97:698-701.

92. Hirrsham C, Bergman N. Halothane and enflurane protect against bronchospasm in an asthma dog model. *Anesth Analg* 1978; 57:629-632.

93. Klide A, Aviado DM. Mechanism for the reduction in pulmonary resistance induced by halothane. *J Pharmacol Exp Ther* 1967; 158:28-35.

94. Canny GJ, Bohn DJ, Levison H. Severe asthma. *Recent Adv Pediatr* 1992; 10:161-171.

31

ARDS in Children

Soonu Udani and Tanu Singhal

INTRODUCTION

Acute respiratory distress syndrome (ARDS) and its milder form, acute lung injury (ALI) results from a pulmonary or systemic insult causing breakdown of the alveolar-capillary barrier leading to an acute inflammatory response and protein rich pulmonary edema. The consequent refractory hypoxemia and respiratory failure that ensue, offer the intensivist one of the greatest challenges of the discipline of critical care.

DEFINITION

Various definitions have been proposed since ARDS was first described in 1967. The latest American-European Consensus Criteria for the standardization of reporting and clinical trial coordination were published in 1994 [1] and are shown in the Box:

Consensus criteria for ALI/ARDS [1]

- Acute onset of respiratory distress
- Severe arterial hypoxemia resistant to oxygen therapy *alone* (PaO_2/FiO_2 ratio < 200 for ARDS and PaO_2/FiO_2 ratio < 200-300 for ALI)
- Diffuse pulmonary inflammation (bilateral infiltrates on chest radiograph)
- No evidence of left atrial hypertension, pulmonary artery occlusion pressure (PAOP) $\leq$ 18 mm Hg

---

This definition is simple, easy-to-use and differentiates the less severe acute lung injury from the more severe ARDS. However, prognostic factors such as etiology and involvement of other organ systems and allowance for ventilator settings at the application of the P: F ratio values are not included. Additionally, the criterion of bilateral lung infiltrates is quite non-specific and subject to significant inter-observer disagreement among radiologists [2].

INCIDENCE

Data from developed countries suggests that the incidence of ARDS in adults is roughly 75 cases per 100,000 people per year [3]. Population based data in children is lacking. A tertiary care center in northern India reported 16 cases of ARDS/1000 pediatric intensive care unit (PICU) admissions, whereas one from the south reported an incidence of 22.7/1000 admissions [4,5]. More children will be ventilated in the PICU (Pediatric Intensive Care Unit) for supportive care and other indications put together than for ARDS.

ETIOLOGY

Common clinical conditions associated with risk of development of ARDS are listed in Table 31.1 [2,6] Severe sepsis, pneumonia, severe trauma and massive transfusions are recognized predisposing factors of ARDS [6]. Severe sepsis is associated with the highest risk of progression to ARDS, roughly 40% [2,7]. The recent increase in occurrence of viral pneumonias and the H1N1 epidemic worldwide have increased the burden of ARDS [8]. In tropical countries like India, infections such as malaria (both vivax and falciparum), leptospirosis, dengue, tuberculosis and rickettsia are additional causes of ARDS [9-14].

PATHOGENESIS

Pneumonia is the most common cause of direct injury causing ARDS and it tends to predominate in most studies. The reason for distinguishing between direct and indirect injury is the difference in the pathogenesis and outcome; the latter being much worse in patients with direct injury. Direct injury causes regional consolidation and destruction of the alveoli. Indirect injury is associated with more pulmonary vascular congestion, interstitial edema and less alveolar involvement. Regardless of the cause, the progress of the condition is through distinct stages where the pathophysiology, clinical, radiological and

Table 31.1 Clinical disorders associated with the development of ARDS[6]

Direct lung injury	Indirect lung injury
Common causes	
o Pneumonia o Aspiration of gastric contents	o Severe sepsis/shock o Severe trauma with shock and multiple transfusions
Less common causes	
o Pulmonary contusion o Toxic gas inhalation o Near-drowning o Reperfusion injury after pulmonary embolectomy and lung transplant	o Burns o Acute pancreatitis o Drug overdose o Transfusion of blood products o Post cardiac bypass

histological features run parallel and treatment is tailored to the stage of the disease.

ALI and ARDS are both characterized by damage to the microvascular endothelium and the alveolar epithelium leading to influx of protein rich edema fluid in the air space. Damage to the type I and type II cells of the alveolar epithelium leads to disruption of normal epithelial fluid transport followed by impairing of the reabsorption of edema fluid, reduced production of surfactant, septic shock and disorganized repair with fibrosis[2]. Neutrophils, a complex network of proinflammatory cytokines and the coagulation system initiate and amplify the inflammatory response in ALI and ARDS. Ventilator-induced lung injury (VILI) due to high fractions of inspired oxygen, alveolar overdistension and cyclic opening and closing of atelectatic alveoli adds insult to injury and causes increased permeability with pulmonary edema in the uninjured lung, increased edema in the injured lung as well as multiorgan dysfunction (Figure 31.1).

After the acute phase, a subset of patients with ALI and ARDS progress to fibrotic lung injury. Fibrosis can be observed histologically as early as 5-7 days after the onset of the disorder and correlates with increased risk of death. Fibrosing alveolitis is initiated by the proinflammatory cytokines such as interleukin-1 and the alveolar space becomes filled with mesenchymal cells, their products and new blood vessels. Patients who die of this condition have marked amounts of collagen and fibronectin in the lungs at autopsy.

Resolution of illness is marked by resorption of edema fluid, which in certain individuals occurs within the first few hours of mechanical ventilation. Removal of soluble protein occurs by diffusion in between the epithelial cells and the interstitium and

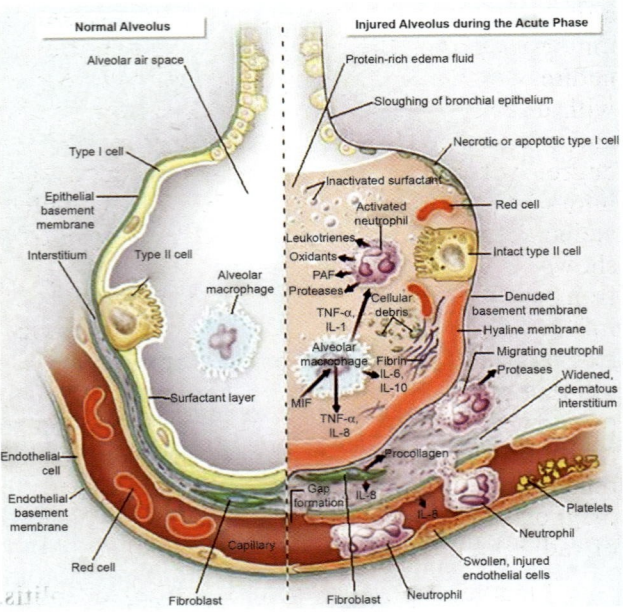

Figure 31.1 Mechanism of alveolar injury in ARDS/ALI[2]

that of insoluble protein by endocytosis and transcytosis of epithelial cells and phagocytosis by macrophages. The mechanism of clearance of the inflammatory cell infiltrate and fibrosis is unclear but the former is attributed to apoptosis. The alveolar type II cells initiate re-epithelialization and restore normal alveolar architecture. The sequence of events in ARDS are summarized in the Box.

Sequence of events in ARDS

- Microvascular injury to the endothelium
- Alveolar epithelium is also injured
- Type II pneumatocytes are damaged
- Surfactant dysfunction and deficiency occurs
- Alveolar fluid clearance hampered, resulting in pulmonary edema
- Macrophages are activated
- Stimulate chemotaxis and activate neutrophils
- Cytokines (TNF, IL 6-8) and oxidants are released

CLINICAL PRESENTATION

The acute stage is characterized by rapid onset of respiratory failure in a patient with predisposing condition(s). The patient becomes anxious, agitated and dyspneic. Stiffening of the lung with decreased compliance leads to increased work of breathing and worsens the dyspnea. Hypoxemia refractory to supplemental oxygen and hypocarbia is present. In later stages acidosis and hypercarbia occurs. At this stage of the disease, the compliance is steadily decreasing but the lung is still amenable to inflation and "recruitment". Hence it is important to understand that the disease is homogenous in nature, with areas of unaffected alveoli interspersed with densely affected alveoli with various grades and severity of involvement. This gives varying degrees of compliance in the lungs, open units interspersed with partially closed or completely atelectatic units. The radiographic picture usually shows bilateral infiltrates, often indistinguishable from cardiogenic pulmonary edema (Figure 31.2). Infiltrates may be patchy or asymmetric and may be associated with pleural effusion. When associated with pneumonia, the picture of the primary pathology may predominate. However, radiographic findings are non-specific; a study reported only 43% agreement among 21 experts in diagnosis of 28 patients of ALI/ARDS on the basis of radiographs of chest[16].

In patients progressing to fibrosing alveolitis, there is persistent hypoxemia, increased alveolar dead space and decreasing lung compliance. Pulmonary hypertension due to obliteration of the capillary bed may be severe and lead to right ventricular failure. Chest radiographs show linear opacities consistent with fibrosis. Incidence of pneumothorax is around 10-13% and is not directly related to airway pressure or positive end expiratory pressure[15].

The clinical course parallels the histological stages. In the initial phase of the illness (first 5-7 days) areas of normal lung are seen between abnormal lung (on CT) and therefore PEEP works. Beyond 5-7 days, the amount of abnormal lung increases, hence PEEP is less effective and hypercarbia is pronounced. The fibroproliferative phase is marked by slow recovery and ventilator dependency.

The resolution phase is characterized by gradual recovery of hypoxemia, improved lung compliance as well as radiographic resolution. The degree of histologic resolution of fibrosis is not well studied but in most patients the lung functions return back to normal[2].

MANAGEMENT

I. Control of underlying disease

Patients with infection should be treated aggressively with appropriate antibiotics intravenously and drainage of pus as and when needed. Blood products should be used with caution.

II. Respiratory support

This is the mainstay of the management and deserves detailed discussion.

1. Basic ventilation strategies. The goal of respiratory support is to maintain adequate oxygenation with minimal ventilator-induced lung damage or ventilator associated lung injury (VILI/VALI). The most revolutionary change in the management of ARDS has been adoption of the "lung protective strategies" wherein lower tidal volumes and appropriate higher positive end expiratory pressures (PEEP) are used to minimize lung injury[17] (Box).

Lung Protective Ventilation Strategies (LPVS)
• Avoid regional over distension (Baby lung concept)
• Avoid repeated opening/closing of airways (Open lung concept)
• Permissive hypercapnia
• Permissive hypoxemia

2. Baby lung concept[18]. This concept originated when multiple CT scan examinations showed in most patients with ARDS that normally aerated tissue has the dimensions of the lung of a 5-6 years old child (300–500 gm aerated tissue). The respiratory system compliance is

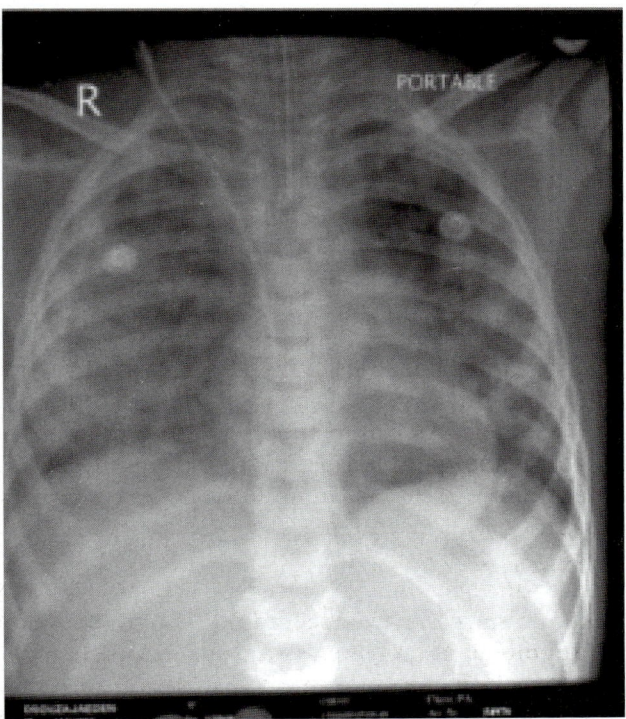

Figure 31.2 Typical skiagram of chest in ARDS

linearly related to the baby lung quantity, suggesting that the ARDS lung is not only stiff but also small, with nearly normal intrinsic elasticity in the early phases. This is a functional, not anatomical concept and provides a rationale for gentle lung ventilation. The smaller the baby lung, the greater is the potential for damage and VALI (ventilator associated lung inury) is attributable in part to the application of physiological tidal volumes of >8-10 ml/kg to the reduced area of non-consolidated alveoli (Figure 31.3).

3. *Initiation of mechanical ventilation.* Amato et al[19] in 1998 first demonstrated the benefits of using low tidal volumes, low plateau pressures and optimal PEEP on mortality in ARDS. The ARDS Net trial (2000) which randomized 861 adult patients with ALI / ARDS to either traditional ventilation (V_t 12 ml/kg and peak pressures of 50 cm of H_2O) or lung protective ventilation (V_t 6 ml/kg or peak pressures of < 30 cm of H_2O) reported significantly reduced mortality in the lung protective ventilation group (31% vs 39.5%).[9] The patients with the worst lung compliance at randomization had the greatest reduction in mortality with the low V_t strategy. The lung protective group also had larger number of ventilator free days and lower end organ complications such as cardiac failure, renal failure and disseminated intravascular coagulation.

Though no specific conventional mode has been shown to be superior to the other, the preferred ventilation mode is volume controlled, pressure-limited and time-cycled ventilation. Controlled mandatory ventilation (CMV) with sedation and neuromuscular blockade (fentanyl, midazolam and pancuronium infusion) to suppress the respiratory drive and reduce oxygen requirements of respiratory muscles is preferred in a sick patient. The initial ventilator setting are shown in the Box.

Initiatial Ventilator Settings

- Non-invasive ventilation is successful in very early and mild ARDS.
- Ventilator mode: PRVC > PCV >VCV (HFOV whenever indicated)
- Tidal volume: < 6 ml/kg (adjusted according to plateau pressure)
- Plateau pressure: <30 cm H_2O
- Rate: 6 to 35
- I: E ratio: 1:1 to 1:3
- PEEP and FiO_2 is set according to predetermined combinations (PEEP range 5 to 24 cm H_2O), limit FiO2 less than 0.6 whenever possible.
- Oxygenation target: PaO_2 55-80 mmHg/ SpO_2 88 to 95%

It is advisable to start with FiO_2 of 1.0, tidal volume 6 ml per kg, PEEP of 5 cm H_2O and inspiratory flow rates ~ 60 L/min. Subsequent adjustments are made to achieve arterial oxygen saturation of >90% with FiO_2 < 0.6 and peak airway pressures of 30 to 35 cm H_2O. However, in severe disease, this goal may be unrealistic and at the cost of severe VILI. Hence, if hemodynamics, tissue perfusion and metabolic acidosis are not serious issues, lower levels of SpO_2 (85%) and PaO_2 values of 55mm Hg may be acceptable. The oxygen carrying capacity of the blood should be maintained with hemoglobin of at least 10 gm/dl.

Most of these ventilator adjustments focus on achieving optimal PEEP settings. PEEP improves oxygenation by promoting movement of fluid from alveolar to interstitial space, recruitment of small airways and collapsed alveoli and increasing the functional residual capacity. Potential detrimental effects of PEEP include barotrauma due to alveolar overdistension and hemodynamic derangements due to impaired venous return and reduced cardiac output. Current practice is to increase PEEP by 2 to 5 cm of H_2O every 5-10 breaths, watching for hemodynamic derangements. There is no evidence that recruitment maneuvers such as sigh, CPAP or BiPAP influence outcome in pediatric ARDS. It is important to remember that only if the lung is "recruitable", will PEEP be optimally effective.

4. *Selection of PEEP.* A high PEEP and low FiO_2 strategy is preferred in all patients. The FiO_2 and PEEP are titrated as shown in the bottom half of the Table 31.2. There will be a cohort of patients that will not tolerate this and will

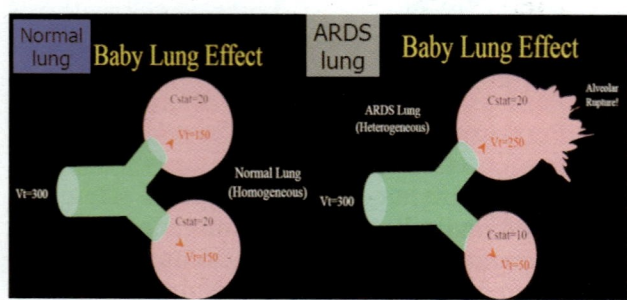

Figure 31.3 Baby lung concept where pressure and volume are transmitted to the "normal" alveoli

respond poorly to high PEEP and will not allow reduction in the FiO₂. These patients may need to go on the low PEEP high FiO₂ (top panel) or may need to go on another form of support like HFOV (Figure 31.4).

Since high FiO₂ may result in cellular toxicity and reabsorption atelectasis, efforts should be made to keep the FiO₂ below 0.6 as soon as possible. No clinical trial has addressed the issue of inspiratory time; the I: E ratio may be increased to 1:1 or 2:1 (inverse ratio ventilation) to improve oxygenation. However, reversed ratios are uncomfortable for the patient, result in increased plateau pressure and are best avoided.

5. *Open lung concept (OLC).* An increased initial inflation pressure recruits collapsed alveoli, which then require minimal pressure to stay open. Early recruitment (< 72 hr) gives a better response. This is probably related to the change from the exudative to a fibroproliferative process, when worsening of compliance will make the lung non-recruitable. Recruitment at the early stage of severe lung injury may dramatically improve oxygenation and maintain integrity of the newly recruited lung. Percentages of recruitable lung vary from negligible to >50% in ARDS patients. Both Pressure and Time are important for alveolar recruitment. The goal of this concept

is to decrease atelectasis and increase optimal gas exchange [20,21,22,23] (Figure 31.4).

The pressure volume loop illustrates how to open the lung at high inflation pressures but in order to keep it open at the same volume, requires much lower pressure. The lung usually opens to a volume of 45 cm of water which is in the unsafe zone. As the pressures are decreased, even at a pressure of about 25 cm, the lung maintains that volume keeping the ventilation process within the safe zone.

A randomized controlled trial with concealed allocation and blinded data analysis conducted on 983 patients between August 2000 and March 2006 in 30 intensive care units in Canada, Australia, and Saudi Arabia demonstrated no significant difference in all-cause hospital mortality or barotrauma using the open lung concept compared to an established low-tidal-volume ventilation strategy. The "open-lung" strategy, however, did appear to improve secondary end points related to hypoxemia and use of rescue therapies.[24]

6. *Recruitment maneuvers (RMs).* Recruitment maneuvers use brief elevations of airway pressures considerably higher than those that result from tidal ventilation. A recruitment maneuver (RM) and high PEEP intend to aerate collapsed and flooded alveoli, which

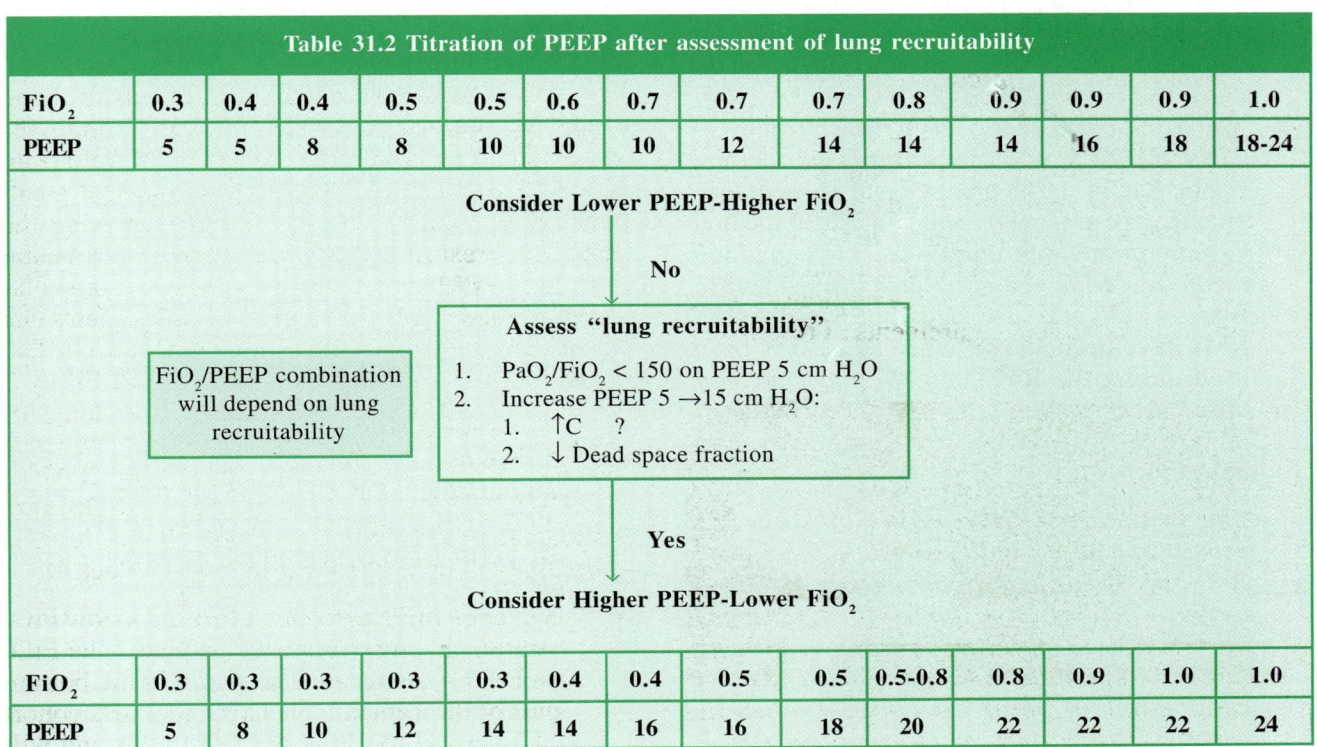

Table 31.2 Titration of PEEP after assessment of lung recruitability

FiO₂	0.3	0.4	0.4	0.5	0.5	0.6	0.7	0.7	0.7	0.8	0.9	0.9	0.9	1.0
PEEP	5	5	8	8	10	10	10	12	14	14	14	16	18	18-24

Consider Lower PEEP-Higher FiO₂

No

FiO₂/PEEP combination will depend on lung recruitability

Assess "lung recruitability"
1. PaO₂/FiO₂ < 150 on PEEP 5 cm H₂O
2. Increase PEEP 5 →15 cm H₂O:
   1. ↑C ?
   2. ↓ Dead space fraction

Yes

Consider Higher PEEP-Lower FiO₂

FiO₂	0.3	0.3	0.3	0.3	0.3	0.4	0.4	0.5	0.5	0.5-0.8	0.8	0.9	1.0	1.0
PEEP	5	8	10	12	14	14	16	16	18	20	22	22	22	24

Section 4

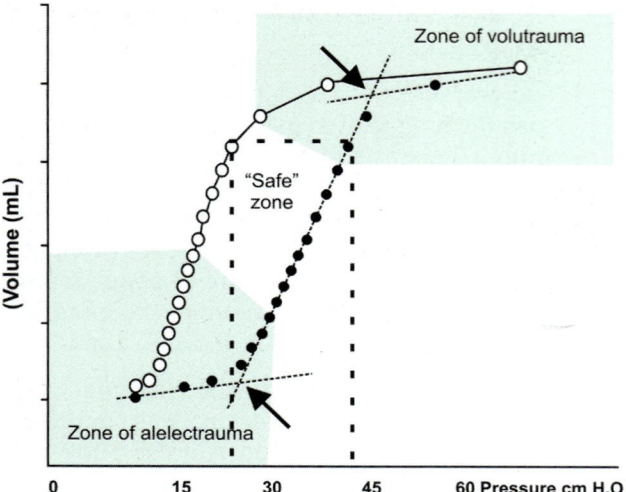

Figure 31.4 Pressure volume loop in patients with ARDS to promote the concept "open the lung and keep it open"

may improve oxygenation, decrease ventilator-induced lung injury from the shear stress forces of repetitive opening and closing of alveoli, and improve compliance of the system in some patients.

A commonly used RM was first described by Grasso et al[25] in 22 patients by using a PEEP of 40 cm for 40 secs. If the lung is recruitable, there is an improvement in lung and chest wall compliance by as much as 175%. This in simple terms at the bedside translates into an improvement in SpO_2, PaO_2, and reduction in FiO_2 within about 2 minutes. *Patients with non-recruitable lungs respond with little change or actually show deterioration in these parameters or in their hemodynamics; which indicates that a switch in strategy to early HFOV may be required.* This method is popular in adult practice but in pediatric practice, the gradual incremental PEEP method is more commonly employed. Two common methods used in pediatrics are outlined below. Better results and sustained improvement with RMs have been shown when PEEP has been used during the RM along with any method chosen (Figure 31.5). The recruitment maneuvers in ARDS are summarized in Table 31.3.

The need for a fluid bolus or inotrope should not be an indication to abandon an RM but sustained hypotension or high inotrope and poor response to fluids must be taken as a definite adverse event and further RMs should be done with greater caution and at lower pressures. As there is a long inspiratory pause or high PEEP

Table 31.3 Recruitment maneuvers in ARDS
Suggested Method 1
1. Sedate and paralyse the patient
2. Increase the inflation pressure to 40 cm of H_2O for 40 sec (or 1.5 times the current pressure)
3. No RR delivered during the period
4. Reduce pressure gradually by 5 cm every 5 breaths till SpO_2 starts to fall below 90-92%.
5. Raise inflation pressure to 2-5 cm above the level at which SpO_2 fell
Suggested Method 2
1. Start increasing PEEP 2-5 cm at every 2-5 breaths
2. Reach the level at which SpO_2 reaches 90-92%
3. Continue till the SpO_2 falls (over distension reached)
4. Start dropping pressure as shown in method 1
5. Drop to 2-5 cm below the best level and see if SpO_2 falls
6. If it falls raise the pressure back to best level
Monitoring during/after RMs (hemodynamics should be carefully monitored during and immediately after)
• P/F ratio, compliance, dead space ventilation
• It is important to assess improvement in oxygenation and compliance immediately after the intervention and again within 6 to 12 hr.
• If dead-space ventilation increases after the RM, this suggests alveolar over distension; therefore, the PEEP should be decreased.
Disadvantages of RMs
• VILI/barotrauma and hemodynamic compromise
• Translocation of pulmonary bacteria/sepsis
• Release of cytokines into the systemic circulation (Partial recruitment)
• Paradoxically oxygenation may worsen by over distending aerated lung units and redistributing pulmonary blood flow to areas of consolidation.
• Persistent decrease in gastric mucosal perfusion following RMs.

during this procedure, it is uncomfortable for the patient and therefore sedation and paralysis needs are increased during the period of the RM.

7. *Permissive hypercapnia.* The earlier goal of maintaining a $PaCO_2$ within the normal range at all costs has been replaced by the principle of "permissive hypercapnia" wherein arterial pH of 7.15-7.25 and $PaCO_2$ of upto 80 mm Hg are fairly well tolerated. Sodium bicarbonate may be used if there is significant respiratory acidosis. The patient's pH status and tissue perfusion play an important role in the decision to allow the CO_2 to rise. When

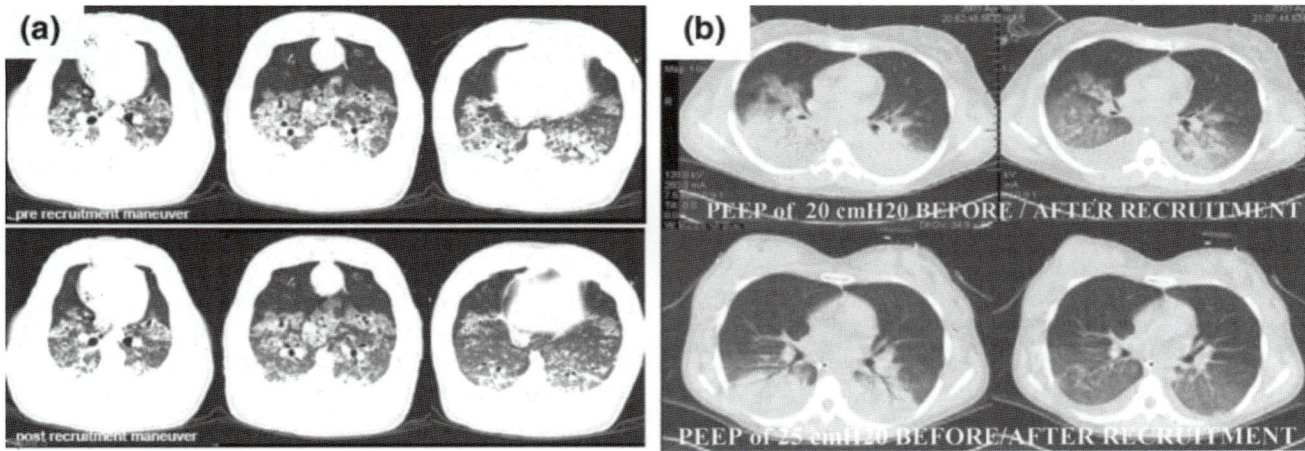

Figure 31.5 CT scans of the chest showing the effect of (a) recruitment maneuvers without PEEP and (b) recruitment maneuvers with PEEP on lung volumes. The expansion of lung is much better when PEEP is employed along with an RM

the lung is the only organ under fire, this is easier to accept but in a septic patient with high CO_2 production, metabolic acidosis and poor tissue perfusion, it is important to correct acidosis to improve the outcome.

Acidosis may constitute a protective adaptation in the context of cellular stress, and may in fact contribute beneficial effects in the setting of acute organ injury. It is hypothesized that hypercapneic acidosis may down-regulate inflammatory cell activity, and may inhibit xanthine oxidase, thus reducing oxidant stress. It is contraindicated in pediatric traumatic brain injury and relatively contraindicated in severe cardiac disease/dysfunction. Stepwise management of hypercapnia and acidosis is mentioned in the box. The disadvantages of permissive hypercapnia include intrapulmonary shunting, decrease in myocardial contractility, risk of arrhythmia and increase in cerebral blood flow.

Stepwise treatment of hypercapnia and acidosis

- Slow respiratory rate upto 35/min
- Respiratory rate increased beyond 35/min followed by buffer therapy
- Persistent acidosis or hypernatremia or hyperchloremic metabolic acidosis
- Needs recruitment
- Recruitment maneuvers and ECMO

---

8. *Stepwise treatment of hypoxemia*[26]. The stepwise correction of hypoxia is shown in the Box.

Stepwise correction of hypoxemia*

- PIP/PEEP titration
- Prone positioning
- High frequency oscillatory ventilation (HFOV)
- Surfactant
- Inhaled nitric oxide (iNO)
- Corticosteroids
- Extracorporeal membrane oxygenation

*   Monitor SpO_2, PaO_2, static compliance and dead space.

(a) Prone positioning. Prone positioning has been shown to improve oxygenation in patients with ALI/ARDS. Potential mechanisms include better recruitment of atelectatic dorsal regions of lungs, decrease in abdominal compression of thorax and optimizing and removal of secretions. There are several disadvantages of prone positioning like increased venous pressure in the head, increased intra abdominal pressure, unplanned extubations and dislodgement of various catheters and the nursing staff needs to be experienced and trained in this maneuver.

Several case reports have documented benefits of prone positioning in adult patients with ARDS. Jolliet et al[27] reported improvement in the PaO_2/FiO_2 ratio by 20 mm Hg in 96% of adults with ARDS following prone positioning. The effort was most dramatic at one hour, continued to show improvement over the next 12 hours and was sustained even when the patients were made supine. A randomized controlled trial in pediatric patients also showed significant improvement of oxygenation following prone positioning without any complications. However, a study that evaluated the impact of prone positioning on mortality from ARDS did not show any significant benefit[28, 29].

Section 4

(b) High frequency oscillatory ventilation (HFOV). The likely advantages for HFOV in ARDS include the use of low Vt with improved lung recruitment and avoidance of alveolar shearing injury and maintenance of near normal $PaCO_2$ with improved minute ventilation. Arnold et al[30] in a randomized controlled trial of pediatric patients with acute respiratory failure (55% of whom met the ARDS criteria) reported significant improvement in oxygenation and better outcome in the HFOV arm patients as compared to the lung protective conventional ventilated patients. When HFOV was instituted before the oxygenation index (OI) rose above 30, the outcome was better and the results were best when the OI was below 20 before HFOV was started.[31]

HFOV for ARDS

- Lung recruitment can be achieved with minimal peak-trough pressure changes.
- It should be considered for use in patients requiring high MAP on conventional ventilation.
- FiO_2 requirements exceed 60% and plateau pressure (Pplat) cannot be maintained ≤ 30 cm H_2O.
- Failure to improve the oxygenation index within the first 24-48 hours is likely to be associated with a poor response to HFOV.
- In most children with ARDS, non-responders to HFOV are likely to have extremely high mortality.

With growing experience with this modality, it is being more frequently used in Indian units with ever increasing success. The advantages of HFOV for ARDS are listed in the Box.

(c) Surfactant. It has been demonstrated that surfactant is functionally and quantitatively deranged in patients with ARDS. Studies on surfactant use in adults with ARDS patients failed to demonstrate any benefit on oxygenation or mortality. Poor delivery of surfactant to the lungs was cited as a possible reason. Both randomized and retrospective studies on surfactant use in pediatric hypoxic respiratory failure (ARDS and non ARDS) have demonstrated rapid and sustained improvement in oxygenation, faster weaning from mechanical ventilation and shorter ICU stay but no difference in mortality. Surfactant use may thus be considered as an adjuvant in only selected children with ARDS.

(d) Glucocorticoids and other anti-inflammatory agents. A seven year study showed that methylprednisolone improved cardio-pulmonary physiology and altered the course of ARDS with 3-7 days of therapy. It also increased the number of ventilator free days, ICU free days and shock free days on evaluation at 28 days. However, this group was also more likely to return back to assisted ventilation and this seems to account for the lack of mortality benefit at 60 days. This study did not show an added incidence of infection whereas others have shown high incidence of nosocomial infection with high doses of steroids. The problem of neuromyopathy with high dose steroid use in children with critical illness must not be ignored.[32] However, a larger randomized controlled trial demonstrated no survival benefit for corticosteroids in persistent ARDS and suggested increased mortality for those who received corticosteroids for more than 14 days after the onset of ARDS[33]. At present, short course of low-moderate dose glucocorticoids can be considered as a rescue therapy in severe non-resolving ARDS between 7-14 days.

(e) Nitric oxide. Since ARDS is inevitably accompanied by pulmonary hypertension, the role of inhaled nitric oxide (iNO) has been extensively evaluated[7, 34]. Data suggest that iNO improves short-term oxygenation in pediatric ARDS patients, but there is little impact on long-term oxygenation index or mortality[34]. iNO is also not available in most units in India and therefore not a therapeutic option in pediatric ARDS. When this modality is available, a short term iNO may be used as salvage therapy in patients with refractory ARDS.

(f) Extra corporeal membrane oxygenation (ECMO). The rationale behind use of ECMO is to support oxygen delivery while lung healing takes place. Retrospective studies on use of ECMO in children with severe respiratory failure, some of which were ARDS related, have shown survival of the critically sick children at high-predicted risk of dying[7,35]. This modality is now available in some centers in India.

III. Supportive care[2, 4]

1. Monitoring hemodynamics and intra-vascular volume. Invasive monitoring of central venous pressure and arterial blood pressure is crucial for management of critically sick children. When high PEEP values are needed, hemodynamic monitoring is essential to assess the response to therapy. Appropriate fluid management is important. It has been shown in animal models that alveolar edema fluid is reduced if left atrial pressures are reduced. The objective is, therefore, to maintain the intravascular volume at the lowest level that is

Table 31.4 Management strategies for pediatric ARDS[2,6,9]

1 Early ARDS (Non-invasive ventilation)

- Administer 40 to 60% inspired oxygen with a tight fitting mask and peak inspiratory flow rates of >70 L/min
- If the patient is well oxygenated on < 60 % inspired oxygen and apparently stable without CO_2 retention, continue non-invasive ventilation with close observation (15 to 30 min)

2. Indications for mechanical ventilation

- Clinical signs of incipient respiratory failure
- Inadequate oxygenation (PaO_2 < 60 mm Hg on FiO_2 > 0.6)
- Rising or elevated $PaCO_2$ (> 45 mm Hg)

3. Initiation of mechanical ventilation

- Ventilator mode: PRVC >PCV >VCV/(HFOV whenever indicated)
- Tidal volume: < 6 ml/Kg (adjusted according to plateau pressure)
- Plateau pressure < 30 cm H_2O
- Rate: 6 to 35
- I: E ratio: 1:1 to 1:3
- PEEP and FiO_2: Set according to predetermined combinations (PEEP range 5 to 24 cm H_2O), limit FiO2 less than 0.6 whenever possible.
- Oxygenation target: PaO_2 55- 80/SpO_2 88 to 95%

4. Subsequent adjustments

- Goal is to maintain PaO_2 between 55-80 mm Hg and pH of >7.15
- Increase PEEP by 2 cm H_2O, watch for hypotension
- Simultaneously reduce FiO_2 to less than 0.6
- Titrate PEEP and FiO_2 based on Table 31.2
- Limit plateau pressures to <30 cm H_2O
- Watch oxygenation index for any worsening demanding a change in strategy

5. Supportive care

- Sedation, analgesia and paralysis for optimum ventilation. Avoid paralysis at a later stage
- Central line and invasive arterial blood pressure monitoring
- Blood transfusion to maintain hemoglobin >10 gm/dl
- Appropriate fluids and if needed inotropes
- Broad spectrum antibiotics if indicated
- Feeding (enteral favoured if possible)
- Monitoring and management of complications such as pneumothorax
- Prevention of nosocomial infections
- Restrict fluids as soon as feasible

6. Options for refractory ARDS

- Glucocorticoids (short course)
- Surfactant
- High frequency oscillatory ventilation if OI rise despite above efforts (early switch desirable)
- Inhaled nitric oxide (iNO)
- ECMO

7. Weaning is done as per individualized protocol of the unit

consistent with adequate systemic perfusion as indicated by renal function and metabolic acid-base balance. The fluid and catheter treatment trial (FACTT study) showed a clear difference between a liberal fluid strategy and a conservative fluid strategy. More ventilator free days and a 2.9% reduction in mortality was seen in the patients managed with a conservative approach to fluids and early institution of diuresis[36]. It does not imply that patients in shock should be fluid restricted. The goal directed therapy should be applied as per shock protocols[37] and only when the hemodynamics are stable and the patient is off inotropes or on less than 5 mcg/k/min of dopamine for > 12 hr, diuresis should be achieved with low dose furosemide infusion (0.05-0.1 mg/kg/hr) and titrated to a urine output of 1.0- 1.5 ml/kg/hour.

Section 4

2. Analgesics and sedatives. They should be used to minimize physical and mental discomfort and optimize respiration. Early in the course of illness neuromuscular blocking agents may be needed to overcome the discomfort of the high PEEP and RMs being given. Asynchrony will add to work of breathing and worsen the clinical status and outcome.

3. Feeding. Adequate nutrition should be ensured to prevent catabolism. Intralipids favourably impact the respiratory quotient but carry risk of infection. Enteral feeding is associated with lower risk of infection, preserves integrity of gut mucosa but may not be tolerated at times due to ileus.

4. Antibiotics. Sepsis is a common precipitating factor for ARDS and trial of broad spectrum antibiotics is advocated. It is, however, important to remember that fever, leukocytosis, raised CRP are usually present in ARDS and may not indicate sepsis. The choice of antibiotics depends on the primary infection that has triggered ARDS, the likely microbial etiology and resistance patterns. For community acquired pneumonia, a combination of a 3rd generaion cephalosporin and macrolide is usually indicated. For gastrointestinal or urinary tract sepsis, third generation cephalosporins with/without aminoglycosides may be given. When multi-drug resistant infections (nosocomially acquired or community acquired in patients with recent history of antibiotic use) are suspected, beta lactam–beta lactamase inhibitor combinations or carbapenems are recommended.

5. Miscellaneous issues. Sudden deterioration in a patient with ARDS may occur due to a number of causes including pneumothorax, bronchial plugging, displaced ET tube, aspiration of gastric contents, cardiac tamponade, arrhythmia, GI stress ulcer etc. and should be managed appropriately. All efforts should be made to prevent nosocomial infection.

The management of pediatric ARDS is summarized in Table 31.4.

PROGNOSIS

The predictors of adverse outcome are listed below:

(i)   Multiorgan failure
(ii) Failure of oxygenation to improve within 6 days[2, 4, 7].
(iii) Profound hypoxemia (high oxygenation index)
(iv) Presence of pneumothorax and air leaks.

The long-term outcome of survivors of pediatric ARDS is good; but follow-up studies are limited to 25% of the survivors with considerable loss of patients to follow-up[7].

Conclusions and Key Messages

(i)   Pediatric ALI/ARDS is an illness with high mortality and requires excellent supportive care in a PICU.

(ii)   Severe sepsis and pneumonia are the main predisposing conditions and should be aggressively treated.

(iii) Mechanical ventilation should be initiated early.

(iv)   Lung protective strategies including use of low tidal volumes and optimal PEEP are imperative.

(v)   Recruitment maneuvers may help decide lung recruitablity and implementation of appropriate strategy.

(vi)   The impact of prone positioning on mortality is uncertain, it does improve oxygenation, has virtually no complications and should be tried.

(vii) HFOV should be instituted early and not as a last resort.

(viii) Supportive care including invasive monitoring, restricted fluid management, attention to multiorgan dysfunction and prevention of nosocomial infection are crucial to improve the outcome.

REFERENCES

1. Bernard GR, Artigas A, Brigham KL, *et al.* The American–European Consensus Conference on ARDS. Definitions, mechanisms, relevant outcomes, and clinical trial coordination. *Am J Respir Crit Care Med* 1994; 149: 818-824.

2. Ware LB, Matthay MA. The acute respiratory distress syndrome. *N Engl J Med* 2000; 342:1334-1349.

3. Hudson LD, Steinberg KP. Epidemiology of acute lung injury and ARDS. *Chest* 1999; 116:S74-S82.

4. Vasudevan A, Lodha R, Kabra SK. Acute lung injury and acute respiratory distress syndrome. *Indian J Pediatr* 2004; 71:743-750.

5. Chetan G, Rathisharmila R, Narayanan P, Mahadevan S. Acute respiratory distress syndrome in pediatric intensive care unit. *Indian J Pediatr* 2009; 76:1013-1016.

6. Hudson LD, Milberg JA, Anardi D, *et al.* Clinical risks for development of the acute respiratory distress syndrome. *Am J Respir Crit Care Med* 1995; 151: 293-301.

7. Anderson MR. Update on pediatric acute respiratory distress syndrome. *Respir Care* 2003; 48:261-276.

8.   Ramsey C, Kumar A. H1N1: viral pneumonia as a cause of acute respiratory distress syndrome. *Curr Opin Crit Care* 2011; 17: 64-71.

9.   Sarkar S, Saha K, Das CS. Three cases of ARDS: An emerging complication of *Plasmodium vivax* malaria. *Lung India* 2010; 27: 154-157.

10. J Murthy GL, Sahay RK, Srinivasan VR, Upadhaya AC, Shantaram V, Gayatri K. Clinical profile of falciparum malaria in a tertiary care hospital. *Indian Med Assoc* 2000; 98:160-162.

11. Kamath SR, Ranjit S. Clinical features, complications and atypical manifestations of children with severe forms of dengue hemorrhagic fever in South India. *Indian J Pediatr* 2006; 73: 889-895.

12. Pandey D, Sharma B, Chauhan V, Mokta J, Verma BS, Thakur S. ARDS complicating scrub typhus in Sub-Himalayan region. *J Assoc Phys India* 2006; 54: 812-813.

13. Mohan A, Sharma SK, Pande JN.Acute respiratory distress syndrome (ARDS) in miliary tuberculosis: a twelve year experience. *Indian J Chest Dis Allied Sci* 1996; 38:157-162.

14. Ittyachen AM, Krishnapillai TV, Nair MC, Rajan AR. Retrospective study of severe cases of leptospirosis admitted in the intensive care unit. *J Postgrad Med* 2007; 53: 232-235.

15. Gattinoni L. Pelosi P, Sutter PM. ARDS caused by pulmonary and extrapulmonary disease. Different syndromes? *Amer J Resp Crit Care Med* 1998; 158: 3-11.

16. Rubenfeld GD, Caldwell E, Granton J, Hudson LD, Matthay MA. Interobserver variability in applying a radiographic definition for ARDS. *Chest* 1999; 116:1347-1353.

17. The Acute Respiratory Distress Syndrome Network. Ventilation with lower tidal volumes as compared with traditional tidal volumes for acute lung injury and the acute respiratory distress syndrome. *N Engl J Med* 2000; 342:1301–1308.

18. Gattinoni L, Pesenti A. The concept of "baby lung." *Intensive Care Med* 2005; 31:776–784.

19. Amato MB, Barbas CS, Medeiros DM, Magaldi RB, Schettino GP, Lorenzi-Filho G, *et al*. Effect of a protective-ventilation strategy on mortality in the acute respiratory distress syndrome. *N Engl J Med* 1998; 338:347–354.

20. Amato MB, Barbas CS, Medeiros DM, *et al*. Beneficial effects of the 'open lung approach' with low distending pressures in acute respiratory distress syndrome. A prospective randomized study on mechanical ventilation. *Am J Respir Crit Care Med* 1995; 152: 1835-1846.

21. Lachmaan B. Open up the lung and keep the lung open. *Intensive Care Med* 1992; 18:81-85.

22. Gattinoni L, Caironi P, Cressoni M, *et al*. Lung recruitment in patients with the acute respiratory distress syndrome. *N Engl J Med* 2006; 354:1775–1786.

23. Borges JB, Okmato GFJ, Matos M, *et al*. Reversibility of lung collapse and hypoxemia in early respiratory distress syndrome. *Am J Respir Crit Care Med* 2006; 174: 268-278.

24. Lung Open Ventilation Study Investigators Ventilation Strategy Using Low Tidal Volumes, Recruitment Maneuvers, and High Positive End-Expiratory Pressure for Acute Lung Injury and Acute Respiratory Distress Syndrome. A Randomized Controlled Trial. *JAMA* 2008; 299: 637-645.

25. Grasso S, Mascia L, Del Turco M, *et al*. Effects of recruiting maneuvers in patients with acute respiratory distress syndrome ventilated with protective ventilatory strategy. *Anesthesiology* 2002; 96:795-802.

26. Janet V. Diaz, Roy Brower, Carolyn S. Calfee, *et al*. Therapeutic strategies for severe acute lung injury. *Crit Care Med* 2010; 38:1644 –1650.

27. Jolliet P, Bulpa P, Chevrolet JC. Effects of the prone position on gas exchange and hemodynamics in severe acute respiratory distress syndrome. *Crit Care Med* 1998; 26:1977–1985.

28. Kornecki A, Frndova H, Coates AL, Shemie SD. A randomized trial of prolonged prone positioning in children with acute respiratory failure. *Chest* 2001; 119:211–218.

29. Gattinoni L, Tognoni G, Pesenti A, Taccone P, Mascheroni D, Labarta V, *et al*. Effect of prone positioning on the survival of patients with acute respiratory failure. *N Engl J Med* 2001; 345:568–573.

30. Arnold JH, Anas NG, Luckett P, Cheifetz IM, Reyes G, Newth CJ, *et al*. High-frequency oscillatory ventilation in pediatric respiratory failure: a multicenter experience. *Crit Care Med* 2000; 28:3913–3919.

31. Slee- Wiffels FY, *et al*. High-frequency oscillatory ventilation in children: a single-center experience of 53 cases. *Crit Care* 2005; 9: R274-9. Epub 2005 Apr 8.

32. Efficacy and safety of corticosteroids for persistent acute respiratory distress syndrome. The National Heart, Lung, and Blood Institute Acute Respiratory Distress Syndrome (ARDS) Clinical Trials Network *N Engl J Med* 2006; 354:1671-1684.

33. Steinberg K, Hudson L, Goodman R, *et al*. Efficacy and safety of corticosteroids for persistent acute respiratory distress syndrome. *N Engl J Med* 2006; 354:1671–1684.

34. Sokol J, Jacobs SE, Bohn D. Inhaled nitric oxide for acute hypoxemic respiratory failure in children and adults. *Cochrane Database Syst Rev* 2003; (1): CD002787.

35. Chauhan S, Malik M, Malik V, Chauhan Y, Kiran U, Bisoi AK. Extra corporeal membrane oxygenation after pediatric cardiac surgery: a 10 year experience. *Ann Card Anaesth* 2011; 14:19-24.

36. ARDS Network comparison of two fluid management strategies in ALI. *New Engl J Med* 2006; 354: 2564-2575.

37. Rivers EP (Editorial). Fluid management strategies in ALI. Liberal, conservative or both? *New Engl J Med* 2006; 354:2564-2575.

Section 4

32

Congestive Heart Failure

S Garg, JPS Narula and R Tandon

Congestive heart failure (CHF) is defined as a pathological state in which heart is unable to maintain an output necessary to meet the metabolic requirements of the body or when the heart can do so only with elevated filling pressures. Low cardiac output characterizes most forms of heart disease. However, certain high cardiac output states like anemia, arteriovenous fistulae, beriberi and thyrotoxicosis may also lead to heart failure. Low cardiac output may be due to inadequate cardiac filling and/or insufficient contraction and emptying. Both systolic and diastolic dysfunctions of the heart can lead to abnormal filling of the heart. Systolic dysfunction is the predominant form of heart failure in children and most of the discussion below pertains to it.

ETIOPATHOGENESIS

Pediatric patients with CHF are characterized by tremendous heterogeneity with respect to age and mechanisms of disease in various regions of the world. The commonest cause of CHF in infants is congenital heart disease. In older children it is rheumatic fever and rheumatic heart disease in the developing world; and cardiomyopathy and myocardial dysfunction after repair or palliation of congenital heart defects in the developed world.

Congenital Heart Disease

Congenital heart disease is the commonest cause of heart failure in newborns and infants. Older children may present with sequel of repair or palliation. Congenital cardiac defects that are most commonly associated with CHF in order of frequency are; transposition of great arteries, coarctation of the aorta, ventricular septal defect, aortic atresia, common atrio-ventricular canal, transposition of pulmonary veins, single ventricle without pulmonic stenosis and patent ductus arteriosus[1]. Some of the mechanisms by which congenital heart disease may lead to heart failure are discussed below.

1. **Increased pulmonary blood flow**. These lesions produce an excessive workload on the myocardium as a result of volume overload. Left-to-right shunt lesions including ventricular septal defect, atrioventricular septal defect and large patent ductus arteriosus are the main causes of increased pulmonary blood flow without cyanosis. Infants with left-to-right shunt tend to develop congestive heart failure around six to ten weeks of life. At birth the pulmonary vascular resistance is high but there is a gradual fall during the first few weeks of life. The size of left-to-right shunt reaches its maximum around the age of six to ten weeks when pulmonary vascular resistance is lowest. The chances of further increase in the shunt after a few months of life are minimal. Therefore, congestive cardiac failure in older children is unlikely to occur unless there are associated additional complications.

Cyanotic heart diseases with increased pulmonary blood flow include transposition of great arteries with or without a ventricular septal defect, truncus arteriosus, total anomalous pulmonary venous drainage, malposition complexes and tricuspid atresia without obstruction to pulmonary blood flow. Patients with transposition of great arteries or of the pulmonary veins manifest congestive heart failure within the first two to three months of life. Congestive cardiac failure begins within the first week of life in patients with transposition of great arteries without a ventricular septal defect and those with obstructive total anomalous pulmonary venous connection. In transposition of great arteries with a ventricular septal defect and unobstructed total anomalous pulmonary venous connection, CHF develops by the age of six to eight weeks following the physiological fall in pulmonary vascular resistance.

2. **Obstructive lesions.** Obstructive lesions produce an excessive workload on the myocardium because of pressure overload. These include critical or severe aortic stenosis, mitral stenosis or pulmonary stenosis; coarctation of the aorta and, interrupted aortic arch. In congenital obstructive lesions of the heart, CHF is a relatively late phenomenon. However, atresia or critical stenosis of aortic, mitral or pulmonary valves can result in CHF within the first few days of life. Coarctation of the aorta may result in CHF within the first few months of life. However, if these patients do not manifest CHF in the first year, collaterals develop and prevent the onset of failure by decompressing the aortic obstruction.

3. **Coronary anomalies.** Coronary anomalies can cause acute or chronic myocardial ischemia leading to myocardial dysfunction. Common congenital coronary anomalies are anomalous origin of the left coronary artery from pulmonary artery and coronary-cameral fistulae.

4. **Other conditions.** Valvular regurgitations especially mitral regurgitation or tricuspid regurgitation can present with heart failure by causing volume overload. Other uncommon conditions like vein of Galen or hepatic arterio-venous malformations can also cause high output heart failure.

Around 90 percent of all cases of CHF in children occur before the end of first year of life[1, 2]. Patients with congenital heart disease have a relatively healthy myocardium and if they do not develop heart failure within the first year of life, they are not likely to do so in the next 10 years, unless complicated by anemia, infection or bacterial endocarditis. Table 32.1 lists the developmental conditions causing CHF during early infancy.

Cardiomyopathies

Three pathophysiologic forms of cardiomyopathies are recognized; dilated, hypertrophic and restrictive. Dilated cardiomyopathy accounts for 90 percent of cases. Dilated cardiomyopathy may be idiopathic or the end result of a number of causative factors some of which are listed in Table 32.2.

In Duchenne and Becker's muscular dystrophies, abnormal amounts of dystrophin in the cardiac myocytes leads to necrosis and fibrosis with resultant cardiomyopathy[3, 4]. In utero HIV (Human immunodeficiency virus) exposure can result in abnormalities in left ventricular function irrespective of the infant's HIV status. Children with vertically transmitted HIV infection can have abnormal left ventricular shortening fraction and increased left ventricular wall mass[5].

Anthracyclins have gained widespread use in the treatment of childhood leukemia and solid tumors. Upto 5% of patients develop anthracyclin related CHF and patients treated with a cumulative dose of higher than 300 mg/m^2 are at the highest risk[6]. The risk increases further with female sex, younger age at the start of chemotherapy, type of tumor, black race, presence of trisomy 21, radiation therapy involving the heart and exposure to cyclophosphamide, ifosfamide or amsacrine.

Hypertrophic and restrictive cardiomyopathies lead to predominant diastolic dysfunction; systolic dysfunction supervenes in the later stages.

Myocarditis

Myocarditis is defined as inflammation of the heart muscle. The commonest cause of myocarditis in North America and Europe is viral with coxsackie B and adenovirus infections accounting for over 80% of cases[7]. Chagas disease is the most frequent cause in Central and South America[8]. In the past a

Section 4

Table 32.1 Time of onset of congestive failure in congenital cardiac diseases

Age	Conditions
Birth to 72 hours	Pulmonary, mitral and aortic atresias or critical stenosis.
4 days to 1 week	Hypoplastic left and right heart syndromes, transposition and malposition of great arteries with poor mixing
1 to 4 weeks	Transposition and malposition complexes, endocardial fibroelastosis, coarctation of the aorta.
1 to 2 months	Transposition and malposition complexes, endocardial cushion defects, ventricular septal defect, patent ductus arteriosus, total anomalous pulmonary venous connection, anomalous left coronary artery from pulmonary artery.
2 to 6 months	Transposition and malposition complexes, ventricular septal defect, patent ductus arteriosus, total anomalous pulmonary venous connection, aortic stenosis, coarctation of the aorta.

Table 32.2 Causes of dilated cardiomyopathy or dilated cardiomyopathy like presentation in children

1. **Primary genetic conditions**
   - Familial isolated dilated cardiomyopathy
   - Neuromuscular disorders: Duchenne/Becker muscular dystrophy, Friedreich's ataxia,
   - Inborn errors of metabolism: Glycogen storage disease, mucopolysaccharidosis, fatty acid oxidation defects, systemic carnitine deficiency

2. **Primary non-genetic conditions**
   - Congenital heart disease: Coarctation of aorta, dysplastic mitral valve, anomalous origin of left coronary artery from pulmonary artery
   - Infections: Coxsackie B, human immnunodeficiency virus, Echo, mumps and Epstein-Barr viruses, *Trypanosoma cruzii, Borrelia burgdorferi*
   - Hypertension: Primary or secondary
   - Cardiac arrhythmia: Supraventricular tachycardia, atrial flutter/fibrillation
   - Pulmonary Disease: Primary pulmonary hypertension, chronic lung disease
   - Toxins or drugs: Anthracyclins, cyclophosphamide, iron overload, cocaine
   - Collagen vascular diseases: Rheumatic carditis, juvenile rheumaoid arthritis, systemic lupus erythematosus, Kawasaki's disease
   - Hematological diseases: Thalassemia, sickle cell disease
   - Endocrine disorders: Hypo/Hyperthyroidism
   - Malnutrition: Kwashiorkor, pellagra, thiamine or selenium deficiency
   - Malignancy: Leukemia, lymphoma, neuroblastoma
   - Post-cardiac surgery
   - Radiation exposure

---

large number of cases of acute myocarditis were attributed to rheumatic heart disease and diphtheria. In the Indian subcontinent diphtheria is being controlled aggressively and has become rare.

Although viral infection is the initial trigger for myocarditis, the current understanding is that the host's immuno-inflammatory response to infection is the major contributing factor to myocardial damage[9, 10]. Of all the patients presenting with acute viral myocarditis, one-third recover normal cardiac function, one-third show signs of chronic heart failure and one-third either die or require heart transplantation.

Arrhythmias

Three-fourth of patients with supraventricular tachycardias and CHF are below four months of age. Heart rates that are persistently above 180/ minute for more than 48 hours tend to precipitate CHF. There is a tendency for the recurrence of arrhythmia if the onset is after 4 months of age. Fetal bradycardia can cause hydrops fetalis or infantile CHF. Non-sinus supraventricular tachycardia is a known cause of reversible symptomatic cardiomyopathy in older children and young adolescents[11].

Anemia

In children with a normal heart, protracted hemoglobin levels of around 5g/dl can result in CHF. While in a heart compromised by disease, cardiac failure may be precipitated even with higher hemoglobin levels of 7 or 8 g/dl. Younger infants are more susceptible to develop cardiac failure due to anemia. The heart compensates for chronic tissue hypoxia by remodeling and elevation of cardiac output only when hemoglobin level becomes as low as 7g/dl[12]. Till that level, compensation is accompanied by an increase of erythrocyte 2,3 diphosphoglycerate activity and the increased peripheral oxygen extraction.

Heart complications are common and remain the leading cause of mortality in beta-thalassemia[13]. Before the introduction of intensified transfusions and iron chelation therapy, multiple transfused patients with thalassemia major died most commonly in the second decade of life because of heart failure[14].

Rheumatic Fever and Rheumatic Heart Disease

The commonest cause of congestive cardiac failure in older children in certain parts of the world is acute rheumatic fever with carditis and rheumatic heart disease. Acute rheumatic fever may be associated with pancarditis which includes pericarditis, myocarditis and endocarditis ; the latter causing chronic rheumatic heart disease due to valvular involvement. Both stenotic and regurgitant valvular lesions may be seen. Mitral valve is the most commonly affected valve followed by aortic and tricuspid valves in that order. More than one valve may be involved in a given patient. CHF in acute rheumatic fever is due to an acute volume load from mitral and/or aortic regurgitation and not due to myocarditis *per se*.

Hypertension

Systemic hypertension due to acute glomerulonephritis or nonspecific obstructive aortitis is not an infrequent cause of CHF in older children.

Postoperative

Ischemia-reperfusion injury associated with cardiopulmonary bypass and aortic cross-clamping is a common cause of acute myocardial dysfunction in the pediatric population. Cardiopulmonary bypass is associated with an activation of inflammatory cascade that can result in myocardial dysfunction.

PATHOPHYSIOLOGY

Congestive heart failure is a complex clinical syndrome that defies simple definition. Myocardial dysfunction, the pivotal abnormality is characterized by a decrease in the myocardial contractility. Because of myocardial dysfunction, the reserve of the ventricles as a pump becomes insufficient to meet body requirements. Congestive heart failure is thus the systemic manifestation of the inadequate pump function of the heart. Sympathetic and renin-angiotensin system (RAS) activation and release of a number of vasodilatory molecules occurs in an attempt to improve the cardiac output and maintain perfusion to vital organs as a compensatory mechanism. Unfortunately the compensatory mechanisms over react[15]. This results in a further impairment of cardiac contractility, establishing a vicious cycle of failure begetting failure (Figure 32.1).

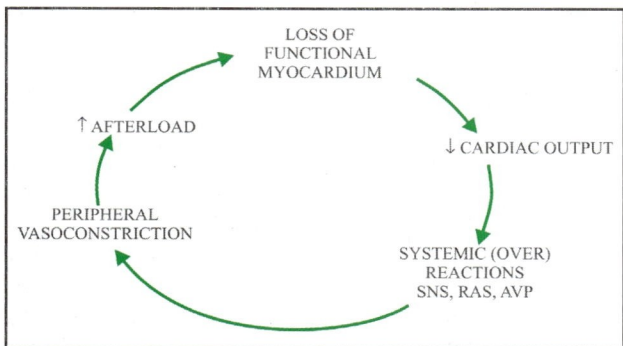

Figure 32.1 the loss of functional myocardium results in reduction of cardiac output, perpetuating activation of sympathetic (SNS), renin angiotensin (RAS) and antidiuretic systems (AVP). The resultant increase in peripheral impedance initiates a vicious cycle worsening the cardiac performance

Myocardial component. The myocardial failure appears to be directly due to myocyte loss. Compensatory or reactive hypertrophy occurs in the remaining viable myocytes to sustain the higher load per cell. Progressive hypertrophy produces impaired contractility and changes in ventricular compliance. Widespread fibrosis involving the myocytes or the connective tissue affects both the systolic and the diastolic function. Decreased myocardial function leads to compensatory ventricular dilatation that enhances myocardial wall stress, leading to further impairment of the myocardial function. The inappropriately high levels of circulating catecholamines result in 'down regulation' of beta-1 adrenergic receptors[16]. The recognition of cellular and molecular abnormalities in CHF has lead to the trial of newer therapeutic modalities like angiotensin, endothelin, peptide growth factor, nitric oxide (NO) and prostacyclin[17].

Peripheral components. CHF is characterized by high levels of circulating norepinephrine as well as an increased plasma renin activity (PRA) and plasma arginine-vasopressin[18]. As mentioned earlier these supporting mechanisms for the failing circulation contribute to further burden on the myocardium that is already operating inefficiently[15]. These compensatory systems probably have different trigger mechanisms as the correlation between plasma levels of these protective mechanisms is relatively modest[19, 20]. However, they facilitate each others biological effects and share the common outcome i.e. vasoconstriction and antidiuresis.

Cardiac output is the key reflection of cardiac activity and must be maintained to meet the metabolic requirements of the tissues of the body. The cardiac output is essentially determined by (i) the available (end-diastolic) volume to be ejected *(preload);* (ii) the capacity of the myocardium to contract (inotropic state or *contractility);* (iii) the impedance to be ejected against *(afterload);* and (iv) the frequency of ejections *(heart rate)[21].* Though these four factors are intimately inter-related, they can operate independent of each other.

Preload is basically a function of venous return as well as the compliance of ventricles and thus determines the end-diastolic volume and pressure. According to the Starling's law an increase in the resting muscle fiber length augments the force of contractions[22]. An increase in the volume of the cardiac chamber would enhance the systolic wall stress and the stroke volume. Preload, in fact, does not alter the inotropic status (contractility) but mechanically stretches the sarcomeres allowing more effective overlapping of the actin and myosin filament[23]. Clinically the left and right atrial pressures measured as pulmonary artery wedge and central venous pressures are the best guides of preload to the ventricular chambers[24]. Afterload represents the resistance to ventricular emptying. It can be described as the ventricular wall stress that develops during ejection and is determined by ventricular pressure, diameter and wall-thickness[25].

Myocardial contractility represents the inherent capacity of the heart muscle to increase the force and magnitude of contraction independent of loading conditions. It is dependent to a large extent on the availability of calcium ions to the contractile proteins of the heart muscle[26]. The myocardial contractility can be increased or decreased by hormonal stimuli, drugs, autonomic stimuli and myocardial diseases[27]. Assessment of contractility is useful to find out the status of the myocardium which determines the long-term prognosis of a patient following correction of a structural abnormality. The heart rate is directly related to cardiac output and is used as a compensatory mechanism by the body to maintain optimal cardiac output by increasing or decreasing the heart rate. The cardiac output is the net product of heart rate and the stroke output per beat. If the stroke output falls, the heart rate increases in response to increased catecholamine secretion, to compensate for the fall in cardiac output.

CLINICAL FEATURES

The clinical presentation is determined largely by the cause of the CHF and the age of the patient.

Fetus. Disorders of cardiovascular system are the most frequent underlying cause of non-immune hydrops fetalis[28]. These disorders are either structural malformations like hypoplastic left heart syndrome and endocardial cushion defect or fetal arrhythmias.

Newborn. In newborn infants, CHF interferes with the ability to breathe and feed. Feeding may be labored or impossible because of rapid breathing. The infant may take 45-60 minutes or more to finish the feeding. The child remains perpetually hungry and becomes irritable with bouts of crying. There may be profuse sweating, particularly while feeding. Crying, defecation and sleeping may be affected. Common signs of CHF in the neonate in the order of their frequency include tachypnea, tachycardia, liver enlargement, and cardiomegaly. Less common signs include pulmonary rales and rhonchi, peripheral edema, elevated systemic venous pressure, inappropriate diaphoresis, gallop rhythm, pulsus alternans and ascites[29]. Pleural and pericardial effusions due to CHF are rare. Tachycardia may be a cause or an effect of CHF; primary tachy-cardias must be considered if the heart rate remains rapid and constant. Poor perfusion as manifested by pallor, sallow, cyanotic or gray complexion and poor capillary refill is ominous and a late sign of CHF.

Blood pressure measurement should be performed on all four extremities in the neonates/infants with heart failure. A systolic blood pressure that is more than 10 mmHg higher in the upper body relative to the lower body is abnormal and suggests coarctation of the aorta, aortic arch hypoplasia or interrupted aortic arch. Measuring oxygen saturations at both the preductal and postductal sites is an important part of initial evaluation. Differential cyanosis is seen in persistent pulmonary hypertension of the newborn and left-heart abnormalities (aortic arch hypoplasia, interrupted arch) when associated with a right-to-left shunt through a patent ductus arteriosus. Patients with critical coarctation or interrupted arch may present with CHF or shock when the ductus closes.

Some patients with CHF may have bounding pulses; this should lead to consideration of arteriovenous malformations, ductus arteriosus, coronary fistulae or other aortic runoff lesions. Peripheral cyanosis occur due to poor perfusion in CHF. Central cyanosis is suggestive of congenital heart disease with increased pulmonary blood flow.

Abnormal precordial activity may be an important clue towards cardiac pathology. Systolic murmur may be heard in many forms of congenital heart disease. A diastolic murmur is less common but can be heard in truncus arteriosus with truncal insufficiency, coronary-cameral fistulae and absent pulmonary valve syndrome. A diastolic rumble or gallop occurs in many types of heart failure, especially those with pulmonary overcirculation.

Infants. Infants with CHF also often present with poor feeding, lethargy, diaphoresis and tachypnea. Slow weight gain in an infant may be because of small feeds due to easy fatigability and excessive loss of calories from increased work of breathing associated with CHF. Rarely there may be an unusual sudden gain in weight due to fluid retention, manifesting as facial puffiness or edema over sacrum or feet. Cyanosis, hypotonia and shock are late findings. Two congenital cardiac malformations that can present in later infancy are certain forms of total anomalous pulmonary venous drainage and the anomalous origin of left coronary artery from pulmonary artery.

Children and adolescents. Toddlers and older children typically manifest symptoms of fatigue, exercise intolerance and growth failure. School going children may be asked about their performance in gym class. Tachypnea and tachycardia are usually present. Abdominal pain and distension may occur due to hepatomegaly. In older children, venous distension and peripheral edema is usually present.

Functional Assessment of CHF in Infants and Children

New York Heart Association (NYHA) classification is the most commonly used method for functional assessment in adults. Modifications of the system have been devised for infants and children, but their prognostic importance has not been assessed.

CHF classification for infants with LV dysfunction is given below (Ross *et al. Pediatr Cardiol* 1992, 13:72-75).

NYHA I: No signs

NYHA II: Respiratory rate >50, with and without hepatomegaly

NYHA III: Respiratory rate >50, hepato-megaly, with rib retractions

NYHA IV: Respiratory rate >60, heart rate >160 bpm, hepatomegaly, rib retractions, with or without poor perfusion

Modified NYHA classification for children is given below:

Class I: No limitations or symptoms, school-age child takes gym class and keeps up with peers.

Class II: Slight limitation of physical activity, comfortable at rest, but ordinary activity can cause fatigue, palpitations, or dyspnea, school-age child takes gym class but dose not keep up with peers, secondary growth failure is likely.

Class III: Marked or severe limitation of physical activity, less than ordinary activity such as walking less than one block can cause fatigue, palpitations, or dyspnea, school-age child is unable to take gym class, and secondary growth failure is likely.

Class IV: Symptoms at rest with tachypnea, retractions, grunting or diaphoresis, unable to perform any physical activity without discomfort, symptoms are present at rest and increase with any activity, secondary growth failure is common.

Recently, The New York University Pediatric Heart Failure Index has been devised to assess severity of chronic heart failure in children[30]. A scoring system from 0-30 has been designed based on symptoms, signs, medications and other treatment methods being received by the child.

INVESTIGATIONS

Common investigations for evaluation of a patient with heart failure are listed below:

1. **Chest X-ray**. It may reveal cardiomegaly, pulmonary venous congestion, pulmonary edema or pleural effusion. Chest X-ray may give information regarding the underlying etiology.

2. **Electrocardiogram (ECG)**. It may show tachycardia, bradycardia or ventricular hypertrophy. Certain specific ECG patterns are associated with certain forms of congenital heart disease.

3. **Echocardiography**. Because manifestations of CHF and primary pulmonary diseases may be similar in infants, recognition of CHF is often difficult. ECG and X-ray findings are also nonspecific. Echo is the most accurate way to confirm the presence of heart disease. It provides information about the structure and function of the heart and great vessels. Echo is extremely useful for deciding the therapeutic options even for a complex congenital heart disease.

4. **B-type natriuretic peptide (BNP)**. The cardiac natriuretic hormones play an important role in the regulation of extracellular fluid volume and vascular tone. They can counter the effects of the renin-angiotensin-aldosterone peptide hormones and induce natriuresis, diuresis and vasodilatation. Plasma BNP elevation is a reliable test in recognizing ventricular dysfunction in children with various kinds of congenital heart diseases[31]. BNP levels are normal in patients with heart disease without ventricular dysfunction. BNP is secreted from the cardiac ventricular myocytes in response to an increase in ventricular wall tension[32]. Human pro-BNP consists of 108 amino acids. Processing of the molecule releases the biologically active 32-amino acid peptide and an amino-terminus fragment (N-BNP)[33]. N-BNP is not only a sensitive and specific marker of ventricular dysfunction, but remains stable in the whole blood for >24 hours at 20°C. Plasma N-BNP levels may reflect the severity and the impairment of cardiac function in children with CHF[34].

5. **Cardiac catheterization**. It is useful not only for the diagnosis of the underlying cardiac disorder but also for carrying out certain

Section 4

palliative or curative interventional therapeutic procedures at the same time. Cardiac catheterization may have to be delayed until the acute heart failure state is controlled.

6. **Endomyocardial biopsy**. Some experts consider it as an essential part of investigation of myocarditis and cardiomyopathy. Recent evidence suggests that endomyocardial biopsy may be a valuable diagnostic tool and should be included in the evaluation of patients with initially unexplained cardiomyopathy[35]. Biopsy has historically been the 'gold standard' in diagnosing myocarditis[36]. The degree of inflammation and the degree of fibrosis can be easily assessed and will affect treatment decisions. If available, routine PCR (polymerase chain reaction) for at least coxsackie B and adenovirus should be done on all biopsy specimens with acute myocarditis.

Work-up for unexplained cardiomyopathy

Work-up for unexplained cardiomyopathy should include investigations for a metabolic cause. A detailed family history, blood studies, including pH, bicarbonate, electrolytes, glucose, ammonia, lactate, pyruvate, alanine and other amino acids, creatine kinase and liver function tests; mitochondrial DNA studies; plasma or tissue carnitine (total, free and acyl); acylcarnitine derivatives in blood; and urine studies for acylglycine derivatives and quantitative organic acids may be helpful. Hypoglycemia, metabolic acidosis or hyperammonemia may be an indicator for an underlying metabolic disorder[37]. Hyperketotic hypoglycemia may suggest an organic acidemia and non-ketotic hypoglycemia indicates a fatty acid oxidation defect. Elevated creatine kinase, MB fraction and cardiac troponin levels are markers of myocardial injury.

Work-up for suspected viral myocarditis

Viral myocarditis is generally associated with elevated CRP, elevated WBC count with a lymphocyte predominance and positive viral titers[38]. Traditionally, a fourfold rise in acute and convalescent antibody titers to a virus establishes the diagnosis of viral myocarditis[9, 39]. Endomyocardial biopsy is still considered to be the standard by many investigators though it is far from ideal[40]. Antimyosin scintigraphy, contrast-enhanced magnetic resonance angiography and echocardiographic digital image processing are some of the newer up-coming techniques for assessment of myocarditis[39].

MANAGEMENT

The medical management of CHF is directed towards improving cardiac performance, augmenting peripheral perfusion and decreasing systemic and pulmonary venous congestion. Aggressive measures should be taken to minimize the workload on the heart and to avoid unnecessary demands for increased cardiac output.

Recognition and treatment of precipitating and aggravating factors. Precipitating and aggravating factors for CHF include poor compliance, anemia, hypertension, infective endocarditis, myocarditis, thyrotoxicosis, drug toxicity, fever, infections, arrhythmias, ischemia and pulmonary embolism[41]. If the patient is not responding well, the precipitating and aggravating factors should be diligently looked for and appropriately managed.

General measures. Acute stage management includes attention to fluids, electrolytes and acid-base status, treatment of anemia and chest infections, and oxygen inhalation to correct hypoxemia[42]. Calorie and protein requirements of children with CHF are high while the intake is usually inadequate[43]. Infants with CHF may lack sufficient strength for effective sucking due to rapid respirations and easy fatigability. Nasogastric feeding with a calorie-dense formula (0.8 kcal/ml) is recommended to reduce fluid intake and provide extra energy to meet the enhanced metabolic requirements. Because of its long half-life, serum prealbumin is a more reliable parameter of nutritional status compared to albumin or transferrin levels[44].

Use of extra salt and high sodium containing foods should be avoided. Availability of potent diuretics has obviated the need for rigorous restrictions on salt and fluid intake. Enforced bed rest is impractical and probably unnecessary. Adequate oxygen delivery is dependent on an adequate level of hemoglobin. Iron supplementation or blood transfusion are helpful in anemic children. Glucose should be administered as soon as intravenous access is attained because hypoglycemia is common in the setting of CHF. Evaluation and treatment of additional organ system dysfunction, particularly pulmonary, renal, hepatic and central nervous system should be carried out simultaneously. Dialysis may be required in patients with renal insufficiency.

Respiratory support. When respiratory distress, low cardiac output or poor perfusion are present, emergency evaluation and treatment in an intensive care unit (ICU) is required. An adequate venous access should be obtained as soon as possible. Arterial line assists in monitoring blood pressure, acid-base status and oxygenation. If respiratory distress is marked, support of airway and breathing is critical. A stable airway is essential for adequate oxygenation and mechanical ventilation should be instituted early when indicated.

Oxygen. Patients with respiratory distress and/or hypoxia may benefit from oxygen inhalation. Administration of oxygen must be considered carefully in neonates because supplemental oxygen may lead to pulmonary overcirculation in cases of duct-dependent pulmonary or systemic blood flow.

Diuretics. Diuretics are the main stay of therapy for acute heart failure in children. Immediate treatment with an intramuscular dose of furosemide (even while in doctor's office) may be indicated if the patient seems to be in respiratory distress from pulmonary edema. However, if perfusion is poor, a diuretic may be contraindicated without intravenous access. Diuretics reduce the circulating blood volume, the venous return is decreased causing a reduction in the preload and the ventricular end-diastolic volume. Decrease in dilatation of the ventricles moves them to a more favorable position on the pressure-volume curve, thereby increasing efficiency. Diuretics also decrease peripheral and pulmonary edema and ease the work of breathing. Moreover, loss of sodium and water results in decrease in blood pressure and thus the afterload. It must be kept in mind, however, that the decrease in blood volume by diuretics leads to decreased renal perfusion. If diuresis is achieved vigorously it may result in hypotension and increase in blood urea nitrogen. Additional adverse effects may be hyponatremia, hypokalemia, acidosis, hyperglycemia, hyperuricemia and hypercalciuria. It is necessary to monitor the blood pressure, electrolytes and blood urea when potent diuretics are being used.

The diuretic of choice is furosemide either alone or in combination with a potassium sparing diuretic like spironolactone or amiloride. It has been shown that the combination of furosemide with a potassium sparing diuretic is better than furosemide with potassium supplementation in preventing hypokalemic arrhythmias. The usual dose for furosemide or ethacrynic acid is 1-2 mg/kg intravenously, and dose may be repeated 2-4 times per day

A small, randomized trial in children has demonstrated the safety and efficacy of spironolactone, but its potential impact on mortality has not been examined. In adults it has been shown to reduce the mortality by as much as 27%[45]. The exact reason for this remarkable survival benefit is still being investigated. Possibilities include the beneficial effect of spironolactone on attenuation of the aldosterone-induced myocardial fibrosis, or catecholamine release, or both. Recent evidence suggests that angiotensin converting enzyme inhibitors may potentiate the diuretic effect of spironolactone[46].

Digitalis. The two primary indications for the use of digitalis in infants and children are congestive heart failure and paroxysmal tachycardia of supraventricular origin. Even after two centuries of its discovery, digitalis continues to arouse controversies[47]. The unusual effect of the drug in stimulating myocardium while depressing the sinoatrial and atrioventricular nodes, is an advantage over other inotropic agents. Evidence of increased contractility, however, does not consistently correlate with clinical improvement. There is evidence for increased parasympathetic cardiac and arterial baroreceptor activity with cardiac glycosides, which decrease central sympathetic outflow and thus exert a favorable neurohormonal response. Most of the available data on digoxin relates to acute heart failure, and the beneficial results are often extrapolated to chronic CHF.

Section 4

Table 32.3 Recommended doses of digoxin in children		
Age	Total digitalizing dose (mcg/kg)	Daily maintenance dose (mcg/kg)
Premature infants	20 IV	5 IV
Full term neonates (up to 3 months)	30 IV	8-10 IV or PO q 12 hr
Infants <2 yr	40-60 PO	10-12 PO q 12 hr
Children >2 yr	30-40 PO	8-10 PO q 12 hr
Higher doses may be used in supraventricular tachycardia		

Though several studies have demonstrated protracted positive inotropic effects of digitalis in chronic CHF, equally large number of studies have shown lack of any observable worsening of the patient when the drug is discontinued[48]. Digitalis is a potentially dangerous drug, the incidence of digitalis toxicity varies between 15 to 20 percent because of its low therapeutic to toxic dose index. The currently recommended dosage schedule of digitalis is depicted in Table 32.4.

Although rarely necessary rapid digitalization of infants with CHF can be carried out intravenously. One-half of the total digitalizing dose is given immediately, and one-fourth dose at 8 and 16 hours later. The ECG must be monitored for any evidence of digitalis toxicity and dysrhythmias before administering each fraction of digitalizing dose. Maintenance digitalis therapy is started 12 hours after full digitalization and administered in two divided doses daily. The oral maintenance dose is approximately 25 percent higher than the parenteral dose. In children with mild to moderate CHF or those already receiving digitalis, initiation of a maintenance of digoxin schedule, without a loading dose, will achieve full digitalization in 7 to 10 days. An estimation of serum digoxin levels is useful when a standard dose of digoxin is not producing beneficial response or when toxicity of digitalis is suspected. The blood digitalis level should be maintained between 2-4 ng/ml in an infant and 1-2 ng/ml in older children. Myocarditis, prematurity and serum electrolyte abnormalities such as hypokalemia or hypercalcemia, potentiate the effects of digitalis toxicity. Hypokalemia deserves special attention as it is extremely common in this setting. The development of any cardiac arrhythmia during the course of digitalis therapy must be considered to be related to digoxin toxicity until proven otherwise[49]. Digoxin may not be helpful and may even be deleterious in acute myocarditis[50].

Vasodilators. Despite different mechanisms of actions, all vasodilators favorably alter the short term hemodynamic response[51]. Long term trials of some of these drugs has shown continued benefits. Captopril[52] and isosorbide dinitrate[15, 53] improve symptomatic status and exercise capacity. Hydralazine[54] and prazosin[55], however, have not been found to be more effective than placebo during long-term use. The vasodilators also redistribute the blood flow to regional beds. Reduced hospitalization and mortality has been shown with angiotensin converting enzyme (ACE) inhibitors as vasodilator therapy. ACE inhibitors produce their effects through at least three mechanisms; inhibition of the angiotensin-converting enzyme, inhibition of bradykinin degradation and inhibition of norepinephrine release from sympathetic nerve endings. In pediatric practice, patients of CHF not showing adequate response with diuretics and digoxin should receive ACE inhibitor as the third drug. Uncommonly dry, irritating cough can be a significant and troublesome side effect of ACE inhibitor therapy. Children who are intolerant to ACE inhibitor therapy may be given a trial of angiotensin receptor blocker such as losartan. Table 32.3 summarizes the site of action, dose and mode of administration of common vasodilators.

Several small trials have shown at least a short-term reduction in neurohormonal markers as well as clinical improvement in infants with heart

Agent	Site of action	Dose	Tolerance
Table 32.4 Doses and mode of administration of vasodilators			
Nitroglycerine	Venous	0.05-20 mcg/kg/min IV infusion	Common
Isosorbide dinitrate	Venous	0.1 mg/kg q 6 hr PO (maximum dose 2 mg/kg/day)	Common
Nitroprusside	Venous + arteriolar	0.5-1.0 mg/kg/IV q 6 hr	Rare
Hydralazine	Arterial	0.5-1.0 mg/kg/IV q 6 hr, 1.7 mg/kg/day PO in 3-4 doses	Occasional
Prazosin	Venous + arterial	5-25 mcg/kg/dose PO q 6 hr	Common
Nifedipine	Venous + arterial	0.3 mg/kg/dose q 6 hr PO	Rare
Captopril	Venous + arterial	Neonate: 0.4-1.6 mg/kg/day PO Infants: 0.5-6.0 mg/kg/day in 3 div doses PO Children: 12.5 mg q 12 hr PO	
Enalapril	Venous + arterial	0.1- 0.5 mg kg/day in two div doses, PO	
Losartan	Venous + arterial	0.5 mg/kg/day once daily PO	
Minoxidil	Arterial	0.2 mg/kg/day initial dose, increase slowly upto 1.0 mg/kg/day PO	Occasional

failure secondary to left-to-right shunts[56, 57]. One retrospective study showed reduced mortality in children with dilated cardiomyopathy treated with ACE inhibitors compared with the standard treatment (digoxin and diuretics)[58.] However, there are no randomized controlled trials to determine whether ACE inhibitor therapy has an overall benefit in terms of long-term morbidity, mortality and quality of life for children with left ventricular dysfunction. Aspirin may attenuate the useful effects of ACE inhibitors; simultaneous use of these two agents should be avoided[59].

Beta-blockers. It is widely recognized that myocardial cell loss irrespective of the basic cause precipitates a vicious cycle where excessive sympathetic activity causes myocardial beta receptor "down regulation" in addition to the peripheral vasoconstriction. The adverse effects of sympathetic activation include increased ventricular volumes and pressures caused by peripheral vasoconstriction, cardiac hypertrophy and coronary vasoconstriction leading to ischemia, increased programmed cell death and increased risk of arrhythmias. The prognosis of patients with CHF is inversely related to the circulating catecholamine levels. If catecholamines indeed contribute to pathogenesis of CHF, it must be worth while trying a beta blocker in this situation. Beneficial effects of beta blockers in dilated cardiomyopathy have been demonstrated[60-62]. The improvement in ventricular function occurs slowly over a period of months.

Vasodilator beta-blockers have now become available for use in CHF. Carvedilol a new beta blocker being used extensively has b1, b2, a1 blocking properties in addition to an antioxidant effect. Carvedilol blocks the deleterious effects of chronic adrenergic over stimulation of the myocardium and improves myocardial function. As an antioxidant, carvedilol blocks oxidation of norephinephrine, expression of several genes involved in myocardial damage and cardiac remodeling thus protecting the myocardium[63, 64]. It has been combined with diuretics, digitalis and ACE-inhibitors as the fourth drug with benefit in terms of reduced hospitalization as well as mortality[65, 66]. A multicenter retrospective report of carvedilol in children has demonstrated a potential improvement in ventricular performance and symptoms[67]. The average initial dose is 0.08 mg/kg and is uptitrated to maintenance dose of 0.46 mg/kg over nearly 10 weeks. In a multi center trial in children, after 3 months on carvidilol, there were improvements in modified NYHA class in 67% of patients and improvement in mean shortening fraction from 16.2 % to 19%. Side effects, mainly dizziness, hypotension, and headache, occurred in 54% of patients but by and large they were well tolerated.

Beta-blockers have been shown to be efficacious in children with congenital heart disease, anthracycline-induced cardiomyopathy and dilated cardiomyopathy, and before heart transplant[68-70]. In children with dilated cardiomyopathy, two nonrandomized trials have shown improvement in left ventricular function, improved exercise tolerance, and a decreased need for heart transplantation[70, 71]. One small case series showed that the addition of propranolol to diuretics and digoxin improved the clinical symptoms and reduced neurohormonal markers in infants with CHF due to large left-to-right shunts[59]. The use of beta-blockers in pediatric patients with either asymptomatic or symptomatic left ventricular dysfunction can potentially slow the progression of left ventricular dilation and reduce all-cause mortality. There is no reliable predictor to the beneficial response and temporary deterioration may occur in some patients. Beta-blockers should be commenced under supervision and titrated up from a low dose. Common side-effects include bradycardia, myocardial depression and exacerbation of bronchial asthma. Beta blockers should be avoided in the setting of decompensated heart failure when associated with bradycardia and bronchospasm.

Calcium channel blockers. Calcium channel blockers like nifedipine and diltiazem have also been used in CHF. However, most studies do not favor use of calcium channel blockers in CHF since they do not improve short term or long term exercise capacity[65] and have been found to increase mortality in CHF due to systolic dysfunction.

Carnitine. It is a naturally occurring compound in the body and is present in a high concentration in the myocardium and other muscle tissues. It is an essential factor in the transport of long chain fatty acids from the cytoplasm to the interior of the mitochondria where β-oxidation occurs. Carnitine deficiency has been shown to result in cardiomyopathy which responds to carnitine supplementation. Myocardial ischemia results in a deficiency of myocardial carnitine. Left ventricular failure due to valve dysfunction has been shown to be associated with myocardial carnitine deficiency. Although supplementation with carnitine has been shown to improve myocardial dysfunction in primary carnitine deficiency, use in the absence of deficiency is debatable. Since it is well tolerated and has little side effects (nausea, vomiting,

Section 4

abdominal cramps and diarrhea) supplements of carnitine to patients responding poorly to the standard treatment may be tried[72].

Some authors suggest that a trial of L-carnitine is warranted in all cases of cardiomyopathy. By offering a route for removal of accumulating toxic intramitochondrial acyl CoA derivatives, L-carnitine offers the possibility of improving overall mitochondrial energy metabolism. Usual oral or intravenous dose of 50-300 mg/kg per day has been shown to be safe and efficacious for treatment of inborn errors of metabolism in children. In such patients, treatment may be lifesaving.

Immune-modulators. In pediatrics, it is a common practice to treat new onset heart failure with high doses of methyl-prednisone and/or immune globulins. Both of these options can result in fluid retention that can lead to worsening of cardiac failure. There was no long term survival benefit following immunoglobulin therapy in a large controlled study[73, 74].

MANAGEMENT OF REFRACTORY HEART FAILURE

When significant symptoms persist despite optimum doses of diuretics, ACE inhibitors and digoxin, steps need to be taken to identify and treat any precipitating factors such as infection or anemia, and to evaluate compliance to therapy, before instituting more aggressive or invasive measures.

1. **Additional diuretics**. The diminished absorption and waning action of diuretics can be partially overcome by parenteral administration of furosemide. An alternative approach is sequential segmental nephron blockade by combining metolazone, with furosemide[75]. The use of this combination can produce profuse diuresis and requires close monitoring of fluid and electrolyte status.

2. **Intravenous inotropes**. Beta-agonists dopamine and dobutamine can temporarily improve myocardial function and partly reverse the abnormal neuroendocrine profile of CHF. The inotropic agents do not correct the basic myocardial abnormality. It is presumed that in the normal as well as the failing heart, the myocardium is only partially activated by inotropic agents and that sufficient reserve cardiac contractility can still be stimulated to raise cardiac output.

Dopamine predominantly a beta receptor agonist acts on dopamine receptors in low doses and alpha receptors in higher serum concentrations The positive inotropic effect of dopamine is aided by increased renal cortical flow and diuresis[76]. The peripheral vasoconstriction which occurs at a higher dose is a limiting factor as it increases afterload and wall stress[77]. It has several deleterious side effects namely tachycardia, arrhythmias and increased myocardial oxygen demand[76]. Dobutamine (DBA) is another predominant beta receptor agonist. Short term intermittent once or twice a week infusion of dobutamine in ambulatory patients is one of the most popular regimens currently being used[78]. Dopamine in low doses can be used concomitantly to further reduce the afterload[79].

Noncatecholamine-nonglycoside inotropic agents like amrinone and milrinone appear to selectively and potently inhibit the cAMP specific cardiac phosphodiesterase[80]. All the agents belonging to this category have similar action though the degree of inotropic and vasodilating activity may differ. These drugs have mostly been studied in patients with severe CHF and have been shown to increase the cardiac output, reduce the ventricular filling pressure, and enhance the systolic emptying of the ventricle[81]. However, no significant change occurs in the heart rate or blood pressure which is an advantage over catecholamine inotropic agents. At a low dose they augment cardiac contractility that tends to level off as the dose is increased and substantial vasodilation occurs with larger doses[19]. These drugs do not prolong life, and have been found to increase the mortality and thus not recommended for long term use (Table 32.5).

3. **Anti-arrhythmic agents and ablation therapy**. Arrhythmia is a major cause of morbidity and mortality in pediatric patients with end stage heart failure. In patients with dilated cardiomyopathy, between 50-63% of children who die have ventricular arrhythmias at presentation[82, 83]. The technological advances in ablation and improved understanding of tachyarrthymias over the past 15 years have greatly improved the ablative treatment of tachyarrthymias in children[84]. In most cases this method of treatment is the preferred first-line approach for treatment of symptomatic tachyarrhythmias in children.

Table 32.5 Dose of non-digitalis inotropic agents and diuretics

Agent	Route of administration	Dose
Inotropic agents		
1. Isoproterenol	IV	0.05 - 0.5 mcg/kg/min infusion 0.5-20.0 mcg/kg/min infusion
2. Dopamine	IV	(maximum dose 50 mcg/kg/min) 5.0-10.0 mcg/kg/min infusion
3. Dobutamine	IV	(maximum dose 40 mcg/kg/min) 0.75 mg/kg bolus over 2 min
4. Amrinone	IV	then 5-10 mcg/kg/min infusion (maximum dose 10 mg/kg/day)
Diuretics		
1. Hydrochlorthiazide	PO	2-5 mcg/kg/day (1-2 doses)
2. Furosemide	IV	1-2 mg/kg/dose upto 6 mg/kg/day
	PO	1-4 mg/kg/day (1-2 doses)
3. Spironolactone	PO	2-4 mg/kg/day (2 doses)
4. Metolazone	PO	0.1-0.2 mg/kg/day

4. **Resynchronization therapy**. Uncoordinated ventricular contraction resulting from prolonged intra-ventricular conduction (bundle branch block) can significantly depress systolic function, reduce cardiac output and increase end-systolic volume[85-87]. Improved systolic function, smaller ventricular dimensions, a more normal ventricular wall motion pattern and a more favorable profile for autonomic tone can be achieved with resynchronization therapy. Clinical benefits of ventricular resynchronization are well maintained over intermediate follow-up and include improvement in exercise tolerance and reduced hospitalizations[88]. This is usually accomplished with a specialized generator equipped with three dedicated ports that connect to a standard right atrial lead, along with two separate ventricular leads. Recent case reports of the use of this therapy in pediatric population with heart failure appear quite encouraging[89, 90].

Multisite ventricular pacing was found to have beneficial hemodynamic effects in patients with QRS prolongation or bundle branch block after operation for congenital heart disease[91]. It could be used as an effective adjunct therapy in both weaning from cardiopulmonary bypass and post-operative cardiac dysfunction. In a retrospective review of 7 patients who developed ventricular dysfunction after surgical correction of congenital heart disease, a significant improvement in ejection fractions were noted following cardiac resynchronization therapy[92]. Left ventricular dimensions also improved. It is being tested in patients with right bundle branch block following tetralogy repair.

Chronic right ventricular pacing can cause adverse effects on LV performance and can lead to the development of cardiomyopathy[93, 94]. This group of patients are the ideal candidates for resynchronization therapy. The major constraints of device therapy in children include small size of cardiac chamber and difficult vascular access.

5. **Extra corporeal membrane oxygenator (ECMO)**. Extracorporeal membrane oxygenation is used near the end of the therapeutic algorithm for low cardiac output and is reserved for patients who are believed to have little chance of surviving without support. In children, unlike in adults, mechanical circulatory support can reduce the risk of death in the short-term but has not proven useful for long-term support. Moreover, these devices do not allow for any patient mobilization and are not suitable for longer-term support.

6. **Other mechanical support devices**. External left ventricular assist devices (LVADs) are now available for children of all sizes but their use is restricted to a small number of centers[95]. None of the existing LVADs are suitable for long-term support in children with CHF, although recent reports suggest that LV recovery is possible in off-loaded patients with dilated cardiomyopathy and viral myocarditis[96, 97]. The LVAD normalizes LV pressure-volume relations, increases myocardial and systemic perfusion,

and reverses neurohormonal changes and cytokine release in heart failure. Although there is no prospective data to support device therapy in pediatric patients, several large, retrospective studies suggest that pediatric patients are likely to get the same reduction in mortality as adult patients, with a slightly higher rate of complications from the device implant.

7. **Cardiac transplant**. Survival as high as 77% at 1 year and 65% at 5 years has been reported with pediatric cardiac transplant[98]. Patients are considered for transplant when, despite optimum medical therapy, they show progressive deterioration in symptomatology or ventricular function, profound growth failure, develop life-threatening arrhythmia, require ongoing intravenous support or exhibit an unacceptably poor quality of life[99]. Key pediatric issues after transplantation include psychosocial support for the patients and family with regard to schooling, physical growth, neuromotor development, and future expectations.

Management of Heart Failure associated with Specific Conditions

1. *Ductus dependent circulation*. Neonates who present with CHF in first few weeks of life have ductal-dependent systemic flow until proven otherwise and resuscitation of the infant is not successful until the ductus is opened. Prostaglandin E1 (PGE$_1$) has been successfully used for this purpose. The usual starting dose is 0.025-0.1 mg/kg/min. Once therapeutic effect has been achieved, the dose may be decreased to 0.025mg/kg/min or less without loss of therapeutic effect. Common side effects associated with administration of PGE$_1$ include hypotension, rhythm disturbances, peripheral vasodilation, seizures, respiratory apnea or hypoventilation, diarrhea and necrotizing enterocolitis.

2. *Rheumatic carditis*. Bed rest is generally advised for patients in heart failure during the early days of their illness. Patients are initially treated with steroids. Steroids positively affect the outcome in patients with rheumatic pancarditis and acute heart failure.

3. *Kawasaki disease*. Treatment of patients with Kawasaki's disease in the first 10 days of illness with 2 g/kg dose of IVIG (intravenous immunoglobulin) and aspirin 80 to 100 mg/kg/d,

reduce the risk of coronary abnormalities from 20-25% to 2-4%[100].

4. *Anthracycline toxicity*. Dexrazoxane, a potent iron chelator can reduce free radical formation and may prevent the cardiotoxicity of anthracycline cancer therapy[101].

5. *Patent ductus arteriosus*. Indomethacin therapy may be useful in neonatal period in assisting ductus closure upto the age of two to three weeks.

6. *Acute viral myocarditis*. Enteroviral and adenoviral antibody titers, and isolation of EBV, CMV and HIV agents provide non-specific circumstantial evidence of viral infection. The coxsackie B virus and CMV can be cultured from the buffy coat and attempts should be made to culture enterovirus from a rectal swab and CMV from urine. Amlodipine has had beneficial effects in models of viral myocarditis through the inhibition of nitric oxide synthase. Several studies have suggested that patients with myocarditis secondary to either coxsackie virus or adenovirus may benefit from ribavirin if treatment is started early in the course of the disease. There is some evidence that immunosuppressive therapy may be useful in patients with active myocarditis[102]. Immunoglobulins may reduce level of cytokines in heart failure and short term echocardiogram improvement may be attributable to this, but resolution of myocarditis is not affected[21].

7. *Muscular dystrophy*. Deflazacort is an oxazolone derivative of prednisone. In a retrospective cohort study of patients with Duchenne's muscular dystrophy and myocardial dysfunction, patients who had been receiving deflazacort for >3 years were more likely to have preserved cardiac function compared to the controls[103]. Preservation of cardiac muscle function was associated with better pulmonary and cardiac muscle function.

Newer Agents Under Trial

Nesiritide is the recombinant form of human BNP available for therapeutic use. Its use in adult patients with CHF has been successfully demonstrated. Its safety and efficacy in children with decompensated heart failure has recently been reported[104]. Treatment with nesiritide resulted in decreased thirst, improved appetite, improved urine output, and improved functional status. Patients are started at a dose of 0.01 mcg/kg/min and titrated to a maximum dose of 0.03 mcg/kg/min in escalating doses of 0.005 mcg/kg/min.

Human growth hormone stimulates myocardial hypertrophy and increases myocardial contractility. Initial trials have confirmed beneficial effects on energy efficiency and echocardiographic indices[105].

L-thyroxine and taurine have been shown to have positive inotropic action and reduce peripheral vascular resistance[106, 107].

Nitric oxide (NO). Supplemental oral L-arginine, the precursor of NO and low dose nitroglycerine infusion have been shown to enhance endothelium-dependent vasodilatation[108].

Calcium sensitizers increase inotropy by increasing the affinity of troponin C for calcium and thus increase contractility of the heart without increasing intracellular calcium load. They also produce peripheral vasodilation through the vascular K-ATPase channels. Levosimendan is one of the calcium-sensitizing agents being used in clinical trials, and initial reports show beneficial effects on cardiac hemodynamics and clinical symptoms[109, 110].

Endothelin antagonists. Both oral and parenteral agents are being investigated. Tezosentan has been reported to significantly increase cardiac index and decrease pulmonary capillary wedge pressure[111].

Vasopressin antagonists. Vasopressin stimulation results in vasoconstriction and fluid retention, both of which may worsen CHF. In heart failure, vasopressin levels have been shown to be markedly elevated and may be associated with adverse cardiovascular outcome. Tolvaptan, a vasopressin antagonist was found to be effective in weight reduction but no difference was found in the in-hospital mortality[112].

Batista procedure. It involves partial left ventriculectomy and mitral valve repair or replacement[113]. This surgery has been done mainly in patients with dilated cardiomyopathy, where it is thought that restoration of normal LV dimensions will improve myocardial performance.

Surgical Management

Medical management has a limited role in pediatric patients with structural heart defects because, for most defects, effective surgical therapy is available. Digitalis, diuretics, and ACE inhibitors are used as temporizing therapy to improve the condition of the patient before surgical repair. Only in case of a few defects is long-term medical therapy attempted, either because of the propensity for the defect to regress spontaneously (ventricular septal defect) or because the surgical treatment is problematic (congenital mitral stenosis). In these instances, surgical repair is usually postponed as long as the infant is growing normally and when the risk of pulmonary vascular disease is minimal. Types of operations may be divided into three broad groups; palliative, reparative and cardiac transplantation. Details of these are beyond the scope of this chapter.

Interventional Approach to Congenital Heart Disease

Surgical procedures are being partially replaced by percutaneous interventions or hybrid approaches. Coarctation of aorta beyond the neonatal period as well as muscular ventricular septal defects can be successfully managed by transcatheter approach. Effective percutaneous treatment is also available for children with critical aortic and pulmonary stenoses, patent ductus arteriosus, atrial septal defects and branch pulmonary artery stenosis.

In pediatric patients stents are being used for a variety of diagnoses, such as systemic venous obstruction pathways (Mustard, Fontan baffle, or bi-directional cavopulmonary connections), pulmonary artery, right ventricular to pulmonary conduits, aortic coarctation, the arterial duct, aortoplumonary collaterals, or postoperative systemic to pulmonary shunts[114].

Stepwise Guidelines for the Management of CHF

Step 1. Rest, propped up position, humidified oxygen, diet with sodium restriction.

Step 2. Start digoxin and diuretics. It is better to use furosemide combined with spironolactone instead of furosemide alone with potassium supplementation.

Step 3. Add ACE-inhibitor. If not acceptable due to cough, change to angiotensin receptor blocker.

Step 4. Add isosorbide dinitrate if ACE inhibitors or angiotensin receptor blockers are not tolerated. Do not use hydralazine since it has been shown to increase the mortality.

Step 5. In the presence of inadequate response especially if the patient has tachycardia start carvedilol.

Section 4

Step 6. Consider use of once or twice weekly dobutamine infusion in patients who continue to deteriorate in spite of steps 1 to 5 and add carnitine as a supplement.

Step 7. Consider cardiac transplantation if the patient shows continued deterioration.

Diastolic Dysfunction

Diastolic dysfunction is the abnormality of ventricular relaxation. Diastolic dysfunction caused by poor myocardial compliance or relaxation has been recognized as an important cause, or contributor of CHF. Despite normal or decreased LV end-diastolic volume, compliance is decreased. The isovolumic relaxation time is usually prolonged, with a delay in opening of the mitral valve. The common causes of diastolic dysfunction are left ventricular hypertrophy, hypertension, myocardial ischemia and restrictive cardiomyopathy. Treatment with calcium channel blockers and beta blockers has been helpful in some cases. Restrictive cardiomypathy is probably best managed with beta blockers and a low dose of diuretics; anticoagulation may be required as there is a high incidence of embolic complications in these patients.

REFERENCES

1. Nadas AS, Hauck AJ. Pediatric aspects of congestive heart failure. *Circulation* 1960:424-29.

2. Talner NS. Congestive heart failure in the infant. A functional approach. *Pediatr Clin N Amer* 1971; 18: 1011-29.

3. Ortiz-Lopez R, Li H, Su J, Goytia V, Towbin JA. Evidence for a dystrophin missense mutation as a cause of X-linked dilated cardiomyopathy. *Circulation* 1997; 95:2434-40.

4. Saito M, Kawai H, Akaike M, Adachi K, Nishida Y, Saito S. Cardiac dysfunction with Becker muscular dystrophy. *Am Heart J* 1996; 132:642-67.

5. Lipshultz SE, Easley KA, Orav EJ, Kaplan S, Starc TJ, Bricker JT, Lai WW, Moodie DS, Sopko G, Schluchter MD, Colan SD, Cardiovascular status of infants and children of women infected with HIV-1 (P(2)C(2) HIV): a cohort study. *Lancet* 2002; 360:368-73.

6. Kremer LC, van Dalen EC, Offringa M, Ottenkamp J, Voute PA. Anthracycline-induced clinical heart failure in a cohort of 607 children: long-term follow-up study. *J Clin Oncol* 2001; 19:191-96.

7. Batra AS, Lewis AB. Acute myocarditis. *Curr Opin Pediatr* 2001; 13:234-39.

8. Stiller B, Dahnert I, Weng YG, Hennig E, Hetzer R, Lange PE. Children may survive severe myocarditis with prolonged use of biventricular assist devices. *Heart* 1999; 82:237-40A-44A.

9. Kawai C. From myocarditis to cardiomyopathy: mechanisms of inflammation and cell death: learning from the past for the future. *Circulation* 1999; 99: 1091-100.

10. Liu P, Aitken K, Kong YY, Opavsky MA, Martino T, Dawood F, Wen WH, Kozieradzki I, Bachmaier K, Straus D, Mak TW, Penninger JM. The tyrosine kinase p56lck is essential in coxsackie virus B3-mediated heart disease. *Nat Med* 2000; 6:429-34.

11. Horenstein MS, Saarel E, Dick M, Karpawich PP. Reversible symptomatic dilated cardiomyopathy in older children and young adolescents due to primary non-sinus supraventricular tachyarrhythmias. *Pediatr Cardiol* 2003; 24:274-79.

12. Stone RM, Bridges KR, Libby P. Hematological – oncological disorders and cardiovascular disease. In: Heart Disease, Braunwald E, (ed.). 6th ed. *Philadelphia: WB Saunders,* 2001: 2226-7.

13. Borgna-Pignatti C, Rugolotto S, De Stefano P, Piga A, Di Gregorio F, Gamberini MR, Sabato V, Melevendi C, Cappellini MD, Verlato G Survival and disease complications in thalassemia major. *Ann N Y Acad Sci* 1998; 850:227-31.

14. Engle MA, Erlandson M, Smith CH. Late cardiac complications of chronic, severe, refractory anemia with hemochromatosis. *Circulation* 1964; 30:698-705.

15. Friedman WF, George BL. New concepts and drugs in treatment of congestive heart failure. *Pediatr Clin N Amer* 1984; 31:1197-227.

16. Bristow MR. Myocardial beta adrenergic receptor down regulation in heart failure. *Int J Cardiol* 1984; 5:648-52.

17. Balaguru D, Artman M, Marcelo A. Management of heart failure in children. *Curr Prob Pediatr* 2000; 30:5-30.

18. Cohn JN, Levin TB. Fancis GS, Goldsmith SR. Neurohumoral control mechanisms in congestive heart failure. *Am Heart J* 1981; 102:509-14.

19. Fowler MB, Bristow MR, Minobe WA, Ginsburg R, Laser JA. Correlation between human myocardial beta receptor density and left ventricular failure in heart transplant recepients (abstr.). *J Am Coll Cardiol* 1983; 3:544.

20. Lee JC, Downing SE. Development aspects of the myocardial staircase phenomenon. *J Mol Cell Cardiol* 1978; 10:953-66.

21. Mason DT. Afterload reduction and cardiac performance. Physiological basis of systemic vasodilators as a new approach in treatment of congestive heart failure. *Am J Med* 1978; 65:106-25.

22. Goldsmith SR, Francis GS, Cowley AW, Levine TB, Cohn JN. Increased plasma arginine vasopressin levels

in patients with congestive heart failure. *J Am Coll Cardiol* 1982; 1:1385-90.

23. Little RC, Little WC. Cardiac preload, afterload and heart failure. *Arch Intern Med* 1982; 142:819-22.

24. Grose RM, Strain JE, Bergman MJ, McGinnis J, Greenberg MA, Lejetmal TH. Milrionone vs dobutamine (abstr.). *Circulation.* 1984; 70:II-11.

25. Milnor WR. Arterial impedence as ventricular afterload. *Circul Res* 1975; 36:565-70.

26. Levine TB. Role of vasodilators in the treatment of congestive heart failure. *Am J Cardiol* 1985; 55:32A-35A.

27. Dyke SH, Urschel CW. Sonnenblick EH, Gorlin R, Chohn PF. Detection of latent function in acutely ischemic myocardium in dog. *Circ Res* 1975; 36: 490-97.

28. Bukowski R, Saade GR. Hydrops fetalis. *Clin Perinatol* 2000; 27:1007-31.

29. Bristow JD, Metcalfe J. Physical signs in congestive heart failure. *Prog Cardiovasc Dis* 1967; 10:236-45.

30. Connolly D, Rutkowski M, Auslender M, Artman M. The New York University Pediatric Heart Failure Index: a new method of quantifying chronic heart failure severity in children. *J Pediatr* 2001; 138:644-48.

31. Law YM, Keller BB, Feingold BM, Boyle GJ. Usefulness of plasma B-type natriuretic peptide to identify ventricular dysfunction in pediatric and adult patients with congenital heart disease. *Am J Cardiol* 2005; 95:474-78.

32. Troughton RW, Frampton CM, Yandle TG, Espiner EA, Nicholls MG, Richards AM. Treatment of heart failure guided by plasma aminoterminal brain natriuretic peptide (N-BNP) concentrations. *Lancet* 2000; 355:1126-30.

33. Karl J, Borgya A, Gallusser A, Huber E, Krueger K, Rollinger W, Schenk J. Development of a novel, N-terminal-proBNP (NT-proBNP) assay with a low detection limit. *Scand J Clin Lab Invest* 1999; 230 (Suppl):177-81.

34. Mir TS, Marohn S, Laer S, Eiselt M, Grollmus O, Weil J. Plasma concentrations of N-terminal pro-brain natriuretic peptide in control children from the neonatal to adolescent period and in children with congestive heart failure. *Pediatrics* 2002; 110:e76.

35. Ardehali H, Kasper EK, Baughman KL. Diagnostic approach to the patient with cardiomyopathy: whom to biopsy? *Am Heart J* 2005; 149:7-12.

36. Drucker NA, Newburger JW. Viral myocarditis: diagnosis and management. *Adv Pediatr* 1997; 44: 141-71.

37. Schwartz ML, Cox GF, Lin AE, Korson MS, Perez-Atayde A, Lacro RV, Lipshultz SE. Clinical approach to genetic cardiomyopathy in children. *Circulation* 1996; 94:2021-38.

38. Levi D, Alejos J. Diagnosis and treatment of pediatric viral myocarditis. *Curr Opin Cardiol* 2001; 16:77-83.

39. Feldman AM, McNamara D. Myocarditis. *N Engl J Med* 2000; 343:1388-98.

40. Chow LH, Radio SJ, Sears TD, McManus BM. Insensitivity of right ventricular endomyocardial biopsy in the diagnosis of myocarditis. *J Am Coll Cardiol* 1989; 14:915-20.

41. Hamer J. Modern management of congestive heart failure. *Recent Adv Cardiol* 1985; 9:275-288.

42. O'Laughlin MP. Congestive heart failure in children. *Pediatr Clin N Amer* 1999; 46:263-73.

43. Forchielli ML, McColl R, Walker WA, Lo C. Children with congenital heart disease: a nutrition challenge. *Nutr Rev* 1994; 52:348-53.

44. Barton JS, Hindmarsh PC, Scringeour CM, *et al*. Energy expenditure in congenital heart disease. *Arch Dis Child* 1994; 70:5-9.

45. Pitt B, Zannad F, Remme WJ, Cody R, Castaigne A, Perez A, Palensky J, Wittes J. The effect of spironolactone on mortality in patients with severe heart failure. *N Engl J Med* 1999; 341:709-17.

46. Bauersachs J, Fraccarollo D, Ertl G, Gretz N, Wehling M, Christ M. Striking increase of natriuresis by low-dose spironolactone in congestive heart failure only in combination with ACE inhibition: mechanistic evidence to support RALES. *Circulation* 2000; 102:2325-28.

47. The Digitalis Investigaton Group. The effect of digoxin on mortality and morbidity in patients with heart failure. *N Engl J Med* 1997; 336: 525-33.

48. Applefeld MM, Roffman DS. Digitalis and other positive catecholamine-like inotropic agents in the management of congestive heart failure. *Amer J Med* 1986; 80:40-45.

49. Park MK. Use of digoxin in infants and children with specific emphasis on dosage. *J Pediatr* 1986; 108: 871-7.

50. Sole MJ, Liu P. Viral myocarditis: a paradigm for understanding the pathogenesis and treatment of dilated cardiomyopathy. *J Am Coll Cardiol* 1993; 22 (Suppl A):99A-105A.

51. Levine TB, Francis GS, Goldsmith SR, Simon AB, Chon JN. Activity of the sympathetic nervous system and renin angiotensin system assessed by plasma hormone levels and their relation to hemodynamic abnormalities in congestive heart failure. *Am J Cardiol* 1982; 49: 1659-66.

52. Captopril Multicenter Research Group. A placebo-controlled trial of captopril in refractory congestive failure. *J Amer Coll Cardiol* 1983; 2:755-63.

53. Leier CV, Huss P, Magorien RD, Unverferth DV. Improved exercise capacity and differing arterial and venous tolerance during chronic isosorbide dinitrate

therapy for congestive heart failure. *Circulation* 1983; 67:817-22.

54. Goldberg LI. Dopamine-clinical uses of an endogenous catecholamine. *N Engl J Med* 1974; 291:707-10.

55. Markham EV, Corbett JR, Gilmore A, Pettinger WA. Firth BG. Efficacy of prazosin in the management of congestive heart failure. *Amer J Cardiol* 1983; 51: 1346-52.

56. Montigny M, Davignon A, Fouron JC, Biron P, Fournier A, Elie R. Captopril in infants for congestive heart failure secondary to a large ventricular left-to-right shunt. *Amer J Cardiol* 1989; 63:631-33.

57. Rheuban KS, Carpenter MA, Ayers CA, Gutgesell HP. Acute hemodynamic effects of converting enzyme inhibition in infants with congestive heart failure. *J Pediatr* 1990; 117:668-70.

58. Lewis AB, Chabot M. The effect of treatment with angiotensin-converting enzyme inhibitors on survival of pediatric patients with dilated cardiomyopathy. *Pediatr Cardiol* 1993; 14:9-12.

59. Nawarskas JJ, Spinler SA.Update on the interaction between aspirin and angiotensin-converting enzyme inhibitors. *Pharmacotherapy* 2000; 20:698-710.

60. Buchhorn R, Bartmus D, Siekmeyer W, Hulpke-Wette M, Schulz R, Bursch J. Beta-blocker therapy of severe congestive heart failure in infants with left to right shunts. *Am J Cardiol* 1998; 81:1366-68.

61. Swedberg K, Hjalmarson A, Wasgenstein F, Vallentin I. Prolongation of survival in congestive cardiomyopathy by beta blockers. *Lancet* 1979; 1:1374.

62. Waagstein F, Hjalmarson A, Varnauskas E, Wallentin 1. Effect of chronic beta receptor blockade in congestive cardiomyopathy. *Br Heart J* 1975; 37: 1022-36.

63. Feuerstein GZ, Ruffolo RR Jr. Carvedilol, a novel multiple action antihypertensive agent with antioxidant activity and the potential for myocardial and vascular protection. *Eur Heart J* 1995; 16 (Suppl F):38-42.

64. Rossig L, Haendeler J, Mallat Z, Hugel B, Freyssinet JM, Tedgui A, Dimmeler S, Zeiher AM. Congestive heart failure induces endothelial cell apoptosis: protective role of carvedilol. *J Am Coll Cardiol* 2000; 36:2081-9.

65. Packer M, Bristow MR Cohn JN, Colucci WS, Fowler MB, Gilbert EM, Shusterman NH. The effect of carvedilol on morbidity and mortality in patients with chronic heart failure. *N Engl J Med* 1996; 334:1349-55.

66. Yoshikawa T, Port JD, Asano K, *et al*. Cardiac adrenergic effects of carvediol. *Eur Heart J* 1996; 17 (Suppl B):8-16.

67. Bruns LA, Chrisant MK, Lamour JM, Shaddy RE, Pahl E, Blume ED, Hallowell S, Addonizio LJ, Canter CE. Carvedilol as therapy in pediatric heart failure: an initial multicenter experience. *J Pediatr* 2001; 138:505-11.

68. Shaddy RE. Beta-blocker therapy in young children with congestive heart failure under consideration for heart transplantation. *Amer Heart J* 1998; 136:19-21.

69. Shaddy RE, Olsen SL, Bristow MR, Taylor DO, Bullock EA, Tani LY, Renlund DG. Efficacy and safety of metoprolol in the treatment of doxorubicin-induced cardiomyopathy in pediatric patients. *Amer Heart J* 1995; 129:197-99.

70. Shaddy RE, Tani LY, Gidding SS, Pahl E, Orsmond GS, Gilbert EM, Lemes V. Beta-blocker treatment of dilated cardiomyopathy with congestive heart failure in children: a multi-institutional experience. *J Heart Lung Transplant* 1999; 18:269-74.

71. Ishikawa Y, Bach JR, Minami R. Cardioprotection for Duchenne's muscular dystrophy. *Am Heart J* 1999; 137:895-902.

72. Pepine CJ. The therapeutic potential of carnitine in cardiovascular disorders. *Clin Therap* 1991; 13:2-21.

73. McNamara DM, Holubkov R, Starling RC, Dec GW, Loh E, Torre-Amione G, Gass A, Janosko K, Tokarczyk T, Kessler P, Mann DL, Feldman AM. Controlled trial of intravenous immune globulin in recent-onset dilated cardiomyopathy. *Circulation* 2001; 103:2254-9.

74. McNamara DM, Rosenblum WD, Janosko KM, Trost MK, Villanueva FS, Demetris AJ, Murali S, Feldman AM. Intravenous immune globulin in the therapy of myocarditis and acute cardiomyopathy. *Circulation* 1997; 95:2476-78.

75. Kramer BK, Schweda F, Kammerl M, Riegger GA. Diuretic therapy and diuretic resistance in cardiac failure. *Nephrol Dial Transplant* 1999; 14 (Suppl) 4:39-42.

76. Fisher ML, Plotnick GD, Peters RW, Carliner NH. Beta blockers in congestive cardiomyopathy. *Amer J Med* 1986; 80 (2B):59-66.

77. Beregovich J, Binachi C, Rubler C, Lomnitz E, Cagin N, Levitt B. Dose related hemodynamic and renal effects of dopamine in congestive heart failure. *Am Heart J* 1974; 87:550-57.

78. Hodgson JM, Aja M, Sorkin RP. Intermittent ambulatory dobutamine infusions for patients awaiting cardiac transplantation. *Am J Cardiol* 1984; 53:375-76.

79. Richard C, Picome JL, Rimailho A. Bottineau G, Auzepy P. Combined hemodynamic effects of dopamine and dobutamine in cardiogenic shock. *Circulation* 1983; 67:620-26.

80. Kariya T, Wille LJ, Dage RC. Biochemical studies on the mechanisms of cardiotonic activity of MDL-17, 043. *J Cardiovasc Pharm* 1982; 4:509-14.

81. Sonnenblick EH, Mancini DA. Lejetmel TH. New positive inotropic drugs for the treatment of congestive heart failure. *Am J Cardiol* 1985; 55:41A-44A.

82. Griffin ML, Hernandez A, Martin TC, Goldring D, Bolman RM, Spray TL, Strauss AW. Dilated

cardiomyopathy in infants and children. *J Am Coll Cardiol* 1988; 11:139-44.

83. Lewis AB, Chabot M. Outcome of infants and children with dilated cardiomyopathy. *Am J Cardiol* 1991; 68:365-69.

84. Samii SM, Cohen MH. Ablation of tachyarrhythmias in pediatric patients. *Curr Opin Cardiol* 2004; 19:64-67.

85. Frias PA, Corvera JS, Schmarkey L, Strieper M, Campbell RM, Vinten-Johansen J. Evaluation of myocardial performance with conventional single-site ventricular pacing and biventricular pacing in a canine model of atrioventricular block. *J Cardiovasc Electrophysiol* 2003; 14:996-1000.

86. Leclercq C, Kass DA. Retiming the failing heart: principles and current clinical status of cardiac resynchronization. *J Am Coll Cardiol* 2002; 39: 194-201.

87. Verbeek XA, Vernooy K, Peschar M, Cornelussen RN, Prinzen FW. Intra-ventricular resynchronization for optimal left ventricular function during pacing in experimental left bundle branch block. *J Am Coll Cardiol* 2003; 42:558-67.

88. Linde C, Braunschweig F, Gadler F, Bailleul C, Daubert JC. Long-term improvements in quality of life by biventricular pacing in patients with chronic heart failure: results from the Multisite Stimulation in Cardiomyopathy study (MUSTIC). *Am J Cardiol* 2003; 91:1090-95.

89. Janousek J, Tomek V, Chaloupecky VA, Reich O, Gebauer RA, Kautzner J, Hucin B. Cardiac resynchronization therapy: a novel adjunct to the treatment and prevention of systemic right ventricular failure. *J Am Coll Cardiol* 2004; 44:1927-31.

90. Janousek J, Vojtovic P, Hucin B, Tlaskal T, Gebauer RA, Gebauer R, Matejka T, Marek J, Reich O. Resynchronization pacing is a useful adjunct to the management of acute heart failure after surgery for congenital heart defects. *Am J Cardiol* 2001; 88: 145-52.

91. Zimmerman FJ, Starr JP, Koenig PR, Smith P, Hijazi ZM, Bacha EA. Acute hemodynamic benefit of multisite ventricular pacing after congenital heart surgery. *Ann Thorac Surg* 2003; 75:1775-80.

92. Strieper M, Karpawich P, Frias P, Gooden K, Ketchum D, Fyfe D, Campbell R. Initial experience with cardiac resynchronization therapy for ventricular dysfunction in young patients with surgically operated congenital heart disease. *Am J Cardiol* 2004; 94:1352-54.

93. Tantengco MV, Thomas RL, Karpawich PP. Left ventricular dysfunction after long-term right ventricular apical pacing in the young. *J Am Coll Cardiol* 2001; 37:2093-100.

94. Tse HF, Yu C, Wong KK, Tsang V, Leung YL, Ho WY, Lau CP. Functional abnormalities in patients with permanent right ventricular pacing: the effect of sites of electrical stimulation. *J Am Coll Cardiol* 2002; 40:1451-58.

95. Hetzer R, Loebe M, Potapov EV, Weng Y, Stiller B, Hennig E, Alexi-Meskishvili V, Lange PE. Circulatory support with pneumatic paracorporeal ventricular assist device in infants and children. *Ann Thorac Surg* 1998; 66:1498-506.

96. Levin HR, Oz MC, Chen JM, Packer M, Rose EA, Burkhoff D. Reversal of chronic ventricular dilation in patients with end-stage cardiomyopathy by prolonged mechanical unloading. *Circulation* 1995; 91:2717-20.

97. Muller J, Wallukat G, Weng YG, Dandel M, Spiegelsberger S, Semrau S, Brandes K, Theodoridis V, Loebe M, Meyer R, Hetzer R. Weaning from mechanical cardiac support in patients with idiopathic dilated cardiomyopathy. *Circulation* 1997; 96:542-49.

98. Canter C, Naftel D, Caldwell R, Chinnock R, Pahl E, Frazier E, Kirklin J, Boucek M, Morrow R.Survival and risk factors for death after cardiac transplantation in infants. A multi-institutional study. The Pediatric Heart Transplant Study. *Circulation* 1997; 96:227-31.

99. Costanzo MR, Augustine S, Bourge R, Bristow M, O'Connell JB, Driscoll D, Rose E. Selection and treatment of candidates for heart transplantation. A statement for health professionals from the Committee on Heart Failure and Cardiac Transplantation of the Council on Clinical Cardiology, American Heart Association. *Circulation* 1995; 92:3593-612.

100. Rowley AH, Shulman ST. Kawasaki syndrome. *Pediatr Clin North Am* 1999; 46:313-29.

101. Wexler LH. Ameliorating anthracycline cardiotoxicity in children with cancer: clinical trials with dexrazoxane. *Semin Oncol* 1998; 25(Suppl 10):86-92.

102. Kereikas DJ, Parmley WW. Myocarditis and cardiomyopathy. *Am Heart J* 1984; 108:1318-26.

103. Silversides CK, Webb GD, Harris VA, Biggar DW. Effects of deflazacort on left ventricular function in patients with Duchenne muscular dystrophy. *Am J Cardiol* 2003; 91:769-72.

104. Marshall J, Berkenbosch JW, Russo P, Tobias JD. Preliminary experience with nesiritide in the pediatric population. *J Intensive Care Med* 2004; 19:164-70.

105. Fazio S, Sabatini D, Capaldo B, Vigorito C, Giordano A, Guida R, Pardo F, Biondi B, Sacca L. A preliminary study of growth hormone in the treatment of dilated cardiomyopathy. *N Engl J Med* 1996; 334:809-14.

106. Azuma J, Sawamura A, Awata N, Ohta H, Hamaguchi T, Harada H, Takihara K, Hasegawa H, Yamagami T, Ishiyama T, *et al*. Therapeutic effect of taurine in congestive heart failure: a double-blind crossover trial. *Clin Cardiol* 1985; 8(5):276-82.

107. Klein I, Ojamaa K. Thyroid hormone and the cardiovascular system: from theory to practice. *J Clin Endocrinol Metab* 1994; 78:1026-7.

108. Rector TS, Bank AJ, Tschumperlin LK, Mullen KA, Lin KA, Kubo SH. Abnormal desmopressin-induced forearm vasodilatation in patients with heart failure: dependence on nitric oxide synthase activity. *Clin Pharmacol Ther* 1996;60:667-74.

109. Follath F, Cleland JG, Just H, Papp JG, Scholz H, Peuhkurinen K, Harjola VP, Mitrovic V, Abdalla M, Sandell EP, Lehtonen L; Steering Committee and Investigators of the Levosimendan Infusion versus Dobutamine (LIDO) study. Efficacy and safety of intravenous levosimendan compared with dobutamine in severe low-output heart failure (the LIDO study): a randomised double-blind trial. *Lancet* 2002; 360: 196-202.

110. Kivikko M, Lehtonen L, Colucci WS. Sustained hemodynamic effects of intravenous levosimendan. *Circulation* 2003; 107:81-6.

111. Torre-Amione G, Young JB, Colucci WS, Lewis BS, Pratt C, Cotter G, Stangl K, Elkayam U, Teerlink JR, Frey A, Rainisio M, Kobrin I. Hemodynamic and clinical effects of tezosentan, an intravenous dual endothelin receptor antagonist, in patients hospitalized for acute decompensated heart failure. *J Am Coll Cardiol* 2003; 42:140-47.

112. Gheorghiade M, Niazi I, Ouyang J, Czerwiec F, Kambayashi J, Zampino M, Orlandi C; Tolvaptan Investigators. Vasopressin V2-receptor blockade with tolvaptan in patients with chronic heart failure: results from a double-blind, randomized trial. *Circulation* 2003; 107:2690-96.

113. Suma H, Isomura T, Horii T, Sato T, Kikuchi N, Iwahashi K, Hosokawa J. Two-year experience of the Batista operation for non-ischemic cardiomyopathy. *J Cardiol* 1998; 32:269-76.

114. Okubo M, Benson LN. Intravascular and intracardiac stents used in congenital heart disease. *Curr Opin Cardiol* 2001; 16:84-91.

Section 4

33

Cardiac Arrhythmias

Rajnish Juneja and Anita Saxena

Cardiac arrhythmias in infants and children are assuming increasing importance and pediatricians are now truly on the 'front line' for their diagnosis and emergency treatment. An apparent increase in the frequency of cardiac arrhythmias may be partly related to increasing awareness and improved recognition by newer diagnostic and therapeutic modalities; whereas a "true" increase in incidence is also due to increasing open heart procedures that predisposes these patients to various atrial and ventricular arrhythmias. Similarly, drug effects and drug interactions are increasingly being recognized to be proarrhythmic as was seen with terfenadine (an antihistaminic used for common cold) leading to Torsades-de-pointes and subsequent withdrawal of this drug. Cisapride, a prokinetic agent, was also withdrawn due to risk of QT prolongation and development of life-threatening ventricular arrhythmia. In contrast to adults presenting with arrhythmias, there are several features unique to children that include age-dependent presentation, different natural course of arrhythmias presenting in infancy and early childhood, association with structural heart defects and influence of previous heart surgery in the genesis of arrhythmias.

Arrhythmias form an important, potentially treatable cause of morbidity and mortality; they may be the primary cause for the emergency or may be seen in the intensive care unit secondary to various metabolic and electrolyte disturbances or due to drugs. Arrhythmias are an important cause of sudden cardiac death, though the majority of supraventricular arrhythmias are benign and more of a nuisance rather than being dangerous. This chapter predominantly addresses the recognition and management of primary arrhythmias in infants and children and the issue of syncope and sudden cardiac death (SCD).

INCIDENCE

Around 5% of all deaths in children are sudden cardiac deaths, that makes it equivalent to 1.5-8 deaths/100,000 patient years[1]. In the US alone, there are 5 to 7000 asymptomatic children who would have a sudden cardiac death (SCD). This is against an annual adult SCD rate of 300,000 to 400,000[2]. Given our population the estimated number of sudden cardiac deaths in children would be close to 50,000 in a year. The issue becomes even more pertinent when one realizes that most of these children would be otherwise healthy and 1 in 50,000 to 100,000 deaths would be during competitive sports. A comparative estimate of the risk of sudden death due to an arrhythmia in select congenital heart diseases is provided in Table 33.1 to highlight the relative magnitude of the problem[3].

Table 33.1 Incidence of arrhythmias/SCD in congenital heart diseases (CHD)		
Anomaly or procedure	**Arrhythmia**	
TOF	VT	10% (SCD 2.25%)
VSD, AVSD	SCD	5.8% (?heart block)
Ebstein anomaly	SCD	2.5-20%
AS	SCD	1%
S/P Senning procedure	SCD	2.8%
Fontan procedure	SCD	3%
Eisenmenger complex	SCD	10-47%

VT: Ventricular tachycardia, SCD: Sudden cardiac death, VSD: Ventricular septal defect, AVSD: Atrioventricular septal defect, AS: Aortic stenosis, S/P : Status post

CLASSIFICATION

Arrhythmias are broadly classified into bradyarrhythmias and tachyarrhythmias depending on the heart rate appropriate for the age of the child (Table 33.2). The physiological variations in heart rate are very wide and a high index of suspicion is necessary for the diagnosis and conversely one should avoid over diagnosis and use of relatively toxic drugs like amiodarone. Further classification is either based on the type of arrhythmia or the possible site and cause of the arrhythmia.

Table 33.2 Normal resting and exercise heart rates for various ages

Age	Resting (sleeping)	Resting (awake)	Exercise or fever
Newborn	80-160	100-180	Upto 220
1 week-3 months	80-200	100-220	Upto 220
3 months-2 years	70-120	80-170	Upto 200
2 years-10 years	60-90	70-110	Upto 200
10 years-adult	50-90	55-90	Upto 200

BRADYARRHYTHMIAS

They may occur due to either defective formation or conduction of cardiac impulse.

Disorders of impulse formation

Sick sinus syndrome (Sinus pauses, sinus arrest)

- Non-specific, scar-like degeneration of the heart's conduction system, often age-related (not common in children)

- Familial and hypothyriodism

- Postoperative e.g., following a Glenn shunt, Senning operation

- Drug interactions and medications

Disorders of impulse conduction

- Sinus node conduction abnormalities (sinoatrial block)

- Atrioventricular blocks: First degree, second degree and complete heart block. It may be congenital, postoperative, associated with congenital heart disease (CHD) e.g. with cTGA,

- Ebstein's anomaly, AV septal defects, drug induced leading to bundle branch block and hemiblocks

Bradyarrhythmias are discussed in detail later in the chapter.

TACHYARRHYTHMIAS

Tachyarrhythmias are broadly defined as resting heart rates that are beyond the range of normal heart rate for the age. Thus in a neonate a rate >160/min would qualify for a tachycardia whereas a child in his teens would be considered to have tachycardia if resting heart rate is beyond 100/min. Heart rate limits appropriate for the age are listed in Table 33.2. It is important to distinguish sinus tachycardia from a true supraventricular tachycardia, that can sometimes be very difficult especially when the rates are beyond 180-200 bpm and the P wave gets superimposed on the T wave or may just appear as a notched T wave, giving an impression of "junctional tachycardia" (Figure 33.1). The sinus node in a normal solitus heart is typically situated anterior to the SVC margin and comes down the crista terminalis for 1-1.5 cm. The P wave thus has a typical ECG pattern, with a totally negative aVR, positive inferior and chest leads from V3–V6; biphasic or positive V1 and V2 with an initial component always being positive and lead I and aVL also being mostly positive. The salient differences between sinus tachycardia and supraventricular tachycardia (SVT) are listed in Table 33.3.

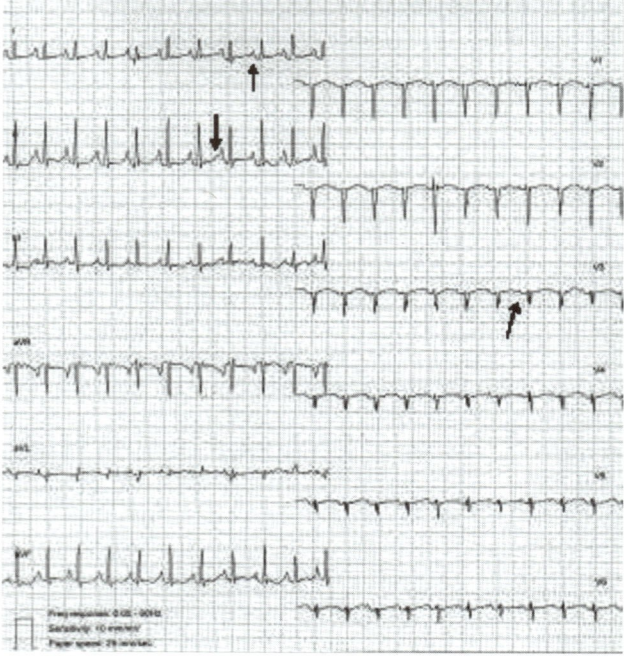

Figure 33.1 12-Lead Holter recording of a 7-year-old child showing sinus tachycardia > 150/min. The T waves are usually not so peaked and hence in the limb leads there is a definite evidence of P on T; this is also evident in the chest leads as a small notch on the T wave (arrows). If such P waves are not recognized, a mistaken diagnosis of junctional tachycardia can be made

Table 33.3 Sinus tachycardia versus supraventricular tachycardia (SVT)

☐ P waves with a morphology not commensurate with the pattern described above suggest an abnormal origin.

☐ Gradual onset and offset of tachycardia

☐ Concomitant illness that could explain the sinus tachycardia e.g., meningitis or encephalitis

☐ Presence of sinus arrhythmia (heart rate changes associated with breathing), though this may be blunted.

☐ Variability in heart rates depending on the autonomic tone (sleep, crying, carotid sinus massage, gag reflex)

☐ PR prolongation during tachycardia would go against sinus tachycardia as sympathetic stimulation should improve normal AV conduction leading to an appropriate PR shortening

☐ "Adenosine challenge": Sinus tachycardia would rarely show an AV block with adenosine while atrial tachycardias are likely to show a transient AV block. Furthermore the slowing/transient block would allow P wave morphology to be seen properly thus establishing its origin.

There are three basic determinants of an arrhythmia and more than one mechanism is often responsible. These determinants are the need for an arrhythmogenic substrate (e.g., presence of a accessory pathway for AVRT or dilated LA for an atrial fibrillation), the modulating factors (changes in the autonomic tone e.g., exercise may precipitate a ventricular tachycardia in congenital Long QT syndrome) and the occurrence of triggers that initiate the arrhythmia (e.g., an atrial premature beat is needed to set off an AVRT or a pulmonary vein ectopic to trigger atrial fibrillation). Traditionally tachycardias were called as PAT (paroxysmal atrial tachycardia), junctional and ventricular tachycardias. However, it is now well known that most of the so called junctional tachycardias are AV re-entrant or AV nodal re-entrant tachycardia and we now broadly group them under supraventricular (mostly narrow QRS) and ventricular (mostly wide QRS; however width of QRS is also dependent on the age and fascicular VT's have a relatively narrow QRS). A better method to classify them is based on the mechanism

of the tachycardia (Table 33.4). The three mechanisms that underlie an arrhythmia are re-entry, enhanced automaticity and triggered activity.

Table 33.4 Classification of tachyarrhythmias

Re-entrant

• AV Re-entrant tachycardias (AVRT)	(73.2%)
▪ Concealed bypass, WPW, PJRT, Mahaim fibers	
• AV nodal reentrant tachycardia (AVNRT)	(12.5%)
• Atrial flutter and IART	
• Atrial fibrillation	
• Ventricular tachycardias	
• Fascicular VT, postoperative VT's,? Torsades-de-pointes	

Enhanced automaticity

• Ectopic atrial tachycardias (EAT)	(14.3%)
• Chaotic atrial rhythm	
• Junctional ectopic tachycardias	
▪ Congenital	
▪ Postoperative	
• Ventricular tachycardias	
▪ Hamartomas, rhabdomyomas	
• Inappropriate sinus tachycardia	

Triggered activity

• RV outflow tachycardia
• Digoxin toxicity

WPW: Wolff-Parkinson-White syndrome, AV: Atrioventricular, PJRT: Permanent junctional reciprocating tachycardia, IART: Intra-atrial re-entrant tachycardia

Re-entrant tachycardias form the majority of tachycardias. A typical example is an accessory pathway mediated tachycardia or a typical atrial flutter. The onset, offset and mechanism of an AVRT is shown in Figure 33.2 A and B. An atrial ectopic gets blocked somewhere in the accessory pathway (longer effective refractory period) and renders it refractory for a short duration (200 to 300 msec). The impulse goes down the AV node-His bundle axis and reaches the accessory pathway from the ventricular end. This delay allows the pathway to recover its conduction and the impulse can now go retrograde into the atrium and reaches the AV node again, conducts orthodromically and sustains a "circus movement". In case the delay has been insufficient for the AV node/His bundle axis to recover conductivity then the impulse gives only one extra P wave and no QRS and therefore no tachycardia. This P wave because of the retrograde conduction through the pathway (or in typical AVNRT due to the fast pathway) is called an "echo beat". All re-entrant circuits therefore have to have a critical area of slow conduction that allows recovery of myocardial excitability to allow the circus movement to perpetuate.

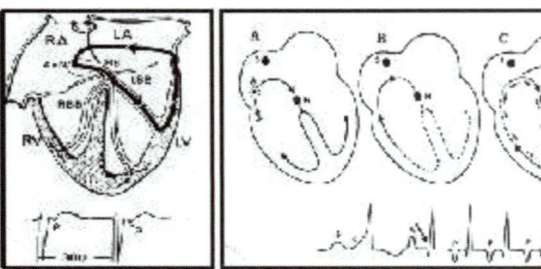

Figure 33.2A Depiction of an orthodromic AVRT. An atrial ectopic blocks in the accessory pathway because of its longer ERP and conducts antegradely via the AV node-His Pukinje axis, thus showing a normal QRS without preexcitation (A, arrow on ECG). The depolarization then reaches the ventricular end of the pathway and finds it excitable and conducts to the atrium (B). The P wave morphology depends on where the pathway is located. If the AV node has recovered by then it travels down again, thus leading to a tachycardia (C). The tachycardia circuit for a left sided pathway is shown in the left figure. If the AV node/HPS has not recovered then it leads to a single echo

An automatic tachycardia on the other hand is a focal area that starts firing at a rate that is more rapid than the normal rate. Automatic tachycardias are called as incessant when they occupy > 50% of the day and can lead to a "dilated cardiomyopathy", that is reversible, called as tachycardiomyopathy. Triggered activity is relatively uncommon and is a term used to describe impulse initiation in cardiac fibers due to the occurrence of after depolarizations. Electrophysiologically they are somewhat like an automatic focus but the focus can be triggered only if the ectopic falls after a critical time of the preceding P/QRS.

Etiology

1. Most supraventricular tachycardias have a structurally normal heart and are due to an accessory pathway or enhanced automaticity. Persistent arrhythmia may result in left ventricular dysfunction or a cardiomyopathy like picture.

2. Transient or permanent atrioventricular block, primary atrial tachycardia, atrial flutter, junctional ectopic tachycardia and ventricular tachycardia may sometimes occur after surgery.

3. Following 'atrial' surgery, bradycardia, primary atrial tachyarrhythmia may occur late after Fontan surgery, atrial switch operation, atrial septal defect closure etc.

4. Following 'ventricular' surgery, ventricular arrhythmias and sudden deaths are known to occur long after the surgical repair of tetralogy of Fallot, and double outlet right ventricle.

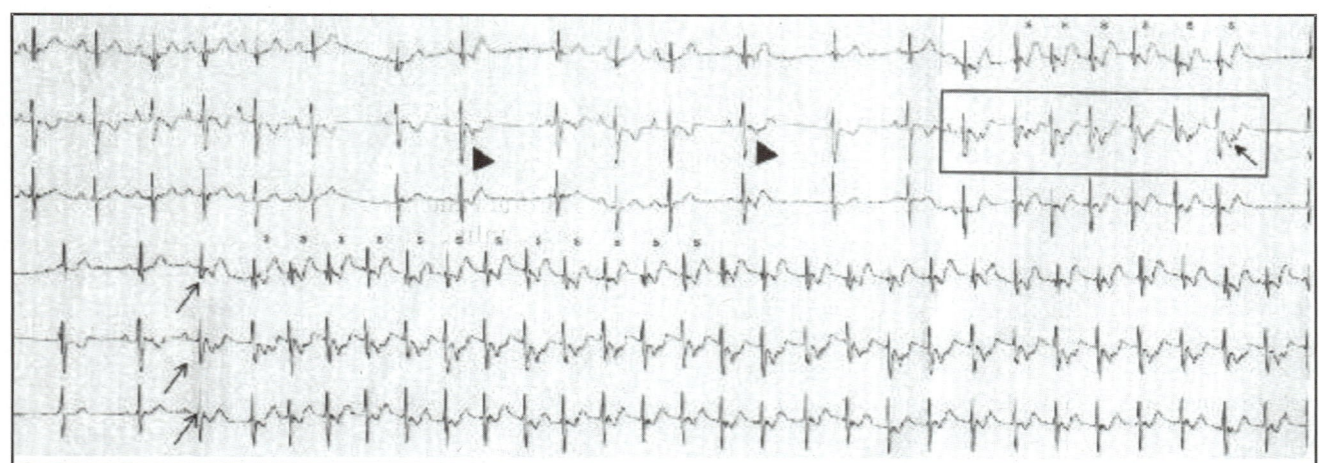

Figure 33.2B Single lead recording of a concealed pathway showing single echoes, a non sustained SVT (in the block) and more sustained SVT in the lower part. Arrowheads shows the echo beats and the thin arrow shows the tachycardia onset. Tachycardia terminates if it finds any structure refractory as seen in the part put in a block and the arrow shows a P and no subsequent QRS showing that the AV node was still refractory

5. Cardiomyopathies like dilated and hyper-trophied variants are associated with atrial and ventricular arrhythmias leading to sudden death at times.

6. Chronic valvular regurgitation/stenosis can result in atrial flutter or atrial fibrillation.

7. Cardiac tumors like rhabdomyoma (commonest cardiac tumor in children) can present with atrial/ventricular arrhythmias.

8. Maternal connective tissue disorders like systemic lupus erythematosus are well known to produce fetal complete heart block.

9. Acute metabolic and electrolyte derangements such as hyperkalemia, hypokalemia, hypothermia, myocardial ischemia, hypoxia, increased intracranial pressure may result in atrial and ventricular arrhythmias.

10. Drugs like digoxin, adrenergic agonists, anti-arrhythmics and drugs producing prolongation of QT interval can also cause arrhythmias (called as proarrhythmia).

Clinical Presentation and Diagnosis

Clinical symptomology depends on age of the child, underlying structural heart disease if any, duration of the tachycardia and parental education/awareness about the disease. Different modes of presentation depending upon the age of the child are summarized below:

Neonates and Infants

- Cardiovascular collapse
- Congestive heart failure
- Tachypnea
- Poor feeding, irritability, unusual behaviour or excessive crying, and listlessness
- Pallor, lethargy, and vomiting
- Syncope and rarely stroke
- Dilated cardiomyopathy (Tachycardiomyo-pathy)
- SIDS (sudden infant death syndrome)

Children over 2 years of age

- Palpitations, often perceived as chest pain by a child
- Pallor
- Syncope, sudden cardiac death, stroke

- Dilated cardiomyopathy (Tachycardiomyo-pathy)

History, Physical Examination and Clinical Course

Older children are more likely to give a history of palpitations while younger children may complain of chest discomfort, headache or stomach ache during an episode of paroxysmal tachycardia. Symptoms of dizziness, pre-syncope or syncope are more ominous and early work-up for arrhythmia is warranted. A detailed family history is also important as some of the arrhythmias may be familial and a family history of sudden death may be a pointer towards serious diseases like congenital LQTS, Brugada syndrome etc.

A careful physical examination should rule out any underlying structural heart disease. Often the examination will be normal, but if the child is seen during arrhythmia, abnormal heart rate and rhythm will be evident. When seen in the "interval period" the child would be absolutely normal; however a thorough clinical, radiographic, ECG, Holter and echocardiographic examination is a must if symptoms are suggestive, more so, if they have caused syncope.

Intraatrial re-entrant tachycardias (IART) and post operative atrial flutter may be detected incidentally on a routine ECG during follow-up. However, if it has been present for a long duration it would lead to ventricular dysfunction and congestive heart failure. IART is basically a re-entrant tachycardia around surgical incisions or scarred areas in the atrium. The scarred areas provide the slowing and also a barrier to the electrical impulse that promotes re-entry. The tachycardia is essentially a macro-reentrant flutter but differs from a usual typical flutter in terms of the circuit, presence of sizeable areas of scarred myocardium and having an isoelectric line between P waves unlike the saw-tooth pattern of a typical flutter.

SVTs are generally benign except for the symptoms that they produce. However, even orthodromic SVT in infants and children can occasionally be very rapid (ventricular rates of 250 to 300/min) and may lead to syncope and death. Antidromic tachycardia (orthodromic conduction through an accessory pathway that returns to the atrium via the AV node) can be associated with a very fast rate and lead to VF and death (Figure

33.3). Spontaneous atrial fibrillation is rare in children less than 10 years and therefore the risk of VF is predominantly due to degeneration of an orthodromic SVT into AF with rapid antidromic conduction (Figure 33.4) or due to antidromic conduction of an accessory pathway with a short refractory period. The other reasons that may lead to death in an SVT could be inappropriate use of drugs to manage and prevent SVT e.g., use of verapamil in a neonate with SVT could lead to cardiogenic shock; delay in management in a hemodynamically unstable child and fear of using DC cardioversion, dangerous proarrhythmias especially after intake of certain drugs that may potentiate 1:1 conduction from atrium to ventricle.

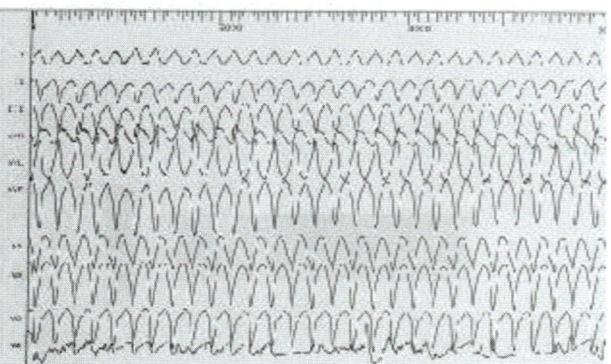

Figure 33.3 12 lead ECG showing a wide QRS tachycardia at a rate of 300/min (the scale on top is in msec and the RR duration is 200 msec giving a rate of 300/min, V6 has artifacts). The QRS is wide with a slow onset and appears like a ventricular tachycardia. The relatively slow onset and a QRS morphology not fitting into a typical LBBB suggests this to be either a VT or SVT with antidromic conduction. Differentiation between the two may be difficult in the absence of a previous ECG. Immediate DCCV should be done rather than waiting for the exact diagnosis – preexcitation would manifest itself once the tachycardia terminates

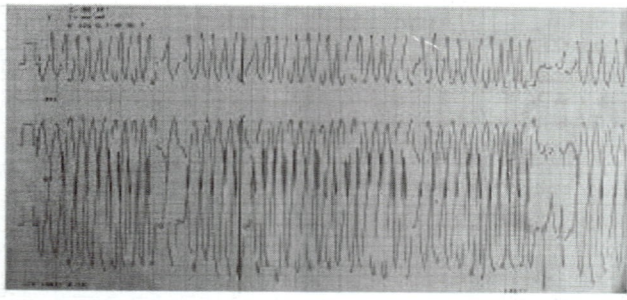

Figure 33.4 Simultaneous 3 channel recording of an irregularly irregular tachycardia with varying QRS morphology and two narrow QRS beats. The irregularity is diagnostic of AF and the varying degree of fusion suggests this to be an AF with antidromic conduction. The RR intervals are as short as 200 msec i.e., rate over 300/min. Arrhythmia may be associated with severe hypotension leading to sudden cardiac death if not treated immediately

ECG Abnormalities

In a child with tachycardia, it is imperative to get a 12 lead ECG (preferably a simultaneous 12 channel ECG) unless the child is in cardiogenic shock and the monitor shows the rhythm to be the cause for the collapse. It is rare to have a situation wherein a full ECG cannot be recorded. The 12 lead ECG is a must as it tells us about the mechanism of the tachycardia which is important not only in immediate management but is desirable in guiding future prophylactic therapy.

The first thing is to check the hemodynamic status for example blood pressure, evidences for congestive heart failure or shock and assess the respiratory status and overall condition of the child. If there is a previous ECG available it should be seen to check for manifest preexcitation. If the child is hemodynamically unstable, DC cardioversion should be done immediately. In a narrow QRS tachycardia one can give adenosine 0.2 mg/kg from a peripheral line while preparing for DC cardioversion. It is probably better to use a larger dose straightaway because of the need to be successful with the first dose itself as it saves time, and reduces the cost and unpleasant symptoms.

The ECG tells the clinician whether the tachycardia is associated with a narrow or wide QRS ; though the QRS width is dependent on the age, broadly a QRS > 120 msec is a wide QRS tachycardia. Some ventricular tachycardias can be narrow, arising typically from the left ventricle fascicles (called as fascicular VT) but have a typical morphology) (right bundle branch block with left axis deviation (Figure 33.5). An SVT can be broad because of several reasons listed below, though all these, especially aberrancy, is rare in children.

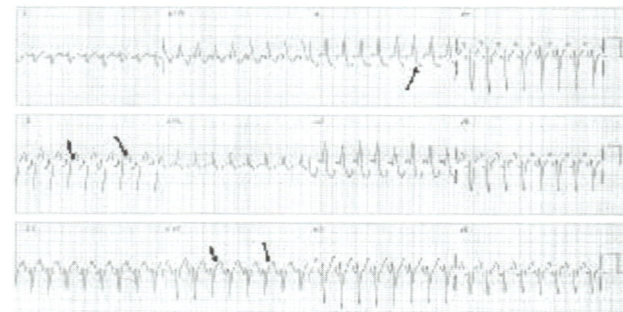

Figure 33.5 Idiopathic LVVT (fascicular VT); QRS is only 120 msec and has a typical morphology in the form of RBBB with left axis. The RBBB pattern suggests LV origin and the superior axis shows the origin to be from the inferior surface. The sharp onset is a pointer to the fascicular origin as opposed to myocardial origin wherein the QRS onset will be slow as ventricular myocardium conducts much slower than the fascicles. The VT will have a right axis if it arises from the anterior fascicle. The arrows show the P waves that are intermittent and not related to the QRS consistently i.e. VA dissociation, a hallmark of VT

1. Underlying conduction disorder e.g., post TOF repair is commonly associated with RBBB.

2. Antidromic tachycardia i.e., an SVT with antegrade conduction via the accessory pathway.

3. SVT over a Mahaim fiber

4. Aberrancy due to fast heart rate (uncommon in children)

When trying to interpret a tachycardia on ECG examination the most important point is to identify the P waves and their relationship to the QRS. Deciphering P wave may be difficult when it falls on the T wave or at the end of the QRS (Figures 33.6 and 33.7) wherein it may be seen as subtle notches on the T wave or a pseudo S/pseudo R waves. Subsequently we need to classify the tachycardia into a short RP i.e., from onset of QRS to the P wave (onset of P may not be apparent, so the P wave is taken wherever seen best, generally Lead II and V1 show the best P wave) or a long RP tachycardia. The common causes for a long RP tachycardia are an ectopic atrial tachycardia, permanent junctional reciprocating tachycardia (PJRT) and atypical AVNRT.

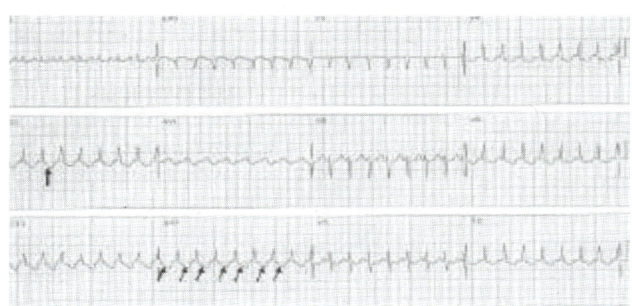

Figure 33.6 12 lead ECG of an AVRT at the rate of approximately 200 bpm. The arrows show the slight slur on the T wave that is the P wave. Note the consistent RP relationship and the RP interval is shorter the PR interval. P waves seen on the T waves are against a typical AVNRT and mostly due to an AVRT. Morphology of the P wave is difficult to make out and hence the location of the pathway cannot be judged in such an ECG

Children with structural heart disease especially Ebstein's anomaly may have multiple accessory pathways, and are predisposed to develop atrial flutter and fibrillation and also have a high propensity for developing ventricular tachyarrhythmias. Table 33.5 highlights ECG clues differentiating the 3 principle varieties of SVT (AVRT, EAT and AVNRT).

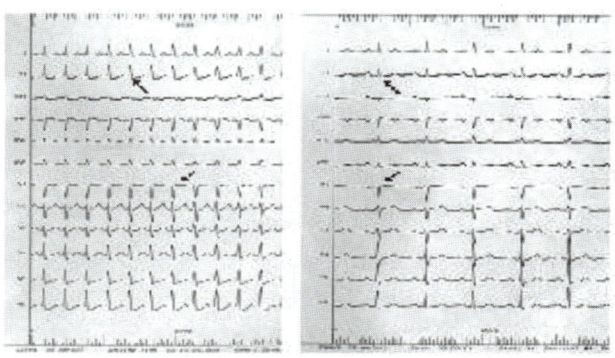

Figure 33.7 12 lead ECG (in stacked format) showing tachycardia on the left and normal sinus rhythm on the right. Arrows show the typical pseudo S and pseudo R because they are formed by the P waves and are not seen in the basal sinus ECG. This sign is > 95% specific for a typical slow fast AVNRT and is a retrograde P wave that is negative in the inferior leads as the atrial depolarization spreads upwards

Additional Investigations

The paroxysmal nature of most arrhythmias makes the diagnosis and management difficult in the absence of a documented ECG. Additional investigations may also be necessary in patients with complete heart block wherein high risk patients can be identified based on 24-48 hour recordings of ECG. Several investigations can therefore help in the diagnosis and planning management and are listed below.

Holter monitoring

Continuous ambulatory 24 to 48 hour ECG recordings with advanced diagnostic features are now available in most Holter recorders. Most Holters are nowadays capable of providing 12 lead recordings (the electrogram maybe somewhat different from the routine ECG as the electrode placement is different for Holter recordings), detecting pacemaker spikes, analyzing QT interval and providing measures of heart rate variability and more recently microvolt T wave alternans and heart rate turbulence. Heart rate variability is a useful tool for analyzing autonomic function and has been extensively used in adult patients for risk stratification for sudden cardiac death. Analysis of these recordings has to be done carefully as subtle findings can be overlooked and sometimes motion artifacts can be interpreted as polymorphic ventricular tachycardia. These recordings do not have a very high pick up rate as the event has to occur while the Holter recorder is on the patient. Holter monitors may be particularly useful in

Table 33.5 Broad clues to differentiate between three common causes of SVT

Features	AVRT	EAT	AVNRT
▪ Onset	Abrupt	Warm-up	Abrupt with PR prolongation
• Heart rate	180-250	120-220	180-250
• AV Block	Never	More than 2:1 is diagnostic	Transient at onset only
• QRS alternans	Likely	Rare	Occasionally at fast rate
• ST-T wave changes	>50%	Occasionally	<50%
• Rate variability	Minimal	May change with autonomic tone	minimal
• Offset	Abrupt; no P after QRS	May show gradual termination or with no P after QRS	Abrupt with a P and no QRS
• Baseline ECG	May show preexcitation	Normal	Normal

AVRT: AV re-entrant tachycardia, EAT: Ectopic atrial tachycardia, AVNRT: AV nodal re-entrant tachycardia

documenting slow heart rate events and in the assessment of asymptomatic bradycardia e.g. congenital complete heart block.

Echocardiography

Echocardiography has a limited role in the diagnosis and management of arrhythmias. It is very useful in the diagnosis of fetal arrhythmias, wherein the exact rhythm can be picked by examining the AV relationship. In children with supraventricular arrhythmias it is usually done to rule out structural heart defects like Ebstein's anomaly, hypertrophic or dilated cardiomyopathy. It can diagnose "tachycardiomyopathy" i.e., LV dysfunction because of incessant tachycardia but echo assessed ventricular function should be interpreted carefully if done during tachycardia. It is mandatory in all patients with ventricular tachycardia as these are often due to underlying structural heart defects.

Cardiac event recorders

Event recorders are more useful in capturing intermittent arrhythmia events. The availability of patient or parent activated recorders during symptomatic events and subsequent transtelephonic transmission has greatly improved the ability to document the etiology of cardiac symptoms. The limitation of an event recorder is the availability of only a single or two channels and the necessity for activation by parents, teachers, friends, etc., if the arrhythmia leads to a syncope without any premonition or occurs in a child too small to realise the abnormality. Most of these recorders capture a minute before the switch is put on and will continue to record for another 5 minutes (these durations are programmable as needed). If the child is

intelligent he/she can activate the recording at the onset of tachycardia that may be useful in the diagnosis. Implantable loop recorders are more sophisticated wherein a small device (REVEAL®, Medtronic Inc.) is implanted underneath the skin beneath the clavicle. These devices are capable of providing a record for 1-2 years and can be evaluated just like a pacemaker from outside. The high cost of these devices has limited its application in the developing countries.

Exercise testing

Some arrhythmias may be triggered by exercise e.g., catecholaminergic VT, Torsades-de-pointes in the setting of a congenital long QT syndrome and VT in patients with hypertrophic cardiomyopathy. Also the nature or extent of patient's bradycardia (secondary to sinus node incompetence or atrioventricular node disease) may be evaluated with graded exercise testing. Exercise testing can be easily performed on a treadmill in children more than 6 years old and is useful for diagnosis and also for assessing efficacy of a drug, e.g. adequate β-blockade, flecainide overdosage, etc.

Transesophageal atrial pacing and recording studies

Transesophageal pacing and recording is a useful relatively non-invasive method for evaluation of arrhythmias depending on the atrium for initiation or sustenance. The recording provides left atrial events and has been used for risk stratification in the presence of WPW syndrome. The procedure is done under sedation and the presence of a competent pediatrician/anesthetist as small children may not tolerate the pain associated with pacing. A routine soft bipolar/quadripolar catheter or specially designed transesophageal catheter may be used.

Intracardiac electrophysiological studies

In some cases where diagnosis is not clear by noninvasive testing, invasive electrophysiologic (EP) studies are necessary. EP study helps in checking sinus node function, atrioventricular conduction, presence of accessory pathways and the risk associated with them and also prior to radiofrequency ablation. These studies entail insertion of 3 to 4 catheters via the femoral vein/ internal jugular vein that are placed in the right atrium, beside the His bundle, into the right ventricle and in the coronary sinus in some patients. Stimulation techniques for inducing tachyarrhythmia (usually reentrant types are inducible), mapping for the site of the pathway or ectopic focus can all be combined in one session. These studies may at times be associated with serious complications like cardiac perforation and tamponade and therefore must be done under proper supervision in a center capable of handling such complications. The safety of these studies in infants and children is now well established and the threshold for performing such studies is now much lower than earlier.

MANAGEMENT

General Principles

The following general principles should be kept in mind when dealing with a possible arrhythmia in a child.

1. Symptoms of arrhythmia vary at different ages. The classical symptoms like palpitation, dizziness and syncope etc. may not be present in younger children. Some of the young children may complain of discomfort in the chest during episodes of tachycardia.

2. Diagnosis of specific arrhythmia cannot be based on history and examination alone. The arrhythmia must be documented on EKG before starting therapy.

3. Prompt work-up and treatment must be initiated for arrhythmias associated with dizziness or syncope, compromised cardiac function or in children involved in competitive sports.

4. Physical examination of children who have no underlying heart disease is likely to be normal in-between the episodes of arrhythmia.

5. If the patient presents with cardiogenic shock or loss of consciousness, check the rhythm. If there is tachycardia or rhythm is disorganised use of DC cardioversion is recommended, but if there is bradycardia or asystole, start cardiopulmonary resuscitation.

Emergency Management

The acute management of an SVT, once the diagnosis is established, would depend on underlying structural heart disease, preexcitation, age of the child, likely mechanism of tachycardia and the hemodynamic status. In a hemodynamically stable child with mild CHF, vagal maneuvers could be tried before pharmacologic therapy.

Vagal Maneuvers

- Pressure on infant's abdomen

- Carotid sinus massage or gagging

- Ocular pressure is contraindicated in infants and children less than 2 years and in general should be avoided in all children. It is usually ineffective in children < 5 years.

- Diving reflex: Icebag application on the face in infants

Icebag application if done properly has been shown in some studies to have a 90% efficacy rate[4]. A plastic bag of sufficient size to cover the entire face should be filled with ice cubes and water and applied on the child's face for 10 seconds. Inability to breathe for 10 seconds does not matter. It can be reapplied after a minute or so if the first application fails. After the procedure the infant's face should be wiped with warm water as cold panniculitis may occur. The traditional method of immersing the child's face into cold water should not be attempted and application of a cold wet towel to the face is not effective. Our own experience has not shown this technique to be very effective and is rather cumbersome.

Pharmacological Therapy

Adenosine

In general, intravenous adenosine is now considered as the treatment of choice for SVT because of its ultra-short duration of action and therefore a low incidence of complications. It has a 95% efficacy in re-entrant SVT's that is slightly higher than calcium channel blockers that are also

Section 4

effective in over 90% of cases. Adenosine, however, is atleast 10 times costlier than IV verapamil and diltiazem and therefore in the absence of specific situations (mentioned underneath), calcium channel blockers can be used as a cost-effective measure.

The specific indications for use of adenosine are listed below:

- Hemodynamic instability

- Child on oral β-blockers

- Undiagnosed wide QRS tachycardia

- Infants and children <2 years.

- To clarify the diagnosis/mechanism of tachycardia

The success rates in neonates may be lower, around 60%, than reported in older children and adults. PSVT recurrence up to 30% can be seen and frequent VPB's following termination may reinitiate the tachycardia[5]. Adenosine produces a very unpleasant feeling of impending doom and older children should be told about it before pushing in the drug. Serious adverse effects like apnea/bronchospasm, accelerated and prolonged ventricular rhythm, prolonged asystole, proadrenergic effect enhancing AV conduction and shortening of the ERP of the pathway leading to VF may occur accasionally. It is important that the drug is pushed as a bolus followed by administration of 5-10 ml of saline. Although a dose of 0.05mg/kg may be effective but most texts recommend using 0.1/mg/kg and escalating the dose if tachycardia is non responsive. We prefer to use a bolus dose of 0.2 mg/kg, that is more predictable and saves on the cost and unpleasantness of repeated administrations. Adenosine should be administered under ECG control as the mechanism of termination and its effect on AV blockade provides a useful aid to the diagnosis and the P waves seen in isolation (away from QRS and T waves) help in localizing the origin of dysrhythmia (Figure 33.8). The usual effect of adenosine is mediated through AV block and slowing of sinus followed by sinus tachycardia because of sympathetic stimulation. In an emergency when no IV line is available the drug can be given intraosseus[6]. Figure 33.9 shows an algorithm for termination of SVT after administration of IV adenosine.

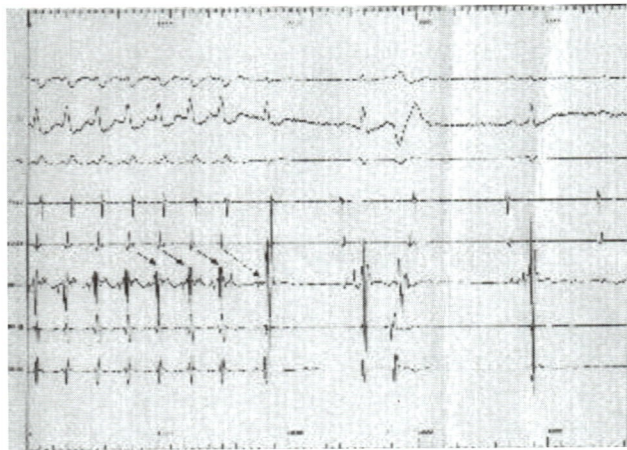

Figure 33.8 Intracardiac recording showing termination of an SVT with Intravenous adenosine. The top 3 channels are surface ECG recordings followed by 2 channels showing intracardiac recordings of right atrium, followed by His Bundle and the last two right venticular recordings 1:1 AV conduction is seen in the first 7 beats followed by abrupt AV prolongation/non conduction (dashed arrow) and termination of tachycardia. Tachycardia termination is followed by a VPB that may reinitiate tachycardia

Verapamil/Diltiazem

Verapamil/diltiazem has more than >90% efficacy rate in terminating a routine re-entrant SVT i.e., AVNRT and AVRT. The drug should be given slowly unlike adenosine because a rapid intravenous push can lead to unstable hemodynamics. It is contraindicated in infants (<2 years of age), presence of CHF/prolonged tachycardia, manifest preexcitation and previous β-blocker therapy. It may be useful when tachycardia is reinitiating after adenosine and in stable patients, because it is far cheaper and cost-effective.

Digoxin

Digoxin has practically no role at present in the acute treatment of an SVT. Its onset of action is slow and efficacy is low (50-90%) and it can lead to serious ventricular arrhythmias when used before DC cardioversion, and in cases of manifest preexcitation. It may be useful in patients with resistant supraventricular tachycardias especially in the postoperative setting wherein an intraatrial re-entrant tachycardia with 1:1 conduction could lead to serious hemodynamic consequences. Another situation wherein it may be useful (often in combination with other drugs) is when there is ventricular dysfunction due to or in association with

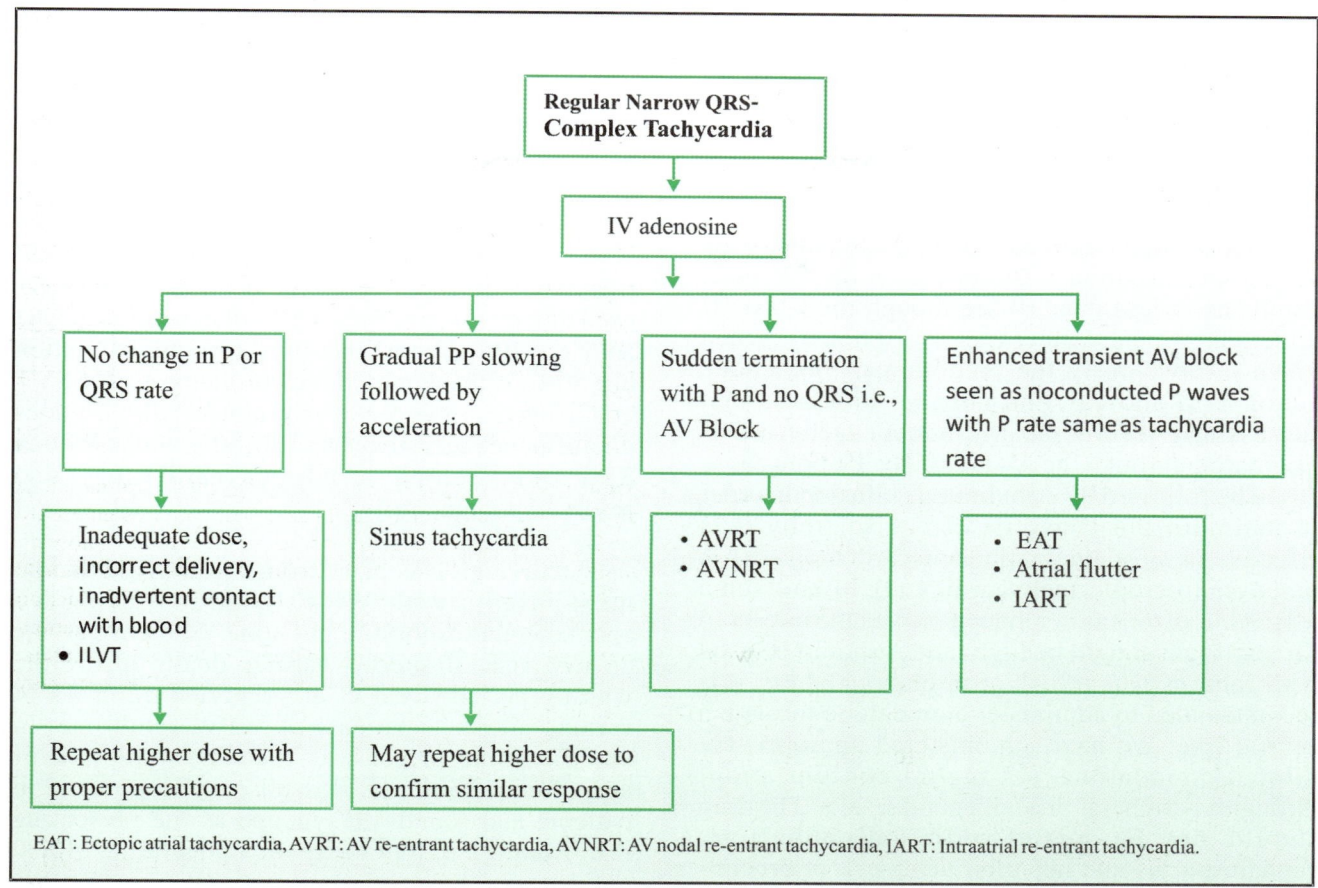

EAT : Ectopic atrial tachycardia, AVRT: AV re-entrant tachycardia, AVNRT: AV nodal re-entrant tachycardia, IART: Intraatrial re-entrant tachycardia.

Figure 33.9 Algorithm showing response to IV adenosine for termination of various supraventricular arrhythmias

tachycardia. Its utility is predominantly due to its AV nodal blocking properties that lead to slowing of the ventricular rate. Intravenous rapid digitalization should be avoided and the drug should be started in maintenace oral doses.

Overdrive Pacing

Overdrive pacing, i.e., pacing at a rate faster than the tachycardia from the atrium or ventricle is highly effective in terminating re-entrant tachycardias. Overdrive pacing can be done by placing a pacing catheter either in the esophagus or by the transvenous route in the atrium or the ventricle. It acts by rendering tissue ahead of the tachycardia refractory, thus stopping the circus movement responsible for the tachycardia.

Some studies have shown transesophageal electrophysiological studies to be highly accurate means of diagnosing and characterizing various mechanisms of supraventricular tachycardia in pediatric patients[7]. Transvenous pacing may be used alternatively through the femoral vein. This route becomes necessary in patients with atrial flutter

that is often resistant to pharmacological therapy and is treated preferably by DC shock. Pacing is done slightly faster than the atrial/ventricular rate that stops the tachycardia either by blocking the reentry or depolarizes a critical area of the circuit ahead of the wavefront.

DC Cardioversion

DC cardioversion is the treatment of choice for all hemodynamically unstable arrhythmias and for other SVT's not responding to all other techniques/medications. Cardioversion facilities should be available wherever medical termination is being attempted because of the rare occurrence of ventricular fibrillation due to enhanced conduction over the accessory pathway. Biphasic shock is now considered more efficacious and needs less energy for cardioversion. The largest size paddles that can be accommodated should be used. Most SVT's and atrial flutter will respond to as low as 0.25 to 0.5 Joules/kg whereas chronic atrial fibrillation may need 1 to 4 Joules/kg. Adequate sedation should be ensured during the shock to minimize pain and optimal skin-paddle contact with adequate jelly to avoid skin burns. Most tachycardias will respond to DC version though automatic foci may be unresponsive in over 50-70% or recur immediately after converting.

Amiodarone

Intravenous amiodarone is useful in a wide variety of arrhythmias. Its effect on the AV node manifests in less than 10 sec though the Class III effect takes much longer (nearly 10 hours). When given intravenously the predominant immediate action is β and calcium channel blockade that successfully reverts most re-entrant tachycardias originating through the AV node. The IV bolus dose has to be followed by a continuous infusion in order to maintain the Class III effect whereby it is effective in most automatic tachycardias like EAT, junctional ectopic tachycardias (JET) and some VTs. Amiodarone is not innocuous and the threshold for starting it should be high; and it should be used with caution. Due to risk of thrombophlebitis, it is recommended to administer amiodarone through a central line. We have administered appropriately diluted amiodarone (<2 mg/ml concentration) through a peripheral line with good results. The drug should not be mixed with aminophylline, cephalosporins and heparin due to risk of precipitation. The other side effects include hypotension, Torsades-de-pointes, ventricular tachycardia, bradycardia, congestive heart failure, fulminant hepatitis and ARDS[8].

Prophylaxis for SVT

The following factors should be taken into consideration for prophylaxis of SVT:

- Type of tachycardia e.g., EAT, AVRT etc.
- Risk of AF and fast response that could be fatal
  - Maximum risk of mortality in patients of WPW between 8-20 years age group
  - Digoxin use in WPW is controversial and should be avoided in children above 8 years.
  - AVNRT/concealed bypass tracts
- Syncope or hemodynamic collapse necessitates aggressive therapy
- Underlying heart disease
- Lack of access to medical care
- Frequency and severity of symptoms
- Parental education, their availability at home and ability to pick up an SVT
- Participation in competitive sports

Natural History of SVT in Infancy

Recurrence of SVT is influenced by the age at presentation. About 40-70% infants do not need treatment after stoppage of medications at one year, even though many of these will still have an inducible SVT on EPS. Almost one-third lose pre-excitation but 30% of these may develop recurrence of SVT at 8-10 years of age[9]. Structural heart disease does not influence recurrence and 20-50% of uncommon SVT's i.e., ectopic atrial tachycardia may also resolve spontaneously[10].

Although it is clear from the above data that most infants with WPW syndrome can have spontaneous resolution, but some of them may be at high risk of sudden cardiac death during the waiting period. Deal et al[11] reported 42 cases of cardiac arrest in patients of WPW syndrome. In 48%, cardiac arrest was the first symptom of arrhythmia. Similarly, Russell et al[12] reported 256 patients and found VF/syncope as the presenting manifestation in four cases. In a population of 690 patients with Wolff-Parkinson-White (WPW) syndrome referred to a tertiary care center, 15 patients (2.2%) had an aborted sudden death episode before reporting to the hospital. VF was the first manifestation of the WPW syndrome in 8 patients and was significantly more frequent in males. Ten of the 15 patients were either doing vigorous exercise or were under emotional stress at the time of aborted sudden cardiac death[13]. In children and adolescents, SCD as the first manifestation is more common than in adults. How to stratify the risk of SCD in these children remains an enigma and even though Pappone et al[14] have proposed newer guidelines, their data are not in agreement with previously published observations.

Choice of Drugs

Choice of drugs for SVT prophylaxis would depend on the mechanism of tachycardia, age of the child, associated structural heart disease/left ventricular function and familiarity with the drug. In general, amiodarone should not be the first line therapy in children because of the high incidence of organ toxicity with prolonged and continuous administration. Thus in most settings radiofrequency ablation would be preferred over amiodarone. Infants and smaller children (less than 15 kg) who are resistant to all other drugs or having severe left ventricular dysfunction, short term administration of amiodarone (1 to 2 years) can be tried till the child can be safely taken up for radiofrequency ablation.

Digoxin

Traditionally, digoxin has been used as the drug of first choice in prevention of recurrent SVT. In view of its property of enhancing AV conduction through the accessory pathway, some authors believe that digoxin can increase the risk of SCD and should not be used. This is predominantly based on data from Deal et al[15] and some anecdotal reports of occurence of VF in children with WPW syndrome on digoxin therapy[16]. However, no cause and effect was established directly by digoxin levels, and a majority of pediatric electrophysiologists continue to use digoxin as the first line drug with reasonable success rates[17].

Digoxin toxicity remains an important concern even though infants and children usually tolerate higher doses. A simple method of administering oral digoxin is to add a decimal before the body weight e.g. 8 kg child can take 0.8 ml BD as 10 mg/kg/day equals 80 mg/day and that translates to 1.6 ml/day. We prefer to keep the dose between 5.0 to 7.5mg/kg in older children and when simultaneously using other antiarrhythmics (even β-blockers) usually administer digoxin 6 days in a week. Children mostly present with blocks and bradycardia rather than tachyarrhythmias and practically any arrhythmia can be seen due to digoxin toxicity. Extracardiac manifestations like nausea, vomiting, and drowsiness are important clues for early manifestation of digoxin toxicity.

β-Blockers

β-blockers are useful and safe for prophylaxis of SVT. Though most people have a tendency to use propranolol because of the multiple strengths available, but the frequency of administration, (3 times a day) makes it cumbersome. Metoprolol and atenolol are easier to give but efficacy rates are not known[18]. In general their efficacy rate is close to 60-70% and they can be safely combined with digoxin. *They should not be combined with calcium channel blockers and IV calcium channel blockers should never be given to children on β-blockers*

Class I and III Drugs

Flecainide (Class Ic) is highly effective in the prophylaxis of most supraventricular tachycardias while propafenone (another class Ic agent) has been found to be particularly more useful for treatment of automatic atrial and junctional ectopic tachycardias. Sotalol (class III) is useful for prophylaxis of atrial flutter, postoperative intraatrial re-entrant tachycardias and ventricular tachycardia but has a 2-4% incidence of Torsades-de-pointes (Tdp) even in normal hearts. These drugs are best given by electrophysiologists familiar with their usage because of the small but definite risk of proarrhythmias[19].

Pediatricians should be familiar with the effects of these drugs so that they can monitor for any complications. Any syncope or unusual behaviour like a change in the eating habits of the child in terms of dairy products should be monitored closely. QRS width or a new onset bundle branch block/hemiblock should be watched for when treating with class Ic agents and QT monitoring for children on class III agents. All these drugs have to be used with utmost caution in children with structural heart disease especially in the presence of hypoxia, ischemia and heart failure.

Amiodarone

The safety and efficacy of amiodarone in the treatment of neonates, infants and children is well established. Most physicians are well aware of its chronic toxicity to the liver, eyes, lungs and hematological system. But its more dangerous and fatal acute hepatic and pulmonary toxicity is not well appreciated. There is a false sense of security in the minds of most cardiologists and the drug is considerably overused in India, where it is often used as a first line drug for treatment of arrhythmias that can be easily controlled with safer drugs.

Nevertheless, it is one of the most versatile antiarrhythmics that can be used intravenously to terminate life-threatening acute arrhythmias and prevent a variety of atrial/junctional and ventricular arrhythmias, whether they are re-entrant or ectopic. When given intravenously in patients with poor left ventricular function, chances of hemodynamic compensation do exist as it has a significant β and calcium channel blocking effect.

Radiofrequency Ablation

Radiofrequency ablation (RFA) has revolutionized the treatment of various arrhythmias during the past 15 years. The concept behind RFA is to do an electrophysiological study, identify the arrhythmic substrate (may be an accessory pathway, ectopic focus or a re-entrant circuit), place a catheter capable of delivering RF energy at the identified site and deliver RF energy at the precise site. The RF energy heats up the tissue in the vicinity of the RF electrode to the preset temperature (55°C to 60°C) and burns irreversibly a small part of the myocardium, whose depth varies with the type of RF electrode. Thus conduction in an accessory pathway can be destroyed by a single burn while in a re-entrant circuit like atrial flutter, multiple burns are required to interrupt the circuit. The procedure has gained widespread acceptance because of its curative nature and is used for all varieties of SVT, atrial flutter and post operative tachycardias, including some forms of ventricular tachycardia and atrial fibrillation. Several advanced mapping tools that give a 3-dimensional picture of the heart (CARTO, ENSITE, CARDIAC PATHWAYS etc) are now available and are very useful for ablation of complex arrhythmias. The high cost of the equipment and the catheters prevents its widespread use in the developing world.

In the pediatric population there were initial reservations about possibility of recurrence of the lesions treated by RF energy. Over the last decade, experience in infant and pediatric population has increased substantially with success and complication rates similar to adult patients. Thus keeping in mind the natural regression of accessory pathways and ectopic foci in a substantial number, indications for RFA have become more liberal in the western world. Our approach has been to try and manage most infants and children less than 4-5 years with drugs unless symptoms are refractory to medications. Several factors govern our policy regarding RFA and some of these are listed in Table 33.6. Table 33.7 gives possible management options for chronic prophylaxis of SVT.

PRIMARY ATRIAL TACHYCARDIAS

These tachycardias are relatively uncommon and can occur even in the presence of AV block because they do not need the ventricle for sustainance.

Table 33.6 Factors that may govern the choice of RFA in our country

- Drug refractory SVT, safety and cost of using multiple antiarrhythmics or amiodarone on a long term basis

- Patient (Parent's) choice

- Risk stratification of SCD in WPW syndrome

- Lack of antiarrhythmic drugs like flecainide, sotalol etc.

- Social factors: Patients from remote areas and illiteracy complicates drug administration/decision for RFA

- Increased risk associated with cardiac anatomy, arrhythmia substrate, patient size, and physician variables etc.

- Threat of coronary damage is real and temptation to ablate annular structures needs restraint

- ECG localization /mechanism often guide the selection of procedure

- Tachycardiomyopathy

- Risk of long fluoroscopy times

Table 33.7 Management options for long-term prophylaxis of SVT

- No treatment

- Pill in the pocket: Treat the episode with oral medications. Combination of propranolol (80 mg) with diltiazem (120 mg) is found to be highly effective in terminating an SVT in an adult population with infrequent episodes. However, these results cannot be extrapolated to children in whom no such data is available (Alboni)

- Drugs

  - Digoxin and propranolol : 70% efficacy in AVRT and AVNRT

  - Flecainide/Propafenone/Sotalol (effective, not easily available, risk of proarrhythmias)

  - Verapamil ? – use only in children over 2-3 years.

  - Amiodarone: Toxicity and efficacy need to be balanced in every case

  - Class IA: Procainamide and disopyramide are rarely used now

- RF Ablation

  - Tachycardia mechanism, frequency, pathway location and likely risk of complications like AV nodal block, embolism, etc.

  - Age and weight of the child

  - Experience of electrophysiologist

  - Availabilty of proper hardware for children

Atrial Flutter

It is a re-entrant tachycardia and usually occurs in the presence of structural heart disease in an older child. It rarely, however, occurs in the presence of normal heart, especially in fetal life and at birth[20]. The re-entrant circuit is usually confined to the right atrium wherein the circuit goes around the tricuspid annulus.

Atrial flutter occurring several years after any surgery involving atrial resection like Senning, Mustard, Fontan or atrial septal defect closure is termed as "intraatrial re-entrant tachycardia", as discussed earlier. In our country, atrial flutter is sometimes seen in children with chronic rheumatic valvular lesions. Onset of atrial flutter in children with underlying heart disease results in deterioration of their hemodynamic status.

The electrocardiogram shows dot regular, fast flutter waves (saw-tooth like P waves) at a rate of 250-350 per minute often with a fixed AV block (2:1 or 4:1) leading to a slower ventricular rate. A ventricular rate of 150/min with the P wave falling right in the middle of the 2 QRS complexes should arouse suspicion of a flutter.

Treatment

Atrial flutter is not easily amenable to drug therapy and therefore transesophageal pacing or DC cardioversion may be necessary. This is often the case in neonates in view of their hemodynamic instability, wherein once terminated it usually doesn't recur. In older children, after conversion to sinus rhythm, long-term drug therapy is needed that is best given by electrophysiologists. In case sinus rhythm is not achieved, rate control should be the goal by increasing AV block, using drugs like digoxin, calcium channel blockers and β-blockers. Radiofrequency ablation is a useful therapeutic modality and is often used as first line treatment especially in cavotricuspid isthmus-dependent flutters.

Atrial Fibrillation

Atrial fibrillation almost always occurs in the presence of structural heart disease, chronic rheumatic valvular lesion being the commonest cause in India. Other causes are the same as for atrial flutter. This arrhythmia is characterized by an extremely fast atrial rate (350-600 per minute) with an irregularly irregular ventricular response.

These fine fibrillatory waves are best seen in precordial leads V4R, V1 and V2.

Treatment

Atrial fibrillation (or flutter) may be associated with atrial thrombus due to relative stagnation of blood in the low pressure atria. Oral anticoagulants for 3-4 weeks are recommended before giving anti-arrhythmic agent or DC cardioversion to achieve sinus rhythm. Recurrences are, however, common and hence chronic therapy for control of ventricular response rate with digoxin, propranolol or calcium channel blockers is necessary. Class Ic and class III drugs are useful drugs to prevent recurrences but should only be used under the supervision of a cardiac electrophysiologist. More recently paroxysmal and persistent atrial fibrillation is increasingly being ablated in the adult patient; this cannot become a practise in the pediatric population due to its complexity and risk of complications.

Chaotic Atrial Rhythm

Previously called as multifocal atrial tachycardia (MAT), a term which should be best avoided as one cannot definitely say that there are multiple foci responsible for the abnormality. A relatively uncommon arrhythmia (0.2% of all pediatric cardiac arrhythmias), it is seen in early childhood (mostly <3 years of age). It generally has a benign course and may be seen in children with cardiomyopathy. Unlike adults this arrhythmia is not associated with hypoxia or respiratory disease. The ECG shows an atrial rate of 250 to 700 bpm, irregular rhythm with > 3 morphologies of P wave and varying PP, PR and RR intervals. There is no dominant atrial rhythm and unlike atrial flutter there is an isoelectric baseline between the P waves. It differs from atrial fibrillation as distinct P waves are visible unlike fibrillatory waves. The tachycardia is often refractory to medical treatment but can be ablated when incessant and refractory to drugs.

VENTRICULAR TACHYCARDIA

Ventricular tachycardia (VT) is rare in children when compared to SVT. It classically presents as a wide QRS tachycardia. However, in infants the widening of QRS is very subtle and may be missed. The presence of AV dissociation in the presence of fast heart rate is diagnostic of VT (atrial activity may be discernible on the ECG by small P waves having no correlation to the QRS). A sustained VT can rapidly result in hemodynamic compromise and ventricular fibrillation. Ventricular tachycardia can be either due to primarily an electrical disorder (now called as channelopathy) or due to a structural heart defect.

The common causes of VT are listed below:

1. Myocarditis, myocardial injury, or ischemia.

2. Arrhythmogenic right ventricular dysplasia in which myocardial thining occurs with replacement by fibrous tissue and fat. Typically RV is involved and the VT is generally monomorphic with a propensity for ventricular fibrillation and SCD. MRI is very useful for the diagnosis and the VT is typically a LBBB with left axis.

3. Cardiac tumors like rhabdomyomas, myocardial hamartomas (Purkinje cell tumors) and histiocytic tumors. Most of these occur in infants and nearly 10% cases of VT in children are due to rhabdomyomas or tuberous sclerosis.

4. Postoperative settings e.g., after TOF repair wherein wide QRS has been found to be an important marker for VT.

5. Cardiomyopathies both dilated and hypertrophied types and in non-compaction of left ventricle, a rare anomaly wherein the ventricular myocardium fails to get compacted.

6. Primary electrical disorders like long QT in the ECG. It may be a congenital abnormality or induced due to certain drugs, resulting in recurrent ventricular tachycardia particularly of Torsades-de-pointes type. This is a specific form of VT in which wide undulating QRS wave form appears to spiral around a single point and the QRS keeps changing its axis (Figure 33.10).

7. Drug toxicity e.g. digitalis, catecholamines, and theophyllines etc.

8. Brugada syndrome is a relatively new concept wherein polymorphic VT or VF occurs and a sinus rhythm shows incomplete RBBB alongwith ST elevation in V1-3.

9. Idiopathic (Fascicular VT) and right ventricular outflow tachycardia is the most typical VPC arising from the RVOT and is easily recognised in the ECG by an LBBB morphology with inferior axis. This VT is typically responsive to adenosine and β-blockers. Sustained VTs are generally fascicular VTs that arise form the left posterior fascicle and have a typical morphology of a

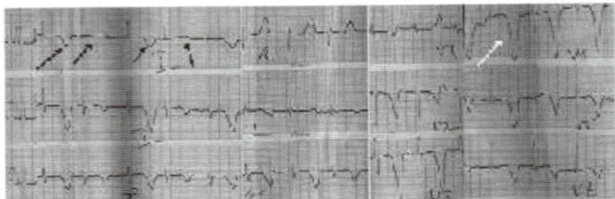

Figure 33.10 12 Lead ECG of a 7 year old child with congenital long QT syndrome. Note that apart from the QTc that is prolonged, the bizzare T waves (white arrow) are also a useful clue to the syndrome. Black arrows show the T wave alternans seen in Leads I and II, that is an important prognostic marker for SCD

relatively narrow QRS (100 msec) with a RBBB pattern and left axis. This is typically a verapamil sensitive VT and is the only wide QRS tachycardia wherein calcium channel blockers can be used.

10. Catecholaminergic VT is typically triggered by sympathetic discharge and is a bidirectional VT.

11. Short QT syndrome is a recently proposed entity wherein a QTc less than 300 msec has been associated with sudden cardiac death and inducible ventricular fibrillation[21].

Treatment[22]

In case patient is unconscious or is hemodynamically unstable, VT must be treated rapidly with synchronized DC cardioversion (1.0 joules/kg). In a relatively stable patient, drugs like lidocaine (1.0 mg/kg/dose over 1-2 minute) may be given followed by lidocaine infusion. Bretylium tosylate is an antifibrillatory drug that may be used in case of recurrence after VF or hemodynamically unstable VT. This drug is extremely expensive and is not easily available in India. One should also look for any cause for VT which can be reversed, like hypokalemia and hypoxia. For emergency treatment of Torsades-de-pointes, an infusion of isoproterenol or infusion of magnesium sulphate is very useful. In selected cases with recurrent VT, an implantable cardiovertor/defibrillator (ICD) may be useful. The ICD is a metallic device quite similar to a pacemaker except that it is more bulky and has thick leads with multiple coils. The device has an algorithm to detect ventricular tachycardia and ventricular fibrillation and treat it with antitachycardia pacing or internal cardioversion/defibrillation as deemed necessary. The device is implanted like a pacemaker and has a battery life of 6-8 years costing from Rs 2–7 lakhs (depending upon its features). Indications for its implantation are expanding rapidly as the device improves survival in many disorders that lead to sudden cardiac death.

Ventricular Fibrillation

This terminal lethal arrhythmia is characterized by bizarre QRS complexes of varying sizes and configurations with a rapid irregular rate. It is always associated with hemodynamic collapse and leads to death if not terminated within 4 minutes (preferably within the first minute). It is the terminal event due to a wide variety of causes and is better termed as a mode of death (like cardiac arrest) rather than a ventricular tachyarrhythmia. Treatment must be immediately instituted with electric cardioversion. Intravenous amiodarone should also be used if VF recurs after cardioversion or is resistant to cardioversion.

Premature Beats

Premature or ectopic atrial and ventricular beats are common in children and are mostly benign when the underlying heart is normal[23]. Incidence of premature atrial beats is as high as 50% in infants and children. Most of these children are asymptomatic and the abnormality is discovered incidentally. Premature ventricular contractions may sometimes be seen in children with structural heart disease like postoperative congenital heart disease and cardiomyopathy. When seen in structural heart disease and especially when it occurs in couplets, triplets or non sustained VT, it signifies a poor long term outcome. No specific treatment is required for isolated premature contractions with structurally normal heart.

Channelopathies

Ion channels are a diverse group of pore-forming proteins that cross the lipid membrane of cells and selectively conductions across this barrier. Ionic movement across cell membranes is critical for several essential physiological processes. Electrochemical gradients across cell membranes can either depolarize cells, by moving positively charged ions in, or repolarize cells, by moving positively charged ions out. These channels thus coordinate electrical signals in diverse tissues that are responsible for every heartbeat, every movement, our thoughts and perceptions, regulation of insulin secretion by pancreatic β-cells, to name a few. Diseases caused by disturbed function of ion channel subunits or the proteins that regulate them are now grouped under channelopathies. These

diseases may be either congenital (mostly passed down by parents and occasionally resulting from a mutation in the encoding genes) or acquired. Cardiac diseases falling into this group were earlier referred to as primary electrical disorders, as these hearts were structurally normal macroscopically. Two of the most important diseases in this category are the Long QT syndrome and Brugada syndrome, that are discussed below.

Long QT Syndrome

Long QT syndrome deserves special mention as it is an important cause of syncope and sudden death in children, adolescents and possibly "crib deaths". It often masquerades as seizures as the child during the polymorphic VT that gets prolonged may get a seizure and present to a neurologist who may not entertain this diagnosis. It is a highly underdiagnosed entity in our country largely because of lack of awareness amongst pediatricians and physicians. A typical presentation in a child is of getting unconscious whenever there is intense sympathetic stimulation (one of our patient used to faint whenever she would be attending a marriage ceremony and the band would suddenly play loud music !) and of having an unexplained death in the family. Such a patient is often found to be on antiepileptic and continue to have episodic fainting attacks despite adequate therapy. A scoring system widely used for the diagnosis of LQTS is shown in Table 33.8.

Table 33.8 Diagnostic criteria for long QT[24]	
ECG	**Score**
QTc > 480 msec	3
450-470 msec	2
< 450 msec (males)	1
Documented Torsades-de-pointes	2
T wave alternans	1
Notched T waves in > 3 leads	1
Low heart rate for age	0.5
Family history	
Definite LQTS	1
Unexplained SCD under age 30	0.5
Syncope	
With stress	2
Without stress	1
Congenital deafness	0.5
High probability of LQT when score is > 4, intermediate 2-3 score and low probability when score is < 1.	

An important point that needs to be understood is that QT may not be always increased and therefore a single ECG showing normal QT does not exclude the possibility of LQTS. Highest risk of death due to LQT is seen in patients with QTc >500 msec, LQT 1 and 2, and males with LQT3. The type of LQT to some extent can be found from the ECG but ultimately genotyping is essential, that is not possible even in most of the developed world. Management of long QT syndrome entails measures to prevent the adrenergic surge by drugs like β-blockers or left cervical sympathetic denervation. Permanent pacing is often resorted to in order to allow high doses of β-blockers and in cases at a very high risk for SCD when an ICD implantation is necessary. Several drugs can potentiate the QT prone patient and unravel LQT or even lead to Torsades-de-pointes. A list of commonly used drugs that can lead to overt LQT is given in Table 33.9.

Table 33.9 Mdications which are dangerous in LQTS
• Phenothiazines
• Macrolides
• Antifungals (ketoconazole)
• Antihistamines
• Other drugs
▪ Cisapride, chloroquine, quinidine, serteraline, sparfloxacin,
• Drugs that may potentiate LQT by drug interaction
▪ Carbamazepine, imipramine, thioridazine, sotolol, amiodarone, cimetidine, diltiazem, metoprolol, nifedipine, phenytoin, verapamil, and warfarin etc.

Brugada Syndrome

Brugada syndrome is a genetic disorder associated with sudden death due to ventricular fibrillation (VF) occurring in patients with a structurally normal heart and a resting ECG showing right bundle branch block with a typical ST elevation in anterior precordial leads V1-V3 (Figure 33.11). The disease is inherited in an autosomal dominant fashion and is more common in young males especially of Asian descent. Abnormal function of either sodium (commonly SCN5A) or calcium channels leads to a transmural and epicardial dispersion of repolarization that precipitates malignant ventricular tachyarrhythmias. The ECG changes may not be present all the time but can manifest during fever or vagal stimulation or be triggered by sodium channel blockers like flecainide and ajmaline. Currently no pharmacologic treatment

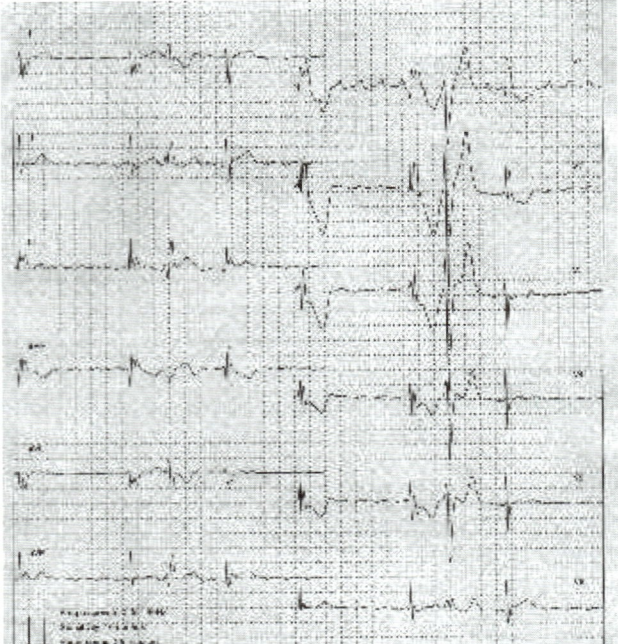

Figure 33.11. 12-lead Holter record showing the Brugada pattern in Lead VI. Baseline rhythm is atrial flutter. The beat following the long pause (arrow) shows an incomplete RBBB pattern with a down sloping elevated ST segment and a negative T wave. A shart coupled VPB follows this beat landing just at the end of T wave. The next beat shows the fused QRS and ST segment, masking the ST elevation

can reliably prevent VF and ICDs are the only option for these patients. The disease is also seen in children and can be very difficult to manage at times as reported by us following ASD closure.[25]

BRADYARRHYTHMIAS

Sick sinus syndrome (SSS) is the inability of the sinus node to generate adequate impulses consistently and is manifest by the absence of regular P waves on the ECG. SSS is an uncommon cause of bradycardia in infants and children compared to atrioventricular blocks that are discussed below.

Atrioventricular Block

A disorder of conduction of impulse from sinus node to ventricles is due to AV block which has been classified according to the severity of conduction abnormality. In mild cases, only prolongation of PR interval occurs (first degree AV block), in more severe cases, some of atrial impulses are not conducted into the ventricles (second degree AV block) and in most severe cases, none of the atrial impulses are conducted to the ventricles (complete AV block).

First Degree AV Block

Prolongation of PR interval occurs due to delay in conduction within atrium, AV node or His-Purkinje system. The common causes of first degree AV block include congenital heart disease like atrial septal defect, Ebstein's anomaly, acute rheumatic fever (functional block), hyperkalemia, hypokalemia, and digoxin effect. It can also occur as a normal finding in some children. Generally no treatment is required for this condition.

Second Degree AV Block

This is subdivided into two types, Mobitz type I and II.

Mobitz Type I. This is also called Wenckebach AV block. The PR interval in the ECG gets progressively prolonged until one QRS complex is dropped completely. The R-R intervals get shortened progressively. This type of block is sometimes seen in otherwise healthy children (during sleep) and at times with myocarditis, cardiomyopathy, cardiac surgery and digoxin toxicity. Treatment is directed at the underlying cause.

Mobitz Type II. This is a more advanced block wherein the AV conduction is all or none. This type of block is generally considered to be below the Bundle of His and can sometimes progress to complete heart block. The diagnosis is made when there is no change in the RR/PR intervals before a dropped QRS. The causes are the same as for Mobitz type I, except, it is not seen in normal healthy children. Treatment includes insertion of a permanent pacemaker, in the absence of a transient reversible cause like hyperkalemia, and severe hypoxia. A 2:1 AV block may be a difficult problem to diagnose as it could be either Mobitz Type I or II. This may give very slow ventricular rates of 60-70/min in a neonate/infant and may be an indication for pacing in a symptomatic child.

Complete Heart Block

Complete heart block (CHB) is the commonest bradycardia (after sinus bradycardia) in a child and is diagnosed on the ECG by atrioventricular dissociation with the atrial beats exceeding ventricular beats and no PR relationship on the surface ECG (Figure 33.12). Congenital complete heart block (CCHB) occurs in 1 in 20,000 births. In about half of these cases, heart is structurally

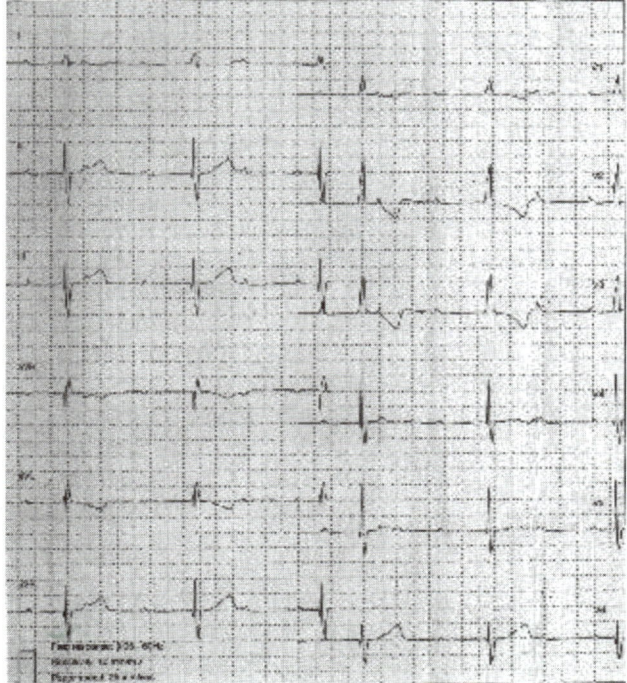

Figure 33.12 Holter trace of an infant with congenital complete heart block. The sleep heart rate is 39 bpm and the QRS is 100 msec that is wide for an infant. The P waves are seen at a rate of 84/min (sleeping sinus rate expectedly low) with no constant PR relation suggesting AV dissociation. Mean awake rates are an important criteria for pacing while sleep rates of less than 30/min is also an indication for pacing

normal. Structural heart diseases associated with CHB include corrected transposition, and endocardial cushion defect. Complete heart block can be detected in-utero with echocardiography by picking AV block by either M-mode echo or Doppler that would show more atrial than ventricular activity, their being no consistent A-V relationship. Fetal electrocardiology is still in infancy and has not yet reached the clinical realm. An important aspect of congenital CHB is the presence of manifest connective tissue disorder or having antiRo/antiLa antibodies in the mother. Almost 50% of mothers with children having CCHB will show evidences of manifest connective tissue disease especially SLE. The incidence of CHB is 1-2% in these mothers that increases markedly if the mother has hypothyroidism. The risk of recurrence in a subsequent child increases to 10-16%. The CHB usually occurs in the 2nd or 3rd trimester and may be preventable by immunosuppressants, though their long-term effects are unknown and there are no definite guidelines. Once CHB has occurred, it does not resolve, though the ventricular rate maybe increased by sympathomimetics. Neonates with congenital lupus erythematosus may also suffer from sinus bradycardia, long QT and a dilated cardiomyopathy.

The newborn with CCHB may have varied manifestations but is often asymptomatic. Uncommonly, especially with structural heart disease the child may have significant cardiomegaly and congestive heart failure. Symptoms like congestive heart failure, seizures due to intermittent asystole, failure to thrive are obvious indications for pacing. The decision to pace becomes more difficult when the child is asymptomatic. In such patients 24 hour Holter is essential and several ECG findings need to be scanned when analyzing the Holter (Table 33.10). Since over 75% of children with asymptomatic CCHB would eventually need a pacemaker by the age of 20, it is often argued why not pace all of them early in life. The main difficulty in this approach is of the logistics of pacing in children because the length of lead needs to be changed as the child grows, danger of venous thrombosis and loss of venous access, faster battery depletion and special pacemaker in neonates and infants because of the need for higher heart rates. In view of the current evidence that long term right ventricular pacing is bad for left ventricular function, it is prudent to stick to conventional guidelines and intervene only when indicated.

Table 33.10 Indications for pacing in asymptomatic congenital complete heart block (CCHB)

- QRS of the junctional escape is wide for the age of the child
- QTc >480 msec and an absolute QT over 600 msec should be regarded with suspicion. At a rate of 30/min if the absolute QT is 600 msec, the corrected QT by Bazzett's formula would be only 430 msec (considered normal); however an absolute QT of 600 msec would still predispose to Torsades-de-pointes
- Mean or lowest daytime awake ventricular rate of < 50/min in infants and children and 55/min in neonates and 65/min in the presence of structural heart disease. Sleep heart rates < 30/min are also considered as an indication for pacing by some authors.
- Cardiomegaly
- Frequent ventricular ectopy, NSVT and presence of short coupled VPBs
- Poor chronotropy

Pacing is also needed in nearly all post-operative heart blocks that do not recover in two weeks. Surgical blocks are commonest with VSD closure (because of the sheer numbers of VSD) and is due to trauma to the Bundle of His during surgery. It may be due to trauma to the AV node in operations like Ebstein or AVSD repair. Congenital or acquired sick sinus in children is uncommon. Surgeries that need extensive atrial incisions like Senning's, Fontan etc. predispose to sick sinus and may need a pacemaker. Table 33.11 summarizes the indications for pacemaker implantation in infants and children.

Table 33.11 Indications for implant of pacemaker in children

Sinus node

- Familial SSS
- Post operative e.g., Glenn, Fontan, atrial rerouting
- Prevention of syncope/drug induced bradycardia
  - LQTS
  - Neurocardiogenic syncope
  - Breath holding spells with documented correlation of bradycardia with seizures
  - Treatment of tachyarrhythmias after congenital heart surgery

AV node/His Bundle

- Congenital CHB
- Acquired CHB
  - Post operative
  - Myocarditis
  - Toxin induced (uncommon like diphtheria, Lyme disease)
  - Post cardiac interventions, radiofrequency ablation for tachyarrhythmias

Permanent pacemaker implantation in neonates and children is a highly specialized domain of pediatric cardiology and cannot be discussed at length in this chapter. Pacemakers as small as 13 gm and implants in neonates less than 1 kg are feasible. These can pace single or both the AV chambers, can vary the rates as per activity, log various events and treat tachyarrhythmias if required. The cost of these may vary from Rs 50,000 to over Rs 2 lakhs and need replacement every 10 - 12 years. In India a life-term warranty is given for these pacemakers i.e., they are replaced free of cost at the end of battery life. The battery in pacemakers cannot be changed or replaced as these are sealed units. The leads may need to be replaced because of the stretch as the child overgrows the length of lead inside the vascular system. No child with a congenital CHB should die for want of a pacemaker and a pacemaker dependent child should not be considered as handicapped in any way.

Syncope and Sudden Cardiac Death

Syncope is defined as an abrupt but transient loss of consciousness associated with absence of postural tone (usually due to reduced cerebral blood flow), followed by rapid, usually complete recovery without any need for an intervention to treat the episode. While alarming, the symptom is relatively nonspecific and is often triggered by a process that results in abrupt, transient (5-20 seconds) interruption of cerebral blood flow especially to the reticular activating system. It is associated with postural collapse and spontaneous recovery. Presyncope is characterized by feeling of faintness and associated symptoms (dizziness without vertigo, feeling of warmth, nausea, sweating and visual blurring progressing to blindness) which may resolve prior to loss of consciousness if the cerebral ischemia is corrected. Syncope always occurs when the patient is in an upright position either sitting or standing. Syncope in children is often benign with more than 25% children having fainted at least once in life. It may be life-threatening in the presence of structural heart disease or when it is due to arrhythmia when it can lead to sudden cardiac death. Some important causes of syncope in children are listed in Table 33.12.

Table 33.12 Common causes of syncope in children
Cardiac syncope
• Obstructive lesions: AS, HCM, PPH, Eisenmenger complex
• Myocardial dysfunction: Dilated cardiomyopathy, neuromuscular disorders, anomalous coronaries, Kawasaki disease
• Dysrhythmias: SVT, LQTS, Brugada syndrome, ARVC, sick sinus syndrome, atrial flutter and fibrillation (especially with structural heart disease and WPW syndrome), ventricular tachycardias and AV blocks
Autonomic syncope
• Neurocardiogenic (vasovagal), and dysautonomia
Non-cardiac syncope
• Breath holding spells, seizures, psychogenic, drug-related, metabolic and situational

Sudden cardiac death (SCD) is a natural death from cardiac causes heralded by abrupt loss of consciousness within one hour of the onset of acute symptoms. Prexisting heart disease may or may not have been known but the time and mode of death are unexpected. SCD accounts for nearly half of all deaths due to cardiac causes in adults, the coronary artery disease being the commonest cause in vast majority. However, causes of SCD are different in children and are listed in Table 33.13.

Table 33.13 Causes of sudden cardiac deaths (SCD) in children
Known heart disease
• Congenital
▪ Tetralogy of Fallot
▪ Transposition of great arteries
▪ Fontan procedure
▪ Aortic stenosis
▪ Marfan syndrome
▪ Eisenmenger complex
▪ Complete heart block
• Acquired
▪ Kawasaki disease
▪ DCM, myocarditis
• Aortic dilatation
Unrecognized heart disease
▪ HCM
▪ Congenital coronary anomalies
▪ ARVC
Without structural heart disease
▪ LQTS
▪ WPW syndrome
▪ Primary VT and VF
▪ PPH
▪ Commotio cordis

Syncope may be seen in several of the diseases mentioned in Table 33.12 and is often a precursor of sudden death in these patients. However, the commonest cause of syncope is the neurocardiogenic syncope also called as vasovagal syncope. The syncope may be either cardio-inhibitory (increased vagal discharge leading to severe bradycardia or transient asystole) or vasodepressor (inappropriate vasodilatation due to sympathetic withdrawal) or both. It is often precipitated by signs of autonomic hyperactivity like diaphoresis, nausea, pallor, and hyperventilation. Other precipitating factors are a hot or crowded environment, extreme fatigue, severe pain, hunger, prolonged standing or the sight of blood etc. It always occurs in an upright position and is preceded with prodromal symptoms and the child would be seen to be sweating, ashen pale and have a feeble or impalpable pulse. The pathophysiology of this syncope is related to a sudden increase in peripheral venous pooling leading to a reduction in the venous return to the heart. This leads to overvigorous ventricular contractions and activation of myocardial C fibers with a sudden surge of neural traffic to the brainstem signalling that the patient is "hypertensive". This leads to sympathetic withdrawal and hypotension with bradycardia. The fall in blood pressure is protective as it restores cerebral blood flow immediately and thus restores consciousness. It is important to let the child remain recumbent for sometime as immediate standing may lead to recurrence of symptoms. At times, the fall in vasovagal syncope may be dangerous enough to lead to severe injury and such a syncope is called as malignant syncope.

Neurocardiogenic syncope are fairly typical in nature and the diagnosis can be generally made with a good history corroborated by a head up tilt test (HUTT). The head up tilt test is a fairly simple investigation wherein the child is made to stand on a plank attached to the bottom of a table that can be tilted from 0 to 90 degrees. The test is done by tilting the table from 60 to 80 degrees for 20 minutes to half an hour and using provocative measures like IV isoprenaline or sublingual nitroglycerin. The child with a vasovagal attack typically has a similar syncope during the tilt that can be rapidly reversed by making the table horizontal. It is not mandatory to do a HUTT after a single faint but should be done if syncope recurs or is malignant. Most of these children do not need any treatment but if they recur then simple measures like normal salt and water intake, maintaining toe movements during prolonged standing, crossing legs and tensing muscles for 30 seconds, intense gripping of hands and tensing arms during the prodrome , "tilt training" can help in aborting or decreasing the severity of attacks. In children, fludrocortisone has been found to be very useful in preventing these episodes. The other options include use of midodrine (alpha-1 adrenergic stimulator) or fluoxetine (antidepressant, SSRI). β-blockers have not been found to be useful in randomized clinical trials and therefore are not the first option. Rarely permanent pacemakers maybe needed when the condition leads to injuries and is not responsive to drug therapy. Most often the cause of syncope can be made out with good history, examination and simple tests but in some situations a more detailed evaluation is warranted.

Another important fact while elucidating the cause of syncope/SCD is the relationship to exercise as sympathetic discharge leads to several changes in the genetically prone patient and therefore, apart from the history, an exercise test is often indicated to identify the cause of SCD or induce an arrhythmia in a controlled setting.

CONCLUSIONS

There has been a paradigm shift in the last decade in the management of arrhythmias. Apart from understanding the proarrhythmic effects of antiarrhythmic drugs and dangers of overtreating arrhythmias, significant progress has been made in the genetic map and the associated "channelopathies", that finally translate into clinical syndromes. A lot of this knowledge comes from adult population following the advent of radiofrequency ablation. However, children remain a different subset and as in several other disciplines cannot be just considered as mini adults. Treatment of arrhythmias in infants and children needs to be done by cardiologists trained in arrhythmias or pediatric cardiologists with a background of electrophysiology. It probably belongs to the realm of a super-super cardiac speciality. There is a need for more specialists with this background, since the incidence of arrhythmias is likely to increase as more and more children with heart disease get operated. It is extremely distressing to see mortality in infants and children because of a readily treatable and reversible disorder. Perhaps more intensive education programs, sensitization of pediatricians towards this eminently curable but fatal disorder is the need of the hour. Rather than looking at complex ECG's with a detached mind that these are too complex and not very treatable, a beginning has to be made to get the pediatricians involved in the care of these children.

REFERENCES

1. Driscoll DJ, Edwards WD. Sudden unexpected death in children and adolescents. *J Am Coll Cardiol* 1985; 5:118B-121B.

2. Myerburg RJ, Interian A Jr, Mitrani RM, *et al*. Frequency of sudden cardiac death and profiles of risk. *Am J Cardiol* 1997; 80:10F-19F.

3. Berger S, Dhala A, Friedberg DZ. Sudden cardiac death in infants, children, and adolescents. *Pediatr Clin North Am* 1999; 46:221-234.

4. Sreeram N, Wren C. Supraventricular tachycardia in infants: response to initial treatment. *Arch Dis Child* 1990; 65:127-129.

5. Sherwood MC, Lau KC, Sholler GF. Adenosine in the management of supraventricular tachycardia in children. *J Paediatr Child Health* 1998; 34:53-56.

6. Friedman FD. Intraosseous adenosine for the termination of supraventricular tachycardia in an infant. *Ann Emerg Med* 1996; 28:356-358.

7. Samson RA, Deal BJ, Strasburger JF, Benson DW Jr. Comparison of transesophageal and intracardiac electrophysiologic studies in characterization of supraventricular tachycardia in pediatric patients. *J Am Coll Cardiol* 1995; 26:159-163.

8. Daniels CJ, Schutte DA, Hammond S, Franklin WH. Acute pulmonary toxicity in an infant from intravenous amiodarone. *Am J Cardiol* 1997; 80:1113-1116.

9. Perry JC, Garson A Jr. Supraventricular tachycardia due to WPW syndrome in children: early disappearance and late recurrence. *J Am Coll Cardiol* 1990; 16:1215-1220.

10. Mehta AV, Sanchez GR, Sacks EJ, Casta A, Dunn JM, Donner RM. Ectopic automatic atrial tachycardia in children: clinical characteristics, management and follow-up. *J Am Coll Cardiol* 1988; 11:379-385.

11. Deal BJ, Dick M, Beerman L. Cardiac arrest in young patients with Wolff-Parkinson-White syndrome. *Pacing Clin Electrophysiol* 1995; 18 (pt II):815.

12. Russel MW, Dorostkar PC, Macdonald D II. Incidence of catastrophic events associated with the Wolff-Parkinson-White syndrome in young patients: diagnostic and therapeutic dilemma. *Circulation* 1993; 88:2608.

13. Timmermans C, Smeets JL, Rodriguez LM, Vrouchos G, van den Dool A, Wellens HJ. Aborted sudden death in the Wolff-Parkinson-White syndrome. *Am J Cardiol* 1995; 76:492-494.

14. Pappone C, Manguso F, Santinelli R, Vicedomini G, Sala S, Paglino G, Mazzone P,Lang CC, Gulletta S, Augello G, Santinelli O, Santinelli V. Radiofrequency ablation in children with asymptomatic Wolff-Parkinson-White syndrome. *N Engl J Med* 2004; 351:1197-1205.

15. Deal BJ, Keane JF, Gillette PC, Garson A Jr. Wolff-Parkinson-White syndrome and supraventricular tachycardia during infancy: management and follow-up. *J Am Coll Cardiol* 1985; 5:130-135.

16. Byrum CJ, Wahl RA, Behrendt DM, Dick M. Ventricular fibrillation associated with use of digitalis in a newborn infant with Wolff-Parkinson-White syndrome. *J Pediatr* 1982; 101:400-403.

17. O'Sullivan JJ, Gardiner HM, Wren C. Digoxin or flecainide for prophylaxis of supraventricular tachycardia in infants? *J Am Coll Cardiol* 1995; 26:991-994.

18. Ko JK, Ban JE, Kim YH, Park IS. Long-term efficacy of atenolol for atrioventricular reciprocating tachycardia in children less than 5 years old. *Pediatr Cardiol* 2004; 25:97-101. Epub 2003 Dec 4.

19. Wong KK, Potts JE, Etheridge SP, Sanatani S. Medications used to manage supraventricular tachycardia in the infant: A north American survey. *Pediatr Cardiol* 2006; 27:199-203.

20. Casey FA, McCrindle BW, Hamilton RM, Gow RM. Neonatal atrial flutter: significant early morbidity and excellent long-term prognosis. *Am Heart J* 1997; 133:302-306.

21. Gaita F, Giustetto C, Bianchi F, Wolpert C, Schimpf R, Riccardi R, Grossi S,Richiardi E, Borggrefe M. Short QT syndrome: a familial cause of sudden death. *Circulation* 2003; 108:965-70. Epub 2003 Aug 18.

22. Zeigler VL, Gillette PC, Crawford FA Jr, *et al.* New approaches to treatment of incessant ventricular tachycardia in the very young. *J Am Coll Cardiol* 1990; 16:681-685.

23. Yabek SM. Ventricular arrhythmias in children with an apparently normal heart. *J Pediatr* 1991; 119:1-11.

24. Schwartz PJ, Moss AJ, Vincent GM, Crampton RS. Diagnostic criteria for the long QT syndrome. An update. *Circulation* 1993; 88(2):782-784.

25. Mehrotra S, Juneja R, Naik N, Pavri BB. Successful use of quinine in the treatment of electrical storm in a child with Brugada syndrome. *J Cardiovasc Electrophysiol* 2011; 22:594-597.

Section 4

Acute Kidney Injury

34

Arvind Bagga and Mukta Mantan

Acute renal failure (ARF) is characterized by an abrupt decline in renal functions, resulting in a sustained rise in blood levels of urea and creatinine[1]. The incidence of ARF in neonatal and pediatric units varies, depending upon the criteria used for its definition[2]. Despite advances in therapy, the mortality is 30-40%, and a proportion of patients show chronic kidney disease and dialysis dependency[1,3,4]. Multiple definitions of ARF are proposed, based on age-dependent levels of serum creatinine and urine output. During the last few years, experts representing multiple specialties have proposed the term *acute kidney injury* (AKI) to denote sudden deterioration of kidney function.

Definition and Staging of AKI

AKI is diagnosed if there is an abrupt (within 48 hr) reduction in kidney function, defined as an absolute increase in serum creatinine of either ≥ 0.3 mg/dl *or* a percentage increase of $\geq 50\%$ *or* reduction in urine output (documented urine output of <0.5 ml/kg/hr for >6 hr). These criteria include both an absolute and a percentage change in creatinine to accommodate variations related to age, gender and body mass index and reduce the need for a baseline level of serum creatinine.

Patients meeting the definition of AKI can be staged from stage 1 to 3 (Table 34.1). This staging system corresponds to the RIFLE stages proposed previously. The **R**isk, **I**njury and **F**ailure classes match to stages 1, 2 and 3 respectively. **L**oss and **E**nd stage kidney disease were removed from the staging system, since they represent outcomes. Given the variability in indications and resources for commencing renal replacement therapy, patients receiving such therapy are classified as stage 3 AKI.

Occasionally patients with AKI may show normal or marginally reduced urine output (non-oliguric renal failure); elevated blood levels of creatinine suggest the diagnosis in these cases. Abnormalities of fluid and electrolyte homeostasis are frequently associated. While AKI usually occurs in patients with previously normal renal function, it might be superimposed on pre-existing renal disease (acute-on-chronic renal failure).

Classification

In the absence of a universally accepted definition and recognition that ARF actually includes a spectrum of clinical conditions, the term AKI has been proposed for the entire spectrum of the syndrome. Diagnostic criteria for AKI include an abrupt (within 48 hr) reduction in kidney function, defined as 50% or greater increase in serum creatinine or oliguria (<0.5 ml/kg/hr for >6 hr). Staging of AKI based on glomerular filtration rate, serum creatinine and urine output has been proposed (Table 34.1), but requires validation in children[5]. This staging will enable uniformity in reporting and comparisons of outcome.

CAUSES

Acute deterioration of kidney function occurs due to prerenal, intrinsic renal or postrenal causes[1,4]. Prerenal failure occurs due to inadequate systemic and/or renal circulation, due to either systemic hypovolemia or renal hypoperfusion. Prerenal failure is reversible if treated promptly. If the hypovolemia persists, sustained renal hypoperfusion results in acute tubular necrosis (ATN). Postrenal failure occurs as a consequence of mechanical obstruction in the urinary collecting system. Both pre- and postrenal categories can, if prolonged, lead to parenchymal injury to the kidneys (intrinsic renal failure).

Important causes of AKI are listed in Table 34.2. The epidemiology of the condition is changing worldwide. While in developed countries more cases are being reported from surgical and

Table 34.1 Staging of acute kidney injury (AKI)*

The criteria proposed by the AKI Network (AKIN) and the pediatric modified RIFLE (R, risk; I, injury; F, failure; L, loss; E, end stage) pRIFLE) classification

AKIN Stage	Serum creatinine criteria	Urine output criteria
1	Increase in serum creatinine of ≥0.3 mg/dl from baseline or increase by ≥150% to 200% (1.5-2 fold)	Less than 0.5 ml/kg per hour for >6 hr
2	Increase in serum creatinine to more than 200% to 300% (>2-3 fold) from baseline	Less than 0.5 ml/kg per hour for >12 hr
3**	Increase in serum creatinine to more than 300% (>3 fold) from baseline (or serum creatinine of ≥4.0 mg/dl with acute increase of ≥0.5 mg/dl)	Less than 0.3 ml/kg per hour for 24 hr, or anuria for 12 hr
pRIFLE Stage	Serum creatinine criteria	Urine output criteria
Risk (R)	Decrease in estimated creatinine clearance (eCCl) by ≥25%	Less than 0.5 ml/kg per hour for >8 hr
Injury (I)	Decrease in estimated creatinine clearance (eCCl) by ≥50%	Less than 0.5 ml/kg per hour for >16 hr
Failure (F)**	Decrease in estimated creatinine clearance (eCCl) by ≥75% or eCCl <35 ml/1.73 m^2/minute	Less than 0.3 ml/kg per hour for 24 hr, or anuria for 12 hr
Loss (L)	Persistent failure >4 weeks	
End stage (E)	Persistent failure >3 months (End stage renal disease)	

*Only one criterion (creatinine or urine output) should be fulfilled to qualify for a stage
**Patients receiving renal replacement therapy (RRT) are considered in stage 3 or F

oncological units, the profile in developing countries is still related to infections. The most common cause of AKI in developing countries is ATN secondary to multiple factors including dehydration, shock, septicemia and administration of nephrotoxic drugs. AKI related to overwhelming sepsis or following major surgery (especially cardiac) is common in hospitalized children. Diarrhea associated hemolytic uremic syndrome (HUS) is an important cause of intrinsic renal failure in young children in south Asia[6], though reduced incidence and appropriate management of Shigella dysentery has resulted in its decline during the last few years. Recent epidemics of D+ HUS continue to emphasize the importance of this condition. Acute glomerulonephritis (GN) is a significant cause of acute renal failure in older children. While appropriate use of antibiotics has resulted in a decline of poststreptococcal GN, other infections may result in a similar clinical syndrome. ATN due to snakebite and leptospirosis is frequent in coastal areas of Orissa, Tamilnadu and Kerala. Acute intravascular hemolysis following exposure to oxidant drugs in G6PD deficient subjects and falciparum malaria is important in certain regions. AKI consequent to vivax malaria is also reported[7]. Epidemics of severe renal failure from diethylene glycol-contaminated glycerin, used to manufacture expectorants and antipyretics, have occasionally been reported[8].

Neonatal AKI

Better chances of survival of sick and low birth weight babies has resulted in increasing recognition of neonatal AKI in NICUs[2]; perinatal asphyxia is an important cause in preterm and term babies. Other causes include hypovolemia, septicemia, respiratory distress syndrome and intravascular volume depletion following surgery. Bilateral renal artery thrombosis may occur after umbilical artery catheterization. Commonly used medications, e.g., aminoglycosides, vancomycin, amphotericin B, indomethacin, captopril and furosemide contribute to the occurrence of renal dysfunction. Use of NSAIDs or ACE inhibitors during the antenatal period may cause hypotension and AKI in the newborn. Urinary tract abnormalities, *e.g.,* posterior urethral valves, bilateral pelviureteric junction obstruction and renal dysplasia may also present in the neonatal period.

CLINICAL FEATURES

The presenting symptoms of AKI include oliguria with peripheral or pulmonary edema.

Section 4

Table 34.2. Important causes of acute kidney injury

Prerenal failure

- Hypovolemia (dehydration, blood loss, diabetic ketoacidosis)
- Third space losses (septicemia, nephrotic syndrome)
- Congestive heart failure
- Perinatal asphyxia
- Drugs (ACE inhibitors, NSAIDs, diuretics)

Intrinsic renal failure

- *Acute tubular necrosis*
  - Prolonged prerenal insult *(vide supra)*
  - Medications: aminoglycoside, radiocontrast, NSAIDs
  - Exogenous toxins: diethylene glycol, methanol
  - Intravascular hemolysis, hemoglobinuria
  - Tumor lysis syndrome
- *Hemolytic uremic syndrome*
  - Diarrhea associated (D+) and atypical (D-) forms
- *Glomerulonephritis (GN)*
  - Postinfectious GN
  - Systemic disorders: SLE, Henoch-Schonlein syndrome, microscopic polyangiitis, membranoproliferative GN
- *Interstitial nephritis:* Drug-induced and idiopathic
- *Bilateral renal vessel occlusion:* Arterial or venous

Postrenal failure

- Posterior urethral valves
- Urethral stricture
- Bilateral pelviureteric junction obstruction
- Ureteral obstruction: stenosis, stone, ureterocele
- Neurogenic bladder

ACE: angiotensin converting enzyme; NSAIDs: non-steroidal anti-inflammatory drugs; SLE: systemic lupus erythematosus

---

Patients may show altered sensorium and seizures due to uremia, dyselectrolytemia or severe hypertension. Features suggesting an underlying cause include a history of fluid or blood loss with severe dehydration (ATN); edema, hematuria and hypertension (acute GN); dysentery, pallor and petechiae (HUS); sudden pallor, cola-colored urine and jaundice (acute intravascular hemolysis). A history of poor urinary stream and palpable kidneys and bladder suggests obstruction, while abdominal colic, hematuria and dysuria suggest urinary calculi. Anuria is unusual and its presence indicates bilateral urinary tract obstruction, renal cortical necrosis, bilateral vascular obstruction, severe GN or vasculitis.

Children with renal failure secondary to acute interstitial nephritis, aminoglycoside toxicity and perinatal asphyxia show normal urine output (non-oliguric renal failure). Patients with non-oliguric ARF are often asymptomatic and the diagnosis might be missed if renal function tests are not performed[9].

Acute on Chronic Renal Failure

AKI is occasionally superimposed on chronic renal disease. Urinary tract infection, hypertension, hypovolemia and use of nephrotoxic drugs may cause deterioration of renal function in patients with pre-existing renal damage. The presence of short stature, anemia, hypertensive target organ damage, osteodystrophy and small contracted kidneys on ultrasonography suggest chronic kidney disease. In patients with underlying renal disease, an acute increase of serum creatinine by 0.5 mg/dL from baseline is considered as *acute on chronic renal failure*.

DIAGNOSIS

A careful history provides useful clues to underlying cause of AKI. Conditions resulting in decreased intravascular volume are associated with oliguria and prerenal failure. In a child having oligoanuria, it is important to assess for prerenal factors that lead to renal hypoperfusion. A history of diarrhea, vomiting, fluid or blood loss should be sought and an assessment of fluid intake in the previous 24 hr made.

In prerenal AKI, renal blood flow and glomerular filtration rate decline, but tubular reabsorption of salt and water continues. Thus, there is oliguria with low urine sodium, high urine osmolality, increased blood urea to creatinine ratio and low fractional excretion of sodium. The rise in blood urea to creatinine ratio occurs because oliguria with decreased tubular flow results in greatly increased urea reabsorption while that of creatinine is not affected. The level of blood urea and urea to creatinine ratio is also elevated when there is increased urea production (*e.g.*, due to excessive breakdown, infections or high-dose steroid therapy). ATN is characterized by diminished tubular function with high urine sodium and dilute urine. Of the several indices that differentiate prerenal from established renal failure, fractional excretion of sodium is the most sensitive and reliable (Table 34.3). These indices are, however, not useful in patients with non-oliguric renal failure and those receiving diuretics.

Recent research has focused on identifying early and more specific indicators of AKI, e.g., plasma neutrophil gelatinase-associated lipocalin (NGAL) and cystatin C and urinary NGAL, interleukin 18 (IL-18), and kidney injury molecule 1 (KIM-1) which get upregulated in proximal tubules after ischemic injury[10]. A rise of NGAL up to 10 fold has been seen within 6-hr of cardiac surgery in those patients that later developed AKI. The specificity and clinical utility of these markers, however, remains to be established.

In prerenal AKI, expansion of the intravascular volume leads to improved renal perfusion and increase in urine output. Dehydration is corrected by infusion of 20-30 ml/kg of isotonic saline or Ringer's lactate over 30-45 minutes. During this period, the child's vital signs are monitored and care taken to avoid overhydration. Central venous pressure (CVP) should be measured to determine the adequacy of fluid replacement if clinical assessment of hypovolemia is difficult. If urine output increases and CVP is still low, infusion may be continued. Once fluid replacement is accomplished, furosemide (2-3 mg/kg) may be given intravenously. This should normally induce diuresis (urine flow of 2-4 ml/kg over the next 2-3 hr if renal tubular function is intact). If these measures fail to induce diuresis, a diagnosis of intrinsic renal failure is made[11,12].

INVESTIGATIONS

Important investigations in patients with AKI are listed in Table 34.4. Investigations are aimed at identifying the severity of AKI, complications of the condition and determine the etiology. Regular monitoring of body weight, electrolytes, urea and creatinine is extremely important to assess the out come.

Kidney biopsy

A kidney biopsy is not needed in most patients with AKI and is rarely necessary in the first 2 weeks of illness. A biopsy is indicated in patients suspected to have rapidly progressive GN, nonresolving acute GN or interstitial nephritis where appropriate specific therapy might be beneficial. The procedure is also necessary in patients with clinical diagnosis of ATN or HUS if significant renal dysfunction persists beyond 4 weeks, to determine renal histology as an aid to diagnosis and prognostication. Finally, a kidney biopsy is also useful in patients where the underlying cause of AKI is not apparent on clinical features and investigations.

Patients with severe azotemia (blood urea >180 mg/dL, creatinine >3-4 mg/dL) are at risk of bleeding following renal biopsy. These patients

Table 34.3. Indices to differentiate pre-renal from established (intrinsic) acute kidney injury

Parameter	Pre-renal azotemia	Intrinsic renal failure
Urinary sodium (mEq/L)	<20	>40
Urinary osmolality (mOsm/kg)	>500	<300
Blood urea-creatinine ratio	>20	<20
Urine-plasma osmolality ratio	>1.5	<1.0
Fractional excretion of sodium* (%)	<1	>3

$$*FeNa\,(\%) = \frac{\text{urine sodium} \times \text{serum creatinine}}{\text{serum sodium} \times \text{urine creatinine}} \times 100$$

Table34.4. Investigations in patients with acute kidney injury

Blood

- Complete blood counts
- Urea, creatinine, sodium, potassium, calcium, phosphate, pH, bicarbonate

Urine

- Urinalysis; culture (if symptoms of urinary infection)
- Sodium, osmolality, fractional excretion of sodium
- Chest X-ray for fluid overload and cardiomegaly
- Ultrasonography of KUB (identify obstruction, dilatation, small kidneys)

Investigations to determine the cause

- Peripheral smear examination, platelet and reticulocyte count; LDH levels; stool culture (suspected hemolytic uremic syndrome)
- Blood ASLO, complement (C3), antinuclear antibody (ANA), antineutrophil cytoplasmic antibody (ANCA) (suspected acute, rapidly progressive GN)
- Doppler ultrasonography (suspected arterial or venous thrombosis)
- Renal biopsy (rapidly progressive GN; determine severity of injury; cause of AKI not clear)

should be dialyzed, either peritoneally or by hemodialysis, to reduce the severity of azotemia. Hypertension should be adequately controlled; platelet count and bleeding, clotting and prothrombin time should be normal before under taking the biopsy. Intravenous (0.3 µg/ kg) or nasal (2-3 µg/ kg) desmopressin, administered 60-90 minutes prior to the procedure, reduces the risk of bleeding.

MANAGEMENT

Treatment of complications

Immediate attention should be directed towards detection and management of life-threatening complications. Clinical evaluation includes measurement of blood pressure, fundus examination and search for signs of congestive heart failure, fluid overload, acidosis and anemia. Investigations include estimation of blood levels of hemoglobin, urea, creatinine, sodium, potassium and bicarbonate. An electrocardiogram (ECG) is done to detect potassium toxicity and an X-ray film of the chest for pulmonary edema. Table 34.5 summarizes the management of complications that might be present.

Hyperkalemia is a serious emergency as the resultant cardiac toxicity may cause sudden death. Urgent treatment is instituted depending on blood potassium levels and ECG changes. Concomitant metabolic acidosis should be corrected. While sodium bicarbonate, glucose, insulin and salbutamol reduce the extracellular concentration of potassium by moving the ion into the cells, calcium infusion decreases membrane irritability without altering serum potassium levels. The action of kayexalate (sodium polystyrene sulfonate) or calcium resonium, which exchange potassium for sodium or calcium ions, is slow and therefore not useful in emergency. Peritoneal or hemodialysis is the most effective method to remove excess potassium from the body.

Overhydration, pulmonary edema and congestive heart failure result from excessive amount of fluid administration. These patients are treated using the standard guidelines. Hypertension is commonly observed in cases of GN and HUS. The symptoms of hypertensive encephalopathy are generally related to rapidity of rise rather than absolute value of the blood pressure. They include headache, blurring of vision, convulsions, papilledema, cranial nerve palsies (especially facial), vomiting and altered sensorium. Blood pressure should be reduced with appropriate medications (Table 34.5).

Hyponatremia (sodium <130 mEq/L) is usually the result of excessive fluid administration rather than salt loss. The condition is best managed by fluid restriction; patients with resistant hyponatremia can be satisfactorily managed by dialysis. Treatment with hypertonic saline (3%) is reserved for those with symptomatic hyponatremia (encephalopathy, lethargy and seizures), but should be used cautiously because of potential complications of fluid overload, hypertension and intraventricular hemorrhage.

Standard Supportive Care

In a child with AKI in whom serious complications are absent or have been adequately treated, standard supportive care is instituted[13]. Management is based on close attention to the intake of fluids and electrolytes, provision of proper nutrition, prevention and treatment of infections, careful monitoring and dialysis.

Fluid and electrolyte balance

Fluid and electrolyte intake in a patient with AKI should be regulated. The daily fluid requirement

Table 34.5 Management of complications

Complication	Treatment	Remarks
Fluid overload	*Fluid restriction* : Insensible losses (400 ml/m²/d); add urine output and other losses; 5% dextrose for insensible losses; N/5 saline for urine output	Monitor other losses and replace as appropriate, consider dialysis
Pulmonary edema	Oxygen; furosemide 2-4 mg/kg iv	Monitor CVP; consider dialysis
Hypertension	*Symptomatic:* Sodium nitroprusside 0.5-8 mg/kg/minute by infusion; furosemide 2-4 mg/kg iv; nifedipine 0.3-0.5 mg/kg oral/sublingual *Asymptomatic :* Nifedipine, amlodepine, prazosin, labetalol, clonidine	In emergency, reduce blood pressure by one-third of the desired reduction during first 6-8 hr, 1/3rd over next 12-24 hr and the final 1/3rd slowly over 2-3 days
Metabolic acidosis	Sodium bicarbonate (IV or oral) if bicarbonate levels <18 mEq/l	Watch for fluid overload, hypernatremia, hypocalcemia; consider dialysis
Hyperkalemia	Calcium gluconate (10%) 0.5-1 ml/kg over 5-10 minutes iv Salbutamol 5-10 mg nebulized Sodium bicarbonate (7.5%) 1-2 ml/kg over 15 minutes Dextrose (10%) 0.5-1 g/kg and insulin 0.1-0.2 U/kg Calcium or sodium resonium (Kayexalate) 1 g/kg per day	Stabilizes cell membranes; prevents arrhythmias Shifts potassium into cells Shifts potassium into cells Requires monitoring of blood glucose Given orally or rectally, can be repeated every 4 hours
Hyponatremia	Fluid restriction; if sensorial alteration or seizures occur, administer 3% saline 6-12 ml/kg over 30-90 minutes	Hyponatremia is usually dilutional; 12 ml/kg of 3% saline raises sodium by 10 mEq/L
Severe anemia	Packed red cells 3-5 ml/kg; consider exchange transfusion	Monitor blood pressure, fluid overload
High phosphate	Phosphate binders (calcium carbonate, acetate; aluminum phosphate)	Avoid high phosphate products like milk products and high protein diet

Modified from Pediatric Nephrology; Srivastava RN, Bagga A (Eds) *Jaypee Bros, New Delhi* 5th edn, 2011.

Section 4

amounts to insensible water losses (300-400 ml/m²), urinary output and non-renal or insensible fluid losses. Insensible fluid losses are replaced with 5-10% dextrose solution. Urine output should be monitored without resorting to catheterization. Urinary losses and those from extrarenal sources should have their composition analyzed and replaced accordingly. It is preferable to administer the required amounts of fluids by mouth. If there is persistent vomiting, intravenous route may be necessary. *Potassium containing fluids should not be given to patients with oliguria.*

Ongoing treatment is guided by intake-output analysis, daily weight, physical examination and serum sodium. If fluid in an appropriate volume and composition has been given, the patient should lose 0.5-1% of his body weight every day. This weight loss is a result of caloric deprivation and not inadequate fluid therapy. The serum sodium concentration should stay within the normal range.

A rapid weight loss and increasing level of serum sodium suggest inadequate free water replacement. On the other hand, an absence of weight loss and hyponatremia indicate excessive free water replacement.

Diet

Patients with AKI are catabolic and have increased metabolic needs. Adequate nutritional support is desirable with maximization of caloric intake. However, volume restriction necessary during the oliguric phase often imposes severe limits on the caloric intake. A diet containing 0.8-1.2 g/ kg of protein in infants and 0.6-0.8 g/kg in older children and a minimum of 50-60 kcal/kg should be given. The latter requirement can be met by adding liberal amounts of carbohydrates and fats to the diet. Once dialysis is initiated, dietary fluid and electrolyte restrictions can be made more liberal. Vitamin and micronutrient supplements are provided.

Management of infections

Patients with AKI are susceptible to infections because of depressed immunity induced by azotemia, associated malnutrition and invasive procedures. Various infections (respiratory and urinary tract, peritonitis and septicemia) are the immediate cause of death in majority of patients. All procedures must be performed with strict aseptic techniques, intravenous lines carefully watched, and skin puncture sites cleaned and dressed. Oral hygiene should be ensured.

Sepsis is suggested by hypothermia, persistent hypotension, hyperkalemia and a disproportionate rise of blood urea compared to creatinine. The patient should be frequently examined to detect infection, which may be present without fever. Once infection is suspected, specimens are taken for culture studies and appropriate antibiotics are started.

Use of medications

Drugs that increase severity of renal damage or delay recovery of renal function (*e.g.* aminoglycosides, radiocontrast media, NSAIDs, amphotericin B) should be avoided. Medications that reduce renal perfusion *e.g.,* ACE inhibitors and indomethacin should be used cautiously. The dose and dosing interval of antibiotics particularly those, which are nephrotoxic, should be modified depending on the severity of renal failure[11].

Role of diuretics, mannitol and dopamine

Diuretics may be useful in instances where a high urine flow is required to prevent intratubular precipitation as with intravascular hemolysis, hyperuricemia and myoglobinuria. Inappropriate use of loop diuretics may cause ototoxicity, interstitial nephritis, hypotension or persistence of patent ductus arteriosus in the newborn. There is no evidence that treatment with diuretics improves renal function or the long-term outcome in patients with intrinsic renal failure[14]. Mannitol has been used, as a diuretic, but no clear benefits of its use are demonstrated. Intravenous administration of mannitol, in patients with volume overload and oliguria, might be detrimental and result in congestive heart failure.

There is no evidence that administration of low dose dopamine (1-3 µg/kg/min) improves renal function, reduce need for dialysis or enhance survival.[14,15] Rather it may be detrimental and cause

complications like arrhythmias. Its use is currently not recommended. Other experimental therapies including calcium channel blockers, antioxidants, thyroxin, peptide growth factors and cytokines have been used in order to attenuate renal injury or enhance recovery of renal function, but results of clinical trials are disappointing[16].

Specific Therapy

Intensive immunosuppression with high dose intravenous methylprednisolone followed by oral or intravenous cyclophosphamide is indicated in patients with crescentic GN, lupus nephritis and vasculitis. A brief course of treatment with oral corticosteroids is useful in patients with acute interstitial nephritis. Treatment in patients with D+ HUS is chiefly supportive. Intensive plasmapharesis is recommended for patients with D- (atypical) HUS, and selected patients of crescentic GN and severe lupus nephritis.

Postrenal ARF

The management is to bypass the obstruction *e.g.,* catheterization or vesicostomy in children with posterior urethral valves or percutaneous nephrostomy in bilateral obstruction at the pelviureteric junctions. If the patient is sick or the diagnosis of obstruction unclear, intermittent peritoneal dialysis is done initially and nephrostomy undertaken at a later stage.

Monitoring

It is extremely important to record the fluid intake, output and body weight daily. A close monitoring is done for blood levels of urea, creatinine and electrolytes. On fluid restriction and inadequate calorie intake most patients lose weight by 0.5% daily. Patients should be regularly screened for the presence of hosptial acquired infections.

Renal Replacement Therapy

Severe AKI requiring dialysis can be managed with a variety of modalities, including peritoneal dialysis, intermittent hemodialysis, and continuous hemofiltration or hemodiafiltration. The choice of dialysis modality to be used in managing a specific patient is influenced by several factors, including the goals of dialysis, the unique advantages and disadvantages of each modality and institutional resources.

Indications for initiating renal replacement therapy include severe or persistent hyperkalemia

(>7 mEq/L), fluid overload (pulmonary edema, severe hypertension), uremic encephalopathy and severe metabolic acidosis (tCO$_2$ <10-12 mEq/L), hyponatremia (<120 mEq/L) or hypernatremia (>150 mEq/L). The decision to start dialysis should be based on an overall assessment of the patient keeping in mind the likely course of AKI.

Intermittent Peritoneal Dialysis (IPD)

The initial renal replacement therapy of choice in sick and unstable patients is often IPD[17]. It is popular because of the ease of doing the procedure and its effectiveness in children of all ages. Peritoneal access, in most centers in India, is obtained using a stiff catheter and trocar. These catheters should be removed after 48-72 hr, beyond which the risk of infection is very high. The risk of injury to the viscera and infections is less with soft silastic catheters (Tenckhoff or Cook), which can be used for repeated dialysis for prolonged periods. The standard Tenckhoff catheter needs to be placed surgically but a temporary catheter is available for bedside insertion.

The composition of dialysate and speed of procedure depends upon the clinical condition of the patient. The fill volume varies from 30-50 ml/kg (800-1200 ml/m²). Commercially available dialysates are lactate based, with a dextrose concentration of 1.7%. In patients with fluid overload, peritoneal dialysis solution with 2.5-3% dextrose is used to increase ultrafiltration[18]. The initial dialysis cycles are of short duration (20-30 minutes). It is important to correctly measure indwell and the drain fluid to estimate the ultrafiltrate. Once potassium levels are normal, potassium chloride (2-3 mEq/L) is added to the dialysate. Patients who are sick and have severe lactic acidosis are dialyzed using a bicarbonate dialysate. The dialysate effluent is checked for clarity and cell count after the first 10 cycles.

Complications of PD are related to insertion of the stiff catheter. Bleeding, bowel and bladder perforation are uncommon. Catheter blockage occurs occasionally and may require maneuvering. The incidence of peritonitis is between 20-30% when the catheter is used for less than 72 hr, but increases significantly thereafter[19]. If the duration of renal failure is prolonged and there is a need for renal replacement therapy, chronic PD may be performed, either manually (continuous ambulatory peritoneal dialysis; CAPD) or with the use of an automated device (continuous cycling peritoneal dialysis; CCPD).

Hemodialysis (HD)

HD is more efficient for correction of fluid and electrolyte abnormalities. However it is expensive to establish, requires expertise and skilled nursing and is not available at most centers in our country. It is not suited for patients with hemodynamic instability, bleeding tendency and in very young children where vascular access might be difficult.

The equipment required is the HD machine, pediatric dialyzer with tubings and dialysate fluid (Figure 34.1). The hollow fiber dialyzers are made of cellophane, cuprophane or cellulose acetate, and are available in sizes ranging from 0.5-1.5 m². The extracorporeal volume of the circuit should not exceed 10% of patient's blood volume and the dialyzer should be 70-80% of the total body surface. An appropriate vascular access is necessary for removing and returning large quantities of blood required for the procedure. The most common vascular access for children is a double lumen venous catheter (sizes 8-12F) inserted into internal jugular, femoral or subclavian vein. Ideal dialysates have composition similar to extracellular fluid to prevent electrolyte imbalance. Their sodium concentration varies between 135-140 mEq/L, potassium concentration 0-4 mEq/L, calcium 3-3.2 mEq/L, magnesium 1-1.5 mEq/L and acetate/bicarbonate 35-40 mEq/L.

The blood pump in the dialysis machine regulates the flow of blood from the patient to the dialyzer. The heparinized blood flows (4-5 ml/kg/min) on one side of the semipermeable membrane of the dialyzer, while the dialysate flows at a rate 1.5-2 times the blood pump rate on the other side. After dialysis the blood is returned to the patient's circulation. The hemodialysis machine has an ultrafiltrate controller, which determines removal of free water. Most children are well maintained

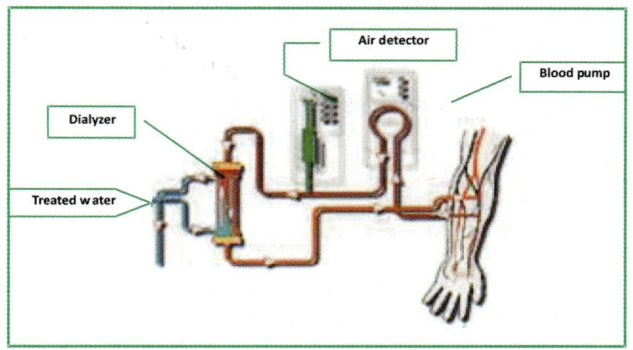

Figure 34.1 Hemodialysis circuit

on dialysis for a duration of 3-4 hr, three times a week. Due to higher metabolic needs children require more dialysis in relation to their body size as compared to adults. Sick patients with fluid overload and hypertension often benefit from daily dialysis[20].

Continuous Renal Replacement Therapies (CRRT)

CRRT is an extracorporeal blood purification therapy intended as a substitute for impaired renal function over an extended period of time and applied for 24 hr a day. These therapies are gaining increasing popularity for treatment of critically ill patients with severe AKI in developed countries. Modalities include CAVH (continuous arteriovenous hemofiltration), CVVH (continuous venovenous hemofiltration), continuous venovenous hemodiafiltration (CVVHD) and slow continuous ultrafiltration (SCUF). These therapies are useful when large amount of fluids have to be removed in sick and unstable patients[21]. CVVH is also preferred in AKI secondary to major surgical procedures, burns, heart failure and septic shock especially when conventional HD or PD is not possible. Continuous hemofiltration provides smoother control of ultrafiltered volume and gradual correction of metabolic abnormalities in unstable patients. Special equipment and trained staff is necessary to provide CRRT in children. Large volumes of replacement fluids are required that increase the cost of therapy.

Prognosis

Despite advances in dialysis techniques, the morbidity and mortality of AKI is high[22]. The eventual recovery and outcome of patients with AKI depend on the underlying condition. While the prognosis in ATN and acute interstitial nephritis is satisfactory, patients with multiorgan failure and cortical necrosis fare poorly. The outcome in crescentic GN and vasculitis depends on severity of the renal injury and promptness in initiation of specific therapy. AKI secondary to septicemia, D-HUS and following cardiac surgery is associated with high mortality. The prognosis is poor in neonates with structural abnormalities and disseminated intravascular coagulation. Those in whom the recovery of renal function is incomplete might develop progressive renal failure.

REFERENCES

1. Hui-Stickle S, Brewer ED, Goldenstein SL. Pediatric ARF epidemiology at a tertiary care center from 1999-2001. *Am J Kidney* Dis 2005; 45: 96-101.

2. Agras PI, Tarcan A, Baskin E, Cengiz N, Gurakan B, Saatci U. Acute renal failure in the neonatal period. *Renal Failure* 2004; 26: 305-309.

3. Arora P, Kher V, Rai PK, Singhal MK, Gulati S, Gupta A. Prognosis of acute renal failure in children: A multivariate analysis. *Pediatr Nephrol* 1997; 11: 153-155.

4. Srivastava RN, Bagga A, Moudgil A. Acute renal failure in north Indian children. *Indian J Med Res* 1990; 92: 404-408.

5. Mehta RL, Kellum JA, Shah SV, Molitoris BA, Ronco C, Warnock DG. Acute Kidney Injury Network (AKIN): Report of an initiative to improve outcomes in acute kidney injury. *Crit Care* 2007; 11:R31

6. Srivastava RN, Moudgil A, Bagga A, Vasudev AS. Hemolytic uremic syndrome in children in northern India. *Pediatr Nephrol* 1991; 5: 284-288.

7. Kanodia KV, Shah PR, Vanika AV, Kasat P, Gumber M, Trivedi HL. Malaria induced acute renal failure: a single center experience. *Saudi J Kidney Dis Transpl* 2010; 21: 1088-1091.

8. Singh J, Dutta AK, Khare S, Dubey NK, Harit AK, Jain NK, Wadhwa TC, Gupta SR, Dhariwal AC, Jain DC, Bhatia R, Sokhey J. Diethylene glycol poisoning in Gurgaon, India, 1998. *Bull World Health Organ* 2001; 79: 88-95.

9. Moghal NE, Brocklebank JT, Meadow SR. A review of acute renal failure in children: incidence, etiology and outcome. *Clin Nephrol* 1998; 49: 91-95.

10. Nguyen MT, Devarajan P. Biomarkers for the early detection of acute kidney injury. *Pediatr Nephrol* 2008; 23: 2151-2157.

11. Filler G. Acute renal failure in children: etiology and management. *Pediatr Drugs* 2001; 3: 783-792.

12. Flynn JT. Causes, management approaches, and outcome of acute renal failure in children. *Curr Opin Pediatr* 1998; 10: 184-189.

13. Dursum B, Edelstein CL. Acute renal failure. *Am J Kidney Dis* 2005; 45:614-618.

14. Kellum JA. The use of diuretics and dopamine in acute renal failure: a systematic review of the evidence. *Crit Care* 1997; 1: 53-59.

15. Chertow GM, Sayegh MH, Allgren R, Lazarus JM. Is the administration of dopamine associated with adverse or favourable outcomes in acute renal failure? Auriculin Anaritide Acute Renal Failure Study Group. *Am J Med* 1996; 101: 49-53.

16. Schena FP. Role of growth factors in acute renal failure. *Kidney Int Suppl* 1998; 66: S11-S15.

Section 4

17. Srivastava RN, Bagga A. Renal replacement therapy. In: Pediatric Nephrology, *New Delhi, Jaypee Brothers* 5th edition 2011; pp 174-186.

18. Flynn JT, Kershaw DB, Smoyer WE, Brophy PD, Mc Bryde KD, Bunchman TE. Peritoneal dialysis for management of pediatric acute renal failure. *Perit Dial Int* 2001, 21: 390-394.

19. Sharma RK, Kumar J, Gupta A, Gulati S. Peritoneal infection in acute intermittent peritoneal dialysis. *Ren Failure* 2003; 25: 975-980.

20. Sciffl H, Lang SM, Fischer R. Daily hemodialysis and the outcome of acute renal failure. *N Engl J Med* 2002; 346: 305-315.

21. Pannu N, Klarenbach S, Wiebe N, Manns B, Tonelli M. Alberta Kidney Disease Network. Renal replacement therapy in patients with acute renal failure: A systematic review. *JAMA* 2008; 299: 793-805.

22. Radhakrishnan J, Kiryluk K. Acute renal failure outcomes in children and adults. *Kidney Int* 2006; 69: 17-19.

Section 4

35

Acute Liver Failure

Pankaj Vohra

Acute liver failure (ALF) is a clinical syndrome due to severe hepatocyte dysfunction that occurs in the absence of a prior liver disease. If recovery does not occur, it usually culminates into multi-organ failure and death. On the other hand, if the patient survives, the liver usually recovers completely especially if the cause is known to be a drug or infection.

DEFINITION

There is no universally accepted nomenclature for hepatic failure. Currently the most widely accepted definition of acute liver failure includes the following features[1]:

1. Biochemical evidences of liver disease.
2. Vitamin K corrected INR of > 2 without evidence of encephalopathy or INR of more than 1.5 with evidences of encephalopathy.
3. No evidence of chronic liver disease.

Alternatively, it is defined as development of hepatic necrosis with encephalopathy within eight weeks of the onset of liver disease[2]. Some of the other definitions have used the time interval between the onset of jaundice (and liver disease) and development of encephalopathy as follows:

(i) *Hyperacute liver failure.* Onset of ALF within one week of appearance of jaundice. These patients have the best outcome.

(ii) *Acute liver failure.* Onset of encephalopathy between 8 to 28 days of jaundice.

(iii) *Sub-acute liver failure.* Onset of encephalopathy between 29 days to 12 weeks of jaundice. This group has the worst survival rate[3].

The diagnosis of acute hepatic failure in neonates is difficult due to a number of reasons as listed below[4]:

- Bilirubin is elevated in most ill neonates (sepsis being the most common cause of acute liver failure in this age group) and occasionally in severe neonatal liver failure the increase in bilirubin may be of the indirect type because there are just not enough hepatocytes to conjugate bilirubin!

- Prothrombin time is prolonged even in normal infants.

- Ammonia may be elevated in several types of metabolic disorders other than liver failure.

- Disseminated intravascular coagulopathy is common in neonates and complicates assessment of coagulation profile.

- Encephalopathy is difficult to diagnose as sepsis, meningitis, hypoglycemia etc. may have the same clinical picture.

ETIOLOGY

With the exception of paracetamol toxicity, the etiology of liver failure rarely has any implications on the management of the patient with ALF. In neonates, infections or inborn errors of metabolism are common, while hepatotropic viruses (singly or combined) are more likely to cause ALF in older children. In a study from Delhi, Hepatitis A virus and Hepatitis E virus (singly or combined) were responsible for almost 65% of all cases[5]. *Hepatitis A remains the most common cause of acute liver failure in children[6]*. Hepatitis C alone is a rare cause of acute liver failure.

Hepatitis A on the other hand is a rare cause of acute liver failure in infants. Hepatitis B infection usually produces a chronic liver disease if contracted vertically or during early neonatal period. Rarely, it can result in acute hepatic failure at about 12 weeks of age following vertical infection from the mother who is HBsAg positive and HBeAg negative. Dengue has been reported as an important cause of acute hepatic failure especially in infancy[7]. Metabolic liver disease is a common cause of liver failure in neonates followed by herpes, neonatal hemochromatosis, mitochondrial disorders, fatty acid oxidation defects and hemophagocytic lymphohistiocytosis[8].

Paracetamol toxicity in young children shows a bimodal age distribution. An early peak during 1 to 4 year olds occurs due to accidental overdose. In children over 11 years, ingestion is more likely to be deliberate or suicidal. Maximal liver injury occurs 2-4 days after ingestion. Sodium valproate causes microvesicular steatosis and may precipitate fulminant hepatic failure especially in infants and children getting multiple antiepileptic drugs or with mitochondrial defects[9]. Nimesulide has also been found to be hepatotoxic due to idiosyncratic reactions even when taken in therapeutic doses[10]. Mushroom poisoning, rodenticide poisoning and malignancy especially leukemia are some of the other rarer causes of acute liver failure. The common causes of acute liver failure are listed in Table 35.1.

However, in any child who presents as acute hepatic failure, the possibility of an underlying chronic liver disease should be seriously considered. Acute liver failure may develop in a patient with an underlying liver disease due to a superimposed insult (Table 35.2). The clinical features that may point towards the presence of an underlying chronic liver disease are listed below:

- Past history of liver disease
- Growth failure
- Presence of a hard liver
- Splenomegaly
- Moderate or large ascites
- Spider nevi
- Presence of portal hypertension
- Low serum albumin

CLINICAL PRESENTATION

The typical pediatric patient with acute liver failure is often a previously healthy child with no history of any major medical problem. As the disease is most commonly due to a water-borne virus, history of recent blood transfusion or surgery is rarely elicitable. Initially the child has non-specific prodromal symptoms such as malaise, nausea, fatigue, fever and loss of appetite. This is followed 5-7 days later by dark colored urine and jaundice. These children are usually diagnosed to have viral hepatitis at this stage. High grade fever

Table 35.1 Etiology of acute liver failure

Viral hepatitis (Isolated/mixed)
- Hepatitis A, B, C, D, E
- Herpes simplex
- Epstein-Barr virus
- Parvovirus B19
- Varicella zoster
- Cytomegalovirus
- Adenovirus
- Echovirus
- Coxsackie virus
- Dengue virus

Other infections
- Leptospirosis
- Malaria

Drug induced
- Paracetamol
- Sodium valproate
- Phenytoin
- Isoniazid
- Nimesulide

Metabolic causes
- Tyrosinemia Type 1
- Mitochondrial disorders
- Hereditary fructose intolerance
- Niemann–Pick disease C
- Fatty acid oxidation defects

Hypo-perfusion
- Acute Budd-Chiari syndrome
- Veno-occlusive disease
- Right sided congestive heart failure
- Cardiogenic shock
- Ischemia

Miscellaneous causes
- Autoimmune hepatitis especially Type 2 AIH
- Hemophagocytic lymphohistiocytosis
- Malignancy e.g. acute leukemia
- Amanita (poisonous mushroom)
- Rodenticide
- Unknown causes

HCV alone rarely causes acute hepatic failure.

may occur due to hepatitis or super added infection or due to an alternative infection like severe malaria (*P. falciparum*), enteric fever, and leptospirosis, etc. However, in children who ultimately develop acute liver failure, there is rapid onset of altered mental status heralding the onset of hepatic

Table 35.2 Chronic liver diseases that may present as acute hepatic failure

- Wilson's disease	- Reactivation of latent hepatitis B infection after immunosuppression or chemotherapy
- Autoimmune hepatitis	
- Super infection with hepatitis D virus (or any other virus) in a child with hepatitis B carrier state	- Hepatitis A or E super-infection in a cirrhotic child

Section 4

encephalopathy. It is difficult to identify the patient who is likely to develop liver failure but children with following features are more likely candidates for ALF[11].

- Persistent vomiting.
- Small or shrinking liver size.
- Rapidly falling transaminases in the absence of other evidences of improvement.
- Very high transaminases >10,000 u/l.
- Pregnancy (especially with HEV infection).

As a part of evaluation of the child, the liver size is critical. Large hepatomegaly is associated with better prognosis while a shrinking liver is indeed ominous. Hence liver span must be checked and recorded daily.

Every clinician should carefully ask and/or look for early manifestations of hepatic encephalopathy in all children with acute hepatitis and if there is a suspicion, these children should be admitted to the hospital for observation. The clinical features of hepatic encephalopathy are variable. Patients with hepatic encephalopathy are traditionally divided into stages or grades that often correlate with the clinical severity and prognosis. Table 35.3 summarizes the stages of encephalopathy based on the signs and symptoms. Initial symptoms of encephalopathy may be subtle and are likely to be passed off as a behavioral aberration of the child. Change in personality is one of the earliest signs of hepatic encephalopathy. On the other hand, children may pass through various stages of encephalopathy so rapidly that the parents may not notice the early phase. A child with acute onset of combative behavior or being irritable without reason should always be screened for hepatic encephalopathy. There may be associated asterixis (flapping tremor), rigidity, hyperreflexia, extensor plantar response and fetor hepaticus. EEG may show symmetric high-voltage, triphasic slow wave (2 to 5 per sec) pattern. In Reye's syndrome, liver failure may occur with no or minimal jaundice and in hyperacute liver failure, encephalopathy may precede development of jaundice[13]. Grade 3 and 4 encephalopathy is usually accompanied with cerebral edema and this

Table 35.3 Staging of hepatic encephalopathy

Grade 1.	Altered mood or behavior, sleep disturbances, irritability
Grade 2.	Drowsy, inappropriate behavior, minimal confusion
Grade 3.	Stupor, somnolence, inarticulate speech, marked confusion and combative behaviour; usually due to cerebral edema
Grade 4.	Coma

is the most common cause of death in acute liver failure[14]. However, death from acute liver failure may occur without the development of encephalopathy or cerebral edema and on the other hand a rapidly increasing grade of encephalopathy should alert the physician to shift the child to a liver transplant center. The presence of focal neurological signs should alert the pediatrician to an alternative diagnosis.

Other clinical and laboratory features of acute liver failure are summarized in Table 35.4.

Table 35.4 Clinical features of acute hepatic failure

Jaundice	Hepatic encephalopathy
Coagulopathy	Cerebral edema
Hypoglycemia	Hepato-renal syndrome
Metabolic acidosis	Increased risk of sepsis
Shrunken liver	Multi-organ dysfunction

GENERAL PRINCIPLES

Acute liver failure is a medical emergency and is often associated with an unpredictable and at times a fatal outcome. Recovery occurs if the liver gets adequate time to regenerate with supportive therapy. Every child with acute hepatic failure, must be cared for in an ICU setting, either in a hospital with facilities for liver transplantation or having facilities for transportation to a liver transplant center. The aim of therapy is to prevent complications like encephalopathy and cerebral edema, sepsis, GI bleed and renal failure while assessing etiology of ALF and preparing the patient for liver transplantation in the event of lack of spontaneous recovery despite intensive care.

There are limited randomized controlled trials to assess various therapeutic options in the management of ALF. Most of the therapies employed in acute liver failure are non-specific and are usually directed to prevent or control complications of the disease. Therapeutic modalities are largely based on protocols developed with clinical experience and retrospective studies. There is no known therapy that helps to regenerate the liver faster. However, liver transplantation has changed the bleak outlook of advanced hepatic failure[12].

One of the most important components of management of acute liver failure is counseling of the parents and relatives. Unfortunately the disease is unpredictable and in most situations with advanced failure it is associated with high mortality rates. The progression of the disease and likely morbidity and mortality rates should be discussed early in the course of the illness and if feasible communication with transplant center should be initiated. In addition, family surveys may be undertaken for Wilson's disease or Hepatitis B antigen in the family members. Hepatitis A vaccine should be given to the siblings of the index patient. Broad guidelines for monitoring of a child with ALF are listed in Table 35.5. These may be modified as per the clinical presentation.

LABORATORY INVESTIGATIONS

The initial work-up of the child should include; assessment of severity of disease, etiology of ALF and institution of specific therapy (if available) and identification of complications. The single most important clinical marker in acute hepatic failure is encephalopathy and the most important laboratory parameter is prothrombin time. INR (Internationational normalized ratio) is a more useful parameter rather than prothrombin time (PT) alone as it is easily comparable across various testing kits. Levels of transaminases are not of prognostic significance except when their levels fall precipitously in the absence of clinical improvement. Recently phosphate levels have been considered to have prognostic significance. If the serum phosphate levels are low that is a good prognostic marker as it signifies its uptake by the regenerating hepatocytes[13].

Table 35.5 General principles of care and monitoring

- Ensure complete asepsis (strict handwashing)
- Establish adequate IV access (preferably CVP line)
- Continuous monitoring of vital signs
- Pulse oximetry
- Neurological/coma grading every 2 hourly
- Blood sugar estimation 2-6 hourly
- Na/K, arterial blood gases, prothrombin time, liver function tests, and serum creatinine every 12-24 hours
- Blood counts, blood culture, urine culture, ESR, CRP and X-ray chest every 24-72 hours
- Nasogastric tube for feeding/drainage
- Urinary catheter
- Care of bowel, bladder, back, skin, eyes etc.

What all should be avoided in acute liver failure?
- Paracetamol
- NSAIDs
- Aminoglycosides
- Sedation
- Aggressive diuresis
- Hypokalemia
- Aggressive fluid therapy
- Corticosteroids (except in certain circumstances)

Table 35.6 Investigations to be ordered in a child with acute hepatic failure

- Complete blood counts
- Liver function tests
- Ammonia level[@]
- Prothrombin time and INR
- Blood sugar level
- Electrolytes[†]
- Kidney function tests[$]
- Serum phosphate levels
- Urine analysis
- Blood culture
- Blood gas and acid-base parameters
- Blood grouping and cross matching
- X-ray chest
	- Viral hepatitis markers including
	  • HAV IgM antibody
	  • HEV IgM antibody
	  • HBsAg
	  • Anti HBc IgM antibody
	- Store sera prior to administration of any blood products for future investigations if needed

In presence of hemolysis or severe anemia - Malarial parasite, malarial antigens - G6PD screening - Ceruloplasmin/urine copper - Leptospira antibodies	**In selected patients** - NS1 antigen, dengue serology - Autoimmune markers - Ceruloplasmin/urinary copper - Paracetamol level - Drug screen - Urine succinylacetone - Metabolites for fatty acid oxidation defects

@ Ammonia levels correlate poorly with encephalopathy
† When bilirubin levels are high, special filters fitted in the automated machines are required for reliable assessment of electrolytes and creatinine
$ Urea is a poor marker of renal function
# With ongoing hemolysis and blood transfusion falsely elevated levels of G6PD can occur

Investigations that need to be sent in a child with acute liver failure to assess the severity, possible etiology and complications are shown in Table 35.6.

Checking the serum paracetamol level 4 hours after ingestion can assess the risk of developing liver damage. Standard nomograms are available to determine the risk of liver toxicity. There is negligible risk of liver damage if the paracetamol level is less than 120 mg/l at 4 hours after ingestion. Blood levels taken before 4 hours of ingestion are not useful. Usually a paracetamol dose in excess of 150 mg/kg is considered as potentially toxic though this does not hold true if multiple agents are taken together or a child is getting excess dose of paracetamol continuously over several days[14].

There is virtually no role of obtaining a liver biopsy in a child with acute liver failure. This is a dangerous procedure in the presence of coagulopathy and is likely to show only necrosis of hepatocytes. Liver biopsy rarely alters the therapy in acute liver failure. However, if it is imperative to obtain a liver biopsy (e.g. autoimmune hepatitis presenting as an acute liver failure), transjugular biopsy may be performed.

MANAGEMENT

The treatment of ALF is mostly supportive to prevent complications and prolong survival in order to give chance to hepatocytes for spontaneous recovery. There are no specific or reliable drug to promote regeneration of hepatocytes. There is no standard recommended antiviral therapy for any of the hepatotropic viruses including HBV causing acute liver failure. However, for some conditions that may present as acute liver failure, specific therapy is available as shown in Table 35.7. Therefore, all these conditions must be aggressively looked for and appropriately managed.

Table 35.7 Conditions that may present as acute liver failure and have a specific therapy

Condition	Therapy
Acetaminophen toxicity	N-acetyl cysteine
Amanita (mushroom) poisoning	Penicillin
Herpes simplex	Acyclovir
Autoimmune hepatitis	Corticosteroids
Malaria	Quinine/Artemether
Enteric encephalopathy	Cefotaxime/Ceftriaxone
Wilson's disease	D-Penicillamine
Tyrosinemia	NTBC
Leptospirosis	Penicillin, doxycycline or tetracyclines

While managing children with ALF, certain medications or procedures must be avoided to prevent precipitation or worsening of the complications (Table 35.8).

Table 35.8 Medications and procedures to be avoided in a child with ALF

- Benzodiazepines and narcotics
- NSAIDs and paracetamol
- Aminoglycosides
- Contrast media
- Steroids
- Excessive diuresis or large volume paracentesis
- Fluid overload
- Excessive dietary protein
- Surgery

The supportive management of children with ALF is summarized in Table 35.9.

Table 35.9 Standard protocol for management of acute liver failure

- Raise head end (30°-45°) and maintain head in neutral position
- Inj. cefotaxime and cloxacillin
- IV fluids N/2 saline in 10% dextrose at two-third of maintenance after initial resuscitation (in presence of cerebral edema) to maintain serum sodium between 145-155 mEq/l
- KCL to be added as per serum potassium level
- Lactulose through NG tube
- Mannitol 20% 3-5 ml/kg/dose IV slow bolus 4-6 hourly for 6-8 doses in grade 3-4 encephalopathy
- Ranitidine 2 mg/kg IV 12 hourly
- Inj. vitamin K 5 mg SC or IV
- Adequate nutrition

Fluid and Metabolic Disturbances

Fluid disturbances. Initially aggressive volume resuscitation with normal saline, Ringer's lactate, plasma or blood is required in a significant proportion of patients. Most experts recommend two-third maintenance fluids along with CVP monitoring to achieve a dextrose concentration above 100 mg/dl and prevent or treat cerebral edema.

Metabolic acidosis. This is seen in approximately 30% of patients of acute liver failure following acetaminophen overdose, but occurs in only 5% of patients with acute liver failure due to other causes. Correction of fluid deficit will automatically correct the metabolic acidosis in most patients but in cases where this does not happen, sepsis or severe liver failure should be suspected.

Hypokalemia. Hypokalemia is common in patients with ALF. Hypokalemia can precipitate as well as worsen the severity of hepatic encephalopathy in patients with acute liver failure.

In addition, serum potassium levels often overestimate total body potassium because of leakage of potassium from the intracellular compartment and hence higher amounts of potassium need to be administered.

Metabolic alkalosis. Correction of hypokalemia often leads to correction of metabolic alkalosis.

Hyponatremia. Dilutional hyponatremia is common. SIADH and hepatorenal syndrome can further aggravate hyponatremia. Dilutional hyponatremia requires fluid restriction.

Hypernatremia. Lactulose and mannitol may contribute to increase in free water loss. Increased administration of fluids including via NG tube corrects the abnormality.

Hypoglycemia. Symptomatic hypoglycemia is common in most cases of ALF. Hypoglycemia should be promptly treated with 1 ml/kg of 50% dextrose intravenous infusion followed by preparation of maintenance fluids in 10% dextrose. The aim is to maintain blood glucose levels between 100 to 150 mg/dl. In situations where fluid restriction prevents maintenance of blood sugar, a 20% dextrose solution via a central line may have to be administered.

Super-added Infections

Nosocomial and super added bacterial infections are common in patients with acute liver failure. Almost two-thirds of patients develop intercurrent infections which are an important cause of death. Most infections are by 'gut' organisms and include *E. coli,* Salmonella, Klebsiella, Staphylococcus, and at a later stage fungal infections. Fungal infections are more common in patients on prolonged broad spectrum antibiotics and renal failure.

Patients with acute liver failure require ongoing monitoring for signs of infection, because bacteremia does not always manifest with typical clinical and laboratory features. Presence of fever, leukocytosis, positive cultures, unexplained drop in blood pressure, reduced urine output, worsening encephalopathy, severe acidosis and DIC are important correlates of sepsis and warrant aggressive investigations to identify the site and nature of pathogens. Septicemia may lead to multi-organ failure in patients with acute liver failure.

Although the initial investigations should be able to identify possible infections, prophylactic antibiotics form a major and important part of treatment regimen for acute liver failure because subtle or uncontrolled infections worsen the prognosis. Strict hand washing and all aseptic precautions must be strictly followed to reduce risk of nosocomial infections in patients with acute hepatic failure. The first line combination of antibiotics include a 3rd generation cephalosporin and cloxacillin. The change in antimicrobials and antifungals are guided by culture results and the nature of PICU flora.

Cerebral Edema

Cerebral edema is a major cause of mortality in patients with acute liver failure. Cerebral edema can lead to cerebral hypoxia, tonsillar herniation and death. A sustained rise of intracranial pressure (ICP) to 30 mmHg or more is suggestive of raised ICP. Most patients in grade III-IV encephalopathy will have raised ICP. Cerebral edema supervenes in 50-80% patients with ALF.

Cerebral edema presents as paroxysmal or sustained systemic hypertension and increase in the tone of the muscles of the arms and/or legs. Impaired or absent pupillary reflexes, bradycardia, increased reflexes and finally decerebrate posturing are other signs of raised ICP. In final stages marked hyperventilation, trismus, opisthotonos and respiratory arrest occurs. Headache and vomiting are uncommon. Unfortunately, there is poor correlation between the intracranial pressure and clinical signs. Papilledema is uncommon and CT scan is indicative of cerebral edema in only 30-60% patients.

Body movements, excessive and frequent handling of the patient, frequent suctioning or noxious stimuli tend to increase the intracranial pressure. Sustained severe hypoxemia or hypercapnia also raises the ICP, as does seizure activity. Management of cerebral edema is summarized in Table 35.10.

Mannitol, an osmotic diuretic, is used to lower the ICP. It is effective only in those patients in whom initial ICP is less than 60 mmHg. Serum osmolality should be monitored in patients receiving mannitol. The drug is contraindicated if serum osmolality exceeds 320 mOsm/kg. If renal failure develops, mannitol should be used only in combination with ultra-filtration. Steroids are not useful for treatment of cerebral edema in patients with ALF.

ICP monitoring device can be placed either in the epidural or subdural space. The aim of therapy is to keep the ICP below 20 mm Hg and cerebral

---

Table 35.10 Protocol for management of cerebral edema in acute liver failure

- Raise head end of the bed by 30°
- Place head in neutral position
- Ensure minimum handling of the patient
- Maintain serum sodium level between 145-155 mEq/l
- Elective ventilation (maintain $PaCO_2$ between 25-30 mm Hg)
- Mannitol 3 to 5 ml/kg/dose of 20% solution by rapid IV push; maximum 6-8 doses can be given at 4-6 hourly interval
- If there is no beneficial effect, thiopental infusion can be given to patients on ventilator and continuous blood pressure monitoring
- Prevent hyponatremia, acidosis and hypoglycemia

---

perfusion pressure above 50 mm Hg (Cerebral perfusion pressure = BP – ICP). Bleeding and infection are the main risk factors of this procedure. Hence it is rarely used in most settings but may be useful in centers where liver transplantation is performed. Transcranial Doppler has been found to be useful in assessing intracranial pressure but there is limited experience for its use.

Hepatic Encephalopathy

Hepatic encephalopathy has been defined as a complex neuropsychiatric syndrome characterized by a global depression of CNS functions, which may progress to impaired consciousness and coma. Irritability, restlessness and sleep disturbances are the most common early manifestations of hepatic encephalopathy. It is reversible and occurs due to exposure of the brain to various toxins that are not being excreted by the liver. Associated conditions that may result in neurological deterioration include hypoglycemia, sepsis, hypoxemia, occult seizures and cerebral edema.

The clinical presentation of hepatic encephalopathy may be variable and is summarized in Table 35.3. Progression from the early stages of hepatic encephalopathy to coma may occur in a matter of hours, despite therapy. Hence it is imperative that all children with ALF or those manifesting any features of encephalopathy are monitored closely.

Table 35.11 shows the guidelines for management of hepatic encephalopathy. Role of neomycin and L-dopa is limited and no longer recommended. Oral ampicillin and lactulose has been used with efficacy in the past and continues to be used; however no clear guidelines are available. There is good data for the use of rifaximin in adults but there is no experience of its use in children till date.

Table 35.11 Management protocol for hepatic encephalopathy

Lactulose
- 0.5 ml/kg/dose (maximum 30 ml/dose) oral or through NG tube four times/day at a rate adjusted to produce 2-4 loose stools per day; can be given as retention enema in case of GI bleed. Need to watch for dehydration and hypernatremia

Enteral feedings
- No restriction of proteins for Grade I and II encephalopathy; vegetable proteins are preferred.
- Micronutrients like vitamins B complex, C, E and zinc are recommended

Anticonvulsants (if seizures occur or in deep coma to control occult seizures)
- Phenytoin sodium 2-3 mg/kg/day

Combative behaviour
- Restrain the child to avoid injury, small doses of midazolam or haloperidol may be given

Bowel wash
- To be avoided unless patient is constipated as it may increase intra-cerebral pressure

Steps to prevent worsening of encephalopathy
- Avoid GI bleed or remove any blood that may be present in the GI tract
- Avoid sedatives as far as possible
- Avoid excessive handling and diuresis
- Watch and treat sepsis aggressively
- Watch and treat seizures (occult seizures are common in advanced hepatic encephalopathy)

Coagulopathy

Clinical and laboratory manifestations of coagulopathy include bruising and bleeding from mucosal surfaces, intracranial hemorrhage, as well as excessive bleeding associated with any invasive procedure. Prothrombin time is prolonged. Disseminated intravascular coagulation (DIC) is a common accompaniment of acute liver failure. Estimation of factor VIII level may be useful to distinguish between acute hepatic dysfunction and DIC. Direct measurement of factor VII has also been found to be useful in assessing prognosis.

The conventional approach for treatment of severe coagulopathy associated with acute liver failure includes administration of vitamin K in doses of 5-10 mg intravenously or subcutaneously per day to increase the concentration of vitamin K-dependent coagulation factors. Administration of fresh frozen plasma is recommended if invasive procedures are planned or if there is active bleed or when the INR exceeds 2 (or PT >60 seconds)[15]. To prevent gastrointestinal bleed, parenteral ranitidine or proton pump inhibitors should be administered. The use of NSAIDs and nasal intubation should be avoided.

Renal Failure

Renal failure can occur due to pre-renal azotemia as a result of decreased circulating blood volume, acute tubular necrosis (ATN), pigment nephropathy and functional renal failure also commonly referred to as "hepato-renal syndrome". Hepato-renal syndrome is defined as an unexplained progressive renal dysfunction without obvious histological lesions. Hepato-renal syndrome has a variable clinical course, but risk of mortality is uniformly high. There is enough evidence to suggest that events accompanied by absolute or relative hypovolemia due to septicemia, excessive use of diuretics, large volume paracentesis, and gastrointestinal bleeding, may predispose to the development of hepato-renal syndrome. Hepato-renal syndrome is suspected when there is decreasing urine output with increasing blood urea and creatinine. It is characterized by avid sodium retention and negligible urinary sodium loss. The urine analysis does not show any casts, proteins or cells and oliguria is unresponsive to volume expansion. In hepato-renal syndrome urinary sodium is less than 10 mEq/L, in contrast to ATN, where urinary sodium is more than 20 mEq/L.

The management of hepato-renal syndrome is unsatisfactory and therefore it is important to avoid nephrotoxic drugs (aminoglycosides, NSAIDS). Recovery occurs when hepatic dysfunction improves or when liver transplantation is performed. However, restricting sodium and water intake to two-thirds or less depending upon urine output, dialysis, terlipressin and low dose dopamine (2-5ug/kg/min) are recommended. Continuous hemo-filtration is recommended if there is renal failure. It must be remembered that high bilirubin levels interfere with creatinine estimation and may actually under-estimate it.

Nutrition

Nutrition is an important component of therapy for acute liver failure as the patient is in a catabolic state. Provision of adequate calories is imperative while supplying at least 0.8 g/kg/d of protein. Restriction of dietary proteins with subsequent progressive increments while assessing clinical tolerance is the cornerstone of nutritional therapy in acute liver failure. However, protracted nitrogen restriction must be avoided. A positive nitrogen balance may have beneficial effect on encephalopathy by promoting hepatic regeneration and increasing the capacity of muscles to detoxify ammonia. Modifying the composition of the diet and increasing the calories to nitrogen ratio may improve tolerance to proteins. At isonitrogen levels, vegetable and dairy products produce less encephalopathy than non-vegetarian sources of protein because of a higher content of branched chain amino acids. Fiber may be added to the diet as it increases the elimination of nitrogen products in the stools. Enteral administration of nutrients is preferable to parentral route because it lessens volume overload and risk of infection. Commercial formulas are now available with supplements of branched chain amino acids that may be useful.

Newer Therapies

N-acetyl cysteine. N-acetyl cysteine is a sulphahydryl group provider. It has traditionally been used for treatment of acetaminophen-induced acute liver failure where it is considered as a specific antidote. However, there are reports of its use in non-acetaminophen induced liver failure with some success[16,17]. It is now recommended in all liver failure.

L-Ornithine L-aspartate. L-Ornithine L-aspartate reduces the production of ammonia. It may be administered orally or parenterally but variable results have been noted. However, randomized controlled trials in children are not available and is not used in our unit.

Bioartificial liver. Bioartificial livers are recent advancements in the management of ALF but essentially remain experimental especially in children with liver failure.

Liver Transplantation

Liver transplantation is the therapy of choice for advanced liver failure and is fast becoming a possibility in India. In this context the prognostic factors in a child with acute liver failure assumes importance since one needs to decide which child is likely to benefit and survive following liver transplant. In addition, 'timing' of the transplant is crucial and a team of doctors need to decide it. Liver transplantation should be carried out only if the likelihood of survival following transplant is higher than recovery due to spontaneous regeneration in the diseased liver[18].

When a child with ALF manifests with following adverse features, he should be transferred to the Transplantation Center[15]. In India, because there is lack of insurance and awareness, the family should be mentally and monetarily prepared before the transfer.

- Hepatic coma Grade 2-3
- Prothrombin time >60 seconds
- Sudden decrease in transaminases without clinical improvement
- Bilirubin >20 mg/dl
- Decreasing or shrinking liver size
- Hypoglycemia
- Blood pH <7.3
- Wilson's disease presenting as acute liver failure

A number of prognostic factors of ALF have been proposed by many workers from all over the world including India[19]. A recent study from United Kingdom has shown that children with fulminant hepatic failure with severe coagulopathy, low alanine aminotransferase on admission and prolonged duration of illness before the onset of hepatic encephalopathy are more likely to require liver transplantation. Clinical and biochemical parameters that are incriminated with a high probability of death in patients of acute liver failure include prolonged prothrombin time, low factor V levels, high bilirubin levels, grade III/IV hepatic encephalopathy and electrolyte disturbances. A prolonged duration of jaundice (>2 weeks) before development of encephalopathy is a recognized poor prognostic factor.

King's criteria have been followed by several transplant centers which basically differentiate between acetaminophen (paracetamol) related and non-acetaminophen related hepatic failure[20]. The emphasis on the former is blood pH, prothrombin time and serum creatinine while in the latter group, age of the child, bilirubin level, duration of jaundice before onset of encephalopathy and coagulopathy are taken into consideration for making a decision.

Contraindications and complications of liver transplantation

The contraindications for emergency liver transplantation in patients with ALF include irreversible brain damage, severe ARDS, cerebral perfusion pressure (CPP) <40 mm Hg for more than 2 hours, sustained elevation of ICP of more than 50 mm Hg, septic shock, severe cardio-pulmonary disease, mitochondrial disorder, malignancy and AIDS.

The major constraints to the success of liver transplant in our country include extremely high cost and non-availability of donor (cadaveric) liver. In most centers in India live related donors are most commonly used for liver transplantation in children. The common complications following liver transplant include rejection, infections due to immuno-suppression, adverse reactions to drugs, reappearance of primary disease (e.g. Hepatitis B), tumors etc. However, the quality of life in most post transplant patients is quite good.

Following recovery from acute liver failure with or without transplantation, most children show complete recovery unless they have had irreversible brain damage or when acute disease occurred in a child having underlying chronic liver disease. Rarely, there have been instances of development of bone marrow failure after several weeks to months of the procedure and therefore transplant patients need a regular follow-up[21].

CONCLUSIONS

In summary, acute liver failure in children is rare but it is associated with high mortality. Most cases in our country are due to water-borne hepatotropic viruses HAV and HEV. The clinician must be aware of the early and the subtle signs of acute liver failure. The focus of therapy should be on prevention, early recognition and appropriate management of complications. Despite good intensive care, only 20%–30% children with advanced liver failure survive. Liver transplantation is the only effective therapy for this conditions. Family therapy including counseling, not giving false hope and administration of specific therapy for condition like Wilson disease, Hepatitis B and prevention of Hepatitis A among contacts are recommended.

REFERENCES

1. Squires RH, Shneider BL, Bucavalas J, *et al*. Acute liver failure in children: The first 348 patients in the pediatric acute liver failure study group. *J Pediatr* 2006; 148(5): 652-658.

2. Polson J and Lee WM. AASLD Position paper: The management of acute liver failure. *Hepatology* 2005; 41: 1179-1197.

3. O'Grady JG, Schalm SW, Williams R. Acute liver failure: redefining the syndromes. *Lancet* 1993; 342: 273-275.

4. Vohra P. Approach to metabolic liver disease in infants. *Pediatr Today* 2004; 7: 259-264.

5. Arora NK, Nanda SK, Gulati S, *et al*. Acute viral hepatitis types E, A, and B singly and in combination with acute liver failure in children in north India. *J Med Vir* 1996; 48: 215-221.

6. Chadha MS, Walimbe AM, Chobe LP, Arankalle VA. Comparison of etiology of sporadic acute and fulminant

viral hepatitis in hospitalized patients in Pune, India during 1978-81 and 1994-97. *Indian J Gastroenterol* 2003; 22:11-15.

7. Poovorawan Y, Hutagalung Y, *et al.* Dengue virus infection: A major cause of acute hepatic failure in Thai children. *Ann Trop Pediatr* 2006; 26: 17-23.

8. Durand P, Debray D, Mandel R, Baujard C, Branchereau S, Gauthier F, Jacquemin E, Devictor D. Acute liver failure in infancy: a 14-year experience of a pediatric liver transplantation center. *J Pediatr* 2001; 139:871-876.

9. Schwabe MJ, Dobyns WB, Burke B, Armstrong DL, Valproate-induced liver failure in one of two siblings with Alpers disease. *Pediatr Neurol* 1997; 16:337-343.

10. Medani G, Fox M, Oehen HP, *et al.* Fatal hepatotoxicity secondary to nimesulide. *Eur J Clin Pharmacol* 2002; 57: 919-920.

11. Fulminant Hepatic Failure In: Diseases of the Liver and Biliary System. Sherlock S, Dooley J (Eds), Ninth Edition, *Blackwell Scientific Publications.*

12. Dhawan A, Cheeseman P, Mieli-Vergani G. Acute liver failure in children. *Pediatric Transplant* 2004; 8:584-588.

13. Ozturk Y, Berktas S, Soylu OB, *et al.* Fulminant hepatic failure and serum phosphorous levels in children from the western part of Turkey. *Turk J Gastroenterol* 2010; 21: 270-274.

14. Savino F, Lupica MM, Tarasco V, *et al.* Fulminant hepatitis after 10 days of acetaminophen treatment at recommended dosage in an infant. *Pediatrics* 2011; 127(2):e 497-7.

15. Kelly DA. Managing liver failure. *Postgraduate Med J* 2002; 78: 660-667.

16. Ben Avi Z, Vaknin H, Tur-Kaspa R. N-acetylcysteine in acute hepatic failure (non-paracetamol induced). *Hepato Gastroenterol* 2000; 47: 786-789.

17. Sklar GE, Subramaniam M. Acetylcysteine treatment for non-acetaminophen induced acute liver failure. *Ann Pharmacother* 2004; 38:498-500.

18. Pinelli D, Spada M, Lucianetti A, *et al.* Transplantation for acute liver failure in children. *Transplant Proc* 2005; 37: 1146-1148.

19. Srivastava KL, Mittal A, Kumar A, *et al.* Predictors of outcome in fulminant hepatic failure in children. *Indian J Gastroenterol* 1998; 17:43-45.

20. O'Grady JG, Alexander GJ, Hayllar KM, Williams R. Early indicators of prognosis in fulminant hepatic failure. *Gastroenterology* 1998; 97:439-445.

21. Tung J, Hadzic N, Layton M, *et al.* Bone marrow failure in children with acute liver failure. *J Pediatr Gastroenterol Nutr* 2000; 31:557-561.

Section 4

36

Acute Gastrointestinal Bleeding

Surender K Yachha and Anshu Srivastava

Gastrointestinal bleeding is a common problem in children that may manifest as hematemesis, melena or hematochezia. Due to its alarming nature medical attention is sought early, which is helpful in prompt management. Children usually tolerate bleeding better due to non-existence of co-morbid conditions. However, their management has to be efficient and timely due to their small blood volumes and rapid depletion. The bleeding can occur from anywhere in the gastrointestinal tract and the following terms are used to describe it.

Upper gastrointestinal bleeding (UGIB) is defined as bleeding from a site proximal to the ligament of Trietz (at the level of duodenojejunal flexure).

Lower gastrointestinal bleeding (LGIB) is defined as bleeding from a site distal to ligament of Trietz.

Hematemesis refers to passage of blood in vomiting and suggests an UGI site of bleeding. The vomitus may be bright red or altered coffee-ground in color depending upon the severity of hemorrhage and the duration it stayed in contact with gastric juice.

Melena refers to passage of black tarry stools and suggests an UGI or small bowel site of bleeding. The combination of hematemesis and melena indicates that the bleeding is from the upper gastrointestinal tract and significant in amount.

Hematochezia is passage of bright red blood in stools and usually originates from colon. The site of bleeding may also be from small bowel if the bleeding is massive.

Hemobilia refers to bleeding from biliary tree.

Hemosuccus pancreaticus is a bleeding from the pancreas.

Obscure GI Bleed (OGIB) is defined as bleeding from gastrointestinal tract (GIT) that persists or recurs without any obvious etiology after a diagnostic esophagogastroduodenoscopy (OGD) and colonoscopy. It accounts for ~5% of all GI bleeds and is classified into two types:

Occult OGIB manifests with stool occult blood positivity and/or iron deficiency anemia.

Overt OGIB manifests as visible blood in stool and/or vomitus

UGIB is more common and often massive than LGIB in children. For the purpose of a better understanding we shall discuss them separately although it should be remembered that the initial resuscitation and supportive treatment is the same irrespective of the site of bleeding. Also patients with coagulopathy or thrombocytopenia can have both UGIB and LGIB at the same time.

UPPER GASTROINTESTINAL BLEEDING

The causes of hemorrhage from UGI tract vary in different age groups and can be broadly divided into neonatal-infant and older child groups as shown in Table 36.1. There are very few Indian studies on UGIB in children (Table 36.2)[1, 2]. Differences in the etiology between the two centers is perhaps due to the fact that one is a specialist gastroenterology center and the other is a general pediatric hospital. Also in the second study only UGI endoscopy was done to find out the cause of bleeding. Varices, esophagitis and gastritis are the commonest causes of UGIB in Indian children.

CLINICAL FEATURES

A detailed history and clinical examination along with resuscitation and evaluation of the etiology of bleed should be done simultaneously as shown in the flow chart (Figure 36.1). The aims of clinical evaluation are listed below:

Determine that the patient has really bled and the bleeding is from the gastrointestinal tract. In patients with minor bleed and no hemodynamic changes especially if the history appears unreliable one should differentiate bleed

Table 36.1 Causes of upper gastrointestinal bleeding

Neonate/Infant	Children >2 years
▫ Swallowed maternal blood	▫ Esophagitis due to reflux, drugs, infections
▫ Hemorrhagic disease of the newborn (HDN)	▫ Mallory-Weiss tear
▫ Esophagitis	▫ Caustic ingestion
▫ Gastritis	▫ Trauma, foreign body
▫ Gastroduodenal ulceration	▫ Portal hypertension causing esophageal/gastric varices; congestive gastropathy; gastric antral vascular ectasia (GAVE)
▫ Vascular malformation	▫ Gastritis
▫ Esophageal duplication	▫ Peptic ulcer (duodenal/gastric ulcer)
▫ Sepsis/coagulopathy	▫ Vascular malformation, Henoch-Schonlein purpura, sepsis/coagulopathy
▫ Rare: Antral/duodenal webs, gastric cardia prolapse, heterotopic pancreatic tissue	▫ Tumors: Leiomyoma, lymphoma. Rare: gastrointestinal duplication, hemobilia, radiation gastritis, Munchausen's syndrome by proxy

Table 36.2 Indian series on upper gastrointestinal bleeding

Cause	Mittal et al 1994 (n = 236)[2]	Yachha et al 1996 (n = 75)[1]	Yachha et al SGPGI 2000-10 experience (n= 235)
Varices (esophageal or gastric)	39.5%	95%	81.7%
Esophagitis	23.7%	-	-
Gastritis/gastric erosions	7.2%	1.3%	6.8%
Gastric ulcer/duodenal ulcer	1.6%	-	3%
Esophageal ulcer	0.5%	-	0.4% (drug related)
EST/EVL related ulcer	-	-	4.3%
Henoch-Schonlein purpura	-	1.3%	-
Idiopathic thrombocytopenic purpura	-	1.3%	0.9%
Splenic/pancreaticoduodenal artery aneurysm	-	1.3%	0.9%
Cow's milk allergy	-	-	0.4%
Unknown	27.5%	none	1.7%

from coloring agents (beetroot, drugs like iron and bismuth). It is important to differentiate GI bleed from epistaxis, hemoptysis or oromucosal bleeding by history and examination.

Assess the hemodynamic status and extent of intravascular volume depletion. Heart rate, blood pressure, pulse volume, poor peripheral perfusion, peripheral cyanosis and urine output are important parameters to be monitored. Oliguria can develop secondary to reduced renal perfusion. Increase in heart rate by 20 beats per minute and drop in systolic blood pressure by 10 mm Hg from basal level are reliable markers of significant blood loss in children. Measurement of central venous

pressure if possible is very helpful in selected situations e.g. persistence of hemodynamic compromise despite volume correction and renal failure.

Identify the site of bleeding i.e. UGIB versus LGIB. This is essential to identify the site of bleeding as the investigative protocol and management differs in the two conditions. Presence of hematemesis and melena with hemodynamic instability suggests an UGI source while passage of bright red blood in stools points to LGIB. But sometimes brisk or massive bleed from an UGI source may also lead to passage of bright red blood in stools. Elevation of BUN secondary to absorption

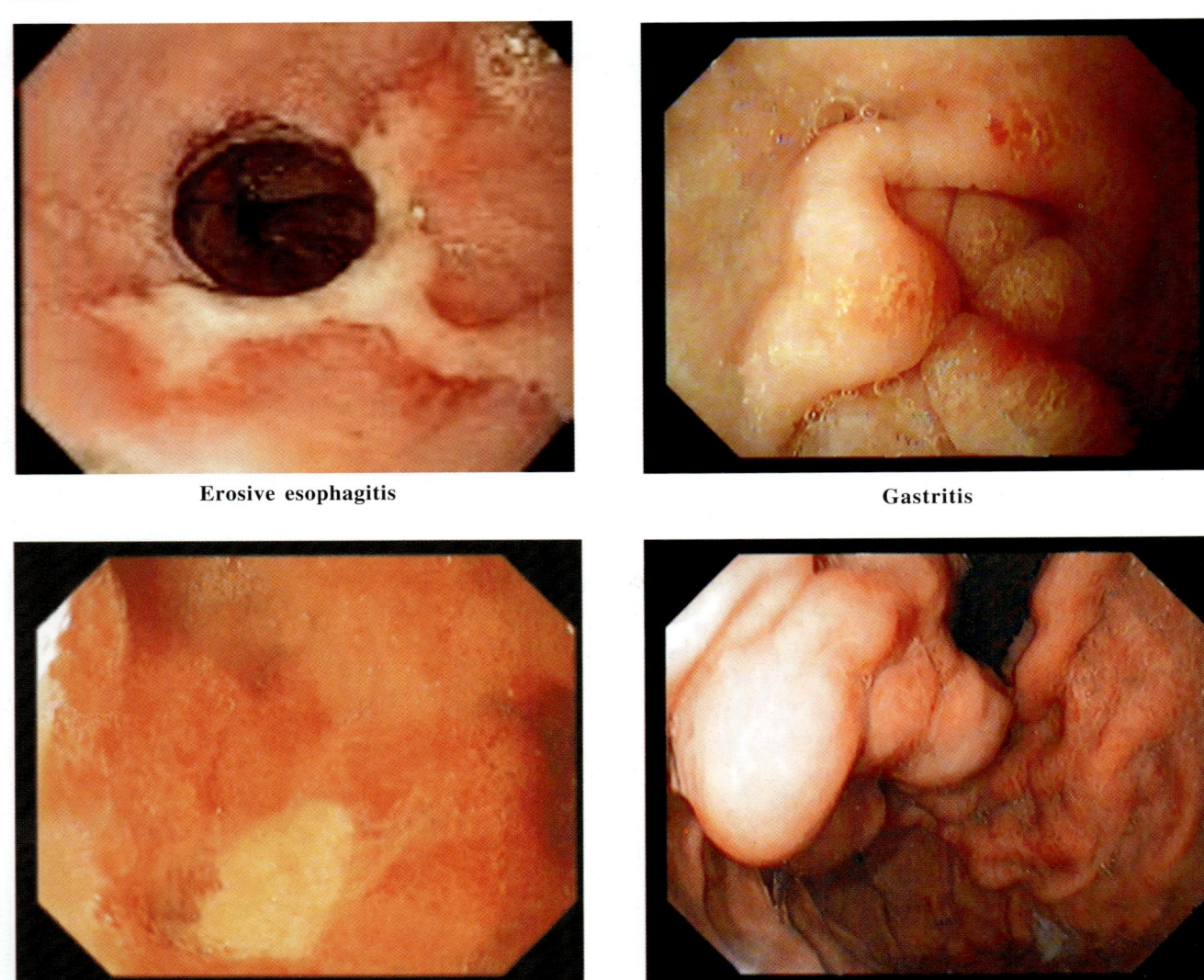

Figure 36.1 Endoscopic appearance of common causes of upper gastrointestinal bleeding

of intestinal blood also points to an UGI cause. In a child with massive bleeding, UGIB is more likely and it should be ruled out by placement of a nasogastric (NG) tube and subsequently confirmed by upper gastrointestinal endoscopy before proceeding to other invasive investigations. *It is important to remember that absence of blood in the NG aspirate does not rule out an UGI source of bleed.* Nasogastric tube should be left *in-situ* for gravity drainage to detect any recurrence of bleeding for 24 hours and vigorous NG suction should be avoided to prevent mucosal trauma[3].

Determine the likely cause of bleeding. Ask for history of ingestion of aspirin, NSAID, steroids or anticoagulants, presence of heart burn, regurgitation, abdominal pain, foreign body ingestion,

corrosive intake, jaundice, blood transfusion, surgery in the past, previous episodes of hematemesis, family history of peptic ulcer and inflammatory bowel disease. *Painless passage of large amount of blood in vomitus points towards variceal bleeding.* One should always look for features of liver disease like splenomegaly, jaundice, ascites, etc. In portal hypertension (PHT) the spleen may reduce in size, just after a bout of massive hematemesis and thus missed on examination. In coagulopathy and thrombocytopenia there will be evidences of bleeding from multiple sites.

LABORATORY INVESTIGATIONS

Investigations are aimed at establishing the site, severity and cause of bleeding. These can be broadly divided into two groups:

To determine the severity of bleeding

- Hematocrit (HCT) and hemoglobin should be monitored frequently to assess the severity of blood loss. Fall in hemoglobin (Hb) is documented after a few hours once hemodilution has occurred.

To determine the cause of bleeding

- Coagulation profile (PT/APTT) may be deranged in DIC/liver disease.

- Platelet count is reduced in idiopathic thrombocytopenic purpura and in portal hypertension (PHT) secondary to hypersplenism.

- Liver function tests, urea, creatinine, and electrolytes.

- In a neonate Apt test is useful to differentiate between fetal bleeding and swallowed maternal blood.

- UGI endoscopy under conscious sedation or general anesthesia is done after the patient is hemodynamically stable. Protection of airway is very important as the risk of aspiration is high when the patient is actively bleeding. UGI endoscopy is extremely useful for evaluating the cause and site of bleeding and also for treating the lesion.[4,5] A complete examination of esophagus, stomach and duodenum with retroflexion to inspect the fundus and gastroesophageal junction is essential. The main reasons for missing a lesions are (i) delayed endoscopy when the lesion is not actively bleeding, (ii) lesion being obscured by blood and (iii) pallor of lesion due to anemia and volume contraction. One should always make an attempt to adequately evaluate the commonly missed sites on endoscopy like upper part of fundus, posterior and inferior wall of duodenum, high lesser curvature, anastomotic site (gastrojejunostomy) and hiatus hernia.

- Ultrasound examination of abdomen is useful for confirming the existence of PHT in subjects with hematemesis and evaluation of mass lesions.

- Selective angiography of celiac trunk may be done occasionally when vascular lesions are suspected as discussed below.

- Once the cause of bleeding is identified, the management is done accordingly as discussed below along with general supportive measures.

MANAGEMENT

It is largely dependant upon the severity and site of bleeding. Patients with minor bleed have normal cardiovascular status, those with moderate bleed have orthostatic hypotension and tachycardia whereas presence of shock, tachycardia and altered mentation is a feature of massive bleed. Urgent management is required for patients with massive GI bleed.

General Supportive Measures

- Good venous access (2 intravenous lines in subjects with massive bleed), intake output monitoring, oxygen inhalation and charting of vitals is mandatory.

- Hemodynamic resuscitation with blood transfusion and crystalloid/colloid infusion for maintenance and to replace the ongoing losses.

- Correction of coagulopathy and thrombocytopenia by fresh frozen plasma (FFP) and/or platelet transfusion.

- Correction of electrolytes and acid base abnormalities.

Specific Treatment

It can be broadly subdivided into two groups; variceal and non-variceal.

Variceal Bleeding

In a child with portal hypertension, esophageal varices are the commonest cause of UGI bleeding. Gastric varices, congestive gastropathy and gastric antral vascular ectasia (GAVE) can also present with hematemesis. The various therapeutic options to stop bleeding are discussed below[6]. It is important not to overtransfuse a patient with variceal bleeding and a target hemoglobin of about 7-8 g/dl or HCT of 22-24% should be maintained because over-transfusion can cause a rebound increase in portal pressure and precipitate early rebleeding. Fresh frozen plasma and platelets (platelet count of <50,000/ ml) are often used to correct coagulopathy but its exact role needs to be studied further[7]. Short-term antibiotic prophylaxis (third generation cephalosporin for 7 days), a measure that reduces bacterial infections, variceal rebleeding, and death should be used in every child with cirrhosis admitted with gastrointestinal hemorrhage.

The choice of treatment for controlling the bleed in any given patient depends upon the availability of therapeutic options, condition of the patient at presentation and the expertise of the available personnel.

Pharmacological Therapy

Somatostatin and octreotide. These drugs decrease the splanchnic and azygous blood flow thus reducing the pressure in the varices and they also reduce the gastric secretions. Overall this therapy is well tolerated, with mild side effects like hyperglycemia, abdominal discomfort, nausea and diarrhea which often resolve spontaneously. Somatostatin and octreotide are both equally effective. Limited studies in children have shown control of bleeding in 64-71% children [8,9]. The doses are as shown in Table 36.3. Infusion should be given for at least 24-48 hours after the bleeding has stopped to prevent recurrence and care should be taken not to stop the infusion abruptly. In adults the infusion is usually continued for 5 days to prevent early rebleeding.

Vasopressin. It acts by increasing the splanchnic vascular tone and thus reducing portal blood flow [10]. It has a half life of 30 minutes and usually is given as an initial bolus followed by continuous intravenous infusion. When vasopressin infusion is unable to control the bleeding or serious side effects such as hypertension, seizures or cardiac arrhythmia occur; the infusion of vasopressin should be abandoned. It is effective in about 50% of children with variceal bleeding.

Terlipressin is a synthetic analogue of vasopressin. It acts by reducing portal pressure and blood flow through collaterals. It is given as 2 mg intravenous injection every 4 hours in adults till a bleed free period of 24-48 hours is obtained. It is preferred over vasopressin as it needs no infusion, cardiac side effects are minimal and it has been shown to reduce mortality in adults [11]. But pediatric data is not available regarding the utility and safety of the drug.

Nitroglycerine. It is a potent vasodilator and is useful in reducing the side effects of vasopressin. Trials in children are not available.

In adult patients with variceal bleed, two meta-analyses have shown that EST is not superior to vasoactive drugs for control of acute bleeding, reduced transfusion needs, deaths or adverse events [12] and that a combination of endoscopic therapy (sclerotherapy or band ligation) plus vasoactive drugs (somatostatin, octreotide or vapreotide) is better than endoscopic therapy alone in controlling the bleeding both initially and at day 5 although the mortality remained the same [13]. Both these trials are in adults with cirrhosis and no similar data is available for children. In children, octreotide (which is less expensive) therapy should be started

Table 36.3 Drugs and their dosages for GI bleeding	
Drug	**Dose and comments (ref 33)**
Antacids	0.5-1.0 ml/kg q 4 hr PO, titrate to keep gastric pH >4
Ranitidine	2-4 mg/kg/day PO q 8-12 hr, max 10 mg/kg/d (300 mg per day) 2-4 mg/kg/day IV q 8-12 hr
Sucralfate	0.5-1.0 g PO q 6 hr
Proton pump inhibitors (PPI)	Omeprazole 0.7-3.3mg/kg/day single or 2 div doses Lansoprazole 15 mg/day if weight <30 kg; 30 mg if weight >30 kg. Esomeprazole 10 mg/d if weight <20 kg; 20 mg if weight >20 kg. PPI infusion for ulcer bleed: intravenous pantoprazole 2 mg/kg (max 80 mg) loading followed by 0.2 mg/kg/hr infusion (max 8 mg/hr)
Vasopressin	IV bolus 0.33 u/kg over 20 min and then same amount every hour as a constant infusion
Octreotide	1μg/kg bolus and then 1μg/kg/hr infusion, max 5 μg /kg/hr
Somatostatin	250 μg bolus and then 250 μg/hr infusion in adults. Pediatric dose is not established
Anti-*H. pylori* (PPI+ 2/3 antibiotics) PPI Amoxycillin Clarithromycin Metronidazole	 As above 50 mg/kg/day (max dose 2 g) in BD doses PO 20 mg/kg/day (max dose 1g) in BD doses PO 20 mg/kg/day (max dose 1g) in BD doses PO

urgently for control of variceal bleeding and endoscopic treatment should be offered at the earliest possible after resuscitation.

Tamponade of Varices

Sangstaken-Blakemore tube (SBT) is a triple lumen tube with connection to an esophageal balloon, a gastric balloon and one perforated distal end which helps in aspiration of the stomach contents. Experience, choice of appropriate size of tube and observation of simple precautions ensures success of this procedure[3, 14]. An appropriate sized, pediatric SBT is passed through the nose and allowed to reach the stomach, gastric balloon is then inflated with 75-150 ml of air depending on the size of the patient (stomach) and tube is gently pulled outwards till it sits snugly against the upper dome of stomach and diaphragm. Care should be taken to avoid any respiratory embarrassment. Plain X-ray film should be done to check the proper placement of gastric balloon in the stomach. If the bleeding persists, the esophageal balloon should be inflated with an air pressure of 20 mm Hg that can be maintained and monitored with the help of a sphygmomanometer. Gastric contents should be allowed to drip under the effect of gravity and without the application of negative suction. Above the esophageal balloon, the secretions tend to accumulate which should be removed with a catheter. The esophageal balloon should be deflated after 12-24 hours and the stomach irrigated to watch for further bleeding. If bleeding continues, the balloon compression is re-instituted for another 8-12 hours.

Failure to control the bleeding with SBT may be due to gastric varices or duodenal varices and unusual causes of bleeding. The SB tube is relatively cheap, requires little skill vis-à-vis EST and has efficacy of above 75 percent in controlling acute variceal bleeding. Adequate sedation is important both for patient comfort and compliance. Esophageal necrosis and perforation, pulmonary aspiration and rebleeding on deflation of balloon are important complications. Linton-Nachlas tube has a larger gastric balloon and is used for tamponade of gastric varices.

Endoscopic Therapy

Esophageal Varices

Sclerotherapy of varices (EST). Skill in performing the procedure and availability of proper sized fiberoptic endoscopes and appropriate sclerosing agents are essential for the success of the procedure. The varices are inspected and their location, size and extent are documented with a fiber-optic endoscope. A flexible needle is inserted through the endoscope to inject 2-3 ml of sclerosant (1 per cent ethoxysclerol) into the engorged vessel. At each session, 5-8 injections are given at various sites beginning at the gastroesophageal junction (Figure 36.2). Following emergency EST, the varices are then sclerosed at intervals of 2-3 weeks until all varices are obliterated. Emergency EST is very effective (>90 percent) in controlling esophageal variceal bleeding[8, 15]. Transient fever and retrosternal discomfort are the commonest complaints after sclerotherapy and is seen in nearly one-third of subjects. Major complications include esophageal ulceration (13-32%), perforation (1.0-1.4%), and stricture of esophagus (4.3-18%)[16-18].

Endoscopic variceal ligation (EVL) is done with a device called multiple band ligator. The band ligator has an outer cylinder that is fitted with multiple bands (4-6 in number in different brands) on the inner side along with an attached trip wire for firing the bands on to the varix. The whole assembly of multiple band ligator is fitted on to the endoscope that is passed into the esophagus of the patient. First a diagnostic UGI endoscopy is done to note the details of the varices and thereafter the scope is removed, banding apparatus is loaded on the scope and the scope is reintroduced. The variceal column is sucked into the outer cylinder and the band is deployed by pulling the trip wire around a part of mucosa containing the offending varix (Figure 36.3). Ligations are repeated around the circumference of the esophagus in a spiral fashion. One or two bands are applied to each varix in the distal esophagus. Subsequently, at each ligation site, a superficial ulcer develops when the rubber band and necrotic ligated tissue sloughs. These ulcers are not as deep as those seen after EST. Due to the size of the currently available ligators (not available for pediatric scope), EVL can easily be performed in children >2 years of age and it is desirable to give sedation in order to minimize the risk and increase the ease of performing the procedure.

Although experience in children is limited, but EVL has been shown to have a 90-100% efficacy in controlling acute bleeding.[19] McKiernan et al[20] found re-bleeding in 2/26 (7.6%) children and complications in 6/28 (21%) subjects in the form of bleeding close to the site of banding in 2 and retrosternal discomfort in 4 subjects. The bleeding was stopped in the same endoscopy session by application of another band. EVL is also not feasible

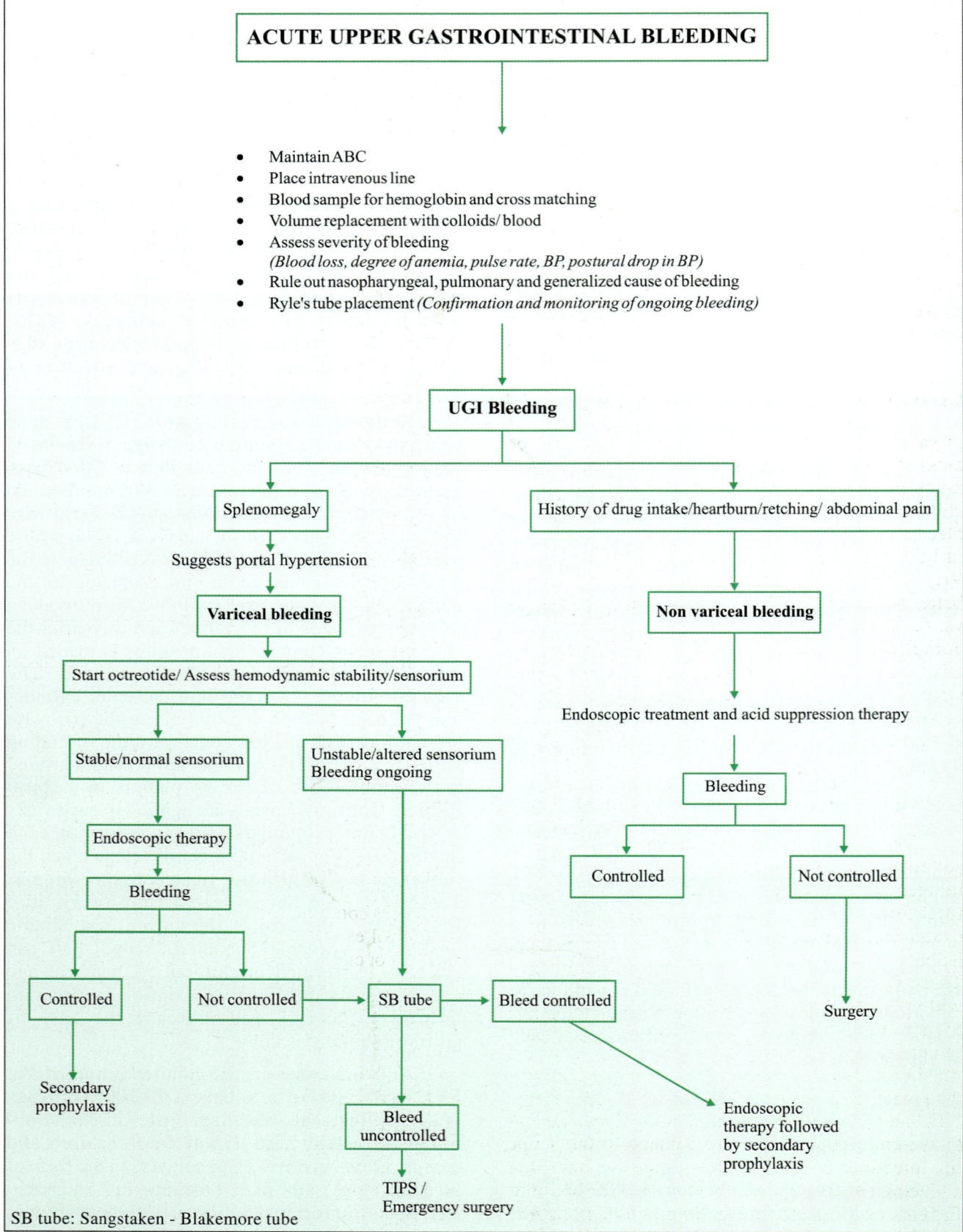

Figure 36.2 Algorithm for management of acute upper G1 bleeding

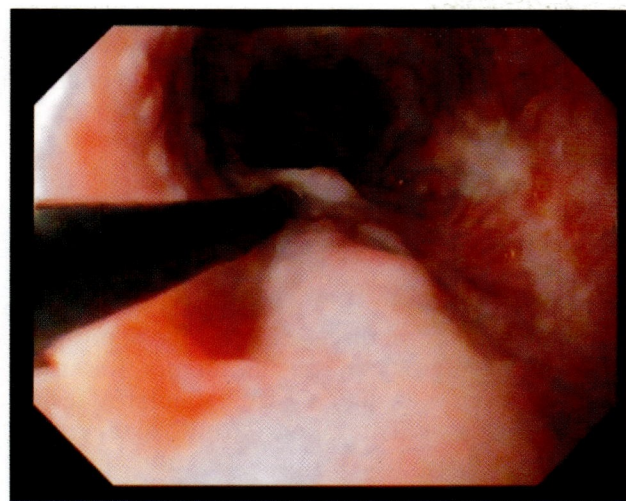

Endoscopic sclerotherapy (EST)

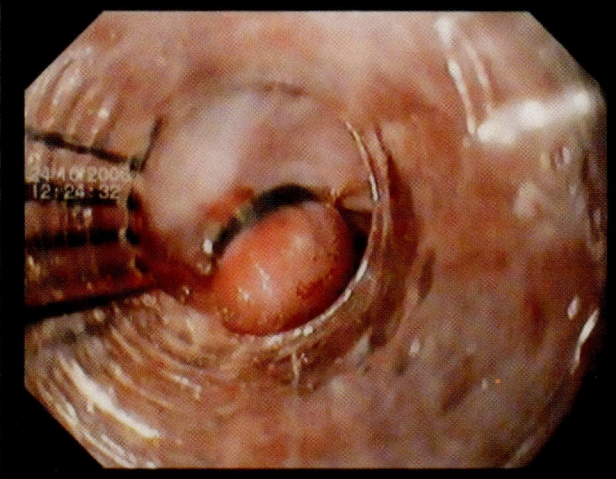

Endoscopic variceal ligation (EVL)

Figure 36.3 Endoscopic treatment of esophageal varices [Sclerotherapy (EST) and band ligation (EVL)]

in small varices (grades I/II) and these should be tackled by EST during eradication therapy. In a randomized controlled trial of EST versus EVL in children by Zargar et al [8], the efficacy of controlling bleeding and rate of variceal eradication was similar in both groups (100% in both) and (96% EST vs 91.7% EVL.) respectively but overall EVL was better as it required lesser number of sessions (3.9 vs. 6.1), had lower re-bleeding (4% vs. 26%) and complication rate (4% vs. 25%). EVL has the advantage that it does not lead to esophageal stricture formation. One study, using clipping apparatus has shown 99.3% success rate of ligation at first attempt with no recurrence and rebleeding on follow-up of 9-48 months [21].

Gastric Varices

The gastric varices are known to bleed more severely than esophageal varices, though the incidence of bleeding is much less. Endoscopic injection of tissue adhesive (glue) N-butyl 2 cyanoacrylate (marketed in India as Nectacryl) or isobutyl 2 cyanoacrylate is used for gastric varices. These two agents are tissue adhesives that harden within 20 seconds of contact with blood, and lead to more rapid control of active bleeding compared to conventional EST. The technique has a risk of causing damage to endoscope directly by glue if the precautions are not taken during the procedure. Silicone oil should be smeared along the distal end of the endoscope to prevent damage to the scope tip. Injections of 0.1 to 1.0 ml of glue are made into a bleeding varix depending upon the size of varix. Patients may develop rebleeding due to sloughing and ulceration after glue injection which may require surgical intervention. Although this has been established as an effective treatment modality in adults [22], there are very few studies of efficacy of glue injection for gastric varices in children [23]. In the experience of authors glue injection is safe and highly effective for control of bleeding from gastric varices.

Transjugular Intrahepatic Portosystemic Shunt (TIPS)

It involves insertion of a multipurpose catheter through the jugular vein and superior vena cava with the aid of the puncture device. The catheter is passed via hepatic vein into a branch of portal vein through the hepatic parenchyma. The passage is dilated by a balloon and an expansile metallic mesh prosthesis is placed to maintain the communication directly between the portal vein and hepatic vein. This procedure results in bypassing liver resistance and consequently decreases the portal pressure. Experience of this procedure in children is limited [24]. The most common indication for TIPS is inability to control esophageal/gastric variceal bleeding by medical or endoscopic measures in cirrhotic patients who have a patent spleno-portal axis. This procedure is not feasible in patients with extrahepatic portal venous obstruction (EHPVO) due to thrombosed portal vein. Overall success rate is 75-85% in children [25] and an abnormal vascular anatomy is the most common cause of failure. Adverse events include precipitation of encephalopathy and shunt occlusion. TIPS placement is expensive and needs expertise which is available only in a few centers in India. Fortunately this procedure is needed less often in children who mostly have EHPVO and in whom the bleeding is usually controlled easily. TIPS is

Section 4

mostly used as a bridging measure in children with cirrhosis and complicated portal hypertension awaiting liver transplantation.

Surgical Management

Emergency surgery is the only option available in situations where endoscopic and medical therapy fails. It is also required when bleeding is from ectopic varices that cannot be effectively controlled by endoscopic procedures. Hepatic disease and dysfunction should be assessed before contemplating shunt surgery. Surgery can be done either in the form of portocaval shunt (selective or nonselective) or devascularization with esophageal staple transection. The results of shunt surgery have improved in the last couple of years and reports have confirmed feasibility and efficacy of shunt surgery in children with portal hypertension[26]. Rex shunt is done by placement of a jugular auto graft between the left branch of portal vein and superior mesenteric vein in subjects with EHPVO. It has the advantage of maintaining the hepatopetal blood flow[27]. But as the procedure needs expertise and lacks long term follow-up data, its use is still limited.

Nearly two-thirds of subjects with PHT develop a re-bleed after the first variceal bleed, therefore secondary prophylaxis is a must after initial control of bleeding. alpha-blockers, EST and EVL are all effective in reducing the risk of re-bleeding. There is limited data regarding the use of propranolol in children and at present endoscopic treatment with EVL is preferable compared to EST especially for older children. A useful strategy in children would be to start with EVL and thereafter to do EST when the varices are small and difficult to band, so as to ensure faster variceal eradication with less side effects[28]. As there is a risk of esophageal variceal recurrence in ~10%, with appearance of new gastric varices and/or portal hypertensive gastropathy, these patients should be under regular follow up.

To summarize, acute variceal bleeding (AVB) is a dreaded complication of patients with PHT. Initial management includes appropriate fluid replacement, blood transfusion to attain a target hemoglobin level of ~ 8 g/dl and antibiotic prophylaxis in cirrhotics. Standard of care mandates for early administration of vasoactive drug therapy followed by EVL or EST (if EVL cannot be performed) within the first 12 hours of the index bleed. The use of pharmacologic agents may be prolonged for up to 5 days. Patients who fail endoscopic therapy may require balloon tamponade followed by TIPS or surgical management if the bleed is still uncontrolled. All patients surviving an episode of AVB should undergo further secondary prophylaxis to prevent rebleeding.

Non-variceal Bleeding (NVB)

The causes of non-variceal UGI bleeding include peptic ulcer, Mallory-Weiss tears, erosions secondary to stress, medications and trauma from foreign bodies etc, esophagitis, gastritis, inflammatory bowel disease like Crohn's, prolpase gastropathy, angiodysplasia and tumors. Rarer but important causes include CMA[29], dieulafoy lesion (submucosal "caliber-persistent" artery that protrudes through a minute 2-5 mm mucosal defect)[30], arteriovenous malformations, hemobilia, hemosuccus pancreaticus, and aortoenteric fistulas developing secondary to foreign bodies in GI tract[31]. In children esophagitis, ulcers or erosions are important causes of non-variceal bleeding. The majority of nonvariceal upper gastrointestinal bleeds will not rebleed once treated successfully.

Duodenal and gastric ulcers occur in children secondary to *H. pylori* infection, NSAID and other drugs, stress, Crohn's disease etc[32]. In a pediatric series of 67 cases with peptic ulcer; 32 (47.7%) had *Helicobacter pylori* infection and 11 (16.5%) had previous use of non-steroidal anti-inflammatory drugs (NSAIDs). Non-*H. pylori,* non-NSAID peptic ulcer disease was found in 24 (35.8%) patients. The, *H. pylori*-related peptic ulcer disease was associated with familial peptic ulcer and the presence of duodenal ulcer. However, short-term NSAID use was correlated highly with gastric ulcers[33]. The overall outcome of childhood peptic ulcer disease is good if treated adequately. A recent population-based survey from France in children showed that UGIB could be attributable to the use of NSAIDs, including ibuprofen and aspirin, in approximately one third of cases[34]. The findings of this study call for more caution in prescribing NSAIDs to children and use of drugs like acetaminophen for antipyretic and analgesic action, particularly in patients with medical risk factors for UGIB.

Intravenous proton pump inhibitors (PPI) should be initiated in any patient suspected to have non-variceal bleeding from the upper gastro-intestinal tract[35]. Intravenous PPIs are available as various preparations (e.g. omeprazole, pantoprazole, esomeprazole) and there is no current consensus about the drug of choice. High-dose infusion PPI is thought to promote clot stability and facilitate hemostasis by raising the intragastric pH.

An early and meticulous UGI endoscopy done after resuscitation of the patient is essential both for finding the cause of NVB and offering therapy. A prokinetic is a useful adjunct to endoscopy in patients who have large amounts of blood clots in their stomach (as seen endoscopically or suspected when persistent hematemesis occurs) and in patients who have recently consumed food and require urgent endoscopy.

Endoscopic biopsy should be taken in esophagitis/gastritis. In peptic ulcer disease, antral and corpus biopsies are taken for diagnosis of *H. pylori* that includes tissue diagnosis using combination of rapid urease test, culture, Gram staining and histology. In subjects with diffuse mucosal bleeding, the aim is to increase the pH of the stomach. Neutralizing the acid with various drugs as shown in Table 36.3 is the main stay of therapy in this condition[36]. Anti-*H. pylori* medications are given for eradication of infection to prevent ulcer recurrence in subjects with *H. pylori* positive ulcer disease. Specific antifungals and anti-viral therapy is required for infectious esophagitis. Stoppage of an offending drug like NSAID is a must for prompt recovery.

Endoscopic treatment is effective in patients with focal sites of bleeding[37]. Injection, electro coagulation and heater probes are all equally effective and can be used for peptic ulcers with active bleeding/visible vessel or adherent clot[38]. Adrenaline and hypertonic saline are preferred for injection therapy and care should be taken to avoid alcohol injection in children as it can lead to necrosis and ulceration[39]. Hemoclips can be applied on vessels e.g. Dieulafoy's lesion to stop the bleeding.

Argon plasma coagulation (APC) which is a non contact form of monopolar coagulation, has the advantage of limited depth of penetration. In a study of 12 children with GI bleeding, the bleeding was controlled in 8 (66%) and transfusion requirement was decreased in 3 (25%) patients[40]. It is a very useful method for controlling bleeding from vascular lesions, gastric antral vascular ectasia (GAVE) and radiation gastritis. Step-wise management of acute upper GI bleeding is summarized in Figure 36.1.

PREVENTION

In the following high risk situations it is useful to institute certain therapeutic measures to prevent occurrence of first episode of bleeding or its recurrence:

- Nearly 10% of ICU subjects have evidence of UGI bleeding but clinically significant bleeding is seen in <2%. Patients with coagulopathy, respiratory failure and high PRISM (pediatric risk of mortality score >10) are at an increased risk of bleeding[41]. Prophylactic acid neutralizing therapy may be helpful in reducing the risk of bleeding in this high risk group.

- Secondary prophylaxis for variceal bleeding as discussed above.

- *H. pylori* eradication therapy to prevent recurrence of peptic ulcer.

LOWER GASTROINTESTINAL BLEEDING

The causes of LGIB are divided into two groups; neonatal–infants and older children as shown in Table 36.4. Studies regarding etiology of

Section 4

Table 36.4 Causes of lower gastrointestinal bleeding	
Neonates/Infants	**Children >2 years**
❑ Anorectal fissure	❑ Polyps
❑ Infectious colitis	❑ Solitary rectal ulcer syndrome (SRUS)
❑ Allergic colitis	❑ Anal fissure
❑ Necrotizing enterocolitis	❑ Hemorrhoids
❑ Hirschsprung's enterocolitis	❑ Rectal varices/colopathy
❑ Intussusception/duplication cyst	❑ Inflammatory bowel disease (ulcerative colitis, Crohn's disease)
❑ Arteriovenous malformation	❑ Pseudomembranous colitis
❑ Rectal prolapse	❑ infectious colitis
❑ Meckel's diverticulum	❑ Henoch Schonlein purpura, Hemolytic uremic syndrome
❑ Coagulopathy, disseminated intravascular coagulopathy, hemorrhagic disease of the newborn	❑ Arteriovenous malformation
	❑ Meckel's diverticulum
	❑ Disseminated intravascular coagulopathy

LGIB in children from India show that colitis, polyps and solitary rectal ulcer syndrome (SRUS) constitute the main causes of LGIB (Table 36.5).

CLINICAL EVALUATION

History and physical examination helps in narrowing down the differential diagnosis of LGIB. A sick preterm infant with abdominal distension, blood in stools, feed intolerance and systemic instability is likely to have necrotizing enterocolitis (NEC). Delayed passage of meconium followed by constipation, abdominal pain and distension is seen in Hirschsprung's disease. Allergic colitis is mostly seen in infants who are top fed with cow's milk and usually present with anemia and loose stools mixed with blood. Crampy abdominal pain and stool mixed with blood and mucus, suggests infectious, inflammatory or ischemic colitis. Onset of bloody diarrhea after antibiotic use points towards pseudomembranous colitis. It is important to remember that community-acquired antibiotic associated bloody diarrhea (CABD) is not uncommon even in infants and highlights the importance of rational use of antibiotics[44].

Presence of extraintestinal manifestations like aphthous ulcers, joint pains and iritis are recognized extra intestinal manifestations of inflammatory bowel disease (IBD). History of painful defecation and passage of hard stools along with blood streaking of stools is seen in anal fissure. In a patient with history of constipation, straining at stools and digital evacuation, the most likely cause of bleeding is SRUS. Intussusception is characterized by episodes of pain, vomiting and red currant-jelly stools i.e. mixture of blood, mucoid exudates and stool. Painless bleeding is seen commonly in polyps, Meckel's diverticulum, ulcer or vascular anomaly. Venous malformations and hemangiomas are commonly associated with LGIB. Presence of typical cutaneous lesions as seen in blue rubber bleb nevus syndrome often suggests the diagnosis. Children with HIV infection or immunosuppression secondary to chemotherapy can develop CMV enterocolitis or polymicrobial inflammation of cecum (typhlitis), both of which can lead to significant rectal bleeding.

Presence of fissure and fleshy anal tags suggests IBD whereas characteristic oro-buccal pigmentation is seen in Peutz-Jegher's syndrome. Abdominal examination is useful in detecting sausage shaped mass in intussusception. A gentle per rectal examination can detect polyps in the rectum and also stool impaction. Presence of palpable purpura in lower limbs with abdominal pain suggests a diagnosis of Henoch-Schönlein purpura (HSP). Asking the child to strain will show the presence of rectal prolpase.

LABORATORY INVESTIGATIONS

The aim of investigations in a child with LGIB is to localize the site of bleeding i.e. small bowel or colon and also to determine the etiology in order to manage it appropriately. The general investigations are similar to that of UGIB and specific investigations are listed below (Table 36.6).

- *Hemogram* may show neutrophlic leukocytosis in patients with infectious colitis and anemia, raised ESR with thrombocytosis in children with IBD.

Table 36.5 Indian series on lower gastrointestinal bleeding			
Cause	Yachha et al[1] (n = 64)	Khurana et al[42] (n = 85)	Mandhan[43] (n = 207)
Colitis	42%	Amebic 23.5%	18%
Polyps	41%	54.1%	75%
Solitary rectal ulcer syndrome	4.5%	4.7%	3.5%
Enteric bleeding	4.5%	-	-
Portal colopathy	3%	1.2%	-
A-V malformation	1.5%	-	-
Hemorrhoids	1.5%	-	-
Others	–	Pseudomembranous colitis 1.2%, Henoch-Schönlein purpura 2.4%	Lymphonodular hyperplasia 3%, foreign body 0.5%
Unknown	1.5%	12.9%	-

Table 36.6 Specific investigations for the diagnosis of lower gastrointestinal bleeding

Condition	Investigations and findings
Allergic colitis	Sigmoidoscopy for aphthous ulcers. Rectal mucosal biopsy for eosinophils
Hirschsprung's disease with enterocolitis	Transition zone on barium enema. Absence of recto-anal inhibitory reflex on manometery. Biopsy showing absence of ganglion cells
Necrotizing enterocolitis	Pneumatosis intestinalis on plain X-ray abdomen and perforation of gut
Hemorrhagic disease of the newborn	Prolonged prothrombin time, corrected by vitamin K
Pseudomembranous colitis	*C. difficile* toxin in stools. Sigmoidoscopy showing yellowish membrane with colitis
Amebic dysentery	Hematophagous trophozoites in stool and ulcers on sigmoidoscopy
Bacillary dysentery	Blood and pus cells on stool examination
Hemorrhoids	Proctoscopy
Rectal prolapse	Perianal examination during straining
Portal colopathy/rectal varices	Colonoscopy: Rectal varices, colopathy showing erythematous mucosa with cherry red spots
Solitary rectal ulcer syndrome	Sigmoidoscopy shows ulcer/s and hyperemia on anterior rectal wall. Biopsy shows fibrous obliteration/ edema of lamina propria
Polyps	Colonoscopy
Duplication/Meckel's diverticulum	Tc99m scan/small bowel barium study
Intussusception	Ultrasound abdomen
Henoch-Schonlein purpura	Endoscopy may show erosions in duodenum and small bowel, skin biopsy from lesions for IgA deposits and urine examination for hematuria/proteinuria
Arterio-venous malformation	Colonoscopy, angiography
Radiation proctitis	Sigmoidoscopy shows hyperemia, ulcers and telangiectasia

- *Complete stool examination* for trophozoites, cysts, stool culture and sensitivity if indicated, clostridium difficile toxin assay and eosinophils are helpful in suspected cases of allergic colitis.

- *Proctosigmoidoscopy* is useful in children with LGIB. Enema is given 20-30 minutes before the procedure. It is useful for detecting presence of colitis, polyps, SRUS, hemorrhoids and rectal varices. A flexible sigmoidoscope is used in children and many of the lesions can be treated in the same session. Hemorrhoids are best seen on rigid proctoscopy. In the study by Khurana *et al*[42] 69/85 (81.2%) cases with LGIB could be diagnosed by flexible sigmoidoscopy alone.

- *Colonoscopy* is the investigation of choice for proximal colonic bleeds. It is often difficult to get a proper view in subjects with active bleeding. Bowel preparation is done by standard polyethylene glycol electrolyte solution. Examination of the terminal ileum should be attempted to detect active bleeding from the small bowel. Polyps are a major cause of LGIB in children and they are often situated in the left colon and therefore sigmoidoscopy is usually enough. But in subjects with multiple polyps, family history of polyposis or recurrence of bleeding after polypectomy, a complete colonoscopy should be done. Poddar et al[45], reported that 15% of polyps are seen in proximal colon and 17% subjects have multiple polyps which suggests the importance of a complete colonoscopy in these subjects.

- *Tc* ^{99m} *pertechnate* scan is done to detect ectopic gastric mucosa present in Meckel's diverticulum or gastric duplication. As 90% of the bleeding Meckel's has gastric mucosa, it is very useful for diagnosing Meckel's diverticulum.

- *Technetium 99m red blood cell scan* (Tc RBC scan). In this test, small amount of subject's blood is withdrawn, tagged with Tc ^{99m} and then re-injected into the patient. 93% of the Tc activity is confined to intravascular space,

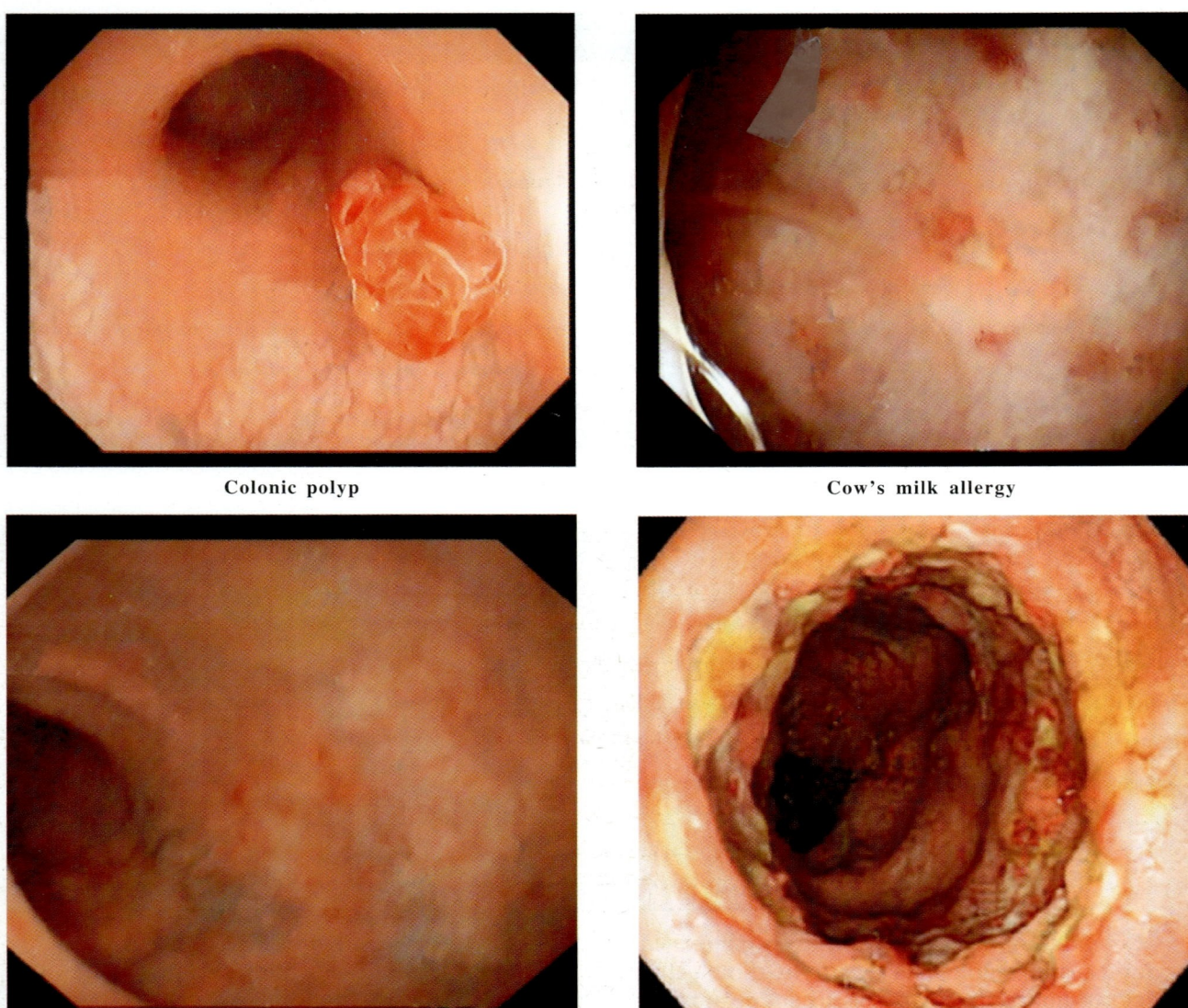

Colonic polyp

Cow's milk allergy

Rectal varices and colopathy

Transverse ulcers in colonic TB

Figure 36.4 Endoscopic appearance of common causes of lower gastrointestinal bleeding

thus any activity seen in the gut suggests the site of bleeding. It requires a minimum of 0.1 ml/minute of blood loss in order to detect the site of bleed. It is often used before selective angiography as it is non-invasive and helps in choosing the artery [celiac trunk, superior mesenteric (SMA) or inferior mesenteric (IMA)] for selective angiography according to site of bleeding on Tc RBC scan.

- *Angiography.* Catheter is negotiated through the femoral artery for selective cannulation of the desired vessel e.g. celiac trunk, SMA, and IMA. It requires at least 0.5 ml/minute of blood loss for a positive result. Extravasation of dye into the gastrointestinal tract indicates a bleeding lesion. Mucosal blush represents a vascular lesion and an early venous return

suggests an AV malformation. Injection of sclerosant or embolisation of the vessel with coils or gel foam can be done to stop the bleeding.

- *Plain X-ray abdomen* has a limited utility in children with GI bleeding. In cases with rectal bleeding with abdominal pain, it may show air fluid levels, pneumatosis intestinalis in NEC or focal/generalized bowel thickening (thumb printing) in conditions like Henoch-Schölein purpura.

- *Barium study* has a negligible role in a patient with active bleeding. It can be used for detection of colitis, polyposis, diverticulosis, etc. in the quiescent stage of a child with intermittent bleeding.

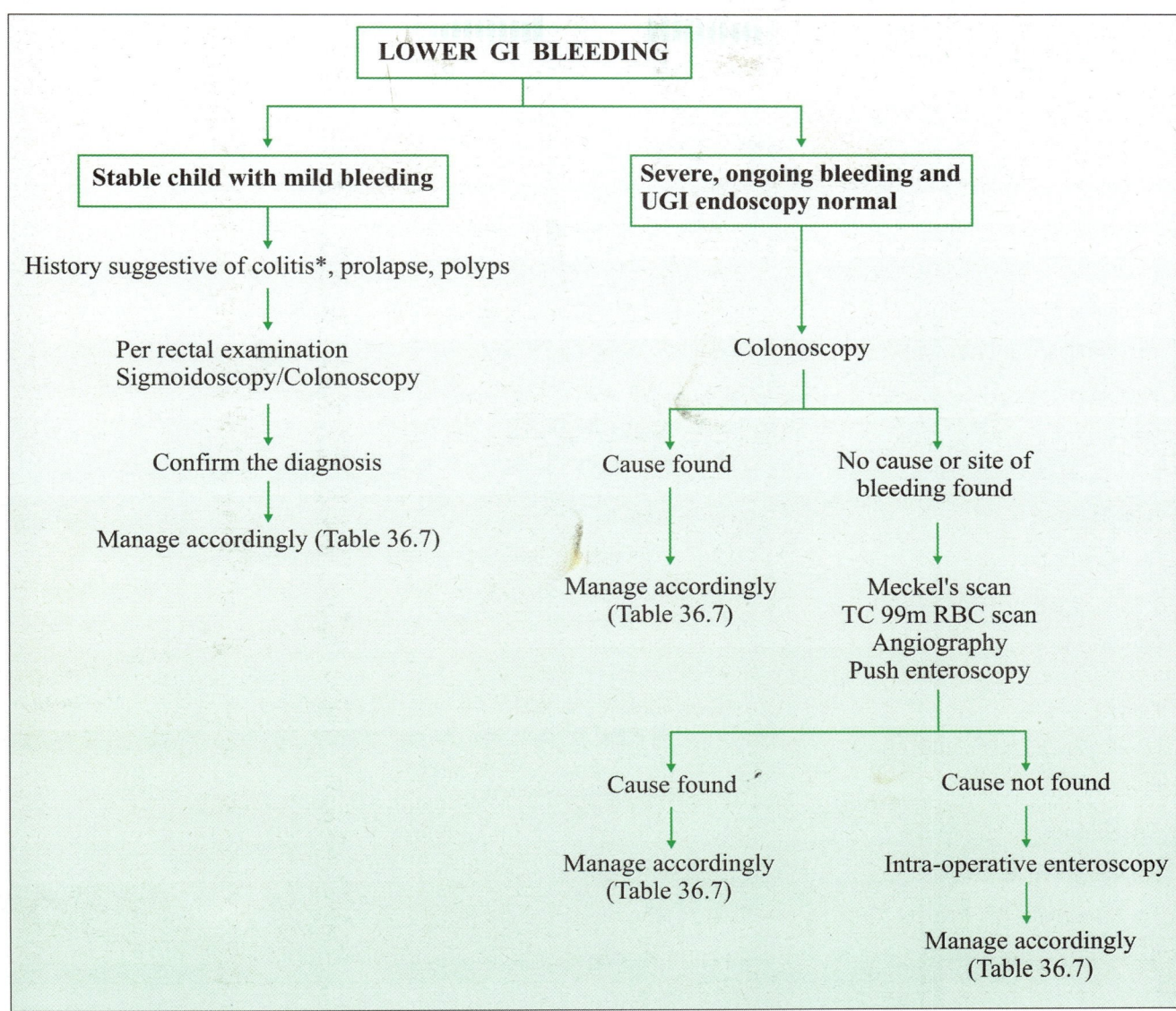

Figure 36.5 Algorithm for management of acute lower GI bleeding

- *Ultrasound examination* of abdomen is useful for making a diagnosis of intussusception in a child with bleeding per rectum.

- *CT and MRI scan* are generally reserved for evaluation of mass lesions or complex vascular anomalies.

A stepwise approach for the management of lower GI bleeding is summarized in Figure 36.5. At times when the above investigations fail to localize the site of bleeding then it is essential to evaluate the small bowel. Wireless capsule endoscopy (WCE), double balloon endoscopy (DBE) and push endoscopy are the main methods for visualization of the small bowel.

Capsule endoscopy. It can be done safely even in small children of 2-3 years of age. The child either swallows the capsule or it is placed in the stomach with the help of special placement devices. The capsule records images during its transit and is finally passed out in the stools. The images are then analyzed to detect the site and cause of bleeding. Capsule endoscopy is contraindicated in subjects with suspected intestinal obstruction as the capsule can get impacted. It is an expensive but non-invasive tool and can help in making a diagnosis in large number of cases of obscure gastrointestinal

Table 36.7 Management strategies for lower gastrointestinal bleeding	
Cause	**Treatment options**
Allergic colitis	Withdrawal of milk/milk products
Hirschprung's disease with enterocolitis	Antibiotics followed by definitive surgical treatment
Necrotizing enterocolitis	Antibiotics, supportive therapy and surgery if needed
Hemorrhagic disease of the newborn	Vitamin K and supportive therapy
Pseudomembranous colitis	Stop offending antibiotic, vancomycin or metronidazole
Amebic dysentery	Metronidazole
Bacillary dysentery	Nalidixic acid or quinolones and 3rd generation cephalosporins
Inflammatory bowel disease	Steroids, immunosuppression and 5 ASA
Anal fissure	Treatment of constipation, local nitroglycerine ointment application, sitz bath
Hemorrhoids	Banding, injection and surgery
Rectal prolapse	Treatment of precipitating cause, colonoscopic injection, surgery
Portal colopathy/rectal varices	Beta blockers, injection therapy and shunt surgery
Solitary rectal ulcer syndrome	Treatment of constipation, 5 ASA or sucralfate enema, local APC (argon plasma coagulation) treatment
Polyps	Polypectomy
Duplication/Meckel's diverticulum	Surgical excision
Intussusception	Radiologic reduction or surgery
Arteriovenous malformation	Endoscopic treatment, hormone therapy, surgery
Henoch-Schönlein purpura	Supportive therapy and steroids
Thrombocytopenia/DIC	Platelets, fresh frozen plasma
Radiation proctitis	Argon plasma coagulation and sucralfate enema

bleeding.[46,47] The disadvantages of WCE include uncontrollable movement of the capsule in the intestine, which may result in some valuable video images being overlooked and inability to perform therapeutic interventions.

Push enteroscopy is done with a pediatric colonoscope or adult gastroscope and detects bleeding sites in the proximal jejunum.

Double balloon enteroscopy (DBE) is a useful diagnostic and therapeutic tool for small bowel bleeding in children. The DBE is similar to the regular endoscope except that it has two balloons connected to an air pump–one is attached to the tip of the endoscope and the other to the distal end of an overtube. By using these balloons to grip the intestinal wall, the endoscope can be inserted further into the small bowel without forming redundant loops. Sequential inflation and deflation of the two anchoring balloons at the distal end of the enteroscope allows the enteroscope to proceed forward, which makes thorough examination of the small intestine possible. Trans-oral and if required subsequent trans-anal DBE allows visualization of entire small bowel and therapeutic interventions like hemostasis, polypectomy and biopsies[48]. It is a laborious, time consuming and invasive method which requires expertise and is best done under general anesthesia or deep sedation. In a recent pediatric study, the bleeding source was found in 21 of 27 patients with obscure gastrointestinal bleeding (detection rate of 77.8%)[49]. DBE is useful in conjunction with WCE for optimizing diagnostic potential in the small bowel. Complications reported in literature with DBE include intestinal perforation, pancreatitis and paralytic ileus[50].

Peroperative enteroscopy is the last resort and is done at the time of surgery, if the patient continues to bleed and none of the investigations have revealed the cause.

MANAGEMENT

Apart from supportive treatment which is similar to that of UGIB, the specific treatment is dependent upon the cause as shown in Table 36.7. Gastrointestinal hemorrhage is common in children and it is amenable to treatment if managed properly and in time. Prompt resuscitative measures, efforts to identify the cause of bleeding and timely referral to a specialized center are the key to reduce morbidity and mortality due to acute gastrointestinal bleeding. A multidisciplinary team of pediatrician, pediatric gastroenterologist, radiologist and surgeon is required to have the best patient outcome without any sequelae.

REFERENCES

1. Yachha SK, Khanduri A, Sharma BC, Kumar M. Gastrointestinal bleeding in children. *J Gastroenterol Hepatol* 1996; 11:903-907.

2. Mittal SK, Kalra KK, Aggarwal N. Diagnostic upper gastrointestinal endoscopy for hematemesis in children: Experience from a Pediatric Gastroenterology Centre in north India. *Indian J Pediatr* 1994; 61:651-654.

3. Brodoff M, Conn HO. Esophageal tamponade in the treatment of bleeding varices. *Dig Dis Sci* 1980; 25: 267-272.

4. Conn HO, Bordoff M. Emergency endoscopy in the diagnosis of gastro-intestinal hemorrhage. *Gastroenterology* 1964; 47:500-512.

5. Beppu K, Inokuchi K, Koyanagi N. Prediction of variceal hemorrhage by esophageal endoscopy. *Gastrointest Endosc* 1981; 27:213-218.

6. Molleston JP. Variceal bleeding in children. *J Pediatr Gastroenterol Nutr* 2003; 37: 538-545.

7. Sarin SK, Ashish Kumar A, Angus PW, Baijal SS, Baik SK, Bayraktar Y, et al. Diagnosis and management of acute variceal bleeding: Asian Pacific Association for Study of the Liver Recommendations. *Hepatol Int* 2011; 5(2):607-24.

8. Zargar SA, Javid G, Khan BA, *et al.* Endoscopic ligation compared with sclerotherapy for bleeding esophageal varices in children with extrahepatic portal venous obstruction. *Hepatology* 2002; 36:666-672.

9. Eroglu Y, Emerick KM, Whitingon PF, Alonso EM. Octreotide therapy for control of acute gastrointestinal bleeding in children. *JPGN* 2004; 38:41-47.

10. Nadar A, Grace ND. Pharmacologic intervention during the acute bleeding episodes. *Gastrointestinal* Endoscopy *Clin North Amer* 1999; 9:287-299.

11. Ioannou GN, Doust J, Rockey DC. Systematic review: terlipressin in acute esophageal variceal hemorrhage. *Aliment Pharmacol Ther* 2003;17:53–64

12. D' Amico G, Pietrosi G, Tarantino J, *et al.* Emergency sclerotherapy versus vasoactive drugs for variceal bleeding in cirrhosis: a Cochrane meta-analysis. *Gastroenterology* 2003; 124:1277-1291.

13. Banares R, Albillos A, Rincon D, *et al.* Endoscopic treatment versus endoscopic plus pharmacologic treatment for acute variceal bleeding: a meta-analysis. *Hepatology* 2002; 35:609-615.

14. Pitcher JL. Safety and effectiveness of the modified Sangstaken-Blakemore tube. A prospective study. *Gastroenterology* 1971; 61:291-298.

15. Yachha SK, Sharma BC, Kumar M, Khanduri A. Endoscopic sclerotherapy for esophageal varices in children with extrahepatic portal venous obstruction: a follow-up study. *J Pediatr Gastroenterol Nutr* 1997; 24:49-52.

16. Poddar U, Thapa BR, Singh K. Endoscopic sclerotherapy in children: experience with 257 cases of extrahepatic portal venous obstruction. *Gastrointest Endoscopy* 2003; 57(6):683-686.

17. Supe AN, Mathur SK, Borwankar SS. Esophageal endoscopic sclerotherapy in children using 3% aqueous phenol. *Indian J Gastroenterol* 1994; 13(1):1-4.

18. Zargar SA, Yattoo GN, Javid G, *et al.* 15 year follow-up of endoscopic injection sclerotherapy in children with extrahepatic portal venous obstruction. *J Gastro Hepatol* 2004; 19:139-145.

19. Price MR, Sartorelli KH, Karren FM, *et al.* Management of esophageal varices in children by endoscopic variceal ligation. *J Pediatr Surg* 1996; 31:1056-1059.

20. Mc Keirnan PJ, Beath SV, Davison SM. A prospective study of endoscopic esophageal variceal ligation using a multiband ligator. *JPGN* 2002; 34:207-211.

21. Ohnuma N, Takahashi H, Tanabe M, *et al.* Endoscopic variceal ligation using a clipping apparatus in children with portal hypertension. *Endoscopy* 1997; 29:86-90.

22. Bleau BL. Endoscopic management of the acute variceal bleeding event. Gastroenterol Endoscopy *Clin North Amer* 1999; 9:189-206.

23. Fuster S, Costaguta A, Tobacco O. Treatment of bleeding gastric varices with tissue adhesive (histoacryl) in children. *Endoscopy* 1998; 30:S39-S40.

24. Hackwarth CA, Leef JA, Rosenblum JD, *et al.* Transjugular intrahepatic portosystemic shunt creation in children: initial clinical experience. *Radiology* 1998; 206:109-114.

25. Fox VL. Gastrointestinal bleeding in infancy and childhood. *Gastroenterol Clin N Amer* 2000; 29:37-66.

26. Shun A, Delaney DP, Martin HC, *et al.* Portosystemic shunting for pediatric portal hypertension. *J Pediatr Surg* 1997; 32:489-493.

27. Bambini DA, Superina R, Almond PS, Whitington PF, Alonso E. Experience with Rex shunt (mesenterico-left

Section 4

portal bypass) in children with extrahepatic portal hypertension. *J Pediatr Surgery* 2000; 35:13-18.

28. Poddar U, Bhatnagar S, Yachha SK Endoscopic band ligation followed by sclerotherapy: Is it superior to sclerotherapy in children with extrahepatic portal venous obstruction? *Gastroenterol and Hepatol* 26 (2011) 255–259.

29. Aanpreung P, Atisook K. Hematemesis in infants induced by cow milk allergy. *Asian Pac J Allergy Immunol* 2003;2:211-216.

30. Itani M, Alsaied T, Charafeddine L, Yazbeck N. Dieulafoy's lesion in children. *J Pediatr Gastroenterol Nutr* 2010;51:672-674.

31. Hill SJ, Zarroug AE, Ricketts RR, Veeraswamy R. Bedside placement of an aortic occlusion balloon to control a ruptured aorto-esophageal fistula in a small child. *Ann Vasc Surg* 2010; 24: 822.e7-9.

32. Mouzan MI, Abdullah AM. Peptic ulcer disease in children and adolescent. *J Trop Pediatr* 2004; 50: 328–330.

33. Huang SC, Sheu BS, Lee SC, Yang HB, Yang YJ. Etiology and treatment of childhood peptic ulcer disease in Taiwan: a single center 9-year experience. *J Formos Med Assoc* 2010;109:75-81.

34. Grimaldi-Bensouda L, Abenhaim L, Michaud L, Mouterde O, Jonville-Béra AP, Giraudeau B, *et al.* Clinical features and risk factors for upper gastrointestinal bleeding in children: a case-crossover study. *Eur J Clin Pharmacol* 2010; 66:831–837.

35. Wee E. Management of nonvariceal upper gastrointestinal bleeding. *J Postgrad Med* 2011; 57: 161-167.

36. The Harriet Lane Handbook. Sixteenth edition, 2002. *Mosby* (An Imprint of Elsevier).

37. Spolidoro JV, Kay M, Ament M, *et al.* New endoscopic and diagnostic techniques: working group report of the First World Congress of Pediatric Gastroenterology, Hepatology and Nutrition: Management of GI bleeding, dyspepsia screening and endoscopic training- Issues for the new millennium. *J Pediatr Gastroenterol Nutr* 2002; 35:196-204.

38. Wyllie R, Kay MH. Therapeutic intervention for non variceal gastrointestinal haemorrhage. *J Pediatr Gastroenterol Nutr* 1996; 22:123-133.

39. Kay MH, Wyllie R. Alcohol is not for kids: endoscopic hemostasis of bleeding peptic ulcers in pediatric patients. *J Pediatr* 1998; 133:802.

40. Khan K, Schwarzenberg SJ, Sharp H, Weisdorf-Schindele S. Argon plasma coagulation: clinical experience in pediatric patients. *GI Endoscopy* 2003; 57:110-112.

41. Chaibou M, Tucci M, Duggas MA, *et al.* Clinically significant upper gastrointestinal bleeding in a pediatric intensive care unit: a prospective study. *Pediatrics* 1998; 102: 933-938.

42. Khurana AK, Saraya A, Jain N, Chandra M, Kulshreshtha R. Profile of lower gastrointestinal bleeding in children from a tropical country. *Tropical Gastroenterol* 1998; 19:70-71.

43. Mandhan P. Sigmoidoscopy in children with chronic lower gastrointestinal bleeding. *J Pediatr Child Health* 2004; 40:365-368.

44. Barakat M, El-Kady Z, Mostafa M, Ibrahim N, Ghazaly H.Antibiotic-associated bloody diarrhea in infants: clinical, endoscopic, and histopathologic profiles. *J Pediatr Gastroenterol Nutr* 2011;52(1):60-64.

45. Poddar U, Thapa BR, Vaphei K, Singh K. Colonic polyps: experience of 236 Indian children. *Amer J Gastroenterol* 1998; 93:619-622.

46. Tokuhara D, Watanabe K, Okano Y, Tada A, Yamato K, Mochizuki T, Takaya J, Yamano T, Arakawa T.Wireless capsule endoscopy in pediatric patients: the first series from Japan. *J Gastroenterol* 2010 ;45:683-691.

47. Fritscher-Ravens A, Scherbakov P, Bufler P, Torroni F, Ruuska T, Nuutinen H, Thomson M, Tabbers M, Milla P.The feasibility of wireless capsule endoscopy in detecting small intestinal pathology in children under the age of 8 years: a multicentre European study. *Gut* 2009; 58:1467-1472.

48. Thomson M, Venkatesh K, Elmalik K, van der Veer W, Jaacobs M. Double balloon enteroscopy in children: Diagnosis, treatment, and safety. *World J Gastroenterol* 2010; 16: 56-62.

49. W Liu, C Xu, J Zhong. The diagnostic value of double-balloon enteroscopy in children with small bowel disease: Report of 31 cases. *Canad J Gastroenterol* 2009; 23:635-638.

50. Ohmiya N, Yano T, Yamamoto H, Arakawa D, Nakamura M, Honda W, *et al.* Diagnosis and treatment of obscure GI bleeding at double balloon endoscopy. *Gastrointest Endosc* 2007; 66: S72-S77.

37

Viral Encephalitis and Encephalopathies

Rashmi Kumar

The term 'encephalitis' literally means inflammation of the brain parenchyma, part or all of the 'encephalon'. It is an important cause of death and permanent neurologic disability in both adults and children. The invasion by a viral agent causing direct neuronal injury is the most common cause of encephalitis, when it is called 'viral encephalitis' (VE). Direct injury by viral invasion may result in acute, subacute or chronic manifestations. Sometimes the inflammation is not due to invasion but is an indirect immunologically mediated injury.

Noninflammatory diffuse cerebral dysfunction is termed as 'encephalopathy' and common causes include metabolic, toxic or ischemic disorders. The term encephalopathy is also used for altered mentation due to any cause. This chapter will focus only on acute encephalitis and encephalopathies which may present as a medical emergency in children.

Encephalitis and meningitis are overlapping syndromes. Pathologically, some degree of both meningeal and parenchymal inflammation is found in most patients with viral and nonviral invasion of the brain[1]. Therefore, many workers prefer the term 'meningoencephalitis' to meningitis or encephalitis. Clinically there is a spectrum of manifestations, but by and large two distinct patterns are seen[2]. When the illness is associated with prominent sensorial alterations, the clinical syndrome is believed to be 'encephalitis', and when meningeal irritation is prominent, it is called 'meningitis'. The term aseptic or viral meningitis is used for a self-limited illness with a predominantly meningitic presentation with little or no sensorial alteration.

VIRAL ENCEPHALITIS

The magnitude of the problem of viral encephalitis is difficult to assess because of lack of uniform definition. The burden of encephalitis-associated admissions among all age groups in the United States during 1988-1997 was analysed and was found to be substantial with nearly 19,000 admissions annually[2]. In India, the incidence is not known largely because a wide variety of central nervous system disorders may mimic encephalitis. At the Childrens' Hospital of the the CSM Medical University, Lucknow, a total of 150-200 patients are admitted annually with the clinical diagnosis of VE. However, the prevalence may vary from region to region in the country due to geographical differences and also from center to center depending on the definition used and extent of the diagnostic work-up.

ETIOLOGY

Table 37.1 shows the viral agents that can cause encephalitis. These include primary neurotropic viruses such as arboviruses, herpesviruses and rabies virus as well as other 'incidental' nervous system pathogens such as enteroviruses, orthomyxoviruses, paramyxoviruses and adenoviruses, which primarily cause disease elsewhere in the body, and involve the CNS in a small proportion of patients only[4]. Worldwide, Japanese encephalitis (JE) is held to be the single largest cause of VE[3]. The relative importance of different agents in producing encephalitis varies from region to region.

A large number of viruses are known to cause encephalitis but virological diagnosis is complex, expensive and time consuming. Even in advanced centers, etiological diagnosis is possible in only a small proportion of clinically suspected cases. The responsible virus may be detectable only in the brain itself, and is either absent or transiently found in blood or CSF. Specimens are often not collected early enough during the course of illness. Etiological studies have consistently revealed pathogens in only a proportion of patients. The California Encephalitis Project enrolled 1570 patients with suspected encephalitis over a 7 year period (1998-2005). A core battery of tests for 16 viral agents and selective testing for other agents on the basis of epidemiologic and clinical features were performed. A confirmed or probable etiologic agent was

Section 4

Table 37.1 Viral agents that are known to cause acute encephalitis[3, 4]

Arboviruses, togaviruses, and alphaviruses
- Western equine encephalitis virus
- Eastern equine encephalitis virus
- Venezuelan equine encephalitis virus

Flaviviruses (Mosquito borne)
- Japanese encephalitis virus
- St Louis encephalitis virus
- West Nile virus
- Murray valley encephalitis virus
- Non arthropod borne togavirus (rubella virus)

Bunyaviruses
- California encephalitis virus

Reoviruses
- Colorado tick fever encephalitis virus

Herpesviruses
- Herpes simplex 1 and 2
- Varicella zoster virus
- Ebstein-Barr virus
- Cytomegalovirus
- Human Herpesvirus – 6
- B virus

Enteroviruses
- Polioviruses
- Coxsackie viruses
- Echoviruses
- Enteroviruses 70 and 71

Orthomyxoviruses
- Influenza viruses

Paramyxoviruses
- Measles virus
- Mumps virus
- Parainfluenza viruses
- Nipah virus

Adenoviruses

Rhabdoviruses

identified in 16%, of which 69% were viral, 20% were bacterial, 7% prion, 3% parasitic and 1% fungal. An additional 13% had possible etiologies identified, of which many agents were not hitherto implicated as a cause of encephalitis[5]. In a large Finnish study, polymerase chain reaction (PCR) in cerebrospinal fluid (CSF) was used for diagnosis in over 3000 patients with suspected viral CNS disorders[6]. *Varicella zoster* virus was found to be the commonest virus associated with encephalitis comprising 29% of all confirmed or probable etiologic agents while *Herpes simplex* virus and enteroviruses accounted for 11% each and *Influenza A* in 7% of cases. A nationwide study of etiology of acute encephalitis in adults was conducted in France in 2007. Of 253 patients enrolled, cause of the encephalitis was determined

in 131 (52%); *Herpes simplex virus* 1 (42%), varicella-zoster virus (15%), *Mycobacterium tuberculosis* (15%), and *Listeria monocytogenes* (10%) being the most frequently identified agents[7]. Of 5,296 patients studied in Australia over an 18 year period (1990-2007), the etiology was identified in 30.6% and herpes simplex (12.9%) was the commonest agent[8]. In a study on 322 adults and children with clinical encephalitis in Egypt, *N. meningitidis, S. pneumonia* and *M. tuberculosis* were the most frequently detected bacterial agents, while Enteroviruses, herpes simplex viruses and varicella zoster viruses were the most common viral agents encountered[9].

Studies from Asia reveal a different picture. In a study from Beijing on 97 children with acute encephalitis, viral etiology could be established in 35 cases. The most frequently identified pathogens were enteroviruses (15.4%), mumps (7.2%), rubella (6.2%), JE (5.1%), human herpesvirus 6 (2.0%), *Herpes simplex* encephalitis (2.0%), and *Ebstein-Barr* virus (1.0%)[10]. A study from Penang, Malaysia reported etiologic diagnosis in 13 of 195 children with viral encephalitis. Of these 8 had evidences of JE, one had mumps encephalitis and 4 were IgM positive for cytomegalovirus infection[11]. In a study of clinically diagnosed JE in Guizhou Province, China, between April and November 2006, JE infection was confirmed in 1,210 of 1,382 (87.6%) while other viral pathogens responsible for encephalitis, including echovirus, mumps virus, herpes simplex virus, and cytomegalovirus, were identified in 67 of 172 (38.9%) JE-negative cases[12]. In Vietnam, children less than 16 years of age presenting with acute encephalitis were subjected to viral culture, serology and real time (RT)-PCRs. A confirmed or probable viral causative agent was established in 41% of 194 enrolled patients. The most commonly diagnosed causative agent was JE virus (n = 50, 26%), followed by enteroviruses (n = 18, 9.3%), dengue virus (n = 9, 4.6%), herpes simplex virus (n = 1), cytomegalovirus (n = 1) and influenza A virus (n = 1)[13].

In India, there have been few comprehensive studies looking into the etiology of VE. JE is probably the commonest form and occurs in epidemics over large parts of the country, especially the south and east. Rabies is another form of viral encephalitis which poses a public health problem in our country. A study from Lucknow showed that of 394 children admitted to hospital with an illness consistent with encephalitis, 93 had one or more indicators of JE. Of the remainder 187 children who underwent investigations for enteroviruses and respiratory viruses, 14 had laboratory indicators for these viruses[14]. In a recent study on 87 children in western Uttar Pradesh, the most common etiology of VE was enterovirus 71 (42.1%), followed by measles (21.1%), varicella zoster virus (15.8%), herpes simplex virus (10.5%), and mumps (10.5%). JE virus was not found in any case[15]. An outbreak of viral encephalitis was reported from April to October 2006 from Gorakhpur area after the JE vaccination campaign. Using reverse transcription–PCR in cerebrospinal fluid, enteroviruses (EV) were detected in 66 (21.6%) of 306 patients. Sequencing and phylogenetic analyses of PCR products from 59 (89.3%) of 66 specimens showed similarity with EV-89 and EV-76 sequences[16]. Outbreaks of childhood encephalopathy syndrome with high case-fatality were a recurrent annual seasonal feature in Saharanpur in western Uttar Pradesh (UP) for the last few years. A case control study implicated ingestion of beans of *Cassia occidentalis* as the cause with 44.4% of cases compared to 5.6% controls having a definite history of eating the weed before falling ill (odds ratio 12.9 (95% CI 2.6-88.8, $P<0.001$)[17].

In addition, outbreaks of VE are often caused by emerging and re-emerging pathogens. Unexpected neurovirulence from hitherto benign viral agents and freak epidemics have been encountered[18]. Investigation of a severe outbreak of acute encephalopathy without rash in children in north India (adjoining areas of Haryana, Punjab and Uttar Pradesh) in 1997 confirmed that measles virus was responsible for this epidemic[19]. Enterovirus 71, which was hitherto considered a causative agent for herpangina and hand-foot-and-mouth disease produced a large epidemic of encephalitis with high mortality rate in Taiwan in 1998[18]. In 1999, an outbreak of encephalitis occurred in New York City and the causative agent was identified as the West Nile virus,[20,21]. Since then the infection is endemic in eastern states of America. The Chandipura virus was identified as the cause of the 2003 epidemic of encephalitis in Andhra Pradesh[22]. Nipah virus, a newly described agent belonging to the paramyxovirus family was the cause of an outbreak of encephalitis in Malaysian pig farmers[23]. Dengue hemorrhagic fever is known to produce neurologic manifestations including encephalopathy but dengue is now recognised as a cause of viral encephalitis due to actual viral invasion of the brain[24,25].

EPIDEMIOLOGY

Several factors such as age, geographical location, season, climate and host immune status affect the epidemiology of encephalitis. Arboviruses or arthropod borne viruses have their life cycle in insect vectors and vertebrate animals, occasionally infecting man who is a 'dead end' host. Different arboviral encephalitides have their own specific geographical distribution depending on the activity of their insect vectors. For example, arboviral encephalitides prevalent in the United States are Western equine encephalitis, eastern equine encephalitis, Californian encephalitis, St Louis encephalitis, etc. Venezuelan encephalitis is found in South America and Japanese encephalitis in Asia. These encephalitides tend to occur in epidemics or outbreaks. Occasionally, a fresh viral pathogen when introduced into a susceptible population produces an explosive outbreak. HSE tends to occur sporadically worldwide with little seasonal variation[3, 26]. Mumps, measles and rabies encephalitis have been largely eradicated from many developed countries due to effective vaccination program[3].

PATHOGENESIS

The illness begins with entry of the infecting agent and replication at an extraneural site. Factors such as mucosal integrity, pH and secretory immunoglobulins affect the ability of the virus to invade the host and replicate effectively[1]. Most viruses reach the nervous system hematogenously and the probability of an encephalitis depends on the degree of viral amplification at the extraneural site and the ensuing viremia[3, 4]. Hematogenously borne viruses such as arboviruses invade the brain through the choroid plexus or through the endothelium of cerebral blood vessels. Other viruses gain access to the brain by the neuronal route. For example, the rabies virus replicates locally at the site of animal bite, then enters nerve endings and travels retrograde via axons to the brain. Similarly, transmission through the neural route is believed to play an important role in the pathogenesis of HSE. Herpes simplex virus type 1 causes encephalitis beyond the neonatal period which may result both from reactivation of latent virus in the trigeminal ganglion and from primary infection[4]. Upon reaching the brain, the virus replicates in neurons and may lead to cell death. There are varying degrees of parenchymal and meningeal inflammation, edema and necrosis[1]. Some viruses may have a predisposition to involve specific areas of the brain such as temporal lobe in *Herpes simplex* and hippocampus in rabies[3, 4].

CLINICAL FEATURES

Even when the diagnosis of viral encephalitis is suspected, identification of the etiologic agent is a daunting task for reasons already mentioned. Geographic and seasonal factors, history of recent travel, contact with animals, animal bite and occupation need to be considered. JE occurs in post monsoon epidemics in southern and eastern parts of the country. A setting of immunodeficiency may point to specific agents like cytomegalovirus[3].

Clinical manifestations depend on whether the brain parenchyma or meninges are predominantly involved producing an encephalitic or meningitic syndrome respectively. The same virus may produce a meningitic picture in one and encephalitic picture in another patient[4]. The severity of manifestations may vary widely either as a mild febrile illness associated with headache to a severe disorder with convulsions, coma, neurological deficits and death[1]. Usually the onset is abrupt with fever and declining mental status. There may be irritability, agitation, screaming spells, confusion, delirium, drowsiness, stupor or coma. Headache may be complained of in older children. Typical features include an initial stage of fever, headache and vomiting lasting for less than a week followed by convulsions, coma and neurological deficits with or without signs of meningeal irritation. Severe cases may be associated with life-threatening rise in intracranial tension, decerebration or flaccid coma. Typically this stage lasts for 7-10 days after which there is gradual recovery with or without sequelae[26]. Some patients may have a biphasic course. Occasionally VE may be subacute in onset or present as stroke, a movement disorder or a behavioral disturbance (as seen with HSE)[3]. Chronic encephalitis can present like a degenerative brain disorder.

Examination should include a search for skin rash often seen with enteroviral encephalitis, measles, dengue and varicella zoster. Parotitis often occurs with mumps. Mucous membrane lesions like 'cold sore' believed to be a manifestation of herpes simplex infection, have little diagnostic value[27]. Concurrent upper respiratory infection is characteristic of influenza. Patients with rabies may have the characteristic hydrophobia or aerophobia.

Neurological signs in acute encephalitis do not reliably identify the underlying etiology despite the propensity of certain neurotropic viruses to affect specific focal areas of the nervous system. A constellation of frontotemporal signs with aphasia, personality change and focal deficits or focal seizures is characteristic of HSE[26]. With the availability of newer noninvasive techniques of diagnosis, milder, atypical cases and an 'expanded' spectrum of HSE in children with multifocal or diffuse brain involvement has been described[28,29]. Rabies may present as an ascending paralysis simulating Guillain-Barré syndrome[30]. JE is associated with prominent extrapyramidal or basal ganglia signs in the form of rigidity and abnormal movements especially in the convalescent stage[31].

INVESTIGATIONS

1. *Complete blood counts.* In the acute stage, blood counts usually reveal a polymorpho-nuclear leukocytosis. Low platelet counts and high packed cell volume in patients from endemic areas may point towards dengue infection.

2. *Cerebrospinal fluid (CSF) examination.* This is an essential part of the investigation of encephalitis but should be done when considered safe. CSF in viral encephalitis typically shows a pleocytosis of upto 300 cells per cu mm which can be either predominantly lymphocytic or polymorphonuclear, with normal to slightly raised protein and normal or raised sugar level. CSF pleocytosis (>5 cells/cu mm) is present in >95% cases of acute viral encephalitis[32] and exceeds 500 /cu mm in 10% cases of acute viral encephalitis (AVE)[33]. The CSF in AVE is indistinguishable from aseptic or viral meningitis. Any significant reduction of CSF glucose as a ratio of the corresponding plasma glucose is unusual in VE[34].

3. *Culture studies.* Samples for viral culture from respiratory secretions, throat swab, CSF, blood, urine and stool taken as early as possible in the course of illness should be collected in appropriate transport media and sent to the reference laboratory[35].

4. *Serological investigations* in acute serum for specific IgM antibody level or in paired sera for 4-fold rise in IgG level. Japanese encephalitis is commonly diagnosed by the antibody capture ELISA for IgM antibody in acute phase serum and CSF[36], with CSF being more sensitive and specific. IgM antibody in both may be absent in the first few days of the illness. Specific IgG ratios in serum and CSF can be used to identify infection with specific viruses but these are seldom useful in early stages of the illness[35]. A CSF to serum ratio of anti HSV-IgG antibodies of greater than 20 was earlier used for the diagnosis of HSE but is usually seen only after 5-6 days of illness[37].

5. *Polymerase chain reaction* (PCR) is being developed to provide a rapid, and accurate diagnostic tool for a host of pathogens and is the mainstay of diagnosis[35]. This is widely used for diagnosis of HSE with high sensitivity (>90%) and specificity (100%)[38,39]. Reverse transcriptase PCR assay (RT-PCR) is used for the diagnosis of enteroviral meningo-encephalitis[40]. More recently, the technique of multiplex PCR is being used to detect any of several agents in a single test[41].

6. No single test is pathognomonic for ante-mortem diagnosis of human rabies. Saliva can be tested by virus isolation or reverse transcription followed by polymerase chain reaction (RT-PCR). Skin biopsy specimens are examined for rabies antigen in the cutaneous nerves at the base of hair follicles. Immuno-fluorescent staining of corneal smears and skin biopsy specimen do not have a high yield. Serological assays are not suitable for diagnosis of rabies as virus-specific antibodies in serum tend to appear on an average 8 days after the onset of clinical symptoms. The fluorescent antibody test is considered the gold standard for the post mortem diagnosis in animals[42].

7. *Neuroimaging of brain* is now a standard investigation in patients with suspected VE. Neuroimaging is often normal, may reveal cerebral edema, diffuse low attenuation, patchy hypodensities or specific abnormalities as in HSE[26,34]. Cranial neuroimaging may also be useful in ruling out other treatable intracranial disorders as well as acute disseminated encephalomyelitis (ADEM). Magnetic resonance imaging (MRI) is the procedure of choice but cranial computed tomography is a good alternative if MRI facility is not available or if patient is very restless. Characteristic abnormalities are found in HSE which shows early changes of focal edema in the medial aspects of the temporal lobes, orbital surfaces of the frontal lobes, insular cortex and cingulate gyrus[3] (Figure 37.1). CSF PCR has been shown to have a good correlation with MRI. In one study reported from Brazil, 17 patients with focal encephalitis were evaluated by both Herpes simplex-1 PCR and MRI. MRI lesions involving the inferomedial region of one or both temporal lobes were observed in all but one PCR positive patient. No PCR negative patient had abnormal MRI findings. The presence of hemorrhagic encephalitis suggests a severe illness. MRI was also useful in establishing an alternative

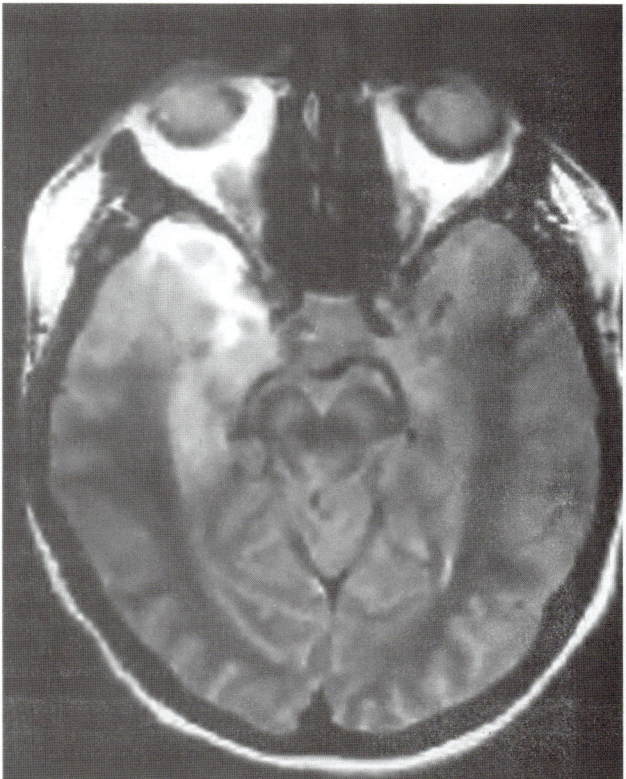

Figure 37.1 MRI brain showing temporal lobe changes seen in Herpes simplex encephalitis (HSE)

diagnosis in 3 of the 8 MRI negative patients[43]. Computed tomography shows focal changes (reduced attenuation over one or both temporal and/or frontal regions) in about 50% cases in later stages but it may be within normal limts in the first 4-5 days[44]. The presence of typical deep white matter changes on MRI are suggestive of acute disseminated encephalomyelitis (Figure 37.2). In JE, neuroimaging is reported to show distinct hypodensities in the thalamus, basal ganglia and brain stem[45,46].

8. *Electroencephalography* shows diffuse slow waves as a nonspecific finding in VE[3]. In HSE, EEG is always abnormal [27]. In early stages, nonspecific changes may be seen. More characteristic changes of 2-3 Hz periodic lateralised epileptiform discharges (PLEDs) originating from the temporal lobes, are seen in less than half the cases in later stages[47,48] (Figure 37.3).

9. *Functional neuroimaging* studies using technitium labelled hexamethylpropylene amineoxime (99 Tc-HmPAO) single photon emission computed tomography (SPECT) showing bitemporal hyperperfusion is a sensitive marker of HSE[49].

Section 4

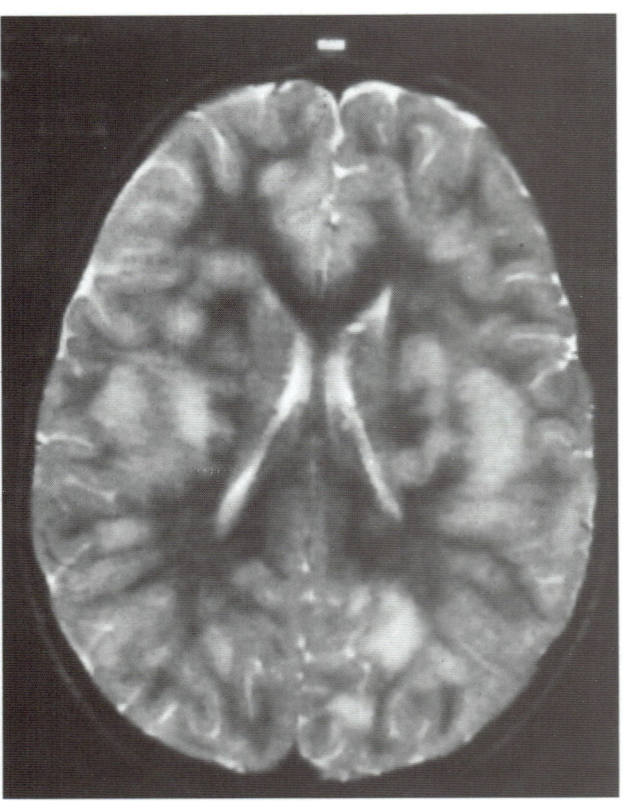

Figure 37.2 MRI brain showing typical deep white matter changes of acute disseminated encephalomyelitis (ADEM) in T2-weighted image.

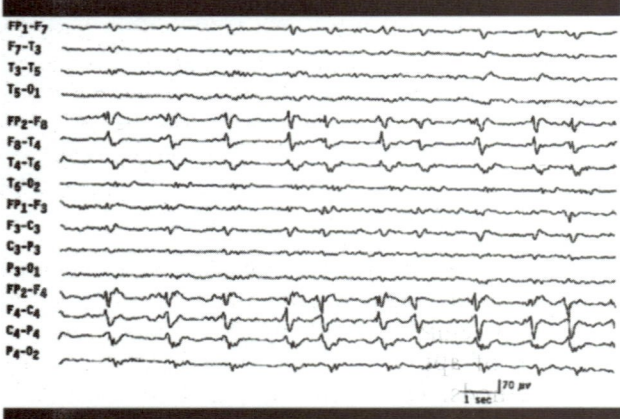

Figure 37.3 EEG showing characteristic 2-3 Hz periodic lateralized epileptiform discharges (PLEDs)

10. *Brain biopsy.* This is rarely indicated to establish etiology except in severely affected patients with unknown etiology who deteriorate despite acyclovir [34].

DIFFERENTIAL DIAGNOSIS

In practice, since specific investigations are time consuming, the diagnosis of encephalitis is presumptive based on clinical assessment and exclusion of other possibilities. The diagnosis of acute encephalitis is suspected in a febrile patient who presents with altered consciousness and signs of diffuse cerebral dysfunction. The term *acute febrile encephalopathy* is used for a febrile illness with altered sensorium of 2 weeks or less duration in a previously well child[50]. Acute viral encephalitis therefore may need to be distinguished from (a) other infectious (nonviral) encephalomeningitides, (b) non-infectious but inflammatory cerebral disorders such as acute disseminated encephalomyelitis and (c) encephalopathies. Human slow viral infections such as subacute sclerosing panencephalitis, progressive rubella panencephalitis, Cruetzfeldt Jacob disease, Kuru and progressive multifocal leukoencephalopathy produce a chronic progressive illness. HIV-AIDS *per se* causes a subacute or chronic encephalitis but the associated immuno-suppression may predispose to encephalitis by other pathogens.

Infectious Encephalomeningitides

The differential diagnosis of viral encephalitis includes a large number of infections depending upon geographical, seasonal and epidemiological factors. Table 37.2 gives a list of these pathogens.

Bacterial meningitis. This also has an acute onset and an overlapping clinical picture with VE. The most common pathogens are Gram-negative bacilli and *Staphylococcus aureus* in newborns, *H. influenzae* in infancy and *Streptococcus pneumoniae* and meningococcus beyond 2 years of age. Onset is abrupt with fever and headache,

Table 37.2. Non-viral infectious causes of encephalitis[62]
• Rickettsia : Rocky mountain spotted fever, endemic and epidemic typhus, Coxiella burnetii, Ehrlichiosis
• Bacterial:
o   Pyogenic and tuberculous meningitis
o   *Mycoplasma pneumoniae*
o   *Listeria monocytogenes*
o   Spirochetes: Syphilis, leptospirosis, lyme disease
o   Brucellosis
o   Legionella
o   *Salmonella typhi*, cat scratch disease (Bartonellosis)
• Fungi: Cryptococcus, Histoplasma, Aspergillus, mucormycosis, Candida, Coccidioidomycosis
• Protozoa: Plasmodium, Trypanosoma, Naeglaria, acanthamoeba, *Toxoplasma gondii,* schistosomiasis, *Echinococcus granulosus*
• Metazoa: Trichinosis, Echinococcus, Cysticercus, Schistosoma

followed by convulsions, altered mentation and neurological deficits. It may be distinguished on the basis of prominent meningeal signs, marked polymorphonuclear pleocytosis and reduced sugar in the CSF. Gram staining of smear and culture studies may show bacterial pathogens. Complications such as subdural collections and infarcts may be seen on imaging studies and these are not usually seen with VE.

Tuberculous meningitis (TBM). This continues to be fairly common in developing countries and may be differentiated from VE by its subacute or insidious onset. The prodromal stage i.e. period between onset of first symptom to development of neurological manifestations is usually more than one week[51]. CT scan in later stages shows basal enhancement (82.7%) with hydrocephalus (80.6%)[52]. In fact, a normal scan in a comatose child almost rules out TBM.

Other infectious agents. These include *Naegleria fowleri* (primary amebic meningo-encephalitis), toxoplasmosis, cysticercosis, trypanosomiasis, cat scratch disease (Bartonellosis), brucellosis, scrub typhus, human monocytic ehrlichiosis, *Mycoplasma pneumoniae* and fungal infections[4]. An epidemic of scrub typhus was recently reported from Tamil Nadu[53]. Lyme disease and leptospirosis may be associated with aseptic meningitis syndrome. Brain abscess caused by pyogenic bacteria can also occasionally mimic VE. HIV-AIDS, subacute sclerosing panencephalitis (SSPE) and progressive rubella panencephalitis cause a chronic encephalitis. The infectious agent identified requires specific treatment.

Postinfectious or Postvaccinal Acute Disseminated Encephalomyelitis (ADEM)

Viral encephalitis due to actual viral invasion of the CNS should be differentiated from post infectious or post vaccinal acute disseminated encephalomyelitis (ADEM). Common post-infectious causes include measles, rubella, mumps, varicella zoster, influenza A & B, Rickettsia and *Mycoplasma pneumoniae* while vaccines associated with this syndrome include rabies, vaccinia, measles and yellow fever. The illness is monophasic with altered consciousness, convulsions and multifocal neurological signs affecting cerebellum, optic nerves, long tracts, spinal cord and peripheral nerve roots. Fever, is usually absent at the onset of symptoms[54]. A history of a viral exanthem or vaccine in the recent past is usually available. CSF may reveal a mild pleocytosis. Characteristic plaque like lesions are seen in deep white matter and other areas of the neuraxis. Treatment options include high dose pulse steroids, intravenous immunoglobulins and plasmapheresis. In a study of 52 consecutive children in Chandigarh, the mean age at presentation was 6.14 +/- 3.17 years, 73.1% were male. A history of antecedent infectious illness or vaccination was present in 17 children. Sudden onset motor weakness (76.9%), seizures (36.5%), altered sensorium (55.8%) and pyramidal signs (80.7%) were the common findings. Characteristic subcortical hyperintense lesions in T2-weighted sequences on MRI were seen in the parietal (53.8%), frontal (30.17%), thalamic (30.7%), basal ganglia (17.3%), and callosal (13.46%) regions. The response to methyl-prednisolone was good, with dramatic recovery in 26.9% and marked improvement in 51.9% at discharge. Follow-up of 44 children revealed residual smaller MRI lesions in 30. These lesions either disappeared or were further reduced after 6 months in 75% of cases. Four children had relapse of ADEM with new lesions on MRI, all of whom responded to methylprednisolone. None of the clinical or radiologic features at presentation had any significant correlation with relapse[55].

TREATMENT

Supportive treatment is the mainstay of therapy for a child with presumed viral encephalitis. A severe case should be managed in an intensive care unit. An active search for treatable causes of acute encephalopathy should continue side by side along with measures to protect the brain from further insult. The following management steps are taken depending upon the clinical status and underlying etiology.

1. Excellent supportive care should be provided to maintain airways, breathing and circulation. Body temperature should be brought down by use of appropriate antipyretic and cooling methods. Hydration, electrolyte status and acid-base parameters should be maintained within normal range. It is prudent to use appropriate parenteral antibiotics until a bacterial cause is excluded with certainty.

2. Convulsions are best managed with intravenous anticonvulsants such as phenytoin or valproate which do not depress the sensorium.

3. Tube feeding may be started once the patient is stabilised and convulsions are controlled. Care must be taken to prevent aspiration and the protocol for management of a

comatose patient should be followed (Refer to Chapter 17).

4. Intracranial pressure lowering agents such as mannitol infusion (0.25 to 1.0 gm/kg every 4–6 hours) or intravenous furosemide may be needed. Hyperventilation to keep arterial CO_2 tension between 25–30 mm Hg may be used to combat raised intracranial tension. When facilities are available, monitoring of intracranial tension is useful[56]. In the case of rapidly increasing intracranial tension with clinical deterioration unresponsive to medical treatment, surgical decompression can be life saving[27].

5. Gastric hemorrhage (stress ulcer) is a common event and should be managed with antihistamines, antacids, ranitidine and if necessary, a blood transfusion.

6. The role of steroids in acute viral encephalitis is debatable. Theoretical arguments exist for and against their use. On the one hand, life threatening rise in intracranial tension may be relieved by steroids while on the other there is a risk of flaring up of the viral infection with steroids. A study that evaluated high dose dexamethasone in JE found no benefit of steroid therapy[57]. Their efficacy in the setting of AVE is unproven and they should preferably be avoided.

7. Specific therapy is recommended in encephalitis due to Herpes group of viruses. Acyclovir in a dose of 10 mg/kg administered as an intravenous infusion over one hour every 8 hours for 14 days (21 days in immuno-compromised) is indicated in HSE. Success of antiviral therapy depends on early institution of therapy. In many centers in the west, in the absence of an epidemic, acyclovir is started as soon as VE is suspected clinically, whether or not any evidence of localisation is present[35]. In the Indian context, no hard criteria can be laid down since the relative importance of HSE in different regions of the country is not really known. It seems reasonable to start acyclovir if focal features are present or neuroimaging studies reveal temporal lobe involvement. The toxicity and side effects of acyclovir include bone marrow suppression, vomiting and hypotension after intravenous administration and, occasionally, non-oliguric renal failure in dehydrated patients[58]. Confusion, hallucinations, seizures and coma are rare. Blood counts and relevant biochemical parameters should be closely monitored. Caution should be exercised in the presence of renal impairment as 80% of the drug is excreted unchanged in the urine[59]. Relapses may occur in as high as 5% cases[54]. Foscarnet is a new drug which is used for acyclovir-resistant HSE[60]. Acyclovir is also recommended for varicella–zoster encephalitis, with ganciclovir being an alternative drug. A combination of ganciclovir and foscarnet is recommended for cytomegaloviral encephalitis[3]. Pleconaril is a investigational agent for enteroviral infections, which acts by inhibiting viral attachment and uncoating[61]. Oseltamivir can be considered for influenza (H1N1) encephalitis.[62] Trials with α interferon and nasogastric ribavirin in JE in children have revealed no benefit[63,64].

ENCEPHALOPATHIES

The presence of fever in itself is not sufficient to make a diagnosis of infective or inflammatory encephalitis since encephalopathy may be precipitated by systemic infection or sepsis without cerebral inflammation (infective encephalopathy) or some other cause of fever may co-exist. Clues must be sought to differentiate encephalopathy from encephalitis, but the distinction is not always possible on clinical grounds. General features of encephalopathies are listed below:

- Absence of fever or meningeal signs
- Absence of focal neurologic signs or focal seizures
- No peripheral leukocytosis
- Normal CSF
- Diffuse slowing on electroencephalography
- Normal imaging studies

Examples of encephalopathies that should be considered in the differential diagnosis of AVE are listed below:

Infectious Encephalopathies

Cerebral malaria. It is characterized by sudden onset with fever, anemia, splenomegaly and occasionally hemoglobinuria. Smear for malarial parasites and rapid tests for malaria are positive. CSF examination is essentially normal and low glucose level may be due to hypoglycemia. Cerebral malaria is considered by some to be an example of infective encephalopathy rather than true encephalitis since the neurological symptoms of cerebral malaria result from brain hypoxemia and metabolic complications (hypoglycemia and acidosis) due to heavy parasitic load leading to capillary occlusion[65].

Enteric encephalopathy. This entity is an important consideration in India. A step ladder pattern of fever with encephalopathy developing in the second week of illness with normal CSF are characteristic features.

Shigella encephalopathy. A history of dysentery with blood and mucus in the stools is usually present with fever and toxicity. Neurologic manifestations include convulsions, headache, lethargy, confusion, nuchal rigidity or hallucinations. The cause of the neurologic symptoms is not clear. In the past, these were attributed to neurotoxicity caused by Shiga toxin[66].

Sepsis syndrome. Overwhelming sepsis with organ failure may also present as febrile encephalopathy.

Reye's Syndrome

This syndrome of acute encephalopathy with fatty infiltration of the liver usually presents with a history of a preceding viral infection (upper respiratory infection in 90%; varicella in 5-7%). A history of preceding intake of salicylates may be present. Abrupt onset of protracted vomiting is followed by delirium, combative behavior and stupor. Most children have a mild course but rapid progression to seizures, coma and death may occur. Focal neurologic signs are absent and CSF is normal except for elevated pressure. Mild hepatomegaly and hypoglycemia are common. Hepatic dysfunction is suggested by raised liver enzymes (>3 fold), raised serum ammonia and abnormal coagulogram but serum bilirubin is usually normal. Liver is yellow to white because of high triglyceride content and biopsy reveals diffuse microvesicular fatty infiltration without any evidence of inflammation or necrosis[67]. Reye's syndrome has been reported from different parts of India[68,69].

Heat Stroke

Severe heat injury is characterised by body temperature over 104°F and altered mental status. Heat stroke is a medical emergency and occurs in the setting of competitive sports or in elderly chronically ill patients exposed to summer heat waves. Sports related heat stroke is associated with intense physical exertion and profuse sweating in contrast to classic heat stroke with hot, and dry skin[70]. There is history of prolonged exposure to hot environment, hyperpyrexia, mental changes and marked elevation of hepatic transaminases.

Neuroleptic Malignant Syndrome

This may occur even after the offending neuroleptic agent has been withdrawn. It is characterized by high grade fever, altered sensorium, nuchal rigidity and 'lead pipe' stiffness of the extremities. Creatine phosphokinase level is markedly elevated[71].

Miscellaneous Conditions

Hypertensive encephalopathy, hepatic coma, dyselectrolytemia, accidental or intentional poisoning, inborn errors of metabolism, lead encephalopathy, diabetic ketoacidosis, brain tumors and vascular disorders if associated with fever due to any cause may also produce a picture of acute febrile encephalopathy.

REFERENCES

1. Prober CG. Central nervous system infections. In: Nelson Textbook of Pediatrics, Behrman RE, Kleigman RM (Eds.). *WB Saunders Co, Pennsylvania,* 16th edn 2000, pp 751-760.

2. Khetsuriani N, Holman RC, Andeson LJ. Burden of encephalitis associated admissions in the United States 1988-1997. *Clinical Infect Dis* 2002:35:175-182.

3. Bale JF Viral encephalitis. *Med Clin N Amer* 1993: 77(1); 25-41.

4. Cherry JD. Encephalitis. In: Nelson Textbook of Pediatrics, Behrman RE, Kleigman RM (Eds.). *WB Saunders Co, Pennsylvania,* 14th edn 1993; pp 666-669.

5. Gles K, Schuster FL, Christie LJ, Tureen JH. Beyond viruses: clinical profiles and etiologies associated with encephalitis. *Clinical Infect Dis* 2006; 43: 1565-77.

6. Koskineimi M, Rantalaiho T, Piiparinen H. Infections of the central nervous system of suspected viral origin: a collaborative study from Finland. *J Neurovirol* 2001; 7:400-408.

7. Mailles A and Stahl JP, Steering Committee and the Investigators Group. Infectious Encephalitis in France in 2007: A National Prospective Study. *Clin Infec Dis* 2009; 49:1838–1847.

8. Clare H, David ND, Christopher L, Craig D, David W, Mark SC and Paul MK. Etiology of encephalitis in Australia, 1990–2007. *Emerg Infect Dis* 2009; 15(9):1359-1365.

9. Selim HS, El-Barrawy MA, Rakha ME, Yingst SL, Baskharoun MF. Microbial Study of Meningitis and Encephalitis Cases. *J Egypt Public Health Assoc* 2007; 82 (1&2):1-19.

10. Xu Y, Zhaori G, Vera S, *et al.* Viral etiology of acute childhood encephalopathy in Beijing diagnosed by

analysis of single samples. *Pediatr Infect Dis J* 1996; 15(11):1018-1024.

11. Yong YK, Chong HT, Wong KT, Tan CT, Devi S. Aetiology of viral central nervous system infection, a Malaysian study. *Neurology Asia* 2008; 13 : 65 – 71

12. Xufang Y, Huanyu W, Shihong F, Xiaoyan G, Shuye Z, Chunting L, Minghua L, Yougang Z and Guodong L. Etiological spectrum of clinically diagnosed Japanese encephalitis cases reported in Guizhou Province, China, in 2006. *J Clin Microbiol* 2010; 48(4):1343-1349.

13. Tan LV, Qui PT, Quang Ha D, Hue NB, Bao LQ, Cam BV, Khanh TH, Hien TT, Chau NVV, Tram TT, Hien VM, Nga TVT, Schultsz C, Farrar J, Doorn HR, de Jong MD. Viral etiology of encephalitis in children in southern Vietnam: Results of a one-year prospective descriptive study. *PLOS Negl Trop Dis* 2010; 4(10): e854.

14. Kumar R, Mathur A, Kumar A, *et al*. Virological investigations of acute encephalopathy in India. *Arch Dis Child* 1990; 65:1227-1230.

15. Beig FK, Malik A, Rizvi M, Acharya D, Khare S. Etiology and clinico-epidemiological profile of acute viral encephalitis in children of western Uttar Pradesh, India. *Indian J Infect Dis* 2010; 14: e141—e146.

16. Sapkal GN, Bondre VP, Fulmali PV, Patil P, Gopalkrishna V, Dadhania V, Ayachit VM, Gangale D, Kushwaha KP, Rathi AK, Chitambar SD, Mishra AK and Gore MM. Enteroviruses in patients with acute encephalitis, Uttar Pradesh, India. *Emerg Infect Dis* 2009; 15(2): 295-298.

17. Vashishtha VM. Acute febrile encephalopathy: more stringent criteria needed to make a correct diagnosis. *Indian J Pediatr* 2009; 76:1185.

18. Whitley RJ, Gnann JW. Viral encephalitis: familiar infections and emerging pathogens. *Lancet* 2002; 359:507-514.

19. Wairagkar NS, Shaikh NJ, Ratho RK, Ghosh D, Mahajan RC, Singhi S, Gadkari. Isolation of measles virus from cerebrospinal fluid of children with acute encephalopathy without rash. *Indian Pediatr* 2000; 38:589-595.

20. Center for Disease Control and Prevention Update: West Nile like viral encephalitis in New York 1999. *JAMA* 1999; 282(18):714.

21. Fine A, Layton M. Lessons from the West Nile virus encephalitis outbreak in New York City 1999. *Clin Infect Dis* 2001; 32(2):277-282.

22. Rao BL, Basu A, Wairagkar NS, Gore MM, Arankalle VA, Thakare JP, Jadi RS, Rao KA, Mishra AC. A large outbreak of acute encephalitis with high fatality rate in children in Andhra Pradesh, India, in 2003, associated with Chandipura virus. *Lancet* 2004; 364(9437):869-874.

23. Chua KB, Goh KJ, Wong KT, Kamarulzaman A, Tan PS, Ksiazek TG, Zaki SR, Paul G, Lam SK, Tan CT. Fatal encephalitis due to Nipah virus among pig farmers in Malaysia. *Lancet* 1999; 354(9186):1257-1259.

24. Lum LC, Lam SK, Choy YS, *et al*. Dengue encephalitis a true entity? *Am J Trop Med Hyg* 1996; 54:256-259.

25. Kumar R, Tripathi S, Tambe JJ, Arora V, Srivastava A, Nag VL.Dengue encephalopathy in children in northern India: Clinical features and comparison with non dengue. *J Neurol Sciences* 2008; 269(1):41-48.

26. Whitley RJ. Viral encephalitis. *New Engl J Med* 1990; 323(4):242-249.

27. Kennedy PGE. Viral encephalitis: causes, differential diagnosis and management. *J Neurol Neurosurg Psychiatr* 2004; 75:110-115.

28. Klapper PE, Cleator GM, Longson M. Milder forms of Herpes simplex encephalitis. *J Neurol Neurosurg Psychiatr* 1984; 47:1247-1250.

29. Schlesinger Y, Buller RS, Brunstrom J, *et al*. Expanded spectrum of Herpes simplex encephalitis in childhood. *J Pediatr* 1995; 126:234-241.

30. Plotkin SA. Rabies. In: Nelson's Textbook of Pediatrics, Behrman RE, Kleigman RM (Eds). *WB Saunders Co, Philadelphia,* 14th Edn; 1993 pp 832-835

31. Kumar R, Senthilselvan A, Mathur A, *et al*. Clinical predictors of Japanese encephalitis. *Neuroepidemiology* 1994; 13:97-102.

32. Davis LE. Diagnosis and treatment of acute encephalitis. *The Neurologist* 2000; 6:145-159.

33. Tyler KL. Aseptic meningitis, viral encephalitis and prion diseases. In: Harrison's Principles of Internal Medicine. Faici AS, Braunwald E, Isselbacher KJ (Eds). 14th Edn *New York McGraw Hill* 1998: 2439-51

34. Chaudhuri A, Kennedy PGE. Diagnosis and treatment of viral encephalitis. *Post Graduate Med J* 2002; 78: 575-583.

35. Kennedy C. Acute viral encephalitis in childhood. *BMJ* 1995; 310:139-140.

36. Reuben R, Gajanana A. Japanese encephalitis in India. *Indian J Pediatr* 1997; 64:243-251.

37. Ho SH, Harter DH. Herpes simplex virus encephalitis. *JAMA* 1982; 247:337.

38. Aurelius E, Johansson B, Skoldenberg B, *et al*. Rapid diagnosis of Herpes simplex encephalitis by nested polymerase chain reaction assay of cerebrospinal fluid. *Lancet* 1991; 337:189-192.

39. Troendle-Atkins J, Demmler GJ, Buffone GJ. Rapid diagnosis of Herpes simplex virus encephalitis by using the polymerase chain reaction. *J Pediatr* 1993; 123: 376-380.

40. Stellrecht KA, Harding I, Woron AM, Lepow ML, Venezia RA. The impact of an enteroviral RT-PCR assay on the diagnosis of aseptic meningitis and patient management. *J Clin Virol* 2002; 25(Suppl 1): S19- S26.

41. Ferrari S, Toniolo A, Monaco S, Luciani F, Cainelli F, Baj A, Temesgen Z and Vento S. Viral encephalitis: etiology, clinical features, diagnosis and management. *Opin Infect Dis J* 2009; 3:1-12.

42. http://www.cdc.gov/rabies/diagnosis/animals-humans.html accessed 22nd April 2011

43. Domingues RB, Fink MC, Tsanaclis AM, *et al.* Diagnosis of Herpes simplex encephalitis by magnetic resonance imaging and polymerase chain reaction of cerebrospinal fluid. *J Neurol Sci* 1998; 157:148-153

44. Zimmermann RD, Russell EJ, Leeds NE, *et al.* CT in early diagnosis of Herpes simplex encephalitis. *Am J Neuroradiol* 1980; 134:61-66.

45. Misra UK, Kalita J, Jain SK, *et al.* Radiological and neurophysiological changes in Japanese encephalitis. *J Neurol Neurosurg Psychiatr* 1997; 54:1484-1487.

46. Shaji H, Kido H, Hino H. Magnetic resonance imaging findings in Japanese encephalitis. *J Neuroimaging* 1994; 57:206-211.

47. Ito Y, Ando Y, Kumino H, *et al.* Polymerase chain reaction proven Herpes simplex encephalitis in children. *Pediatr Infect Dis J* 1998; 17: 29-32.

48. Misra UK, Kalita J. Neurophysiological studies in Herpes simplex encephalitis. *Electromyography Clin Neurophys* 1998; 38(3):177-182.

49. Launes J, Siren J, Valanne L, *et al.* Unilateral hyperperfusion in brain-perfusion SPECT predicts poor prognosis in acute encephalitis. *Neurology* 1997: 48: 1347-1351.

50. Kalra V. Acute febrile encephalopathy. In: Practical Paediatric Neurology. Gupta V, Gupta D (Eds.). *Avichal Publishing Co.* 2nd Edn 2008. *Arya Publications* pp 112.

51. Kumar R, Singh SN, Kohli N. A diagnostic rule for tuberculous meningitis. *Arch Dis Child* 1999; 81: 221-224.

52. Kumar R, Kohli N, Kumar A, Sharma B. Value of CT scan in diagnosis of meningitis. *Indian Pediatr* 1996; 33(6):465-468.

53. Mathai E, Rolain JM, Varghese GM, Abraham OC, Mathai D, Raoult D. Outbreak of scrub typhus in southern India during the cooler months. *Ann NY Acad Sci* 2003; 990:359-364.

54. Coyle PK. Post infectious encephalomyelitis. In: Infectious Diseases of the Nervous System. Devis LE, Kennedy PGE (Eds.). *Oxford, Butterworth–Heinemann* 2000; p 83-108.

55. Singh RR, Chaudhary SK, Bhatta NK, Khanal B, Shah D. Clinical and etiological profile of acute febrile encephalopathy in eastern Nepal. *Indian J Pediatr* 2009; 76(11):1109-11011.

56. Kumar R. Viral encephalitis. *Pediatr Today* 2000; 3: 34-42.

57. Hoke GH, Vaughn DW, Nisalak A. Effect of high dose dexamethasone on the outcome of acute encephalitis due to Japanese encephalitis virus. *J Infect Dis* 1992; 164:631-637.

58. Handa SK, Das CP, Prabhakar S. Acyclovir induced extrapyramidal symptoms. *Neurol India* 2002; 50: 109-110.

59. de Miranda P, Blum MR. Pharmacokinetics of acyclovir after intravenous and oral administration. *J Antimicrob Chemother* 1983; 12 b (Suppl):29-37.

60. Kohl S. Herpes simplex virus. In: Nelson's Textbook of Pediatrics. Behrman RE, Kleigman RM (Eds.). *WB Saunders Co, Philadelphia* 15th Ed, 1996 pp 885-889.

61. Tunkel AR. Double-blind placebo-controlled trial of pleconaril in infants with enteroviral meningitis. *Curr Infect Dis Rep* 2004; 6(4):295-296.

62. Tunkel AR, Glaser C, Block KC, Sejvar JJ, Marra CM, The management of encephalitis: clinical practice guidelines by the Infectious Diseases Society of America. *Clinical Infect Dis* 2008; 47: 303-327.

63. Solomon T, Hart IJ, Beeching NJ. Viral encephalitis: a clinician's guide. *Pract Neurol* 2007; 7: 288–305.

64. Kumar R, Tripathi P, Baranwal M, Singh S, Tripathi S, Banerjee G. Randomized, controlled trial of oral ribavirin for Japanese encephalitis in children in Uttar Pradesh, India. *Clin Infec Dis* 2009;48:400-406.

65. White NJ, Ho M. The pathophysiology of cerebral malaria. *Adv Parasitol* 1992; 31:84-94.

66. Cleary TG. Shigella. In: Nelson's Textbook of Pediatrics, Behrman RE, Kleigman RM (Eds.). *WB Saunders Co, Pennsylvania* 17th Edn 2004, pp 919-920.

67. Rudolph JA, Balisteri WF. Reye's syndrome and the mitochondrial hepatopathies. In: Nelson Textbook of Pediatrics, Behrman RE, Kleigman RM (Eds.). *WB Saunders Co, Pennsylvania,* 17th edn 2004, pp 1335-1337.

68. Benakappa DG, Das S, Shanker SK, Sridhara Rama Rao BS, Prakash GS, Aswath NSC, Benakappa A. Reye's syndrome in Bangalore. *Indian J Pediatr* 1991; 58: 805-810.

69. Ghosh D, Dhadwal D, Aggarwal A, Mitra S, Garg SK, Kumar R. Investigation of an epidemic of Reye's syndrome in northern region of India. *Indian Pediatr* 1999; 36:1097-1106.

70. Behrman RE, Kleigman RM (Eds). In: Nelson's Textbook of Pediatrics 17th Edn *WB Saunders Co, Pennsylvania* 2004, pp 2314-2315.

71. Dalton R. In: Nelson's Textbook of Pediatrics, Behrman RE, Kleigman RM (Eds.). *WB Saunders Co, Pennsylvania* 17th Edn 2004, pp 96.

Section 4

38

Status Epilepticus

Sheffali Gulati and Meharban Singh

Status epilepticus (SE) is an acute, life-threatening neurological emergency that may lead to permanent neurological damage or even death. It poses a therapeutic challenge to the treating physician. Status epilepticus is estimated to affect approximately 1:150,000 people per year in United States[1]. The figure must be higher in our country. It is more frequent in children, following acute neuroinfections, dysmetabolic states, hypoxia, brain damage and sudden withdrawal of antiepileptic drugs (AEDs). It is estimated that 1.3% to 16% of all patients with epilepsy will develop SE at some point in their lives[2]. The management of a patient with SE requires early recognition, timely intervention and a series of important decisions based on an accurate clinical assessment[3, 4].

DEFINITION

In 1997, the International League Against Epilepsy defined status epilepticus as "a single epileptic seizure of >30 minute in duration or a series of epileptic seizures during which consciousness is not regained between ictal events in a >30-min period."[5] Based on the fact that continuous seizures lasting 45-83 minutes result in neuronal injury in animal models, the proposed 30 minute cut-off seems reasonable. Lately it is being increasingly recognized that seizures lasting for more than 10 minutes may cause brain damage and therefore the duration of seizure activity in the definition of status epilepticus is being reduced. The typical generalized tonic-clonic seizures in adults rarely last longer than 5 minutes. The seizures lasting beyond 5 minutes are less likely to cease without medical intervention. These facts have been highlighted by some authors to propose an "operational definition" by which one can identify the patients who are at a higher risk of progressing to status epilepticus and who require aggressive initial and ongoing management. Few authors recommend an operational definition of status epilepticus; either continuous seizures lasting for at least 5 minutes or two or more discrete seizures between which there is incomplete recovery of consciousness[6]. Status epilepticus equivalents include five minutes of continuous convulsive seizures; three discrete convulsions within one hour; thirty minutes of continuous seizures or lack of recovery between discrete seizures which may be focal, complex partial seizures, absences and other non-convulsive seizures[6].

Practically speaking, any patient who exhibits persistent seizure activity or who does not regain consciousness for five minutes or more after a witnessed seizure should be considered to have status epilepticus. Also any patient who is brought to the emergency room with continuing seizure activity should be assumed to have SE.

CLASSIFICATION

There is no consensus regarding the classification of SE. The classification based on the origin of seizures is most commonly used[7]. Status epilepticus may be generalized (tonic-clonic, myoclonic, absence, atonic, akinetic) or partial (simple or complex). Treiman[8] has proposed that SE may be classified into generalized convulsive status (overt or subtle) and non-convulsive status epilepticus (simple partial, complex partial, absence). Some workers have classified SE on the basis of age of the patient[9].

Status epilepticus is generally broadly classified as shown in Table 38.1[10]. Of these, generalized tonic-clonic seizures are the most common. It has the highest potential for complications or death. Status epilepticus conventionally implies generalized convulsive status epilepticus.

Table 38.1 Classification of status epilepticus

- Convulsive (includes tonic-clonic, tonic, clonic and myoclonic)
- Non-convulsive (includes absence status)
- Partial status epilepticus (includes elementary, somatomotor seizures, dysphasia)
- Complex partial (includes fugue states, psychomotor seizures)
- Unilateral status (hemiclonic, hemiconvulsion-hemiplegia)

Convulsive Generalized Status Epilepticus

Grandmal status epilepticus. It is manifested by generalized tonic-clonic activity that is characterized either by seizures that are generalized from the onset, or seizures that get secondarily generalized after a partial onset. It occurs five to six times more frequently in patients with symptomatic seizures than in those with seizures of unknown cause (idiopathic). The majority of patients with symptomatic seizures have brain tumor, head trauma, cerebrovascular disease or a metabolic disorder.

Tonic status epilepticus. It is almost always seen in children with secondary generalized epilepsy associated with varying degrees of intellectual disability/mental retardation (Lennox-Gastaut syndrome). Seizure activity is characterized by brief attacks of bilateral tonic spasms.

Clonic status epilepticus. It occurs almost exclusively in infants and children below five years of age and accounts for half the cases of generalized convulsive status in children. About 50 percent of patients with clonic status belong to the idiopathic group; while in the other 50 percent a specific cause such as chronic encephalopathy, infection or a metabolic disturbance can be found. Clinically, the patient has bilateral jerking which is usually asymmetrical and asynchronous and may recur irregularly.

Myoclonic status epilepticus. It is most frequently seen in association with secondary generalized epilepsy in children. Clinically it is characterized by clouding of consciousness and irregular, rapid muscle jerks which are bilateral but asymmetrical. In the rare instance myoclonic status occurs in the presence of primary generalized epilepsy. The myoclonic status can occasionally occur as a manifestation of a diverse group of diseases, such as acute or sub acute encephalopathy (metabolic, viral, toxic) and some neurodegenerative diseases. This acquired variant of myoclonic epilepsy is often associated with a poor outcome.

Nonconvulsive Generalized Status Epilepticus

Although convulsive generalized status epilepticus is often life-threatening, the different forms of non-convulsive status epilepticus (NCSE) such as complete partial status and absence status epilepticus are rarely fatal. The NCSE is less commonly recognized and often missed in children.[11]The electroencephalogram documents continuous epileptiform abnormalities in the absence of overt clinical signs. The common situations in which NCSE may be encountered include patients with atypical absence seizures who have prolonged unresponsiveness, comatose patients following post-traumatic or post-anoxic brain injury, and patients with convulsive SE whose convulsions are controlled but have prolonged altered sensorium.

NCSE, like convulsive status epilepticus, is a state of continuous or intermittent seizure activity without a return to baseline lasting more than 30 minutes. In general, NCSE differs from convulsive status epilepticus by the lack of a predominant motor component. The hallmark of NCSE is a change in behavior or mental status that is associated with diagnostic EEG changes. The common types of nonconvulsive status epilepticus (SE) by age are listed below.

Nonconvulsive SE confined to childhood
(i)   Electrical SE during slow-wave sleep
(ii)   Landau-Kleffner syndrome

Nonconvulsive SE occurring in childhood and adult life
(i)   Absence SE
(ii)   SE in coma
(iii) Specific forms of SE in patients with learning difficulties
(iv)   Nonconvulsive simple partial SE
(v)   Complex partial SE

Nonconvulsive SE confined to adult life
● *De novo* absence status of late onset

The precipitating factors that are implicated in NCSE include metabolic abnormalities, CNS infection, drug toxicity, alcohol intoxication/withdrawal, pregnancy, central nervous system disturbances, and electroconvulsive treatment. Different series have indicated that a precipitating factor can be identified in 15% to 70% of cases, emphasizing the importance of detailed history in the evaluation of these patients.

Elementary Partial Status Epilepticus

There is a wide spectrum of elementary partial seizures. Of these, somatomotor status and dysphasic status account for a majority of the cases. Somatomotor status epilepticus typically consists of constant and repetitive clonic twitchings of the contralateral muscles of the body (focal body seizures) which are followed by transient hemiparesis (Todd's paralysis). Several seizures may occur in a day but consciousness remains intact. Jacksonian seizures have a tendency to spread or "march" as for instance from the arm to the face and onto the leg. The activity may spread to the other side of the body with accompanying loss of consciousness. When constant clonic activity persists and remains limited to one body region, it is known as *epilepsia partialis continua*. Focal motor status is usually due to ischemia, trauma, inflammation or a structural lesion. In about half the cases, a history of epilepsy is present. Absence status epilepticus account for 10 percent of the attacks and usually occurs in children who have severe primary generalized epilepsy or Lennox Gastaut syndrome. This is one of the most difficult types of status to control.

Erratic Status Epilepticus

This clinical type of status epilepticus is seen only in neonates (Table 38.2) and has characteristics different from status epilepticus observed in older children and adults. Status epilepticus in the newborn period is almost always followed by poor outcome, particularly when it occurs in the first three days of life. The prognosis is related to the underlying etiology rather than the occurrence of seizures. Some of the etiological factors that should be considered include; trauma, hypoxic-ischemic encephalopathy, hypoglycemia, infections (especially meningitis and sepsis), CNS developmental defects, drug withdrawal, aminoacidopathies, pyridoxine dependency and kernicterus.

ETIOLOGY

The causes of SE in children can be grouped into prolonged febrile seizures, acute symptomatic seizures, remote symptomatic seizures, acute on remote symptomatic seizures, idiopathic/cryptogenic causes, and unknown causes. The commonest etiology for pediatric SE in most of the prospective studies is prolonged febrile seizures. This is followed by acute symptomatic seizures, remote symptomatic seizures and cryptogenic seizures in variable proportions in different studies. The causes of status epilepticus in various series are detailed in Table 38.3[13-15].

Table 38.2 Neonatal seizures types[12]

I. Subtle seizures
Premature and full-term infants
- Tonic horizontal deviation of eyes and jerking
- Eyelid blinking or fluttering
- Sucking, smacking, drooling and other oral-buccal-lingual movements
- "Swimming", "rowing", "pedaling" movements

II. Generalized tonic seizures
Primarily premature infants
- Tonic extension of upper and lower limbs (mimics decerebrate posturing)
- Tonic flexion of upper limbs, extension of lower limbs (mimics decorticate posturing)

III. Multifocal clonic seizures
Primarily full-term infants
- Multifocal clonic movements (simultaneous or in sequence)
- Nonordered ("non-Jacksonian") migration

IV. Focal clonic seizures
Full-term and premature infants
- Well-localized clonic jerking
- Infant is usually not unconscious

V. Myoclonic seizures
Premature and full-term infants
- Single or several synchronous flexion jerks of upper and lower limbs
- May precede hypsrrhythmia

Table 38.3 Causes of status epilepticus by etiology

Acute neurological (26%-49%)
- CNS* infections (meningitis, encephalitis, cerebral malaria, sepsis syndrome)
- Electrolyte disorders (hyponatremia, hypocalcemia, hypomagnesemia)
- Toxins/ metabolic causes (Reye's syndrome, IEM**, lead, uremia)
- Trauma (including surgery)
- Acute anoxic insults
- Cerebrovascular accidents

Chronic CNS disorders (11%-21%)
- Neonatal nonprogressive insult
- Space occupying lesions (tumors, abscess, neurocysticercosis, bleed)
- CNS malformations
- Progressive encephalopathy

Cryptogenic or idiopathic (46%-58%)
- Febrile
- Afebrile

---

* **CNS:** Central nervous system.
** **IEM:** Inborn error of metabolism

The causes can be effectively grouped into three broad categories: (i) prolonged febrile seizures, (ii) idiopathic status epilepticus (seizures develop in the absence of an underlying CNS lesion or insult) and (iii) symptomatic status epilepticus (seizures occur as a result of underlying CNS insult or metabolic abnormality).

Status epilepticus occurs most frequently in children aged 5 years or younger (85%)[16]. Although individuals with a history of epilepsy are particularly at risk of developing status epilpeticus, while approximately 50% of cases occur in the absence of previous known epilepsy[17]. Among children with a first unprovoked seizure, 9% have been reported to manifest as status epilepticus[18-19]. The causes of SE are age-dependent and are listed in Table 38.4.

The search for a precipitating factor is of fundamental importance, as it will guide appropriate therapy. The important risk factors for SE include history of epilepsy, low antiepileptic drug (AED) level, younger age, genetic predisposition and acquired brain insult[22]. The important precipitating factors include febrile illness, inadequate or irregular AED therapy, sudden discontinuation of AED, sleep deprivation, fatigue, emotional upset, metabolic abnormalities, intake of drugs (theophylline, amphetamines, isoniazid, organophosphorous

Table 38.4 Causes of status epilepticus (age-wise)[20-21]

Neonates (first month of life)
- Birth injury (anoxia, hemorrhage) and congenital abnormalities
- Metabolic disorders (hypoglycemia, hypocalcemia, hyponatremia, hypernatremia) and inborn errors of metabolism (lipidoses, aminoacidurias, pyridoxine dependency)
- Infection (meningitis)
- Drugs/ drug withdrawal

Early childhood (<6 years)
- Birth injury
- Febrile convulsions (1 month to 6 years)
- Infections
- Metabolic disorders
- Trauma
- Neurocutaneous syndromes
- Cerebral degenerative diseases
- Tumors
- Toxins
- Idiopathic

Children and adolescents (>6 years)
- Birth injury
- Trauma
- Infections
- Epilepsy with inadequate drug levels
- Cerebral degenerative diseases
- Tumor
- Toxins
- Idiopathic

compounds), hyperventilation, intermittent photic stimulation, and AED over dose (carbamazepine in non-convulsive SE). In a study at AIIMS on 30 children with SE, sixteen patients (53.3%) presented with SE as a first manifestation without any prior history of seizure activity. Among these 16 patients, 11 patients (68.7%) were less than 5 years of age[23].

PATHOPHYSIOLOGY

Status epilepticus results from inability to normally abort an isolated seizure due to ineffective inhibition or due to abnormally persistent and excessive excitation. The studies in animal models of status epilepticus using broad-spectrum glutamatergic agonist kainic acid (KA model) and the muscarinic agonist pilocarpine (Pilo model) have shown that a progressive reduction in γ-aminobutyric acid (GABA) mediated inhibition is an important component of SE. This is the reason that the drugs that are effective early in the course of SE often fail to control seizures in later stages of SE. The self-sustaining nature of SE has been suggested due to activity-dependent trafficking of GABA-A receptors. Excessive activation of excitatory amino acid receptors or excessive release of glutamate can also cause prolonged seizures[24]. Drugs and compounds that antagonize the effects of GABA, the main inhibitory neurotransmitter of the brain may cause status epilepticus[25]. The most vulnerable areas include the limbic system, cerebellum, middle cortical area and the thalamus. Prolonged seizure activity (lasting more than 1 hour) may lead to hypotension, hyperkalemia, hypoglycemia, lactic acidosis, myoglobinuria, acute tubular necrosis and death.

CLINICAL FEATURES

The child may present to the emergency department with frank and persistent seizures. With passage of time, the clinical manifestations become subtle and the child may have only small amplitude twitching movements of the face and limbs or nystagmoid jerking of the eyes. The child may have tachycardia, hypertension and features of raised intracranial pressure (ICP). The differential diagnosis of convulsive status epilepticus includes rigors due to sepsis, myoclonic epilepsy, dystonias and pseudostatus epilepticus. In the latter the consciousness is often retained during convulsions[26].

Clinical manifestations of NCSE

In nonconvulsive status epilepticus, clinical features include altered sensorium that may fluctuate, agitation, abnormal eye movements (including ocular deviation and nystagmus), aphasia and abnormal limb posturing. Clinical manifestations may vary considerably, ranging from subtle changes recognizable only to family members, to psychotic or affective states, all the way to delirium or coma The variety of presentations described in the literature are listed below.

- Mild cognitive disturbances
- Prolonged confusional states
- Mood disturbances
- Cortical blindness
- Speech disturbances (verbal perseveration to reduced verbal fluency, muteness, speech arrest, aphasia, echolalia or confabulations)
- Bizarre behaviour which is uncharacteristic and deviates from usual (eg, laughing, dancing, and singing inappropriately)
- Clear psychotic states
- Autonomic disturbances such as belching, borborygmus, flatulence
- Sensory and psychic phenomena
- Motor activity usually normal in most cases; however, decreased response time, clumsiness, apraxia, focal jerks, twitching of facial muscles (in particular of the eyelids) and automatisms such as licking, chewing, or picking have been noted[11].

Diagnosis therefore requires a high degree of suspicion and can only be confirmed definitively by electroencephalography (EEG)[26]. In a recent study, 8% of patients in coma were diagnosed to have non-convulsive status epilepticus[27].

DIAGNOSTIC EVALUATION

The clinical setting in which SE has occurred, including history and clinical examination is the crucial factor that determines the extent of investigations in an individual patient. In an emergency and intensive care setting, much of this evaluation can occur once the child is stabilized and the seizures are controlled partially or fully. Table 38.5 summarizes the investigations in specific clinical situations.

Blood is obtained for complete blood count (CBC), determination of electrolytes, blood glucose, calcium and magnesium levels, creatinine, liver function tests (LFT), arterial lactate, creatine kinase and anticonvulsant drug levels. If indicated, blood and urine may be obtained for metabolic studies and toxicology. Hypoxia and acidosis should be ruled out by doing an arterial blood gas (ABG).

Cerebrospinal fluid (CSF) examination is mandatory if meningitis or encephalitis is considered. It should be performed after exclusion of raised ICP. It is important to remember that approximately 20% of patients have CSF pleocytosis with a white blood cell count of upto 80 x 10^6/l following SE, so called benign post-ictal pleocytosis. These patients should be treated for suspected meningitis until the diagnosis is excluded by culture or other studies[5].

Fundus examination is done for papilledema (a sign of raised ICP) and retinal hemorrhages. Computerized tomography (CT) or magnetic resonance imaging (MRI) scan is obtained on an emergent basis if seizures are refractory to treatment, progressive neurological findings are present on serial examination, partial seizures, worsening focal findings on the EEG, suspicion of increased ICP, after head trauma and in cases in whom surgery is being considered. The yield of CT or MRI scan in a child with normal neurologic examination and EEG is less than 5%[10].

Electroencephalography (EEG) is extremely useful, but underutilized, in the diagnosis and management of status epilepticus. Although overt

Table 38.5 Basic investigations in patients with SE		
Category	**Always recommended**	**Individualized**
New-onset SE	<ul><li>Serum electrolytes</li><li>Blood glucose</li><li>Neuroimaging (CT/MRI as feasible)</li><li>EEG</li></ul>	<ul><li>Complete blood counts</li><li>Lumbar puncture</li><li>Metabolic testing</li><li>Toxicology screen of blood and urine</li></ul>
SE in a known case of epilepsy	<ul><li>Anti-epileptic drug levels</li><li>EEG</li></ul>	<ul><li>Complete blood counts</li><li>Serum electrolytes</li><li>Blood glucose</li><li>Neuroimaging (CT/MRI as feasible)</li></ul>

convulsive status epilepticus is readily diagnosed, EEG can establish the diagnosis in less obvious cases. Privitera *et al*[28] showed that EEG monitoring was useful to diagnose status epilepticus in 37 percent of patients with altered consciousness in whom diagnosis was unclear on the basis of clinical criteria. EEG can also help to confirm that an episode of status epilepticus has ended. DeLorenzo *et al*[29] monitored patients for at least 24 hours after clinical signs of status epilepticus had ended. They found that nearly one-half of their patients continued to demonstrate electrographic seizures that had no clinical correlation. The investigators concluded that EEG monitoring after presumed control of status epilepticus is essential for optimal management.

Patients with status epilepticus who fail to recover rapidly and completely should be monitored with EEG for at least 24 hours after an episode to ensure that recurrent seizures are not missed. This is also useful in patients with prolonged altered sensorium following control of convulsive seizures to rule out NCSE. Monitoring is also advised if periodic discharges appear in the EEG of a patient with altered consciousness who has not had obvious seizures. Periodic discharges in these patients suggest the possibility of preceding status epilepticus, and careful monitoring may clarify the etiology of the discharges and allow the detection of recurrent status epilepticus. Continuous EEG monitoring is also required in cases of pyridoxine dependency.

It is crucial that pharmacotherapy is not delayed while investigations are being conducted. Tests and procedures required for evaluation of SE are summarized in Table 38.6.

Table 38.6 Tests and procedures for evaluation of status epilepticus (modified)[30]	
Advised in all cases	**To be considered when indicated**
• Pulse oximetry • Cardiac monitoring • CBC • Blood glucose • Electrolytes • Calcium • Magnesium • ABG	• Lumbar puncture • Antiepileptic drug levels • Toxicology screen • LFT/RFT* • Ammonia level, arterial lactate, urine for metabolic screen • Creatine kinase • Blood culture • EEG • CT/MRI
* Liver function tests/renal function tests	

Diagnostic approach in NCSE

Because of the wide range of presentations of NCSE, the diagnosis is often missed, confused for a psychiatric disorder or a neurologic insult. A detailed history, including change from baseline status, onset and duration of the events, presence or absence of lucid interval, timing in relation to the sleep/wake cycle, and presence or absence of motor activity or automatisms, needs to be obtained. Past medical, neurologic, psychiatric history, family history, social history and medication history are additional important components of the diagnostic evaluation. The emergency physician should be familiar with protean manifestations of NCSE and consider EEG monitoring and a therapeutic trial of antiepileptic drugs in clinical conditions associated with agitation, bizarre behaviour, staring, increased muscle tone, mutism or subtle myoclonus.[11]

COMPLICATIONS

The consequences of status epilepticus are considerable in terms of neuronal damage and loss of life. There is evidence to suggest that more that 60 minutes of convulsive status epilepticus may produce irreversible brain damage due to multiple factors. The mortality rate in patients with status epilepticus ranges from 6 to 18 percent[31-32]. The mortality is partly due to cardio-respiratory arrest, but more often as a result of the underlying illness (tumor, trauma, infection). In some reports, death was also related to untoward effects of excessive intravenous anticonvulsants. Medical complications that have been reported to occur in status epilepticus are enumerated in Table 38.7. Hyperpyrexia commonly occurs due to sustained motor activity. A prompt and profound fall in blood pH may occur due to lactate production. Due to metabolic acidosis, shift of potassium from intracellular compartment may lead to hyperkalemia and cardiac arrhythmia. Respiratory insufficiency and hypoxia needs careful monitoring and management.

MANAGEMENT

The main objective of therapy is to abort the seizures and treat the provoking or precipitating condition. The vital signs should be monitored by attaching the patient to a multi-channel monitor. Input-output (condom or catheter) should be maintained. Ensuring patent airway, adequate ventilation and oxygenation, normoglycemia and normothermia are the most important initial steps. It has been shown in experimental animals that the

Table 38.7 Medical complications of status epilepticus[33]	
1. **Cardiovascular complications** • Tachycardia, bradycardia, cardiac arrest • Hypertension, hypotension, shock • Cardiac failure • Cardiac arrhythmias 2. **Respiratory system failure** • Apnea, tachypnea, bradypnea Cheyne-Stokes breathing • Pulmonary congestion (may be neurogenic) • Pneumonia, aspiration • Airway obstruction 3. **Kidney failure** • Oliguria, uremia • Acute tubular necrosis • Lower nephron nephrosis • Rhabdomyolysis, myoglobinuria	4. **Autonomic disturbances** • Hyperpyrexia • Excessive sweating, vomiting, dehydration, electrolyte loss • Hypersecretion (salivary, tracheobronchial) 5. **Metabolic and biochemical derangements** • Acidosis (metabolic, respiratory) • Azotemia • Hyperkalemia • Hypoglycemia • Hyponatremia • Hepatic failure 6. **Infections** • Pulmonary, bladder, skin, nosocomial sepsis

risk of permanent brain damage is directly related to the duration of the status epilepticus[5]. The broad principles and clinical approach towards management are outlined in Table 38.8.

General Principles

Prompt and appropriate pharmacological therapy can reduce mortality and morbidity. It includes initiating ABC of life support, prompt administration of effective antiepileptic drugs in adequate doses and identifying and treating the underlying cause. Initial treatment begins with institution of the standard measures like supporting and securing the airway. Excessive oral secretions are removed by gentle suction. Oxygen should be provided by nasal cannula or mask. Endotracheal intubation should be considered if there are signs of respiratory failure. It also prevents the pulmonary aspiration of gastric contents. Nasogastric tube is placed in position and IV access is established by inserting two IV catheters to allow for fluid therapy and pharmacotherapy.

If hypoglycemia is confirmed or a blood glucose determination is unavailable, a rapid infusion of 5 ml/kg of 10% dextrose or 2 ml/kg of 25% dextrose is administered. In order to maintain cerebral perfusion pressure, systolic blood pressure should be maintained at normal or high normal levels during prolonged seizures, using vasopressors if needed[5].

Table 38.8 Goals and initial management of status epilepticus	
The goals of treatment	**Initial management steps**
• Ensure adequate oxygenation of brain and cardiorespiratory function • Terminate seizures clinically and electrically as rapidly as possible • Prevent seizure recurrences • Identify precipitating factors • Correct metabolic abnormalities • Prevent systemic complications • Manage underlying cause of status epilepticus and its complications	• Assess and secure airway • Give oxygen by nasal cannula or mask • Consider intubation if respiratory assistance is needed • Monitor vital signs (pulse, respiration, blood pressure, temperature); and control any abnormalities as needed • Establish two IV lines • If hypoglycemia is established or a blood glucose estimation is unavailable, administer 5 ml/kg of 10% dextrose or 2 ml/kg of 25% dextrose • Perform laboratory investigations • Administer anticonvulsants while taking a quick history and doing physical examination

All patients with SE have some degree of cerebral edema and raised ICP. Raised intracranial pressure was historically managed by fluid restriction in an effort to avoid increasing brain water. It was later discovered that hypovolemia may lead to decreased cerebral perfusion with aggravation of global hypoxic ischemic injury. Also there is no evidence that fluid restriction improves cerebral edema. Thus hypovolemia must be assiduously avoided. Hypotonic intravenous fluids should be avoided because they may lead to fluid shift into the brain compartment and exacerbate cerebral edema. Dextrose 5% solution with half normal saline, normal saline, or Ringer's lactate is preferred. The patient should be monitored closely for the syndrome of inappropriate secretion of antidiuretic hormone (SIADH), with measurements of serum and urine osmolality. Fluid intake should be kept at the usual maintenance levels but lowered if the syndrome of inappropriate secretion of antidiuretic hormone begins to appear. Bicarbonate should only be given if it is low enough to be of immediate concern. It can be given to half correct the acidosis when the pH is less than 7.2.

A quick physical examination including neurological assessment should be done concurrently to detect evidences of trauma, raised ICP (papilledema, bulging anterior fontanel or focal neurological signs), manifestations of sepsis or meningitis, retinal hemorrhages (subdural hematoma), irregular respirations (brainstem dysfunction), and pupillary size abnormalities suggesting toxin or drug ingestion or uncal herniation. Further investigations can be planned after taking a detailed history and systemic examination.

Therapeutic approach and options are guided by prehospital treatment, drugs available, duration of SE, cardiopulmonary status and intensive care support available.[34-35] The proposed algorithm for pharmacotherapy of SE is detailed in Figure 38.1[36]

Over one-half of the patients with SE will respond to therapy with a single antiepileptic drug. It is difficult to predict at presentation who will respond to the initial drug treatment. When a patient has refractory status, the search for an acute or progressive cause should be intense. Experimental data indicate that delay in the treatment of SE increases the likelihood that the patient will not respond to one or even two medications[5]. The commonly used drugs with their doses and infusion rates are summarized in Table 38.9. If seizures are

Table 38.9 Doses, infusion rates and side effects of various drugs used in status epilepticus

Drugs	Dose	Rate of administration	Time taken to stop seizures (min)	Maximum single dose	Duration of action	Side effects
Diazepam	0.1-0.3 mg/kg IV	5 mg/min	1-3	10 mg	15-30 min	Respiratory depression, sedation, hypotension
Lorazepam	0.05-0.1 mg/kg IV	2 mg/min	1-5	4 mg	12-24 hr	Respiratory depression, sedation, hypotension
Phenytoin	20 mg/kg IV	1 mg/kg/min upto maximum of 50 mg/min	10-30	1500 mg/day	24 hr	Cardiovascular collapse, hypotension, cardiac arrhythmia
Fosphenytoin	20 mg/kg PE*, IV	3 mg/kg/min upto maximum of 150 mg/min	–	1500 mg PE*/day	–	There is less risk for hypotension and phlebitis
Phenobarbital	20 mg/kg IV	2 mg/kg/min upto maximum of 100 mg/min	20-30	1000 mg/day	>48 hr	Respiratory depression, hypotension especially if used after benzodiazepines

PE*: Phenytoin equivalents: 150 mg fosphenytoin equals 100 mg of phenytoin

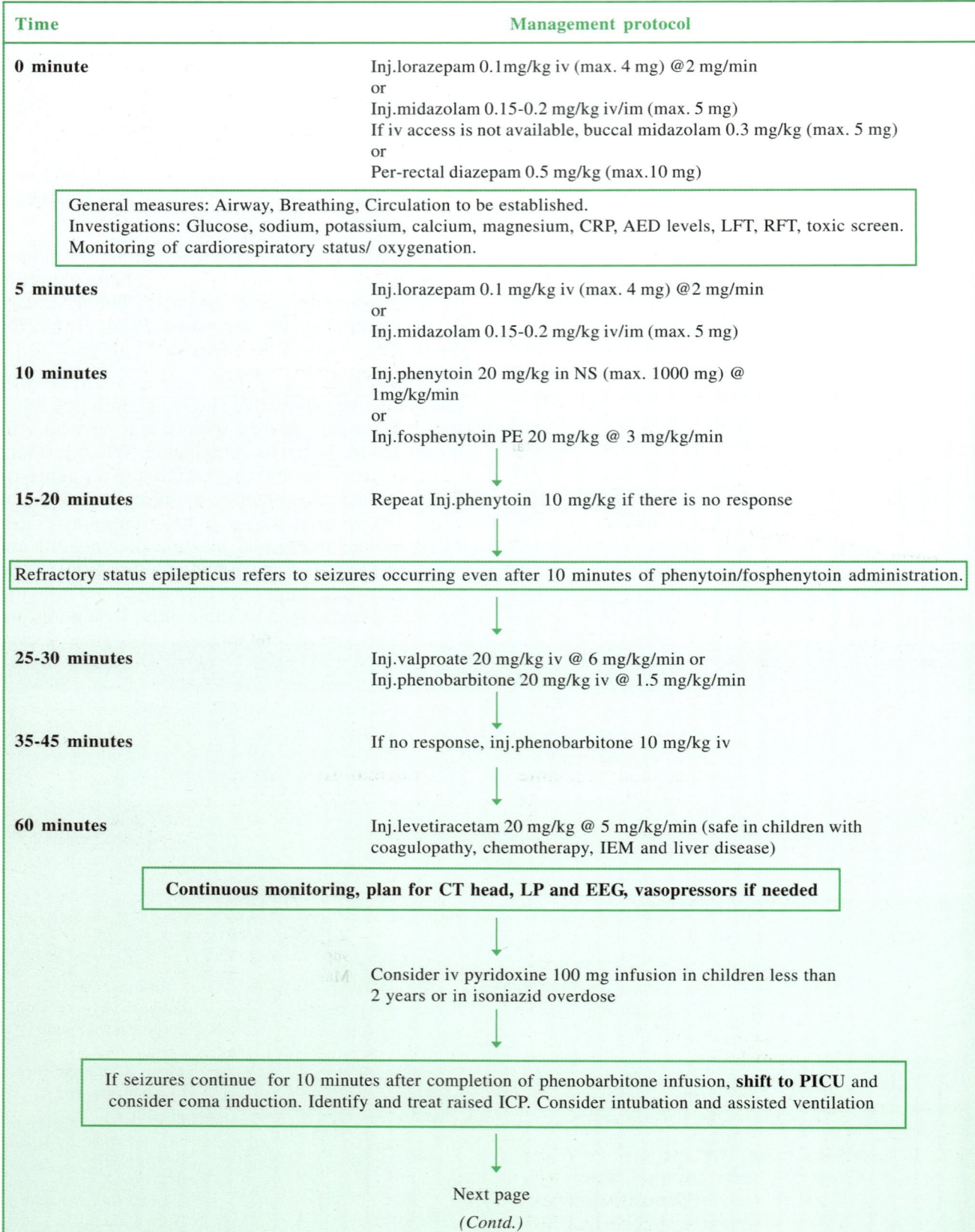

Time	Management protocol
0 minute	Inj.lorazepam 0.1mg/kg iv (max. 4 mg) @2 mg/min or Inj.midazolam 0.15-0.2 mg/kg iv/im (max. 5 mg) If iv access is not available, buccal midazolam 0.3 mg/kg (max. 5 mg) or Per-rectal diazepam 0.5 mg/kg (max.10 mg)

General measures: Airway, Breathing, Circulation to be established.
Investigations: Glucose, sodium, potassium, calcium, magnesium, CRP, AED levels, LFT, RFT, toxic screen.
Monitoring of cardiorespiratory status/ oxygenation.

Time	Management protocol
5 minutes	Inj.lorazepam 0.1 mg/kg iv (max. 4 mg) @2 mg/min or Inj.midazolam 0.15-0.2 mg/kg iv/im (max. 5 mg)
10 minutes	Inj.phenytoin 20 mg/kg in NS (max. 1000 mg) @ 1mg/kg/min or Inj.fosphenytoin PE 20 mg/kg @ 3 mg/kg/min
15-20 minutes	Repeat Inj.phenytoin 10 mg/kg if there is no response

Refractory status epilepticus refers to seizures occurring even after 10 minutes of phenytoin/fosphenytoin administration.

Time	Management protocol
25-30 minutes	Inj.valproate 20 mg/kg iv @ 6 mg/kg/min or Inj.phenobarbitone 20 mg/kg iv @ 1.5 mg/kg/min
35-45 minutes	If no response, inj.phenobarbitone 10 mg/kg iv
60 minutes	Inj.levetiracetam 20 mg/kg @ 5 mg/kg/min (safe in children with coagulopathy, chemotherapy, IEM and liver disease)

Continuous monitoring, plan for CT head, LP and EEG, vasopressors if needed

Consider iv pyridoxine 100 mg infusion in children less than 2 years or in isoniazid overdose

If seizures continue for 10 minutes after completion of phenobarbitone infusion, **shift to PICU** and consider coma induction. Identify and treat raised ICP. Consider intubation and assisted ventilation

Next page

(Contd.)

Figure 38.1 Algorithm for management of convulsive status epilepticus (Contd.)

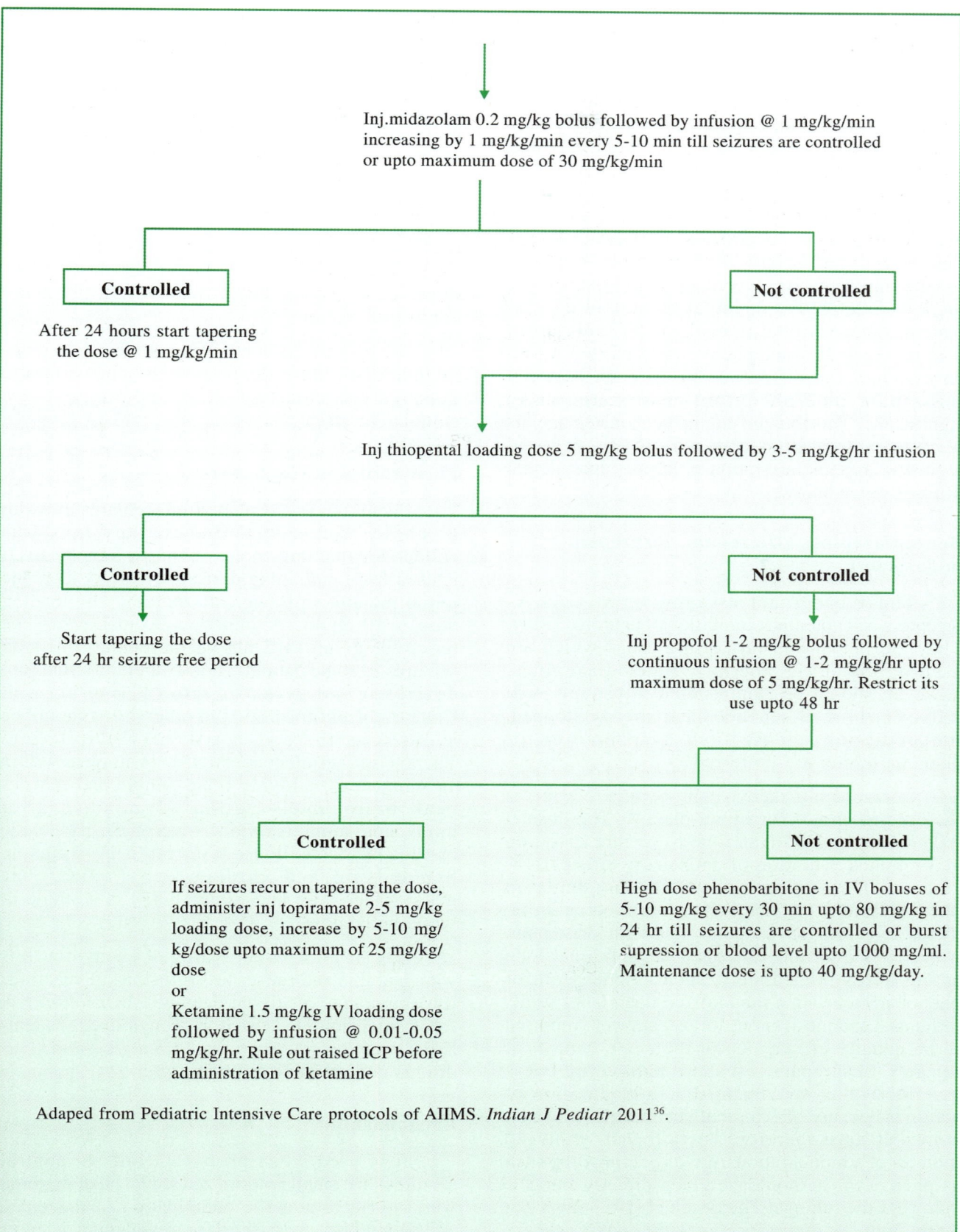

Inj.midazolam 0.2 mg/kg bolus followed by infusion @ 1 mg/kg/min increasing by 1 mg/kg/min every 5-10 min till seizures are controlled or upto maximum dose of 30 mg/kg/min

Controlled

After 24 hours start tapering the dose @ 1 mg/kg/min

Not controlled

Inj thiopental loading dose 5 mg/kg bolus followed by 3-5 mg/kg/hr infusion

Controlled

Start tapering the dose after 24 hr seizure free period

Not controlled

Inj propofol 1-2 mg/kg bolus followed by continuous infusion @ 1-2 mg/kg/hr upto maximum dose of 5 mg/kg/hr. Restrict its use upto 48 hr

Controlled

If seizures recur on tapering the dose, administer inj topiramate 2-5 mg/kg loading dose, increase by 5-10 mg/kg/dose upto maximum of 25 mg/kg/dose
or
Ketamine 1.5 mg/kg IV loading dose followed by infusion @ 0.01-0.05 mg/kg/hr. Rule out raised ICP before administration of ketamine

Not controlled

High dose phenobarbitone in IV boluses of 5-10 mg/kg every 30 min upto 80 mg/kg in 24 hr till seizures are controlled or burst supression or blood level upto 1000 mg/ml. Maintenance dose is upto 40 mg/kg/day.

Adaped from Pediatric Intensive Care protocols of AIIMS. *Indian J Pediatr* 2011[36].

Section 4

Figure 38.1. Algorithm for management of convulsive status epilepticus

refractory to the frontline anticonvulsants, continuous EEG monitoring is advocated.

Drugs should always be administered intravenously. In case of difficult access, per rectal diazepam, lorazepam, valproate or paraldehyde may be used. Midazolam can be given intranasally and bucally. Intranasal or sublingual lorazepam may be used. There is no ideal drug and a compromise between effective therapy and its inevitable side effects has to be accepted. A recent 5-year randomized multicentric trial compared 4 options for the initial intravenous therapy. Lorazepam 0.1 mg/kg was effective as initial therapy in 65% of patients, phenobarbital 15 mg/kg in 58%, diazepam 0.15 mg/kg in 56% and phenytoin 18 mg/kg in 44% cases. Only the difference in efficacy between lorazepam and phenytoin was statistically significant[37]. This trial did not include lorazepam plus phenytoin treatment arm which is a favored regimen[34]. A brief description of various antiepileptic drugs is given below:

Benzodiazepines (Diazepam, lorazepam, midazolam)

These drugs act as agonists at $GABA_A$ receptors and potentiate inhibition of neuronal firing. They are potent and fast acting drugs which are used as the initial therapy. Benzodiazepines, however, should be administered to patients with active seizures. If seizures have already stopped, longer acting agents such as phenytoin or phenobarbitone are preferred[5].

Lorazepam is increasingly being preferred as the drug of choice for initial therapy. The dose is 0.05-0.1mg/kg IV. Mean time to seizure cessation is 3 minutes. Duration of antiseizure effect is 12-24 hours. It has recurrence rates almost similar to phenobarbitone or phenytoin when used as initial therapy.[37] If seizures are controlled with lorazepam, it becomes less imperative to use additional long acting drugs immediately, such as phenytoin or phenobarbitone. In a randomized open label study, intranasal and intravenous lorazepam were reported to be equally efficacious in the acute control of seizures.[38] Diazepam is a short acting drug but is as effective as lorazepam. Its short duration of action is because of rapid redistribution to body fat stores. It must therefore be followed within 20 minutes of administration by a long acting drug such as phenytoin. It should be given directly into the vein (not the tubing). The dose is 0.1-0.3 mg/kg at a rate upto 2 mg/min for a maximum of 3 doses. Midazolam may also be used as the initial drug. The dose is 0.2 mg/kg and it is short acting. It can

be administered by the intravenous, intranasal, buccal, rectal or intramuscular routes. Whether midazolam is a suitable first line agent in the treatment of SE is not clear. Its potent antiepileptic effect, relative safety record, and ease of administration by various routes clearly makes midazolam a potentially important and useful drug in the treatment of SE. Buccal midazolam (0.2-0.5 mg/kg/dose) has been shown to be effective for acute treatment of febrile or afebrile seizures in children[39]. In a study comparing intranasal midazolam with rectal diazepam, both were observed to be equally efficacious in the acute control of seizures[40].

Adverse effects of intravenous benzodiazepines include respiratory depression, hypotension and impaired consciousness. Repeated doses have a cumulative effect.

Phenytoin and fosphenytoin

Phenytoin (or fosphenytoin) remains the drug of choice for second-line therapy in status epilepticus that does not respond to lorazepam. It is used for maintaining antiseizure effect after the initial therapy with benzodiazepines. The loading dose is 20 mg/kg. As much as 30 mg/kg may be required (given in 5 mg/kg increments) to stop seizures in some patients. It is diluted in saline (not dextrose) and given at rate of 1mg/kg/min. Concurrent administration of other drugs should be avoided as there is a risk of precipitation. Therapeutic serum concentration is attained within 10 minutes. It is highly lipid soluble and reaches peak brain levels within 15 minutes after intravenous administration. Adverse effects include cardiovascular collapse with rapid IV infusion, hypotension and cardiac arrhythmias. The maintenance dose is 5-8 mg/kg/day in a single or two divided doses.

Fosphenytoin is a prodrug of phenytoin. It is water soluble and causes less infusion site reactions (phlebitis and soft tissue damage). It has less risk for hypotension The dose is in phenytoin equivalents (PE). It can be given at a rate of 3 mg/kg/min. This drug is not available in India as yet.

Phenobarbital

It is used when phenytoin fails to control seizures. In a small randomized study, phenobarbital was as effective as the combination of diazepam and phenytoin[41]. It is useful for treatment of seizures in neonates. It is given as a loading dose of 15-20 mg/kg over 10-30 min. The maintenance dose is

3-5 mg/kg/day in one or two divided doses. It may depress respiration and level of consciousness especially if benzodiazepines have also been given.

Valproic acid

Intravenous valproic acid has been recently introduced in the market and has been found to be effective in controlling status epilepticus[42]. The dose is 25 mg/kg (3 mg/kg/hr). Per rectal valproate can be given in a dose of 20 mg/kg. Limdi *et al*[43] reviewed 63 patients with SE treated with IV valproate (average dose 31.5 mg/kg). The drug was well tolerated and effective in 63.3 percent patients. Peters *et al*[44] studied 102 adult patients who received standardized high dosage intravenous valproate in various emergency situations, including status epilepticus They concluded that intravenous administration of valproate seems to be an easy-to-use, safe and effective formulation as an alternative to phenytoin in all emergency seizure situations including status epilepticus.

Paraldehyde

It is relatively safe for administration in children. The loading dose is 150-200 mg/kg IV slowly over 15-20 min and maintenance dose is 20 mg/kg/hr in 5% concentration in a glass bottle. A 5% solution is prepared by adding 1.75 ml of paraldehyde to 5% dextrose solution to a total volume of 35 ml. The rectal dose of paraldehyde is 0.3 –0.5 ml/kg (max 5ml) diluted 1:1 in a vegetable oil. This dose can be repeated at 20 minute intervals if seizures persist[5]. *Glass syringes should be used while administering the drug as it is not compatible with plastics.*

Tiagabine

Tiagabine has been found to be safe and effective in adults but no trials have been conducted in children[45].

General anesthesia

It can be used as an adjunct to the management of status epilepticus if conventional drug therapy fails to control seizures and when barbiturate coma is not an option. Continuous EEG monitoring is desirable to ensure effective and rational therapy.

Treatment of non-convulsive status epilepticus (NCSE)

General principles for the management of NCSE include early identification of causative and precipitating factors so that they can be corrected as soon as possible. Physiologic stresses including infections, toxins, metabolic abnormalities, structural lesions, drug interactions or withdrawal, and pregnancy may present with either a new seizure or exacerbation of a known disorder. It is unclear whether the morbidity that can occur in NCSE is due to the NCSE *per se* or is it due to the underlying conditions. There is no consensus to guide the timing of interventions and treatment is tailored to the individual situation after careful assessment of risk-benefit ratio. Treatment of NCSE is summarized in Table 38.10.

Treatment of Refractory Status Epilepticus

The classical definition of refractory status epilepticus includes seizures that occurs even after

Section 4

Type	Treatment choice	Other drugs
Typical absence SE	BZD oral or IV	Acetazolamide, valproic acid
Complex partial SE	BZD oral, IV or rectal	Lorazepam and phenytoin/fosphenytoin or phenobarbitone
Electrical SE	Clobazam oral	Other BZD, corticosteroids or subpial transection
Atypical absence SE	VPA oral or IV	BZD, lamotrigine, topiramate
Tonic SE	Lamotrigine oral	Methyl phenidate, corticosteroids, phenytoin
NCSE in coma	BZD, phenytoin, phenobarbitone IV	Concomitant anesthesia with thiopental sodium (thiopentone sodium), pentobarbital (pentobarbitone), propofol or midazolam

Table 38.10 Treatment of NCSE

BZD: Benzodiazepines,   VPA: Valproic acid

10 minutes of phenytoin/fosphenytoin administration. The more widely used definition is seizures (clinical or electrographic) persisting despite administration of two or more antiepileptic drugs. The management options are detailed in Table 38.11.

<table>
<tr><td colspan="2">

Table 38.11 Management of refractory status epilepticus[34]

</td></tr>
</table>

- Intubate and ventilate the patient
- Attach to EEG monitor
- CVP lines may be inserted
- Administer any one of the following drugs:
  Midazolam 0.2 mg/kg IV stat followed by continuous infusion at a rate of 0.75 to 32 µg/kg/minute

  or

  Propofol 1 to 2 mg/kg stat followed by 1-2 mg/kg/hr and titrated to a maximum of 5 mg/kg/hr. The infusion is maintained for 12-24 hours.

  or

  Pentobarbital 10-15 mg/kg as initial IV bolus followed by 2-5 mg/kg boluses every 5 minutes till seizures are controlled followed by continuous infusion 1-3 mg/kg/hr

  or

  Thiopental infusion loading dose 3-5 mg/kg followed by further boluses of 1-2 mg/kg every 3-5 minutes till cessation of seizures (maximum dose of 10 mg/kg) followed by continuous infusion of 3-5 mg/kg/hr.
- Continue maintenance doses of phenytoin/valproate/ levetiracetam and phenobarbitone
- Use vasopressors (dopamine) to treat hypotension

Midazolam infusion has been shown to be effective in terminating refractory status epilepticus in children with an average time to control seizures within 47 minutes when administered at a mean infusion rate of 2.3µg/kg/min (range 1-32 µg/kg/min)[46]. When midazolam is not available, diazepam infusion can be used in a dose of 0.02-0.04 mg/kg/min[47]. Intravenous valproic acid has also been used in refractory SE in a loading dose of 20-40 mg/kg diluted 1:1 in normal saline or 5% dextrose solution administered over 1 to 5 minutes (repeat after 10-15 minutes if necessary) followed by an infusion at a rate of 5 mg/kg/hr[48].

Thiopental is a rapidly acting intravenous barbiturate used in refractory SE. Peak brain levels are reached after 30 seconds but the drug rapidly redistributes to the lipid-dense tissues and brain levels of drug are therefore difficult to manage. Pentobarbital is one of the major metabolites of thiopental. Thiopental causes hypotension, often necessitating lowering of the infusion rate and/ or

vasopressor administration. Propofol has gained popularity as an alternative. It has barbiturate-like and benzodiazepine-like effects at the $GABA_A$ receptor and has a potent anticonvulsant action at clinical doses. Its infusion may cause hypotension but this can be minimized by adequate intravascular filling and the use of modest doses of vasopressor drugs. The use of propofol before thiopental has been suggested for refractory status epilepticus (RSE) in children in a recent study conducted by van Gestel *et al*[49.]

Other drugs used in refractory SE include paraldehyde, lidocaine, clonazepam and chlormethiazole. Anesthetic agents used include thiopental, pentobarbitone sodium, isoflurane, etomidate and propofol[49].

Ambulatory Management

Status epilepticus is frequently encountered in the out patient department, ambulatory clinic or at home. Rectal, intranasal, buccal and sublingual routes of drug administration may be used.[38-40] Midazolam can be given intranasally (0.2 mg/kg) and bucally (0.2-0.5 mg/kg/dose). Rectal administration of diazepam (0.5-1.0 mg/kg/dose upto maximum of 10 mg) and lorazepam (0.1-0.4 mg/kg/dose) are safe and effective. Intranasal and sublingual lorazepam in a dose of 0.05-0.1 mg/kg may be used. The tablet is placed under the patient's tongue by taking due care to prevent aspiration and choking.

Management of Complications

Management of complications is symptomatic and supportive and includes ventilatory support, control of hyperthermia, optimal fluid management, use of vasopressors, treatment of arrhythmias, and management of raised intracranial pressure. Forced diuresis and urinary alkalinisation should be considered in the presence of myoglobinuria, in an attempt to prevent acute tubular necrosis and renal failure. At times seizures may continue unabated, despite seemingly adequate AED therapy, until specific cerebral edema therapy is given (mannitol 0.25 gm/kg stat dose). In patients in whom SE is a symptom of underlying brain insult, regular mannitol or even neurosurgical decompression may be necessary.

Long-term use of antiepileptic drugs

The use of anticonvulsant therapy after status epilepticus is controversial. Long-term therapy is desirable in children with progressive neurological disorder, structural brain lesions or patients with known epilepsy[5, 52]. Chronic AED therapy is not indicated in patients with SE solely due to transient metabolic disturbances or in febrile SE. However, the parents should be guided regarding intermittent febrile seizure prophylaxis in the latter case scenario. Between these two extremes, whether treatment is necessary or not is debatable. When SE is the first or sole seizure in a child and no cause is found, the decision to initiate long term AED therapy should be individualized. When underlying risk factors for seizures are identified, it is preferable to start AEDs. In view of poor follow-up and nonavailability of medical facilities in our country, it is preferable to start antiepileptic therapy after control of SE.

Refractory and Super refractory Status Epilepticus

Refractory convulsive status epilepticus is diagnosed when seizures are not controlled with initial benzodiazepine therapy or a subsequent anticonvulsant drug. Typically drug-induced anesthesia is then pursued with propofol, midazolam or a barbiturate[54]. This results in prolonged, intensive care, which requires meticulous attention to medical management to minimize complications. When seizures persist other options must be considered. These include (i) other medications, (ii) surgery, (iii) the ketogenic diet, (iv) hypothermia, (v) inhalational anesthetic agents, and (vi) immune modulating therapy.

Super-refractory status epilepticus is defined as SE that has continued or recurred despite 24 hours of general anesthesia[54]. It is encountered typically, but not exclusively, in two quite distinctive clinical situations: (1) patients with severe acute brain injury and (2) in patients with no history of epilepsy in whom SE develops as a bolt from the blue with no overt cause. This latter situation has been considered by some to be a "syndrome" entitled NORSE i.e. new-onset refractory status epilepticus. There are no randomized or controlled studies of therapy. The published evidence base consists largely of case reports or small series, and therefore any recommendations on therapy must be considered anecdotal at best. Although efforts are made to control the seizures, it is vital that the therapy is directed where ever possible at the underlying condition.

The therapeutic modalities include electro-convulsive therapy (ECT), transcranial magnetic stimulation, vagus nerve stimulation and drainage of the cerebrospinal fluid (CSF). Other modalities like neurosurgery and ketogenic diet has also been reported to be successful (Figure 38.2).

ROLE OF SURGERY IN REFRACTORY STATUS EPILEPTICUS

Refractory status epilepticus (RSE) (ie, status epilepticus that fails to respond to pharmacologic treatment) is associated with high mortality and deleterious sequelae. Estimates of mortality in children is around 50%. In previously healthy children who develop RSE, some studies have documented high rates of long-term development of epilepsy and deterioration of neurologic function. In the past 2 decades, surgical treatment has emerged as a therapeutic option for RSE in both adult and pediatric patients.[55] Children can tolerate major resections such as hemispherectomies, and partially regain verbal memory after temporal resections[56].

The criteria for surgical treatment of epilepsy are listed below[57].

1. Pharmacoresistance: Children who do not respond to the first line 2 or 3 medications are not likely to benefit from a trial of additional drugs including new AEDs. In addition to pharmacoresistance, children with disabling AED's side effects are surgical candidates.

2. Absence of serious adverse consequences from the surgery, and ability of the remaining brain to carry on normal motor and social functions.

3. Delineating the epileptogenic zone if a curative targeted resection is contemplated.

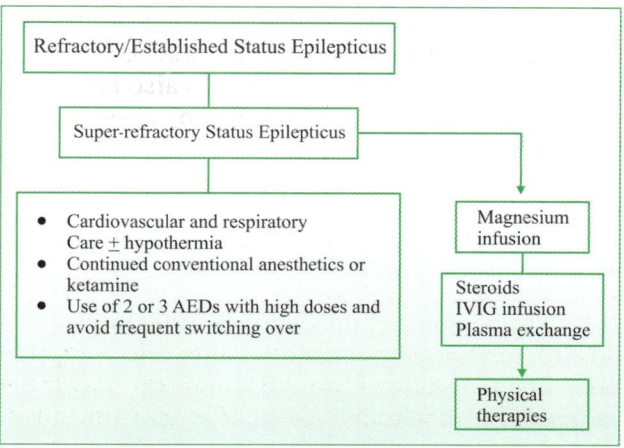

Figure 38.2 Protocol for management of super-refractory status epilpeticus

Presurgical Evaluation

A detailed structural (EEG, CECT, MRI) and functional imaging studies like PET (FDG, AMT, Flumazenil), SPECT (ictal, interictal, subtractional), fMRI and MEG (magneto-encephalography) should be undertaken before taking a decision for surgery.

Epileptogenic lesion. Anatomical abnormality visible on gross inspection or on imaging, which is able to produce seizures,and should be included in the resection to achieve seizure control.

Epileptogenic zone. The area is responsible for the generation of focal seizures, its removal is necessary and sufficient to achieve seizure freedom. It usually includes, but can be larger than the epileptogenic lesion.

Symptomatogenic zone. The area is necessary to produce clinical symptoms, but whose removal is not necessary for seizure freedom.

Irritative zone. The area is involved in administration of IEDs, but whose resection is not necessary for seizure freedom.

Ictal onset zone. The area from which seizures originate on ictal EEG.

Functional deficit zone. An area showing hypometabolism on functional imaging, usually much larger than the epileptogenic zone.

Ideal surgical candidate with status epilepticus[55]

Patients with covulsive or noncovulsive RSE who have a high degree of concordance between semiology, imaging, functional imaging with PET or SPECT and EEG (scalp and invasive) indicating a single epileptogenic zone,with focal cortical dysplasia as the underlying pathology, appear most likely to benefit. However, the optimal time for surgery is unclear. Substantial morbidity and mortality are likely to occur with increasing duration of RSE. Some workers have suggested a two week period of failed medical treatment as sufficient justification for surgery.

Outcome of Surgery

Surgical resection should be undertaken only in children with intractable seizures and refractory SE unresponsive to pharmacotherapy. In experienced hands the surgical procedure is safe and associated with good outcome. Seizures are controlled in over 75% patients. There is striking improvement in behaviour, increased attention span and disappearance of defiant aggressive behaviour. The improvement in speech is variable and depends upon the nature and site of lesion. The operative mortality with newer hemispherectomy technique is under 1%. The reported risk of permanent surgical morbidity depends upon the surgical procedure and varies from 1.1% for temporal lobe surgery to about 5% for frontal lobe resection.

PROGNOSIS

The consequences of convulsive SE are related to etiology, duration, associated systemic abnormalities, age of the patient, type of seizures and mode of therapy[5]. The prognosis of prolonged febrile seizures and idiopathic status epilepticus is good. Status epilepticus due to other causes have a much higher mortality rate. Prolonged uncontrolled seizures for more than 45 minutes and presence of septic shock are associated with high mortality[23]. The overall mortality rate of status epilepticus is approximately 5%. Long term sequelae include epilepsy in 20-40%, encephalopathy in 6-15% and focal neurological deficits in 9-11%. Aicardi and Chevrie[20] found that permanent neurologic sequelae occurred in 20% and mental retardation in 33%. Refractory epileptic seizures may occur in 26% of children with SE[51].

CONCLUSION

The mortality and morbidity associated with status epilepticus has decreased with early and aggressive management. The use of intramuscular, rectal, intranasal, and buccal routes for administration of AED may circumvent vascular access problems in children. Promotion of domiciliary management is likely to decrease the burden of status epilepticus in the community and thus will help in reduction of childhood neuromorbidity and mortality

REFERENCES

1.   DeLorenzo RJ, Pellock JM, Towne AR, Boggs JG. Epidemiology of status epilepticus. *J Clin Neurophysiol* 1995; 12(4):316-325.

2.   Hanhan UA, Fiallos MR, Orlowski JP. Status epilepticus. *Pediatr Clin North Am* 2001; 48(3): 683-694.

3.   Barbosa E and Freeman JM. Status epilepticus. *Pediatr Rev* 1982; 4: 185.

4.   Delgado-Escueta AV, Westerlain C and Treiman DM. Current concepts in neurology. Management of status epilepticus. *N Engl J Med* 1982; 306:1336.

5. ILAE Commission Report. The Epidemiology of the Epilepsies: Future directions. *Epilepsia* 1997, 38(5): 614-618.

6. Heidi LR, Frank WD. Seizures. *Neurol Clin North Am* 1998; 16:257-284.

7. Gastaut H. Classification of status epilepticus. *Adv Neurol* 1983; 34:15-35.

8. Treiman DM. Electroclinical features of status epilepticus. *J Clin Neurophysiol* 1995; 12:343-362.

9. Shorvon SD. Status epilepticus: its clinical features and treatment in children and adults. *Cambridge University Press,* 1994.

10. Gastaut H. Classification of status epilepticus. In: Status Epilepticus: Mechanisms of Brain Damage and Treatment. Delgado AV, Porter RJ, Wasterlain CG (eds). *New York; Raven Press,* 1982; pp 15-36.

11. Kaplan PW. Non convulsive status epilepticus in the emergency room. *Epilepsia* 1996; 37:643-650.

12. Neonatal Seizures. In: Neurology of the Newborn. Volpe J. (Ed.).5th edition. 2008 *WB Saunders*; pp 211-218.

13. Aicardi J, Chevrie JJ. Convulsive status epilepticus in infants and children: A study of 239 cases. *Epilepsia* 1970; 11:187-197.

14. Phillips SA, Shanahan RJ. Etiology and mortality of status epilepticus in children. A recent update. *Arch Neurol* 1989; 46:74-76.

15. Shinnar S, Maytal J, Krasnoff L, Moshe SL. Recurrent status in children. *Ann Neurol* 1992; 31:598- 604.

16. Moe PG, Seay AR. Neurologic and muscular disorders. In: Current Pediatric Diagnosis and Treatment. Hay WW (Ed.). *New York: Lange Medical Books,* 16 edn. 2003; 717-792.

17. Hesdorffer DC, Logroscino G, Cascino G, Annegers JF, Hauser WA. Incidence of status epilepticus in Rochester, Minnesota 1965-1984. *Neurology* 1998; 50:735-741.

18. Shinnar S, Berg AT, Moshe SL, *et al.* The risk of seizure recurrence following a first uprovoked seizure in childhood: a prospective study. *Pediatrics* 1990; 85:1076-1085.

19. Shinnar S, Berg AT, Moshe SL *et al.* The risk of seizure recurrence following a first unprovoked seizure in childhood: an extended follow up. *Pediatrics* 1996; 98:216-225.

20. Maytal J, Shinnar S. Febrile status eplepticus. *Pediatrics* 1990; 86:611-616.

21. Shinnar S, Pellock JM, Moshe SL, *et al.* In whom does status epilepticus occur?: Age related differences in children. *Epilepsia* 1997; 38:907-913.

22. Fountain NV. Status epilepticus: Risk factors and complications. *Epilepsia* 2000; 41(suppl 2): 23-30.

23. Gulati S, Kalra V, Sridhar MR. Status epilepticus in Indian children in a tertiary care centre: Clinical profile and immediate outcome. *Indian J Pediatr* 2005; 72: 105-108.

24. Kothman E. The biochemical basis and pathophysiology of status epilepticus. *Neurology* 1990; 40(suppl 2): 13-23.

25. Kapur J, Macdonald RL. Rapid seizure-induced reduction of benzodiazepine and Zn^{2+} sensitivity of hippocampal dentate granule cell GABA receptors. *J Neurosci* 1997; 17:7532-7540.

26. Chapman MG, Smith M, Hirsch NP. Status Epilepticus. *Anaesthesia* 2001; 56: 648-659.

27. Towne AR, Waterhouse EJ, Boggs JG, Garnett LK, Smith JR, De Lorenzo RJ. Prevalence of nonconvulsive status epilepticus in comatose patients. *Neurology* 2000; 54:340-345.

28. Privitera M, Hoffman M, Moore JL, Jester D. EEG detection of nontonic-clonic status epilepticus in patients with altered consciousness. *Epilepsy Res* 1994; 18:155-166.

29. DeLorenzo RJ, Waterhouse EJ, Towne AR, Boggs JG, Ko D, DeLorenzo GA, *et al.* Persistent nonconvulsive status epilepticus after the control of convulsive status epilepticus. *Epilepsia* 1998; 39:833-840.

30. Tunik MG, Young GM. Status epilepticus in children: The acute management. *Pediatr Clin North Am* 1992; 39:1007-1030.

31. Aicardi J and Chevrie JJ. Consequences of status epilepticus in infants and children. *Adv Neurol* 1983; 34: 115.

32. Towne AR, Pellock JM, Ko D, *et al.* Determinants of mortality in status epilepticus. *Epilepsia* 1994; 35: 27-34.

33. Glaser, Medical complications of status epilepticus. In: Advances in Neurology. Delgado Escueta *et al* (Eds.), *Raven Press, New York,* 1983 Vol. 34, 396;.

34. Treiman DM. Treatment of status epilepticus if first drug fails: Veterans Affairs Status Epilepticus Cooperative Study Group. *Epilepsia* 1999; 40:243.

35. Lowenstein DH, Alldredge BK. Status epilepticus. *N Engl J Med* 1998; 338:970-976.

36. Raj D, Gulati S, Lodha R. Status Epilepticus.*Indian J Pediatr* 2011; Feb;78(2):219-226.

37. Treiman DM, Meyers PD, Walton NY, *et al.* A comparison of four treatments for generalized convulsive status epilepticus. Veterans Affairs Status Epilepticus Cooperative Study Group. *N Engl J Med* 1998; 339:792-798.

38. Arya R, Gulati S, Kabra M, Sahu JK, Kalra V. Intranasal versus intravenous lorazepam for control of acute

seizures in children: a randomized open-label study. *Epilepsia.* 2011 Apr;52(4):788-793.

39. Wiznitzer M. Buccal midazolam is effective for acute treatment of seizures. *J Pediatr* 2006; 148(1):143.

40. Bhattacharya M, Kalra V, Gulati S. Intranasal midazolam vs rectal diazepam in acute childhood seizures. *Pediatr Neurol* 2006;34:355-359.

41. Shaner DM, McCurdy SA, Herring MO, Gabor AJ. Treatment of Status epilepticus: a prospective comparison of diazepam and phenytoin versus phenobarbital and optional phenytoin. *Neurology* 1988; 38:202-207.

42. Yu KT, Mills S, Thompson N, Cunanan C. Safety and efficacy of intravenous valproate in pediatric status epilepticus and acute repetitive seizures. *Epilepsia* 2003; 44:724-726

43. Limdi NA, Shimpi AV, Faught E, Gomez CR, Burneo JG. Efficacy of rapid IV administration of valproic acid for status epilepticus. *Neurology* 2005; 64(2):353-355.

44. Peters CN, Pohlmann-Eden B. Intravenous valproate as an innovative therapy in seizure emergency situations including status epilepticus: experience in 102 adult patients. *Seizure* 2005; (3):164-169.

45. Kalviainen R. Long term safety of tiagabine. *Epilepsia* 2001; 42(suppl 3):46-48.

46. Rivera R, Segnini M, Baltodano A, *et al.* Midazolam in the treatment of status epilepticus in children. *Crit Care Med* 1993; 21:991-994.

47. Singhi S, Murthy A, Singhi P, Jayashree M. Continuous midazolam versus diazepam infusion for refractory convulsive status epilepticus. *J Child Neurol* 2002; 17:106-110.

48. Uberall MA, Trollmann R, Wunsiedler U, *et al.* Intravenous valproate in pediatric epilepsy patients with refractory status epilepticus. *Neurology* 2000; 54: 2188-2189.

49. van Gestel JP, Blusse van Oud-Alblas HJ, Malingre M, Ververs FF, Braun KP, van Nieuwenhuizen O. Propofol and thiopental for refractory status epilepticus in children. *Neurology* 2005; 65(4):591-592.

50. Haafiz Allah, Kissoon N. Status epilepticus: current concepts. *Pediatr Emerg Care* 1999; 15(2): 119-129.

51. Maytal J, Shinnar S, Moshe SL, *et al.* Low morbidity and mortality of status epilepticus in children. *Pediatrics* 1989; 83:323-331.

52. Berg AJ, Shinnar S. The risk of recurrence following a first unprovoked seizure in childhood: A quantitative review. *Neurology* 1991; 41:965-972.

53. Wheeles JW. Treatment of refractory convulsive status epilepticus in children: Other therapies. *Semin Pediatr Neurol* 2010;17:190-194

54. Simon S. Super-refractory status epilepticus: An approach to therapy in this difficult clinical situation. *Epilepsia* 2011 52(Suppl. 8):53–56.

55. Vendrame M, Lodden Kemper T. Surgical treatment of refractory status epilepticus in children: Candidate selection and outcome. *Semin Pediatr Neurol* 2010;17:182-189.

56. Hirsch E, Arzimanoglou A. Children with drug-resistant partial epilepsy: criteria for the identification of surgical candidates. *Rev Neurol* (Paris) 2004;160 (Spec No 1). 5S210-5S219

57. Tellez-Zenteno JF, Dhar R, Wiebe S. Long term seizure outcomes following epilepsy surgery: a systematic review and meta-analysis. *Brain* 2005; 128:1188-1198.

Section 4

39

Acute Flaccid Paralysis

R K Sabharwal

INTRODUCTION

Acute flaccid paralysis (AFP) is a clinical syndrome characterizedby rapid onset of weakness, including (less frequently) weakness of the muscles of respiration and swallowing, progressing to maximum severity within 1 to 10 days[1, 2]. AFP surveillance is a key strategy for monitoring the progress of polio eradication and is a sensitive instrument for detecting potential poliomyelitis cases and poliovirus infection. Highly sensitive surveillance for acute flaccid paralysis (AFP), including immediate case investigation, and specimen collection are critical for the detection of wild poliovirus circulation with the ultimate objective of polio eradication. AFP surveillance is also critical for documenting the absence of polio virus circulation for polio-free certification

Accurate diagnosis of the cause of AFP has profound implications for therapy and prognosis. If untreated, AFP may not only persist but also lead to death due to failure of respiratory muscles. The involvement of respiatory muscles should be identified early so that assisted ventilation is provided without any delay to salvage these patients. With global efforts aimed at interrupting polio transmission, the incidence of paralytic polio has reduced substantially. Consequently, polio is not a common cause of acute paralysis seen in emergency practice. The leading cause of AFP at present is Guillain-Barré syndrome (GBS) in 30-90% cases[5-7]. The most critical task for the physician evaluating a child with paralysis is defining the anatomical level of the underlying abnormality and the likely pathology.

APPROACH

Although AFP is a hallmark of damage to the lower motor neurons, damage to the upper motor neurons may present with flaccid weakness due to "spinal shock". Most cases of acute flaccid paralysis with a preserved sensorium result from diffuse disorder of the motor unit (which may involve anterior horn cells, axons, neuromuscular junctions, or muscle), but when bulbar muscles are spared it is critical first to consider acute lesions of the cervical spinal cord due to myelitis, vascular changes, or trauma. If there is a lesion of the cervical cord, the initial period of spinal shock may be characterized by flaccid paralysis with areflexia below the level of the lesion. Establishing this diagnosis may be particularly challenging in very young children, in whom the tell tale signs of sphincter involvement or sensory loss below a certain level may be difficult to discern. A practical approach to the management of the child with weakness should start with the anatomic localization of the pathological process causing weakness (Table 39.1).

History

A detailed history should be taken by probing following points.

(i) Trauma, animal bite and snake bite should be asked. Paralytic rabies can mimic GBS and several patients with paralysis have undergone plasma exchange because of a misdiagnosis of GBS[8].

(ii) Family history of episodic weakness may indicate a familial periodic paralysis or porphyria.

(iii) Pre-existing systemic disorders like auto-immune vasculitis, inflammatory arthritis and diabetes mellitus, etc.

(iv) Medication use such as anticonvulsants phenytoin, barbiturates (causing osteomalacia); diuretics, chemotherapy, or high dose steroids.

(v) Accidental poisoning with organsphosphates and barium etc.

(vi) Sudden weakness after a large glucose load in a malnourished child may occur due to acute hypophosphatemia.

(vii) Porphyria or myoglobinuria should be suspected when there is history of passing high colored urine.

(viii) Is there a pre-existing neuromuscular disorder or has the condition arisen *de novo?* Several inherited neuromuscular disorders may undergo rapid progression in their final stages and produce respiratory failure (X-linked muscular dystrophies, acid maltase deficiency), while myasthenia gravis may be associated with recurrent episodes of profound weakness in the presence of infection, stress or precipitating drugs.

(ix) Prior episodes of painless weakness is suggestive of familial periodic paralysis; recurrent attacks of exercise intolerance (proximal muscle weakness + muscle cramping and muscle tenderness + myoglobulinuria after performing physical exercise) suggest an inborn error of glycogen metabolism (after a short bout of heavy exercise), or lipid metabolism (after a bout of prolonged exercise in a relatively fasted state).

(x) History of an underlying malignancy suggests the possibility of paraneoplastic neuropathy, or drug-induced neuropathy or myopathy (e.g. cyclosporine, vincristine) and spinal cord compression.

Clues to the Diagnosis

The following clinical features provide important diagnostic clues:

1. *Onset.* Certain disorders may present in an "hyper-acute" onset with weakness developing over minutes or hours. The causes include familial potassium-associated periodic paralysis, psychogenic weakness, and various intoxications. Spinal cord trauma and infarction may have an apoplectic onset. Weakness from motor neuron or peripheral nerve disorders usually develops over days or weeks.

2. *Past history* of vaccination or immunization may precede GBS, transverse myelitis or acute demyelinating encephalomyelitis (ADEM).

3. *Gastrointestinal symptoms.* These accompany porphyria, botulism, sea food poisoning, organophosphate toxicity, and arsenic or thallium ingestion. Acute hypokalemic weakness may follow chronic vomiting or diarrhea.

4. *Pain.* The onset of weakness due to GBS, polio, porphyria or dermatomyositis may be preceded by neck pain, back pain or myalgias. Spinal pain (girdle pains) may result from a caries spine, metastasis or compressive myelopathy. Distal paresthesias or dysesthesias may occur with GBS or toxic neuropathies.

5. *Pattern of limb weakness.* Polio and occasionally porphyria are distinguished by

---

Table 39.1 Conditions to be considered in a patient with AFP

1. **Motor neuron**
   - Poliovirus
   - Other neurotropic viruses

2. **Peripheral nerves**
   - Acute Guillain-Barre syndrome (GBS)
   - Porphyria
   - Toxic neuropathies
     Arsenic, nitrofurantoin, heavy metals, thallium
   - Diphtheria
   - Collagen disorders

3. **Neuromuscular junction (NMJ) disorders**
   - Myasthenia gravis
   - Drug-induced neuromuscular blockade
   - Organophosphorus poisoning
   - Botulism
   - Animal venoms and toxins (snake bite)
   - Hypermagnesemia

4. **Muscle**
   - Periodic paralysis
   - Hypokalemia
   - Rhabdomyolysis
   - Inflammatory myopathies

5. **Critical illness neuropathy and myopathy**

6. **Acute myelopathy**
   - *Spinal cord infection*
     □ Viruses and retroviruses, rabies, herpes simplex virus-2, HIV
     □ Bacteria
        Tuberculosis, Mycoplasma, Borellia
     □ Parasitic
        Neurocysticercosis, hydatid disease
     □ Fungi
   - *Compressive myelopathy*
     □ Trauma
     □ Epidural abscess
     □ Hematomyelia
     □ Spinal cord infarction
     □ Tumors
     □ Idiopathic transverse myelitis (post or para-infectious)

7. **Miscellaneous conditions**
   - Cerebral venous thrombosis
   - Acute stroke
   - Hypoxic-ischemic events
   - Mitochondrial disorders

asymmetric limb weakness. Distal weakness is a feature of peripheral neuropathies.

6. *Bulbar dysfunction.* This is prominent in neuromuscular junction disorders and may be seen in GBS, porphyria, polio and diphtheria.

7. *Ptosis or ophthalmoplegia* suggest a neuromuscular junction disorder, though it may be seen in GBS, Miller-Fisher variant or brainstem pathologies like infarction, Bickerstaff's encephalitis, or central pontine myelinolysis, etc.

8. *Pupillary changes.* Pupillary paralysis is a classic feature of botulism and tick paralysis. Paralysis of accommodation occurs with diphtheria and miosis with organophosphate poisoning.

9. Dengue fever may cause weakness due to severe myositis and myelitis.

10. *Dermatomal vesicles* are suggestive of herpes zoster myelitis and vesicles over hands, feet and mouth may occur in children with enterovirus 71 infection.

Patterns of Weakness

1. Flaccid symmetric weakness with areflexia (+/- bulbar and respiratory involvement): GBS when there are sensory symptoms and minimal sensory loss and familial periodic paralysis when there is no sensory involvement.

2. Symmetric proximal weakness with preserved reflexes is seen in acute myopathy (PM-DM); and osteomalacic myopathy.

3. Flaccid paraplegia or quadriplegia with sensory level, and bowel-bladder dysfunction occurs due to spinal cord pathology.

4. Opthalmoplegia with motor weakness are suggestive of GBS; Miller-Fisher variant, Bickerstaff's encephalitis, myasthenia gravis and tick paralysis.

5. Fatigable muscle weakness with bulbar signs/opthalmoplegia occurs in myasthenia gravis

6. Bulbar predominant involvement:

Botulism, myasthenia gravis, motor neuron diseases and pontine lesions.

7. Prominent autonomic dysfunction:

Guillain-Barré syndrome, paraneoplastic syndromes, organophosphate toxicity (muscarinic cholinergic overstimulation) and botulism.

Laboratory Investigations

The following investigations are useful for establishing the cause of AFP.

- Complete blood counts. Anemia and leukocytosis as useful markers of systemic illness.
- Eosinophil count may be elevated in vasculitic neuropathy, trichinosis and cysticercosis.
- ESR is often elevated in infections and autoimmune disorders.
- CPK and aldolase are elevated in primary muscle diseases.
- BUN is elevated in myoglobinuria, rhabdomyolysis and renal insufficiency.
- Electrolytes, calcium, phosphorus, and magnesium, vitamin B_{12} and vitamin D are useful markers for metabolic disorders and periodic paralysis.
- Thyroid hormone assay is indicated when thyroid related myopathy is suspected.
- AFP surveillance to rule out paralytic poliomyelitis.
- Collagen markers and serology for the diagnosis of vasculitic neuropathy, polymyositis, myasthenia gravis.
- Blood and CSF serology for viruses, *Campylobacter jejuni* and *Mycoplasma pneumoniae.*
- Nerve conduction studies, EMG, and repetitive nerve stimulation for GBS, myopathic disorders, myasthenia gravis and botulism.
- Evoked potentials
- MRI/CT scans of brain, spinal cord and muscles
- Lumbar puncture when transverse myelitis, TB arachnoiditis and GBS are suspected.

AFP Surveillance

The worldwide polio eradication campaign has been successful in achieving a 99% reduction in the global incidence of polio since 1988[3]. WHO recommends that all AFP cases under 15 years of age or with paralytic illness at an age where polio is suspected should be reported immediately and investigated within 48 hours, and two stool specimens should be collected 24–48 hours apart and within 14 days of the onset of paralysis[4]. Specimens arriving in the laboratory must be of adequate volume (approximately 8–10 g), have appropriate documentation (i.e. laboratory request form) and be in good condition, i.e. with no leakage or desiccation and with evidence that the reverse cold chain has been maintained (presence of ice or temperature indicator).

Management

The two most important goals in the management of a child with AFP are (i) stabilization of the patient and attending to ventilatory needs (ii) taking a history and doing complete physical examination to diagnose the underlying disorder, order appropriate tests, and institute specific therapy. The child with AFP should be admitted to the ICU if there is (i) vasomotor and respiratory insufficiency; (ii) rapid progression of disease; (iii) bulbar symptoms; (iv) suspected poisoning, and (v) acute severe systemic illness.

A detailed discussion of common conditions which cause AFP is given below.

A. SPINAL CORD DISORDERS

All patients with suspected acute spinal cord dysfunction require emergency evaluation. These children will often present with rapidly progressive paraplegia or quadriplegia and may be incorrectly diagnosed as GBS. The following steps are useful in assessing the patient with a suspected spinal cord disorder (Figure 39.1)[9].

(a) Initial evaluation of a patient with an evolving myelopathy should determine structural compressive cause of myelopathy by gadolinium contrast MRI of the cervical and thoracic spine.

(b) If no structural cause can be detected, then a lumbar puncture should be performed to exclude an inflammatory cause of the myelitis. The CSF should be examined for biochemistry, cytology, as well as for intrathecal antibody synthesis. A small volume can be stored in the refrigerator for future studies if needed.

(c) If the MRI spine fails to show gadolinium enhancement and there is no pleocytosis in

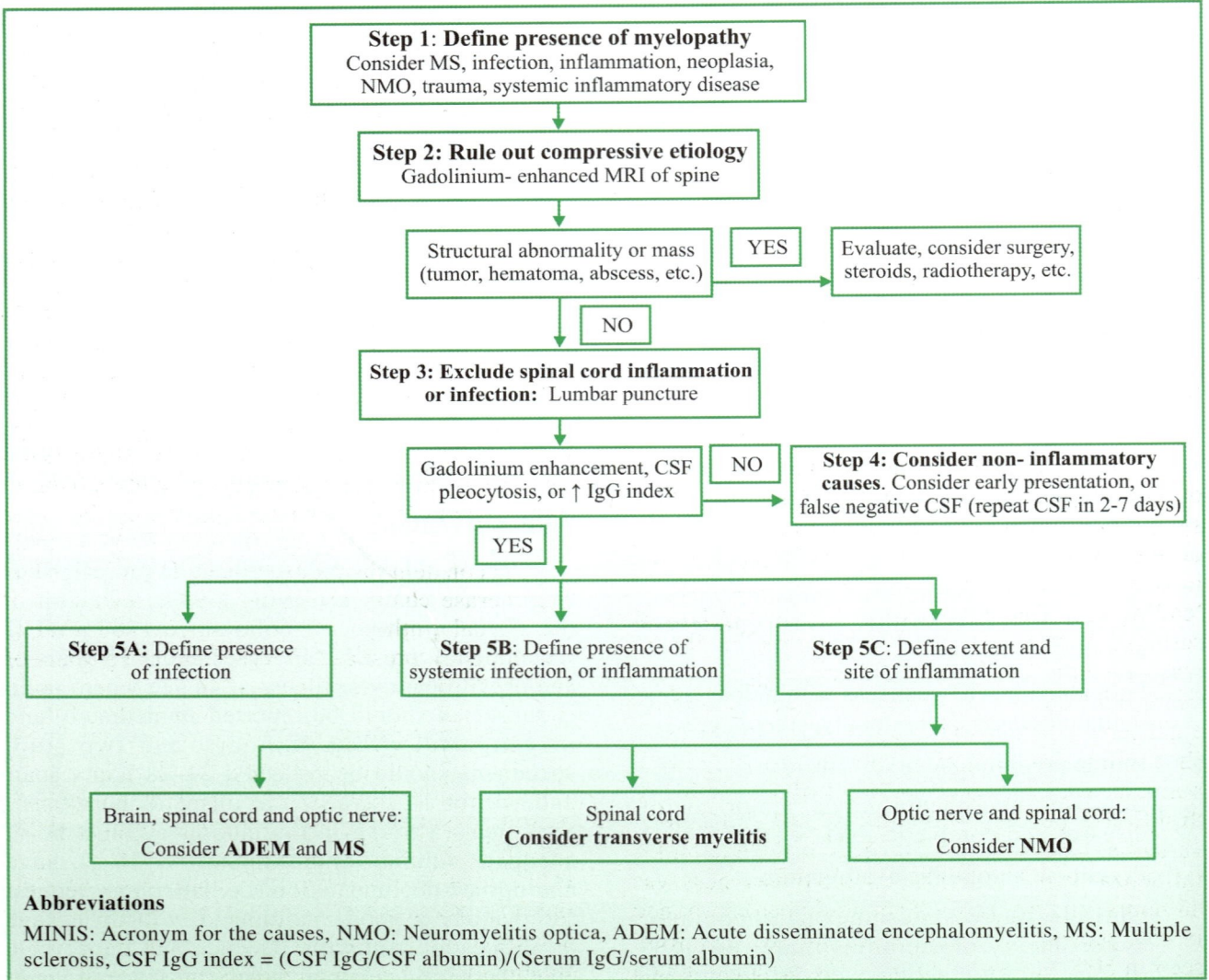

Step 1: Define presence of myelopathy
Consider MS, infection, inflammation, neoplasia, NMO, trauma, systemic inflammatory disease

Step 2: Rule out compressive etiology
Gadolinium- enhanced MRI of spine

Structural abnormality or mass (tumor, hematoma, abscess, etc.) — YES → Evaluate, consider surgery, steroids, radiotherapy, etc.

NO

Step 3: Exclude spinal cord inflammation or infection: Lumbar puncture

Gadolinium enhancement, CSF pleocytosis, or ↑ IgG index — NO → **Step 4: Consider non- inflammatory causes.** Consider early presentation, or false negative CSF (repeat CSF in 2-7 days)

YES

Step 5A: Define presence of infection

Step 5B: Define presence of systemic infection, or inflammation

Step 5C: Define extent and site of inflammation

Brain, spinal cord and optic nerve: Consider **ADEM** and **MS**

Spinal cord **Consider transverse myelitis**

Optic nerve and spinal cord: Consider **NMO**

Abbreviations

MINIS: Acronym for the causes, NMO: Neuromyelitis optica, ADEM: Acute disseminated encephalomyelitis, MS: Multiple sclerosis, CSF IgG index = (CSF IgG/CSF albumin)/(Serum IgG/serum albumin)

Figure 39.1 Algorithm for an approach to a case of myelopathy

the CSF, then a "non-inflammatory" cause is most likely.

(d) If an "inflammatory" myelopathy is identified, then a brain MRI and visual evoked potentials (VEP) should be obtained to determine the extent of the inflammation. The presence of demyelination on VEP but not in the brain, indicates neuromyelitis optica (Devic's disease). If demyelination is detected on MRI of the brain, the diagnosis of ADEM or multiple sclerosis should be suspected.

(e) Patients with an inflammatory myelopathy with absence of demyelination in the brain or optic nerves are likely to have acute transverse myelitis (ATM). Further, evaluation should be done to decide whether ATM is "primary" or "disease-associated".

I.   Acute transverse myelitis (ATM)

The diagnosis of idiopathic ATM is based on following criteria[9]:

(a) Development of sensory, motor, or autonomic dysfunction attributable to the spinal cord pathology.

(b) Bilateral signs and symptoms.

(c) Exclusion of extra axial compressive etiology by MRI.

(d) Inflammation within the spinal cord demonstrated by CSF pleocytosis, increased IgG index, or gadolinium enhancement of lesion on MRI.

(e) Progress to nadir between 4 hours to 21 days following the onset.

The syndrome is characterized by sudden onset of progressive weakness of legs. The earliest symptom is sensory loss or pain in the back, thighs or legs. Bowel and/or bladder involvement occurs in over 70% patients. The weakness may ascend leading to a flaccid quadriplegia. In the largest series of ATM reported in 45 children[10], the illness was clustered between children younger than 3 years, and those between 5 to 17 years. Twenty eight percent patients had a confirmed immunization shot within 30 days. The vaccines included oral polio, measles-mumps-rubella (MMR), hepatitis A, diphtheria-pertussis-tetanus (DPT), influenza, varicella, Japanese B encephalitis, and Hemophilus influenzae type b. Time for maximal weakness was 48 hours, and a sensory level could be determined in 85% patients. Elevated WBC's in the CSF were seen in 50% of cases, but only 5% demonstrated a elevated IgG index.

Treatment involves administeration of methylprednisolone (1g/1.73 m^2 daily for 3-5 days) intravenously, followed by oral prednisolone tapered over 2-3 weeks. Plasmapheresis, intravenous immunoglobulins (IVIG), intravenous cyclophosphamide and other immunosuppressants can be tried in non-responders. Residual disabilities of gait, numbness and bladder dysfunction may persist in 40-75% cases even after several years.

2.   Post-vaccinal or post-infectious myelitis

The condition generally occur within 3 weeks of vaccination or systemic infection and is characterized by severe and symmetrical involvement. The common immunizations associated with this form of myelitis include polio, measles, rubella, pertussis, hepatitis B, rabies, and Japanese B encephalitis.

3.   Viral myelitis

The presence of meningoencephalitic symptoms such as fever, meningismus, and encephalopathy are suggestive of an infection. Viral myelitis results from direct viral infection of the neural elements of the spinal cord. The presence of fever, rash, meningeal signs, herpes eruptions, zoster rash, genital ulcers and adenopathy should arouse the suspicion of a viral etiology. Herpes simplex virus type1 (HSV 1) commonly causes myelitis in children, while HSV 2 causes myelitis in adults. Both forms of disease can vary from mild involvement with full recovery to a severe necrotizing myelitis with severe residual deficits. Genital herpes may precede HSV 2 myelitis by several days. Typical CSF cell counts tend to range between 10 and 200 cells/mm^3. In necrotizing myelitis striking pleocytosis up to 5000 cells/mm^3 with preponderance of neutrophils may be seen. The CSF protein is usually raised. Diagnosis depends on demonstration of HSV DNA in CSF by polymerase chain reaction (PCR) or evidence of intrathecal synthesis of HSV-specific antibodies by detecting the presence of anti-HSV IgM antibodies in the CSF.

Varicella-Zoster virus (VZV) can cause zoster myelitis, with most cases occurring in immunocompromised hosts. Myelitis can occur as a complication of primary varicella infection. Spinal cord involvement follows the onset of zoster by 5 to 21 days, and patients present with a sub-acute onset of asymmetric leg weakness, progressing to a sensorimotor paraparesis. No controlled trials of treatment are available, but acyclovir is given in doses of 30 mg/kg/day for 21 to 35 days.

Section 4

4. Tuberculous myelopathy

Spinal cord is enveloped by pus extruding anteriorly from the affected vertebrae. Myelopathy typically results from pressure on the anterior spinal cord by caseous or granulating tissue, inflammatory thrombosis of the anterior spinal artery, or injury to the cord from spinal instability. The latter may lead to complete spinal cord transection.

5. Other forms of bacterial myelopathy

A number of other bacterial infections have been associated with myelitis. On rare occasion, the spinal cord may be seeded by bacteria leading to a suppurative myelitis with abscess formation. Spinal epidural abscess may present as surgical emergency evolving rapidly over several days or may occur more indolently. Staphylococcus aureus is the etiologic agent in over 50% of acute spinal epidural abscesses, though a number of other organisms may be implicated. The spread of infection may occur directly from a focus of osteomyelitis or hematogenously from a distant site, such as skin furuncles or pulmonary infection. Trauma to the back, typically minor in nature, has been reported in as many as one-third of individuals developing spinal epidural abscess.

Acute onset of irritability, fever, and painful neck movements in a child should alert the clinician to the possibility of infective causes such as meningitis, acute epiduritis, and spinal epidural abscess. Epidural and vertebral tumors may have an apoplectic onset of pain and paraplegia because of vertebral body collapse. If there is a history of occipito-nuchal pain on coughing, sneezing, and neck extension, one should suspect an Arnold-Chiari malformation, cranio cervical anomaly, or posterior fossa pathology. In Lyme disease, the infection due to *Borrelia burgdorfei* may also result in a myelopathy

6. Poliomyelitis

Poliomyelitis usually present as an acute febrile viral meningitis syndrome with meningeal signs, malaise, headache and gastrointestinal symptoms. The lower motor neuron signs develop within 1 to 2 weeks, but may rarely develop early along with other presenting symptoms. The motor signs are maximal during 1-4 days and are usually asymmetric with mostly lumbar involvement and spinal cord being more involved than brain stem. The proximal muscles are affected more than distal. There is no sensory deficit but myalgias may be severe. A CSF neutrophilic pleocytosis common at the onset is replaced after a few days by moderate number of lymphocytes and monocytes. The protein content of CSF is slightly raised, but it rises gradually till the third week in paralytic cases, and returns to normal by the sixth week. Atrophy appears rapidly, usually within 5 to 7 days, and may progress over several weeks.

Electrophysiology studies will help to differentiate poliomyelitis due to poliovirus or other neurotropic viruses from a peripheral neuropathy such as GBS. In difficult situations MRI shows increased T-2 weighted signal in the anterior horns and swelling of spinal cord. Isolation of polio virus from the stools is a reliable method for diagnosis. There is no specific treatment. General supportive measures and intensive care as described under GBS is the mainstay of management.

7. "Polio-like illness" due to non-polio viruses

Small epidemics of acute flaccid paralysis have been caused by non-polio enteroviruses. Coxsackie A7 virus caused outbreaks of paralytic disease in the former Soviet Union, South Africa and Scotland; and enterovirus 71 outbreaks in Southeast Asia in the late 1990s. Japanese B virus is reported to cause an AFP with clinical and pathological findings similar to poliomyelitis, and is considered to be the commonest cause of AFP in South Vietnam[11]. Flaviviruses like Japanese encephalitis (JE), West Nile virus (WNV), St. Louis encephalitis virus; dengue and chikungunya viruses can affect the spinal cord and cause polio-like illness. Other viruses isolated in AFP epidemics in India include Coxsackie B, and Echoviruses 11,12,13,7,8 and 30.

8. Transverse myelitis due to systemic inflammatory diseases

Transverse myelitis may result from systemic inflammatory diseases like Sjogren syndrome, systemic lupus erythematosus (SLE), antiphospholipid antibody syndrome, mixed connective tissue disorder, and sarcoidosis. These disorders should be suspected in the presence of skin rash, oral or genital ulcers, arthritis, livido reticularis, photosensitivity, erythema nodosum, keratitis, conjunctivitis, serositis, anemia, thrombocytopenia, elevated erythrocyte sedimentation rate (ESR), and history of venous or arterial thrombosis. Appropriate serological tests, tests for auto antibodies, coagulation parameters, complement levels etc. should be carried out.

B. PERIPHERAL NEUROPATHIES

Acute onset peripheral neuropathies are rare. Majority of neuropathies have a sub-acute or chronic course. Neuropathies manifesting in days include GBS, vasculitic neuropathies, diphtheria, acute intermittent porphyria, critical illness neuropathy, and toxic neuropathies. Toxic and metabolic neuropathies present as distal symmetrical neuropathies, whilst proximal involvement may occur with GBS, porphyria and diabetes mellitus. Asymmetric presentation as in mononeuritis multiplex should alert the clinician to the possibilities of connective tissue disorders and vasculitic neuropathies.

1. Guillain-Barré syndrome (GBS)

Guillain–Barre´ syndrome is the commonest cause of acute flaccid paralysis in children. Diagnosis is made by pattern recognition of the typical picture of a monophasic symmetric ascending paralysis, areflexia/hyporeflexia progressing during 4 weeks. Leg or back pain occurs at onset in 50–79% of children and adults. Eighty percent of children reach nadir within 2 weeks after onset. At times one sees a hyper acute onset of GBS; the child complaining of tiredness at night and awakening the next morning with a flaccid, symmetrical, quadriplegia accompanied by opthalmoplegia and bulbar involvement resembling a "locked-in-syndrome" similar to Bickerstaff encephalitis or botulism. In botulism, there are gastrointestinal symptoms, dry mouth, descending paralysis, and dilated unresponsive pupils while consciousness is affected in encephalitis.

GBS rarely affects newborn infants, but merits consideration in the differential diagnosis of neonatal flaccid paralysis. Even without any known intrauterine events, GBS may occur shortly after birth, as early as age 3 weeks. These previously healthy babies present with an acute, rapidly progressive, and often severe hypotonia, with respiratory distress and feeding difficulties[12]. *The absence of sensory nerve action potentials (SNAPs) is the most important EMG clue to the diagnosis of neonatal GBS.*

EMG findings of very slow motor nerve conduction velocities, dispersed low amplitude compound muscle action potentials (CMAPs), and absent sensory nerve action potentials (SNAPs) are diagnostic of an acquired demyelinating polyneuropathy (GBS).

GBS has 4 clinical variants that can be distinguished by the clinical findings and nerve conduction studies:

(i) Acute inflammatory demyelinating polyradiculoneuropathy (AIDP)

(ii) Acute motor axonal neuropathy (AMAN)

(iii) Acute motor and sensory axonal neuropathy (AMSAN)

(iv) Miller–Fisher syndrome (MFS) (regional variant).

Much attention has been focused on *C. jejuni* infection as an important association with the AMAN variety of GBS that occurs in epidemics in China[13]. AMAN is not uncommon in India and Bangladesh. The AMAN form is more rapid in onset, often the deep tendon jerks are retained or even brisk and autonomic dysfunction seldom occurs. Two patterns of recovery are noted; rather rapid recovery within days, and quite slow and poor recovery.

Features suggestive of GBS include a definite sensory level, marked symmetry in motor disability and persistent bowel or bladder involvement. The conditions that should be excluded include hexacarbon abuse, porphyria, post diphtheritic neuropathy, lead neuropathy, a pure sensory syndrome and an alternate paralytic disorder.

Cerebrospinal fluid examination shows albumino cytological dissociation with elevated proteins in the absence of significant pleocytosis (< 10 cells/mm^3 of CSF).

Differential diagnosis of GBS includes poliomyelitis, botulism, periodic paralysis, transverse myelitis, meningoencephalitis, brain stem encephalitis, stroke, porphyria, toxic neuropathies and posterior fossa tumors. Vasculitic mononeuritis multiplex may mimic GBS, and a history of disease evolution, systemic symptoms should be sought, and appropriate serological tests for a systemic vasculitis should be done. Salient differences between GBS and poliomyelitis are shown in Table 39.2.

Management

All patients with GBS should be hospitalized due to the risk of respiratory failure and need for intubation and mechanical ventilation. Indications for ICU admission include (a) rapidly progressive weakness, (b) oropharyngeal weakness, (c) dysautonomia, (d) respiratory insufficiency, and (e) evidence of aspiration pneumonia. The need for intubation and assisted ventilation should be determined. In general, one should err on the side

Table 39.2 Salient differences between acute polio paralysis and GBS

Features	Poliomyelitis	GBS
Age (years)	< 5 years	> 3 years
Fever	Fever, headache and meningeal signs	May occur 2-3 weeks prior to onset of paralysis
Progression	Rapid over 24-48 hrs.	Average 12 days for occurrence of maximum weakness
Symmetry	Asymmetrical, monoplegia, para- or quadriplegia	Symmetrical, legs affected more than arms
Atrophy	Rapid, starts within 5-7 days	Slow over weeks
Sensory	Motor dominant	Sensory symptoms in 70% cases
Cranial nerves	May be involved in bulbar polio	Facial weakness in 53%, opthalmoplegia, and bulbar nerves are affected
Electrophysiology	Acute denervation and reduced compound action potentials	Reduced conduction velocity, increased distal latency in demyelinating GBS; sensory nerves are involved

of early intubation rather than late. Tracheostomy should be delayed at least 2 weeks, unless there is evidence of axonal type of GBS or significant bulbar weakness exists.

Intravenous immunoglobulins (IVIG). IVIG is a safe and effective therapy in children with GBS. Side effects are few and include mild flu-like symptoms, nausea, headache and malaise. It should be avoided in children with IgA deficiency and in renal failure. Severe allergic reactions including anaphylaxis, circulatory overload and acute lung injury (pulmonary edema) may occur rarely. We have treated over 50 children with IVIG in a dose of 2 g/kg administered over 2 days with good results. Shahar et al[14] found marked and rapid improvement in 25 of 26 children treated with IVIG. It is ideal if it can be instituted early in the course of disease (preferably within the first few days) so that the morbidity and severity of the disease is ameliorated, the need for assisted ventilation is warded off or shortened and the hospital stay is reduced.

Plasmapheresis. This is as effective as IVIG, but its use is limited due to the size constraints of the patients and lack of availability of the equipment and infrastructure for plasmapheresis. It has limitations for its use in children with autonomic and cardiovascular compromise.

General and supportive care. The following principles of supportive care should be followed:

(i) Positioning and skin care
(ii) Bladder and bowel care
(iii) Eye and mouth care
(iv) *Fluids and nutrition.* Adequate intake of calories and their proportionate increase in infected patients. Parenteral nutrition may be required, and the need for percutaneous gastrostomy considered in selected cases.
(v) Nosocomial infections may occur in up to 25 percent patients. Culture surveillance of urine and sputum once or twice a week may help to provide information regarding the likely pathogens.
(vi) Physical therapy
(vii) *Pain relief.* A substantial number of patients develop significant pain in the thighs, calves, buttocks and trapezii. The pain may be severe in the evenings and at night. Pain near the joints and burning sensations around the thighs, calves and feet may occur. Mild narcotics are effective at night and do not cause dependence. Non-steroidal antiinflammatory drugs are not consistently beneficial. Gabapentin, carbamazepine, and tricyclic antidepressant medications may be helpful in the short-term and long term management of neuropathic pain. At times, intramuscular prednisone given in a single dose of 1mg/kg helps in combating the muscle pains.
(viii) *Autonomic disturbances.* Hypotension may be treated with fluid replacement; vasopressors are rarely required. Hypertension should be treated with short acting alpha-adrenergic blocking drugs, if it is

persistent and severe. Severe bradycardia may require temporary pacing.

(ix) Prevention of deep vein thrombosis

Outcome

The prognosis is excellent with majority of patients making a good recovery over weeks or months. The factors that correlate with poor outcome include rapid progression to severe weakness (7 days or less), need for prolonged ventilator support, mean distal compound muscle action potential amplitude less than 20 percent of normal, and preceding *Campylobacter jejuni* infection. About 90–95% of pediatric cases of GBS recover completely within 6–12 months independent of any therapeutic intervention, compared to 20% risk of persistent disability in adults.

2. Vasculitic neuropathies

They may follow primary or secondary systemic vasculitis. The typical clinical features of vasculitic neuropathy are acute to sub-acute onset of painful neuropathy. The most common presentation is an asymmetric polyneuropathy or mononeuritis multiplex. Commonly, the mononeuritis progresses rapidly so that on presentation the deficits appear confluent. Thus, it is important to obtain a detailed history of the clinical course of the initial and subsequent deficits. Accompanying constitutional symptoms may include myalgias, arthralgias, weight loss, fever, respiratory difficulty, abdominal pain, rash, or night sweats.

Electrodiagnostic studies help to reveal the acute-to-subacute axon loss of motor and sensory nerves, often in a patchy, multifocal distribution. Laboratory evaluation of suspected cases of vasculitic neuropathy should include a complete blood count (CBC), metabolic panel, ESR, C-reactive protein, antinuclear antibodies, rheumatoid factor, antineutrophil cytoplasmic antibody (ANCA), hepatitis B and C markers and cryoglobulins etc.

C. DISEASES OF THE MUSCLES

Acute myopathy does not cause muscle atrophy, and tendon reflexes are usually preserved. The presence of acute or rapid muscle atrophy and areflexia usually suggests a lower motor neuron (anterior horn cell or peripheral nerve) lesion. Acute painless myopathies are suggestive of periodic paralysis or toxic myopathies. Recurrent muscle weakness with myoglobinuria indicates a metabolic myopathy and appropriate genetic tests should be done.

A history of muscle weakness, pain and/or myoglobinuria which is provoked by exercise suggest the possibility of a glycolytic pathway defect. Episodes of weakness which occur in association with fever are supportive of a diagnosis of carnitine palmityl transferase deficiency. Periodic paralysis is characteristically provoked by exercise and ingestion of a carbohydrate meal followed by a period of rest.

1. Polymyositis/Dermatomyositis

Juvenile dermatomyositis (JDM) is the most common condition among the idiopathic inflammatory myopathies in children, accounting for 85% of the pediatric inflammatory myopathy cases. It is characterized by small vessel vasculopathy, involving arterioles and capillaries. Its most obvious effects are seen in skeletal muscles and in the skin, although other organ systems may be involved, including the gastrointestinal tract, heart, and lungs. It is classically characterized by symmetric, frequently progressive, proximal muscle weakness, and inflammatory cutaneous lesions, including but not limited to, erythematous scaly lesions over the metacarpophalangeal and/or interphalangeal joints (Gottron papules), a violaceous hue over the eyelids (heliotrope), with or without periorbital edema, malar erythema, periungual telangiectasia, and erythematous scaly rash over the neck, upper back, and extensor surfaces of the extremities.

Dermatomyositis (DM) is more common than idiopathic polymyositis (PM) in children as compared to adults. It presents more acutely and is often associated with systemic manifestations. The diagnosis is not difficult as the disorder generally has an onset over weeks or months. An acute fulminant course can occur that may need differentiation from GBS. Selective muscle involvement of the neck flexors, hip and pelvic girdle muscles provides an important clue to the diagnosis. There are no sensory symptoms or signs and deep tendon jerks are preserved.

The diagnosis is based on the presence of typical muscle weakness and skin changes, raised CPK (10 to 50 times normal), EMG evidences of an inflammatory myopathy, and typical features on muscle biopsy. A normal CPK does not exclude the diagnosis of DM. MRI of the muscles is a sensitive test to detect muscle inflammation and at times more useful than a poorly conducted or ambiguous EMG. Corticosteroids (prednisolone 1-2 mg/kg/day in a single dose) is the first line of treatment. Methyl prednisolone pulse therapy may be useful in severe and fulminant cases. Once the patient

Section 4

has stabilized or muscle strength has returned to normal (usually 4-6 months), the dose can be reduced gradually every 2-4 weeks. In steroid non-responders methotrexate, azathioprine, IVIG, cyclo-phosphamide, mycophenolate, etc. may be tried.

2. Acute viral myositis and benign acute childhood myositis (BACM)

Although myositis may occur after bacterial, parasitic, or viral infections, the viral myositides are the most commonly seen disorders by the clinician. A number of viruses like coxsackie virus, parainfluenza, mumps, measles, adenovirus etc. may cause myositis. As respiratory symptoms subside, pain, swelling, muscle tenderness signal the onset of myositis. The pain can be so severe that it may interfere with child's ability to walk or perform routine daily life activities. Weakness can be profound, and myoglobinuria may occur. The CPK can be elevated more than 10 times the normal upper limit. Treatment is conservative with bed rest, hydration, and anti-inflammatory medications. Recovery takes place in 7 to 10 days.

Benign acute childhood myositis (BACM) is a transient muscle syndrome classically occurring in children after an influenza virus infection (URI). BACM causes difficulty in walking due to severe bilateral calf pain. The child is reluctant to walk, and tends to walk on toes. The incidence of this well described phenomenon is uncertain but infrequent, and it is usually recognized during times of large influenza outbreaks and epidemics. A number of these children may be suspected to have GBS or a transverse myelitis.

3. Dengue myositis

Dengue virus infection may rarely result in acute pure motor quadriplegia due to myositis. In an endemic area it should be considered in the differential diagnosis of acute flaccid paralysis. In a recent epidemic, seven out of 16 patients with dengue infection presented with quadriplegia[15]. Weakness developed within 3 to 5 days of illness and was moderate to severe. Laboratory tests showed markedly raised CPK, liver enzymes and coagulation disturbances. In another report of 7 patients with dengue fever myositis, myalgia and respiratory distress was prominent[16]. Two of these patients had fulminant myositis requiring ventilation and succumbed to their illness.

4. Periodic paralysis

Paralysis caused by either hereditary hypokalemia or hereditary hyperkalemia usually develops during the course of a day and may be apoplectic. Usually, the limbs are most involved, and the bulbar muscles are relatively spared. The initial episode most often occurs during childhood, and unless other family members are known to have this disorder, it is frequently mistaken for the Guillain–Barré syndrome.

A simple classification of periodic paralysis is based on serum potassium; hypokalemic, hyperkalemic, and normokalemic. In addition, periodic paralysis may be primary (genetic) or secondary. The cause of secondary hypokalemic paralysis is gastrointestinal or urinary loss of potassium. The secondary group may have more severe hypokalemia and need longer time to recover. Patients with severe hypokalemia with acidosis or alkalosis should be investigated for secondary causes as their management differs. Thyrotoxicosis is an important cause of hypokalemic periodic paralysis, especially in Asians.

D. DISORDERS OF NEUROMUSCULAR JUNCTION

1. Myasthenia gravis

Myasthenic crises can occur in undiagnosed myasthenics, where it is important that the condition is considered early and appropriate treatment is instituted. In established patients the weakness may be precipitated by infection or treatment with drugs that interfere with neuromuscular transmission such as an aminoglycoside antibiotic or inadequate immunosuppression.

Patients with myasthenia gravis may become critically ill rapidly, and the severity of exacerbation may be misjudged. It is a medical emergency and requires prompt treatment. The common indication for ICU admission is imminent respiratory failure. It can be extremely difficult to distinguish between worsening of myasthenia gravis or excessive anticholinergic medication when a patient with known myasthenia gravis presents with rapidly increasing muscular weakness, with or without respiratory difficulty. Features suggestive of a cholinergic crisis (too much medication) include muscle fasciculations, pallor, sweating, hypersalivation and small pupils.

Treatment of precipitating factors is frequently sufficient to restore adequate respiratory function. If this has not occurred within 24 to 48 hours, plasma exchange or IVIG should be considered. Endotracheal intubation may be avoided by measures such as nursing in the upright position, using incentive spirometry, and assisted coughing. Administration of IVIG (400 mg/kg/day for 5days) or plasmapheresis (5 plasma exchanges for 2 consecutive days) gives prompt relief and bypasses the need for assisted ventilation.

Pyridostigmine is stopped temporarily during mechanical ventilation, to upgrade the acetylcholine receptors, and also to exclude the possibility of a cholinergic crisis. It can be restarted parenterally after 2-3 days, in doses lower than what were used before the crisis.

2. Botulism

Botulism occurs following ingestion of contaminated seafood (type E toxin) or improperly sterilized bottled or canned food (type A and B toxins). The symptoms may start 12 to 48 hours after ingestion of the contaminated food. Bulbar symptoms, including pupillary paralysis, diplopia, ptosis, blurred vision, impaired speech, and difficulty in swallowing occur initially and are followed by weakness in the upper limbs, followed by involvement of the legs. In severe cases, respiratory failure requiring mechanical ventilation occurs. The descending paralysis may help to clinically differentiate it from GBS. It is important to remember that normal pupils do not exclude the diagnosis of botulism. In infants, this disorder occurs between 6 weeks to 9 months of age. Infants often have an antecedent history of constipation and poor feeding, and a significantly large proportion have been fed honey[17]. Bulbar signs are common and include a poor cry, poor sucking, impaired pupillary responses and external ophthalmoplegia. With progress of the disease, a flaccid paralysis develops. The illness lasts 4-20 weeks and almost all infants recover.

The diagnosis of botulism is difficult to establish as it may mimic viral encephalitis, GBS, sepsis and neonatal myasthenia. The presence of bulbar signs and pupillary abnormalities in an alert child is characteristic of botulism. An EMG will show the striking incremental response at 50 Hz repetitive stimulation. Whilst botulism in older children is due to ingestion of preformed toxins (A, B, or E), infant botulism results from colonization of the gut with type A or type B spores of *C. botulinum.* In most cases, administration of antitoxin is ineffective by the time botulism is diagnosed. Treatment is supportive with mechanical ventilation, nasogastric feeding and care of the paralyzed patient.

E. ACUTE NEUROMUSCULAR WEAKNESS IN THE ICU

Weakness acquired in the ICU due to neuromuscular disease is 2-3 times more common than primary neuromuscular disorders such as GBS, myopathies or motor neuron diseases. Critical illness myopathy (CIM) and critical illness neuropathy (CIP) are being increasingly reported in adults, but in children the diagnosis is probably missed and only the severe ones are reported. CIP and CIM may be just another organ failure (neuromuscular), developing in association with other multiple organ failures in the critically ill patient[18].

1. Critical illness polyneuropathy and myopathy

It is a sensory motor neuropathy developing in critically ill patients affected by sepsis and multi-organ involvement. Sepsis, systemic inflammatory response syndrome (SIRS), and multiorgan failure are important correlates of development of these syndromes. The neuropathy may occur as early as 2 to 5 days in the presence of sepsis and SIRS[19]. The additional factors which may predispose to development of acute sensory motor neuropathy include the use of NMJ blockers, corticosteroids, cytotoxic drugs, and status asthmaticus. The neuropathy may resemble GBS and be severe enough to produce diaphragmatic weakness. However, the facial, bulbar and ocular muscles are not involved in critical illness neuropathy.

CIM has been reported in children admitted to ICUs and is characterized by persistent moderate to severe flaccid, generalized weakness that becomes apparent when neuromuscular blockade therapy is stopped. Distal and proximal muscles may be equally affected. The reflexes may be normal, reduced or absent. The most prominent problem in the ICU is the difficulty in weaning the patient off the ventilator, due to diaphragmatic or intercostal weakness. Most patients recover within 4 to 12 weeks. The laboratory investigations fail to show hypokalemia, hypophosphatemia or hypermagnesemia. The CPK may be increased 2 to 3 times the normal early in the course. Electrophysiological studies show a mixed axonal neuropathic and myopathic pattern[18, 19]. Transplant patients seem to be at greater risk of CIM. Recovery occurs in a stereotyped manner, first in the upper and proximal lower limbs followed by distal lower limbs. Effective treatment of infection, drainage of abscess, fluid resuscitation and physiotherapy all have a role in recovery. IVIG has not been shown to be useful.

2. Neuromuscular blockade (NMB)

Prolonged NMB occurs when synaptic transmission remains impaired and muscle weakness persists after NMB drug has been discontinued. It may be brief, lasting minutes or hours after a single dose of neuromuscular blockage drug. In the ICU, after repeated doses of pancuronium or vecuronium, a flaccid weakness of all four limbs with ptosis and ophthalmoplegia may persist lasting for days or weeks[20, 21]. NMB agent used for mechanical ventilation for at least 2 days may produce prolonged muscular weakness, most likely from accumulation of the metabolites of pancuronium or vecuronium. In addition, the metabolism of these drugs may be affected by multi organ failure, resulting in accumulation of these agents or their metabolites. Such accumulation results in prolonged NMB effect lasting for days after the drug is stopped. Besides, these drugs being amino steroids may be myotoxic, especially when combined with steroids. The disorder can be recognized through repetitive nerve stimulation test and temporarily reversed by neostigmine.

REFERENCES

1. Freemon FR. Hemiplegia and monoplegia. In: Neurology in Clinical Practice. Vol 1, 2nd edn. Bradley WG, Daroff RB, Fenichel GM, Marsden CD (Eds.). *Butterworth Heinemann, Boston* 1996, pp 359-373.

2. Roman GC. Tropical neurology. In: Neurology in Clinical Practice. Vol 2, 2nd edn. Bradley WG, Daroff RB, Fenichel GM, Marsden CD (Eds.). *Butterworth Heinemann, Boston* 1996, pp 2103-2128.

3. Global polio eradication initiative annual report 2007: Impact of the intensified eradication effort. http://www.polioeradication.org/content/publications/Annual Report 2007.

4. WHO-recommended standards for surveillance. Poliomyelitis 2003. pp31-34. http://www.who.int/vaccines-documents/DocsPDF06/843.pdf

5. Saraswathy TS, Zahrin HN, Apandi MY, Kurup D, Rohani J, Zainah S, Khairullah NS. Acute flaccid paralysis surveillance: looking beyond the global poliomyelitis eradication initiative. *Southeast Asian J Trop Med Public Health* 2008; 39:1033-1039.

6. Alcalá H. The differential diagnosis of poliomyelitis and other acute flaccid paralyses. *Biol Med Hosp Infant Mex* 1993; 50:136-144.

7. Wu HS, Liu TC, Lii ZL. Zou LP, Zhang WC, Zhaori G, Zhang J. A prospective clinical and electrophysiologic survey of acute flaccid paralysis in Chinese children. *Neurology* 1997:49:1723-1725.

8. Hemachudha T, Laothamatas J, Rupprecht CE. Human rabies: a disease of complex neuropathogenetic mechanism and diagnostic challenges. *Lancet Neurol* 2002; 1: 101–109.

9. Transverse Myelitis Consortium Working Group. Proposed diagnostic criteria and nosology of acute transverse myelitis. *Neurology* 2002; 59: 499-505.

10. Pidcock FS, Krishnan C, Crawford TO, Salorio CF, Trovato M, Kerr DA. Acute transverse myelitis in childhood. *Neurology* 2007; 68: 1474-1480.

11. McKhann GM, Cornblath DR, Ho TW, Li CY, Bai AY, Wu HS. Clinical and electrophysiological aspects of acute paralytic disease of children and young adults in northern China. *Lancet* 1991; 338:593-597.

12. Jones HR Jr. Childhood Guillain-Barre´ syndrome: Clinical presentation, diagnosis, and therapy. *J Child Neurol* 1996:11:4-12.

13. Griffin JW, Li CY, Ho TW, Xue P, Macko C, Gao CY. Guillain-Barre syndrome in northern China. *Brain* 1995: 577-595.

14. Shahar E, Shorer Z, Roifman CM, Levi Y, Brand N, Ravid S. Immunoglobulins are effective in treatment of severe pediatric Guillain-Barré syndrome. *Pediatr Neurol* 1997; 16:32-35.

15. Kalita J, Misra UK, Mahadevan A, Shankar SK. Acute pure motor quadriplegia: is it dengue myositis? *Electromyogr Clin Neurophysiol* 2005; 45:357-361.

16. Paliwal VK, Garg RK, Juyal R, Husain N, Verma R, Sharma PK, Verma R, Singh MK. Acute dengue virus myositis: a report of seven patients of varying clinical severity including two cases with severe fulminant myositis. *J Neurol Sci* 2011; 300:14-18.

17. Arnon SS. Infant botulism. *Ann Rev Med* 1980; 31:541-560.

18. Maramattom BV, Wijdicks EFM. Acute neuromuscular weakness in the intensive care unit. *Crit Care Med* 2006; 34: 2835-2841.

19. Vondracek P, Bednarik J. Clinical and electrophysiological findings and long-term outcomes in pediatric patients with critical illness polyneuromyopathy. *Eur J Pediatr Neurol* 2006; 10: 176-181.

20. Bizzarri-Schmid ND, Desai SP. Prolonged neuro-muscular blockade with atracurium. *Canad Anaesth Soc J* 1986; 33:209-212.

21. Torres CF, Maniscalo WM, Agostinelli T. Muscle weakness and atrophy following prolonged paralysis with pancuronium bromide in neonates. *Ann Neurol* 1985; 18:403-408.

40

Endocrinal Emergencies

Anurag Bajpai

The endocrine system plays an important role in regulation of metabolism and maintenance of homeostasis. Endocrine disorders are associated with wide variety of disturbances in metabolism resulting in myriad of clinical presentations. The fact that identification of endocrine etiology in an emergency setting is usually followed by initiation of specific treatment emphasizes the need for a high index of suspicion for endocrine disorders in such settings. Contrary to popular belief, resource intensive investigations are not required for diagnosing most endocrine emergencies and a combination of careful clinical evaluation and readily available investigations is sufficient in most cases. It is, however, important to emphasize that while initiation of specific treatment should take precedence over diagnostic workup, collection of appropriate blood samples before initiation of therapy is helpful in subsequent management. Throughout this chapter emphasis has been laid on

identification of features suggestive of an endocrine emergency. Practical approach using readily available investigations and guidelines for management of common endocrinal emergencies (except diabetic ketoacidosis which is discussed in Chapter 41) has been provided.

Common Correlates of Endocrine Emergencies

Non-specific features of endocrine disorders often cause delayed and missed diagnosis in majority of cases with fatal consequences at times. This emphasizes the need for a high index of suspicion for endocrine etiology in all children presenting to the emergency department. Endocrine etiology should be considered in the differential diagnosis of all sick children especially in the presence of seizures, stridor, cardiac failure, encephalopathy and shock. Table 40.1 presents clinical syndromes

Table 40.1 Indications for evaluation of a possible endocrine disorder			
Feature	**Usual diagnosis**	**Endocrine condition**	**Investigations**
Seizures	Meningitis	Hypocalcemia, hypoglycemia, hypernatremia	Serum electrolytes, calcium, blood sugar
Encephalopathy	Meningitis	DKA, hypoglycemia, hypercalcemia, hypernatremia, hyponatremia	Blood sugar, serum calcium, sodium
Shock	Sepsis	Adrenal insufficiency, DKA, acute DI	Sodium, potassium , blood sugar
Dehydration	Diarrhea	DKA, DI, hypercalcemia, adrenal insufficiency	Sodium, potassium, blood sugar, and calcium
Cardiac failure	DCM, CHD	Hypocalcemia, hypoglycemia, hyperthyroidism	Calcium, blood sugar, Free T4, TSH
Acute abdomen	Appendicitis	DKA, hypercalcemia	Blood sugar, calcium
Tachypnea	Pneumonia	DKA	Blood sugar, urine ketones
Bradycardia	Heart block	Hypothyroidism	Free T4, TSH
Hypothermia	Sepsis	Hypothyroidism	Free T4, TSH
Arrhythmia	PSVT	Hyperthyroidism, hypocalcemia, hypercalcemia	Calcium, Free T4, TSH

DI: Diabetes inspidus, DKA: Diabetic ketoacidosis, CHD: Congenital heart disease, DCM: Dilated cardiomyopathy, PSVT: Paroxysmal supraventricular tachycardia

requiring endocrine evaluation along with usually suspected diagnosis and desired investigations.

HYPOCALCEMIA

Hypocalcemia, a common correlate of endocrine disorder in children, may present to the emergency room with seizures, tetany, stridor, cardiac arrhythmia or cardiac failure. Identification of hypocalcemia guides successful management in most cases emphasizing the need for estimation of calcium levels in appropriate settings[1].

Clinical Features

Calcium plays an important role in stabilization of cell membrane and excitation-contraction coupling. Hypocalcemia predisposes the individual to increased neuromuscular irritability (resulting in seizures and muscular spasms) on one hand and decreased muscular contractility (resulting in decreased cardiac contractility) on the other. Calcium has a crucial role to support cardiac function with effects on repolarization and contractility. In the neonatal period subtle clinical features like lethargy, jitteriness and poor feeding are characteristic features of hypocalcemia[2]. Seizures are more common in neonates as compared to post neonatal age group and hypocalcemia is the commonest biochemical abnormality associated with neonatal seizures. In the post-neonatal period the commonest presentation of hypocalcemia is spasm of laryngeal and limb muscles. Severe hypocalcemia has been associated with reversible cardiac failure mimicking dilated cardiomyopathy[3]. Though most commonly observed in the neonatal period; the disorder has been reported in all ages.

Pointers to the Diagnosis

Hypocalcemia should be considered in all neonates with seizures, patients with dilated cardiomyopathy, laryngospasm and cardiac arrhythmias[4] (Table 40.2). In all subjects with suspected hypocalcemia, signs of covert hypocalcemia should be elicited. Chvostek sign involves tapping of facial nerve at the angle of mouth to produce twitching of circumoral muscles. Trousseau's sign is elicited by demonstration of carpal spasm after inflation of blood pressure cuff 20 mm Hg above the systolic pressure for three minutes. It is important to emphasize that tetany may also occur in other metabolic disorders like hypomagnesemia and hypo- and hyperkalemia. Hypocalcemia should be strongly suspected in subjects with unexplained cardiomyopathy in the presence of tetany, rickets and prolonged QT interval. Hypocalcemia causes slowing of repolarization and increased QTc interval. The corrected QoT (QoTc) interval takes into account not only the Q_0T (interval from the beginning of Q wave to the beginning of T wave) but also RR interval (time interval between two R waves). QoTc interval for heart rate is a reliable indicator of hypocalcemia[5]. This is calculated by the formula: $QoTc = Qot \sqrt{RR}$. *QoTc greater than 0.22 is suggestive of hypocalcemia.*

Table 40.2 Pointers to hypocalcemia
Neonatal period
❑ Jitteriness, seizures
❑ Stridor, apnea
❑ Cardiac failure
❑ Setting: Low birth weight babies, infants of diabetic mothers, severe birth asphyxia, sepsis, exchange transfusion with citrated blood, DiGeorge's syndrome, hypomagnesemia, formula-fed babies, etc.
Post-neonatal period
❑ Seizures, tetanic spasms
❑ Stridor, tetany
❑ Arrhythmia with prolonged QT interval
❑ Cardiac failure with decreased ejection fraction
❑ Setting: Rickets, renal failure, malabsorption, anti-epileptic drugs, DiGeorge's syndrome, parathormone deficiency, and hypomagnesemia, etc.

Diagnosis

Presence of signs of hypocalcemia, features of rickets and prolonged QoTc interval should prompt estimation of serum calcium levels. If calcium levels are not available, administration of calcium after obtaining a blood sample is desirable. Total calcium levels are dependent on free calcium, albumin and acid base status. Estimation of ionic calcium level is representative of biologically active calcium and is therefore desirable for the diagnosis of hypocalcemia. If this is not available ionic calcium levels may be deduced from total serum calcium levels and plasma protein levels using the formula given below[6]:

$$\text{Ionic calcium} = \text{Total calcium} - 0.8 \times (\text{Albumin} - 4)$$

Calcium levels are lower in the neonatal period and a cut off of 7.5 mg/dl (1.0 mMol/l = 4 mg/dl) is used as against 8.0 mg/dl for the post-neonatal period. Features of hypocalcemia usually do not develop till the total calcium levels fall below 7.0 mg/dl in neonates and 7.5 mg/dl in the post-neonatal period.

Etiology

Hypocalcemia can result from inefficient action of paratharmone (caused by low levels of PTH or peripheral resistance) and vitamin D (caused by nutritional deficiency, decreased activation or resistance) or increased binding of calcium to plasma protein (due to alkalosis) or chelating agents like phosphates, citrate and drugs. Early-onset neonatal hypocalcemia (within 72 hours of life) is usually observed in pre-term and small-for-dates neonates with birth asphyxia and maternal diabetes mellitus. Children born to mothers with hyperparathyroidism usually present with hypocalcemia in the first week of life[7]. Due to maternal hypercalcemia there is suppression of fetal parathyroid gland leading to self-limited neonatal hypocalcemia which resolves within two weeks. Vitamin D-dependent rickets (caused by decreased 1-alpha hydroxylase action or resistance to calcitriol), renal failure, inefficient PTH action (hypoparathyroidism and pseudohypoparathyroidism) and phosphate load due to formula feeds are important causes of late-neonatal hypocalcemia. Maternal vitamin D deficiency is associated with decreased vitamin D stores in the newborn[8]. Most healthy term children have normal calcium levels at birth; mobilization of calcium during bone mineralization around one month of age, may lead to hypocalcemia (hungry bone syndrome). Late-onset tetany in formula-fed babies usually presents around one month of age with low calcium and high phosphate levels. Renal failure, inefficient PTH action and vitamin D deficiency are important causes of hypocalcemia in late infancy and childhood.

Evaluation

Following initial stabilization, detailed history regarding age of onset, presenting features, frequency of episodes and family history should be obtained. Neonates with hypocalcemia should be screened for prematurity, birth asphyxia, maternal hyperparathyroidism and exposure to formula feeds. Early-onset hypocalcemic rickets suggests the

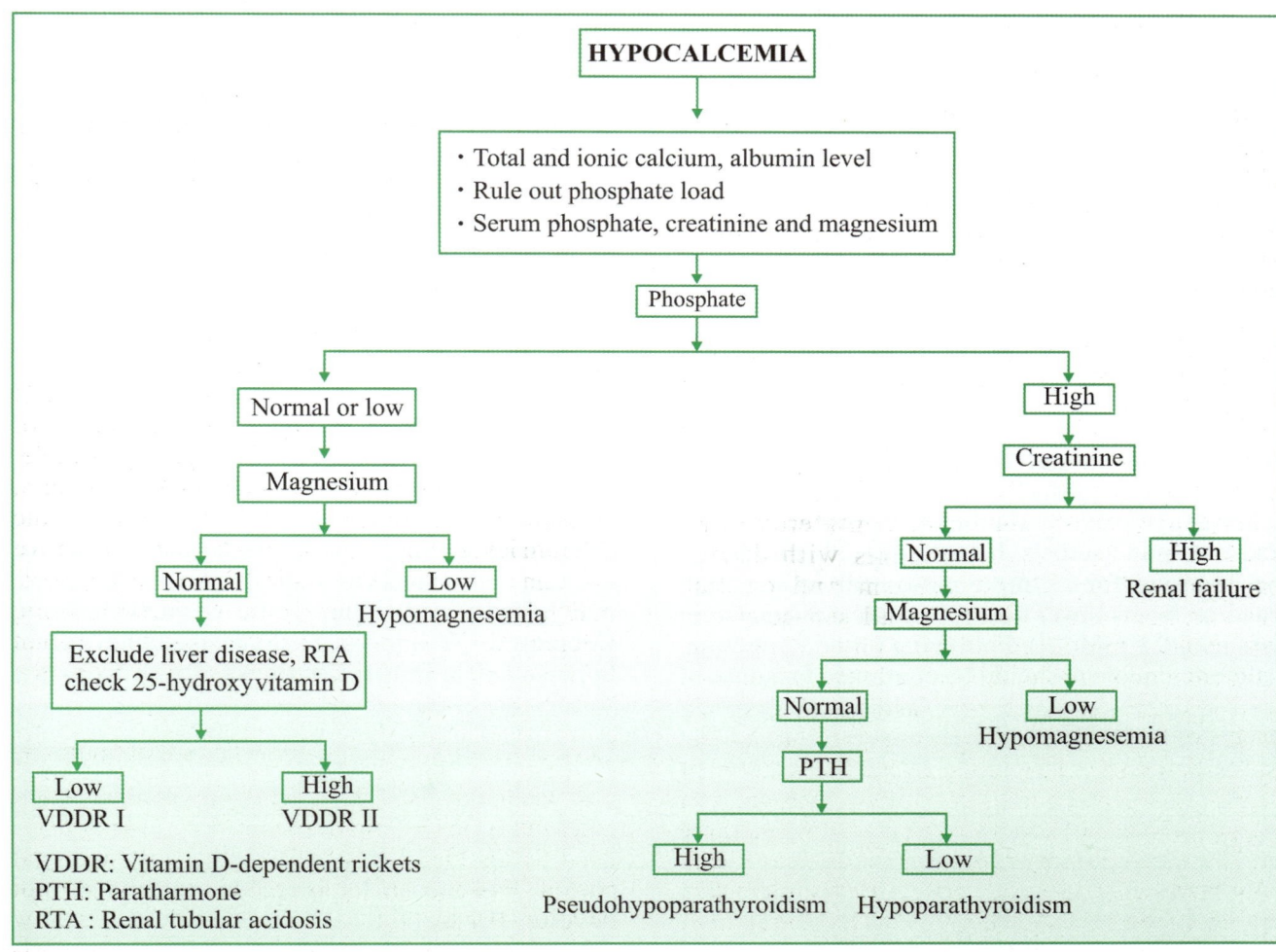

Figure 40.1 Approach to a child with persistent hypocalcemia

diagnosis of vitamin D- dependent rickets. Congestive cardiac failure, recurrent infections and abnormal facies in a child with hypocalcemia suggest the diagnosis of DiGeorge malformation complex.

Initial investigations include serum calcium, phosphate, alkaline phosphatase, renal function tests, and liver function tests[9]. Phosphate regulation is dependent on paratharmone (PTH); inefficient PTH action (as in hypoparathyroidism and pseudohypoparathyroidism) therefore causes elevated phosphate levels. Vitamin D related disorders on the other hand are associated with hyperparathyroidism and consequent hypophosphatemia. Hypocalcemia with hyperphosphatemia and normal renal functions are reliable markers of inefficient PTH action, which should be further evaluated by estimation of PTH levels (Figure 40.1). Infants with severe vitamin D deficiency may, however, have elevated phosphorus levels despite high PTH levels. This is due to transient PTH resistance induced by severe vitamin D deficiency and often results in misdiagnosis of pseudohypoparathyroidism. Hypomagnesemia should be considered in all patients with refractory hypocalcemia. Patients with hypocalcemic rickets should be evaluated with liver function tests, renal function tests, venous blood gas and malabsorption studies. When these investigations are normal, the diagnosis of nutritional rickets and vitamin D-dependent rickets (VDDR) should be considered.

Management

Intravenous calcium should be administered in all children with suspected symptomatic hypocalcemia after obtaining blood sample. Calcium gluconate 2 ml/kg of 10% solution (provides 9 mg Ca++ per ml) should be infused slowly over 10 minutes under cardiac monitoring. Care should be taken to avoid extravasation of calcium as this may cause dermal necrosis. Intravenous calcium should be reserved for asymptomatic individuals with calcium levels lower than 6.0 mg/dl (Ionic calcium less than 0.8 mMol/l). Following initial correction, calcium gluconate should be continued in a dose of 75-80 mg/kg/day (2 ml/kg every 6 hourly). This should ideally be dissolved in maintenance fluids. Care should, however, be taken not to mix calcium gluconate with phosphate or bicarbonate to avoid crystallization in the IV tubing. Intravenous calcium should not be mixed with phosphate or bicarbonate as this may lead to crystallization in the IV tubing. The dose of calcium gluconate is decreased to 75% on day 2 and 50% on day 3. Intravenous calcium should be replaced with oral calcium after stabilization and initiation of specific therapy. Magnesium sulfate (0.1 ml/kg of 50% solution, 12 hourly for four doses IM) is indicated in children with refractory hypocalcemia.

HYPERCALCEMIA

Hypercalcemia is rare but a frequently missed disorder in children. Early diagnosis and management is essential for preventing short and long-term complications of the disease.

Clinical Features

Elevated serum calcium levels results in depressed neuro-muscular activity, increased rate of repolarization of cardiac muscle, release of gastric acid and resistance to action of the antidiuretic hormone (ADH). This results in constipation (decreased muscular contractility), abdominal pain (increased gastric acid production and pancreatitis), polyuria (resistance to ADH) and decreased QT interval (rapid repolarization). Features of hypercalcemia depend on the severity and rapidity of its development (Table 40.3).

Correlates of hypercalcemia

Hypercalcemia should be suspected in all neonates with features of septicemia and meningitis without laboratory evidence of infection. Hypercalcemia should also be considered in the differential diagnosis of acute abdomen, polyuria, unexplained dehydration and hypertension. There may be irritability, failure to thrive and hypotonia. Decreased QT interval on ECG is suggestive of hypercalcemia in these settings.

Table 40.3 Features of hypercalcemia		
Severity	**Calcium level**	**Features**
Mild	10-12 mg/dl	Asymptomatic, irritability
Moderate	12-14 mg/dl	Polyuria with abdominal pain, lethargy, decreased feeding, hypertension
Severe	>14 mg/dl	Altered sensorium, seizures, hypertension and dehydration

Hypercalcemia is diagnosed in the presence of elevated total (>12 mg/dl) or ionic (>1.5 mMol/l) calcium levels. Decreased QT interval is a non-specific indicator of hypercalcemia. In asymptomatic individuals, calcium levels should be repeated at least three times before establishing the diagnosis.

Etiology

Elevated calcium levels are caused by increased release (from bone under the influence of PTH) or absorption (from intestine under the influence of vitamin D) of calcium. Inactivating mutation of calcium sensing receptor presents in the neonatal period with refractory hypercalcemia and parathyroid hyperplasia. Parathyroid adenoma is an important cause of hypercalcemia in older children and adults. Increased vitamin D level due to exogenous administration or endogenous production caused by increased macrophage 1-alpha hydroxylase activity (as in sarcoidosis) is an important cause of hypercalcemia. Hypercalcemia in children with subcutaneous fat necrosis is caused by release of precipitated calcium and increased activity of 1-alpha hydroxylase action. Williams syndrome is characterized by significant hypercalcemia, abnormal facies and supra-valvular aortic stenosis which usually presents in late infancy. Hypercalcemia may be associated with hyperthyroidism, McCune Albright syndrome and administration of certain drugs (Lithium, thiazides, aluminium).

Diagnosis

Details of family history (for calcium sensing receptor defect), features of sarcoidosis and exposure to drugs (vitamin D, lithium, thiazide) should be recorded. Features of Williams syndrome and cutaneous nodules (fat necrosis) should be looked for. Initial investigations should include serum phosphate, alkaline phosphatase and creatinine[10]. Persistent hypercalcemia should be followed up with

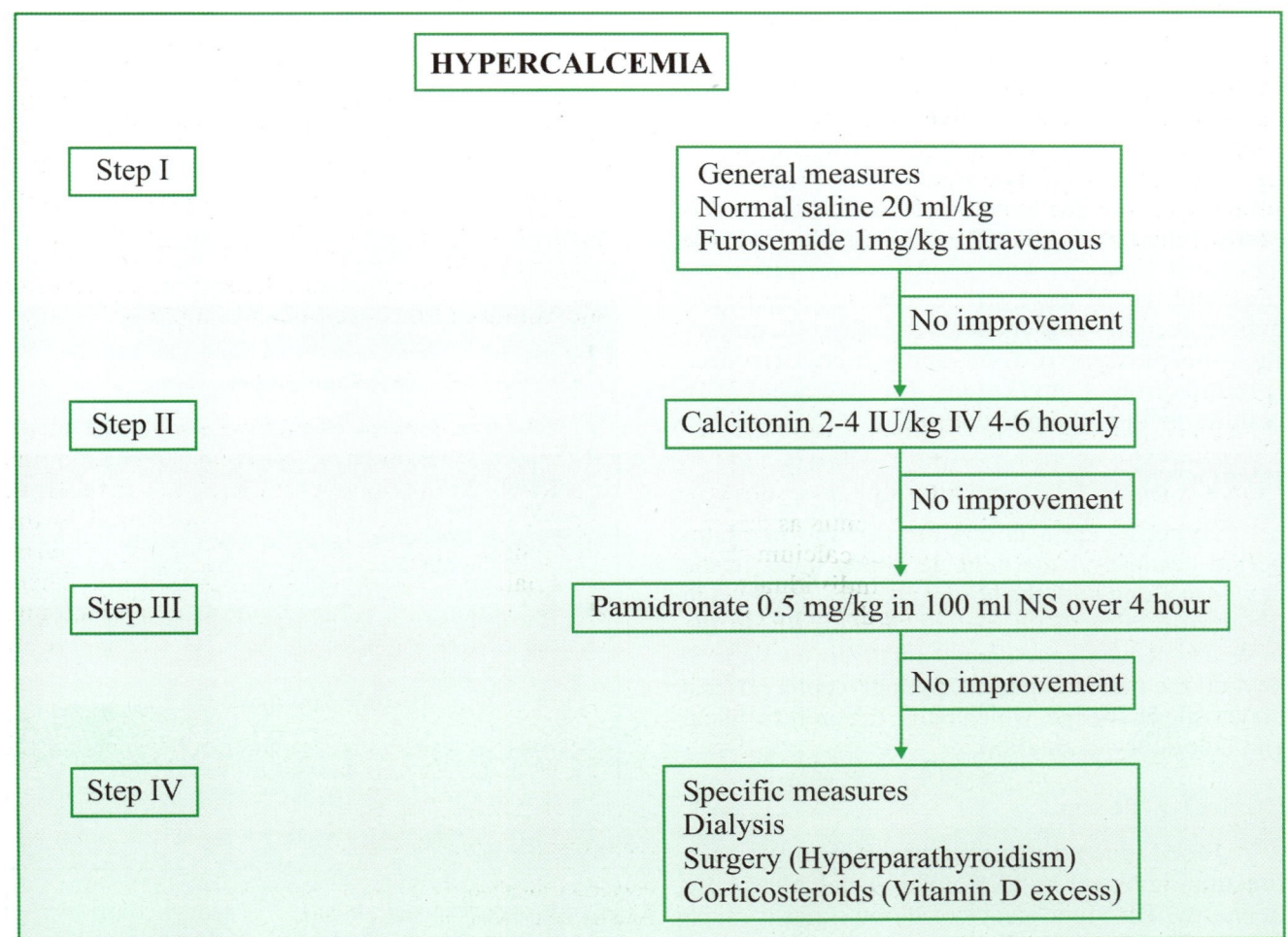

Figure 40.2 Stepwise approach for management of hypercalcemia

estimation of PTH levels. High PTH levels are suggestive of hyperparathyroidism; low or normal levels are indicative of iatrogenic excess of vitamin D (associated with high 25-hydroxyvitamin D levels) or increased 1-alpha hydroxylase activity (associated with low 25-hydroxyvitmain D and high 1, 25 dihydroxyvitamin D levels).

Management

Initial management involves stabilization and correction of hypoxia and dehydration. Hydration is the most important aspect of management of hypercalcemia. This can be achieved by fluid bolus (20 ml/kg of normal saline) followed by twice maintenance intravenous fluids[6]. Hydration alone decreases serum calcium levels by 1-3 mg/d within one to two hours. This should be followed by intravenous furosemide (1 mg/kg). It is important to emphasize that furosemide should be given only after correction of dehydration as it is not only ineffective but likely to be hazardous in the presence of dehydration. Intravenous calcitonin (2-4 unit/kg 4-6 hourly) should be given to children with no improvement with these measures (Figure 40.2). Rapid development of tachyphylaxis limits sustained efficacy of calcitonin. Children with recalcitrant hypercalcemia should receive the anti-resorptive agent pamidronate (0.5 mg/kg in 100 ml normal saline over 2-4 hours). Dialysis is required in subjects with severe hypercalcemia (calcium levels more than 15 mg/dl). These measures provide transient benefits and specific measures are required in almost all cases of persistent hypercalcemia. This includes parathyroid surgery in hyperparathyroidism and glucocorticoids (prednisolone 1 mg/kg/day for two weeks) in children with vitamin D excess.

HYPOGLYCEMIA

Hypoglycemia is common in the neonatal period because of the delicate homeostasis in the newborn along with the abrupt changes involved in the transition from the secure in-utero life to the insecure outside world. Though relatively uncommon beyond the neonatal period, hypoglycemia poses a diagnostic challenge, which requires careful clinical and laboratory evaluation.

Clinical Features

Blood glucose plays an important role in cell functioning by acting as a readily available source of energy. The significance of blood sugar is much greater for the brain because it almost entirely depends on glucose for its energy requirements.

Hypoglycemia leads to impaired central nervous system function (neuroglucopenia) on one hand and stimulation of sympathetic nervous system on the other. Neuroglucopenic symptoms are characterized by headache, impaired concentration, decline in cognitive functions, seizures and impaired consciousness. Stimulation of sympathetic nervous system results in release of catecholamines with symptoms like tachycardia, flushing and perspiration. In most individuals sympathetic symptoms precede the development of neuroglucopenic symptoms except in diabetics. In the neonatal period hypoglycemia presents with nonspecific features including jitteriness, seizures, apnea, hypothermia and hemodynamic instability[11]. Cardiac dysfunction with cardiac failure may also occur in children with hypoglycemia. Blood sugar levels should, therefore, be measured in all sick children.

Clinical Correlates

Considering the wide spectrum of neonatal hypoglycemia, the disorder should be suspected in all sick neonates. In particular alterations in behavioral pattern, temperature instability, decreased feeding and seizures in a previously well child are strong indicators of hypoglycemia. Beyond the neonatal period, hypoglycemia should be considered in all subjects with seizures, encephalopathy, syncope and acute ataxia (Table 40.4). Regular monitoring of blood sugar is mandatory for children with type 1 DM due to high risk of hypoglycemia.

Table 40.4 Correlates of hypoglycemia in children
Neonatal period
❑ Jitteriness, seizures, lethargy
❑ Apnea, cyanotic spells, respiratory distress
❑ Hypothermia
❑ Cardiac failure
❑ Routine monitoring: Large-for-dates, small-for-dates, pre-term, infant of diabetic mother, birth asphyxia, hypothermia, sepsis, exchange blood transfusion, maternal medications, history of sibling death due to inborn error of metabolism
Post-neonatal period
❑ Anxiety, tachycardia, perspiration, tremulousness, headache, mental confusion
❑ Seizures
❑ Acute ataxia
❑ Syncope
❑ Encephalopathy
❑ Bizarre neurological signs
❑ Routine monitoring: Adrenal insufficiency, diabetes mellitus, protein energy malnutrition, starvation

Diagnosis

Hypoglycemia is defined as blood sugar less than 50 mg/dl (1 mMol/l = 18 mg/dl); lower cutoff during the neonatal period (40 mg/dl) has been recommended. From a practical standpoint, blood sugar should be maintained between 60-100 mg/dl. Blood sugar levels can be estimated in the laboratory by the glucose oxidase method or with a glucometer. If these facilities are not available dextrose can be administered after obtaining blood sample. It is important to emphasize that glucometers are usually unreliable at low sugar values and hypoglycemia detected by them needs to be confirmed by a simultaneously performed laboratory value.

Etiology

Hypoglycemia may result from decreased production or increased utilization of glucose[12] (Table 40.5). Differentiation of these disorders is critical as physiological glucose replacement (6-8 mg/kg/min) is sufficient to maintain blood sugar in children with decreased production while significantly higher infusion rates are required in the presence of increased utilization of glucose. Hypoglycemia in the neonatal period is most commonly due to decreased body stores related to intra-uterine growth retardation and pre-term gestation or increased utilization caused by hyperinsulinism, birth asphyxia and septicemia. Common causes of persistent hypoglycemia in neonates include hyperinsulinism, fatty acid oxidation defects and hypopituitarism. Hyperinsulinism is the commonest cause of persistent neonatal hypoglycemia. It could be because of diffuse or focal pathology. Inactivating mutation in the potassium ATP channel and activating glucokinase and glutamase dehydrogenase enzyme are major causes of diffuse hyperinsulinism. Recently prolonged hyperinsulinism has been identified in neonates with small-for-gestational age or birth asphyxia. The condition usually resolves by 3 to 6 months. Ketotic hypoglycemia, glycogen storage disease and hyperinsulinism are important causes during infancy and childhood. Ketotic hypoglycemia is the commonest form of hypoglycemia beyond infancy and presents at the age of 2-5 years with early morning hypoglycemia. Hypopituitarism is a well-known cause of hypoglycemia. Glycogen storage disease (GSD) is characterized by hepatomegaly, ketotic hypoglycemia, lactic acidosis and hypotonia. Fatty acid oxidation defects present with hypoketotic hypoglycemia during infancy.

Table 34.5 Causes of hypoglycemia in children

Neonatal period

Transient
- Low birth weight, pre-term gestation, small-for-dates, discordant twin
- Infant of diabetic mother
- Birth asphyxia
- Sepsis
- Exchange blood transfusion, high position of umbilical artery catheter

Persistent
- Hyperinsulinism: Focal or diffuse hyperinsulinism, transposition of great vessels, Beckwith-Wiedmann syndrome
- Galactosemia, organic acidemias
- Hypopituitarism

Post-neonatal period
- **Systemic disorders.** Sepsis, cerebral malaria, Reye syndrome, PEM, malabsorption, liver failure, renal failure, heart failure, diarrhea, burns, shock
- **Substrate deficiency.** Ketotic hypoglycemia, organic acidemias
- **Counter-regulatory hormone deficiency.** Panhypopituitarism, GHD, adrenal insufficiency
- **Glycogen storage disease.** Type I, III, VI
- **Gluconeogenic defects.** Fructose 1, 6-bisphosphatase, pyruvate carboxylase, galactosemia, hereditary fructose intolerance
- **Fatty acid oxidation defects.** Acyl Co A defect, carnitine deficiency
- **Drugs.** Salicylates, quinine, propranolol, insulin overdose, pentamidine, etc.
- **Hyperinsulinism.** Genetic, factitious, insulinoma, and drugs

Clinical Evaluation

Evaluation of hypoglycemia involves identification of etiology and institution of appropriate management. Post-prandial hypoglycemia is uncommon and should raise the possibility of galactosemia or fructose intolerance. Hypoglycemia occurring 2-4 hours after meals is usually observed in hyperinsulinism and GSD 1 while onset after overnight fast is a feature of gluconeogenic defect and ketotic hypoglycemia. Recurrent diarrhea, jaundice and cataracts are suggestive of galactosemia and fructose intolerance. Family history of sibling deaths points to congenital adrenal hyperplasia or severe form of hyperinsulinism. Child should be examined for dysmorphic features, growth retardation (hypopituitarism), hypogonadism and ambiguous genitalia (congenital adrenal hyperplasia), pigmentation (adrenal insufficiency), hypotonia

(GSD), jaundice (galactosemia, fatty acid oxidation defect), hepatomegaly (GSD) and cardiomyopathy.

Laboratory Investigations

Neonates with persistent (lasting beyond 7 days of life) and severe hypoglycemia (glucose infusion rate requirement greater than 12 mg/kg/min) should be evaluated for etiology of hypoglycemia. Beyond the neonatal period, this workup is indicated in all children with hypoglycemia. Initial investigations should include urine ketones, blood gas, reducing substances in urine and blood lactate. It is important to obtain these crucial samples before initiation of treatment, as restoration of euglycemia alters the profile in most cases.

Stepwise approach to a child with hypoglycemia has been provided in Figure 40.3[13]. All children with hypoglycemia should produce ketones unless fatty acid oxidation is defective or suppressed by high insulin levels or due to accumulation of intermediary metabolites (fructose intolerance and galactosemia). Positive urine reducing substance in the setting of hypoketotic hypoglycemia indicates the diagnosis of fructose intolerance or galactosemia. Insulin levels should be estimated in those children with hypoglycemia who do not have ketones or reducing substances in urine. High insulin levels are diagnostic of hyperinsulinism; low levels favor the diagnosis of fatty acid oxidation defects. Elevated blood lactate in a child with hypoglycemia is suggestive of GSD 1 or fructose 1, 6-bisphosphatase deficiency. Children with features of GSD and normal blood lactate levels are most likely to have type III and VI GSD. Ketotic hypoglycemia in the absence of elevated blood lactate should prompt evaluation of GH and adrenal hormones.

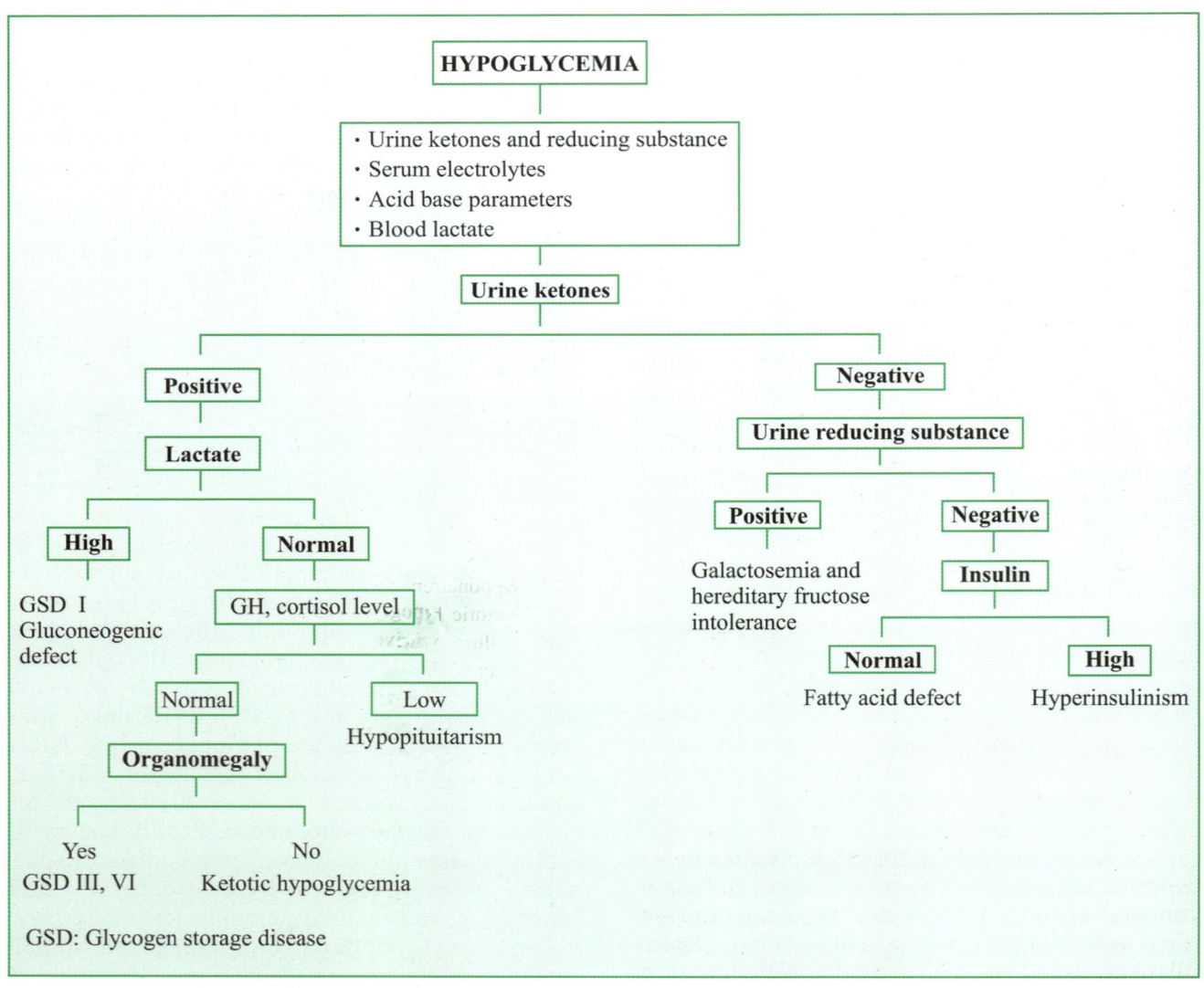

Figure 40.3 Approach to a child with persistent hypoglycemia

Section 4

Management

Hypoglycemia should be managed by bolus of 200 mg/kg dextrose (2 ml/kg of 10% dextrose intravenously) followed by dextrose infusion at a rate of 8 mg/kg/min. Higher dose of dextrose (500 mg/kg or 5 ml/kg of 10% dextrose) is recommended in the presence of seizures. Dextrose concentration required to obtain the desired glucose infusion rate (GIR) can be calculated by the following formula.

$$\text{Dextrose concentration (\%)} = \frac{\text{GIR mg/kg/min} \times 144}{\text{Fluid volume (ml/kg/day)}}$$

Efforts should be made to maintain blood sugar levels above 60 mg/dl. The glucose infusion rate can be increased in increments of 20% after every 15-30 minutes if repeat blood sugar remains low. Fluid with dextrose concentration greater than 12% should be administered using a central line due to the risks associated with infusing hyperosmolar solutions through the peripheral lines. Dextrose infusion should be gradually tapered once the blood sugar is above 60 mg/dl for a period of at least 24 hours.

Specific management is indicated in most children with persistent hypoglycemia. Children with hyperinsulinism have refractory hypoglycemia and may require GIR up to 18-20 mg/kg/minute. Diazoxide (5-15 mg/kg/day in three divided doses) or octreotide (5-20 µg/kg/day subcutaneously 12 hourly) have been used to treat resistant cases of hypoglycemia. Patients who do not respond to drugs should undergo surgery. Children with GSD are treated with regular feeds of uncooked cornstarch (1-2 g/kg every four hours). Hormonal deficiency and ketotic hypoglycemia should be managed with hormonal replacement and regular feeding during intercurrent illnesses respectively.

ACUTE ADRENAL INSUFFICIENCY

Adrenal gland plays a crucial role in maintenance of hemodynamic status and regulation of electrolytes and sugar levels. Untreated adrenal insufficiency is lethal emphasizing the need for early diagnosis and management.

Clinical Features

Mineralocorticoid (aldosterone) deficiency causes increased urinary losses of sodium and water resulting in the clinical syndrome of salt wasting crisis. It is characterized by dehydration, shock, polyuria, hyponatremia and hyperkalemia, and untreated salt wasting crisis is universally fatal[15].

Glucocorticoid (cortisol) deficiency results in impaired stress response, diminished counter-regulatory response to hypoglycemia and disturbed fluid homeostasis. Adrenal insufficiency is usually a chronic insidious process; the diagnosis is missed in majority of cases due to non-specific features. In most cases the condition is diagnosed in the emergency department; inability to identify adrenal insufficiency in this setting may have fatal consequences. Acute adrenal insufficiency is characterized by hyponatremia, hyperkalemia, and hypoglycemia in the setting of shock and polyuria. Primary adrenal insufficiency (Addison's disease) is associated with increased ACTH production and hyperpigmentation, a finding that distinguishes these individuals from those with secondary adrenal insufficiency.

Clinical Correlates

Non-specific symptoms mandates the need for a high index of suspicion for adrenal insufficiency in an emergency setting. The clinico-biochemical picture of shock, hyponatremia, hyperkalemia, and hemoconcentration is characteristic of acute adrenal insufficiency (and salt wasting due to 21-hydroxyalse deficiency in infants) and warrants immediate steroid replacement (Table 40.6). The diagnosis of 21-hydroxylase deficiency although readily established in girls due to genital ambiguity; is often missed in boys with fatal consequences. 21-hydroxyalse deficiency should be considered in all neonates with hyperpigmentation, genital ambiguity, cryptorchidism, polyuria and failure to

Table 40.6 Clinical correlates of adrenal insufficiency in children
Neonatal period
❑ Shock
❑ Hyponatremia with hyperkalemia
❑ Ketotic hypoglycemia
❑ Failure to thrive
❑ Polyuria
❑ Hyperpigmentation
❑ Ambiguous genitalia (21-hydroxyalse deficiency)
❑ Family history of sibling death (21-hydroxyalse deficiency)
Post-neonatal period
❑ Shock
❑ Hyperpigmentation
❑ Hyponatremia, hyperkalemia
❑ Hypoglycemia with ketoacidosis
❑ Catecholamine refractory septic shock

thrive[16]. Family history of sibling death and congenital adrenal insufficiency is another important indicator of 21-hydroxylase deficiency.

Adrenal insufficiency should be considered in the differential diagnosis of all children with shock. Presence of polyuria, hyperpigmentation and characteristic laboratory features (hyponatremia, hyperkalemia or hypoglycemia) are strongly indicative of adrenal insufficiency. It is important to emphasize that while urine output is decreased in all individuals with shock, children with adrenal insufficiency continue to be polyuric even in the presence of hypovolemia. *Polyuria in a child with shock is, therefore, an important indicator of adrenal insufficiency (and also diabetic ketoacidosis and diabetes insipidus).* Covert adrenal insufficiency has been reported in a significant proportion of children with septic shock. This is associated with diminished responsiveness to catecholmaines; a process that is reversible following steroid replacement. Covert adrenal insufficiency should be considered in children with septic shock refractory to catecholamines.

Diagnosis

Low cortisol levels are the hallmark of adrenal insufficiency. Elevated plasma adrenocorticotropin hormone (ACTH) is characteristic of primary adrenal insufficiency; normal levels are observed in secondary adrenal insufficiency. 17-hydroxyprogesterone (17OHP) should be estimated in all infants with suspected 21-hydroxylase deficiency. Elevated 17OHP in the clinical setting of salt wasting is diagnostic of 21-hydroxylase deficiency and estimation of aldosterone, ACTH, plasma renin activity (PRA) and urinary steroids is not required. Hydrocortisone should be administered to all subjects with suspected adrenal insufficiency after obtaining samples for cortisol (or 17OHP in the neonatal period). If these samples cannot be taken, the diagnosis of 21-hydroxylase deficiency may be confirmed later by ACTH stimulation test or measurement of 17OHP levels 48 hours after discontinuation of hydrocortisone[17].

Etiology

Adrenal insufficiency is caused by decreased adrenal steroid production due to defective steroidogenesis, destruction of adrenal gland, suppression of the HPA axis due to prolonged steroid exposure or decreased ACTH production (Table 40.7). Adrenal insufficiency in the neonatal period is most commonly caused by congenital adrenal hyperplasia, adrenal hypoplasia or adrenal hemorrhage. Congenital adrenal hyperplasia (CAH), a group of autosomal recessive defects in steroid synthesis, is characterized by deficiency of adrenocortical hormones on one hand and excess of steroid precursor on the other. 21-hydroxylase deficiency is the commonest form of CAH accounting for 90% cases. This disorder is associated with diminished synthesis of cortisol and aldosterone and elevated androgen levels. Autoimmune destruction, tuberculosis, adrenoleukodystrophy and adrenal hemorrhage are important causes of acquired adrenal insufficiency. Hypothalamic-pituitary axis abnormality is rarely associated with adrenal insufficiency. Adrenal status should, however, be examined in all children with central hypothyroidism before thyroid replacement lest increased metabolism of steroid hormones caused by treatment may precipitate adrenal insufficiency.

Management

Initial management of salt wasting crises includes correction of shock by fluid boluses and management of hyponatremia (3% normal saline), hyperkalemia (calcium gluconate and sodium bicarbonate) and hypoglycemia (10% dextrose). Hydrocortisone should be administered immediately in a dose of 50 mg/m^2 followed by 100 mg/m^2/day[18].

Table 40.7 Causes of adrenal insufficiency

Neonatal period

- Congenital adrenal hyperplasia
  21-hydroxylase deficiency, 17-hydroxylase deficiency, 3-betahydroxysteroid deficiency, StAR protein deficiency
- Congenital adrenal hypoplasia
- Adrenal hemorrhage

Post-neonatal period

- Hypothalamic-pituitary related hypothalamic lesion, panhypopituitarism
- Defective steroidogenesis: CAH
- Anatomical defect: Surgery, trauma, hypoplasia of adrenals
- Autoimmune destruction: Polyglandular endocrinopathy I and II
- Infection: Tuberculosis, HIV, CMV
- Hemorrhage: Waterhouse-Friderichsen syndrome, bleeding disorder
- Miscellaneous conditions: Adrenoleukodystrophy, Tripple A syndrome

StAR: Steroidogenic acute regulatory protein deficiency
CAH: Congenital adrenal hyperplasia

Double-volume maintenance intravenous fluids without potassium should be started after initial stabilization. Frequent monitoring of hemodynamic parameters, urine output and serum electrolytes are mandatory. Once the child is hemodynamically stable, hydrocortisone can be tapered gradually to a dose of 15-25 mg/m²/day (Figure 40.4). Mineralocorticoids (fludrocortisone acetate 0.1 mg/day) should be added once hydrocortisone dose is less than 50 mg/m²/day. Long-term management of adrenal insufficiency requires lifelong replacement of glucocorticoids and mineralocorticoids. Hydrocortisone dose should be increased to 50 mg/m²/day during minor stress (fever >100.4°F, gastroenteritis) and 100 mg/m²/day during severe stress (pneumonia, surgery, shock). The parents should be advised to bring the child to immediate medical attention in case of recurrent vomiting, decreased oral acceptance and shock. Patients with secondary adrenal insufficiency do not require mineralocorticoids and are treated with hydrocortisone alone.

ACUTE DIABETES INSIPIDUS

Antidiuretic hormone (ADH) plays an important role in water regulation. Children with ADH deficiency usually present to the outpatient department with polyuria, polydipsia and failure to thrive. Diffuse damage to the hypothalamic-pituitary region due to any cause may present with acute diabetes insidpius (DI) in an emergency setting.

Clinical Features

Acute DI usually occurs in well-defined settings like neuro-surgery, CNS infections and head trauma. Hypernatremia and polyuria (urine output

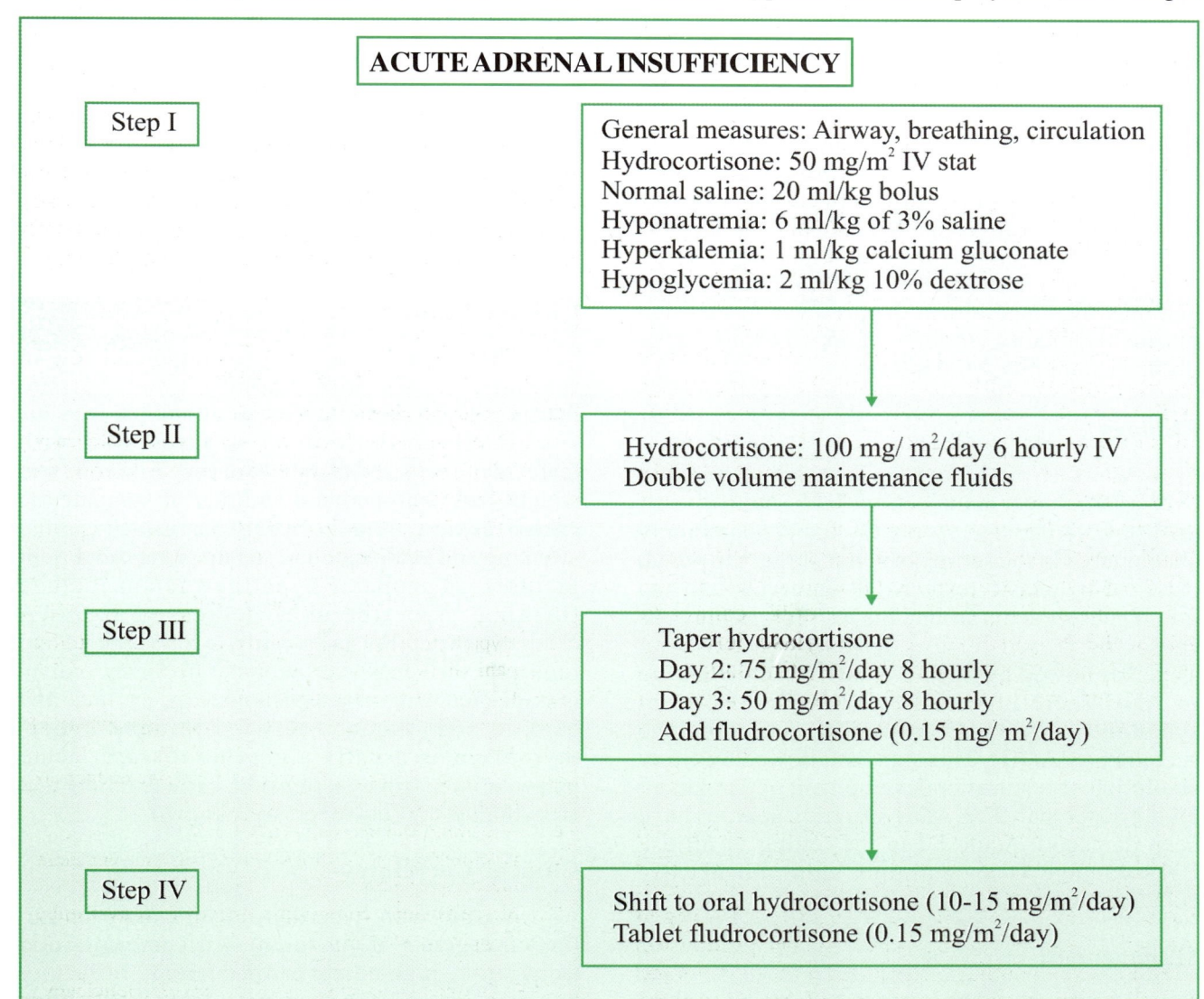

ACUTE ADRENAL INSUFFICIENCY

Step I — General measures: Airway, breathing, circulation
Hydrocortisone: 50 mg/m² IV stat
Normal saline: 20 ml/kg bolus
Hyponatremia: 6 ml/kg of 3% saline
Hyperkalemia: 1 ml/kg calcium gluconate
Hypoglycemia: 2 ml/kg 10% dextrose

Step II — Hydrocortisone: 100 mg/m²/day 6 hourly IV
Double volume maintenance fluids

Step III — Taper hydrocortisone
Day 2: 75 mg/m²/day 8 hourly
Day 3: 50 mg/m²/day 8 hourly
Add fludrocortisone (0.15 mg/m²/day)

Step IV — Shift to oral hydrocortisone (10-15 mg/m²/day)
Tablet fludrocortisone (0.15 mg/m²/day)

Figure 40.4 Stepwise management of acute adrenal insufficiency

up to 20 ml/kg/hour) is characteristic. Close monitoring of urine output is required for early detection of the condition. The diagnosis is, however, usually not established till the development of hypernatremia and hemodynamic instability. Acute DI should be strongly suspected in all children admitted to the ICU with CNS insult who develop polyuria, hemodynamic instability and hypernatremia.

Diagnosis

Polyuria in a child with diffuse CNS insult may be related to central DI, osmotic diuresis caused by mannitol or the syndrome of cerebral salt wasting. Central DI can be readily differentiated from these conditions by the presence of low urine osmolality (as against high urine osmolality in osmotic diuresis and cerebral salt wasting) and high sodium levels (as against low sodium levels in cerebral salt wasting). Dilute urine (urine osmolality <300 mOsm/l) in the presence of increased plasma osmolality (osmolalitiy >300 mOsm/l or serum sodium >146 mEq/L) and response to vasopressin (increase in urine osmolality by more than 50% one hour after 0.5 unit/kg vasopressin) is diagnostic of central DI[19]. Therapeutic trial with vasopressin may be given if these investigations are not available. It is important to emphasize that water deprivation test is not recommended to confirm the diagnosis and may by dangerous in the presence of elevated plasma osmolality (serum sodium >146 mEq/L or plasma osmolality >300 mOsm/l).

Etiology

As ADH producing neurons are distributed over a large area, acute central DI is indicative of diffuse CNS damage. Acute DI is most commonly encountered in the setting of sellar surgery in which classical tri-phasic response is observed[20]. In the initial phase, edema around the ADH secreting cells causes decreased release of ADH and polyuria. This is followed by release of ADH due to damage to ADH-secreting cells resulting in transient syndrome of inappropriate anti-diuretic hormone secretion (SIADH). This state is followed by either resolution of features or development of permanent DI if greater than 95% ADH secreting neurons have been damaged. Acute DI in the setting of diffuse CNS damage is an ominous sign and usually coincides with onset of brain death.

Management

Priority should be given to restoration of fluid status in acute DI. This is usually achieved by administration of isotonic fluids in a bolus of 20 ml/kg. This should be followed by intravenous vasopressin. Inhaled desmopressin should be avoided in acute central DI due to its variable onset and prolonged duration of action. Vasopressin infusion should be started in a dose of 1.5 mU/kg/hour and titrated according to urine output to a dose of 10 mU/kg/hour. It is important to emphasize that fluids should be restricted in a child on vasopressin (400 ml/m²/day plus urine output). Failure to restrict fluids in a child on vasopressin invariably leads to fluid overload. This approach is superior to the approach of replacing urine output with dextrose containing hypo-osmolar solutions. The latter approach requires meticulous monitoring, has the risk of producing dehydration and there is theoretical possibility of worsening polyuria by inducing hyperglycemia due to the use of dextrose containing fluids. The patient should be shifted to desmopressin as soon as consciousness is regained and oral feeding is started. Careful estimation of electrolytes is essential to identify the development of SIADH phase in these subjects.

HYPERTHYROID STORM

Hyperthyroidism is rare in children and non-specific features, however, mandate the need for early diagnosis and appropriate management.

Clinical Features

Thyroid hormones play an important role in regulation of intermediary metabolism, thermogenesis, and integrity of autonomic nervous system. Hyperthyroidism is associated with features of increased metabolism (hyperthermia and weight loss) on one hand and that of sympathetic excess (anxiety, tremors, hypertension, tachycardia, sweating and cardiac failure) on the other. Important features of neonatal hyperthyroidism include flushing, hyperthermia, decreased feeding, excessive irritability, tachycardia, cardiac failure and failure to thrive. Severe neonatal hyperthyroidism is associated with hepatosplenomegaly, jaundice and cardiac arrhythmia[21]. Beyond infancy hyperthyroidism is usually a chronic disease, acute presentations with hypertension, cardiac failure and arrhythmias are, however, well known.

Clinical Correlates

A child with hyperthyroidism can present to the emergency department with unexplained tachycardia, high output cardiac failure, refractory hypertension and hyperthermia (Table 40.8). Wide pulse pressure and increased temperature in a child with cardiac failure should suggest the possibility of hyperthyroidism. Thyroid enlargement, tremors and ocular signs of hyperthyroidism are strong indicators of hyperthyroidism. Hyperthyroidism should be considered in the differential diagnosis of all children with cardiac failure, pheochromocytoma, pyrexia of unknown origin and paroxysmal supra-ventricular tachycardia.

Table 40.8 Clinical correlates of hyperthyroidism
Neonatal period
☐ Anxious wide-eyed stare and alert look
☐ Excessive irritability, hyperthermia
☐ Intrauterine growth retardation
☐ Tachycardia, cardiac failure
☐ Maternal thyroid disorder
☐ Hepatosplenomegaly with thrombocytopenia· Prolonged jaundice
☐ Poor weight gain despite excessive appetite
Post-neonatal period
☐ Irritability, restlessness, altered mood, insomnia
☐ Cardiac failure with wide pulse pressure
☐ Hyperthermia, heat intolerance, warm moist skin and palmar erythema
☐ Unexplained hypertension with tachycardia
☐ Arrhythmia: Sinus tachycardia, atrial fibrillation
☐ Thyromegaly, proptosis and lid lag
☐ Weight loss with increased appetite and stool frequency

Etiology

Common causes of hyperthyroidism have been listed in Table 40.9. Transplacental passage of thyroid stimulating antibody is the commonest cause of neonatal hyperthyroidism. Features are usually present at birth; delayed presentation (after two weeks) has been reported due to concomitant transplacental passage of anti-thyroid medications and TSH receptor blocking antibodies. The disorder is self-limiting with normalization of thyroid functions by three months of age. Graves' disease due to thyroid stimulating antibody is the commonest cause of hyperthyroidism in older children and adolescents[22]. Release of preformed thyroid hormone in sub-acute thyroiditis is associated with hyperthyroidism.

Diagnosis

Clinical features provide important clues to the diagnosis in most cases. Neonatal hyperthyroidism is most commonly caused by transplacental passage of thyroid stimulating antibody; absence of thyroid disease in mother suggests the diagnosis of

Table 40.9 Etiology of hyperthyroidism
Infancy
• Transplacental passage of thyroid antibodies
• Autosomal dominant hyperthyroidism: TSH receptor activating mutation
After infancy
• Central hyperthyroidism: TSH secreting pituitary adenoma
• Graves disease
• Release of preformed thyroid hormone: Sub-acute thyroiditis
• Toxic thyroid nodule, toxic multinodular goiter
• Iatrogenic hyperthyroidism
• Pituitary resistance to T3

autosomal dominant hyperthyroidism. Diffuse non-tender enlargement of thyroid gland is characteristic of autoimmune thyroiditis while tender thyroid enlargement suggests sub-acute thyroiditis. Investigations should include TSH levels and thyroid scan. Low to undetectable TSH is suggestive of Graves disease, while subacute thyroiditis and toxic nodule with high or normal TSH is indicative of central hyperthyroidism. Diffuse increase in uptake on thyroid scan is diagnostic of Graves disease while decreased uptake is observed in sub-acute thyroiditis. Localized increase in thyroid uptake is suggestive of thyroid nodule[23].

Management

Initial management includes supportive care in the form of maintenance of airway, breathing and circulation. Antithyroid drugs are ineffective in the management of thyroid storm due to significant lag in their onset of action. Propylthiouracil (5 mg/kg/day) is superior to methimazole (0.5 mg/kg/day) due to the potential for decreased peripheral conversion of T4 to T3. Beta blockers (propanolol 2 mg/kg/day in two divided does) are effective in amelioration of sympathetic symptoms. Iodinated contrast (idopate 0.001 mg/kg/day) and Lugol's iodine (1 drop 8 hourly) are effective in reversal of features of hyperthyroidism. Prednisolone (1-2 mg/kg/day) inhibits peripheral conversion of T4 to T3 and is indicated in hyperthyroid storm. Cardiac failure refractory to these measures requires treatment with digitalis. Anti-thyroid drugs are ineffective in sub-acute thyroiditis; treatment with propanolol and analgesics is required.

Neonatal hyperthyroidism is treated with propranolol (1-2 mg/kg/day q 8 hr oral), propyl thiouracil (5-10 mg/kg/day q 8 hr oral) and Lugol solution (1 drop every 8 hr). Most cases remit by 3-4 months of age. Some cases of neonatal hyperthyroidism may persist throughout childhood due to mutation in the TSHR gene which leads to constitutive activation of the receptor. Delay in therapy may lead to advanced bone maturation, microcephaly and mental retardation.

REFERENCES

1. Bajpai A, Sharma J, Kabra M, Menon PSN. Approach to a child with hypocalcemia. *Asian J Pediatr Pract* 2001; 4:36-42.

2. Root AW. Disorders of bone mineral metabolism: Normal homeostasis. In: Pediatric Endocrinology. Sperling MA (Ed.). *Saunders Elsevier Philadelphia,* 3rd Edn. 2008, p. 74-126.

3. Gulati S, Bajpai A, Juneja R, Kabra M, Bagga A, Kalra V. Hypocalcemic heart failure masquerading as dilated cardiomyopathy. *Indian J Pediatr* 2001; 68:287-290.

4. Sharma J, Bajpai A, Kabra M, Menon PSN. Hypocalcemia—Clinical, biochemical, radiological profile and follow-up in a tertiary hospital in India. *Indian Pediatr* 2002; 39:276-282.

5. Colleti RB, Pan MW, Smith EWP, Genel M. Detection of hypocalcemia in susceptible neonates: The QoTc interval. *N Engl J Med* 1974; 25:931-935.

6. Root AW, Diamond AW. Disorders of mineral homeostasis in the newborn, infant, child and adolescent. In: Pediatric Endocrinology. Sperling MA (Ed.). *Saunders Elsevier Philadelphia,* 3rd Edn. 2008, p. 686-769.

7. Ip P. Neonatal convulsion revealing maternal hyperparathyroidism: an unusual case of late neonatal hypoparathyroidism. *Arch Gynecol Obstet* 2003; 268:227-229.

8. Mehrotra P, Marwaha RK, Aneja S, Seth A, Singla BM, Ashraf G, Sharma B, Sastry A, Tandon N. Hypovitaminosis D and hypocalcemic seizures in infancy. *Indian Pediatr* 2010 7; 47: 581-6.

9. Bajpai A, Sharma J, Menon PSN (Ed.). Hypocalcemia. In: Practical Pediatric Endocrinology. 1st Edn. *Jaypee Delhi,* 2003, p. 37-42.

10. Bajpai A, Sharma J, Menon PS (Ed.). Hypercalcemia. In: Practical Pediatric Endocrinology. 1st Edn. *Jaypee, New Delhi,* 2003, p. 43-46.

11. Leon DD, Stanley CA, Sperling MA. Hypoglycemia in neonates and infants. In: Pediatric Endocrinology. Sperling MA. (Ed.). *Saunders Elsevier Philadelphia,* 3rd Edn, 2008, p. 165-197.

12. Langdon DR, Stanley CA, Sperling MA. Hypoglycemia in the infant and child. In: Pediatric Endocrinology. Sperling MA (Ed.). *Saunders Elsevier, Philadelphia,* 3rd Edn, 2008, p. 422-443.

13. Bajpai A, Sharma J, Menon PSN (Ed.). Hypoglycemia. In: Practical Pediatric Endocrinology. *Jaypee,* 1st Edn. *New Delhi* 2003, p. 61-67.

14. Narayan S, Aggarwal R, Deorari AK, Paul VK. Hypoglycemia in the newborn. *Indian J Pediatr* 2001; 68:963-966.

15. Miller WL, Achermann JC, Fluck CE. The adrenal cortex and its disorders. In: Pediatric Endocrinology. Sperling MA (Ed.). *Saunders Elsevier Philadelphia,* 3rd Ed, 2008, p. 444-511.

16. Bajpai A, Kabra M, Menon PSN. 21-hydroxylase deficiency: clinical features, laboratory profile and pointers to diagnosis in Indian children. *Indian Pediatr* 2004; 41:1226-1232.

17. Sharma J, Bajpai A, Kabra M. Congenital adrenal hyperplasia presenting as hematuria and acute renal failure. *Indian J Pediatr* 2001; 68:1161-1162.

18. Bajpai A, Sharma J, Menon PSN (Ed.). Adrenal insufficiency. Practical Pediatric Endocrinology. 1st Edn. *Jaypee, Delhi,* 2003, p. 75-78.

19. Muglia LJ. Majzoub JA. Disorders of the posterior pituitary. In: Pediatric Endocrinology. Sperling MA. (Ed.). *Saunders Elsevier Philadelphia,* 3rd Ed., 2008, p. 335-373.

20. Ranadive SA, Rosenthal SM. Pediatric disorders of water balance. *Endocrinol Metab Clin North Am* 2009; 38:663-72.

21. Fisher DA, Grueters A. Disorders of the thyroid in the newborn and infant. In: Pediatric Endocrinology. Sperling MA. (Ed.). *Saunders Elsevier Philadelphia,* 3rd Ed., 2008, p. 198-226.

22. Fisher DA, Grueters A. Thyroid disorders in childhood and adolescence. In: Pediatric Endocrinology. Sperling MA. (Ed.). *Saunders Elsevier Philadelphia,* 3rd Ed, 2008, p. 227-253.

23. Bajpai A, Sharma J, Menon PSN (Ed.). Hyperthyroidism. In: Practical Pediatric Endocrinology. *Jaypee, New Delhi,* 1st Edn. 2003 p. 30-32.

41

Diabetic Ketoacidosis

Anju Virmani

In children with diabetes, diabetic ketoacidosis (DKA) is the most common cause for hospital admission and for death[1]. It is a state of severe metabolic decompensation due to low insulin and high counter-regulatory hormone levels. It is characterized by hyperglycemia, ketonemia and acidosis, which occurs mainly in type 1 diabetes mellitus (T1DM), but can also occur in type 2 diabetes mellitus (T2DM). It is the initial presentation in 20-40% children with T1DM, therefore it should always be considered in the differential diagnosis of any child with coma of acute onset. It also occurs in children known to be diabetic due to deliberate or inadvertent omission of insulin, inadequate doses during a period of illness, interruption of insulin supply in a user of insulin pump, or if insulin gets denatured (e.g. by exposure to high temperatures, say by leaving in a car during summer). The mortality rate varies from 2% in experienced centers, to as high as 24% elsewhere, and has not significantly decreased with advances in management[2]. The prognosis is worse in younger children and in the presence of coma and hypotension. Most deaths are caused by the development of cerebral edema, a poorly understood condition which occurs in 0.3-1% episodes of DKA[3].

DEFINITION

The terms diabetic ketoacidosis, ketosis, and diabetic precoma and coma are used synonymously to describe a state of acute metabolic decompensation comprising of hyperglycemia (blood glucose >11 mMol/l i.e. 200 mg/dl), ketonemia and acidosis (venous pH <7.3 and/or bicarbonate <15 mMol/l or 15 mEq/L). On the basis of the severity of acidosis, DKA is divided into mild (venous pH <7.30, bicarbonate concentration <15 mMol/l), moderate (pH <7.2, bicarbonate <10 mMol/l), or severe (pH <7.1, bicarbonate <5 mMol/l).

There is associated glycosuria, ketonuria, and ketonemia[3]. Rarely, young, partially treated or malnourished children as well as pregnant adolescents may present with near normal glucose values ("euglycemic ketoacidosis")[4]. Conversely, also in this group, ketosis with near normal blood glucose may be due to starvation ketosis. Another variant is coma with mild ketosis but marked hyperglycemia (also referred to as "nonketotic hyperosmolar coma") which may occur in very young children, especially those with brain disorders affecting thirst, and older adolescents with new-onset T2DM.

INCIDENCE

DKA as the first manifestation

Although with increased awareness, frequency of DKA as the first manifestation of T1DM has come down in many regions, it remains 15-67% in Europe and North America[5-7]. The frequency is much higher in regions where T1DM occurs less often; in developing countries and in remote areas; in families with lower socioeconomic status; and in children <4 years of age[8]. High dose glucocorticoids, atypical antipsychotics, diazoxide, and some immunosuppressive drugs may precipitate DKA in predisposed children.

In a known T1DM

In children who are known to have T1DM, the risk of DKA is 1–10% per patient per year. The major precipitating factors include infections and intercurrent illnesses (30-35%), and omission of insulin dose (15-20%) or inappropriate interruption of insulin pump therapy. The most common predisposing infections are pneumonia (40-60%) and urinary tract infections (15%). Other factors include trauma, corticosteroid therapy and pancreatitis. The risk is higher in children with poor metabolic control, previous episodes of DKA, psychiatric disorders (including eating disorders), peripuberty (especially girls), and difficult family circumstances, including lower socioeconomic status and lack of appropriate health facilities.

DIAGNOSIS

In developed countries, most episodes of DKA occur in known T1DM. However, in developing countries, DKA may be the initial presentation (68% in one series), therefore, the diagnosis should be considered in all children who present in coma[9]. Even in new onset patients, a history of progres-sive polyuria and polydipsia, enuresis, and weight loss, is often available. This may be associated with malaise, lethargy, nausea, vomiting, abdominal pain, fruity odor of breath and hyperventilation (Kussmaul's breathing). *In a child with DKA, the severity of dehydration is out of proportion to the severity of vomiting because of the continued fluid losses due to osmotic diuresis.* However, at times it is difficult to distinguish the clinical signs and symptoms of ketosis from the precipitating factors. An acute gastrointestinal infection pre-senting with vomiting and diarrhea may precipitate and merge imperceptibly with the features of DKA. Occasionally, the vomiting and abdominal pain caused by ketosis may be mistaken for a GI infection or for an acute abdomen. Therefore, in all critically sick children blood glucose should be tested by using test-strips.

Physical examination shows moderate to severe dehydration ranging between 5-10% body weight loss. Despite depletion of body water, blood pressure and urine output continue to be maintained till very late stages; DKA should be suspected if dehydration is seen with reasonable urine output. Thus, there is poor correlation between clinical assessment and actual dehydration[10, 11]. The mental status varies from normal to deep coma (10% of cases) although some degree of confusion is present in most cases. Table 41.1 summarizes the salient symptoms and signs of DKA.

DIFFERENTIAL DIAGNOSIS

A child known to have T1DM and presenting with coma or drowsiness should be evaluated for hypoglycemia. There is likely to be a history of excessive insulin or exercise and/ or a missed meal, other symptoms of hypoglycemia, normal respiration, and absence of dehydration.

Table 41.1 Clinical features of DKA	
Symptoms	**Signs**
• Polyuria, nocturia	• Dehydration, low skin turgor
• Polydipsia	• Fruity odor of breath
• Weight loss	• Hypotension
• Weakness	• Tachycardia
• Visual disturbances	• Hyperventilation (Kussmaul's breathing)
• Abdominal pain	• Hypothermia
• Confusion	• Abdominal distension/rigidity
• Drowsiness	• Pneumothorax/ pneumomediastinum
• Coma	

DKA also needs to be differentiated from pre-cipitating factors (e.g. gastroenteritis, appendicitis, pancreatitis, UTI) as well as coma due to other causes (e.g. CNS infections, encephalopathy, drug overdosage, uremia, trauma, seizures, or syncope). Other possibilities include non-ketotic hyperosmolar coma, poisoning (particularly due to aspirin), and inborn errors of metabolism. Occasionally, abdominal distension and tenderness suggest the diagnosis of acute abdomen. Treat-ment of DKA generally corrects the vomiting and pain. If DKA is missed and the child is subjected to laparotomy, the consequences may be disastrous.

Hyperglycemic hyperosmolar nonketotic coma, which is very rare in children, is chara-cterized by the absence of ketonuria and ketonemia, even though the blood sugars are very high (usually 750 mg/dl and above). There is severe dehydration and depressed sensorium, frank coma, various neuro-logical signs and seizures. The serum osmolality is >350 mOsm/kg. It may be due to drug therapy (high doses of glucocortocoids or diazoxide). Plasma osmolality (not the severity of acidosis) is the main determinant of severity and outcome; it can be measured directly by an osmometer or calculated by the formula:

$$\text{Plasma osmolality} = 2 \, (Na^+ + K^+ \, mEq/l) + \frac{\text{Glucose mg/dl}}{18} + \frac{\text{BUN mg/dl}}{2.8}$$

In calculating effective osmolality, urea is excluded as it is freely permeable across the cell membrane.

$$\text{Effective osmolality} = 2\,(Na^+ + K^+\ mEq/L) +$$

$$\frac{\text{Glucose mg/dl}}{18}$$

INVESTIGATIONS

Rapid confirmation of diagnosis and commencement of therapy is essential in reducing morbidity and mortality in DKA. An IV line should be put in immediately, and samples obtained for essential investigations, including the following:

1. Blood glucose, urine glucose and ketones can be tested at the bedside with test strips, which should be available in all emergency areas.

2. Blood samples for glucose, urea, creatinine, electrolytes, hemogram, blood gases, blood culture and antibiotic sensitivity.

3. Urine for ketones, sugar, microsopy (pus cells, bacteria), culture and antibacterial sensitivity.

4. Arterial blood gases.

5. Fundus examination for evidences of raised intracranial tension.

6. ECG for evidence of hypo- or hyperkalemia and cardiac status.

7. X-ray chest to rule out infection.

8. CSF examination if the patient is unconscious, to rule out associated meningoencephalitis, after excluding raised intracranial tension.

Pitfalls in the Diagnosis

The precipitating illness may merge imperceptibly with DKA and should always be carefully evaluated. Moderate leukocytosis (10-15,000/mm^3) caused by the stress is common, and may not indicate infection. However, severe leukocytosis (>25,000/mm^3) is suggestive of infection. Fever may be absent because of the peripheral vasodilatation which causes cooling, so its absence does not rule out infection. Falsely low values of sodium and spuriously high values of potassium, urea, creatinine and amylase may be obtained. The elevated amylase is usually of salivary origin. Elevation of pancreatic enzymes particularly hyperlipasemia, is common but usually not associated with significant symptomatology, and should not be assumed to signify pancreatitis[12]. Urine ketones may be present in only trace amounts, or may even be negative in the presence of severe lactoacidosis but this should not give a false sense of security. After treatment, an apparent rise in ketones should not be confused with worsening of the clinical condition. However, newer sensitive strips for measurement of beta-hydroxybutyric acid (BHBA) are now available for monitoring.

Morbidity and Mortality

In national population based studies from USA[13], Canada[14, 15] and UK[16], mortality rates from DKA are constant at about 0.15%. In areas with poor medical facilities, mortality rates are higher and children may die before definitive diagnosis[17]. For example, the Chandigarh hospital based series reported a mortality rate of 13.2%, serum osmolality being the most important predictor of death[9]. Death is due to cerebral edema in 21-25% cases[15, 16]. Significant neurological sequelae are seen in 10-26% of survivors.

Apart from cerebral edema, mortality and morbidity may be due to hypokalemia, hyperkalemia, hypoglycemia, other CNS complications like hematoma, thrombosis, sepsis, and infections (including rhinocerebral mucormycosis), aspiration pneumonia, pulmonary edema, adult respiratory distress syndrome (ARDS), pneumomediastinum and subcutaneous emphysema, and rhabdomyolysis. Late sequelae are due to cerebral edema and other CNS complications, and these include hypothalamopituitary insufficiency, isolated growth hormone deficiency, and combined GH and TSH deficiency.

PATHOPHYSIOLOGY

DKA develops only if a state of severe insulin deficiency co-exists with exces-sive levels of glucose, counter-regulatory hormones (glucagon, cortisol, catecholamines, and growth hormone). This combination leads to increased hepatic and renal glucose production and impaired glucose utilization in peripheral tissues, which result in hyperglycemia and parallel changes in osmolality of the extracellular space. The hyperglycemia results in glycosuria, and thus osmotic diuresis, with loss of water, sodium, potassium, and other electrolytes. There is also release of free fatty acids into the circulation from adipose tissue (lipolysis) and unrestrained hepatic fatty acid oxidation to ketone bodies (β-hydroxybutyrate [β-OHB] and acetoacetate), with resulting ketonemia and metabolic acidosis. The pH may be further lowered by presence of lactic acidosis due to tissue hypoperfusion (Figure 41.1).

Section 4

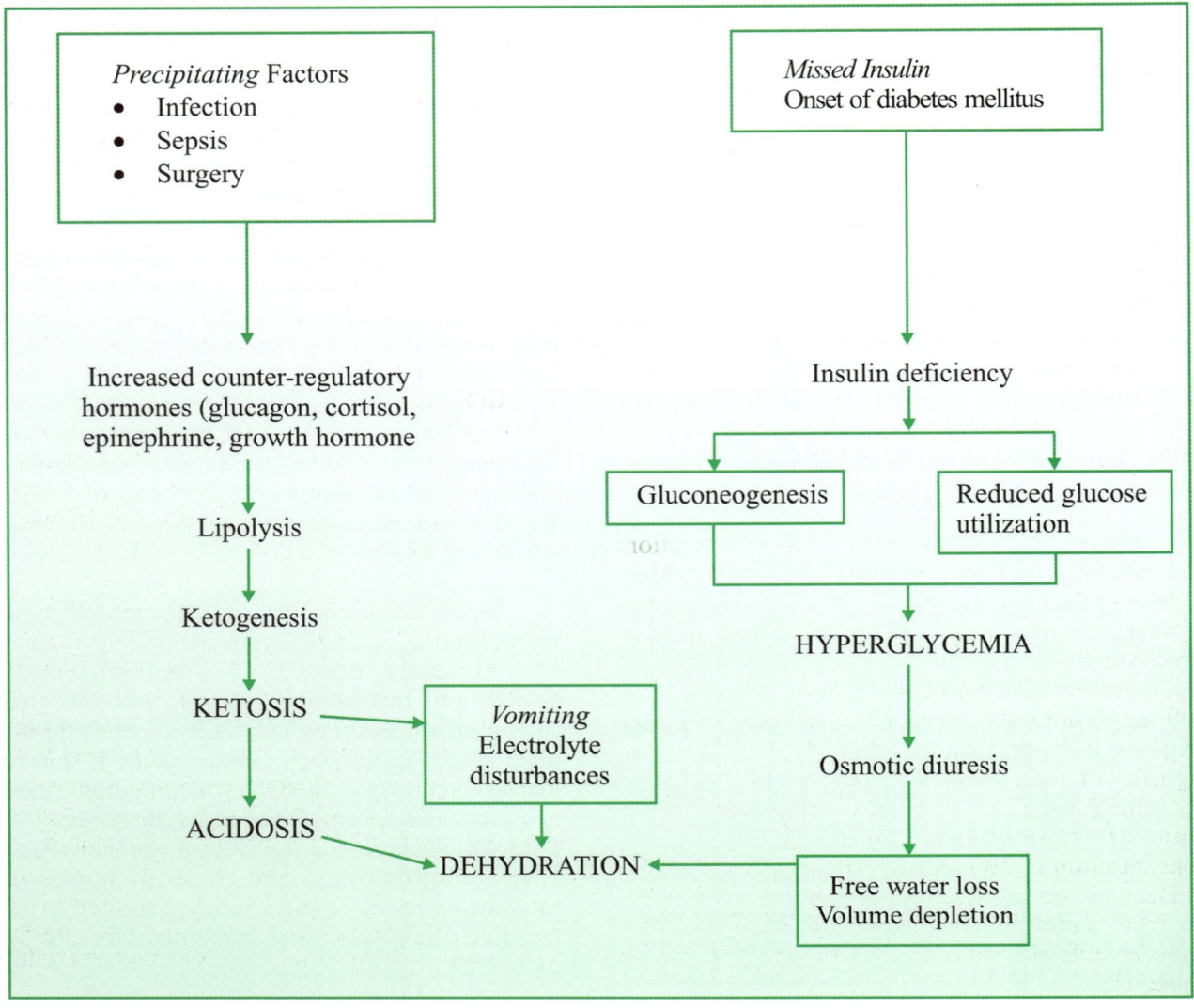

Figure 41.1 Pathophysiology of diabetic ketoacidosis

Role of insulin. Insulin secretion is exquisitely fine tuned to handle metabolic demands and maintain normal physiology. Episodic spikes of insulin release in response to food intake are superimposed on a steady basal rate of insulin secretion. Insulin stimulates anabolic processes in the liver, muscle and adipose tissue to permit glucose utilization and storage of energy from ingested food as glycogen, protein and fat. These actions are mediated by glucose transporters (GLUT), a family of proteins spanning the plasma membrane. GLUT-2, present on the liver cells, is up-regulated by glucose and down-regulated by insulin. In the absence of insulin, it transports excessive glucose out of the cell causing hyperglycemia. GLUT-4, on the skeletal muscle, is inactive in the absence of insulin, reducing peripheral utilization of glucose. The deficiency of insulin leads to glycogenolysis

(to supply glucose, which is the sole energy source for the brain); and lipolysis (to supply free fatty acids and ketone bodies, which are utilized by the cardiac and skeletal muscles). The paradox underlying DKA is the glucose lack at the cellular level, despite high blood glucose levels.

Role of counter-regulatory hormones. These hormones affect catabolic processes directly and also by inhibiting the action of insulin. Glucagon plays a key role in the pathogenesis of DKA. A decrease in the insulin to glucagon ratio tilts the balance of metabolism in favor of gluconeogenesis, glycogenolysis and lipolysis. Epinephrine inhibits insulin release and peripheral uptake of glucose. It also stimulates glycogenolysis, gluconeogenesis and lipolysis. Cortisol decreases peripheral uptake of glucose and plays a facilitatory role in the lipolytic action of epinephrine. Growth hormone reduces insulin secretion and antagonizes peripheral glucose uptake. The counter-regulatory hormone excess, however, cannot produce DKA without the presence of relative or absolute insulin deficiency.

Renal functions. Normally all the glucose filtered through the glomeruli is reab-sorbed by the proximal tubules. When hyperglycemia exceeds the renal threshold for glucose reabsorption, glycosuria, and therefore osmotic diuresis and dehydration occurs. As the increased glucose cannot be transported into the cells in the absence of insulin, an osmotic gradient between the extracellular and intracellular fluids develops. This masks the clinical sever-ity of dehydration by minimizing the hemodynamic consequences.

The dehydration results in volume contraction and reduced glomerular filtration rate (GFR), which reduces glucose clearance, thus augmenting hyperglycemia. Before this state is reached, glycosuria would limit the hyperglycemia to moderate levels. Thus a blood glucose of more than 600 mg/dl not only denotes severe DKA, but also implies dehydration in excess of 10% with significant reduction of renal function. It also accounts for the fact that fluid replacement alone, without insulin therapy, can lower the glucose concentration to 300 mg/dl. The osmotic diuresis of DKA causes passive loss of electrolytes as well as free water. The losses and maintenance requirements of fluids and electrolytes are given in Table 41.2.

Table 41.2 Fluid and electrolyte losses in DKA		
Components	**Losses (mean and range)**	**Maintenance requirements (per day)**
Water	85 ml/kg (60-100)	1500 ml/m^2
Sodium	6 mEq/kg (5-13)	45 mEq/m^2 (3 mEq/kg)
Potassium	5 mEq/kg (4-16)	35 mEq/m^2 (2 mEq/kg)
Chloride	4 mEq/kg (3-9)	30 mEq/m^2 (2 mEq/kg)
Phosphate	3 mEq/kg (2-5)	10 mEq/m^2 (0.7 mEq/kg)

Dehydration. Dehydration is caused by osmotic diuresis, and worsened by rapid deep breathing due to acidosis. Depending on the severity and length of the illness, fluid losses range from 70-150 ml/kg (7-15% of body weight). However, because of the shift of water from the intracellular fluid compartment (ICF) to the extracellular fluid compartment (ECF), shock with hemodynamic compromise is rare. Volume contraction leads to decreased tissue perfusion and lactic acidosis, which may account for about 25% of the acidemia. Rehydration alone reduces blood glucose significantly by improving glomerular filtration and thus clearance of glucose and ketones.

Sodium. About 20% body sodium is lost by osmotic diuresis. Loss of free water exceeds sodium loss, but the serum sodium concentra-tion is not raised because the high serum osmolality and hyperglycemia draw water out from the cells to the extracellular fluid. Each 100 mg/dl elevation of blood glucose lowers the serum sodium by 1.6 mEq/kg. The corrected sodium can be estimated as measured Na$^+$ (glucose in mMol/l − 5.6)/2. The associated hypertriglyceridemia also causes a spurious depression of serum sodium.

Potassium. Excessive loss of potassium (20% body potassium) is due to osmotic diuresis and increased aldosterone activity stimulated by dehydration. Additional losses of potassium may occur due to vomiting. In the early phase of DKA, however, normokalemia or hyperkalemia is the rule due to the intra-to-extravascular shift of potassium as well as the decreased GFR. The mechanisms involved in this apparent elevation of serum K$^+$ are given below:

1. K$^+$ is dragged out of the cells by water moving from the intracel-lular fluid to the extracellular fluid.
2. K$^+$ moves out of cells in exchange with H$^+$ ion.
3. K$^+$ moves out with phosphate to maintain electroneutrality of the cells.
4. K$^+$ leaks from the muscle cells due to glycogen deposition and protein breakdown.

Rehydration invariably leads to hypokalemia. This is due to the dilution of serum K$^+$, improved GFR accelerating renal losses, correction of acidosis, and treatment with insulin leading to the return of K$^+$ into the cells. Cardiac arrhythmias are a major complication seen in association with changes in K$^+$ homeostasis. A delay in potassium therapy during the first 1-2 hours of rehydration may be acceptable, but subsequent replacement should not be deferred even if the serum K$^+$ level is normal or slightly elevated.

Phosphate. The pattern of phosphate concentration closely follows that of potassium.

Phosphate depletion and inhibition of red blood cell oxidative metabolism leads to a decrease in 2, 3-diphosphoglycerate (2, 3 DPG) concentration in the red blood cells. The shift to the left of the oxygen dissociation curve caused by decrease in the 2, 3 DPG is counteracted by the acidosis, which promotes oxygen release from the hemoglobin (Bohr effect). It may lead to muscle weakness, rhabdomyolysis, decreased cardiac contractions and respiratory muscle weakness. Children with DKA repair their 2, 3 DPG level rapidly even without phosphate supplementation, unlike their adult counterparts.[26] Thus, while phosphate supplementation prevents or corrects hypophosphatemia, its need and overall efficacy are not conclusively demonstrated.

Bicarbonate. Although the serum bicarbonate is low, little or no bicarbonate deficit is created as lactic acid and ketoacids are metabolized to bicarbonate in the liver and peripheral tissues during insulin therapy.

Creatinine. Renal dysfunction and increased protein catabolism increase serum BUN and creatinine. The common laboratory method for estimating creatinine also detects acetoacetate, leading to a spurious elevation of serum creatinine.

Anion gap. Anion gap is calculated by the formula: $[Na^+ + K^+] - [Cl^- + HCO_3^-]$. The normal anion gap is 8-12 mEq/l. It is elevated in DKA, lactic acidosis and renal failure. Patients with DKA show varying degrees of hyperchloremic acidosis with pure anion gap or mixed anion gap.

Evaluation of pure metabolic acidosis is calculated by the following formula because there is a predictable relationship between bicarbonate and pCO_2:

$$pCO_2 = 1.5 \times [HCO_3^-] + 8 \pm 2$$

If pCO_2 is less than predicted, the patient has superimposed respiratory alkalosis. Respiratory alkalosis without hypoxemia indicates sepsis, and with hypoxemia suggests pneumonia or adult respiratory distress syndrome (ARDS).

Consequences of Ketoacidosis

Beta-hydroxybutyric acid (BHBA) and acetoacetic acid (AAA) are strong organic acids. Acetone is not a ketoacid. In states of severe dehydration and acidosis, urinary ketones may be less than expected for the degree of ketosis because the AAA to BHBA relationship (reflecting the redox state) is altered in favor of BHBA. The semi-quantitative nitroprusside reaction detects only acetone and AAA, whereas BHBA is the major ketone body in blood and urine (8:1). The ketoacids are completely dissociated at physiological pH and are buffered by bicarbonate. With therapy, AAA and acetone levels increase and this should not be interpreted as worsening of DKA. Profound metabolic acidosis adversely affects functioning of several organs, including the heart. Cardiac function is reduced because of depression of the vasomo-tor center, reduced arterial smooth muscle tone as well as myocardial contractility. Hyperventilation and Kussmaul breathing lead to hypocapnia, which in turn causes cerebral vasoconstriction and reduced cerebral blood flow. Increased prostaglandin synthesis in adipose tissues resulting from insulin deficiency can cause abdominal distension and tenderness, as well as tachycardia and flushed facies. Metabolic acidosis and potassium depletion can result in paralytic ileus.

Cerebral Edema

Cerebral edema (CE) is a dreaded complication of DKA which is associated with a high rate of mortality and neurologic sequelae. It is mainly a pediatric problem, occurring rarely in patients over the age 20 years. Cerebral edema occurs before treatment of DKA is started or later during the course of treatment. The commonest time of onset of cerebral edema is 4–12 hours after start of therapy, when the child appears to be improving. It is more likely to occur in children at onset of T1DM, age <5 years, longer duration of symptoms, marked neurologic depression at admission, severe acidosis, raised blood urea nitrogen, and in those given rapid fluids or high doses of insulin (causing rapid fall in blood glucose levels)[18]. It should be especially looked for in children who have low serum sodium at onset, or a rapid fall in plasma osmolality or serum sodium level. Symptoms and signs include headache, lethargy, irritability, vomiting, gradually deteriorating level of consciousness, convulsions, hypo- or hyperthermia, inappropriate slowing of the pulse rate, increase in blood pressure, and hyperpyrexia. Careful and repeated assessment of these vital signs is important, as reliance cannot be placed solely on the Glasgow coma scale. Moreover, abnormal neurological signs and symptoms are common in children with DKA and do not always demand specific treatment, so careful judgment is required[19].

Mechanisms underlying the development of cerebral edema are not completely understood. The age dependence may point to developmental changes in cerebral metabolism which may be critical in the pathogenesis of CE[19]. The proposed mechanisms include cerebral ischemia/ hypoxia causing generation of inflammatory mediators; increased cerebral blood flow; disruption of cell membrane ion transport; aquaporin channels; generation of intracellular organic osmolytes (myoinositol, taurine) and subsequent cellular osmotic imbalance[20]. Thus, CE may be due to rapid correction of dehydration and hyperosmolality, excessive insulin dose, alkali therapy, or hypoxia. CT or MRI imaging studies in children with DKA show that some degree of cerebral edema may be present even in patients without clinical evidences of raised intracranial pressure. Some researchers suggest that the treatment of DKA may be causally related to the development of CE, while others dispute this[21, 22].

Prevention of cerebral edema is best achieved by using isotonic sodium solutions for correction of hypovolemia; giving replacement fluids slowly; correcting acidemia and hyperglycemia gradually but steadily; and monitoring serum sodium[23].

MANAGEMENT OF DKA

Children with ketosis and hyperglycemia without vomiting or severe dehydration can be managed in the pediatric ward, under the supervision of a pediatric diabetologist. There must be experienced nursing staff trained in monitoring and management; clear written guidelines; and laboratory access for frequent evaluation of biochemical variables. If the family is educated, willing to come for review daily, and can access the diabetes team at any time, the child may even be managed at home.

Children with severe DKA (long duration of symptoms, dehydration, compromised circulation, or altered sensorium) or high risk of development of cerebral edema (age <5 years, new onset T1DM) should be admitted immediately in a pediatric intensive care unit and managed by an experienced diabetes team.

The management of DKA is divided into 3 phases:

(a)   Management of the acute emergency phase;

(b)   Management of the transition from DKA to hyperglycemia and then euglycemia; and

(c)   Guidelines for follow-up, including search for cause of DKA, and prevention of recurrence.

(a)   Treatment during the emergency phase

The following guidelines should be followed:

1.   ABC of resuscitation i.e. maintenance of airways, breathing and circulation.

2.   Expansion of intravascular volume.

3.   Correction of fluid and electrolyte abnormalities.

4.   Provision of adequate insulin to prevent ketosis and reduce hyperglycemia.

5.   Correction of metabolic acidosis only if cardiac depression due to severe acidosis.

6.   Prevention and monitoring of complications (including hypoglycemia, aspiration, congestive cardiac failure, cerebral edema, ARDS, electrolyte imbalance, associated infections including septicemia and fungemia, and renal failure).

Monitoring

Monitoring of the following parameters should be done and documented (Table 41.3):

(i)   Hourly heart rate, respiratory rate, blood pressure.

(ii)   Hourly (or even more frequent) fluid input and output (consider urinary catheterization only if consciousness is impaired).

(iii)   Hourly capillary blood glucose (cross checked against laboratory venous glucose as capillary methods may be inaccurate if the child has poor peripheral circulation and/ or acidosis).

(iv)   Baseline ECG monitoring to assess T-waves for evidence of hyperkalemia/ hypokalemia, and serum electrolytes in severe DKA.

(v)   Neurological observations for warning signs and symptoms of cerebral edema (more frequently than hourly if severe) as listed below:

   •   Headache

   •   Persistence of vomiting

   •   Change in neurological status (restlessness, irritability, increased drowsiness, incontinence)

Table 41.3 Diabetic monitoring sheet													
Hours after admission	0	1	2	3	4	5	6	7	8	8½	9	9½	10
Blood glucose strip test	✓	✓	✓	✓	✓	✓	✓	✓	✓	✓	✓	✓	✓
Lab blood glucose	✓		✓		✓		✓		✓				✓
Ketones	✓		✓				✓		✓				✓
Na/K	✓		✓				✓				✓		
Ca/PO4	✓		✓				✓				✓		
ABG	✓		✓				✓				✓		
BUN	✓		✓				✓				✓		
Creatinine	✓		✓				✓				✓		
Urine glucose	✓		✓				✓		✓				
Urine ketones	✓		✓				✓		✓				
Insulin u/kg													
Fluids IN	✓		✓		✓		✓						
Fluids OUT	✓		✓		✓		✓						
BP	✓	✓	✓	✓	✓	✓	✓	✓	✓	✓	✓	✓	✓
HR	✓	✓	✓	✓	✓	✓	✓	✓	✓	✓	✓	✓	✓
RR	✓	✓	✓	✓	✓	✓	✓	✓	✓	✓	✓	✓	✓
ECG	✓		✓				✓						
General status	✓	✓	✓	✓	✓	✓	✓	✓	✓	✓	✓	✓	✓

✓ Tests are to be done

- Slowing of pulse rate
- Rising blood pressure
- Specific neurological signs (for example cranial nerve palsies, pupillary response)
- Decreased oxygen saturation.

(vi) The following laboratory tests should be repeated 2–4 hourly: Electrolytes, urea, hematocrit, blood glucose, and blood gases. If DKA is severe, electrolytes and blood glucose should be tested hourly.

The initial resuscitation therapy for DKA is summarized in Table 41.4.

Dehydration

The objectives of fluid and sodium replacement are listed below:

(i) Restoration of circulating volume,

(ii) Replacement of sodium and the ECF and ICF deficit of water,

(iii) Restoration of GFR with enhanced clearance of glucose and ketones from the blood, and

(iv) Prevention of cerebral edema.

Dehydration is usually less than 10%. Because of the intra- to extra-vascular shift of water, shock is rare, and serum sodium is unreliable in trying to assess the degree of ECF contraction. Raised blood urea nitrogen and hematocrit is more useful marker of severe ECF contraction. Intravenous fluid administration causes a sharp fall in blood glucose, but it also causes a rise in intracranial pressure (ICP), especially when hypotonic fluids are used. Slow fluid deficit correction with isotonic or near-isotonic solutions results in earlier reversal of acidosis, and reduces the risk of cerebral edema, but may be associated

Table 41.4 Initial resuscitation therapy for DKA

Goal	Time	Approach
1. ABC of resuscitation	First few minutes	• Intubate if comatose • Breathing • Circulation: establish venous access
2. Establish the diagnosis	First few minutes	• Brief history • Sampling
3. Volume repletion	First few minutes	• In shock: 20 ml/kg normal saline bolus • Otherwise as per 8-10% deficit
4. Lowering hyperglycemia, correcting ketosis	After step 3 is achieved	• Start IV insulin therapy 0.1 u/kg/hour
5. Fine-tuning of biochemistry	After step 4	• Change to 0.45% saline, add potassium, adjust according to reports
6. Prevent hypoglycemia	When blood sugar <300 mg/dl	• Add 5% dextrose to infusate

with the development of hyperchloremic metabolic acidosis. Therefore the fluid deficit is replaced over 36-48 hours:

- 20% as normal saline or Ringer's lactate during the first hour
- 40% as N/2 saline during the next 10-12 hours
- Remaining 40% over the next 24 hours.

Maintenance fluids are added in an ongoing manner, with fluid balance and therapy recalculated every 2-4 hours depending on the clinical condition of the child. The guidelines for administration of fluids, electrolytes and insulin are summarized in Table 41.5.

Insulin

Rehydration alone reduces hyperglycemia, but insulin is essential to normalize blood glucose and suppress lipolysis and ketogenesis. The "low dose" intravenous insulin regimen is standard therapy, though subcutaneous and intramuscular routes have been used in the past. Insulin is started after the initial 1-2 hours of fluid expansion intravenously at a dose of 0.1 unit/kg/hour. This achieves steady state plasma insulin levels within an hour, and effectively offsets insulin resistance, inhibits lipolysis and ketogenesis; suppresses glucose production and stimulates peripheral glucose utilization. A lower dose of 0.05 unit/kg/hour may be advisable in

Table 41.5 Fluids, electrolytes and insulin therapy for DKA

Duration	Fluids	Na+	K+	Cl-	PO$_4$	Insulin
Hour 1	20 ml/kg normal saline	4 mEq	-	4 mEq/kg	-	-
Hour 2	Repeat normal saline bolus if in shock	4 mEq	-	4 mEq/kg	-	-
Hours 2-12	30-40% of calculated deficit (i.e. 30-40 ml/kg) of N/2 saline + Maintenance (N/5 saline) + Losses (N/2 saline)	2 mEq/kg	4 mEq/dl	2 mEq/kg	2 mEq/kg	0.1 unit/kg/hr
When blood sugar is <300 mg/dl	5% dextrose in N/2 saline	"	"	"	"	Decrease insulin to 0.05 unit/kg/hr
Next 24 hours	5% dextrose in N/4 saline	1 mEq/kg	4 mEq/dl	1 mEq/kg		Subcutaneous insulin

children <4 years of age. This regimen produces a predictable and slow fall of serum glucose, with lower risk of hypoglycemia or hypokalemia. The aim of insulin therapy in the first 24 hours is reduction of hyperglycemia (to levels of 200-300 mg/dl), and not achievement of euglycemia. When blood glucose falls to 300 mg/dl, 5% dextrose is added to the saline infusion; and when blood glucose falls below 250 mg/dl, the glucose infusion concentration is increased to 10% instead of decreasing insulin infusion rate[24].

Acidosis and ketonemia get corrected more slowly than hyperglycemia. Once acidosis is controlled, and the child is accepting orally, subcutaneous insulin can be started. However, intravenous infusion of insulin should be continued for 30 minutes after the first administration of subcutaneous insulin, giving it enough time to get absorbed and start acting. Subcutaneous insulin regimens cannot be covered in this chapter, but briefly consist of boluses of rapid acting (lispro, aspart) or regular insulin before each meal, and long acting (glargine, levemir) insulin once or twice a day to cover basal needs. NPH insulin can be used to provide basal needs, but its action is very variable, resulting in frequent hypo- and hyperglycemia[25]. The total daily dose of insulin is usually 0.7-1.0 unit/kg, but soon after the DKA episode, higher doses may be needed for a few days. Regular insulin must be given 20-40 minutes before the meal; rapid acting insulin can be given 5-10 minutes earlier. In very small children (e.g. those < 4 years), it may even be given immediately after intake of food so that the quantity of food eaten is known.

Potassium

Potassium shifts from the ICF to the ECF compartment. At presentation serum potassium may be normal, increased (due to reduced renal function) or decreased (prolonged duration of disease). With insulin therapy and correction of acidosis, the potassium is driven back into the cells, causing marked hypokalemia. It is, therefore, important to replace potassium at the rate of 40 mEq/l, once the child has passed urine (should not be given in the presence of renal failure or anuria). If potassium is low even at presentation, it should be given with the initial fluids at the rate of 20 mEq/l, before insulin is started.

Sodium

Hyponatremia (if not artifactual) may be a sign of inappropriate secretion of ADH and a warning for potential CNS complications. If serum sodium levels do not rise slowly in parallel with decrease in blood glucose and lipids during therapy, it should be taken as a warning sign for the development of osmotic cerebral edema. Appropriate and accurate management of fluids is crucial in this situation.

Phosphate

Intracellular phosphate depletion and phosphate loss due to osmotic diuresis leads to fall in total body phosphate level. After treatment is started, plasma phosphate levels further fall as it re-enters cells with severe metabolic disturbances. However, prospective studies have not shown any significant clinical benefit from phosphate replacement. If potassium phosphate is given, careful monitoring is necessary to prevent hypocalcemia[25].

Bicarbonate

Acidosis, even if severe, is reversed by replacement of fluids and administration of insulin. Insulin therapy reduces synthesis of ketoacids and allows excess ketoacids to be metabolized, resulting in regeneration of bicarbonate (HCO_3^-) and spontaneous correction of acidemia. Also, restoration of normovolemia improves tissue perfusion and renal functions, thus increasing the excretion of organic acids and reversing lactic acidosis. In DKA, the anion gap is increased. The major anions retained are beta-hydroxybutyrate (β-OHB) and acetoacetate.

Anion gap = $[Na^+]-[Cl^-] + [HCO_3^-]$ (normal value is 12 ± 2 mMol/l)

The indications for bicarbonate therapy in DKA are unclear. While controlled trials of sodium bicarbonate administration have not shown clinical benefit, there are several reasons for concern about its use[27]. Bicarbonate therapy may cause following metabolic changes:

(i) Paradoxical CNS acidosis. Overzealous use of alkali can lead to a rise in $paCO_2$ (since there is less acidemic stimulus to hyperventilation), resulting in a fall in cerebral pH as the lipid soluble CO_2 crosses the blood brain barrier faster than HCO_3 ions.

(ii) Hypokalemia

(iii) Higher sodium load

(iv) Increased serum hypertonicity

(v) Increased hepatic ketone production, thus slowing the rate of recovery from ketosis

(vi) Overshoot alkalosis due to participation of "alkali reserve" (salts of ketoacids are converted to bicarbonate with initiation of insulin therapy).

Cautious alkali therapy is advocated in patients with severe acidemia (arterial pH <6.9) and patients with potentially life threatening hyperkalemia in whom decreased cardiac contractility and peripheral vasodilatation can further impair tissue perfusion. Sodium bicarbonate 40 mEq/m^2 in N/2 saline is infused over 2-4 hours, aiming to raise the arterial pH above 7.1, a level at which the child is out of danger.

If bicarbonate is to be given, rapid injection should be avoided. It should be administered showly over 2-4 hours under cardiac monitoring. The best method is to add the bicarbonate in the crystalloid solution that is given in the first few hours, at a concentration of 25-50 mEq/l (1 ml of 7.5% sodium bicarbonate will provide approximately 1 mEq of Na and HCO$_3$ each). To put it simply, adding 40 ml of NaHCO$_3$ into 500 ml of 0.45% saline without dextrose will give a solution containing an approximate sodium concentration of 150 mEq/l. The formula used to calculate bicarbonate dose is given below:

0.6 × Weight in kg × Base deficit = mEq HCO$_3$.

Usually, it is recommended to give only one-third of the calculated deficit, i.e. about 1mEq/kg for 15 mMol base deficit, or approximately 1 ml/kg, of a 7.5% NaHCO$_3$.

Supportive Therapy

In unconscious patients, this includes nasogastric tube placement for aspiration of stom-ach contents and collection of urine by condom drainage in boys and bag drainage in girls. Catheterization should be done only in unconscious patients who have not passed urine for 4-6 hours.

Antibiotics

There is no role of routine use of prophylactic antibiotics. The total leukocyte count may be spuriously raised even without infection. Precipitating or associated infections should be looked for and managed appropriately.

Treatment of cerebral edema

Treatment should be initiated as soon as the condition is suspected. The rate of fluid administration should be reduced; either intravenous 20% mannitol (0.25–1.0 g/kg over 20 min) or hypertonic (3%) saline (5–10 ml/kg over 30 min) can be given. A better response is likely if mannitol or hypertonic saline are used early. Intubation and ventilation may be necessary, but aggressive hyperventilation should be avoided as it has been associated with poor outcome. There are no data regarding use of glucocorticoids in DKA-related cerebral edema. After starting treatment for CE, a head CT scan is done to check for any intracranial pathology.

Treatment of other complications

Other complications which can occur include dyselectrolytemia (hyperchloremic acidosis, hyperkalemia, hypokalemia, hypophosphatemic muscle weakness), hypoglycemia, gastric dilatation, pancreatitis, renal failure (especially due to acute renal tubular necrosis because of dehydration), ARDS (usually due to fluid overload), rhabdomyolysis and myoglobinuria, venous thrombosis, septicemia and fungal infections. They should be managed appropriately.

Common Pitfalls in the Management of Diabetic Ketoacidosis

1. Delay in the diagnosis, especially in the very young.

2. Delay in starting treatment.

3. Inadequate monitoring of clinical and laboratory parameters, inadequate supervision of treatment or inexperienced medical team.

4. Non-aspiration of stomach contents in the obtunded patient.

5. Errors in the insulin dosage
   (a) Use of too little and too late insulin delays recovery.
   (b) Too much insulin causes hypoglycemia and hypokalemia.

6. Fluid replacement errors
   (a) Inadequate or delayed fluid therapy may precipitate shock.
   (b) Too much fluid administration precipitates congestive cardiac failure, pulmonary edema, and possibly cerebral edema.

Section 4

7. Potassium replacement errors

   (a) Too little or delay in its administration precipitates lethal hypokalemia.

   (b) Too much and too early potassium therapy precipitates lethal hyperkalemia.

8. Bicarbonate replacement errors

   Too much may lead to metabolic alkalosis, and perhaps cerebral edema.

9. Unrecognized cerebral edema.

10. Failure to monitor and compensate for urine output.

11. Recurrence of ketoacidosis due to early stoppage of intravenous insulin or inadequate subcutaneous insulin after changing to intermittent insulin therapy.

12. Reliance on the electrocardiogram alone as a marker of serum potassium level.

(b) Transition from DKA to hyperglycemia and then euglycemia

Once the child's sensorium returns back to normal, and there is no gastric distension or vomiting, oral fluids can be offered; initially sips of water, then milk, followed by semi-solids. When the child is able to tolerate oral food, subcutaneous insulin can be started. IV insulin should be continued for 1-2 hours after the first subcutaneous injection is given, to avoid a sudden rise in blood glucose. In the initial 24-36 hours, blood glucose should be monitored 30 minutes before and 2 hours after each meal, and maintained between 200-300 mg/dl. Later, glucose level can be checked before each meal, and maintained between 90-130 mg/dl. For the newly diagnosed child, appropriate education to the family regarding insulin administration, and blood glucose monitoring, should begin within 24 hours. After a day or two, education regarding diet and life style modifications should be given.

(c) Prevention of DKA and Follow-up

Increased awareness, especially in high risk groups e.g. family members of T1DM patients, and the public at large can reduce the incidence of DKA by ensuring early diagnosis of diabetes mellitus in children[26,27]. Diabetes education programs, with ongoing emphasis on guidelines to identify sick child, and access to 24 hour telephone helplines can considerably reduce the incidence of DKA[28,29]. This is particularly important for children using insulin pumps. Recurrent DKA poses a potential risk, and is often due to psychopathology in the diabetic child or the parents. A recent study showed that less than 5% patients accounted for 22.5% of all episodes of DKA which can pose a significant financial and emotional burden[30]. Most events are due to omission of insulin. Mental health interventions and emphasis on supervised insulin administration help to reduce the risk of recurrence of DKA. The availability of aerosolized insulin for use in children is likely to improve the compliance and hopefully reduce the risk of DKA.

REFERENCES

1. Edge JA, Ford-Adams ME, Dunger DB. Causes of death in children with insulin dependent diabetes 1990–96. *Arch Dis Child* 1999; 81:318–323.

2. Lebovitz HE. Diabetic ketoacidosis. *Lancet* 1995; 345:767-771.

3. ESPE/LWPES consensus statement on diabetic ketoacidosis in children and adolescents. Dunger DB, Sperling MA, Acerini CL, Bohn DJ, Daneman D, Danne TPA, Glaser NS, Hanas R, Hintz RL, Levitsky LL, Savage MO, Tasker RC and Wolfsdorf JI. Arch Dis Child 2004; 89:188-194.

4. Bell PM, Hadden DR. Ketoacidosis without hyperglycemia during self monitoring of diabetes. *Diabetes Care* 1983; 6:622-623.

5. Levy-Marchal C, Papoz L, de Beaufort C, *et al.* Clinical and laboratory features of type 1 diabetic children at the time of diagnosis. *Diabet Med* 1992; 9:279–284.

6. Komulainen J, Lounamaa R, Knip M, Kaprio EA, Akerblom HK. The Childhood Diabetes in Finland Study Group. Ketoacidosis at the diagnosis of type 1 (insulin dependent) diabetes mellitus is related to poor residual beta cell function. *Arch Dis Child* 1996; 75: 410–415.

7. Neu A, Willasch A, Ehehalt S, Hub R, Ranke MB; DIARY Group Baden-Wuerttemberg. Ketoacidosis at onset of type 1 diabetes mellitus in children: frequency and clinical presentation. *Pediatr Diabetes* 2003; 4(2):77-81.

8. Mallare JT, Cordice CC, Ryan BA, Carey DE, Kreitzer PM, Frank GR. Identifying risk factors for the development of diabetic ketoacidosis in new onset type 1 diabetes mellitus. *Clin Pediatr* 2003; 42:591-597.

9. Jayashree M, Singhi S. Diabetic ketoacidosis: predictors of outcome in a pediatric intensive care unit of a developing country. *Pediatr Crit Care Med* 2004; 5: 427-433.

10. Koves IH, Neutze J, Donath S, Lee W, Werther GA, Barnett P, and Cameron FJ. The accuracy of clinical assessment of dehydration during diabetic ketoacidosis in childhood. *Diabetes Care* 2004; 27:2485-87.

11. Mackenzie A, Barnes G, Shann F. Clinical signs of dehydration in children. *Lancet* 1989; 2:605–607.

12. Haddad NG, Croffie JM, Eugster EA. Pancreatic enzyme elevations in children with diabetic ketoacidosis. *J Pediatr* 2004; 145:122-24.

13. Levitsky L, Ekwo E, Goselink C, Solomon I, aceto T. Death from diabetes in hospitalized children (1970–1988). *Pediatr Res* 1991; 29:A195.

14. Curtis JR, To T, Muirhead S, Cummings E, Daneman D. Recent trends in hospitalization for diabetic ketoacidosis in Ontario children. *Diabetes Care* 2002; 25:1591-96.

15. Cummings E, Lawrence S, Daneman D. Cerebral edema in pediatric diabetic ketoacidosis in Canada. *Diabetes* 2003; 52:A400.

16. Glaser N, Barnett P, McCaslin I *et al*. Risk factors for cerebral edema in children with diabetic ketoacidosis. The Pediatric Emergency Medicine Collaborative Research Committee of the American Academy of Pediatrics. *N Engl J Med* 2001; 344:264–269

17. Virmani A, Ushabala P, Rao PV. Diabetes mortality in a tertiary care referral hospital in India. (Letter to the Editor) *Lancet* 1990; 335:1341.

18. Marcin JP, Glaser N, Barnett P, McCaslin I, Nelson D, Trainor J. Louie J, Kaufman F, Quayle K, Roback M, Malley R, Kupperman N. American Academy of Pediatrics. The Pediatric Emergency Medicine Collaborative Research Committee. Factors associated with adverse outcomes in children with diabetic ketoacidosis-related cerebral edema. *J Pediatr* 2002; 141:793-797.

19. Muir AB, Quisling RG, Yang MCK, and Rosenbloom AL. Cerebral edema in childhood diabetic ketoacidosis. Natural history, radiographic findings, and early identification. *Diabetes Care* 2004; 27:1541-1546.

20. Glaser NS, Wootton-Gorges SL, Marcin JP, Buonocore MH, Dicarlo J, Neely EK, Barnes P, Bottomly J, Kuppermann N. Mechanism of cerebral edema in children with diabetic ketoacidosis. *J Pediatr* 2004; 145(2):164-171.

21. Brown TB. Cerebral edema in childhood diabetic ketoacidosis: Is treatment a factor? *Emerg Med J* 2004; *21:*141-144.

22. Muir A. Cerebral edema in diabetic ketoacidosis: a look beyond rehydration. *J Clin Endocrinol Metab* 2000; 85:509-513.

23. Carlotti APCP, Bohn D, Halperin ML. Importance of timing of risk factors for cerebral edema during therapy for diabetic ketoacidosis. *Arch Dis Child* 2003; 88:170-173.

24. Savage MW, Dhatariya KK, Kilvert A, Rayman G, Rees JA, Courtney CH, Hilton L, Dyer PH, Hamersley MS. Joint British Diabetes Societies Guidelines for the Management of Diabetic Ketoacidosis. *Diabetes Med* 2011; 28:508-515.

25. Umpierrez GE, Jones S, Smiley D, Mulligan P, Keyler T, Tempone A, Semakula C, Umpierrez D, Peng L, Ceron M, Robalino G. Insulin analogs vs. human insulin in treatment of patients with diabetic ketoacidosis: a randomized controlled trial. *Diabetes Care* 2009; 32:1164-69.

26. Fisher JN, Kitabchi AE. A randomized study of phosphate therapy in the treatment of diabetic ketoacidosis. *J Clin Endocrinol Metab* 1983; 57: 177-180.

27. Okuda Y, Adrogue HJ, Field JB, Nohara H, Yamashita K. Counterproductive effects of sodium bicarbonate in diabetic ketoacidosis. *J Clin Endocrinol Metab* 1996; 81:314-320.

28. Vanelli M, Chiari G, Ghizzoni L, Costi G, Giacalone T, Chiarelli F. Effectiveness of a prevention program for diabetic ketoacidosis in children. An 8 year study in schools and private practice. *Diabetes Care* 1999; 22:7-9.

29. Hoffman WH, *et al*. Service and education for the insulin-dependent child. *Diabetes Care* 1978; 1:285–288.

30. Edge JA, Hawkins MM, Winter DL, Dunger DB. The risk and outcome of cerebral edema developing during diabetic ketoacidosis. *Arch Dis Child* 2001; 85:16–22.

Section 4

42

Hematologic Emergencies in Children

Rachna Seth and Namita Gupta

INTRODUCTION

Hematological emergencies may be defined as sudden or unexpected life-threatening events in clinical hematology and oncology which require immediate action predominantly based on clinical judgment and supported by investigations that can be expected to produce rapid results. Some of these may be anticipated with reasonable frequency among pediatric patients particularly in those with known blood disease or who have a systemic disease.

The emergencies may be classified as disorders affecting the erythrocytes (various forms of anemia); leukocytes (disorders of neutrophils primarily); platelets; hemostasis; and defence mechanisms against infections etc. (Table 42.1). This article will focus on issues mainly related to hematologic emergencies some of which will be discussed in detail. For oncologic emergencies please refer to Chapter 43.

DISORDERS OF RED BLOOD CELLS

Children with a red cell volume or hemoglobin concentration that is below the 3rd centile for patient's age is classified as anemic. In general hemoglobin of less than 11gm/dl is consistent with anemia. Anemia is the most common red cell disorder in pediatric intensive care and severe anemia is an emergency that requires rapid evaluation and treatment to prevent hypoxia, congestive heart failure and death. There are a number of red cell disorders, not so serious and are easily managed; these will not be discussed here. However, there are situations in which the anemia is severe and difficult to manage e.g. severe hemorrhage which may necessitate massive transfusion with its attendant risks and complications, sickle cell disease and its known life threatening complications, autoimmune hemolytic anemia (AIHA), G6PD deficiency etc. and will be discussed in detail. Figure 42.1 summarizes a stepwise approach for the diagnosis of anemia in a child.

Table 42.1 Common hematologic emergencies

Disorders affecting the erythrocytes
- o Blood loss
- o Increased red cell destruction
- o Decreased red cell production

Disorders of hemoglobin structure and production
- o Sickle hemoglobin disorders
- o Thalassemia major
- o Methemoglobinemia

Disorders of white blood cells
- o Neutropenia
- o Disorders of neutrophil function

Disorders of platelets
- o Idiopathic thrombocytopenic purpura (ITP)
- o Non immune thrombocytopenia and abnormalities of platelet function

Coagulation disorders
- o Inherited bleeding disorders
- o Inherited hypercoagulable conditions
- o Disseminated intravascular coagulation (DIC)

Other hematologic emergencies
- o Postsplenectomy sepsis
- o Transfusion reaction

Blood Loss

The blood loss may occurs due to trauma, acute or chronic gastrointestinal hemorrhage, bleeding diathesis, surgical procedure and frequent blood sampling.

Bleeding from gastrointestinal tract and other forms of non traumatic bleeding can also be life-threatening. The severity of bleeding is more in the presence of an anatomic lesion like esophageal varices or a bleeding disorder like coagulopathy due to liver failure. Unexplained severe anemia requires a careful search for bleeding in the gastrointestinal tract, retroperitonium or elsewhere[1].

Increased Red Cell Destruction

This may be due to membrane disorders of red blood cells, metabolic abnormalities, autoimmune

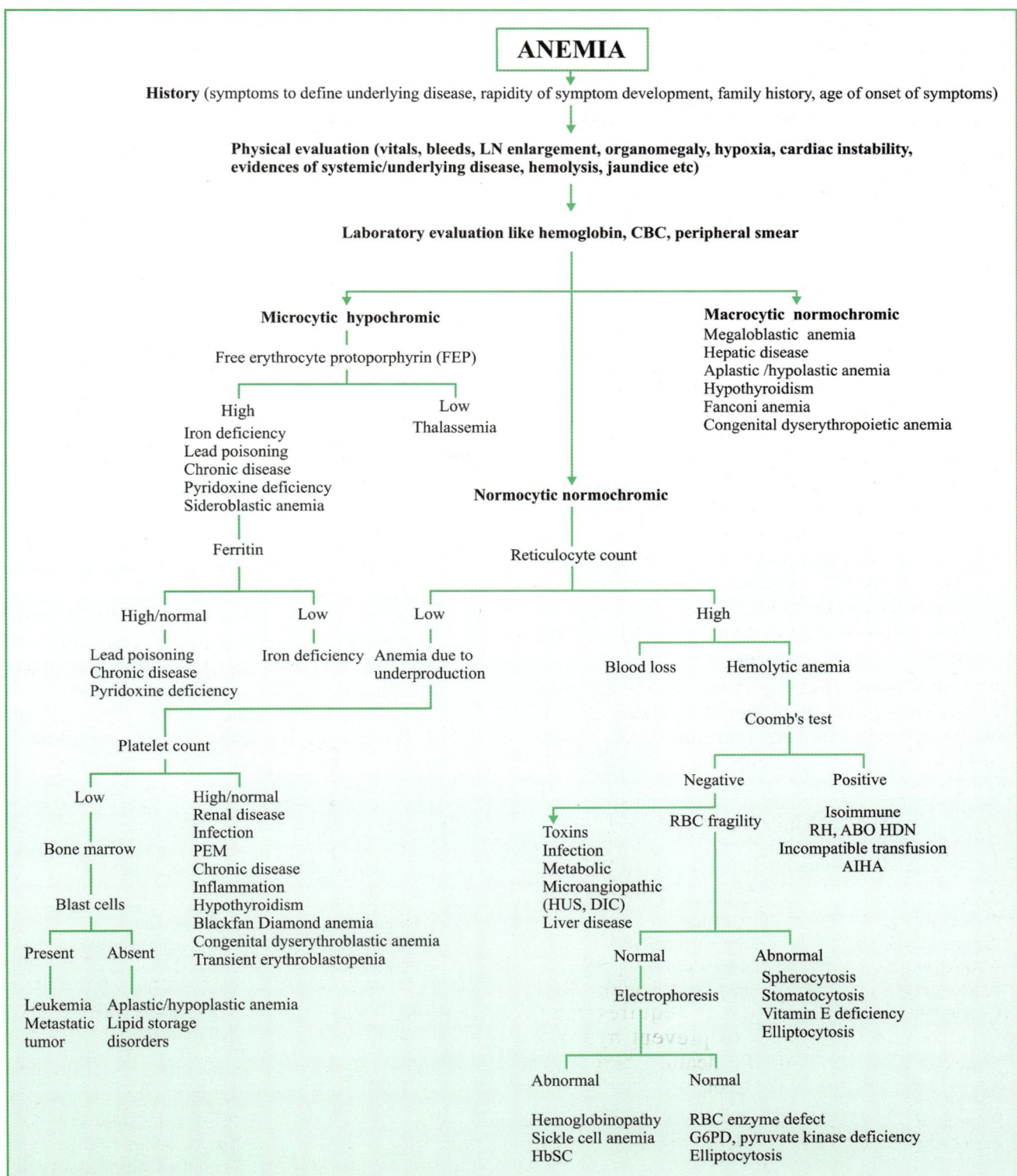

Figure 42.1 Algorithm for evaluation of a child with anemia

hemolytic anemia, non-immune hemolytic anemia or erythrocyte fragmentation syndromes.

(a)   Membrane disorders

The anemia in disorders of the red cell membrane like hereditary spherocytosis, elliptocytosis is rarely severe enough to constitute a hematologic emergency. However, the hemoglobin level may fall further when red cell destruction increases (hemolytic crisis which is associated with acute infections and is self-limiting) or red cell production slows down (aplastic crisis mostly accompanying parvovirus infection). The hemoglobin level and reticulocyte count should be routinely checked when children with a known disorder of red cell membrane develop increasing pallor or jaundice associated with an infectious illness. The hemolytic crisis is characterized by worsening jaundice, falling hemoglobin, and increasing reticulocyte count. The aplastic crisis is associated with slowly increasing pallor, worsening anemia and low or absent reticulocytes.

(b) Metabolic abnormalities

Like the membrane disorders, metabolic abnormalities usually do not cause severe anemia. However, episodes of acute and sometimes life-threatening intravascular hemolysis may occur in the presence of glucose-6-phosphate dehydrogenase (G6PD) deficiency (Table 42.2)[2]. The acute intravascular hemolysis usually occurs within 1-3 days of oxidant exposure and is characterized by pallor, malaise, fever, icterus, abdominal and back pain and dark colored urine.

Laboratory investigations reveal anemia, reticulocytosis and diagnostic blister cells in peripheral smear. Diagnosis of G6PD deficiency is established by G6PD enzyme level assay. Management consists of stabilization, intravenous fluids to prevent renal tubular damage and packed red cell transfusion in severe hemolysis.

(c) Autoimmune hemolytic anemia (AIHA)

AIHA is one of the most serious forms of severe anemia seen particularly in young children. The affected RBCs are lysed intravascularly or removed prematurely from the circulation by macrophages of the reticuloendothelial system. AIHA may be associated with infections, drugs, inflammatory diseases or malignancies. However, a specific cause is not found in most cases[3].

AIHA is usually associated with sudden onset of pallor, jaundice and dark urine. Anemia is usually severe and the child may appear desperately ill with signs of congestive cardiac failure and splenomegaly[4,5].

Laboratory evaluation shows severe anemia with reticulocytosis (may be low at onset). Peripheral smear shows spherocytosis and red cell fragments. Free hemoglobin in urine produces a positive dipstick reaction for blood in the absence of red cells on urine microscopy[2,4]. The direct Coombs' test using broad spectrum Coombs' serum (IgG, IgM and complement) is usually positive in childhood

Table 42.2 Agents causing hemolysis in G6 PD deficient patients			
Analgesics /antipyretics	**Quinocids**	**Nitrofurans**	**Sulphonamides**
Acetanilid	Quinacrine	Nitrofurantoin	N-acetyl sulfanilamide
Phenacetan	Quinine	Furaltadone	Sufapyridine
Acetylsalicylic acid	Pyrimethamine	Nitrofurazone	Sulfamethoxypridazine
Antipyrine	Plasmoquine	Furazolidine	Sulfadiazine
Aminopyrine	Chloroquine		Sulfisoxazole
P-aminosalicylic acid			Sulfathiazole
			Sulfacetamide
Antimalarials	**Sulfones**		**Other agents**
Pentaquine	Thiazolsulfone		Naphthalene
Primaquine	Diaminodiphenylsulfone (dapsone)		Phenylhydrazine
Pamaquine	Sufoxone sodium		Toluidine blue
			Methylene blue
			Acetylphenylhydrazine
			BAL
			Nalidixic acid
			Menadione
			Probenecid
			Chloramphenicol
			Quinidine
			Fava beans

AIHA[1,6]. The management is summarized in Table 42.3.

<table>
<tr><td colspan="1" align="center">**Table 42.3 Management OF AIHA[4,5,7]**</td></tr>
</table>

❑ Hospitalization for careful observation and treatment. Monitor vital signs.

❑ Maintain normal/increased urine output with intravenous fluids

❑ Immediately begin with corticosteroid therapy (Prednisone 2 mg/kg/day or equivalent parenteral dose) till hemoglobin is stable. Alternatively administer gamma globulins (IVIG 1 gm/kg) alone or in combination with corticosteroids.

❑ Administer red cell transfusion only when severe anemia is accompanied by signs of hypoxia/cardiac failure. Give first 5 ml in 10-15 minutes and observe for acute hemolysis. Check plasma layer of a spun hematocrit for pink color indicative of hemolysis of the transfused red cells. If symptoms and signs of worsening hemolysis are present, try a different unit of red cells.

❑ If hemoglobin level does not increase after transfusion, increase steroid dosage to 4 mg/kg/day; or begin plasmapharesis or exchange blood transfusion or emergency splenectomy may be life saving.

(d) *Non immune acquired hemolytic anemia*

Acute hemolytic anemia in children may be caused by infections, chemicals, or drugs that damage the red cells directly. These conditions may mimic AIHA. However, the DCT is negative and the hemolytic anemia is acquired. Infections causing acute hemolysis include malaria, Gram-negative and Gram-positive organisms. Chemicals and drugs similar to those causing bleeding in G6PD deficient children may cause oxidative hemolysis[8].

(e) *Erythrocyte fragmentation syndromes*

Red blood cells may undergo fragmentation and lysis when subjected to excessive trauma within the cardiovascular system. Hemolytic anemia as a result of RBC destruction or fragmentation may be associated with abnormal valves, hemolytic uremic syndrome (HUS), thrombotic thrombocytopenic purpura (TTP), collagen vascular disease, hemangiomas etc. Clinical profile is that of the underlying disease and peripheral smear shows red cell fragments.

Decreased Red Cell Production (Aplastic and hypoplastic anemia, nutritional anemia)

Disorders of red cell production unless accompanied by shortened red cell survival, are characterized by slowly progressive anemia. Aplastic and hypoplastic anemia, usually have a protracted course. After initial stabilization these children require intensive diagnostic evaluation and careful assessment for management. Transfusion must be used with caution in management of aplastic and hypoplastic anemia because exposure to human HLA and other antigens may adversely affect engraftment of transplanted bone marrow. The indications of blood (packed red cells) transfusions in such children include severe anemia (hemoglobin < 3-4 gm/dl), heart failure due to severe anemia or poor oxygenation. Use of filtered red cells from an unrelated CMV seronegative donor should be used[8].

Disorders of Hemoglobin Structure and Production

Sickle cell disease

Sickle cell disease (SCD) is the most common form of hemoglobinopathy and is predominantly found in people from Africa or the middle east. In India the gene frequency for the disease is 4.3% and occurs in tribal populations of Orissa, Maharashtra, Madhya Pradesh and Jharkand[10]. A single amino acid substitution on the chain of hemoglobin causes deformation of the RBCs into a sickle shape when exposed to cold, hypoxia or dehydration. Red cell rigidity leads to reduced tissue blood flow, intermittent vascular occlusion and hemolysis[9-11].

Vasoocclusion crisis due to thrombosis and obstruction of small vessels in the bones, lung, brain, and spleen causes pain and permanent ischemic tissue damage. In homozygous children 90-100% of the hemoglobin is HbS and they develop symptomatic anemia compared to 20-30% in the heterozygous who are asymptomatic except under conditions of severe hypoxia. Sickle cell hemoglobin C disease and sickle beta thalassemia are less common variants with less severe clinical manifestations. Sickle cell disease is diagnosed by electrophoresis[11-14].

Acute splenic sequestration crisis may develop in young children with the homozygous variant because of pooling of a large portion of their peripheral blood in the spleen. They present with left upper quadrant pain, pallor and lethargy, massive splenomegaly and hypovolemic shock. This is generally seen in children before auto infarction has occurred.

Sepsis in sickle cell disease occurs suddenly and is often fatal and the leading cause of death in children with sickle cell disease (SCD). Most SCD patients are asplenic by the age of 12 months owing to repeated splenic infarctions. They are at risk of infection from encapsulated organisms like *Haemophilus influenzae*, *Streptococcus pneumoniae* and salmonella. Any febrile illness in such patients is a medical emergency and intravenous antibiotics must be started immediately and shock must be managed early and appropriately[11].

Aplastic crisis occurs with impairment of RBC production in the bone marrow exacerbating the chronic hemolytic anemia. Hematocrit and reticulocytes are decreased. Parvovirus may be associated with aplastic crisis.

Acute chest syndrome is associated with fever, cough, pleuritic pain, tachypnea and pulmonary infiltrates and pleural effusion on chest radiograph. Pulmonary infarction is difficult to differentiate from pneumonia although in children under 12 years of age, infection with *Streptococcus pneumoniae* or *mycoplasma* is a more common cause of acute chest syndrome.

Table 42.4 Diagnostic features and principles of management of children with sickle cell disease[3, 11-15]

Category	Infant	Child	Adolescent	Management
Vaso-occlusive	Dactylitis			Pain control, hydrate
		Painful crisis	→	Pain control*, hydrate
		Stroke	→	Hospitalize, stabilize, hydrate, treat seizures, partial exchange to reduce HbS below 30% of total hemoglobin, CT/MRI to identify infarction, bleed, aneurysm rupture
		Hematuria	→	Observe
		Autosplenectomy	→	Observe for infection
			Aseptic necrosis of bone	Conservative treatment, arthroplasty
			Acute pulmonary syndrome	Hospitalize, hydrate, prevent hypoxia (oxygen, analgesia*, physiotherapy, CPAP), IV antibiotics (CxR, blood culture), correct dehydration followed by maintenance fluids, exchange transfusion
Increased red cell destruction	Aplastic crisis	→	→	Hospitalize, transfuse to restore RBC mass
		Impaired growth		Observe
			Delayed puberty	Observe
Sequestration and stasis	Splenomegaly			Observe
	Splenic sequestration crisis			Hospitalize, hydrate, support intravascular volume, transfuse to replace sequestered red cells with whole blood/ packed red cells
		Hepatomegaly	→	Observe
		Priapism	→	If severe hospitalize, hydrate, replace sickle cells with normal RBCs (partial exchange) and pain control
Functional asplenia	Sepsis Pneumonia Meningitis Osteomyelitis	→		Hospitalize and give IV antibiotics

* Acetaminophen, codeine or morphine

Hyperhemolytic crisis occurs with acceleration of the hemolytic process and worsening of anemia. Associated G6PD deficiency may be the cause of this complication.

Stroke is usually due to thrombosis of a large vessel (middle cerebral or internal carotid artery) and is uncommon in children less than 1 year of age.

Bone involvement produces pain particularly in the extremities. Dactylitis is particularly common in children under 4 years of age. These children present with hand foot syndrome associated with non pitting edema of the hands and feet, warmth, swelling and tenderness.

The diagnostic features of various complications and their management is summarized in Table 42.4. There is some evidence that hydroxy urea and high dose methyl prednisolone may provide symptomatic relief to patients with sickle cell disease[16,17].

Methemoglobinemia

Methemoglobinemia is an uncommon cause of cyanosis in infants and children but is capable of causing severe problems and even death. The diagnosis of methemoglobinemia should be strongly suspected when cyanosis occurs in the absence of demonstrable cardiac or pulmonary disease and oxygen administration fails to relieve cyanosis[2]. Symptoms depend on the concentration of methemoglobin. As a rapid screening test, a drop of blood is placed on the filter paper. After it is waved off in the air for 30-60 seconds, normal blood appears bright red whereas blood from a patient of methemoglobinemia remains reddish brown. Arterial blood oxygen saturation is low when measured directly by blood oximetry even though PaO_2 is normal. Pulse oximetry devices measure oxygen saturation of only that hemoglobin which is available for saturation. Thus a patient of methemoglobinemia and obvious cyanosis may have normal oxygen saturation by pulse oximeter. Spectrophotometric assays can be used to confirm methemoglobinemia and to determine the level of methemoglobin[1,18-19]. The clinical features and management of methemoglobinemia are summarized in Table 42.5.

DISORDERS OF WHITE BLOOD CELLS

Infection is the most significant complication associated with quantitative or qualitative white cell disorders. These disorders may be associated with repeated local infections leading to severe organ damage or may culminate in fatal disseminated

Table 42.5 Common symptoms and principles of management of methemoglobnemia[6]

Methemoglobin level	Symptoms and signs
10-30%	Cyanosis
30-50%	Dyspnea, tachycardia, dizziness, fatigue, headache
50-70%	Lethargy, stupor
> 70%	Death

Methemoglobin level	Treatment
< 30%	No treatment
30-70%	Methylene blue 2 mg/kg of 1% solution IV over 5 minutes. If there is no response to two doses of methylene blue in a non critically sick child, use 500 mg of ascorbic acid orally if there is no G6PD dificiency.
Severely ill and no response to methylene blue	Hyperbaric oxygen or exchange blood transfusion

Substances and drugs implicated in the formation of methemoglobin in children

(i) Drugs (sulphonamides, quinines, phenacetin, benzocaine)

(ii) Domestic and environmental substances (foods containing nitrites/nitrates, well water containing nitrates, aniline dyes, naphthalene, soap enemas, industrial compounds like nitrobenzene, nitrous gases etc.)

fungal infection. The appropriate emergency management of the child with white cell abnormalities and fever or other signs of infection may have a profound impact on the quality of patient's life.

Neutropenia

Neutropenia is defined as an absolute neutrophil count below 1000/mm^3. When the neutrophil count falls below 500/mm^3, the patients exhibit an increased susceptibility to infections caused by normal skin, respiratory or GI flora. Between 500-1000 cells/mm^3, susceptibility to infection is less significant but the host's ability to combat the typical infections is impaired[6].

A detailed history should be taken in children found to be neutropenic. A history of viral infections, similar history of recurrent infections in the past,

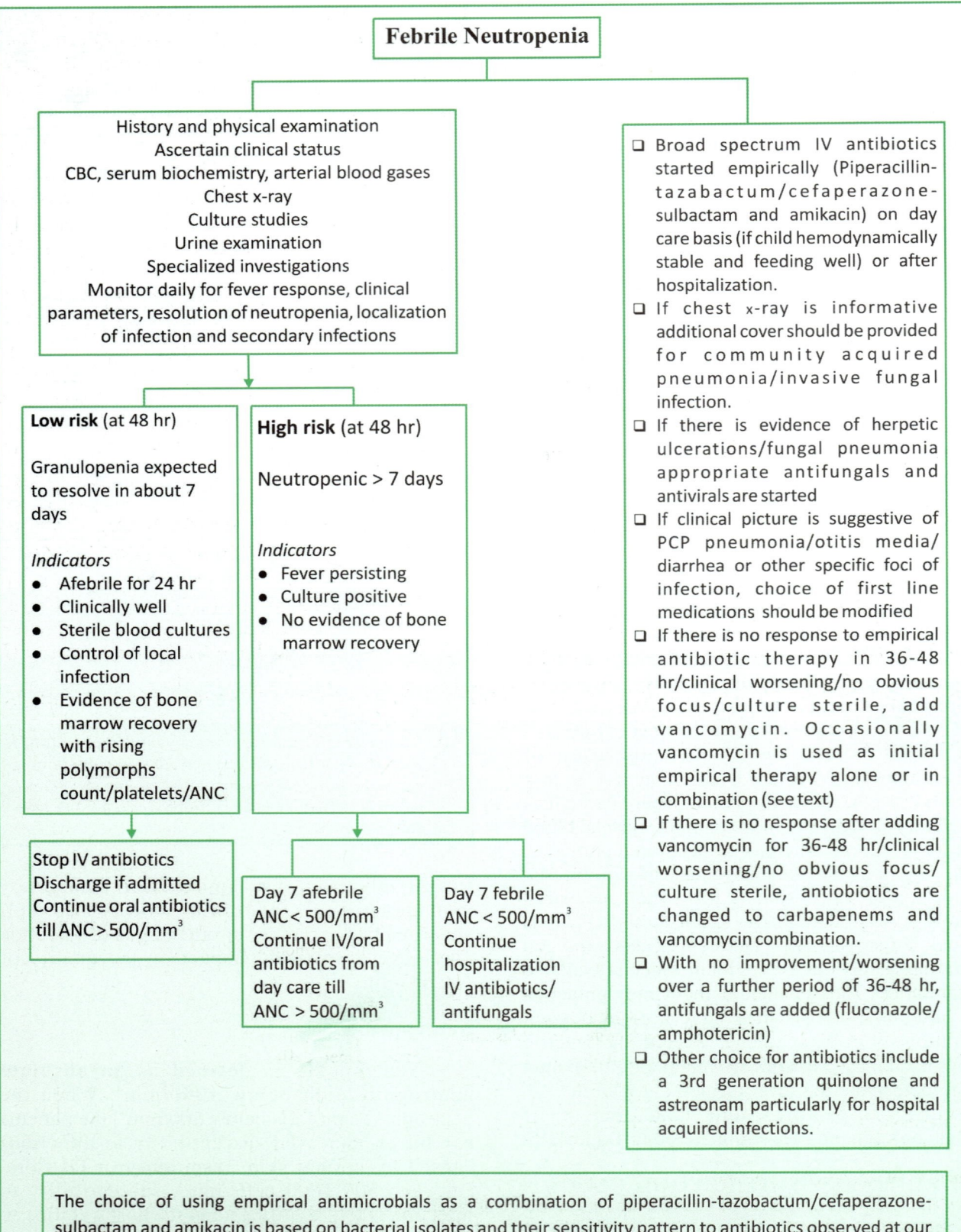

Figure 42.2 Algorithm for management of a patient with febrile neutropenia

history of deaths in the family suggesting a congenital neutropenia, drug history etc. should be taken. Underlying disorders like malignancy or nutritional disorder should be looked for.

Most commonly neutropenia is associated with fever and is known as febrile neutropenia .This is a common entity in children on chemotherapy and is an oncologic emergency. The localizing signs of infection may be absent initially owing to lack of inflammatory cells. A careful history and physical examination should be conducted to identify possible focus of infection to guide the selection of appropriate antimicrobial therapy. It is important to realize that neutropenic patients can have serious life-threatening infections even in the absence of fever and may not present with any localizing symptoms and signs of infection. They should be managed according to the same principles as a neutropenic patient who presents with fever. Numerous disorders of neutrophil function have been described and are associated with severe infections to a variable extent (Table 42.6).

Definition of Febrile Neutropenia

It is usually defined as a single oral/axillary or equivalent temperature of greater than 38.3°C (101 °F) or two consecutive temperatures greater than 38.0°C (100°F) in a 12 hour period lasting for at least 1 hour. Neutropenia is defined as an absolute neutrophil count (ANC) < 500 /mm^3 or < 1,000/mm^3 with an expected decline[20]. At our center we consider ANC < 500/mm^3 as neutropenia.

Evaluation of a patient with febrile neutropenia

(i) History and detailed physical examination. A detailed physical examination conducted daily particularly in those patients who do not show a response to treatment and a search must be made for foci of infection. Areas at risk for infection include the oropharynx, respiratory tract, urinary tract, perianal area, central venous line sites, skin and soft tissues. History of recent invasive procedures should be taken.

(ii) Ascertain clinical status with baseline characteristics of vital parameters. Assess the oral intake. Look for any alteration in sensorium and focal deficit.

(iii) Complete blood count including absolute neutrophil count, arterial blood gas and serum biochemistry should be checked.

(iv) The various samples for cultures include blood, urine and localized collection of pus. Other samples that may be sent are based on clinical

---

Table 42.6 Causes of neutropenia and disorders of neutrophil function in children[1,6]

Neutropenia

- Kostmann's syndrome
- Chronic benign neutropenia (familial)
- Neutropenia associated with immunoglobulin disorders
- Reticular dysgenesis
- Neutropenia associated with phenotypic abnormalities
- Cyclic neutropenia
- Shwachman Diamond syndrome
- Glycogen storage type Ib
- Drugs (chemotherapy, sulphonamides, phenytoin, phenobarbitone, penicillin, phenothiazines)
- Hypersplenism
- Chemicals and toxins
- Infections (bacterial, viral, rickettsial, parasitic)
- Bone marrow infiltration (leukemia, lymphoma, neuroblastoma)
- Nutritional deficiencies (starvation, anorexia nervosa, vitamin B$_{12}$, folate, copper deficiencies)
- Immune neutropenia (collagen vascular disease, Felty's syndrome, etc.)
- Acquired immune deficiency syndrome (HIV)
- Metabolic diseases (Tyrosinemia, methylmalonic aciduria)
- Myelodysplasia

Disorders of neutrophil function

- Cellular defects of chemotaxis (Job syndrome, chronic renal failure, post transplant, malnutrition, infection)
- Secondary defects of chemotaxis (Chediac-Higashi syndrome, hypogamaglobulinemia, Wiskott-Aldrich syndrome
- Complement abnormalities
- Disorders of degranulation
- Defective peroxidative killing of bacteria and fungi (chronic ganulomatous disease)
- Acquired disorders of phagocytic dysfunction (severe iron deficiency, PEM, malignancies, severe burns)

suspicion like stool, central line site, CSF or pus from any site.

(v) Chest X-ray is a mandatory investigation in all children with febrile neutropenia. Initial X-ray chest may be non informative but must be taken as a baseline for comparison with later films. Subtle differences in pneumonic process may become apparent on serial radiographs. CT chest and bronchoscopy are needed in selected cases.

(vi) Specialized investigations for *pneumocystis carinii,* atypical organisms, sinusitis, typhilitis, CNS infections, etc. should be undertaken as and when indicated.

Predominant pathogens associated with episodes of febrile neutropenia

The epidemiology of neutropenic infection varies with the geographic location of the treatment center. Only 10-30% of neutropenic fevers yield a microbiologic diagnosis[20-21]. The common organisms

Table 42.7 Screening tests for a bleeding child

Condition	Platelet count	BT	PTT	PT	TT	Comments
			Screening tests			
Normal	150-400,000/mm^3	4-9 min	25-35 min	12-13 sec	8-10 sec	Fibrinogen 100-400 mg/dl
Hereditary disorders						
Hemophilia (Factor VIII, IX, XI, XII)	Normal	Normal	Raised	Normal	Normal	Factor assay
Factor II, V, X	Normal	Normal	Raised	Raised	Normal	Factor assay
Factor VII	Normal	Normal	Normal	Raised	Normal	Factor assay
von Willebrand disease (many variants)	Normal	Raised	Raised	Normal	Normal	VIII antigen, VIII cofactor, ristocetin cofactor
Platelet dysfunction	Normal/decreased	Raised	Normal	Normal	Normal	Platlet aggregation studies
Acquired disorders						
DIC	Decreased	Raised	Raised	Raised	Raised	Decreased fibrinogen, raised FDPs
ITP	Decreased	Raised	Normal	Normal	Normal	
HSP	Normal	Normal	Normal	Normal	Normal	
Liver failure (severe)	Normal/decreased	Normal/raised	Raised	Raised	Normal/raised	Evidences of liver dysfunction
Uremia	Normal/decreased	Normal	Normal	Normal	Normal/raised	Evidences of renal dysfunction
Anticoagulants	Normal	Raised	Normal/raised	Normal/raised	Normal/raised	
Aspirin toxicity	Normal	–	Normal	Normal	Normal	Platelet dysfunction

Abbreviations

BT : Bleeding time, PTT : Partial thromboplastin time, PT : Prothrombin time, TT : Thrombin time, DIC : Disseminated intravascular coagulation, FDP : Fibrin degradation products, ITP : Immune thrombocytopenic purpura, HSP : Henoch-Schonlein purpura

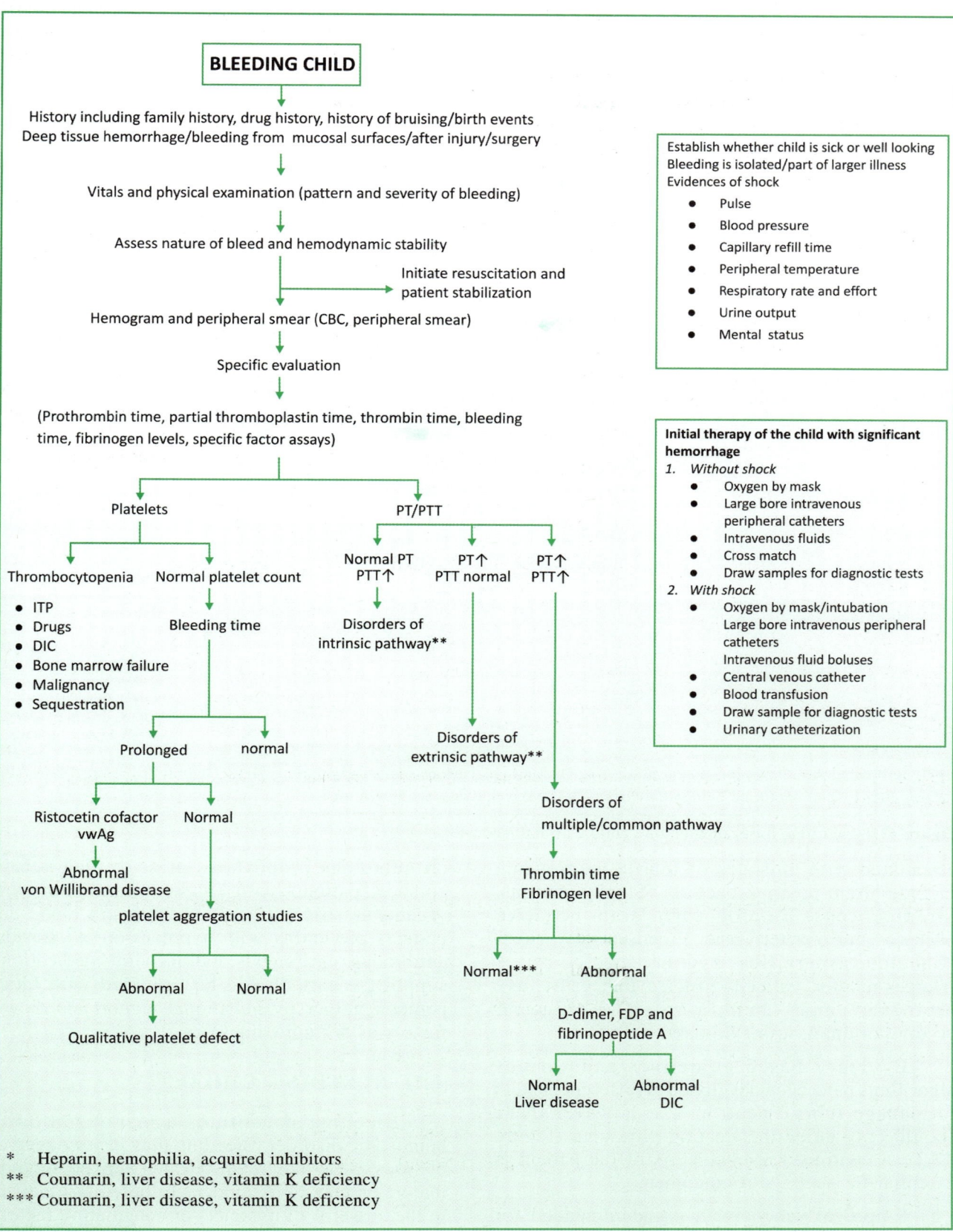

Figure 42.3 Algorithm for diagnostic work up and management of a bleeding child[1,3,6]

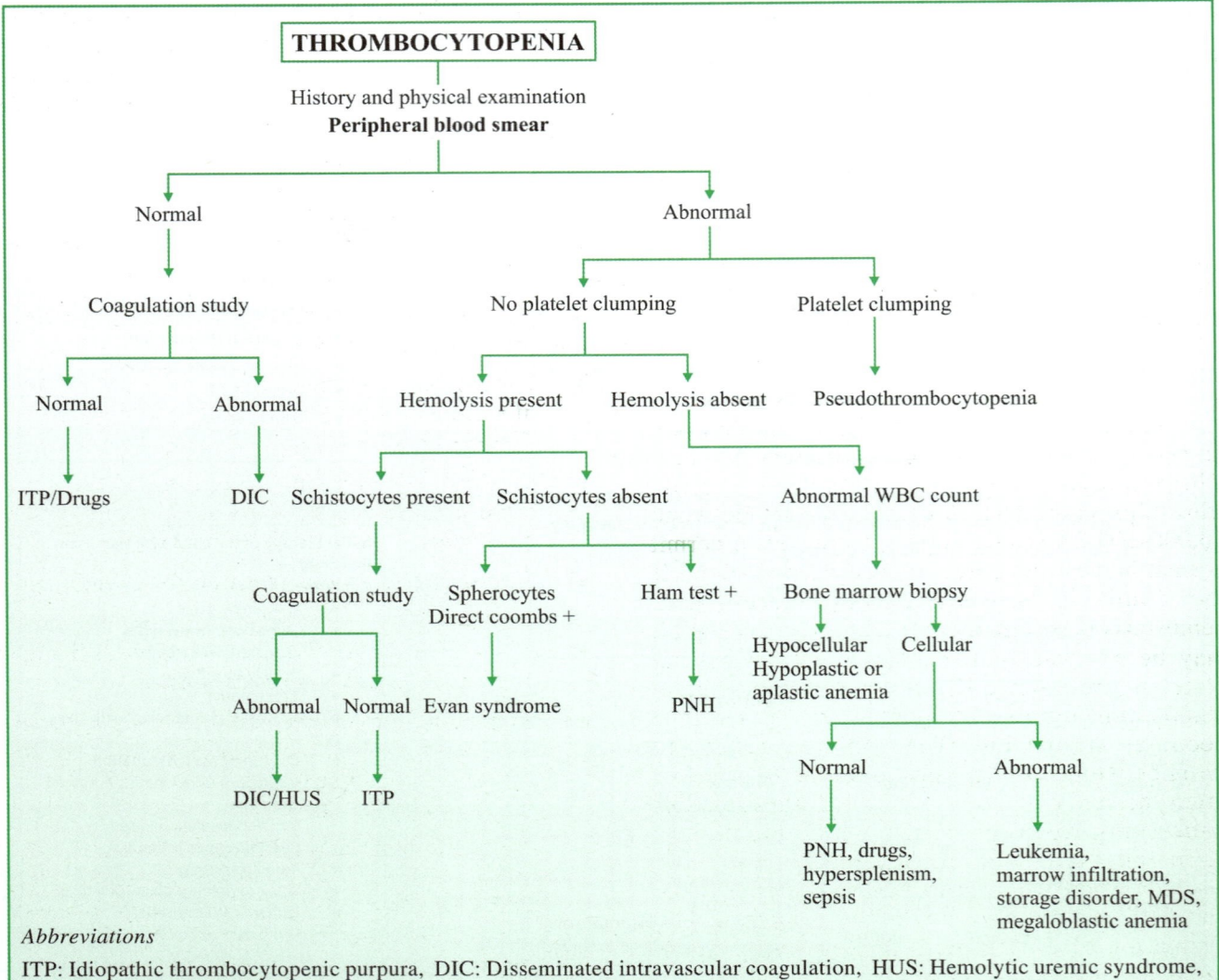

Figure 42.4 Algorithm for evaluation of a child with thrombocytopenia

associated with episodes of febrile neutropenia include Gram-positive bacteria (Staphylococcus, Streptococcus, Enterococci), Gram-negative bacteria (Entrobacteriaceae, Pseudomonas), fungi (Candida, aspergillus, zygomycetes), viruses (Herpes simplex, varicella zoster, cytomegalovirus), protozoa and helminths (Toxoplasma, cryptosporidium, strongyloides).

Evidence based guidelines and various algorithms have been developed at different centers to manage febrile neutropenia; however these should only guide the treating physician (Figure 42.2). A continued re-evaluation of the patient is essential for successful outcome.

Empirical vancomycin is recommended for certain groups of patient like those with obvious central line infections, those receiving intensive chemotherapy leading to severe mucositis, children on quinolone prophylaxis prior to their febrile episode, patients with known colonization with organisms susceptible to vancomycin alone and patients presenting with hypotension[22,23]. Besides antibiotics, antifungals and antiviral medications, supportive care should be provided with blood component therapy, nutritional support and growth factors as per guidelines.

THE BLEEDING CHILD[24-27]

Bleeding constitutes a manifestation of hemostatic disorder. Bleeding may occur due to an obvious cause like trauma (which may be minor or major) or may be secondary to hereditary defects in the vessel wall, platelets or coagulation factors. Based on history, pattern and severity of bleeding, the cause of bleeding can be identified in most children.

Etiologic classification of hemorrhage

1. *Vessel related.* Trauma, surgery and vasculitis
2. *Platelet related.* Thrombocytopenia and thrombocytopathy
3. *Plasma phase related.* Congenital factor deficiency, liver disease and DIC.

Factor assays and mixing studies as required should be done. They are summarized in Table 42.7. Assessment and management of a bleeding children is summarized in Figure 42.3.

Disorders of Platelets

Platelet disorders leading to inadequate homeostasis may be due to insufficient numbers (thrombocytopenia) or defective action (thrombocytopathy). A platelet count between 50,000-100,000/mm^3 is often sufficient to permit normal hemostasis during a surgical procedure. If the count is between 20,000-50,000/mm^3, hemostasis is less likely to be achieved although it may be adequate if the majority of circulating platelets are young. If the counts are less than 20,000/mm^3 the risk of spontaneous hemorrhage becomes significant. The common causes of thrombocytopenia are listed in Table 42.8. Most often thrombocytopenia is a manifestation of an underlying disorder which when adequately managed corrects the platelet count. The discussion here would primarily be restricted to ITP and DIC associated thrombocytopenia. The evaluation of a child with thrombocytopenia is summarised in Figure 42.4.

Idiopathic Thrombocytopenic Purpura (ITP)[25,28]

ITP is the most commonly encountered platelet disorder in children and results from increased destruction of platelets on an autoimmune basis in the spleen leading to thrombocytopenia. ITP is known to be associated with a number of viral infections like measles, rubella, mumps, varicella, infectious mononucleosis, etc. Serious bleeding is rare and occurs in about 2-4% of cases[2]. Most cases are self limiting and symptoms subside in majority in about 6-12 months.

A history of preceding viral illness is present in 50% of children who present with petechiae, purpura and spontaneous bleeding of skin and mucuos membranes. Intracranial bleeds, GIT bleeds and hematuria are rare. The major life threatening complication of ITP is intracranial hemorrhage.

The diagnosis of ITP is made readily in the child with newly acquired petechiae and ecchymosis, thrombocytopenia, normal or increased and lazy megakaryocytes in the bone marrow and absence of any underlying disease.

Management[25,27,29-33]

- Expectant observation with avoidance of trauma

- If a life threatening bleed occurs, platelet transfusions are given.

- Prednisone is given in a dose of 2 mg/kg/day if platelet count is less than 10,000/mm^3 for 2-3 weeks and is tapered over next week.

- Emergent treatment is required if there is severe GI bleeding, epistaxis, hemtauria, headache or intracranial hemorrhage.

- Transfusions may be required for anemia and hypotension.

- IV steroids (hydrocortisone acetate 4-5 mg/kg/dose 6 hourly) in severe cases.

- IV infusion of gamma globulins (0.5 g/kg/dose IV over 4-6 hr for a total of 4 doses) may be given if a rapid rise of platelet is required (life threatening bleeds)

- Anti-D antibodies in a dose of 50 µg/kg by IV infusion is a recent option available to treat ITP. The effect of anti-D is slightly delayed compared to gamma globulin and the peak platelet count may be somewhat lower. Anti-D has the advantage of being administered over minutes rather hours and rarely causes headache.

- In life-threatening bleeds sometimes plasmapharesis and splenectomy have to be considered if patient does not respond to above mentioned treatment.

Management of head trauma in ITP

(i) Mild head trauma without neurologic findings
   - Observe closely
   - Gamma globulin 1.0 g/kg IV infusion or anti-D 50 µg/kg if platelet count is <20,000/mm^3, signs of spontaneous/easy bleeding are present or if follow-up is uncertain

(ii) Severe head trauma or neurologic abnormalities
   - Hydrocortisone 8-10 mg/kg IV every 4-6 hr
   - Gamma globulin 1.0 g/kg IV infusion

Section 4

Table 42.8 Common causes of thrombocytopenia
Increased destruction (Non-immune)

Congenital
  • TORCH infections
  • Giant hemangioma
 	
Acquired
  • HUS, TTP
  • Infection
  • DIC
  • NEC
  • Massive transfusion
  • Prosthetic valves
  • Hypersplenism

Accelerated destruction /loss (Immune)

• Infection
  • ITP
  • Neonatal passive immunization
  • Autoimmune disorders (SLE, Evan's)
  • Drug induced (Table 42.13)

Decreased production of platelets

• Leukemia,
  • Lymphoma
  • Storage disorders
  • Solid tumor
  • Aplastic anemia
  • Congenital: Wiskott Aldrich syndrome
  • Infections (viral, HIV, CMV)
  • Drugs (cytotoxic, anticonvulsants, antibiotics)
  • Congenital amegakaryocytosis

Abbreviations
HUS : Hemolytic uremic syndrome, TTP: Thrombotic thrombocytopenic purpura, DIC: Disseminated intravascular coagulation, NEC: Necrotizing enterocolitis

- Platelet transfusion 0.4 units/kg
- If neurologic signs are severe or progressive, splenectomy, exchange transfusion or, plasmapharesis may be considered

There is no concensus regarding the management of a newly diagnosed patient of ITP[6,29]. The usual benign course of the disease must be weighed against the side effects and cost of corticosteroids, gamma globulins and anti-D antibodies. It would be a rational approach to reserve specific therapy like steroids, gamma globulins and anti-D antibodies for patients with significant bleeding or severe thrombocytopenia (platelet count < 10,000/mm³) several weeks after the diagnosis and patients whose physical activity cannot be restricted[2].

Disseminated Intravascular Coagulation (DIC)

DIC is an acquired coagulation disorder of hemostasis that may occur due to a variety of causes and most commonly accompanies septic shock. Other causes of DIC include malignancy, ischemia or trauma that may trigger the coagulation cascade generating thrombin and simultaneously activating fibrinolysis (Table 42.9). It may be mild and subclinical or severe and life threatening.

Circulating thrombin cleaves fibrinogen to form fibrin monomers which are polymerized in the circulation to form microvascular thrombi in which platelets are trapped. Simultaneously plasmin derived from plasminogen actively cleaves fibrinogen leading to the generation of breakdown products. These products are markers of fibrinolysis and inhibit polymerization of fibrin exacerbating the bleeding tendency created by consumption of coagulant proteins and incorporation of platelets into small vessel thrombi. In essence the normal balance of coagulation and thrombosis is disrupted. DIC results in the deposition of thrombi within the microcirculation, fibrinolysis, consumption of all coagulation factors especially II, V, VIII and platelets. Ultimately DIC is associated with ischemic end organ damage, bleeding manifestations, shock and metabolic acidosis[3,6,7].

Laboratory abnormalities

(i)   The diagnosis is confirmed by a constellation of laboratory abnormalities, most prominently thrombocytopenia, a prolonged PT and aPTT,

Table 42.9 Common causes of DIC
Infection   Gram-negative sepsis, meningococcemia, Gram-positive sepsis (*Streptococcus pneumoniae, Staphyloccus*), viral pathogens (herpes, measles, varicella, CMV, influenza)

Tumor
    Leukemia (APML)
    Solid tumors

Neonatal
    Necrotizing enterocolitis
    Respiratory distress syndrome
    Hemolytic uremic syndrome (HUS)
    Giant hemangioma

Miscellaneous conditions
    Shock (anaphylaxis, heat stroke)
    Snake bite
    Transfusion reactions
    Severe head injury

Table 42.10 Laboratory tests for DIC and liver disease[26,32]

Test	DIC	Liver disease
Blood smear	Fragmented RBCs, decreased platelets	Target cells, occasionally decreased platelets
Platelet count	<1,50,000, may be <50,000/mm³	Variable, rarely < 50,000/mm³
aPTT (intrinsic)	Prolonged	Prolonged
PT (extrinsic)	Prolonged	Prolonged
Fibrinogen	< 150 mg/dl	< 150 mg/dl only if severe disease or fibrinolysis
FDP	> 40 mg/ml	Usually < 40 mg/ml
D-dimers	Present	Absent

a decreased fibrinogen level and presence of FDP in the appropriate clinical setting (Table 42.10).

DIC is a life-threatening disease and its severity can be assessed by DIC score (Table 42.11). The management of DIC is summarized in Table 42.12.

Table 42.11 The disseminated intravascular coagulation score[10]

Investigations	Score
1. Platelet count	
>100,000/mm³	0
50,000-1,00,000/mm³	1
<50,000/mm³	2
2. Elevated fibrin related marker (soluble fibrin monomers/fibrin degradation products like D-dimers*)	
No increase	0
Moderate increase	2
Marked increase	3
3. Prolonged PT	
< 3 sec	0
> 3 but < 6 sec	1
> 6 sec	2
4. Fibrinogen level	
> 1g /L	0
< 1g /L	1

DIC score

(a) If score is ≥ 5 it indicates overt DIC; scoring should be done daily

(b) If score <5 it is suggestive (not affirmative) of DIC.

* D-dimers; a value above the upper limit of normal is considered moderately elevated and a value above 5 times the upper limit of normal is considered as a strong evidence[32].

Table 42.12 Management protocol for DIC

1. **Stabilization**
   - Monitor vital signs
   - Oxygen, IPPV/CPAP for respiratory failure
   - Plasma volume expanders and inotropic drugs for circulatory failure

2. **Interrupt the underlying process**
   Treat the underlying disease (IV antibiotics, antisnake venom)

3. **Replacement therapy**
   Platelet transfusion: 1 unit/5 kg or 10 ml/kg in infants will increase platelet count by 50,000 -100,000/mm³. Repeat if necessary if platelet count is < 20,000/mm³ in a non bleeding child or below 50,000/mm³ in a bleeding child.
   Plasma 10-15 ml/kg in active/impending bleeding. Repeat if child is bleeding and PT/aPTT are deranged. FFP contains factors II, V, and VIII which are usually deficient if hypoxia or acidosis are present.
   Cryoprecipitate (fibrinogen source): 1 unit (bag) of cryoprecipitate per 3 kg in infants and per 5 kg in children (0.2 units/kg) will increase fibrinogen level by 75 – 100 mg/dl thereby promoting hemostasis. Cryoprecipitate has large amount of fibrinogen (FFP is not rich in fibrinogen) and factor VII and may be given if there is no response to FFP.

4. **Pharmacologic intervention**
   Heparin (controversial role): It is useful in purpura fulminans (fibrin deposition in small vessels is of major pathologic significance) and acute promyelocytic leukemia where heparin may normalize coagulation by interfering with action of tissue factor like activity in the granules. It is often started early in children with DIC associated with meningococcemia because of the frequent occurrence of fulminant thrombosis and tissue necrosis. Heparin is administered by continuous IV infusion. 50 units/kg IV is followed by a continuous drip of 10-15 units / kg/hr. A higher dose of 20-25 units kg/hr is used in purpura fulminans.

5. **Exchange transfusion can be done in neonates**

6. **Supportive care**
   Management of renal failure in hemolytic uremic syndrome (HUS).

Section 4

Table 42.13 Drugs associated with immune thrombocytopenia[4,24,29]	
Acetaminophen	NSAIDs
Acetazolamide	Penicillin
Acetylsalicylic acid	Phenothiazines
Benzodiazepines	Phenytoin
Carbamazepine	Propylthiouracil
Cephalosporins	Quinolones
Digoxin	Rifampicin
Dopamine	Streptomycin
Heparin	Sulpha drugs
INH	Tetracyclines
Lidocaine	Thiazides
TCA	Valproate

Platelet function disorders (Thrombocytopathy)

Defective platelet function is a less common cause of significant bleeding in children requiring intensive care. There are many causes of thrombocytopathy. Of these drug induced defects need a special mention since many of the drugs implicated are administered to critically ill children. Since children in the ICU are often at risk for bleeding, these drugs may aggravate the situation. Thrombocytopathy must be suspected when there are bleeding manifestations in a child with a normal platelet count and a normal PT and PTT with a negative FDP assay and a prolonged bleeding time[26]. Drugs inhibiting platelet functions are listed in Tables 42.13 and 42.14.

Management of platelet dependent thrombocytopenia (±bleeding)

❑ Management consists of platelet transfusion and aggressive treatment of any underlying disorder.

❑ Platelet transfusion may be indicated regardless of the number of platelets if there is platelet dysfunction and bleeding.

❑ Transfused platelets should be ABO compatible as ABO antigens are expressed on platelets and matching improves platelet survival.

❑ One unit of platelet (70 ml/5 kg body weight) is likely to increase the platelet count by $50 \times 10^9/L$.

❑ Platelet concentrate is viable for 5 days at 22°C on an agitator but the platelet number and function falls rapidly with time after collection.

Table 42.14 Drugs known to inhibit platelet functions

Antibiotics
Ampicillin, carbenicillin, cephalosporin, methicillin, penicillin G, ticarcillin

Antihistaminics
Chlorpheniramine maleate, diphenhydramine

Non-steroidal anti-inflammatory drugs
Aspirin, naproxen, phenybutazone, sulindac, sulfinpyrazine

Chemotherapeutic drugs
Mithramycin

Ethyl alcohol

Heparin

Macromolecules
Dextran

Nitrofurantoin

Phenothiazines
Chlorpromazine, promethazine

Pseudoephedrine hydrochloride

Pyrimido-pyrimidine compounds

Tricyclic antidepressants
Amitriptyline, imipramine

Triprolidine

Vinca alkaloids

Valproate sodium

(From Nathan DG, Oski FA: Hematology of Infancy and Childhood. *Saunders, Philadelphia*)

❑ Drugs known to adversely affect platelet functions should be avoided.

OTHER HEMATOLOGIC EMERGENCIES

Post-splenectomy Sepsis[6]

Splenectomy may cure or ameliorate several hematologic disorders. However, loss of spleen is associated with an increased risk of sepsis caused by *S.pneumoniae* (commonest), Neisseria *meningitides, E coli, H influnzae* and other bacteria. The infections are particularly severe in children with autoimmune hemolytic anemia and Wiskott Aldrich syndrome. The mortality from sepsis in asplenic patients is high averaging more than 50% and rising to above 80% in the presence of some immunologic abnormalities.

Early detection and aggressive treatment of infection can improve the outcome. The presence of fever in such patients demands a careful evaluation to identify the source of infection. Treatment should be very aggressive after hospitalization with intravenous antibiotics and careful monitoring as these children progress to irreversible shock very rapidly. After splenectomy, the child must be given pneumococcal, meningococcal and H. influenzae type b vaccines, if not already vaccinated.

REFERENCES

1. Cohen A. Hematologic emergencies. *In*: Textbook of Pediatric Emergency Medicine. Fleisher G, Ludwig S, Henretig F (Eds). *Philadelphia: Lippincott Williams & Wilkins;* 4th Ed, 2000. pp. 349-359

2. Vats T. Acute intravascular hemolysis. In: Medical Emergencies in Children. Singh M., (Ed.), New Delhi: 4th Ed. *Sagar Publications; New Delhi* 2007. p. 315-322.

3. Barkin R. Hematologic and oncologic disorders. In: Pediatric Emergency Medicine Concepts and Clinical Practice. Barkin R, Asch S, Knapp J. *et al* (Eds.) *St. louis, Mosby Year Book,* Inc. 1992 pp. 828-844.

4. Sobota A, Neufeld E. Recognition and management of immune thrombocytopenic purpura and autoimmune hemolytic anemia in the emergency department. *Clin Pediatr Emerg Med* 2011; 12:245-252

5. Habibi B, Homberg J, Schaison G, Salmon C. Autoimmune haemolytic anemia in children: A review of 80 cases. *Amer J Med* 1974; 56:61-69.

6. Cohen A. Hematologic Emergencies In: Textbook of Pediatric Emergency. Fleisher G, Ludwig S, Henretig F, (Eds.), *Philadelphia: Lippincott Williams & Wilkins; 4th Ed,* 2000. p. 859-886.

7. Karan E, Paul M. Treatment of autoimmune hemolytic anemia. *Semin Hematol* 2005; 42:131-136.

8. Samuel C, Javier A. Hematologic emergencies: acute anemia. *Clin Ped Emerg Med* 2005; 6:124-137.

9. Macnab A, Macrae D, Henning R. Hematologic problems. In: Care of the Crtically Ill Child. Keeley S, (Ed.) *Churchill Livingstone; London;* 1st Ed 1999. p. 266-274.

10. Seth T. Hematological disorders. In: Essential Pediatrics. Ghai OP, Paul V.K, Bagga A, (Eds.) 7th Ed, *CBS Publishers; New Delhi,* 2010. pp. 296-328.

11. David C, Williams T, Gladwin M. Sickle cell disease. *Lancet* 2010; 376: 2018-2031.

12. Hampton R, Balasa V, Bracey A. Emergencies in patients with inherited hemoglobin disorders - An emergency department perspective. *Clin Ped Emerg Med* 2005; 6:138-148.

13. Zempsky W. Evaluation and treatment of sickle cell pain in the emergency department: Paths to a better future. *Clin Pediatr Emerg Med* 2010; 11:265-273.

14. Rogovik A, Ying Li, Kirby M, Friedman J, Goldman R. Admission and length of stay due to painful vasoocclusive crisis in children. *Amer J Emerg Med* 2009; 27:797-801

15. Carolyn H, Elliott V, Keith Q, Warmerdam V, Jane P, Katie A, Lori S. Use of hydroxyurea in children aged 2 to 5 years with sickle cell disease. *J Pediatr Hematol/Oncol* 2000; 22(4):330-334.

16. Claudia R, Elliott P, Jane W, Lorenzo BS, Diane K, Sidney M, Frans A. Hydroxyurea and arginine therapy: Impact on nitric oxide production in sickle cell disease. *J Pediatr Hematol/Oncol* 2003; 25(8):629-634.

17. Timothy C, Donald M, Bauchanan G. High dose intravenous methylprednisolone therapy for pain in children and adolescents with sickle cell disease. *N Engl J Med* 1994; 330:733-737.

18. Khemri M, Labassi A, Barsaoui S. Severe toxic methemoglobinemia mimicking septic shock in an infant. *Internat Emerg Nursing* 2009;17:181-183

19. Ronald B. An infant with sepsis and methemoglobinemia. *J Emerg Med* 1985; 3:261-264.

20. Meckler G, Lindermulder S. Fever and neutropenia in pediatric patients with cancer. *Emerg Med Clin N Am* 2009; 27:525-544.

21. Pizzo P. Hematologic supportive care of children with cancer. In: Principles and Practice of Pediatric Oncology. Pizzo P, Poplack D, Kluwer W, (Eds.) *Philadelphia: Lippincott Williams & Wilkins;* 6th Ed, 2011.

22. Seth R, Bhatt A. Management of common oncologic emergencies. *Indian J Pediatr* 2011; 78(6):709-717.

23. Hughes WT, Bodey GP, Bow EJ, *et al.* Guidelines for use of antimicrobial agents in neutropenic patients with cancer. *Clin Infect Dis* 2002; 34:730-751.

24. Parthasarathy A. Pediatric hematology. In: IAP Textbook of Pediatrics. Parthasarathy A, Menon PSN, Nair MKC, Eds. *Jaypee Brothers Medical Publishers; New Delhi:* 4th Ed, 2009. p. 767- 871.

25. Mediros D, Buchanan G. Hematology. In: Essentials of Pediatric Intensive Care. Levin D, Morriss F. (Eds.) *Philadelphia:* 2nd Ed, *Churchill Livingstone;* 1997. pp. 473-483.

26. Laurie H, Johnson, Gittelman M. Management of bleeding diathesis: a case-based approach. *Clin Ped Emerg Med* 2005; 6:149-155.

27. Gordan J, Mark L, Bernstein, *et al.* Hematologic disorders in pediatric intensive care unit. In: Textbook of Pediatric Intensive Care. Rogers M, (Ed.) Vol 2, *Williams & Wilkins; USA,* 1987, pp. 1181-1221.

28. Albayark D, IslekI, Gazi K, Gurses N. Acute immune thrombocytopenic purpura: A comparative study of very high oral doses of methylprednisolone and intravenously administered immune globulin. *J Pediatr* 1994; 125(6):1004-1007.

Section 4

29. Watts R. Idiopathic thrombocytopenic purpura: A 10-year natural history study at the childrens hospital of alabama. *Clin Pediatr* 2004; 43(8):691-702.

30. Kocak U, ZiyaY, Kayal Z, Ozturk G, Gursel T. Evaluation of clinical characteristics, diagnosis and management in childhood immune thrombocytopenic purpura: a single center's experience. *Turkish J Pediatr* 2007; 49:250-255.

31. Moser A, Shalev H, Kapelushnik J. Anti-D exerts a very early response in childhood acute idiopathic thrombocytopenic purpura. *Inform Healthcare Pediatr Hematol-Oncol* 2002; 19(6):407-411.

32. Zerella J, Martin L, Lampkin B. Emergency splenectomy for idiopathic thrombocytopenic purpura in children. *J Pediatr Surg* 1978; 13:243-246.

33. Hu Bo, Wang KE. Diagnostic significance of examining the plasma levels of D-dimers and FDP in disseminated intravascular coagulation. *Chongqing Med J* 2004; 11:37.

Section 4

43

Oncological Emergencies

Sameer Bakhshi and Meharban Singh

INTRODUCTION

Advances in the diagnosis and therapy of pediatric cancers has resulted in an increasing number of referrals of children with cancer. This success is accompanied with the need for recognition and proper treatment of emergencies due to various malignancies. Usually, these children are moderately ill at the time of presentation allowing time for an organised work-up. However, they can present occasionally with life-threatening complications either due to the disease or due to cytotoxic and immunosuppressive treatment, which merit urgent attention and intervention. A pathophysiological classification, clinical features and management of common oncological emergencies are discussed.

Broadly speaking, oncologic emergencies can arise in one of the following ways:

1. A solid tumor may invade or compress vital organs (mechanical emergency). Space occupying malignancies in the anterior mediastinum may compress superior vena cava, trachea and esophagus producing mechanical obstruction. Metastasis in the brain may produce raised intracranial tension and tumors compressing the spinal cord can cause irreversible paraplegia. Effusions in the pleural and pericardial cavities may compromise the heart and lung functions.

2. Blood and blood vessel complications such as bleeding, anemia and life-threatening infection may occur due to bone marrow depression. CNS complications may occur due to leukostasis and cerebrovascular accidents due to arteriovenous thrombosis.

3. Malignant disorder or its therapy may produce hormonal or metabolic complications. Hormonal problems can occur because of paraneoplastic secretions. Metabolic problems may develop following rapid lysis of malignant cells and diagnostic procedures or chemotherapy may damage a vital organ.

Table 43.1 lists the common oncologic emergencies. The more frequently encountered complications e.g. superior mediastinal syndrome, febrile neutropenia, acute tumor lysis syndrome and spinal cord compression are discussed in detail.

SUPERIOR VENA CAVA SYNDROME/ SUPERIOR MEDIASTINAL SYNDROME

Superior vena cava syndrome (SVCS) is a symptom complex resulting from compression or obstruction of the superior vena cava. When tracheal compression also occurs, it is called superior mediastinal syndrome (SMS). In children tracheal compression with resultant respiratory difficulty occurs more frequently along with SVC obstruction as compared to adults. These terms, therefore, may be used interchangeably.

Superior vena cava (SVC) is surrounded by lymph nodes draining the right side and lower left side of the chest and the thymus in the anterior superior mediastinum. Enlargement of these structures first compresses the thin walled SVC, which may subsequently develop thrombosis in upto 50 percent of cases. The trachea and the right main bronchus also get readily compressed in children. The relatively small tracheal diameter gets easily compromised and blocked even by minimal edema. The combination of compression and edema result in both reduced airflow and blood flow into thorax.

Malignant tumors which cause SMS are most commonly non Hodgkin's lymphomas (NHL) and T-cell acute lymphoblastic leukemias (ALL)[1]. Germ cell tumors and Hodgkin lymphoma are also implicated. Hodgkin lymphoma is less likely to cause SVCS as it is slow growing and this gives time for the blood vessels to form collaterals. D'Angio reported only 9 cases of SMS among 607 children with cancer[2]. However, in children with malignant anterior mediastinum tumor, SMS is seen in about 12 percent cases[3].

Table 43.1 Common causes of oncologic emergencies

Mechanical compression	Causes
Thoracic	Superior vena cava syndrome/ superior mediastinal syndrome: NHL, T-cell leukemia, Hodgkin's disease Pleural effusion: Lymphoma Cardiac tamponade: Leukemia
Abdominal	Intestinal obstruction: NHL Urinary flow obstruction: Retro-peritoneal sarcoma
Neurological system	CNS metastases, brain tumor Spinal cord compression: Neuro-blastoma, sarcoma, lymphoma
Massive hepatomegaly	Stage IVS neuroblastoma
Hyperleukocytosis (TLC >100,000/ mm³)	CNS leukostasis, pulmonary leukostasis

Blood or blood vessels	
Infections	Febrile neutropenia, catheter-related sepsis, acute typhilitis, perirectal abscess,
Hemorrhage Anemia Leukostasis Venous thromboembolism	L-asparaginase, cisplatin, methotrexate

Metabolic/hormonal	
Metabolic	Acute tumor lysis syndrome Hypercalcemia of malignancy (ALL, NHL, neuroblastoma, Ewing's sarcoma)
Hormonal	Syndrome of inappropriate secretion of antidiuretic hormone (SIADH)

Therapy related	
Hemorrhagic cystitis	Cyclophosphamide, ifosfamide
Cardiomyopathy	Anthracycline
Drug extravasation causing necrosis	Anthracycline, vinca alkaloids
Hemorrhagic pancreatitis	L- asparaginase
Cerebrovascular accidents	Methotrexate, L-asparaginase

Children with SMS/ SVCS may present with cough, orthopnea, headache, hoarseness of voice, difficulty in swallowing, facial swelling and episodes of dizziness. History of worsening of symptoms on Valsalva maneuver may be present. On examination, these children look anxious and may have swelling and plethora of face and neck, conjunctival suffusion, dilatation of veins and edema over neck and upper extremities, papilledema and pulsus paradoxus. Position change may induce changes in respiration and blood pressure. There may be signs of tracheal compression such as decreased air entry, wheezing and stridor. In those with severe compromise, there may be extreme anxiety and restlessness. Symptoms of confusion, irritability, headache, seizures, coma may occur due to raised ICT because of poor venous return from the brain. Right sided pleural effusion may be associated in 20 percent of patients with SMS. Lymphadenopathy in supraclavicular and other areas is often present, but is not invariable.

Investigations

Anteroposterior and lateral chest radiographs are useful to confirm the diagnosis of SMS. They may show widening of superior mediastinum, tracheal deviation to either side and compression which may be anteroposterior or lateral. The history, physical examination and chest radiographs are usually sufficient to generate a differential diagnosis and outline the plan of management. Pericardial tamponade, pleural effusion and congestive cardiac failure should be excluded since they may coexist along with SMS/ SVCS. Serum β-HCG and α-fetoprotein levels may be increased in germ cell tumors.

It is desirable to establish a tissue diagnosis by the least invasive method prior to therapy but at times it is impossible because of the hazards of general anesthesia. Anesthetic procedure entails positioning of the child which may embarrass air and venous return and intubation may be technically difficult. Increase in abdominal muscle tone and decrease in tone of respiratory muscles, relaxation of bronchial smooth muscles and decrease in lung volume may all aggravate SVC compression. The procedure may be associated with uncontrollable hemorrhage; and at times extubation may be exceedingly difficult. Due to these reasons, sincere attempts should be made to obtain the tissue diagnosis from peripheral studies. A peripheral blood count or bone marrow examination often confirms the diagnosis of leukemia. Peripheral lymph node aspiration or biopsy under local anesthesia may confirm the diagnosis of lymphoma. Pleural or pericardiocentesis fluid cytology and flow-cytometry may yield the diagnosis. If the diagnosis is not established by these procedures, computerized tomography (CT) of the chest, upright and supine echocardiography, and a flow volume loop should be evaluated to assess the anesthetic risk. If the patient has low anesthetic risk, a biopsy should be taken under general anesthesia. When despite serious attempts, it is not possible to obtain tissue diagnosis, empirical therapy is advised as depicted in the algorithm (Figure 43.1).

Chemotherapy and radiotherapy may both confound the tissue diagnosis within 48 hours of

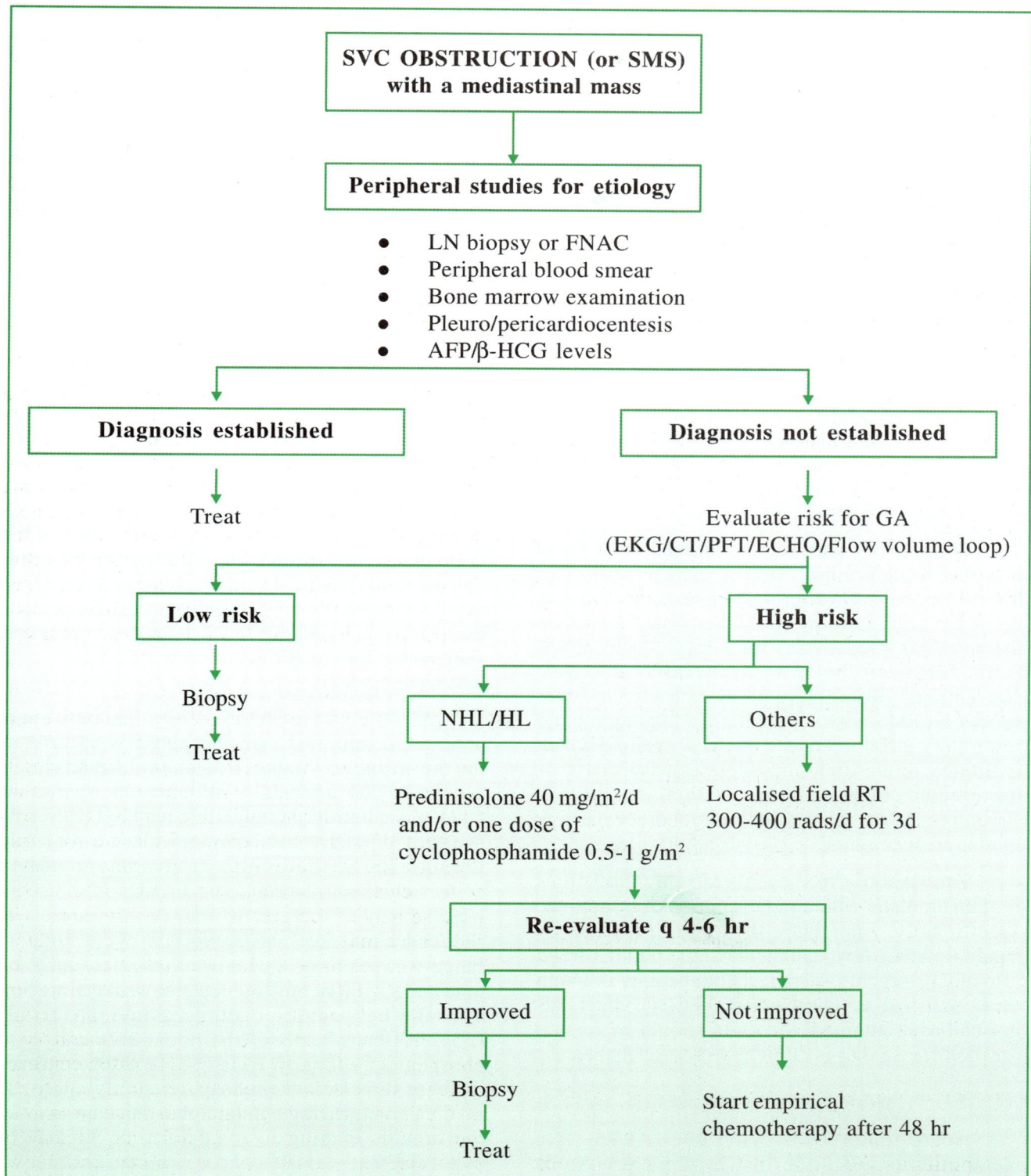

Figure 43.1 Approach to a child with superior mediastinal syndrome

therapy. The biopsy of 8 out of 19 patients were rendered uninterpretable by prebiopsy radiation for mediastinal masses[4]. However, the management of the patient was not altered by the prebiopsy therapy or by continued empirical therapy in the same study.

Management

Children with SMS/SVCS need to be managed under expert guidance. Nursing in propped up position may help in decreasing intracranial pressure. Cautious use of diuretics may provide transient symptomatic relief. It is advisable to avoid IV line insertion in the upper limbs so that no further increase in venous pressure on the upper part of the body occurs. If one is able to make a diagnosis of NHL or Hodgkin's or acute leukemia, steroids alone or in combination with cyclophosphamide may be given to rapidly relieve the symptoms. If a diagnosis of above mentioned possibilities is strongly suspected but cannot be established and the child is not fit for general anesthesia, therapeutic measures outlined in Figure 43.1 may be instituted. In germ cell tumors, a combination of cisplatin and etopopside is administered. Though bleomycin is part of therapy for germ cell tumors, this may be avoided in the setting of SMS because of its potential lung toxicity.

The patient should be reassessed several times in a day to determine whether there is sufficient improvement to allow tissue biopsy. Biopsy should be undertaken as soon as it is feasible. Radiation therapy (300-400 rads/day for 3 days) to a localised field followed by a radiotherapy at lower conventional dosing may be more useful in other causes of SMS/SVCS. Irradiation may aggravate respiratory difficulty due to tracheal swelling which is limited to children and adolescents because of the greater compressibility of their respiratory structures and the inability of their relatively narrow lumina to accommodate post-irradiation edema.

The response to these therapeutic modalities is often dramatic with rapid resolution of symptoms. Traditionally, emergency therapy is provided by irradiation. However, an increasingly popular trend is to initiate urgent systemic chemotherapy, although no established standards exist. If tissue diagnosis is finally not attained, the child should be treated for the disease that is clinically most probable.

ACUTE TUMOR LYSIS SYNDROME (ATLS)

Acute tumor lysis syndrome (ALTS) is a metabolic complication due to rapid release of intracellular metabolites like potassium, uric acid and phosphates in quantities that exceed the excretory capacity[5, 6]. Secondary renal failure and hypocalcemia are common complications following ATLS. The syndrome is most commonly seen following chemotherapy of hematologic malignancies.

Tumor lysis syndrome occurs before therapy or upto 1-5 days after the start of specific chemotherapy in those tumors that have a high growth and marked chemosensitivity. It is most commonly seen in younger age patients with Burkitt's NHL (doubling time 38-116 hours), acute myelomonocytic leukemia (AML-M4), acute monocytic leukemia (AML-MS), T-cell leukemia and in ALL with hyperleukoycytosis (WBC count > 100,000/mm^3). Other factors which are known to predispose to this syndrome include bulky abdominal tumors, tumor infiltration of the kidneys, dehydration, obstructive uropathy, pretherapy raised levels of uric acid, high lactate dehydrogenase, and elevated creatinine with reduced urine output. In the presence of these predisposing factors, aggressive chemotherapy may precipitate the metabolic emergency.

Pathogenesis and clinical features

Hyperleukocytosis and leukostasis may affect intracerebral and pulmonary circulation. CNS manifestation indude headache, confusion, convulsions, focal deficits, sensorial changes, papilledema or retinal venous distension. Pulmonary leukostasis may cause dyspnea, hypoxemia and right ventricular failure. Priapism may occur in severe hyperleukocytosis.

All the three intracellular metabolites; potassium, uric acid and phosphates are excreted by the kidneys. Successful chemotherapy may accelerate the process of spontaneous lysis that takes place before therapy. Uric acid, an excretory product of DNA breakdown (pKa: 5.4), may precipitate in the acidic environment of the collecting tubules, producing urinary obstruction which further increase in urate levels due to its reduced excretion and a vicious cycle ensues. Precursors of purine are known to regulate vascular tone and therefore may reduce glomerular filtration by causing preglomerular vasoconstriction. Lymphoblasts are rich in phosphates; hyperphosphatemia (due to lysis of lymphoblasts) may increase the calcium × phosphate product beyond 60 thus precipitating calcium phosphate crystals in the tubules leading to renal failure. Secondary hypocalcemia may also occur as a consequence of hyperphosphatemia. Hyperkalemia may occur because of its extracellular release (cytosol

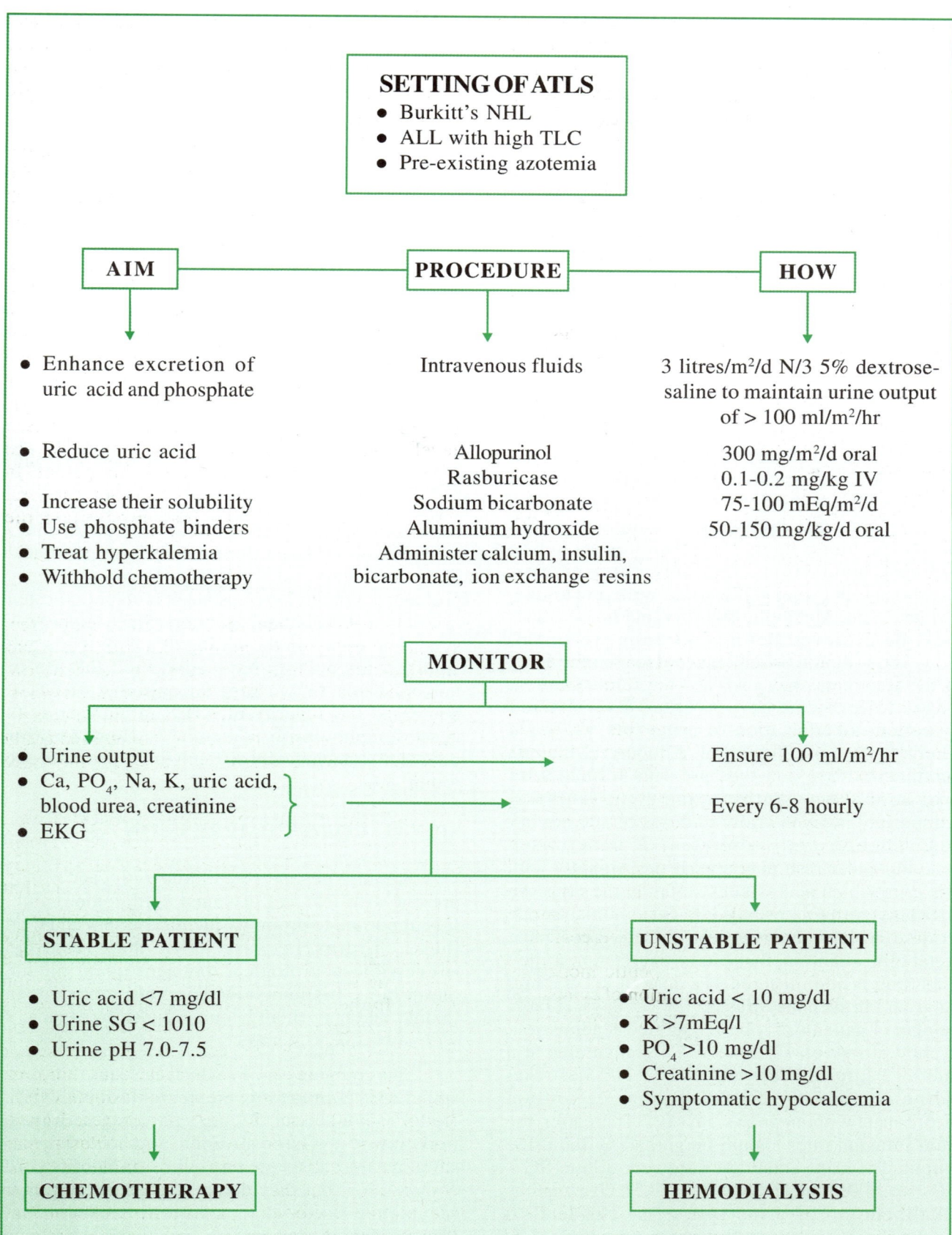

SETTING OF ATLS
- Burkitt's NHL
- ALL with high TLC
- Pre-existing azotemia

AIM — **PROCEDURE** — **HOW**

- Enhance excretion of uric acid and phosphate
- Reduce uric acid
- Increase their solubility
- Use phosphate binders
- Treat hyperkalemia
- Withhold chemotherapy

Intravenous fluids

Allopurinol
Rasburicase
Sodium bicarbonate
Aluminium hydroxide
Administer calcium, insulin,
bicarbonate, ion exchange resins

3 litres/m²/d N/3 5% dextrose-saline to maintain urine output of > 100 ml/m²/hr

300 mg/m²/d oral
0.1-0.2 mg/kg IV
75-100 mEq/m²/d
50-150 mg/kg/d oral

MONITOR

- Urine output
- Ca, PO₄, Na, K, uric acid, blood urea, creatinine
- EKG

Ensure 100 ml/m²/hr

Every 6-8 hourly

STABLE PATIENT
- Uric acid <7 mg/dl
- Urine SG < 1010
- Urine pH 7.0-7.5

UNSTABLE PATIENT
- Uric acid < 10 mg/dl
- K >7mEq/l
- PO₄ >10 mg/dl
- Creatinine >10 mg/dl
- Symptomatic hypocalcemia

CHEMOTHERAPY

HEMODIALYSIS

Figure 43.2 Anticipatory management of acute tumor lysis syndrome

Section 4

breakdown) or due to urate and calcium phosphate nephropathy; which may prove fatal if untreated. Clinical manifestations of hyperuricemia include lethargy, nausea, and vomiting and finally renal failure. Hyperphosphatemia may precipitate hypocalcemia and cause tissue damage due to calcium phosphate precipitation in the tissues. Tissue damage may present as pruritic or gangrenous skin lesions, arthritis, eye inflammation or as renal failure. Hypocalcemia can present as tetany, carpopedal spasms, cramps, seizures, alteration in sensorium or as cardiac arrest. Acute renal failure, cardiac dysrhythmias, neuromuscular symptoms due to hyperkalemia and hypocalcemia may lead to sudden death.

Management

The management of tumor lysis begins with identification of potential high risk patients and institution of aggressive prophylactic measures (Figure 43.2). A child at risk of developing ATLS requires frequent laboratory testing, often 6-8 hourly, of blood counts, electrolytes including sodium, potassium, calcium, phosphorus, bicarbonate and metabolites like urea, creatinine, and uric acid. Metabolic stability and homeostasis must be achieved before initiating treatment. However, it should be remembered that undue delay in the treatment may increase the tumor burden. Renal failure can be prevented by ensuring hydration, alkalinization of urine (pH >7.0) and administration of allopurinol. Allopurinol inhibits xanthine oxidase and thus prevents formation of uric acid from xanthine and hypoxanthine. Allopurinol is given orally in doses of 300 mg/m^2/day. Though well tolerated, a generalised maculopapular rash may appear occasionally with this drug which necessitates stopping the drug. An alternative drug is, rasburicase (recombinant urate oxidase) which converts uric acid to a water soluble metabolite allantoin, that can be excreted in urine[7]. This drug is administered at a dose of 0.1-0.2 mg/kg as an intravenous infusion for 1-5 days. A large number of patients may be dehydrated at admission. A child at risk of ATLS should be rehydrated at a rate of 3 litres/m^2/day with N/3 or N/2 dextrose-saline made with 75-100 mEq/m^2 of sodium bicarbonate without potassium salts. Thereafter, the fluid infusion rates should be guided by the urine output. The urine should be kept very dilute (SG ~ 1.000 to 1.005) and alkaline (pH 7-7.5). Overzealous alkalinization of urine (pH >7.5) can lead to worsening of nephropathy. At a pH above 7.5, xanthine and hypoxanthine stones may form and, at a pH of 8 or above, calcium phosphate may crystallize in the kidneys. The prophylactic measures outlined in Figure 43.2 are sufficient to prevent clinically significant tumor lysis syndrome. Alkalinization is associated with increased risk of development of clinical tetany. Cautious use of diuretics and mannitol is recommended to enhance urinary excretion of uric acid and phosphates.

When hyperkalemia is associated with impending renal failure, potassium intake should be stopped and kayexalate (1 g/kg) with 50% sorbitol should be administered orally. Intravenous calcium gluconate (100-200 mg/kg/dose) is life saving by inducing intracellular shift of potassium. Insulin (1 unit/kg) with 2 ml/kg of 25% glucose as an IV bolus facilitates intracellular influx of potassium.

When frank or impending renal failure cannot be controlled by above mentioned measures, dialysis should be considered. Dialysis would not only improve metabolic problems of hyperkalemia, acidosis, azotemia, and hypocalcemia but would remove uric acid and phosphates. Hemodialysis and continuous hemofiltration are at least 10-20 times more effective than peritoneal dialysis. If peritoneal dialysis is undertaken, it may have to be very prolonged. For obvious reasons, it is contraindicated in children with abdominal tumors. Since tumor lysis syndrome occurs in the setting of a high white cell count, some authors have advocated the use of leukopharesis. In two large uncontrolled studies, it decreased the severity of ATLS in children with acute lymphoblastic leukemia[8, 9]. However, this procedure is technically difficult in the pediatric age group.

SPINAL CORD COMPRESSION

About 4 percent of children with cancer may present with features of spinal cord compression. It is important to promptly identify, assess and treat these children because delay may result in irreversible neurological damage (quadriplegia, paraplegia, bladder/bowel incontinence) even though one may finally "cure" the child of cancer with subsequent therapy.

The common cancers which can cause epidural spinal cord compression are neuroblastoma, NHL, Hodgkin lymphoma, Ewing's sarcoma and acute leukemia[10-14]. Osteosarcoma and rhabdomyosarcoma may also present with extradural cord compression, but they do so as a feature of tumor recurrence rather than at initial presentation. Primary spinal cord tumors such as ependymoma and astrocytoma are rare tumors, and they usually present as intramedullary tumors.

In contrast to adults, most cases of cord compression in children result from extension of paravertebral tumor through the intravertebral foramina into the epidural space rather than extension of tumor into the vertebral column. Once the tumor reaches the extradural space, it may obstruct the vertebral venous plexus due to its mass effect resulting in vasogenic cord edema, myelinolysis, hemorrhagic and ischemic infarction of the cord. The damage to the cord structures is from outer surface towards center. Therefore, posterior columns, anterior horn cells get damaged earlier than the centrally placed micturition centers.

The cardinal symptom of spinal cord compression is back pain. The pain may be radicular, localised to the back or diffuse. The pain was present for a median duration of 14 and 17 days before diagnosis in two large studies[5, 12]. The spine may be involved at any site with no specific predilection. The pain may be aggravated by coughing, Valsalva maneuver, neck flexion, by lying down or by straight leg raising. Sensory loss may occur but is difficult to ascertain in younger children. Variable degree of motor deficits may also occur, but usually start a few days after the onset of pain. Bladder and bowel incontinence are late symptoms and may indicate irreversibility of neurological weakness.

Epidural malignancy is perhaps the next most common cause of non-traumatic spinal cord compression after spinal tuberculosis. Hence, any child with back pain needs a detailed neurological examination and radiological evaluation. There may be local tenderness on percussion. Since spinal involvement in childhood malignancy occurs as a result of spread via the intervertebral foramina, plain radiographs are abnormal in only one third of children. Magnetic resonance imaging (MRI) is the modality of choice since it picks up epidural and paravertebral masses and vertebral metastases without being invasive. Although tuberculosis is a common diagnosis in such situations, sparing of intervertebral discs on MRI is an indicator that the lesion may be non-tubercular. Lumbar puncture for CSF examination is hazardous because it may precipitate neurological deterioration and is best avoided.

Management

All children with back pain and/or neurological deterioration should be investigated and treated on an urgent basis, particularly if the symptoms are progressing rapidly. Therefore, MRI should be planned within the next 24 hours. If a child has neurological weakness, IV dexamethasone 1-2 mg/kg should be given even prior to any imaging study to prevent further deterioration. If pain exists without weakness, oral dexamethasone 1-2 mg/kg/day in 4 divided doses should be given.

If imaging studies demonstrate epidural cord compression, specific therapy should be instituted. Since neuroblastoma, NHL and Ewing's sarcoma are very chemosensitive, specific chemotherapy for these tumors may be as rapidly effective as radiotherapy. Radiation is indicated for radio-sensitive tumors, but care has to be taken to include all tumor sites in the field of irradiation. Laminectomy is recommended for all tumors which do not get relieved with chemo/radiotherapy or for getting a tissue diagnosis in case it is not possible to have a confirmed diagnosis by peripheral studies. These children also require narcotic analgesics to relieve pain.

The prognosis for neurological recovery in children with cord compression is better than in adults, though it depends on the degree and duration of neurological weakness. In a series of 16 patients with neurological deficits who underwent either surgery (8 patients), chemotherapy (6 patients) and/or radiotherapy (4 patients), six (38%) had significant neurological improvement[5]. Children who are ambulatory at diagnosis usually remain ambulatory. As many as one-third to one-half of those who are bedridden begin to ambulate. Thus, it is important to make an early diagnosis and provide prompt treatment.

FEBRILE NEUTROPENIA

Febrile neutropenia is the commonest oncological emergency encountered in children with hematological cancers. Neutropenia, whether it is as a result of routine chemotherapy, underlying cancer itself or due to therapy for bone marrow transplantation, is defined as polymorphonuclear leukocyte count of less than 500 per cubic mm in the peripheral blood[9]. When a patient with neutropenia develops fever (one oral temperature reading of >38.5°C or more than two successive readings of 38°C in a 24 hour period), the child should be promptly examined and an empirical broad spectrum antibacterial regimen started[16]. Each center should strictly adhere to standard criteria for the diagnosis and management of febrile neutropenia. As a rule, even fevers that are observed after administration of blood products or fever-producing antineoplastic agents should be considered potentially infectious in origin, and treated according to a standard protocol (Figure

43.3). In most series, clinical or microbiological infection is documented in only 30 to 50 percent of all such episodes; the rest get labelled as fever of unknown origin.

Diagnosis

Initial evaluation should include a detailed physical examination to screen all possible sites for signs of infection. The usual manifestations of

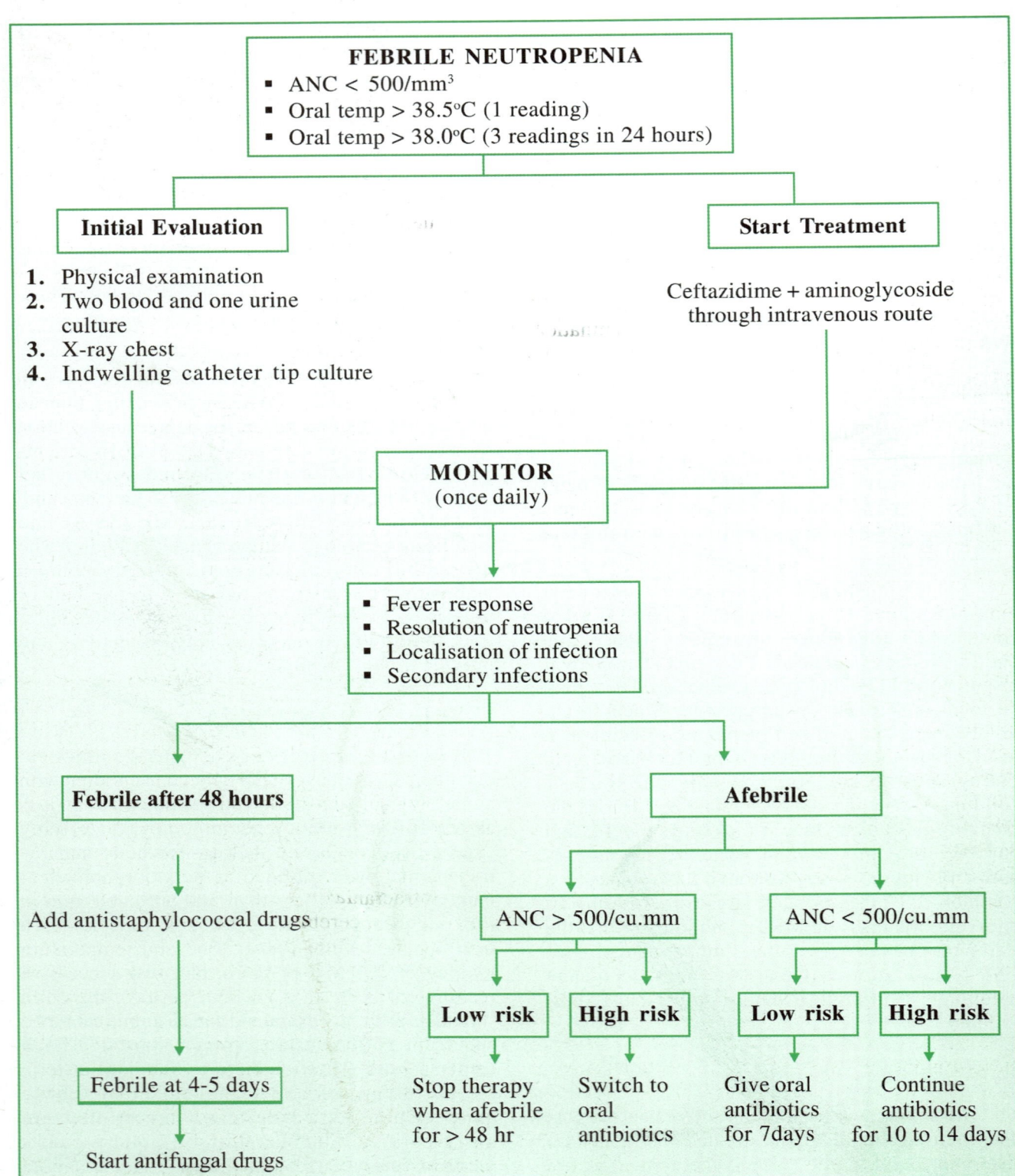

Figure 43.3 Management protocol for febrile neutropenia

infections (except fever) are masked in patients with neutropenia due to inadequate inflammatory response. Special efforts should be made to exclude infections of the ear, nose, throat (tonsillitis, sinusitis), chest, intestines (typhlitis, necrotizing enterocolitis, perirectal abscess) and integument (cellulitis). Subtle signs of meningeal infection should be looked for. Catheter and IV sites are potential sources of infection. The fundus must be examined to exclude candidal endophthalmitis.

It is recommended that at least two blood and one urine sample be taken for culture studies. In a child with an indwelling intravenous catheter, one blood culture should be drawn from the cannula and another from a peripheral vein. If a multiple lumen catheter is inserted, samples for culture should be drawn from all lumens. Urine should also be screened for fungi by microscopic examination for hyphae and culture. A chest radiograph is necessary only if there are respiratory symptoms, it may not be done routinely in all episodes[17]. In those with chest symptoms, persistent fever and an abnormal radiograph, a high resolution CT scan of chest should be done to look for evidences of invasive Aspergillosis. The common radiological signs include ground glass opacities with halo sign and infarcts.

As mentioned earlier, despite advances in diagnostic methods, infection is documented only in 30-40 percent patients[16]. In certain series, presence of fever of >39°C, associated hypotension, absolute neutrophil count of <100/mm^3 and duration of neutropenia for >7 days have been shown to be associated more frequently with bacteremia among all episodes of febrile neutropenia[18, 19]. Low risk febrile neutropenic patients are those in whom the duration of neutropenia is less than 7 days with no obvious focus of infection and they are hemodynamically stable. The low risk patients can be provided routine in-patient care or even managed on ambulatory basis[20].

Management

In all neutropenic patients, barrier nursing should be practised. Hand washing and wearing of gloves should be strictly observed in handling these patients. The predominant infectious agents seen in most centers are Gram-negative organisms (Klebsiella, Enterobacter, Pseudomonas), staphylococci and fungi (candida, aspergillus). Therefore, commonly recommended therapy is a combination of antipseudomonal antibiotic (ceftazidime, cefaperazone/sulbactam) and an

aminoglycoside. Combination of oral amoxicillin-clavulanate with ofloxacin or ceftriaxone with amikacin have been used for low risk febrile neutropenia[20, 21]. Although carbapenems have been used as a single agent for empiric treatment of febrile neutropenia, they are generally used as a second line antibiotic in such patients[22]. If there is an indwelling line *in-situ* or there is no response in 48 hours, antistaphylococcal antibiotic should be added. The choice should be determined by the institutional antibacterial sensitivity data[23, 24]. If fever persists for 4-5 days, antifungal drugs such as amphotericin B should be added empirically[25, 26]. Alternative antifungals specifically for invasive Aspergillosis include voriconazole and caspofungin. In certain clinical situations, co-trimoxazole is administered to cover *Pneumocystis carinii* and anerobes.

When febrile episodes resolve in less than 48 hours, children with leukemia in remission (showing signs of marrow recovery in the form of normalising platelets or improving absolute neutrophil count) and when no evidence of infection is apparent clinically or on microbiology in 48 hours, the antibiotics can be switched off or given orally. The child may be discharged even if the ANC is <500/mm^3.[27, 28] However, if the fever takes longer to respond, the cultures are positive or the ANC is <100/mm^3 on admission, antibiotics are given for 10 to 14 days or till the ANC increases beyond 500/ mm^3.[29] Granulocyte colony stimulating factor in a dose of 5mg/kg/day in addition to antibiotics results in a more rapid neutrophil recovery and relatively fewer days of antibiotic use, though overall response rates are similar[30].

MISCELLANEOUS CONDITIONS

Raised intracranial pressure

Intracranial pressure may be raised due to tumor mass, cerebral edema and obstruction of cerebrospinal fluid pathways by leptomeningeal deposits. The clinical manifestations include headache, vomiting, ataxia, confusion, neurological deficits, seizures and sensorial changes. CT scan and MRI of brain are diagnostic. Apart from general measures (elevation of head, diuretics, mannitol), high dose dexamethasone is useful. Neurosurgical procedures like resection of tumor, decompression or insertion of ventriculoperitoneal shunt may be necessary. Radiotherapy and more recently radiosurgery are useful modalities in selected cases[31].

Neutropenic enterocolitis

Neutropenic enterocolitis or typhlitis is an acute life-threatening inflammation of the small and large bowel, often seen in children with malignancies who are associated with prolonged neutropenia. Apart from mucosal ulcerations due to neutropenic enterocolitis, it may be associated with vincristine induced ileus, L-asparaginase induced pancreatitis, drug induced cholestasis and cholecystitis, intussusception due to bowel tumor or mesenteric lymphnodes and fungal infection.

The early symptoms may be non specific which are followed characteristic features of intestinal perforation, peritonitis and ileus. CT abdomen may show diffusely thickened cecum and ascending colon. The condition is managed by bowel rest, gastric decompression, administration of broad spectrum antibiotics to cover Gram-negative organisum and anerobes and blood component support. Surgery is indicated for intestinal perforation and persistent GI bleeding in the absence of thrombocytopenia. The outcome of these patients is dismal with high mortality rate between 50-100 percent[32].

Venous thromboembolism

Malignant disorders are associated with increased risk of thromboses due to hyper-coagulable state, indwelling central catheters, prolonged immobilization, chemotherapy and surgical procedures[33]. Peripheral venous thrombosis manifests with swollen extremity with evidences of vascular occlusion as suggested by ultrasound flow Doppler. Pulmonary embolism is characterized by sudden onset of dyspnea, pleuritic chest pain, hemoptysis, dizziness or syncope. Skiagram of chest may be normal or show oligemia of the affected segment, linear atelectasis, small pleural effusion or wedge-shaped opacity. ECG shows tachycardia, right ventricular strain pattern or classical $S_1Q_3T_3$ pattern. The diagnosis can be confirmed by spiral CT of thorax, CT pulmonary angiogram or a ventilation/perfusion scan. Cortical venous thromboses may occur in children with ALL and patients on L-asparaginase therapy. Thrombolysis is recommended by administration of unfractionated low molecular weight heparin. Surgical procedures like thrombectomy and placement of IVC filter are recommended in patients with recurrent thromboembolism and when thrombolysis is contraindicated.

REFERENCES

1. Issa PY, Brinhi ER, Janin Y, Slim MS. Superior vena cava syndrome in childhood. *Pediatrics* 1982; 71: 337-341.

2. D'Angio GJ, Mitus A, Evans AE. The superior mediastinal syndrome in children with cancer. *Amer J Roentgenol Radium Ther Nucl Med* 1965; 93: 535-544.

3. King RM, Telander RL, Smithson WA. Primary mediastinal tumors in children. *J Pediatr Surg* 1982; 17:512-517.

4. Klein TS, Neil HS. Lymphadenopathy and aspiration biopsy cytology. *Cancer* 1984; 53:1076-1081.

5. Bouffet E, Marec-Berard P, Thiesse P, Carrie C, Risk T, Jouvet A, Brunat–Mentigny M, Mottolese C. Spinal cord compression by secondary epi- and intradural metastasis in childhood. *Childs Nerv Syst* 1997; 13: 383-387.

6. Cohen LF, Balow JE, Magrath IT, *et al*. Acute tumor lysis syndrome. A review of 37 patients with Burkitt's lymphoma. *Amer J Med* 1980; 68:486-493.

7. Pession A, Barbieri E. Treatment and prevention of tumor lysis syndrome in children. Experience of Associasione Italiana Ematologia Oncologia Pediatrica. *Contrib Nephrol* 2005; 147:80-92.

8. Bunin NJ, Piu Ch. Differing complications of hyperleukocytosis in children with acute lymphoblastic or nonlymphoblastic leukemia. *J Clin Oncol* 1985; 3:1590-1595.

9. Maurer HS, Steinherz PG, Gaynon PS, *et al*. Management of hyperleukocytosis (HL) in children with acute lymphoblastic leukemia (abstract). *Proc Amer Soc Clin Oncol* 1985; 4:172.

10. Aysun S, Topeu M, Gunay M, Topaloglu H. Neurological features as initial presentation of childhood malignancies. *Pediatr Neurol* 1994; 10:40-43.

11. Kataoka A, Shimizu K, Matsumoto T, *et al*. Epidural spinal cord compression as an initial symptom in childhood acute lymphoblastic leukemia: rapid decompression by local irradiation and systemic chemotherapy. *Paediatr Hematol Oncol* 1995; 12: 179-184.

12. Klein SL, Sanford RA, Muhlbauer MS. Pediatric spinal cord metastasis. *J Neurosurg* 1991; 74:70.

13. Lewis DW, Packer RJ, Raney B, *et al*. Incidence, presentation and outcome of spinal cord disease in children with systemic cancer. *Pediatrics* 1986; 78:438.

14. Mora J, Wollner N. Primary epidural non-Hodgkin lymphoma: spinal cord compression syndrome as the initial form of presentation in childhood non-Hodgkin lymphoma. *Med Pediatr Oncol* 1999; 32: 102-105.

15. Hughes WT, Armstrong D, Bodey GP, *et al*. Guidelines for the use of antimicrobial agents in neutropenic patients with unexplained fever: A statement by Infectious Disease Society of America. *J Infect Dis* 1990; 161:381-396.

Section 4

16. Pizzo PA. Evaluation of fever in the patient with cancer. *Eur J Cancer Clin Oncol* 1989; 25:S9-S16.

17. Korones DN, Hussong MR, Gullace MA. Routine chest radiography of children with cancer hospitalised for fever and neutropenia: is it really necessary? *Cancer* 1997; 80:1160-1164.

18. Hann I, Viscoli C, Paesmans M, Gaya H, Glauser M. A comparison of outcome from febrile neutropenic episode in children compared with adults: results from EORTC studies. *Br J Hematol* 1997; 99:580-588.

19. Rackoff WR, Gonier R, Robinson C, Kreissman SG, Breitfeld PB. Predicting the risk of bactermia in children with fever and neutropenia. *J Clin Oncol* 1996; 14: 919-927.

20. Gupta A, Swaroop C, Agarwala S, Pandey RM, Bakhshi S. Randomized controlled trial comparing oral amoxicillin-clavulanate and ofloxacin with intravenous ceftriaxone and amikacin as outpatient therapy in pediatric low-risk febrile neutropenia. *J Pediatr Hematol Oncol* 2009; 31(9):635-641.

21. Malik IA. Outpatient management of febrile neutropenia in indigent pediatric patients. *Ann Acad Med Singapore* 1997; 26:742-746.

22. Riikonen P. Imipenen compared with ceftazidime plus vancomycin as initial therapy for fever in neutropenic children with cancer. *Pediatr Infect Dis J* 1991; 10: 918-923.

23. Ghosh I, Raina V, Kumar L, Sharma A, Bakhshi S, Thulkar S, Kapil A. Profile of infections and outcome in high-risk febrile neutropenia: experience from a tertiary care cancer center in India. *Med Oncol* 2011 Feb 20. (Epub ahead of print).

24. Bakhshi S, Padmanjali KS, Arya LS. Infections in childhood acute lymphoblastic leukemia: an analysis of 222 febrile neutropenic episodes. *Pediatr Hematol Oncol* 2008 Jun; 25(5):385-392.

25. European Organization and Research and Treatment of Cancer (EORTC). International Antimicrobial Therapy Cooperative Group. Empirical antifungal therapy in febrile granulocytopenic patients. *Am J Med* 1989; 86:668-672.

26. Pizzo PA, Robichaud KJ, Gill FA, *et al.* Empirical antibiotic therapy and antifungal therapy for cancer patients with prolonged fever and granulocytopenia. *Am J Med* 1982; 72:101-110.

27. Aquino VM, Buchanan GR, Tkaczewski I, Mustafa MM. Safety of early hospital discharge of selected febrile children and adolescents with cancer with prolonged neutropenia. *Med Pediatr Oncol* 1997; 28:191-195.

28. Lau RC, Doyle JJ, Freedman MH, King SM, Richardson SE. Early discharge of pediatric febrile neutropenic cancer patients by substitution of oral for intravenous antibiotics. *Paediatr Hematol Oncol* 1994; 11:417-421.

29. Pizzo PA, Robichaud KJ, Gill FA, *et al.* Duration of empirical antibiotic therapy in granulocytopenic patients with cancer. *Amer J Med* 1979; 67:194-200.

30. Mitchell PL, Morland B, Stevens MC, *et al.* Granulocyte colony stimulating factor in established febrile neutropenia: a randomized study of pediatric patients. *J Clin Oncol* 1997; 15:1163-1170.

31. Mitera S, Swaminath A, Wong S, Goh P, *et al.* Radiotherapy for oncological emergencies on weekends. Examining reasons for treatment and patterns of practice at a Canadian cancer center. *Current Oncology* 2009, 16: 55-60.

32. Moir CR, Scudamore CH, Benny WB. Typhilitis: selective surgical management. *Amer J Surg* 1986, 151: 563-566.

33. Athale UH, Chan AK. Hematological complications or pediatric hematological emergencies. *Semin Thromb Hemostat* 2007, 33: 408-415.

Section 4

44

Emergencies Due to Inborn Errors of Metabolism

Madhulika Kabra

Inborn errors of metabolism (IEM) are genetic disorders which are caused by deficiency of an enzyme leading to a block in the metabolic pathway. Although individually IEMs are rare but collectively they are not uncommon. They generally present as a life-threatening emergency during newborn period or infancy. The presenting symptoms of these disorders are nonspecific and hence the pediatrician should have a high index of suspicion. There is a need for early diagnosis as timely management can be life saving and specific treatment modalities are available for certain disorders. Moreover, accurate diagnosis is important for prognostication, genetic counseling and prenatal diagnosis in subsequent pregnancies. Most of these disorders have an autosomal recessive inheritance and only a few are X-linked or mitochondrial.

INCIDENCE

Estimated burden of IEM is around 3-4/1000 live births. About 5% of genetic causes of mental retardation are due to IEM[1]. According to various studies from India 0.5 – 2.4% of mentally retarded children have been reported to have an amino acid metabolism disorder. In a study at AIIMS, 2560 cases were screened for inborn errors of metabolism; 49 (1.9%) had amino acid disorders[2]. In a recent study from Hyderabad, screening of 20,000 newborn babies revealed a very high prevalence of congenital hypothyroidism. The next common condition was congenital adrenal hyperplasia followed by G6PD deficiency. Amino acid disorders as a group constituted the next most common disorder[3]. In this chapter we would restrict our discussion on small molecular diseases which present as a life-threatening emergency in infancy and early childhood.

IEMs are primarily classified into two major groups; small molecule diseases and large molecule diseases (Table 44.1)[4]. The major categories of IEMs which can present as an acute emergency can be divided in two major groups . The first group includes disorders that present as acute intoxication usually with encephalopathy like picture but there may be other systemic manifestations or specific organ involvement like liver[5].The examples in this group include aminoacidopathies,organic acidurias (OA), urea cycle disorders (UCD), porphyrias and disorders of sugar metabolism etc. The age of presentation can be neonatal period, infancy, childhood or even later in life. After the neonatal period the manifestations can be intermittent or episodic The second group includes IEMs of intermediary metabolism affecting the cytoplasmic and mitochondrial energy processes. These include disorders of carbohydrate metabolism, mitochondrial

Table 44.1 Clinical classification of inborn errors of metabolism[4]		
Acute onset (generally present in infancy)	**Intermittent onset (precipitated by stress, infection, starvation, diet)**	**Chronic onset (generally present late in childhood)**
Due to small molecular defect (amino acids, organic acids, simple sugars)	Caused by milder metabolic derangements (small molecules)	Due to large molecule defect or storage disorder
Poor feeding, lethargy,vomiting, convulsions, hypotonia, cataract, abnormal body odor. They present like septicemia but sepsis screen is negative.	Repeated episodes ofalterations in consciousness, acidosis or ketosis, hypoglycemia, weakness, ataxia/ spasticity, diarrhea, vomiting and "Reye-like episodes".	Progressive CNS degeneration manifested as seizures, developmental delay or failure to thrive and mental retardation. Hypotonia/spasticity, coarse facies, muscular weakness, organomegaly, and abnormal fundus.

defects, Kreb's cycle and pyruvate oxidation defects and fatty acid oxidation defects (FAOD)

The common presenting manifestations of these disorders is summarized in Tables 44.2 and 44.3[5].

Table 44.2 IEMs presenting as acute illness in neonates and infant <3 months		
Main clinical presentation	**Presenting sign**	**Possible Disorder**
Neurological	Metabolic encephalopathy Seizures + microcephaly	BCAA disorders (MSUD, MMA, PA, IVA, MCD) Glutaric aciduria type II, UCD, Triple H B$_6$-responsive seizures MCD Folinic acid-responsive seizures Cerebral glucose carrier: GLUTI
Hepatic	Encephalopathy	Galactosemia Hereditary fructose intolerance Tyrosinemia type I
Cardiac	Cardiac failure Cardiomyopathy Arrhythmias	Long-chain FAO defects GSD II
Severe hypoglycemia		Glycogenosis type I/III Congenital hyperinsulinism FAO defects Carnitine uptake defect

Modified from reference (5)
Abbreviations : BCAA: Branched chain amino acids, MSUD: Maple syrup urine disease, MMA: Methylmelonic aciduria, PA: Propionic acidemia, IVA: isovaleric acidemia, MCD: Multiple carboxylase deficiency, UCD: Urea cycle defects, GSD: Glycogen storage disorder, FAO: fatty acid oxidation

Table 44.3 Late-onset (late infancy to adulthood) IEMs with acute presentation		
Main clinical presentation	**Important signs/lab abnormalities**	**Possible disorder**
Metabolic coma without focal neurological signs	Acidosis	Multiple carboxylase deficiency, organic acidurias, MSUD
Acute ataxia with lethargy	Hyperammonemia	FAO disorders PDH deficiency Urea cycle disorders, Triple H Lysinuric protein intolerance FAO defects HMGCoA lyase deficiency
	Hypoglycemia	Gluconeogenesis defects Glycogen synthetase deficiency HMGCoA lyase/synthetase deficiency FAO defects
	Hyperlactacidemia	Multiple carboxylase deficiency PDH deficiency Gluconeogenesis defects FAO defects

(Table Contd.)

Table 44.3 Late-onset (late infancy to adulthood) IEMs with acute presentation (Contd.)		
Main clinical presentation	**Important signs/lab abnormalities**	**Possible disorder**
Neurological coma with focal signs, seizures, or intracranial hypertension	Cerebral edema	MSUD OTC deficiency Organic acidurias
	Extrapyramidal signs (dystonia, Parkinsonism)	Glutaric aciduria type I M M A Wilson disease Homocystinuria
	Stroke-like features	UCD Organic acidurias Homocystinurias B_1-respnsive megaloblastic anemias Fabry disease
	Thromboembolic accidents	Homocystinurias (all types)
Hepatic encephalopathy Reye like syndrome	Hypoglycemia, liver dysfunction	Wilson's Disease UCD

Modified from reference (5)
Abbreviations : BCAA: Branched chain amino acids, MSUD: Maple syrup urine disease, MMA: Methylmalonic aciduria, PA: Propionic acidemia, IVA: isovaleric acidemia, MCD: Multiple carboxylase deficiency, UCD: Urea cycle defects, GSD: Glycogen storage disorder, FAO: Fatty acid oxidation, OTC: Ornithine transcarbamylase PDH: Pyruvate Dehydrogenase

When to Suspect an IEM?

1. **History** of consanguinity, developmental delay or sudden infant death syndrome (SIDS), onset of symptoms after institution of feeds, growth failure, recurrent vomiting, poor feeding, seizures especially myoclonic, apnea, and breathlessness are important clues. In the neonatal period the usual manifestations are unexplained lethargy, poor feeding and encephalopathy in a previously normal baby. One should have a high index of suspicion as the picture mimics sepsis or hypoxic-ischemic encephalopathy An early neonatal episode may be precipitated by fetal distress during birth[6]. In infancy and childhood the presentation may be similar and commonly intermittent, precipitated by infection, surgery and dietary alterations, eg protein load in UCD. Disorders like OA, UCD, MSUD, NKH and FAOD commonly present as an acute life threatening illness.

2. **Physical findings**. Clinical findings are nonspecific and include tachypnea, apnea, lethargy, hypertonicity, hypotonicity, hepatosplenomegaly, ambiguous genitalia, jaundice, dysmorphic or coarse facial features, skin rash or patchy hypopigmentation, ocular findings (cataracts, lens dislocation or pigmentary retinopathy), intracranial hemorrhage, and unusual odors. Table 44.4 gives some important clinical markers of acutely presenting IEMs.

Table 44.4 Clinical features of selected IEMs
• **Cutaneous abnormality**. Perioral eruption (multiple carboxylase deficiency), decreased pigmentation (phenylketonuria).
• **Abnormal urinary or body odor.** Musty odor (phenylketonuria), maple syrup (maple syrup urine disease), sweaty feet (isovaleric acidemia, glutaric acidemia type II), cat urine (multiple carboxylase deficiency) and sulphurous smell (homocystinuria).
• **Hair abnormalities.** Alopecia (multiple carboxylase deficiency), kinky hair (Menke's disease, arginosuccinic aciduria, multiple carboxylase deficiency).
• **Dysmorphic features.** Zellweger syndrome, glutaric acidemia type II.
• **Ocular abnormalities.** Cataract (galactosemia, Zellweger syndrome, homocystinuria), iris heterochromia/retinitis pigmentosa (Zellweger syndrome), KF ring (Wilson's disease)
• **Hepatomegaly.** Galactosemia, glycogen storage disease, tyrosinemia
• **Renal enlargement.** Zellweger syndrome, GSD 1, tyrosinemia.

3. **Laboratory findings.** Laboratory findings which which may suggest the possibility of IEM include unexplained metabolic acidosis with increased anion gap, primary respiratory alkalosis, hyperammonemia, hypoglycemia, ketosis or ketonuria, lactic acidosis, non-glucose reducing substance in urine, abnormal liver functions, unexplained neutropenia and thrombocytopenia.

IEMs presenting as an acute emergency may have any one of the following clinical presentations[7,8,9].

Neurologic Syndromes

These can present as acute encephalopathy, chronic encephalopathy, movement disorders and myopathy.

Encephalopathy. This presents as an acute emergency commonly in the neonatal period and needs to be differentiated from many acquired conditions. Encephalopathy of acute onset due to IEM has certain characteristics. It usually occurs with little warning in a previously healthy child and early signs may include behavioral problems. The condition often progresses rapidly and consciousness may fluctuate. It is very unusual to find any associated focal neurological deficits.

The encephalopathy may be recurrent with periods of normalcy in between. Disorders of chronic encephalopathy may also present with acute exacerbations. Examples of acutely presenting IEMs include OA, UCD, FAOD and mitochondrial disorders.

In acute emergencies MSUD, MCAD and UCD can present with features of cerebral edema. Metabolic encephalopathy associated with hemiplegia may be seen in MSUD, MMA, UCD and PA. History or presentation with stroke like episodes may be seen in UCD, OA, MELAS, Fabry's disease and homocystinuria. Thus the presentation may be non specific and features of different disorders can have overlapping manifestations[6].

Movement disorders may occur in a variety of IEMs and are usually associated with other neurologic signs. The manifestations may be intermittent or persistent. Movement abnormalities may be in the form of ataxia, dystonia, choreoathetosis and Parkinsonism. Common examples of IEMs presenting as movement disorder are organic acidurias, neuronal ceroid lipofuschinosis (late onset forms), lysosomal storage disorders and urea cycle disorders etc. These may rarely present as an acute emergency due to status dystonicus.

Myopathy. IEMs presenting with a myopathy are usually due to defects in the energy metabolism. The myopathy may present as progressive muscle weakness. Glycogen storage disease (GSD II & III), exercise intolerance with cramps and myoglobinuria (GSD V, VI) or myopathy as a part of multi-system disease (mitochondrial). Infantile GSD II patients can present with severe muscle weakness involving respiratory muscles or cardiomyopathy and frequently require ventilator support.

Hepatic Syndromes

Liver involvement is seen in a number of IEMs. There are four possible presentations i.e. Jaundice (unconjugated due to G6PD deficiency, Gilbert syndrome, Crigler-Najjar syndrome and conjugated due to galactosemia, tyrosinemia, fructose intolerance), hepatomegaly (GSD, tyrosinemia), hypoglycemia (Galactosemia, GSD) and hepatocellular dysfunction (Galactosemia, GSD III & IV, Niemann-Pick disease type B, α_1 antitrypsin deficiency, etc). Manifestations like hypoglycemia and hepatic failure are indications for admission in the intensive care unit.

Cardiac Syndromes

Serious cardiac disease may be associated particularly with fatty acid oxidation defects, mitochondrial disorders and GSD II. The disorder may present as cardiomyopathy (GSD, FAO defects, mitochondrial disorders, methylmalonic aciduria, Fabry's disease, mucopolysaccharidosis, GM1 gangliosidosis), arrythmias (Kearn Searre syndrome, Fabry's disease, FAO defects) and coronary artery disease (Familial hyper-cholesterolemia).

LABORATORY INVESTIGATIONS

Based on the history and clinical course suggestive of an IEM, an investigational plan should be followed. Initial investigations will help in identification or classification of the defect and institution of presumptive therapy. Figure 44.1 gives a stepwise approach for the diagnosis of a patient suspected to have IEM on the basis screening tests. The algorithmic approach for differential diagnosis of various metabolic abnormalities like metabolic acidosis (Figure 44.2), hyperammonemia (Figure 44.3) and hypoglycemia (Figure 44.4) due to various IEMs provide useful information for making a specific diagnosis[6,7,10].

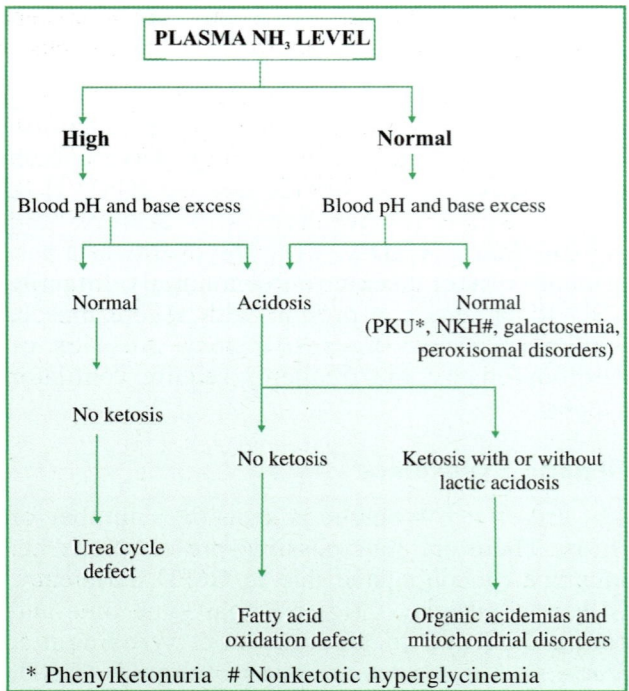

Figure 44.1 Approach to a child with suspected IEM on the basis of blood ammonia level.

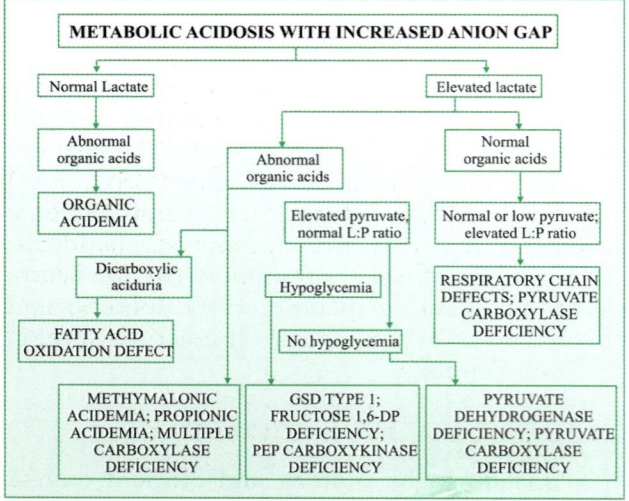

Figure 44.2 Approach to a child with metabolic acidosis

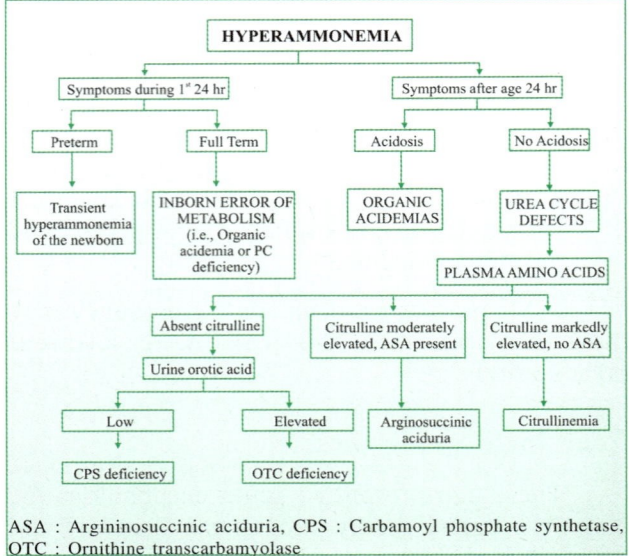

ASA : Argininosuccinic aciduria, CPS : Carbamoyl phosphate synthetase, OTC : Ornithine transcarbamyolase

Figure 44.3 Approach to a child with hyperammonemia

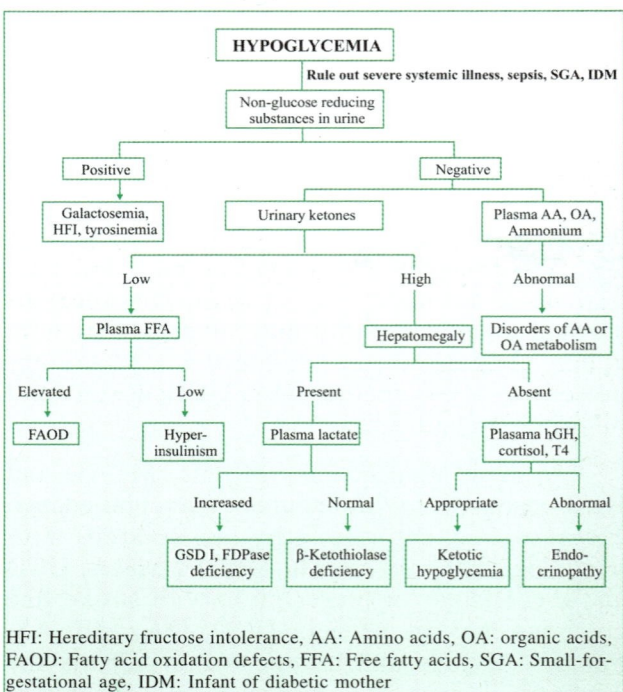

HFI: Hereditary fructose intolerance, AA: Amino acids, OA: organic acids, FAOD: Fatty acid oxidation defects, FFA: Free fatty acids, SGA: Small-for-gestational age, IDM: Infant of diabetic mother

Figure 44.4 Approach to a child with hypoglycemia

Definitive diagnosis may not be possible unless detailed investigations are done, hence treatment has to be started empirically in most situations. Table 44.5 gives details of workup which may be required for acutely presenting IEMs[11]. Routine tests such as blood sugar, serum calcium, liver function tests, blood counts and screening urine tests may give some clues to the diagnosis. Table 44.6 summarizes urinary metabolic screening tests for the diagnosis of common IEMs. Four laboratory tests are particularly useful in broad classification of IEMs and institution of empirical therapy i.e. arterial blood gas, blood lactate, blood ammonia and urine ketones (Table 44.7)[12] Tables 44.8 and 44.9 summarize correlation between clinical features and laboratory investigations in infants presenting as an emergency or encephalopathy due to IEM[13].

Table 44.5 Investigations for life-threatening IEM

Sample	Investigations	Sample collection and storage
Urine	Smell (special odor) Appearance (special color) Acetone Reducing substances Ketoacids (DNPH)	Urine collection: collect sample for each test separately and keep it in the refrigerator. Collect a sample before treatment and freeze at -20°C
Blood	Complete blood cell count Electrolytes (Look for anion gap) Glucose Blood gases (pH, CO_2 HCO_3, O_2) Calcium Uric acid Prothrombin time and liver function tests Ammonia Lactic and pyruvic acids	Plasma, heparinized, 5 ml at -20°C Blood on filter paper ("Guthrie test") Whole blood 10 to 15 ml collected on EDTA and frozen (for molecular biology/enzyme studies) Arterial blood sample
Miscellaneous	Lumbar puncture Chest x-ray Echocardiography, EMG cerebral ultrasound, CT MRI, EEG	Cerebrospinal fluid, 1 ml frozen Postmortem: Liver, muscle biopsies (macroscopic fragments frozen at -70°C) Skin biopsy (fibroblast culture)
Specialized investigations	High performance liquid chromatography (HPLC) Gas chromatorgraphy, Mass spectroscopy (GCMS), Tandem mass spectroscopy (TMS)	

Table 44.6 Urine metabolic screening Tests

Disorder	Ferric chloride	DNPH*	Reducing substances	Nitroprusside test
Phenyl ketonuria	+	+	-	-
Galactosemia	-	-	+	-
Organic aciduria	+	+	-	-
Amino aciduria	-	+	-	-
Homocystinuria	-	-	-	+

DNPH*: Dinitrophenylhydrazine

Table 44.7 Four basic tests for inherited metabolic disorders

Group	Acidosis	ketosis	Lactate	Ammonia	Diagnosis
I	-	+	-	-	MSUD
II	+	+	-	-	Organic aciduria
III	+	+	+	-	Lactic acidosis
IV	-	-	-	+	Urea cycle disorder
V	-	-	-	-	Non ketotic hyperglycinemia, sulfite oxidase deficiency, peroxisomal disorder, phenyl ketonuria and galactosemia

Table 44.8 Acute metabolic disorders in the neonates

Clinical type	Other findings	Most likely diagnosis
"Intoxication" with hyper-ammonemia, no ketonuria	Disturbance of liver function (coagulation defect), temperature-lability, hyperventilation	Urea cycle defects, fatty acid oxidation defects
"Intoxication" with ketoacidosis, with raised ammonia	Dehydration, hypothermia, truncal hypotonia, tremors	Organic acidurias
"Intoxication" without acidosis, and ketonuria	Gradual deterioration	Maple syrup urine disease
"Energy deficiency" with lactic acidosis	Muscular hypotonia, hyperventilation	Respiratory chain defects, PDH/PC deficiencies
Encephalopathy	Seizures, myoclonic jerks, no free interval, normal laboratory findings	Neurotransmitter defects, sulphite oxidase deficiency, peroxisomal disorders
Hypoglycemia	Hepatomegaly, lactic acidosis	Gluconeogenesis defects, glycogen storage disease 1
Liver failure, hepatomegaly	Hypoglycemia	Fatty acid oxidation defects, mitochondriopathies, galactosemia, tyrosinemia type 1

Table 44.9 Investigational approach in a child with acute encephalopathy

Primary lab finding	Secondary lab finding	Likely diagnosis	Differential diagnosis
Metabolic acidosis	Ketosis	Respiratory chain defects, organic acidurias, maple syrup urine disease, PC deficiency, gluconeogenesis defects, ketolysis defects	Diabetes mellitus, poisoning, encephalitis
	No ketosis	PDH deficiency, ketogenesis defects, fatty acid oxidation defects	
Elevated NH_3	Normal blood sugar	Urea cycle defects	Poisoning, Reye syndrome
	Hypoglycemia	Fatty acid oxidation defects, ketogenesis defects, hyperinsulinism variant, some organic acidurias	
Hypoglycemia	Acidosis	Gluconeogenesis defects, glycogen storage disease, maple syrup urine disease, ketogenesis defects	Hypoglycemia due to other causes, endocrine disorders, toxins, drugs
	No acidosis	Fatty acid oxidation defects	
Elevated lactate	Normal blood sugar	Respiratory chain defects, PC deficiency, PDH deficiency	
	Hypoglycemia	Fatty acid oxidation defects, gluconeogenesis defects, glycogen storage disease	

Collection of Blood and Tissue Samples

Samples should be collected before specific treatment is started or feeds are with held, as tests may be falsely normal if the child is off feeds. Samples for serum ammonia and lactate should be immediately tested. Lactate level should be tested on arterial blood which should be collected after 2 hours of fast. Ammonia sample should preferably be collected approximately after 4-6 hours of fasting. Detailed history including intake of drugs should be provided to the laboratory.

Detailed description of all IEMs is beyond the scope of this chapter. Common clinical and laboratory features of acutely presenting IEMs are summarized below:

Urea Cycle Disorders (UCDs)

All UCDs are autosomal recessive except ornithine transcarbamyalase (OTC) deficiency which is X-linked semi dominant. OTC deficiency is the most common UCD. Urea cycle takes place partly within the cytosol and partly in the mitochondria. The essential features of the urea cycle reactions are shown in figure 44.5.

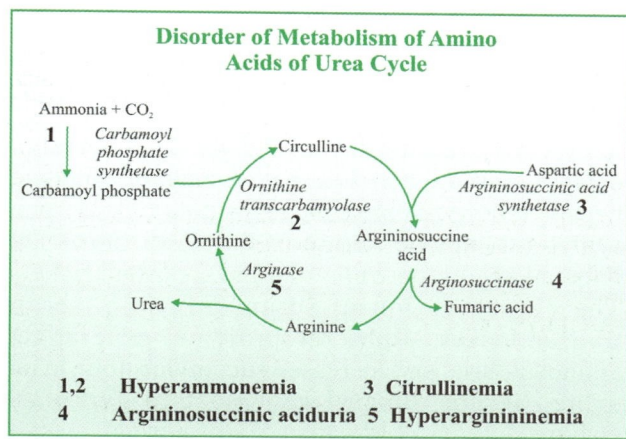

Figure 44.5 Urea cycle defects

The cycle begins and ends with ornithine and urea is the only new compound generated in the cycle; all other intermediates and reactants are recycled. Two moles of ammonia are excreted as 1 mole of urea per cycle. The urea cycle operates to eliminate excess of nitrogen. When dietary proteins increase significantly, enzyme concentrations rise to handle excess of ammonia. Urea cycle disorders (UCD) are characterized by triad of hyperammonemia (blood ammonia >200 mMol/l), encephalopathy and respiratory alkalosis.

Main metabolic abnormalities in UCDs are summarized below:

Hyperammonemia. Plasma ammonia is raised in all UCDs resulting in a similar clinical picture. Hyperammonemia causes accumulation of glutamine in astrocytes resulting in cerebral edema and acute encephalopathy. Severity of hyperammonemia is related to the magnitude of enzyme deficiency, protein intake, rate of endogenous protein catabolism and site of the enzymatic block. Proximal defects in urea cycle pathway result in more severe accumulation of ammonia than in distal defects like arginase deficiency. The normal levels of ammonia are higher in the newborn period. Labs performing the tests should provide age specific cut offs.

Changes in plasma aminoacid levels. The concentration of amino acids immediately proximal to enzyme defect increases and those beyond the block decreases. Plasma alanine and particularly glutamine accumulate while plasma arginine is reduced in all urea cycle disorders except hyperargininemia. Citrulline levels are variable and help to differentiate between proximal and distal UCD. Citrulline is a product of ornithine transcarbamylase and carbamyl phosphate synthetase activity while it is a substrate for distal enzymes. Thus it is increased in argininosuccinic synthetase deficiency and distal blocks. Urinary orotic acid is increased in enzymic blocks distal to formation of carbamoyl phosphate as in OTC deficiency.

Clinical Picture

UCDs may present as an emergency especially in the newborn period and infancy. Older children may present with intermittent exacerbations of symptoms but neonates have a rapid clinical course. Most classical picture is seen in OTC deficiency in male newborns. The infant is normal at birth or till first 24 hours of age with no history of pre or perinatal risk factors. Symptoms appear within a few hours of protein feeding. Common symptoms include lethargy, vomiting, tachypnea, tone changes, loss of normal reflexes, convulsions, hypothermia and rapidly deepening coma. Cerebral edema results in bulging anterior fontanel and this may be mistaken for intracranial hemorrhage. Early transient mild respiratory alkalosis and low blood urea level are important clues.

In older children and adolescents , the clinical features include vomiting, abnormal mental status (lethargy, somnolence, irritability, agitation), disorientation, chronic intermittent ataxia, amblyopia, seizures, developmental delay, learning difficulties, hepatomegaly (most common in argininosuccinic aciduria) and dry brittle hair (argininosuccinic aciduria). Symptoms may progress to acute encephalopathy during stress (infection, anesthesia, puberty, psychological stress and high protein intake). Older patients often control symptoms by decreasing the protein intake. Diagnostic delay is common and these patients are commonly treated as Reye's syndrome, encephalitis, migraine, cyclical vomiting, hyperactivity disorder, epilepsy, hepatitis, psychological problems and poisonings.

Organic Acidurias/Acidemias (OA)

These represent a group of inherited disorders resulting from deficient activity of specific enzymes concerned with catabolism of amino acids, carbohydrates or lipids, leading to tissue accumulation of one or more carboxylic (organic) acids. The majority of the classic organic acid disorders result from abnormal amino acid catabolism of branched chain amino acids (leucine, isoleucine, valine).

Patients affected by organic acidurias predominantly present with neurological symptoms and may have structural abnormalities of brain due to poorly understood etiopathogenesis. Mode of inheritance of the organic acidemias is autosomal recessive. Most OAs become clinically apparent during the newborn period or early infancy. After an initial period of wellbeing, affected children develop a life-threatening episode of metabolic acidosis characterized by an increased anion gap. The usual clinical presentation is that of a toxic encephalopathy and includes vomiting, poor feeding, neurologic symptoms such as seizures and abnormal tone, and lethargy progressing to coma. This non-distinct clinical picture may initially be attributed to sepsis, hypoglycemia or neonatal asphyxia.

In the older child or adolescent, intermittent forms of the organic acidurias can present as loss of intellectual function, ataxia, extrapyramidal manifestations or other focal neurologic signs, Reye syndrome, recurrent keto-acidosis, or psychiatric symptoms. Children with an organic acidemia are susceptible to metabolic decompensation during episodes of increased catabolism, such as intercurrent illness, trauma, or surgery.

Maple Syrup Urine Disease (MSUD)

MSUD is caused by deficiency of branched chain oxo- (or keto-) acid dehydrogenase. Severe forms present with progressive encephalopathy, lethargy, feeding problems, somnolence and coma. Concomitantly with the onset of the symptoms, the patient emits an intense (sweaty, malty, caramel-like) maple syrup-like odor. In general, neonatal MSUD does not display pronounced biochemical abnormalities on routine laboratory tests. There is no significant dehydration, metabolic acidosis, hyperammonemia or changes in blood counts. There is mild elevation of blood lactate level (upto 200 mMol/l). The main laboratory abnormality is the presence of 2-oxo acids detected in urine with 2, 4-dinitrophenylhydrazine (DNPH) test. Qualitative or quantitative aminoacid analysis reveals increased blood levels of branched chain aminoacids; leucine, isolucine and valine.

Nonketotic Hyperglycinemia (NKH)

NKH occurs due to a defect of the enzymes of the glycine cleavage system. It is an autosomal recessive disorder. It usually presents as acute epileptic encephalopathy. The onset may be in the neonatal period, infancy or later. There is no acidosis or ketosis and blood ammonia level is usually within normal range. Plasma and CSF glycine is increased and CSF/plasma glycine ratio is more than 0.08.

Tyrosinemia Type 1

It is caused by the deficiency of the enzyme fumarylacetoacetate hydrolase. There is involvement of the liver, kidneys and central nervous system. In acute form infants are symptomatic by 6 months of age or earlier. Symptoms are nonspecific like failure to thrive, developmental delay, vomiting, diarrhea, hepatomegaly, jaundice, hepatic failure and bleeding manifestations. Chronic symptoms include failure to thrive, cirrhosis and Fanconi syndrome with vitamin D resistant rickets. There is elevation of serum bilirubin, serum transaminases, alpha fetoproteins, generalized aminoaciduria, and increased succinylacetone in the urine. Serum fumaryl acetoacetate hydrolase enzyme activity is less than 5% of normal.

Fatty Acid Oxidation Defects (FAOD)

Inborn errors in mitochondrial fatty acid oxidation represent a group of disorders which affect the metabolism during fasting and metabolic stress. As a consequence, common features include metabolic decompensation associated with fasting, recurrent hypoglycemia, Reye-like syndrome and unexplained sudden infant death. Chronic involvement of fatty acid-dependent tissues may result in myopathy and cardiomyopathy. Neonatal presentation is common with all fatty acid oxidation defects with the exception of primary carnitine deficiency. In the first few days of life, babies may manifest with unexpected cardio-respiratory collapse or rapidly progressive lethargy with profound hypotonia. In most but not all cases, this abrupt deterioration is associated with hypoketotic hypoglycemia. Lactic acidosis, mild to severe hyperammonemia and liver involvement of varying severity are common. Cardiomyopathy with arrhythmia and mild to severe muscular involvement with increased creatine kinase occurs in many long-chain oxidation defects. Unexplained neonatal death occurs in some patients, and there may be a similar history in earlier siblings. The prognosis is variable. Medium chain acyl COA deficiency (MCAD) and long chain acyl COA deficiency (LCAD) are most life-threatening. Many patients who survive the neonatal period, die a few months later due to intercurrent infection or decompensation after an unremitting course with severe encephalopathy.

The late-onset variants of FAOD present with life-threatening episodes of hypoketotic hypoglycemia, coma and multi-organ failure following an intercurrent catabolic state. Despite correction of blood glucose levels, some patients may display persistent lethargy, seizures, dystonic movements or opisthotonos due to concomitant cerebral edema, which suggests that elevated levels of fatty acid intermediates are neurotoxic agents. Liver involvement with hepatic failure, lactic acidosis and hyperammonemia has frequently been misdiagnosed as Reye syndrome. Various degrees of myolysis and or cardiomyopathy are frequently associated. In some cases, rapid unexpected death may suggest sudden infant death syndrome.

Mitochondrial Disorders

Mitochondrial disorders are heterogenous group of disorders that present with various symptoms in a mono or multisystem pattern. The age at presentation is widely diverse. Similar clinical symptoms may be produced by widely different biochemical defects. Genetic respiratory chain defects and the resulting ATP deficiency disturbs numerous cellular functions, especially in organs with a high energy requirement, such as retina, heart or kidneys. Muscle function in particular is regularly affected because of poor supply with ATP and creatine phosphate. Affected children show various combinations of neuromuscular and other symptoms involving different, independent organ systems, sometimes explained by tissue-specific expression of a particular genetic defect. The disease course is variable but often rapidly progressive. Small children frequently suffer from encephalomyopathic disease whilst isolated myopathies predominate in the older patients.

Specific syndromes with overlapping clinical phenotype are reported. Reye syndrome previously recognized as a post infectious encephalopathy has now been recognized as possible disturbance of mitochondrial metabolism. Metabolic disorders other than mitochondrial in nature should also be considered like MCAD deficiency, urea cycle disorders, organic acidurias etc. in patient suspected to have Reye-like syndrome.

Galactosemia

Classical galactosemia caused by the deficiency of galactose-1-phosphate uridyl transferase (GALT) presents with progressive symptoms after initiation of milk feeds. Symptoms usually start on day 3-4 of life and baby may have vomiting, diarrhea, jaundice, liver dysfunction and progressive development of cataracts. Seizures may be caused by hypoglycemia. If untreated child may die of liver failure. These infants are susceptible to develop septicemia especially due to *E. coli*.

Post-mortem Investigations (Biochemical autopsy)

If a child dies of a suspected but undiagnosed metabolic disease or there is sudden infant death without obvious cause, it is essential to collect representative post-mortem samples and discuss their analysis with a metabolic specialist. Genetic counseling of the parents and reliable risk assessment for future children is not possible without a specific diagnosis. The following samples should be collected for post-mortem analyses if a genetic disorder is suspected but no specific metabolic investigations have yet been performed:

- Serum and plasma (5-10 ml frozen in small aliquots)
- Guthrie-card (dried blood spot on a filter paper)
- Urine (10-20 ml, frozen immediately)
- DNA (3-10 ml EDTA whole blood, frozen without centrifuging)
- CSF (small aliquots frozen immediately and stored at -70°C)

Biopsies. The collection of organ biopsies depends on the clinical picture and should be discussed with the laboratory/metabolic specialist. Skin biopsy for fibroblasts can be stored for 1-2 days at 4°C in a culture medium. Muscle (skeletal and heart), liver, kidney and brain tissue should be frozen immediately in liquid nitrogen.

Section 4

MANAGEMENT

The management of IEM requires accurate diagnosis, early intervention, and knowledge of the biochemical basis of the disorder. Specific therapeutic interventions for individual disorders (e.g. dietary therapy) are beyond the scope of this chapter. The principles of management of IEMs are summarized below[14-16].

(i)   Prevention of formation of toxic metabolites by restricting the intake of precursor in the diet.

(ii)   Removal of toxic metabolites by stimulating alternate pathways for removal of accumulated toxic substrate or precursor.

(iii) Enhancing its removal by artificial means.

(iv)   Supplementation of deficient substrate.

(v)   Increasing the activity of deficient enzyme by cofactor therapy in specific diseases, and at times empirically if diagnosis is not established.

(vi)   Supply of essential nutrients or disease specific diet after the diagnosis is established.

(vii) Emergency treatment should be started empirically on suspicion of IEM, and even in the absence of a specific metabolic diagnosis or disease category, since an apparently stable patient with mild symptoms may deteriorate rapidly.

General Measures

Airway, breathing and circulation should be established. Treat precipitating/ associated conditions like septicemia. Seizures should be managed as per the hospital protocol. Pyridoxine should be given to neonates with seizures unresponsive to conventional anticonvulsants. Valproate and phenobarbitone should preferably be avoided as they interfere with mitochondrial metabolism.

Correction of Metabolic Abnormalities

All oral feeds should be stopped to reduce the intake of potentially harmful proteins and sugars.

(a) *Treat hypoglycemia and prevent catabolism.* Hypoglycemia is corrected by IV 25% dextrose 1-2 ml/kg bolus, followed by continuous administration of dextrose. All patients with suspected IEM are given dextrose 10-15% IV at a rate high enough to prevent catabolism (8-10 mg/kg/min). Insulin may be added 0.2-0.3 units/kg, if required, to maintain normoglycemia.

(b) *Maintain fluid and electrolyte balance.* Fluid and electrolytes are added at maintenance concentrations. Necessary adjustments are made to correct any electrolyte or hemodynamic disturbances.

(c) *Treat acidosis.* Acidosis should be corrected slowly by administration of bicarbonate in a dose of 0.35-0.5 mEq/kg/hr (maximum 1-2 mEq/kg/hr). Rapid correction or over-correction of acidosis may have paradoxical deleterious effects on the CNS. For intractable acidosis, hemodialysis or peritoneal dialysis may be required.

Removal of Toxic Metabolites

Abnormal metabolites are removed by restricting the intake of the offending substrate and by promoting renal excretion of toxic metabolites. In severe cases, dialysis (preferably hemodialysis) is desirable. Rapid removal of toxic metabolites can be achieved by exchange transfusion, peritoneal dialysis (PD), hemodialysis, forced diuresis, administration of drugs like sodium benzoate to increase excretion of ammonia by using alternative pathways for the excretion of toxic metabolites, and the use of mega-doses of vitamins/cofactors.

Exchange transfusion is effective in removing toxins that are confined to the vascular space, but has a short-lasting effect, and plays a minor role in the removal of ammonia and amino acids distributed throughout total body water. Clearance of ammonia by peritoneal dialysis (PD) is only 10% compared to its clearance by hemodialysis. Although hemodialysis has advantages over PD, vascular access remains the major technical problem and PD is usually the preferred mode of treatment[17].

Specific Management[14-16]

1. **Hyperammonemia**

Kidneys are not able to clear ammonia effectively. Its removal is hastened by formation of compounds other than urea thus decreasing load on the urea cycle.

(i)   *Sodium benzoate.* It is conjugated with glycine to form hippurate which is excreted in the urine. One mole of benzoate removes one mole of nitrogen. It is administered in a dose of 250–500 mg/kg/d in acute emergency. Major side effects include nausea, vomiting, irritability and incomplete conjugation in neonates with aggravation of unconjugated hyperbilirubinemia.

(ii) *Phenyl acetate.* It conjugates with glutamine to form phenylacetyl glutamine which is excreted in the urine. One mole of phenyl acetate removes two moles of nitrogen.

Emergency Measures

When blood ammonia level goes above 200 mMol/l, urgent measures should be taken to prevent further progression of metabolic abnormalities. Protein intake should be stopped and patient started on 20% intravenous dextrose (along with 0.1-1.0 units of insulin/kg/hr) to maintain blood glucose between 100-150 mg/dl to prevent tissue catabolism. Intralipid in a dose 0.5-1.0 g/kg (upto maximum of 3 g/kg) is administered to maintain anabolic state. Furosemide (2.0 mg/kg oral or 1.0 mg/kg iv every 6 hr) may be given for forced diuresis.

Arginine hydrochloride 350 mg/kg/day is administered to maintain plasma arginine level between 70-150 mMol/l. Sodium benzoate 250-400 mg/kg/day is administered to maintain plasma level upto 2 mMol/dl. Sodium phenyl butyrate or phenyl acetate 250-500 mg/kg/day is recommended to maintain plasma level below 3 mMol/l. Carnitine 100 mg/kg/d in 3-4 divided doses is given to patients with OA presenting as hyperammonemia. Citrulline may be used in a dose of 170 mg/kg/d in infants with carbamyl phosphate synthetase and ornithine transcarbamylase deficiency. Unfortunately intravenous preparations of aforementioned drugs are not readily available in India. Anticonvulsants like sodium valproate should be avoided. Patient should be closely monitored for electrolytes, ABG, blood ammonia, plasma amino acids and lactate levels.

In life-threatening situations, in addition to above measures, extracorporeal detoxification should be started. Hemodiafiltration is ideal when available, otherwise hemofiltration and hemodialysis is satisfactory. Peritoneal dialysis is not effective. Exchange blood transfusion increase protein and ammonia load but may be considered in patients with argininemia. Intravenous preparations of drugs used in treatment of hyperammonemia are not easily available in India and only oral therapy can be instituted in most situations.

Long-term Treatment

Continue low-protein diet containing essential amino acids (distributed over as many meals as is reasonable) to maintain protein synthesis (anabolism). Monitor laboratory values frequently (initially daily) and adjust diet to avoid excessive protein reduction. Maintain anabolic state by providing adequate calories. Ensure daily intake of 1.4 g/kg of protein, 50% should account for mixture of essential amino acids. Administer maintenance oral doses of arginine (100-200 mg/kg/d for OTC/CPS deficiency and upto 600 mg/kg/d for arginosuccinate synthetase deficiency), sodium benzoate (250-400 mg/kg/d) and sodium phenylbutyrate (250-500 mg/kg/d). Supplements of vitamins (e.g. folic acid 500 ug/day) and trace minerals should be provided. If carnitine is low, give supplements in a dose of 30-50 mg/kg (give only intermittently as benzoate may be eliminated as carnitine ester). Consider administration of lactulose as it binds intestinal ammonia to enhance its elimination.

Therapy should be continuously monitored with blood ammonia and amino acid levels. The target value of ammonia is <80 mMol/l. Essential amino acids should be maintained within normal range, particularly during sodium-phenylbutyrate therapy. Serum electrolytes should be monitored and maintained within normal range.

Amino acid and Organic Acid Disorders

In amino acid and organic acid disorders, the accumulated toxic metabolites can be removed by two-volume exchange, or continuous exchange blood transfusion over 15 to 20 hours, peritoneal dialysis (PD), and forced diuresis with furosemide and intravenous fluids. Peritoneal dialysis has been used effectively in the management of acute presentations of MSUD, propionic acidemia, and isovaleric acidemia. The use of bicarbonate in the dialysate may be helpful. Exchange transfusion before and after PD is effective in MSUD, propionic acidemia, and isovaleric acidemia. As the clearance of methylmalonic acid by PD is less than the renal clearance, exchange transfusion and forced diuresis is the treatment of choice in acute decompensation. Glycine (250 mg/kg/day) may be given by nasogastric tube to patients with isovaleric acidemia which results in normalization of plasma isovalerate within three days followed by neurological and hematological improvement after two weeks. During the acute phase, protein restriction and provision of adequate calories is a must to suppress endogenous protein breakdown.

Emergency Treatment

(i) Interrupt catabolic state by intravenous administration of 10-20% dextrose along with insulin.

(ii) Stop protein intake. In some disorders the accumulation of toxic metabolites can be reduced by intestinal antibiotic treatment (metronidazole, colistin).

(iii) Ensure adequate fluid and electrolyte intake and aim for a sodium concentration of around 140 mEq/l to reduce the risk of cerebral edema.

(iv) Carry out detoxifying measures depending on the disease and laboratory findings by forced diuresis, dialysis, hemofiltration.

(v) Consider specific drug treatment (vitamins, carnitine, etc.) depending on the disease and laboratory findings.

Long-term Treatment

(i) Ensure protein restriction and provide semisynthetic mixture of amino acids by eliminating those amino acids whose breakdown is blocked. Supplements of vitamins and trace minerals should be given.

(ii) If indicated give specific vitamins or cofactors, e.g. biotinidase deficiency and holocarboxylase synthetase deficiency, vitamin B_6- or B_{12}-dependent homocysteinemias, vitamin B_{12}-dependent methylmalonic acidurias, vitamin B_2-dependent multiple acyl-CoA dehydrogenase deficiency.

(iii) Carnitine (50-100 mg/kg/day) should be considered in all disorders that cause intra-mitochondrial accumulation of CoA-esters.

(iv) Laboratory monitoring of blood counts, calcium, phosphate, magnesium, iron, liver and kidney function tests, alkaline phosphatase, total protein, albumin, pre-albumin, carnitine, acid-base status, coagulation studies, ammonia, lactate, amino acids in plasma and organic acids in urine is undertaken depending upon the diagnosis.

Disorders of Fatty Acid Oxidation

Mitochondrial oxidation of fatty acids is one of the major sources of energy to the organism. During prolonged fasting, it provides up to 80% of the total energy requirements. The brain (in contrast to the muscle) is unable to fully oxidize fatty acids but adapts to the catabolism of ketone bodies synthesized by the liver. Humans are unable to synthesize glucose from fatty acids and need to catabolize muscle protein for this purpose.

The therapy is directed to prevent fasting and catabolic state. In acute situations, intravenous glucose infusion (8-10 mg/kg/min) should be started without delay. There is no clear evidence that restricting fat is useful in MCAD deficiency. In contrast, in patients with defects in LCAD metabolism, low fat diet supplemented with medium chain triglycerides may be beneficial. In patients with primary carnitine deficiency, carnitine supplementation (100-200 mg/kg/d) improves cardiac and muscle functions within a few months. The role of carnitine supplementation in other beta-oxidation defects is controversial. Some patients with mild variants of MCAD and SCAD deficiencies may respond to oral riboflavin supplementation (100-300 mg/day). Sodium valproate should not be given for control of seizures.

Mitochondrial Disorders[13]

Most therapeutic approaches for the management of mitochondriopathies have not been scientifically evaluated and success is usually limited. If the clinical condition does not improve with a trial of various treatment regimens within six months, it is justified to stop them. General measures include avoidance of drugs that inhibit the respiratory chain, e.g. sodium valproate, barbiturates, tetracyclines and chloramphenicol. L-carnitine 50-100 mg/kg/d (maximum upto 200 mg) should be given in 4 divided doses. Lactic acidosis can be prevented by early control of fever and seizures and avoidance of physical exertion. Acute lactic acidosis due to mitochondriopathy is treated with coenzyme Q_{10}, riboflavin (100 mg/d), vitamin C, carnitine, biotin (20 mg/d), thiamine, tocopherol and vitamins K.

Vitamin/cofactor therapy[15, 16]

In certain IEMs, enhancement of the activity of a mutant enzyme can be achieved by giving mega-doses of a vitamin cofactor required for the enzyme's action (Table 44.10). One-third cases of homocystinuria due to cystathionine β-synthetase deficiency are pyridoxine responsive. Intractable seizures due to pyridoxine dependency (disorder of gamma aminobutyric acid metabolism) respond to oral administration of pyridoxine 10-100 mg/day. Some patients with MSUD may respond to thiamine 10 to 20 mg per day together with a protein-restricted diet. Deficiency of multiple biotin-dependent carboxylases (acetyl CoA carboxylase, propionyl CoA carboxylase, 3-methylcrotonyl CoA carboxylase, and pyruvate carboxylase) appears in two forms, one resulting from deficiency of holocarboxylase synthetase and the other due to biotinidase deficiency. The latter disorder responds

Table 44.10 Vitamin and co-factor therapy in selected IEMs

Cofactor	Function	Cofactor responsive disorders
Thiamine (vitamin B$_1$)	Reactions involving transfer of acetate groups (e.g. transaldolase, transketolase)	• Some cases of lactic acidosis due to PDH deficiency • Thiamine-responsive megalobalstic anemia, diabetes mellitus, deafness • Rare cases of MSUD
Riboflavin (vitamin B$_2$)	Oxidation and reduction reactions	• Some cases of multiple acyl-CoA dehydrogenase deficiency (glutaric aciduria type II)
Pyridoxine (vitamin B$_6$)	Transamination, decarboxylation, rearrangement of many amino acids	• About 50% cases of homocystinuria due to cystathionine b-synthase deficiency • Pyridoxine-responsive seizures of infancy • Cystathioninuria • Xanthurenic aciduria • Hyperomethinemia with gyrate atrophy
Cobalamin (vitamin B$_{12}$)	Methyl group transfer reactions	• Methylmalonic acidemia (cb1A, cb1B) • Homocystinuria and methylmalonic acidemia (cb1C, cb1D, cb1F)
Folic acid	One-carbon metabolism, particularly in nucleic acid synthesis	• Some cases of homocystinuria
Biotin	Reactions involving chemical transfer of CO_2 (e.g. pyruvate carboxylase)	• Biotinidase deficiency • Holocarboxylase synthetase deficiency

to 10 mg of biotin given daily. Some cases of methylmalonic acidemia respond to intramuscular administration of pharmacological doses (1 mg/d) of hydroxycobalamin. A diet low in fat and protein along with a trial of oral riboflavin (200-300 mg per day) and carnitine may be helpful in some patients with glutaric aciduria type I and II. Oral riboflavin may lead to significant clinical improvement in some patients with fatty acid oxidation disorders. Carnitine levels may be low in other organic acidurias and oral carnitine (25-50 mg/kg/day) may improve metabolic control, especially in isovaleric acidemia. Carnitine supplementation has also been recommended for treatment of fatty acid oxidation disorders.

Specific Dietary Restrictions[18]

A galactose-free diet will quickly reverse the clinical symptoms and prevent mental retardation, cataracts, and liver damage in patients with galactosemia. However, recent reports have indicated that despite early diagnosis and treatment, most cases of galactosemia have growth failure, lower intelligence quotient, speech and motor dysfunction, and ovarian failure. Neonates with PKU should be given a protein substitute which is phenylalanine-free but otherwise nutritionally complete.

In patients with glycogen storage disease, deficient hepatic glucose output leads to hypoglycemia. Hypoglycemia can be prevented by frequent feeds during the day and continuous nasogastric feeding at night, in infancy and early childhood. Raw corn starch (2 g/kg every six hours) has been shown to be effective in preventing hypoglycemia in older children with glycogen storage disease type 1 as well as decreasing the risk of hyperlipidemia, hyperuricemia, and lactic acidemia. Corn starch therapy has also been used to manage the hypoglycemic episodes in patients with fatty acid oxidation disorders.

Clinicians must be aware that the special formulae are imcomplete and one should seek the assistance of a dietitian experienced in the care of infants and children with IEM, to ensure adequate intake of essential amino acids and fatty acids, minerals, and vitamins.

Genetic Counseling and Prenatal Diagnosis

The task of the clinician does not end with the accurate diagnosis and management of a patient

Section 4

with IEM. It is important to counsel the family for the risk of recurrence in subsequent pregnancies and possibility of prenatal diagnosis if available.

REFERENCES

1. ICMR Collaborating Centres and Central Coordinating Unit. Multicentric study on genetic causes of mental retardation in India. *Indian J Med Res* 1991; 94: 161-169.

2. Kaur M, Das GP, Verma IC. Inborn errors of aminoacid metabolism in north India. *J Inherit Metab Dis* 1994; 17:1-14.

3. Radharamadevi and Naushad SM. Newborn screening in India. *Indian J Pediatr* 2004, 71:157-160.

4. Carballo EC. Detection of inherited neurometabolic disorders - A practical clinical approach. *Pediatr Clin North Amer* 1992; 39:801-820.

5. Saudubray JM, Sedel F, Walter JH. Clinical approach to treatable inborn metabolic diseases: an introduction. *J Inherit Metab Dis* 2006;29:261-274.

6. Nyhan W.L. When to suspect metabolic disease? In: Inherited Metabolic Diseases, Hoffman G.F., Zschocke J., Nyhan W.L. (Eds.) *Springer* 2010, pp 13-15.

7. Clarke JTR, Neurologic syndromes In : A Clinical Guide to Inherited Metabolic Diseases. Clarke TR Joe (Ed.), *Cambridge University Press.* 2006, pp 28-87.

8. Clarke JTR Hepatic syndromes In: A Clinical Guide to Inherited Metabolic Diseases. Clarke TR Joe (Ed.), *Cambridge University Press.* 2006, pp 116-141.

9. Clarke JTR, Cardiac syndromes In: A Clinical Guide to Inherited Metabolic Diseases. Clarke TR Joe (Ed.), *Cambridge University Press.* 2006, pp 143-159.

10. Bruton BK. Inborn errors of metabolism in infancy; a guide to diagnosis. *Pediatrics* 1998; 102(6):E 69.

11. Saudubray JM, Ogier H, Bonnefont JP. Clinical approach to inherited metabolic diseases in the neonatal period: A 20-year survey. *J Inherit Metab Dis* 1989; 12 (Suppl 1):25-41

12. Gulati S, Vaswani M, Kalra V, Kabra M, Kaur M. An approach to neurometabolic disorders by a simple metabolic screen. *Indian Pediatr* 2000; 37:63-69.

13. Marburg JZ, Marburg GH. Vademecum metabolism, Manual of Metabolic Pediatrics. *Milupa, Schattaner* 1999.

14. Gupta N, Kabra M. Acute management of sick infants with suspected inborn errors of metabolism. *Indian J Pediatr* 2011;78: 854-859

15. Clarke JTR. The management of inherited metabolic diseases: A Review. *Journal Pediatr Obstet & Gynec* 2005; 31:186-196.

16. Low LCK. Inborn errors of metabolism: clinical approach and management. *HKMJ* 1996; 2:274-281.

17. Gortner L, Leupold D, Pohlandt F, Bartmann P. Peritoneal dialysis in metabolic crises caused by inherited disorders of organic acid and amino acid metabolism. *Acta Paediatr Scand* 1989; 78:706-711.

18. Kabra M. Dietary management of inborn errors of metabolism. *Indian J Pediatr* 2002; 69:421-426.

Section 4

45

Otolaryngological Emergencies

Kapil Sikka and Alok Thakur

Life-threatening emergencies due to diseases of ear, nose and throat are uncommon in children except upper airway obstruction due to developmental abnormalities, infections and foreign bodies[1]. Children are more prone to develop upper respiratory tract infections due to a variety of pathogens including vaccine-preventable diseases. Stridor due to upper airway obstruction is more common in children because they have relatively narrow air passages, large tongue, hypertrophy of tonsils and adenoidal tissues, collapsability of upper airways and floppy epiglottis due to lack of supporting cartilage. Children are more vulnerable to develop choking due to inhalation of foreign bodies or insertion of foreign bodies and entry of insects into the nose and ear canal. The common ENT emergencies include epistaxis, ear pain and stridor due to upper airway infection and foreign bodies.

OTOLOGIC EMERGENCIES

Otalgia

Otalgia (ear ache) is a common symptom arising from different structures in and around the ear. The ear ache may be otogenic or non-otogenic. Non-otogenic causes of otalgia include referred pain originating from pathology in the distribution of the V, VII, IX, or X cranial nerves because all of these nerves give sensory branches to the ear. The frequent origin of ear ache from infections in the tonsils and the laryngopharynx emphasizes the need for a complete and thorough ENT evaluation for all cases of otalgia. Younger children may present with excessive crying, fussiness and sleeplessness. ENT examination is mandatory in all children with unexplained fever and crying or fussiness and irritability. The common causes of otalgia in children are enumerated in Table 45.1.

The most common otogenic causes of ear pain are wax in the ear canal, acute otitis media and otitis externa. The common non-otogenic causes shall be discussed under relevant headings later in the chapter.

Impacted Wax

Impacted wax or cerumen is a common cause of otalgia in children[2]. It may present as a mild discomfort or hearing loss, or with severe otalgia closely mimicking infective ear conditions (which may sometimes coexist). The child typically presents with history of ear block for a few days followed by development of severe otalgia. The common predisposing events includes entry of water during head bath and swimming or attempts by the mother

| Table 45.1 Common causes of ear pain ||
Otogenic causes	Non-otogenic causes
External ear • Trauma • Wax • Otitis externa: Bacterial and fungal • Herpes zoster oticus **Middle ear** • Acute suppurative otitis media • Otitis media with effusion • Complicated chronic suppurative otitis media*	• Dental infections and caries • Stomatitis and gingivitis • Temporomandibular joint dysfunction • Tonsillitis and peritonsillar abscess • Sinusitis • Neck abscess • Cervical lymphadenitis • Mumps • Teething
*Uncomplicated CSOM is painless. When pain is present it indicates a complication which may be a simple external otitis, or mastoiditis or an intracranial complication such as an extradural abscess.	

to clean the ear. Diagnosis is simple as impacted cerumen can be seen on otoscopy. Other causes of otogenic otalgia like ASOM and otitis externa may co-exist and should be ruled out.

Treatment is aimed at removing the impacted-wax. This can be done either by suction clearance, cleaning the ear canal with a Jobson's ear probe, or by washing and irrigating the ear canal by syringing. Syringing is suitable for cases with soft wax[3].The pinna is pulled up and backwards, and nozzle of the syringe is aimed slightly upwards and backwards so that the water flows as a cascade along the roof of the canal. The irrigation solution flows out of the canal along its floor, taking out wax and debris with it. Warm water, saline or sodium bicarbonate solution can be used as syringing solutions. Hard impacted wax may require instillation of ceruminolytics for 5-7 days prior to syringing. Various commercially available ceruminolytics or home remedies like olive oil, almond oil, glycerine etc. can be used for softening the wax. Pain relief is usually immediate if cerumen is effectively removed. Analgesia if required can be effectively achieved with oral ibuprofen or paracetamol.

Acute Otitis Media

The spectrum of middle ear inflammatory syndromes which may cause pain include acute otitis media with effusion (OME), non suppurative otitis media (NSOM), acute otitis media (AOM), and acute suppurative otitis media (ASOM). All three conditions are common in childhood and are associated with dysfunction of Eustachian tube and upper respiratory tract infection[4]. These conditions are extremely common in children especially during sudden change of weather and during winter months. The common predisposing conditions include upper respiratory infection, nasal congestion, adenoids, cleft palate and bottle feeding. It is estimated that more than 50% of children will have had atleast one episode of ASOM by the time they achieve the age of nine years.

Otitis media with effusion (OME) or non-suppurative otitis media demonstrates no overt middle ear infection but presents with hearing loss, a retracted and dull tympanic membrane, and middle ear effusion[4]. Intermittent episodes of otalgia may occur. Such episodes of otalgia are classically noted a few hours after the child goes to bed, are ascribed to negative middle ear pressure, and generally respond to paracetamol. Otalgia with OME may, however, also indicate a progression to AOM or ASOM. The pain in these situations is more severe

and associated with signs of inflammation of tympanic membrane.

Acute otitis media (AOM) is an infective condition of the middle ear with more severe pain, mild conductive hearing loss, and redness of the tympanic membrane. AOM may be viral in origin and preceded by coryza, and the use of antibiotics is often not recommended. Acute suppurative otitis media (ASOM) is a more severe infection with manifest suppuration (manifested by a bulging tympanic membrane or a perforated tympanic membrane and otorrhea). The commonly implicated pathogens are *Haemophilus influenzae, Moraxellaa catarrhalis* and *Streptococcus pyogenes*. Anti-biotics are essential and often arrest the progression towards tympanic membrane perforation and a host of other extracranial and intracranial complications including mastoiditis.

ASOM typically presents with a severe crescendo of otalgia in a coryzal child. Other symptoms include hearing loss, fever, excessive crying, irritability, poor feeding and excessive ear pulling. If untreated, it progresses to perforation of the tympanic membrane with a dramatic relief of pain. ASOM is diagnosed by otoscopy, but this may prove difficult in an uncooperative child, obliquity of external auditory canal, or presence of wax in the canal. In the earliest stages the tympanic membrane appears congested, followed by middle ear suppuration with bulging of tympanic membrane and further progression demonstrate a perforation with the egress of pus.

Treatment

Mild otalgia associated with OME/ NSOM does not require antibiotics and is treated with decongestants and analgesics.[5] Manifest ASOM should be treated with appropriate antibiotics (usually co-amoxiclav or cefuroxime/cefaclor), decongestants and analgesics. Nasal congestion should be relieved by local instillation of saline nose drops and steam inhalation. Response to otalgia is immediate, though middle ear effusion and hearing loss may not improve till a few weeks. Myringotomy to release middle ear pus is not commonly performed these days, but may be indicated in emergency situations with a bulging tympanic membrane and severe otalgia, or in cases with complications wherein pus examination for culture studies is considered prudent.

The treatment of AOM is debatable. Clinically, AOM is not easily differentiated from the earliest phase of an acute suppurative otitis media (ASOM) and may even progress to ASOM. This creates a dilemma regarding the use of antibiotics. A recent Cochrane review meta-analysis suggests that antibiotics are not very useful for most children with AOM.[6] Antibiotics marginally decrease the number of children with pain at 24 hours (when most children were better), only slightly reduce the number of children with pain in the few days following but do not reduce the number of children with hearing loss (that can last several weeks). Antibiotics have also been noted to cause unwanted adverse effects and may also increase resistance to antibiotics in the community. The studies included in this review, however, were conducted in high-income countries, and may not represent the situation in other geographical areas wherein the risk of early ASOM masquerading as AOM or of AOM progressing to ASOM may be higher. The decision regarding the use of antibiotics therefore needs to be individualised in different situations and is based on the clinical observations and experience of the physician.

Complications

Acute and chronic suppurative otitis media may be complicated by acute mastoiditis, sigmoid or lateral sinus thrombosis, meningitis, sensorineural deafness, tetanus and facial palsy.

Otitis Externa

Infections of external auditory canal are extremely painful. Otitis externa can be classified as localized otitis externa and diffuse otitis externa. Localized otitis externa (furunculosis) is a localized infection of the ear canal hair follicles. It is caused by Gram-positive organisms, usually *staphylococcal aureus*[7]. It is characterized by a painful swelling in the cartilaginous external auditory canal. Marked tenderness on ear manipulation and pressure over the tragus are characteristic signs. The swelling may also be noted over the conchal bowl or over the tragus. In the latter case, there may be history of ear piercing or pre-existing pre-auricular sinus. Nickel ear-rings may also lead to ear lobe dermatitis.

Diffuse otitis externa involves the entire external auditory canal by the infective agents. These agents may be bacteria, fungi (otomycosis) or viruses (Herpes zoster oticus). Bacterial otitis externa usually presents in warm, humid weather, and may be precipitated by water entering the ears. It is frequent in children when they start swimming (swimmer's ear). Initial symptom is pruritis and scratching of skin leads to superadded bacterial infection. Examination reveals extreme tragal tenderness similar to localized otitis externa. The ear canal is diffusely erythematous with purulent discharge that is thick and non-mucoid. The mucoid component in ear discharge suggests middle ear infection and perforation of tympanic membrane. Necrotizing or malignant otitis externa is rare in children but should be suspected in unresolving cases with immunocompromised status like hematological malignancy, diabetes mellitus, HIV or children receiving chemotherapy.

Otomycosis is the fungal infection of the external auditory canal[7]. The symptoms may mimic bacterial otitis externa and present with otalgia. Most patients complain of pruritis rather than pain. On examination, the canal contains grey, white or blackish debris resembling dirty cotton. The ear canal is edematous. Herpes zoster oticus is the viral infection characterized by painful vesicles over the ear canal, pinna and tympanic membrane. It may be associated with hearing loss and facial nerve palsy.

Treatment

The treatment needs to be tailored to individual patient based upon the diagnosis of etiological agent. The differentiation between viral, fungal and bacterial etiology is fairly straight forward by clinical evaluation. Viral otitis externa (Herpes zoster oticus) requires systemic antiviral therapy along with adequate analgesia. Otomycosis is usually not very painful. These cases require local treatment by removal of debris either by suction cleaning or by syringing. Thereafter, topical antifungal ear drops are prescribed for 7-10 days.

Treatment of bacterial external otitis requires careful inspection and evaluation of ear canal under microscope with adequate analgesia. A pointing abscess is exceedingly painful condition and rapid pain relief may be obtained by local incision and drainage. These cases require oral antibiotics for 7-10 days. The antibiotics should be aimed at covering *Staphylococcus aureus* and *Streptococcus pneumoniae*. Analgesia is an important component of management of otitis externa. NSAIDs usually suffice for pain relief. Small cotton wick medicated with 90:10 glycerol and ichthammol is very helpful in pain relief. It has proven dehydrating and anti-inflammatory properties and antibacterial activity against streptococci and staphylococci. The patient should be instructed to keep the ear dry.

SUDDEN HEARING LOSS

In most situations sudden hearing loss is unilateral, and if this is an isolated symptom, the

Section 4

child may not notice or report it. Sudden hearing loss may be either conductive hearing loss or sensori-neural hearing loss. Tuning fork tests and audiometry are used to differentiate between the two but may be unreliable especially in very young children. Tympanometry is useful for diagnosis of the nature of hearing loss.

Conductive hearing loss with no associated otalgia is almost always secondary to Eustachian tube dysfunction or middle ear effusion. An upper respiratory tract infection may be concurrent. Ear examination may reveal the tympanic membrane to be retracted or dull, and an air fluid level may be seen behind the tympanic membrane. The condition is often self limiting, but resolution may be aided by decongestants and mucolytics.

Sudden sensorineural hearing loss (SSNHL) may be idiopathic and may occur after head or ear trauma. It may be associated with viral illnesses such as acute coryza, mumps, measles or cytomegalovirus infection. Other features of inner ear involvement (vertigo, tinnitus) may or may not be present. No strong evidence exists for the efficacy of any treatment for SSNHL. Oral and intratympanic steroids, hyperbaric oxygen, inhaled carbogen, vasodilators, antivirals etc. have been used with variable results[8]. The usual practice is to prescribe oral prednisolone in dosage of 1 mg/kg/day which is gradually tapered over 10 days.

Ear and head trauma can lead to both conductive and sensorineural hearing loss. Associated ear bleeding may indicate a possible fracture of base of skull and should be evaluated appropriately. Conductive deafness may be secondary to tympanic membrane perforation, ossicular dislocation or hemotympanum. Otoscopy and tuning fork tests are useful to make the diagnosis, though isolated ossicular dislocation may have normal otoscopic findings. Conductive hearing loss, even if due to causes such as tympanic membrane perforation and hemotympanum, usually

does not require any emergency treatment. Post traumatic sensorineural hearing loss is treated in the same manner as described under SSNHL. Associated temporal bone fracture, facial nerve injury or brain injury should be ruled out in such situations.

VERTIGO

Children presenting to the emergency department with complaints of "dizziness" are especially challenging, as they are unable to provide a detailed description of the symptoms. The differentiation between true vertigo originating from inner ear pathology and dizziness due to other causes like anxiety, hypotension and CNS pathologies may prove difficult[9,10].

The differential diagnosis of vertigo is a specialised subject and a comprehensive discussion is not in the purview of this chapter. Other co-existing features indicative of labyrinthine origin (tinnitus, hearing loss) or of central origin (incoordination, tremor, cerebellar signs, known nerve deficits) provide the most definitive clues in differentiating between the two major groups. Nystagmus, if present, can be a useful differentiating sign as labyrinthine nystagmus has very specific features of demonstrating a fast and a slow component usually horizontal and unidirectional and manifests when looking towards the side of lesion, and is enhanced by darkness or removal of fixation.

The common inner ear and central causes of vertigo are listed in Table 45.2. Negative middle ear pressure and middle ear pathology is reported to manifest with poor balance but does not cause severe or rotatory vertigo. Benign paroxysmal vertigo is a migraine related syndrome with short lasting episodes (few minutes) of rotatory vertigo which responds well to anti migraine prophylaxis. Vertigo in association with otorrhea is suggestive of labyrinthitis or a cerebellar abscess and warrants immediate otolaryngological consultation.

Table 45.2 Common causes of vertigo in children	
Inner ear causes	**Central causes**
❑ Labyrinthitis ❑ Eustachian tube dysfunction/ otitis media with effusion (OME) ❑ Ototoxic medications ❑ Trauma ❑ Perilymphatic fistula ❑ Vestibular neuronitis ❑ Endolmphatic hydrops	❑ Migraine/benign paroxysmal vertigo ❑ Motion sickness ❑ Trauma ❑ Cerebellar or brain stem space occupying lesion ❑ Seizures ❑ Meningitis/encephalitis

Treatment

Treatment of acute episodes of vertigo is initially directed at control of symptoms. Children with acute onset severe labyrinthine vertigo should be admitted to the hospital. The child should be nursed in an isolated room in the presence of mother or a relative. The room should be dimly lit and child should be encouraged to relax. Vertigo and vomiting can be effectively handled by providing good labyrinthine sedation. Promethazine hydrochloride in dosage of 6.25 to 12.5 mg intramuscularly is useful and may be coadministered with prochlorperazine 7.5 to 15 mg/day in 3 divided doses. Suppurative labyrinthitis is treated with intravenous antibiotics in anti-meningitic doses as contiguous spread from the labyrinth to the meninges is well known. Early surgical treatment of the middle ear disease is also warranted as vertigo is unlikely to settle unless the pus or cholesteatoma is evacuated.

Facial Nerve Palsy

Acute onset facial paralysis can be a frightening symptom for parents and the affected child. Upper motor neuron paralysis is very rare in children as incidence of stroke is extremely low. The most frequent causes in children include Bell's palsy (acute idiopathic LMN facial paralysis), suppurative otitis media, and trauma[11]. Idiopathic facial palsy (Bell's palsy) presents as a rapid onset lower motor neuron paralysis of facial muscles. Acute onset facial palsy with no other antecedent symptoms and a normal ear examination is diagnostic of Bell's palsy. The prognosis for a complete recovery is excellent, but a follow up over the next few weeks to document such recovery is prudent. Current evidence has linked Bell's paralysis to reactivation of herpes simplex infection[11]. Steroids and acyclovir are generally prescribed, though the evidence supporting their efficacy is considered weak. Local eye care with lubricants and padding is essential to prevent corneal complications.

Facial palsy in association with acute or chronic suppurative otitis media requires emergent treatment. The child should be admitted to the hospital for administration of intravenous antibiotics and for a thorough evaluation to rule out any associated intracranial or extra-cranial complications. An immediate otolaryngologic consultation is mandatory as surgical treatment may be indicated.

Foreign Bodies in the Ear Canal

Foreign bodies in the ear canal are fairly common. Paper bits, cotton buds, tooth picks, beads, stones, button batteries or live insects are frequently encountered foreign bodies. Foreign bodies should be removed immediately to prevent superadded infection, migration, and further complications. Foreign body removal may prove traumatic and should only be undertaken by a trained physician. Most foreign bodies may be easily removed by grasping with forceps as an office procedure or by syringing. Syringing, however, should not be performed in situations with hygroscopic foreign bodies (eg. vegetable foreign body) which may swell and become impacted by instillation of water. Syringing is also contraindicated in patients with pre-existing tympanic membrane perforation and with ventilation tubes. Large impacted foreign bodies and ones deep inside ear canal closely abutting tympanic membrane may require careful retrieval under a microscope, preferably in the operating room. Live insects should always be killed first by instilling mineral oil or alcohol to facilitate their removal.

RHINOLOGIC EMERGENCIES

Foreign Bodies in the Nose

Foreign bodies in the nose are a frequent occurrence in children. Witnessed foreign bodies are easy to diagnose but unwitnessed foreign body insertions may present many weeks or months later as a case of unilateral nasal obstruction, rhinorrhea or epistaxis. The failed attempts at retrieving the foreign body by the guardians or inexperienced practitioners may impact or further push the foreign body so that it may not be visible on anterior rhinoscopy. The view, at times may be obscured by blood or discharge.

All foreign bodies in the nose should be removed. The visible foreign body can be retrieved with the help of a nasal grasping forceps or nasal biopsy forceps on anterior rhinoscopy under head light illumination. Rounded or smooth surfaced foreign bodies are difficult to grasp by biopsy forceps and can be retrieved by passing a curved instrument beyond them and pulling the instrument out. This maneuver may, however, abrade the nasal mucosa and cause epistaxis, which can be easily controlled by pinching the nose and instilling xylometazoline nasal drops. The foreign bodies that are not visible on anterior rhinoscopy, or are impacted and have history of failed retrieval should preferably be retrieved under general anesthesia in the operating room. The availability of a nasal endoscope for such a situation is desirable.

Epistaxis

Epistaxis is fairly common in children, especially in areas and seasons with dry climates. Epistaxis is an alarming symptom for most parents and the volume of blood loss is sometimes overestimated by parents. The anterior most part of the nasal septum is the most frequent site of bleeding as it is especially vascular (Kiesselbach's plexus or Little's area), prone to drying by the dry inspiratory air, and also prone to trauma by nose picking by finger or nail[12].

The common causes of epistaxis in children are listed in Table 45.3. Though it is unusual for epistaxis to be significant in amount or sinister in etiology, a thorough evaluation is mandatory to assess the extent of loss and to ascertain the exact site and cause of bleeding. Fever, if accompanied with epistaxis, should alarm the physician regarding the possibility of thrombocytopenia due to viral fevers e.g dengue hemorrhagic fever.

Treatment

Close inspection of the nasal cavity should be performed under bright light. Most frequently, active bleeders or blood clots are observed over the anterior-inferior part of the septum (Little's area). Such bleeding responds well to gentle pressure by pinching the nostrils and simple first aid measures like elevation of the bleeding site (sitting up and leaning forward) and ice packs/cold water

application on the nose (Figure 45.1). The child and parents should be counselled regarding the nature of disease, with advice to avoid nose picking and to keep fingernails well clipped. Recurrent bleeding may be managed by simple cauterization of the bleeding point/ Little's area under local anesthesia. An oil based ointment may be applied inside the nostrils twice daily for lubrication and to prevent drying.

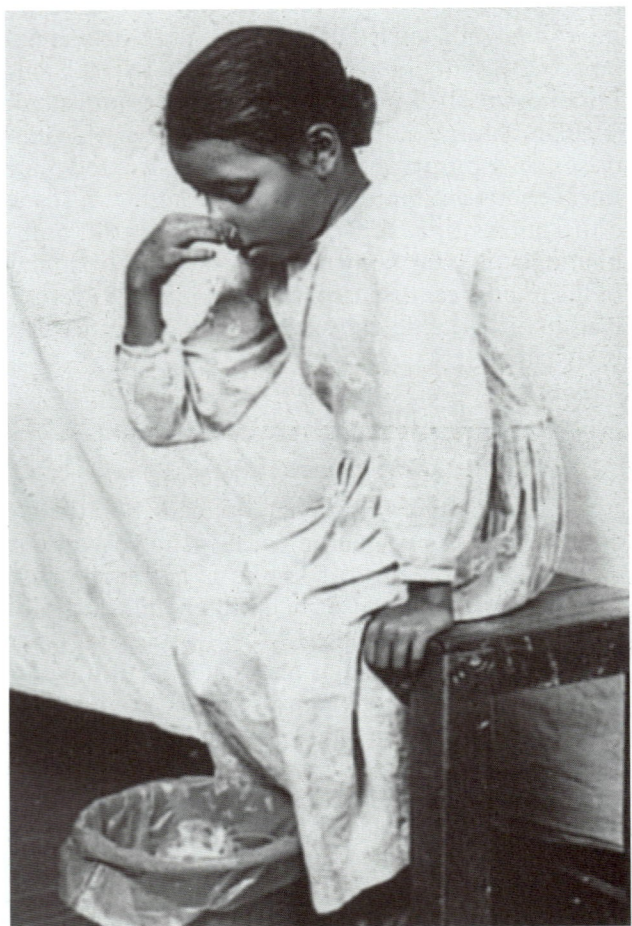

Figure 45.1 The child should be made to sit comfortably, breathe through mouth and pinch the nose firmly at least for 5 minutes to stop bleeding

Severe epistaxis not responding to simple measures may require nasal packing or very occasionally arterial ligation. Nasal packing is traditionally done by sterile paraffin open weave gauze dressing, but this may be traumatic and further abrade the nasal mucosa. Alternatively, Foley's catheter or Simpson inflatable balloon can be inserted in the nose and filled with air or water (Figure 45.2). Prefabricated nasal tampons as currently available are more comfortable and easy to use (Figure 45.3). Significant epistaxis should prompt admission to the hospital and replacement of blood loss. Any underlying cause (rhinitis, tumor,

Table 45.3 Common causes of epistaxis

Local factors

- Little's area crusting/ drying
- Self inflicted trauma e.g. nose picking
- External trauma e.g blow, cricket ball injury
- Foreign body
- Viral or bacterial rhinosinusitis.
- Infected polypi or nasal septum due to tuberculosis, syphilis, leprosy, *Rhinosporidium seebari*
- Telangiectasia (Rindu-Osler-Weber disorder)
- Tumors e.g. Capillary hemangioma, hamartoma, angiofibroma, rhabdomyosarcoma

Systemic factors

- Viral fever
- Hematological disorders e.g. platelet defects or coagulation defects
- Hypertension
- Severe mitral stenosis

Section 4

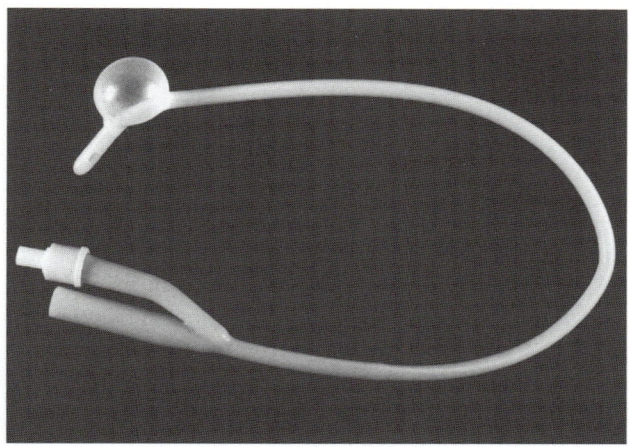

Figure 45.2 Simpson's inflatable balloon which can be filled with air or water to stop the bleeding

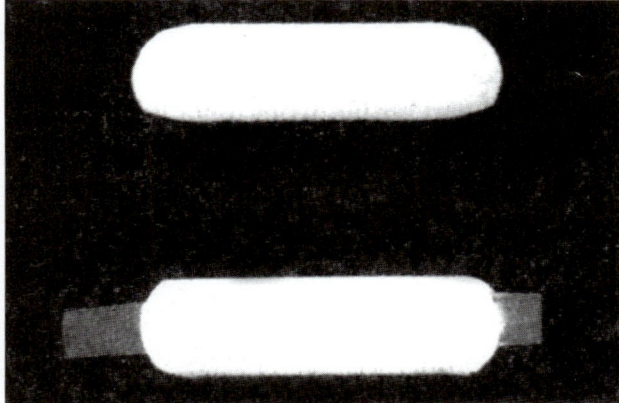

Figure 45.3 Compressed gelfoam nasal pack

vascular malformation, coagulopathy) should be identified and appropriately treated.

Nasal Trauma

Trauma to the face may occur as a result of play ground injuries and road traffic accidents. The nose being the most projected part of face is likely to be affected in most injuries to the face. Patients presenting with facial injuries are also at risk for head injury, cervical spine injury and orbital injury. These injuries can be effectively and judiciously managed if the protocol of careful evaluation of all maxillofacial prominences is followed. History of loss of consciousness, vomiting, ear bleed, CSF leakage, dizziness and seizures gives a clue to the underlying head injury. Visual loss and diplopia provides clue towards possible orbital fractures.

Isolated nasal injuries are usually mild. The patients usually present with edema and swelling over the nose with and without epistaxis. All the facial prominences should be carefully palpated for any swelling or deformity. The nasal skin, nasal skeleton and septum should be carefully assessed. Patients are usually concerned about nasal fractures. They can be counselled that undisplaced nasal fractures do not require any treatment and heal spontaneously. The epistaxis should be managed as described above. The presence of external deformity should caution the clinician about presence of displaced nasal fracture and it should be reduced and fixed as early as feasible. Another condition that warrants immediate attention is the septal hematoma. The presence of a boggy swelling over the nasal septum is suggestive of hematoma and if present, it should be immediately evacuated to avoid infection and pressure necrosis of cartilage.

Infections and Abscesses of Head and Neck

Cellulitis and abscess formation in the fascial spaces of the neck are an important class of emergencies in pediatric practice. Untreated, they may lead to life threatening airway obstruction and may also progress to cause mediastinitis and septicemia.

Pathophysiology

Infections originating in the tonsils and dental spaces are the usual initial sites leading to bacterial neck space infections. Tuberculous cold abscess secondary to liquefaction of a lymph node is not infrequent in children. Abscesses and cellulitis may occur in all the spaces of neck but they most frequently occur in tonsillar space (peritonsillar abscess or quinsy), parapharyngeal space, retropharyngeal space and submandibular or submaxillary space (Ludwig's angina). These neck spaces are intimately related to each other and it is not rare for one space to infect the contiguous areas.

Clinical features

The patient presents with signs and symptoms of sepsis. There is history of neck swelling, muscle spasm, trismus, dysphagia and odynophagia. Fever and sometimes breathing difficulty or stridor may occur. The diagnosis should be made on clinical grounds and treatment initiated immediately. Radiology may help in localising the infection and its spread and in making the distinction between cellulitis and abscess. Ultrasound of neck and CT scan are excellent modalities. CT or ultrasound guided aspiration of pus can provide rapid relief of symptoms and can be a useful alternative to surgical drainage. The status of airway and cervical vertebrae should always be carefully evaluated on CT scan, especially in a case of retropharyngeal

Section 4

abscess. Spinal caries is one of the common causes of retopharyngeal abscess

Treatment

All patients with deep neck abscesses should be admitted to the hospital. Cellulitis may be initially managed by conservative treatment with close monitoring to ascertain clinical response. Broad spectrum antibiotics with coverage for anerobic and aerobic infections should be initially instituted and efforts made to obtain aspirate for culture. Manifest suppuration, lack of response to antibiotics over 48 hours, progressive infection, and airway compromise are all indications for immediate surgical drainage. Maintenance of secure airway is of primary concern in all neck abscesses. Urgent intervention is required if there are signs of airway compromise. Endotracheal intubation is at times risky and may cause rupture of abscess into the airway leading to aspiration. Tracheostomy is a safer option in such cases. Other potentially life-threatening complications include jugular vein thrombosis, descending mediastinitis, sepsis, acute respiratory distress syndrome, and disseminated intravascular coagulation[13].

STRIDOR

Stridor is an audible respiratory noise produced from turbulent flow of air due to narrow or obstructed airway. The presence of stridor indicates significant obstruction in the larynx or trachea. Stridor is usually a high pitched sound which may be inspiratory, expiratory or biphasic. It needs to be differentiated from other "noisy breathing sounds" like stertor and wheeze. Table 45.4 lists the localising value of various airway sounds produced due to obstruction at different sites in the airways.

The presence of airway obstruction, especially in children is governed by the usual laws of physics i.e. Poiseuilie's law which states that resistance is inversely proportional to the fourth power of the radius; and the venturi principle wherein movement of a gas through a partially closed flexible tube leads to fall in lateral pressure causing collapse and narrowing of the tube. The causes of airway obstruction in the pediatric population are listed in Table 45.5.

Table 45.4 Different airway sounds and their localising value

STRIDOR: High pitched sound originating in the larynx or trachea.

- Inspiratory stridor — Obstruction at the level of supraglottis or glottis
- Expiratory stridor — Obstruction at the level of lower trachea
- Biphasic stridor — Obstruction at the level of subglottic or upper trachea

STERTOR: Low pitched snoring sound originating in the pharynx.

WHEEZE: It occurs due to obstruction or spasm of small airways and is seen in bronchial asthma and foreign body inhalation.

*Stridor at other sites may also manifest as biphasic if severe, but would continue to manifest predominantly as inspiratory or expiratory in character as per the site of obstruction.

Table 45.5 Common causes of airway obstruction

CONGENITAL

- Supralaryngeal
  - Nasal piriform stenosis, midnasal stenosis, choanal atresia
  - Nasal mass lesions, encephalocele, meningocele, glioma etc.
  - Micrognathia, macroglossia, midface hypoplasia (Pierre-Robin syndrome)
- Laryngeal
  - Supraglottic: Laryngomalacia, laryngeal cyst
  - Glottic: Web, vocal cord paralysis
  - Subglottic: Sublglottic stenosis, subglottic hemangioma, cleft deformity
- Tracheobronchial
  - Tracheomalacia, tracheal stenosis
  - External compression due to vascular loop, mediastinal tumor

ACQUIRED

- Supralaryngeal
  - Adenotonsillar hypertrophy, retropharyngeal abscess, peritonsillar abscess (Quinsy)
  - Foreign body
- Laryngeal
  - Infections: Epiglottitis, croup, diphtheria, infectious mononucleosis
  - Trauma, intubation
  - Tumors: Hemangioma, adenoma
  - Papillomatosis
  - Foreign body
  - Laryngeal spasm (tetany)
- Tracheobronchial
  - Tracheal stenosis (post intubation)
  - Foreign body
  - Infections (laryngo-tracheo-bronchitis)
  - Extrinsic compression due to mediastinal tumor

Assessment

History, physical examination and resuscitation must be undertaken simultaneously. Stridor is a symptom of underlying pathology but is not a diagnosis. It is important to assess the degree of respiratory distress in relation to the stridor, and assess the likelihood for progression. The time of onset, progression, other associated complaints and past illnesses usually provide useful clues to the diagnosis. The key questions that should be asked on history are listed below.

1. *Time of onset of stridor.* The stridor at birth usually indicates a serious congenital airway obstruction. Laryngomalacia almost never presents at birth but after a few days or weeks of age[14,15].

2. *Progression.* Stridor due to laryngomalacia is usually static and tends to improve with time. Laryngomalacia typically causes stridor that worsens on crying or feeding. All stridors tend to worsen with episodes of upper respiratory tract infection. Sudden onset of stridor with rapid progression indicates upper airway foreign body or infections.

3. *Past history.* History of significant perinatal insult should be sought. Bilateral vocal cord palsy is often preceded by upper respiratory tract infection. History of endotracheal intubation may precede the possibility of subglottic or tracheal stenosis.

4. *Associated symptoms* provide useful clue to the site of obstruction and likely diagnosis. Presence of hoarseness indicates laryngeal pathology, most frequently papillomas. History of cough and aspiration are suggestive of tracheoesophageal fistula and laryngeal cleft. The differences between supraglottic or glottic and infraglottic or tracheal obstruction are summarized in Table 45.6.

5. Fever, dysphagia, hyperextension of neck and drooling indicate epiglottitis or upper airway infections like tonsillitis or peritonsillar abscess.

Examination

The child should be examined with the neck, chest and abdomen uncovered to assess difficult in breathing. Tracheal and suprasternal indrawing, substernal recessions, diaphoresis, signs of exhaustion are all features of severe airway obstruction and necessitate immediate airway management.

Features of systemic infection like fever, tachycardia, tachypnea and cyanosis should be looked for. The site of obstruction can be clinically assessed by carefully analysing the respiratory phase in which stridor is heard. A quick oral and oropharyngeal examination is performed under good illumination. If the child is suspected to have epiglottitis or oropharyngeal and supraglottic edema, this evaluation should be deferred till operating room facilities for emergency airway are available.

On arrival to the emergency room, the child with stridor, especially those with "danger signs" should be monitored with a pulse oximeter. Arterial blood gas analysis is a more reliable measure of oxygenation. If the situation permits, initial clinical evaluation may be supplemented by X-ray neck and flexible nasopharyngoscopy. Plain skiagram of neck, lateral view with neck extended provides an excellent modality for evaluation of the airway from nasopharynx to lower trachea. A constriction of airway due to subglottic stenosis, extrinsic compression of airway, thickened epiglottis in epiglottitis, and dilated ventricle in bilateral vocal cord palsy are useful signs which can be easily identified on plain radiographs.

Flexible endoscopy with a pediatric ultrathin flexible laryngoscope is a reliable method for diagnosing the cause of stridor[16]. The procedure should be performed only in stable patients and with all facilities for airway management at hand. It also has a major advantage over rigid endoscopy for

Section 4

	Table 45.6 Differences between clinical features of supraglottic and tracheal obstruction		
	Symptoms	**Supraglottic obstruction**	**Tracheal obstruction**
❑	Stridor	Inspiratory	Expiratory
❑	Cry and voice	Muffled, weak or hoarse	Normal
❑	Dyspnea	Moderate	Severe
❑	Cough	Occasional or intermittent	Barking or brassy
❑	Dysphagia	Common	Absent

enabling a dynamic evaluation of the larynx in an awake patient. This is especially important as some of the common congenital abnormalities causing stridor like laryngomalacia and bilateral abductor cord paralysis, are easily demonstrated in a spontaneously breathing patient but may be masked when evaluated under anesthesia by rigid endoscopy.

Nevertheless, the gold standard for diagnostic assessment of airway is rigid larygoscopy and bronchoscopy[16]. The procedure is performed under general anesthesia in the operating room. Modern endoscopes and light sources provide excellent visualization of whole larynx, trachea and bronchi. In an emergency situation, bronchoscopy in experienced hands is useful to secure the airway. Rigid endoscopy also allows for simultaneous therapeutic interventions such as removal of foreign body, dilatation of stricture, removal of papillomas, and surgical treatment of laryngomalacia and bilateral vocal cord paralysis.

Treatment

Stridor is merely a symptom and effective treatment is only achieved by establishing a diagnosis and directing treatment for correction of the cause of obstruction. Treatment is aimed at correction of the cause like anti-edema measures like steroids and antibiotics for inflammatory causes or surgical treatment for structural abnormalities due to congenital lesions. Administrations of oxygen, corticosteroids and nebulized epinephrine may provide temporary relief to "buy time" till patient is taken up for definitive surgery. Endotracheal intubation or tracheostomy are effective emergency interventions to secure the airway, but are merely palliative to improve oxygenation till underlying

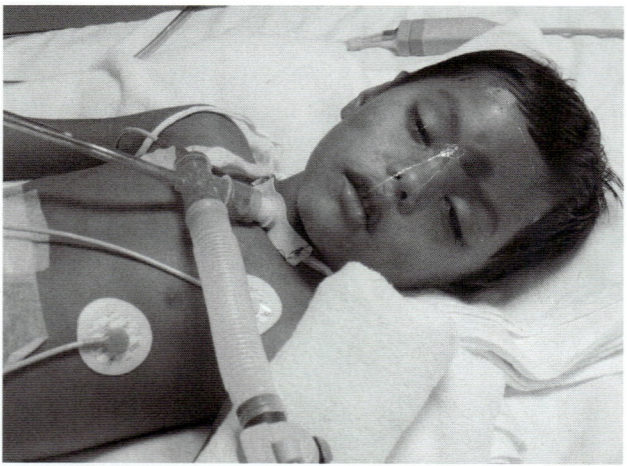

Figure 45.4 Tracheostomy support to a patient with laryngeal diphtheria

cause is tackled and resolved. Tracheostomy may be life saving in a patient with laryngeal diphtheria (Figure 45.4).

Stridor is best managed by a team of specialists including pediatrician, an otolaryngologist, an anesthetist, and at times a pediatric surgeon. The treating team should address the following critical questions in the order as listed below.

(a) The severity of stridor, and the need, if any, for immediate airway support.

(b) The site of obstruction and the exact congenital abnormality.

(c) In cases wherein the stridor is not very severe, the appropriateness of therapeutic intervention vis-à-vis a policy of watchful waiting should be followed. This is especially so, as some cases of congenital stridor are expected to improve with time (laryngomalacia).

(d) If surgical intervention is planned, the possibility of direct surgical correction of the anatomical abnormality should be attempted. This is preferable to the traditional treatment by tracheostomy, as long term tracheostomy poses significant morbidity and developmental limitations on the child.

The options for securing the airway include endotracheal intubation, tracheostomy and rigid ventilating bronchoscopy. Intubation is generally the initial preferred option as it is the quickest and equipment is readily available. In difficult situations, intubation should ideally be undertaken with an otolaryngologist standing by for emergent tracheostomy and rigid bronchoscopy. Emergency tracheostomy in a pediatric patient who cannot be fully anesthetised because of the unsecured airway, however, is a daunting and sometimes dangerous procedure. Rigid bronchoscopy allows for securing the airway under vision and can sometimes prove very useful.

Endoscopic treatment for correction of the underlying pathology may need to be undertaken in emergency situations. Traditional interventions include foreign body removal and surgical debulking of obstructing papillomas. Other airway interventions that have developed recently include endoscopic supraglottopexy and division of aryepiglottic folds for laryngomalacia, endoscopic arytenoidectomy or cordotomy for bilateral vocal cord paralysis, endoscopic laser excision and keel placement for laryngeal web, laser excision and endoscopic steroid injection for subglottic stenosis, and endoscopic closure for grade I/II laryngeal cleft. External single stage techniques include laryngotracheal reconstruction for subglottic stenosis and aortopexy for tracheomalacia[17].

REFERENCES

1. Elden LM, Potsic WP. Otolaryngologic emergencies. In: Textbook of Pediatric Emergency Medicine. Fleisher GR, Ludwig S, (Eds). 6th ed *Lippincott Williams & Wilkins,* 2010.

2. Leung AK, Fong JH, Leong AG. Otalgia in children. *J Natl Med Assoc* 2000; 92(5):254-260.

3. Browning *et al.,* Ear wax clinical evidence 2008; 01:504 (http://clinicalevidence.bmj.com/ceweb/conditions/ent/0504/0504-get.pdf)

4. Paradise JL. Otitis media in infants and children. *Pediatrics* 1980;65(5):917-943.

5. Browning G. Otitis media with effusion. In: Scott-Brown's Otorhinolaryngology, Head and Neck Surgery, Gleeson M, Browning GG, Burton MJ, Clarke R, Hibbert J, Jones NS, (Eds.). 7th ed; *Hodder Arnold;* 2008.

6. Glasziou PP, Del Mar CB, Sanders SL, Hayem M. Antibiotics for acute otitis media in children. *Cochrane Database Syst Rev* 2004; (1):CD000219.

7. Carney AS. Otitis externa and otomycosis. In: Scott-Brown's Otorhinolaryngology, Head and Neck Surgery, Gleeson M, Browning GG, Burton MJ, Clarke R, Hibbert J, Jones NS (Eds.), 7th ed; *Hodder Arnold;* 2008.

8. Buron MJ , Harvey RJ . Idiopathic sudden sensorineural hearing loss. In: Scott-Brown's Otorhinolaryngology, Head and Neck Surgery, Gleeson M, Browning GG, Burton MJ, Clarke R, Hibbert J, Jones NS (Eds.), 7th ed; *Hodder Arnold;* 2008.

9. Veltri RW. Wilson WR, Sprinkle PM, Rodman SM, Kavesh DA. The implication of viruses in idiopathic sudden hearing loss: infection or reactivation of latent viruses. *Otolaryngol Head and Neck Surg* 1981; 89: 137-141.

10. Morrison GAJ. Vertigo in children. In: Scott-Brown's Otorhinolaryngology, Head and Neck Surgery, Gleeson M, Browning GG, Burton MJ, Clarke R, Hibbert J, Jones NS (Eds.), 7th ed; *Hodder Arnold;* 2008.

11. May M, Fria TJ, Blumenthal F, Curtin H. Facial paralysis in children: differential diagnosis. *Otolaryngol Head Neck Surg* 1981; 89: 841-848.

12. Jackson K, Jackson R. Factors associated with active refractory epistaxis. *Arch Otolaryngol Head Neck Surg* 1988; 114: 862-865.

13. Vieira F, Allen SM, Stocks RM, Thompson JW. Deep neck infection. *Otolaryngol Clin North Am* 2008 Jun; 41(3):459-483.

14. Venkatakarthikeyan.C, Thakar A, Lodha R. Ensdoscopic correction of severe laryngomalacia. *Indian J Pediatr* 2005; 72(2):165-168.

15. Nussbaum E, Maggi JE. Laryngomalacia in children. *Chest* 1990; 98: 942-944.

16. Albert D, Boardman S, Soma M. Evaluation and management of the stridulous child. In: Cummings Otolaryngology, Head and Neck Surgery, Flint PW, Haughey BH, Lund VJ (Eds.), 5th ed; *Mosby Elsevier;* 2010.

17. Pradhan T, Sikka K, Thakar A. Posterior cricoid split with costal cartilage augmentation for high subglottic stenosis. *Indian J Otolaryngol Head Neck Surg* 2008; 60: 147-151.

Section 4

46

Dermatological Emergencies

M Ramam and L K Gupta

A significant proportion of children seeking emergency care present with cutaneous lesions as the major or sole complaint. Skin manifestations may be primary in nature or a manifestation of an underlying systemic disorder. Often, a dermatologist is not available for consultation and the management of these patients becomes the responsibility of the family physician or pediatrician. We have attempted here to provide a practical approach for the assessment and initial management of the common dermatological emergencies. The emphasis has been laid on the diagnosis and therapy in the emergency situation. Details of the individual diseases have been deliberately omitted; these can be studied from standard textbooks on the subject. A discussion of the general approach to dermatological emergencies is followed by a fuller description of the individual conditions arranged into groups which share a common management plan. Clinical signs that point towards a particular dermatologic emergency are listed in Table 46.1.

Table 46.1 Common correlates of dermatological emergencies

Clinical parameter	Possible dermatoses
Constitutional symptoms	TEN, SJS, purpura fulminans, sclerema neonatorum
Purpura/ skin necrosis	SJS, TEN, purpura fulminans, necrotising fasciitis
Widespread bullae/ erosions	Pemphigus vulgaris, TEN, SJS, epidermolysis bullosa
Mucosal erosions	Pemphigus vulgaris, TEN, SJS
Generalised exfoliation	SSSS, erythroderma

TEN = Toxic epidermal necrolysis; SJS = Stevens-Johnson syndrome; SSSS = Staphylococcal scalded skin syndrome

APPROACH TO THE CHILD WITH A DERMATOLOGIC EMERGENCY

A quick assessment of the child's condition can be made by asking three questions:

1. Does the eruption involve large areas of the skin?

2. Does the child have blisters or erosions?

3. Does the child appear ill?

Most of the conditions that require immediate intervention involve large areas of the skin. If a child presents early in the disease process, only a few anatomic areas may be affected. However, if the history reveals that the lesions have spread rapidly, the eruption is expected to involve large areas of the skin and would need urgent treatment.

The most serious emergencies are those associated with raw lesions and blisters involving large areas of the skin. These children require immediate hospitalization and intensive care. In newborn babies, sclerema neonatorum (hide-bound skin), subcutaneous fat necrosis (due to cold injury) and purpura fulminans (sepsis) are suggestive of life-threatening disorders with ominous outcome.

Another clue to the severity of a child's disease depends upon how ill the child appears. Though this aspect generally correlates well with the extent of the eruption and the presence of blisters and raw areas, it can be a useful clue in situations where the skin lesions are limited in extent but are associated with complications, e.g. Henoch-Schonlein purpura. Conversely, a child with an extensive eruption may be quite cheerful as in pityriasis rosea or some viral exanthems. These children do not usually need emergency intervention. However, in the latter situation, one must be cautious in ruling out a severe disease because constitutional symptoms may set in later than the skin lesions in some conditions. When in doubt, it is preferable to keep the child under observation.

On the basis of this initial assessment dermatological emergencies can be classified into 3 broad groups:

(a) Diseases with extensive blistering and skin erosions.

(b) Diseases with extensive skin involvement without blisters.

(c) Diseases with localized skin lesions.

These categories are easily recognized and do not require familiarity with the minutiae of dermatological nomenclature. The general approach to diseases within each category is substantially similar and will facilitate initial management till a more specific diagnosis is reached. Each of the following sections begins with the general principles of diagnosis and management of the emergency and is followed by an account of individual conditions, with special focus on specific manifestations.

There is a fourth category of perceived emergencies that are not dealt with in this chapter. In this sub-group, a benign skin disease provokes anxiety in the child or parents prompting them to seek immediate medical attention. The range of conditions that can precipitate this behaviour is too large to deal with but most often the concern is that the child has developed a reaction to a drug or an allergy to a food. If a specific diagnosis of the child's eruption is made, then specific treatment and/ or reassurance is easy. However, if the condition cannot be diagnosed confidently, a quick review of the questions listed at the beginning of this section is a helpful starting point. If the lesions are neither extensive nor troublesome, reassurance may be all that is necessary. However, parents must be asked to report back if they feel the eruption is worsening or if the child appears ill.

EXTENSIVE ERUPTIONS WITH BLISTERING AND RAW AREAS

Diseases with extensive blistering and erosions are characterized by large raw areas of the skin. The development of blisters is followed by rupture and extension to form raw areas. The oral and genital mucosae and the conjunctivae may also be involved. In some patients, severe constitutional symptoms may accompany the eruption.

The prototype of diseases with extensive skin erosions is burn. Though, by convention this is considered a surgical emergency, it exemplifies the problems that occur when the barrier function of skin is severely damaged viz. fluid and electrolyte losses occur and there is increased susceptibility to superadded infections.

Several different conditions, infective and non-infective may lead to this presentation. Some useful diagnostic clues which help differentiate between these conditions include the rapid involvement of extensive areas over a few hours with associated toxemia (toxic epidermal necrolysis (TEN) and Stevens-Johnson (SJ) syndrome), accompanying target lesions (SJ syndrome), necrotic brown lesions (TEN) or large pustules (bullous impetigo), preceding oral mucosal lesions (pemphigus) and history of drug intake (TEN and SJ syndrome).

The treatment of patients with extensive erosions requires immediate hospitalization and excellent nursing and supportive care. The eroded areas need to be cleansed regularly with soap and water followed by application of an antiseptic lotion or cream such as povidone iodine or silver sulfadiazine. In most instances, erosions do not require to be bandaged and can be left open. Paraffin gauze or sofra tulle can be applied on erosions in contact with bed clothes to prevent sticking. Frequent changing of position in bed helps in the healing of erosions on pressure sites. The mucosal lesions in the oral cavity and genitalia should be cleansed by repeated washes with normal saline and antiseptic solutions (povidone iodine mouth wash, diluted Condy's solution). Conjunctival lesions can be cleansed with antibiotic eye drops several times during the day and antibiotic ointment applied at night.

Fluid and electrolyte loss from exuding erosions is a major problem in these patients which may be aggravated by reduced intake due to painful oral lesions. A close record of intake and output should be maintained and patients encouraged to take fluids and semisolids orally. Intravenous fluids should be infused if oral intake is inadequate.

Systemic antibiotics should be instituted if there are signs of cutaneous infection such as pustulation or purulent discharge from the skin lesions or if patients show signs of toxemia such as fever, tachycardia and tachypnea. The organisms responsible for most of the secondary infections are *Staphylococcus aureus* and *Streptococcus pyogenes*. Antibiotics effective against these organisms such as cloxacillin, cephalexin and erythromycin should be administered.

The use of systemic corticosteroids in large doses (1-2 mg/kg of prednisolone equivalent/day) is required in some conditions such as pemphigus, toxic epidermal necrolysis and Stevens-Johnson syndrome.

Toxic Epidermal Necrolysis (TEN)[1-5]

TEN is a severe acute blistering disease that has a high mortality rate without treatment. It is generally considered to be a hypersensitivity reaction to drugs such as thiacetazone, sulphonamides,

Section 4

phenytoin, barbiturates, penicillin, non-steroidal anti-inflammatory agents among the others. The reaction generally develops within 2-3 weeks of starting the drug in a non-sensitized person but may develop within hours if the patient is already sensitized to the drug. TEN can occur at all ages though most patients are young adults.

The eruption begins abruptly as tender, erythematous macules accompanied by vesiculation and bullae. Large areas of the erythematous skin develop a characteristic brown black discoloration (Figure 46.1). The necrotic skin peels off easily (Nikolysky sign) to leave large raw areas. Mucous membrane involvement is invariable and is generally severe. Mucosae of oral cavity, eyes, genitalia, esophagus and bronchial tree may be involved. Ocular lesions carry a high risk of sequelae such as corneal scarring and blindness. There is marked

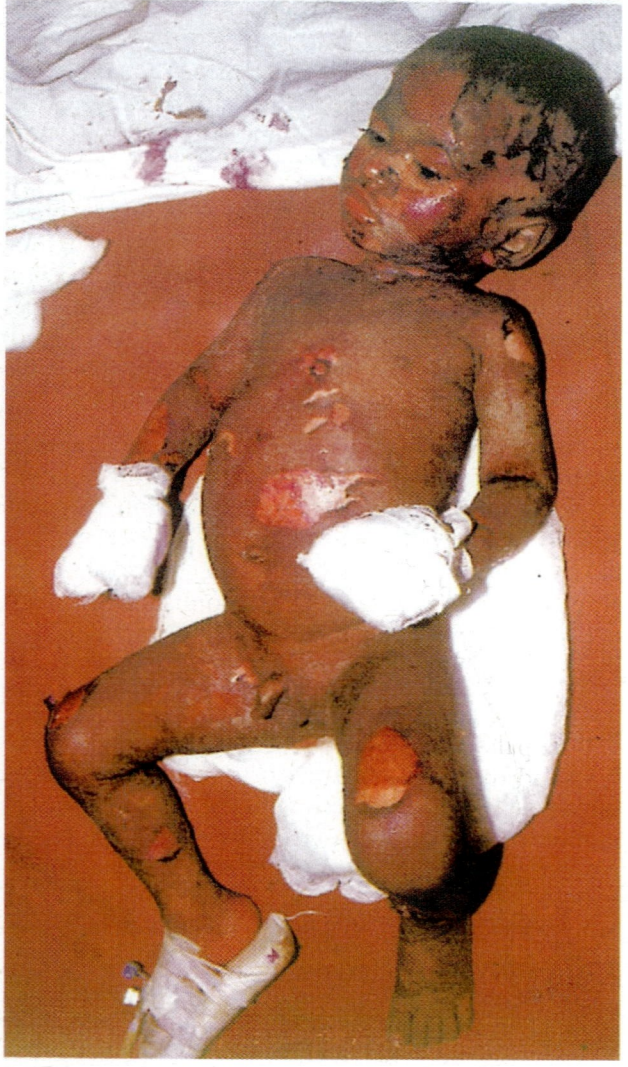

Figure 46.1 Toxic epidermal necrolysis. Characteristic, widespread brown black necrosis and erosions

toxemia and high grade fever. Complications include superadded infections and septicemia, hypovolemic shock, acute tubular necrosis, glomerulonephritis, bronchopneumonia, pulmonary edema and gastrointestinal bleeding.

Management

The immediate stoppage of all the drugs that the patient has been taking is the most important part of the management of TEN. It is emphasised that suspecting and stopping only one of the drugs being taken is extremely dangerous because a mistake in identifying the drug can lead to marked worsening of the condition. If a drug is essential, a chemically unrelated substitute should be used.

Nursing and supportive care is provided as outlined in the section on general principles. Patients who report early during the course of the disease (as manifested by the presence of erythema around skin lesions) benefit from corticosteroid therapy. Those who are seen a few days after onset of disease, show mild or no erythema around skin lesions and/or show peeling of necrotic skin with underlying re-epithelialisation do not require corticosteroids. Prednisolone is administered in an initial dose of 1.5-2 mg/kg daily. The condition of the patient is closely monitored over a period of 24-48 hours for the appearance of new lesions and persistence or appearance of erythema at the periphery of lesions. Erythema on the palms and soles persists much longer than elsewhere and should not be used to titrate therapy. If the signs of activity are present, an increase in the daily dose by 0.5-1 mg/kg of prednisolone equivalent is made and the same dose is maintained for 2-3 days till the disease is controlled. The dose is then abruptly halved every 2-3 days and withdrawn completely over a period of 10-14 days.

Some workers advocate that corticosteroids should be avoided in the treatment of TEN. However, we have had good results with corticosteroid therapy and would advocate a high dose, short duration regime to rapidly control the disease in those with active skin lesions. Other agents that have been described to be effective by some workers include cyclosporine and intravenous immunoglobulins (IVIG).

Stevens-Johnson Syndrome[1,4]

Stevens-Johnson syndrome is an uncommon reaction pattern that is usually triggered by drugs (listed *vide supra* in the section on TEN) or infections (pharyngitis, pneumonitis due to *mycoplasma pneumoniae*, herpes labialis, hepatitis). The clinical picture closely resembles TEN. Target lesions i.e. erythematous lesions with a blue-black center are a distinctive feature (Figure 46.2). In the absence of target lesions, the difference between SJ syndrome and TEN is largely subjective. The management is essentially similar to that of TEN. In addition, a thorough search must be made to look for a focus of infection which may be the cause of the reaction and must be treated appropriately. In patients who have herpes simplex infection, acyclovir 5 mg/kg 8 hourly, intravenously or 200 mg five times a day, orally should be administered.

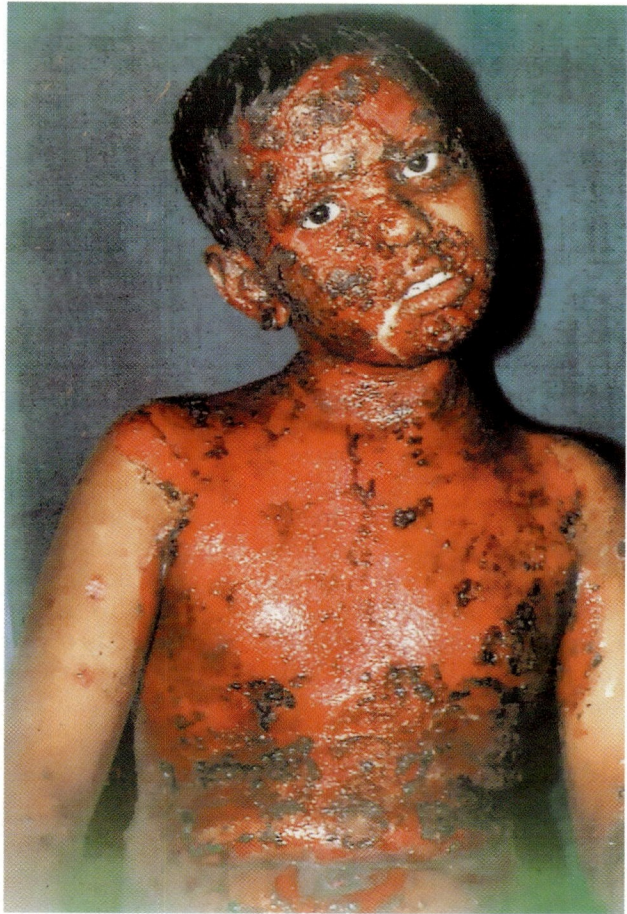

Figure 46.3 Pemphigus vulgaris with extensive erosions and crusting

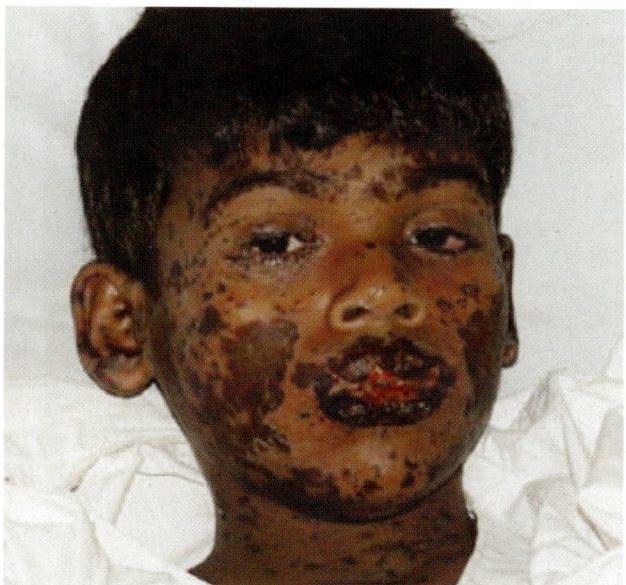

Figure 46.2 Stevens-Johnson syndrome

Pemphigus[3, 6-8]

Pemphigus is an auto-immune blistering disorder that manifests as flaccid bullae which usually occur on apparently normal skin. The bullae rupture easily leaving large, raw areas which have a tendency to extend peripherally (Figure 46.3). Spontaneous healing is very slow. The normal skin can be peeled off easily with gentle pressure (Niklosky's sign). In over half of the patients, ulcers in the mouth precede the appearance of cutaneous lesions and eventually almost all patients develop oral mucosal lesions. Giemsa staining of the scraped material obtained from the base of the freshly ruptured bullae when examined under the microscope (Tzanck smear) reveals the presence of characteristic acantholytic cells i.e. large round epidermal cells with prominent nucleus and loss of contact with surrounding cells. The diagnosis is confirmed by skin biopsy.

Management

The general principles of treatment of diseases with extensive erosions apply to patients with pemphigus. Corticosteroids are the mainstay of therapy. We use dexamethasone 50 mg infused in 5% dextrose on 3 consecutive days, every 4 weeks. In the initial few weeks, most patients will also require a daily dose of oral corticosteroids such as prednisolone 0.5-1 mg/kg. As the disease becomes inactive, the daily dose can be reduced and stopped but the pulses of dexamethasone are continued for a period of 6-9 months after complete clinical remission. In our experience, this regime gives long lasting remissions even after therapy is stopped.

An alternative schedule consists of using 1-2 mg/kg/day or higher dose of prednisolone or equivalent steroid. The daily dose can be increased by 1 mg/kg daily if there is no clinical response as indicated by continued appearance of new lesions, and extension of the old lesions. The dose of steroid should be maintained till all lesions have healed completely. The dose is then gradually tapered and the patient maintained on the minimal required dose.

Most patients also require the use of an additional immunosuppressive agent such as azathioprine, methotrexate or mycophenolate mofetil in order to reduce the requirement of corticosteroids and to maintain a remission. This disease is best managed in association with a dermatologist.

Staphylococcal Scalded Skin Syndrome (SSSS)[9]

SSSS is an uncommon but serious condition caused by the epidermolytic toxin liberated by some strains of *Staphylococcus aureus*. It is characterized by tenderness, erythema and peeling of skin. The condition occurs almost exclusively in infants and young children. It usually begins from perioral areas and flexures and may spread to involve the entire skin (Figure 46.4). Mucosae are not usually affected. The child is usually toxic. The underlying staphylococcal infection is usually occult (conjunctivitis, pharyngitis, otitis media) or sometimes obvious as boils or umbilical sepsis.

Management

The condition is treated by administration of appropriate antibiotics effective against staphylococci, including the penicillinase producing strains. Cloxacillin (100 mg/kg/day) and amoxicillin-clavulanic acid (50-100 mg/kg/day of amoxycillin base) intravenously q 6-8 hours is generally the preferred choice. The use of corticosteroids is contraindicated.

Bullous Impetigo[10]

Bullous impetigo is a contagious, superficial bacterial infection of skin caused by *Staphlylococcus aureus*, *Streptococcus pyogenes* or a mixture of both. The disease commonly affects infants and children. Lesions begin as clear vesicles and flaccid bullae which soon turn into pustules and rupture to form yellow brown crusts (Figure 46.5). Face, especially the area around the nose and mouth and extremities are common sites affected. Extensive areas of the skin may be involved. The lesions remain discrete and even when numerous, generally cause little systemic disturbance. Mucosal lesions do not occur. A Gram stained smear from the blister fluid shows the presence of staphylococci and/or streptococci.

Management

Systemic antibiotics should be administered for a period of 5-7 days. Cloxacillin, amoxicillin-

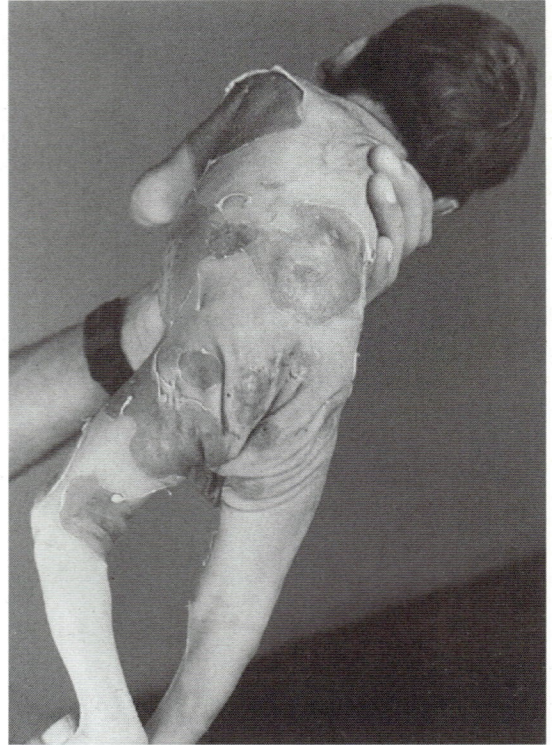
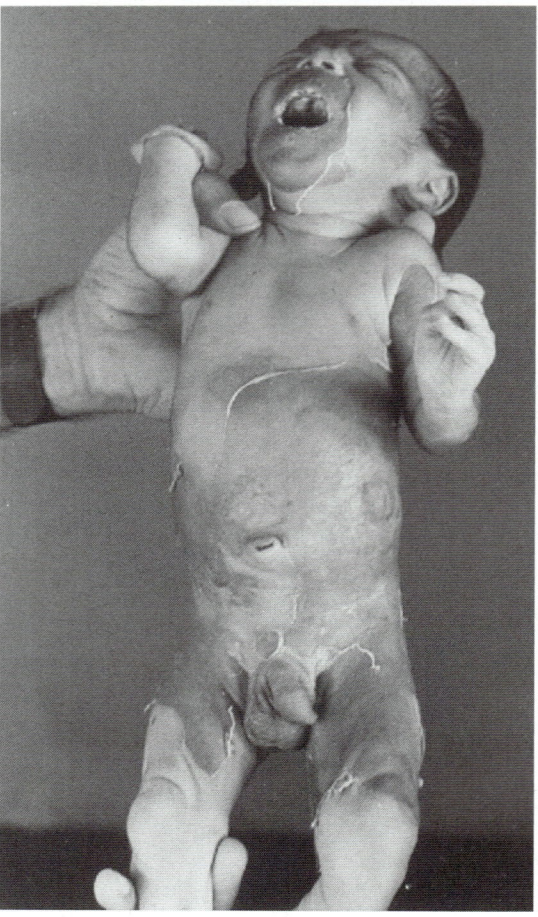

Figure 46.4 Typical appearances of scalded skin syndrome due to staphylococcal infection

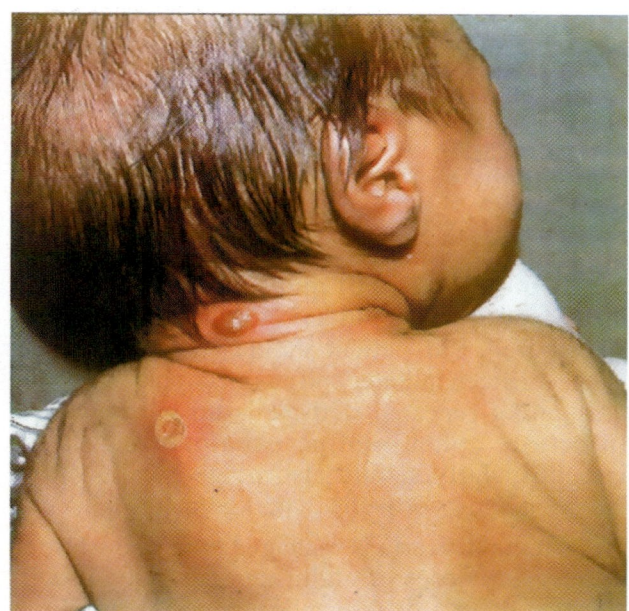

Figure 46.5 Bullous impetigo. Ruptured and intact blisters with turbid fluid on erythematous skin

clavulanic acid, cephalexin and erythromycin are effective choices. The crusts should be removed thoroughly with the help of soap and water. A proper maintenance of hygiene and cleanliness must be emphasised.

Epidermolysis Bullosa[11]

Multiple clear and/or hemorrhagic blisters on the hands and feet and the knees and elbows are suggestive of epidermolysis bullosa. Blisters are present at or soon after birth in severe varieties of the disease and are often accompanied by erosions (Figure 46.6). Extensive erosions of the skin may lead to overwhelming super added infection. In some neonates, epidermolysis bullosa may be accompanied by other anomalies such as pyloric atresia.

Management

Supportive care as detailed in the introductory section is necessary. Associated anomalies should be managed appropriately.

Chronic Bullous Dermatosis of Childhood[3,6,12]

This auto-immune bullous disorder is characterised by tense, clear vesicles and bullae that may develop anywhere on the skin but have a predilection for the peri-oral and genital skin. The blisters often develop in a ring arranged around a central active or healed blister; this is known as the "string of pearls" appearance. The blisters are often impetiginized and may be mistaken for impetigo

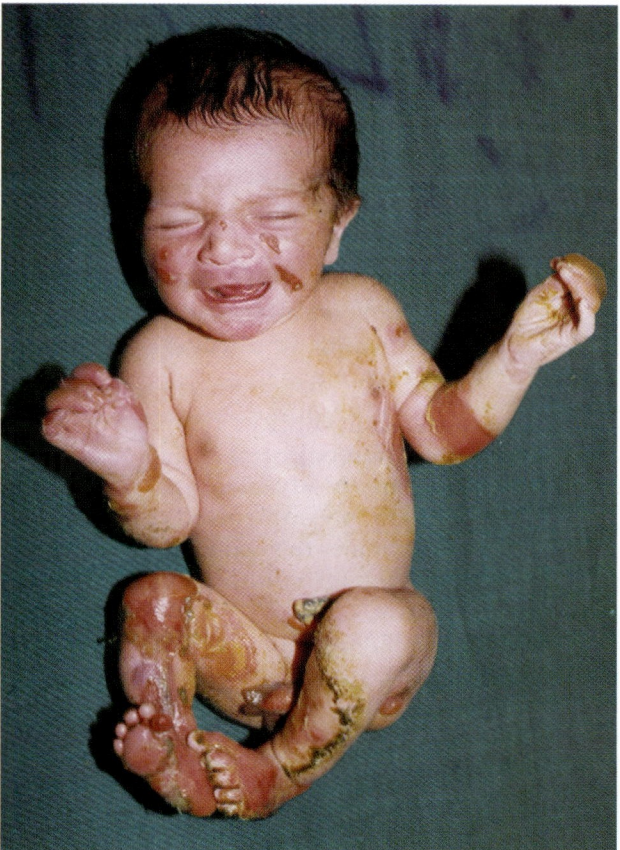

Figure 46.6 Epidermolysis bullosa simplex

contagiosa or infective dermatitis at presentation till a fresh crop of tense vesicles suggests the diagnosis. A biopsy reveals a subepidermal blister and direct immunofluorescence demonstrates a linear band of IgA along the basement membrane zone.

Management

Treatment with dapsone 25-50 mg daily and a low dose of corticosteroids (0.5-1mg/kg) controls the blisters. The corticosteroids may be tapered over 2-4 weeks. Dapsone should be continued for 3-6 months. Recurrences may develop and should be treated similarly. The disease remits spontaneously by puberty in most children.

EXTENSIVE ERUPTIONS WITHOUT BLISTERS/ RAW AREAS

In this group of disorders, patients present with erythema, edema, warmth, tenderness and itching of varying severity. Fever and other constitutional symptoms may accompany the eruption. If lesions persist, secondary changes such as scaling, crusting, thickening, pigmentation and excoriations may appear. Secondary pyogenic infection and

Section 4

generalized lymphadenopathy may occur, following excoriations.

Some useful diagnostic clues to differentiate the dermatoses in this group include duration of individual lesions (few minutes to few hours in urticaria), history of drug intake prior to the development of rash (exanthematous drug eruptions), progressive spread of eruption from one area of skin to another and the occurrence of disease among contacts (viral exanthem) and the presence of pre-existing skin lesions (exfoliative dermatitis).

Immediate intervention in these patients consists of the rapid control of inflammation and relief of symptoms. Many patients have severe itching which can be controlled with oral or parenteral antihistamines (e.g. pheniramine maleate, cetirizine dihydrochloride, cyproheptadine hydrochloride, hydroxyzine hydrochloride). It must be recognized that antihistamines are highly effective in children with urticaria but; they provide only partial symptomatic relief in other conditions. Conventional antihistamines are preferred because their sedative effect contributes to the control of itching. Soothing local applications such as coconut oil or cold water soaks may relieve symptoms. Avoid the use of calamine lotion in undiagnosed rashes because the pink cast of the lotion obscures the cutaneous signs and makes it difficult to evaluate any subsequent changes in the skin. If a drug is suspected to be the cause of eruption further drug intake must be stopped. Efforts should be made to look for any infective focus which should be appropriately treated. Steroids in small doses of 0.5-1 mg/kg of prednisolone equivalent daily are indicated in some conditions such as drug eruption, and exfoliative dermatitis.

Acute Urticaria[13]

This is perhaps the commonest dermatological emergency and is characterized by itchy, erythematous edematous wheals that develop over large areas of the skin. Individual skin lesions usually subside completely in a few minutes to a few hours. However, new lesions may continue to erupt. Mucous membranes may be involved and there may be swelling of the lips, tongue and larynx (angiodema) which can cause respiratory distress. The wheals may be accompanied by abdominal pain, fever and syncope depending on the severity of the attack.

When the process develops very rapidly, it constitutes anaphylactic shock which is characterized by hypotension, bronchoconstriction, urticaria and syncope. The condition is potentially fatal unless managed promptly. Anaphylactic shock usually develops following an injection or an insect bite.

Management

In anaphylactic shock as soon as possible, the patient must be given oxygen inhalation and injection adrenalin (1:1000), 0.01 ml/kg intramuscularly. An intravenous line should be set up, a cut down may be required. The patient should be observed over the next fifteen minutes and an injection of adrenalin 0.01 ml/kg repeated if there is no improvement. Injection pheniramine maleate 25 mg intramuscularly should also be given along with injection hydrocortisone 2 mg/kg im or iv.

Acute urticaria is managed by administration of adequate doses of antihistamines. This usually consists of two different drugs e.g. pheniramine maleate and cetirizine dihydrochloride, given three to four times daily and one to two times daily respectively. There is little to choose among different antihistamines as all work equally well. Parenteral therapy is not usually required. The drugs begin to act within half an hour and peak activity is achieved at 3-4 hours. It is expected that acute urticaria will be substantially controlled within 24 hours. If this does not happen, the dose of antihistamines can be increased, or another antihistamine added to control the symptoms.

Most often, antihistamines are adequate to control the disease. Systemic corticosteroids are often prescribed in acute urticaria but are usually not necessary. Adrenaline should be used only if there is laryngeal edema and respiratory distress.

Once symptoms are controlled, antihistamines should be continued for 7-10 days before stopping therapy. It is important to recognise that most episodes of acute urticaria are self-limited, last for about a week and do not require investigations. When episodes of urticaria persist beyond 6 weeks, it is labeled as chronic urticaria and is beyond the scope of this chapter.

Exanthematous Drug Eruption[14,15]

This is the commonest pattern of drug eruption and can be caused by a number of drugs chiefly sulphonamides, penicillins, anticonvulsants and antitubercular agents. The appearance of the rash does not provide any clues to the causative drug. Characteristically, a symmetrical itchy macular and papular eruption rapidly spreads to involve the entire cutaneous surface including the palms and soles. Initially the lesions are discrete but soon coalesce into large patches (Figure 46.7). The mucosal surfaces may be involved. Fever may sometimes accompany the rash. The rash usually continues to spread if the drug is not stopped. Conversely, it becomes static or begins to regress within 24 hours of stopping the drug. If left untreated, the rash can proceed to exfoliative dermatitis (see below).

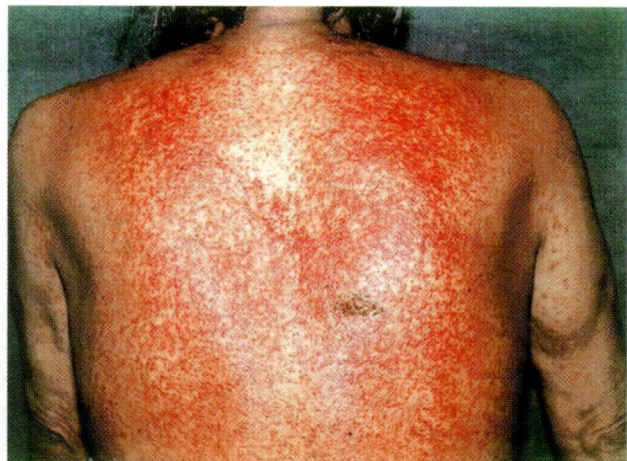

Figure 46.7 Exanthematous drug eruptions. Uniform, erythematous, coalescing papules

The development of a generalised, symmetrical, rapidly progressive, erythematous eruption should prompt a detailed interrogation for drug intake and the timing of the intake in relation to the rash. A system wise questioning for symptoms and the treatment taken is often rewarding as most patients omit to mention over-the-counter preparations and self-prescribed medications unless specifically questioned.

Management

All drugs being taken when the rash developed must be stopped. It is risky to try to guess and stop only one drug because an error may lead to worsening of disease. If a particular drug is essential, a chemically unrelated substitute may be used.

Most patients will require systemic corticosteroid therapy in a dose of 0.5-1mg/kg prednisolone equivalent daily. The rash can be controlled in 24-48 hours as evidenced by fading of erythema and lack of new lesions. The dose of prednisolone can be tapered gradually over a period of 4 weeks; rapid withdrawal may lead to a recurrence of the eruption (even if the drug has been stopped). Antihistamines are not effective in treating exanthematous drug eruptions. They only provide symptomatic relief of itching.

Viral Exanthems[14,16]

Several viral infections are associated with a skin rash. Macular and papular erythematous lesions develop over one part of the skin surface and gradually spread to involve other parts of the body over 2-3 days. Initial lesions may fade while new lesions continue to develop. Mucosal lesions may be seen and occasionally precede the skin eruption. Constitutional symptoms such as fever, myalgia and malaise usually accompany the eruption, but may sometimes precede the rash.

Occasionally, it may be very difficult to differentiate a viral exanthem from an exanthematous drug eruption especially if the patient was taking drug(s) before the onset of the rash. However, spread of the rash in a sequential manner (Figure 46.8) and the development of similar eruptions in other family members or in the community may provide a clue to the cause. Usually, most viral exanthems subside in about 2 weeks with fine scaling and some post-inflammatory pigmentation.

Management

Antipyretics and analgesics may be prescribed for the fever and myalgias. If a drug eruption cannot be reliably excluded, and the patient has already been taking these drugs, chemically unrelated substitutes should be advised.

Exfoliative Dermatitis (Erythroderma)[17,18]

This potentially serious condition can be caused by several diseases including psoriasis, atopic dermatitis, drug eruptions, seborrheic dermatitis and

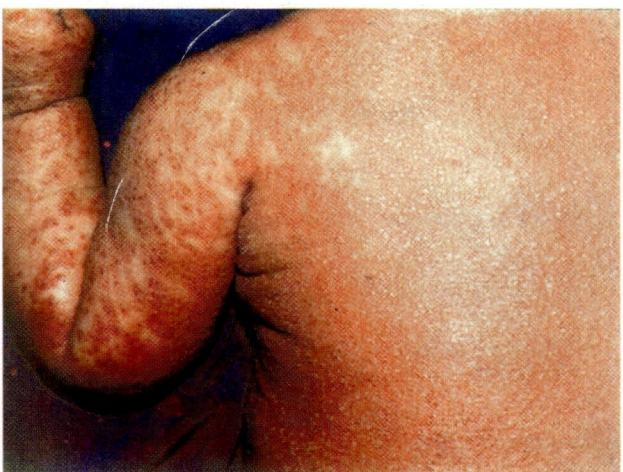

Figure 46.8 Viral exanthem. Papules have coalesced and show subsiding erythema on back while there are fresh, discrete, bright red papules on the arm

ichthyoses among others. Irrespective of the cause, the appearance of these patients is very similar.

The clinical picture is characterised by erythema and scaling involving nearly the entire skin surface. Itching is extremely severe and the nail plates may appear shiny because they are repeatedly polished during scratching. Scaling is often profuse leading to significant protein loss. The patient may be febrile or hypothermic and has difficulty in maintaining a constant body temperature. Generalised lymphadenopathy is usually present.

Management

Antihistamines are required to relieve itching. Sedating conventional antihistamines are preferred. Massage with bland emollients such as petroleum jelly, cold cream or coconut oil will control the scaling and relieve the stretching of the skin. Topical corticosteroids may be added to the emollient to bring about a more rapid resolution. One tube of betamethasone valerate (15 gm) or equipotent steroid cream can be added to 100 gm of vaseline or cold cream and applied all over the body 2-3 times a day. The patient should be well covered to avoid heat loss and hypothermia. A high protein diet is advised to counteract the loss of proteins in scales.

In some patients, these measures are adequate to treat the condition. Others will require therapy with systemic steroids in a dose of 0.5-1.0 mg/kg prednisolone equivalent daily tapered gradually over 4-6 weeks. Corticosteroids should be avoided in erythroderma due to psoriasis. These patients can be treated effectively with methotrexate 0.3-0.5 mg/kg/week.

Harlequin Fetus, Collodion Baby and Other Congenital Ichthyoses[19]

Thick scales over the entire skin is a characteristic feature of some genodermatoses. The degree of scaling and the deformity varies from condition to condition. The most severe cases are examplified by harlequin fetus in which the neonate is encased in a tough sheath of scales (Figure 46.9). Prominent fissures develop between the scales. The stretch produced by the scales leads to ectropion, eclabion and crumpling of the ear. Collodion baby, non-bullous and bullous ichthyosiform erythroderma and lamellar ichthyosis show a similar clinical picture with minor clinical variations in the degree of erythema, stretching of the skin and the presence or absence of blisters.

Management

Severely affected neonates are usually very ill and may be dehydrated and hypothermic. In spite of intensive nursing care, many of these babies die in the first few days of life. In those who survive, emollients such as coconut oil or petroleum jelly may be used to relieve the stretching of the skin. In recent years, oral retinoids such as acitretin, 0.5 mg/kg have been used in these conditions with a significant reduction in scaling and hyperkeratosis. Since the improvement reverses over time once retinoids are stopped, the drug needs to be continued indefinitely or administered intermittently whenever hyperkeratosis recurs. Although the drug is affordable when the patient is a neonate or infant, the high cost and limited availability restricts its use in most patients as the surface area of the body increases. Isotretinoin, a retinoid that is more widely available and significantly less expensive has been found to be as effective as acitretin.

LOCALIZED ERUPTIONS

In the third group of disorders with localized skin lesions, a few or multiple small areas may show varying degrees of erythema, edema, exudation and vesiculation, purpura or gangrene. The clinical picture is determined by the severity and duration

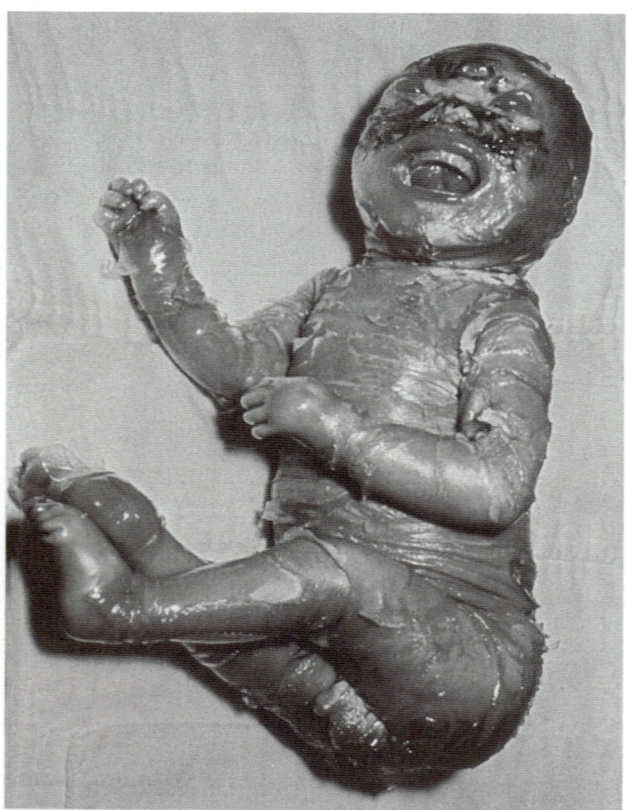

Figure 46.9 Typical appearance of a collodion baby

Section 4

of the insult and the accompanying systemic symptoms.

Therapy of localized skin lesions consists mainly of measures to control inflammation and prevent secondary infection. The associated/underlying systemic disorder should be treated. Application of irritant substances should be stopped and the affected skin washed with soap and water. Topical steroids and antibiotic therapy is required in the dermatitis group. Systemic therapy with antihistamines, steroids and antibiotics may be required if inflammation and infection is severe.

Purpura (syn. petechiae, ecchymosis)[20]

Purpuras represent small bleeds into the skin. Clinically, the lesions are non-blanchable, pink to red spots that fade over 5-7 days with slight hyperpigmentation. They may be caused by a bleeding diathesis or a vasculitis.

Purpura due to a bleeding disorder is recognised by the random distribution of skin lesions determined by the site of skin injury. The purpura itself is bland and unaccompanied by erythema or edema. Mucosal bleeds may also be seen. Large purpuras may be noticed at the sites of injections or venipuncture. The presence of a hematoma at a site of injury or a hemarthrosis provides additional clues. The child may have bleeds from other sites such as the nose or the gut.

Purpura due to a hypersensitivity vasculitis is characterised by the development of lesions mainly on the legs. Lesions also develop on the buttocks and forearms. The trunk, head and face are usually spared. The purpura is bright red, has a blanchable component, and is accompanied by edema and infiltration, which leads to the lesions being, raised i.e. "palpable purpura" (Figure 46.10). In addition, the child may have pain and swelling of the joints, abdominal pain, hematemesis and melena and hematuria. A history of an upper respiratory tract infection or drug intake should be sought.

When purpura is accompanied by fever, the possibility of a septic vasculitis or a hemorrhagic fever must be considered. In septic vasculitis, a few lesions are scattered over the skin in no particular pattern. The skin lesions may have been noticed by the parents but should be looked for in a child with signs of meningeal irritation. The common causes of this syndrome are meningococcemia and dengue hemorrhagic fever (Figure 46.11). In a community experiencing an epidemic, specific treatment should be instituted without waiting for laboratory confirmation of the diagnosis.

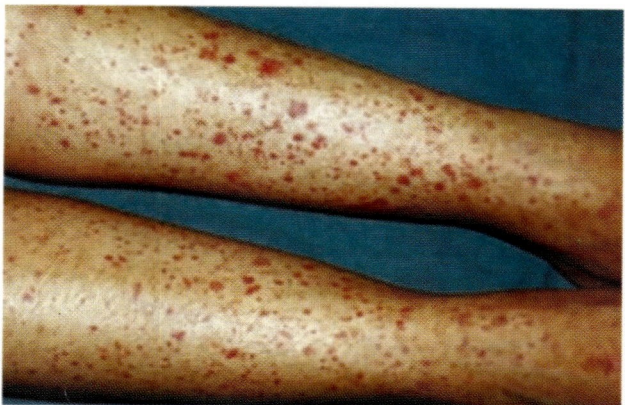

Figure 46.10 Typical vasculitis purpura due to Henoch-Schönlein syndrome ("palpable purpura")

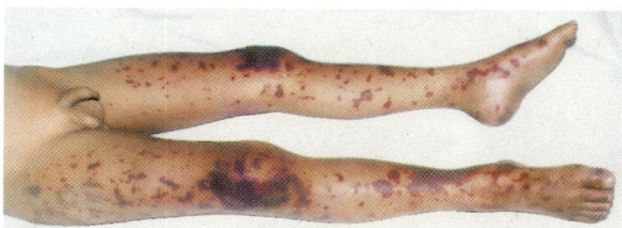

Figure 46.11 Typical irregular purpuric and gangrenous skin rash over the legs in a child with fulminant meningococcemia

In purpura fulminans, several, large ecchymoses develop which progress to hemorrhagic bullae and full thickness necrosis of the skin. Similar lesions may affect the hands, feet and nose (Figure 46.12). There may be bleeds from multiple sites. The condition is usually accompanied by shock which is an extremely grave prognostic sign. The commonest cause is septicemia.

Management

If purpura is due to a bleeding disorder, urgent evaluation and appropriate therapy are recommended (Refer to Chapter 14). Purpura fulminans should be treated with fresh frozen plasma 10 ml/kg, repeated as required. Platelet transfusions may be necessary. The underlying condition should be treated. In patients with septicemia, ceftriaxone or cefotaxime 100-200 mg/kg/day intravenously should be started while awaiting blood culture reports. The antibiotic regime can be modified, if necessary, when the culture reports become available.

Purpura due to hypersensitivity vasculitis requires treatment if the skin lesions are severe, if there is renal involvement or severe articular symptoms. Prednisolone in a dose of 0.5-1 mg/kg/day is administered for 2-4 weeks.

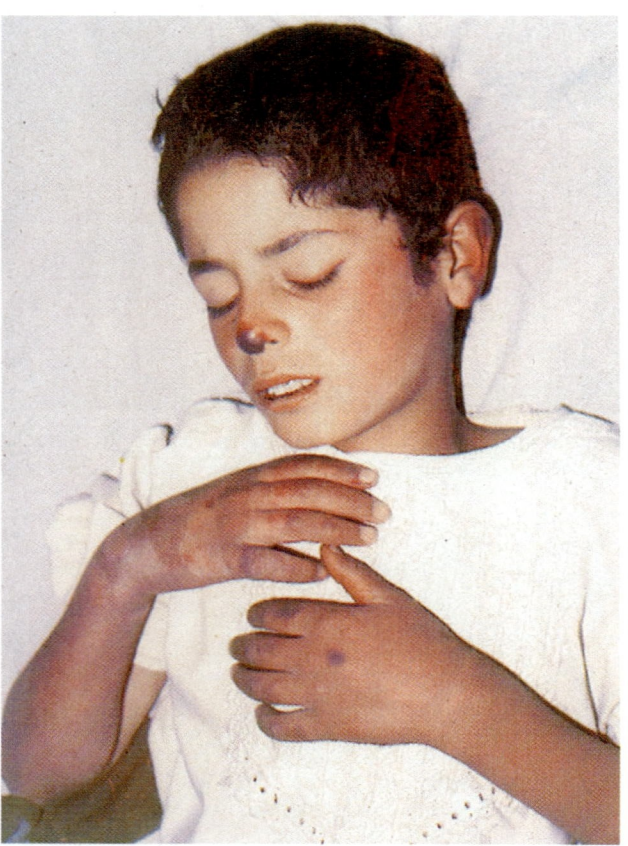

Figure 46.12 Gangrenous lesions over the extremities and nose due to purpura fulminans

In dengue and other haemorrhagic fevers, intravenous fluids and other supportive measures form the mainstay of therapy. For details, please refer to Chapter 29.

Eczema/Dermatitis[21]

Exudative skin lesions accompanied by edema, blisters, papules and papulovesicles are a common reason for seeking urgent medical advice. Commonly, these follow the application of an irritant substance for a banal skin problem. The range of substances applied is large and includes undiluted antiseptics (dettol, savlon), indigenous lotions (zalim lotion, sapat lotion, beetex), acids, plant extracts, and some proprietary preparations (Derobin). An irritant dermatitis occurring in a linear, streaky pattern on exposed skin caused by the vesicating body fluid of insects is seen commonly in the rainy season. Dermatitis may also develop following contact allergy to local medicaments used for dressing and antifungal ointments. Occasionally, dermatitis may develop at the site of a pyogenic infection when purulent discharge and crusting are more prominent.

Irrespective of the cause, the clinical picture is uniform and is determined by the severity of the process. Exudation, edema and blistering are prominent in the acute phase, papulovesicles, and papules in the later phases. There is a tendency for dermatitic lesions to disseminate from the primary site and smaller patches may be found scattered over the rest of the skin.

Management

The most important intervention is to wash the area with soap and water several times a day. Plain corticosteroid cream (e.g. betamethasone valerate, flucinolone acetonide) should be applied twice a day. All other local applications should be avoided. If dermatitis is widespread and severe, a short course of systemic steroids is recommended. Prednisolone 0.5 mg/kg daily usually suffices and can be tapered after 3-4 days. If secondary infection is present, a course of systemic antibiotics should be prescribed.

Photodermatitis

Systemic lupus erythematosus (SLE), a collagen vascular disorder, is characterized by development of classical butterfly erythematous scaly rash involving cheeks and nasal bridge along with progressive systemic manifestations involving practically every organ of the body (Figure 46.13). Skin rash starts as a photo-sensitive erythematous facial blush which progresses to develop thickened epidermis and scaly patches. Additional skin manifestations include painful cutaneous vasculitis of fingers, palms and soles, lacelike bluish or purplish discoloration of skin (livedo reticularis) and Raynaud phenomenon. The disorder is characterized by remissions and relapses and is treated with long term steroid therapy and symptomatic management.

Erythema and burning of sun-exposed areas of skin involving the face (producing butterfly pattern), neck (Casal's necklace), dorsal aspects of hands, forearms and feet are classical features of nicotinic acid deficiency. Pellagra is characterized by a triad of acrodermatitis, diarrhea and dementia that usually occur in communities eating solely a corn based diet which is a poor source of tryptophan. Hartnup disease is a rare autosomal resessive disorder due to inborn error of metabolism with inability to absorb tryptophane leading to deficient synthesis of nicotinic acid with pellagra-like syndrome. There is a dramatic response to administration of nicotinic acid (50-200 mg daily) along with intake of balanced diet and supplements of other B complex vitamins.

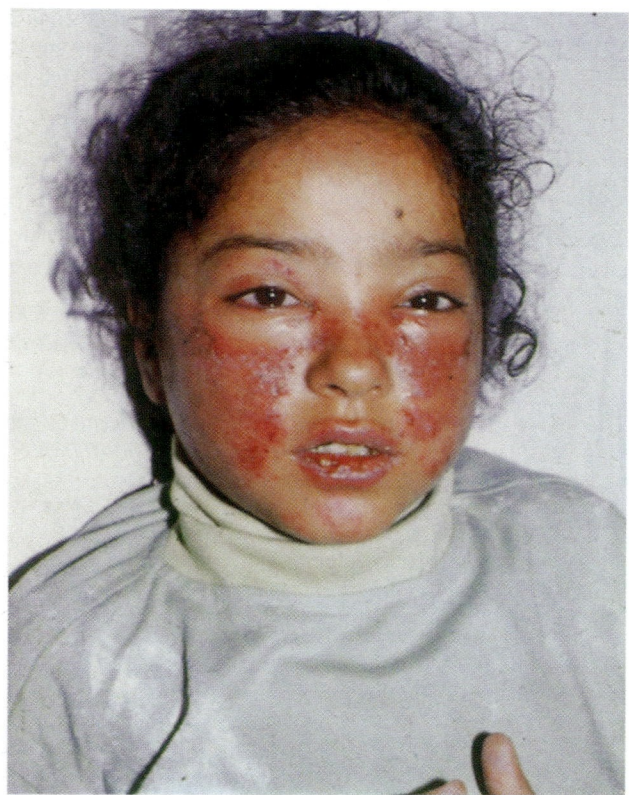

Fig. 46.13 Typical erythematous "butterfly" rash involving malar areas and extending over the bridge of the nose in an adolescent girl with systemic lupus erythematosus. There is intense erythema with papulo-vesicular skin lesions having irregular margins

Cellulitis/Necrotizing Fasciitis[22]

Infection of the deep dermis and subcutaneous tissue by *Staphylococcus aureus* and *Streptococcus pyogenes* leads to cellulitis. This may develop *de novo* or around a pre-existing lesion. Redness, warmth, tenderness and swelling of a localised area usually over the lower limb develops rather rapidly. The area is usually considerably swollen and hot. The overlying skin is red and may show blisters. The draining lymph nodes are tender and enlarged.

Some patients develop more severe damage with necrosis of skin surrounded by inflammatory zone of erythema and blistering. Lesions progress with extension of necrosis. Constitutional symptoms may be severe in these patients.

Management

If seen early, cellulitis can be managed by rest and elevation of the part and systemic antibiotic therapy. Bed rest is advised. The affected limb should be elevated on a pillow and kept immobile

as far as possible. Systemic antibiotic therapy should be aggressive; cloxacillin 100 mg/kg/day or cefazolin 50-100 mg/kg/day are effective initial choices for parenteral therapy. The child may be changed over to oral therapy after the infection is controlled. Treatment should be continued for 10-14 days as the lesions resolve slowly.

Surgical debridement is mandatory when necrosis develops. Early and complete debridement facilitates healing which may require a split skin graft if the excised area is large. Aggressive parenteral antibiotic therapy should be instituted as soon as possible. A suggested combination of intravenous therapy with crystalline penicillin 200,000 units/kg/day, cloxacillin 100 mg/kg/day and metronidazole 30-45 mg/kg/day is recommended.

REFERENCES

1. Bastuji-Garin S, Rzany B, Stern RS, Shear NH, Naldi L, Roujeau JC. Clinical classification of cases of toxic epidermal necrolysis, Stevens-Johnson syndrome and erythema multiforme. *Arch Dermatol* 1993; 129: 92-96.

2. Pasricha JS, Khaitan BK, Shantharaman R, Mital A, Girdhar M. Toxic epidermal necrolysis. *Int J Dermatol* 1996; 35:523-527.

3. Cotell S, Robinson ND, Chan LS. Autoimmune blistering skin diseases. *Am J Emerg Med* 2000; 18:288-299.

4. Forman R, Koren G and Shear NH. Erythema multiforme, Stevens- Johnson syndrome and toxic epidermal necrolysis in children - A review of 10 years' experience. *Drug Safety* 2002; 25: 965-72

5. Chave TA, Mortimer MJ, Hall AP and Hutchinson PE.Toxic epidermal necrolysis: current evidence, practical management and future directions. *Br J Dermatol* 2005; 153: 241-53

6. Yeh SW, Ahmed B, Sami N and Ahmed R. Blistering disorders: diagnosis and treatment. *Dermatol Therapy* 2003; 16 : 214-23

7. Pasricha JS, Khaitan BK, Raman RS, Chandra M. Dexamethasone-cyclophosphamide pulse therapy for pemphigus. *Int J Dermatol* 1995; 34:875-882.

8. De D , Kanwar AJ. Childhood pemphigus. *Indian J Dermatol* 2006; 51(2): 89-95

9. Lyell A. The staphylococcal scalded skin syndrome in historical perspective: emergence of dermopathic strains of *Staphylococcus aureus* and discovery of the epidermolytic toxin. A review of events up to 1970. *J Am Acad Dermatol* 1983; 9:285-294.

10. Tunnessen WW Jr. Practical aspects of bacterial skin infections in children. *Pediatr Dermatol* 1985; 2:255-265.

Section 4

11. Uitto J, Eady R, Fine JD, Feder M, Dart J. The DEBRA International Visioning/Consensus Meeting on Epidermolysis Bullosa: summary and recommendations. *J Invest Dermatol* 2000; 114:734-737.

12. Marsden RA, McKee PH, Bhogal B, Black MM, Kennedy LA. A study of benign chronic bullous dermatosis of childhood and comparison with dermatitis herpetiformis and bullous pemphigoid occurring in childhood. *Clin Exp Dermatol* 1980; 5:159-176.

13. Greaves MW, Sabroe RA. ABC of allergies. Allergy and the skin. I-Urticaria. *BMJ* 1998; 316:1147-1150.

14. Ramam M, Verma KK, Khaitan BK. Exanthematous eruptions. *Nat Med J India* 1998; 11:226-230.

15. Sharma VK, Dhar S. Clinical pattern of cutaneous drug eruptions among children and adolescents in north India. *Pediatr Dermatol* 1995; 12:178-183.

16. Frieden IJ, Resnick SD. Childhood exanthems. Old and new. *Pediatr Clin North Amer* 1991; 38:859-887.

17. Pruszkowski A, Bodemer C, Fraitag S, Teillac-Hamel D, Amoric JC, de Prost Y. Neonatal and infantile erythrodermas: A retrospective study of 51 patients. *Arch Dermatol* 2000; 136:875-880.

18. Sarkar R, Garg VK. Erythroderma in children. *Indian J Dermatol Venereol Leprol* 2010; 76(4): 341-7

19. Akiyama M. Severe congenital ichthyosis of the neonate. *Int J Dermatol* 1998; 37:722-728.

20. Shetty AK, Desselle BC, Ey JL, Correa H, Galen WK, Gedalia A. Infantile Henoch-Schonlein purpura. *Arch Fam Med* 2000; 9: 553-556.

21. Mortz CG, Andersen KE. Allergic contact dermatitis in children and adolescents. *Contact Dermatitis* 1999; 41:121-30.

22. Goldberg GN, Hansen RC, Lynch PJ. Necrotizing fasciitis in infancy: report of three cases and review of the literature. *Pediatr Dermatol* 1984; 2:55-63.

47

Ophthalmic Emergencies

Tanuj Dada and Digvijay Singh

Pediatricians are often the first contact for children having ocular emergencies. For many emergent circumstances such as penetrating injuries, chemical burns and orbital cellulitis, the final outcome depends on the time for the first contact and initiation of treatment. The role of a pediatrician in the management of ocular emergencies, therefore, cannot be overstated.

The common ocular problems faced by the pediatrician in the emergency room include a red eye (both painful and painless), foreign body sensation, sudden diminution of vision, swelling of or around the eyelid and injury (mechanical, chemical or thermal). It is important for the physician to be able to diagnose, provide first aid and appropriately refer most ocular emergencies.[1] Timely intervention and referral goes a long way in minimizing the ocular morbidity especially when expert ophthalmic care is not readily available[1, 2, 3]. Further, it is important for the pediatrician to avoid potentially harmful and improper treatment practices such as bandaging an eye with chemical injury without thorough wash or injudicious and prolonged use of eye drops containing corticosteroids.

APPROACH TO A CHILD WITH AN OCULAR EMERGENCY

Patience and gentle handling are vital for a pediatric ophthalmic examination. Even older children stressed by the injury may vigorously resist any attempt to examine the eye. Forcible examination may exacerbate the damage to the eye especially if it is a penetrating injury. In children older than 3 years, the use of force will make it impossible to elicit any cooperation for further examination. The dictum in pediatric eye examination is to use minimal physical force with the child and maximum observation A few reassuring words and first examining the normal eye may gain the child's confidence. It is best to give children time to calm down after entering the clinic or emergency room (ER) and examine them in the comfort of their parents lap. Examination under anesthesia may be needed in a struggling child and is best left to an ophthalmologist.

The basic equipment required for a elementary eye examination includes a good torch with focal illumination, a magnifying device such as a loupe, Snellen letter and E-chart, a direct ophthalmoscope, some colorful toys and medicines including topical anesthetic agents (xylocaine 4% or proparacaine 0.5%), mydriatic-cycloplegic drops and topical antibiotic drops. Pupillary dilatation if needed may be facilitated by 0.2% cyclopentolate (do not use concentrations of >0.5%), 1% tropicamide or 2.5% phenylephrine which are safe in children. A speculum, Desmarre's retractors and an iris repository should also be available for examination and basic procedures.

The use of mydriatics should be recorded in the patient's record sheet with a mention of the drug and the time of instillation. *Pupillary response to light should be documented before instillation of these drops.*

HISTORY

The first step in evaluating a child in the ER is to obtain an accurate ocular and medical history. The physician should make a note of the presenting complaints, the treatment administered, the circumstances, mode and time of any injury, use of glasses or contact lenses and the status of tetanus toxoid vaccination. History of allergy to medications should be inquired. Any previous ocular disease and treatment should be noted. History of any underlying systemic condition, congenital diseases, vaccination status, dietary intake, exposure to animals (which may require urgent initiation of anti-rabies treatment), sibling rivalry and child abuse should be ascertained.

EXAMINATION

The examination should include an assessment of the general behaviour, a brief systemic and a careful ocular examination. Visual acuity can be assessed in older children using the Snellen's alphabet or tumbling E-chart but toddlers and preschool children require special equipment. A subjective assessment of the visual acuity in infants can be done by indirect means such as checking fixation of each eye to a penlight, checking pupillary responses, documenting any resistance to occlusion of one eye (the better seeing eye) and looking for bilateral red reflexes on distant direct ophthalmoscopy.

Examination should proceed in a systematic manner. The lids and ocular adnexa are examined first using a torchlight as are the ocular movements. Ocular movements in very young children may be noted by Doll's eye reflex or by simply observing the child for a brief period.

The anterior segment may be examined with a torch. Magnification may be obtained by the use of a loupe or the +20D lens of an ophthalmoscope. Look for any signs of bleeding (conjunctiva or anterior chamber), discharge (mucoid or mucopurulent), inflammation (hyperemia, circumcorneal congestion and swelling), foreign body (physical or chemical), corneal or scleral perforation, corneal ulcer (white infiltrates in cornea or sloughing) and cataract (white opaque lens).

The posterior segment of the eye is examined with a direct ophthalmoscope. The physician should try to avoid dilatation of the pupil in every case as it interferes with the assessment of pupillary responses. A note should be made of the digital intraocular tension in intact eyeballs without obvious perforation by gently depressing the superior globe surface through the upper eyelid using one or two fingers while trying to feel if the eye is stony hard or soft. It may be compared with the parent's digital intraocular pressure.

BEYOND THE INITIAL EXAMINATION

If an examination or procedure under anesthesia is required it is best left to an ophthalmologist experienced in handling ocular emergencies. The child should be kept in a fasting state in consultation with the anesthetist till the ophthalmologist is consulted. When indicated, the child may be sedated with oral chloral hydrate (30-50 mg/kg/dose). Care should be taken to protect eyes with penetrating injuries. Excessive crying, straining and vomiting may elevate intraocular pressure and should be treated with sedatives and antiemetics. The child should be effectively restrained to prevent touching or rubbing the

affected eye. A ruptured globe must be protected with a plastic eye shield. If the shield is not available, a disposable styrofoam cup can be cut about 2.5 cm from its base and used for the same purpose. In open globe injuries, depolarizing agents (eg. succinylcholine) should be avoided as they can transiently increase the intraocular pressure and lead to expulsion of intraocular contents[4,5]. Protruding large foreign bodies like knives, pencils or other objects should be stabilized by fluffy bandage material to prevent movements and left in-situ until their surgical removal in the operating room. Saline-moistened guaze can be used to cover lid lacerations.

In addition to the above guidelines, special precautions must be taken while transporting children with eye trauma to the hospital by air or land. Patients with serious eye injuries should have an intravascular access established, the head elevated and body jolts minimized. Hypoxia associated with increased altitude may cause dilatation of retinal choroidal vessels and secondary hemorrhage. The eyes may be bandaged after putting a drop of preservative free antibiotic such as moxifloxacin 0.3%. Antibiotic ointment should not be used in open globe injuries to avoid intraocular penetration[2,3,6]. Instilling eye drops and ointment requires care and the parents should be explained the proper technique for the same[7]. Timely and proper use of topical medications would ensure optimum therapeutic benefit.

INVESTIGATIONS

Radiological and blood investigations may be required, especially in a case of traumatic eye injuries. Plain radiographs can document the presence and number of metallic foreign bodies in the eye and orbit. Ultrasonography is useful for the detection of posterior ocular lesions (vitreous hemorrhage, retinal detachment, and endophthalmitis) which are often obscured by anterior segment disruptions or hyphema. It also provides some clue regarding the status of the lens. Ultrasound examination of eyes with an open globe injury should preferably be deferred until after repair of the perforation.

Computerized tomography delineates the exact extent of orbital wall fractures, associated soft tissue injuries, retro-orbital space collections, intraorbital or intraocular air, radioopaque foreign bodies, injuries of the brain and paranasal sinuses. Magnetic resonance imaging is contraindicated if there are intraocular metallic or magnetic foreign bodies. When possibility of metallic foreign body is

Section 4

ruled out, MRI is useful for delineation of soft tissues, is sensitive to pick up small amount of blood, and is excellent for assessment of posterior fossa, optic nerve and low density objects such as vegetable matter and wooden foreign bodies. In eyes with an external ocular infection, the discharge should be sent for bacterial culture and sensitivity and a topical and oral broad spectrum antibiotic should be administered. Hemogram and urine evaluation should be done if the child is to be subjected to general anesthesia.[5]

TRAUMATIC OCULAR EMERGENCIES

Trauma may be caused by mechanical means, chemical agents or thermal burns and could be penetrating, perforating or a blunt concussion. Ocular trauma is the leading cause of unilateral non-congenital blindness in patients under 20 years of age.[8] According to a report published by National Society for Prevention of Blindness in India, the common causes of injuries in children below 15 years are listed in Table 47.1.

Table 47.1 Common causes of ocular injuries in india[9]
• Sharp and pointed articles 14%
• Bow and arrow 12.5%
• Sports injury 10.7%
• Rural sports like *gulli-danda* 6.7%
• Finger nail injury 1.7%
• Festivals (*Dipawali, Holi*) 2%
• Animals 1.7%
• Accidents 0.36%
• Chemical injury 0.3%

MECHANICAL TRAUMA

Birth trauma

Mechanical trauma to the eyes and eyelids can occur at the time of birth, particularly if the labor is prolonged and difficult or if instrumentation is used for delivery. Some injury to the eye or ocular adnexa occurs in 11 to 59 percent of all births, but fortunately it is usually very mild. A thorough examination of the globe should be performed to rule out any occult ocular injuries in all cases of difficult deliveries. Subconjunctival and even retinal hemorrhages are commonly seen in newborn babies. They spontaneously resolve and do not need any therapeutic intervention.

Child abuse

Ocular trauma may be the first sign and an important component of the symptom complex of child abuse. Approximately 40 percent of children who have been physically abused show evidence of injury in the eyes. The most common ocular findings are retinal or preretinal hemorrhages (Figure 47.1). These are usually caused by a rise in intraocular venous pressure secondary to an increase in the central venous pressure or due to rise in the intracranial pressure. Their discovery in a traumatized child less than 4 years old should make one suspicious about child abuse. Though nothing active needs to be done for the retinal hemorrhages, such children should be admitted to the hospital under the supervision of a pediatrician, and a detailed assessment undertaken. Associated multiple injuries especially fractures of the long bones in different stages of healing, and an inconsistent history is pathognomonic of child battering. Injuries can also occur due to "shaken baby syndrome" (usually associated with severe retinal hemorrhages, vitreous hemorrhage and brain injury) or Munchausen's syndrome by proxy.

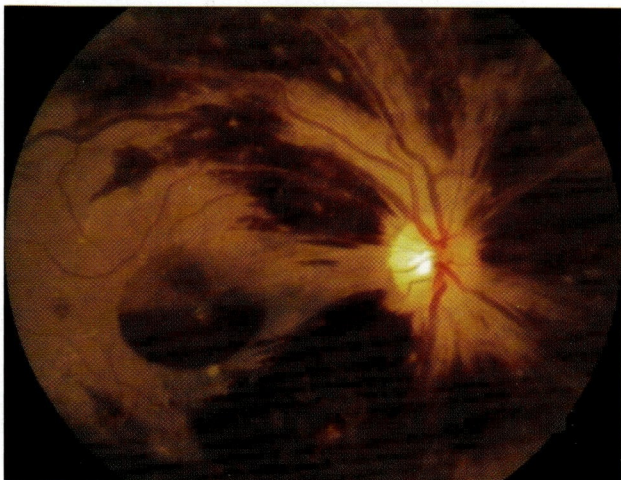

Figure 47.1 Extensive retinal hemorrhages in a shaken infant

Closed Globe Injury

Blunt injury of the eye is potentially very dangerous. It may be produced by diverse causes including injury by fireworks, ball, stone, fist, stick, slingshot among many others (Figure 47.2). Eyelid ecchymoses are treated with ice packs for the initial 48 hours. Concussional injuries often cause a hemorrhage in the anterior chamber (*hyphema*), which can lead to corneal blood staining and secondary glaucoma with subsequent visual loss (Figure 47.3). The child should be advised complete bed rest with the head elevated 30-45 degrees along with a metal or plastic shield over the affected eye. Asprin containing products or other NSAIDs should be avoided. Analgesics, cycloplegics, topical steroids (1% prednisolone acetate, 4-8 times a day)

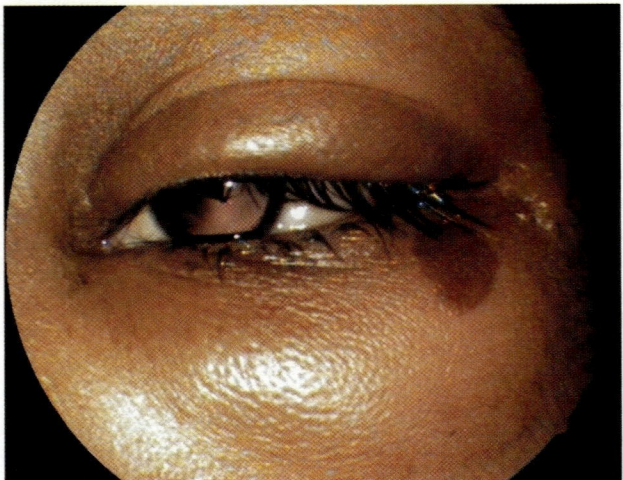

Figure 47.2 Periorbital ecchymosis caused by blunt injury

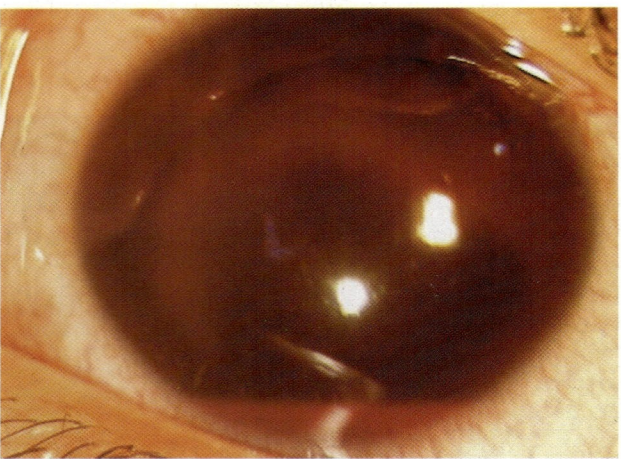

Figure 47.3 Traumatic hyphema

and antiglaucoma medications (0.5% timolol eye drops BD, oral acetazolamide 5 mg/kg/dose, intravenous mannitol 1-2 g/kg) may be required if the intraocular pressure is high. Antiemetics and aminocaproic acid 50 mg/kg, q 4 hr can also be used. The visual prognosis is guarded, as several complications including rebleeding can occur.

Lid lacerations can be caused by severe blunt injuries or sharp objects (Figure 49.4). One should perform a detailed examination to ensure that there is no injury to the globe. Associated canalicular or

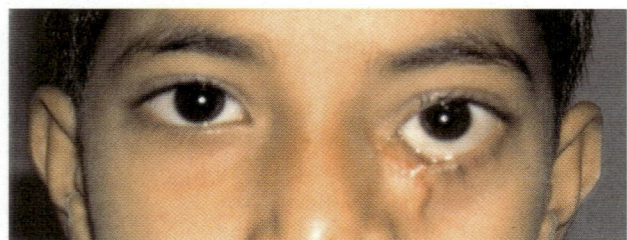

Figure 47.4 Lid laceration of left lower eyelid involving the lid margin

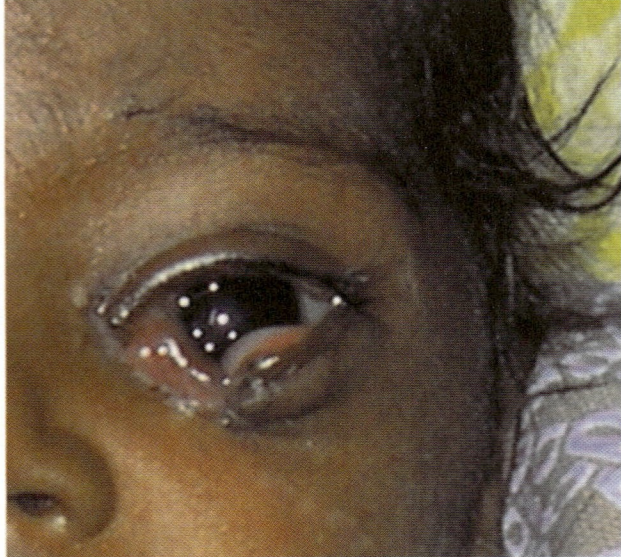

Figure 47.5 Animal claw injury. Lid laceration involving the left lower lacrimal drainage system (punctum and canaliculus)

nasolacrimal duct injuries should also be noted (Figure 49.5). A thorough cleaning of the laceration should be done to remove any foreign matter/debris, tetanus prophylaxis should be given (if indicated) and systemic antibiotics are administered if contamination is suspected. The laceration is best sutured by a trained ophthalmologist especially if associated with a canalicular injury.

Subconjunctival hemorrhage is an extremely common, usually benign cause of red eye. It results from rupture of the small subconjunctival vessels (Figure 47.6). These hemorrhages can be caused by minor trauma or violent valsalva maneuvers, such as spasmodic or whooping cough, vomiting or straining. Less commonly they may be associated with viral infections, uncontrolled hypertension and coagulopathies. The eye should be carefully examined to rule out a retained foreign body, underlying penetrating wound or hyphema. Once coexisting ocular injuries have been excluded, treatment is simple, with cool compresses and reassurance.

Conjunctival foreign bodies. Foreign bodies cause an intense irritation and tearing and need urgent removal. Conjunctival foreign bodies are removed by flushing the eye with a stream of isotonic saline solution or by using a moistened cotton-tip applicator.

Corneal foreign bodies. Foreign bodies embedded in the cornea are potentially serious and need to be removed with a 26-gauge needle under slit lamp examination after using topical anesthesia

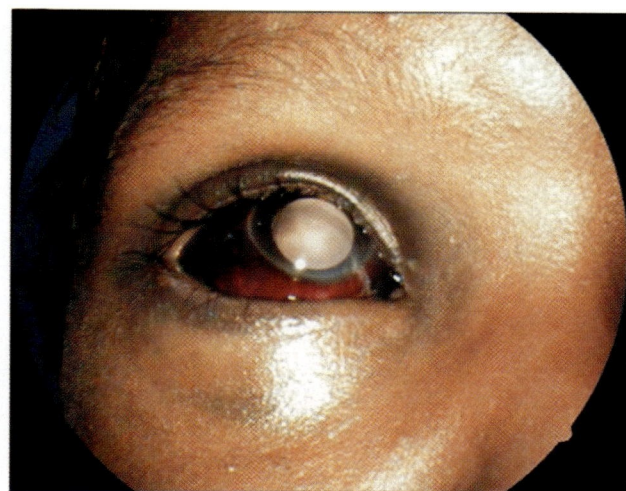

Figure 47.6 Traumatic subconjunctival hemorrhage with cataract

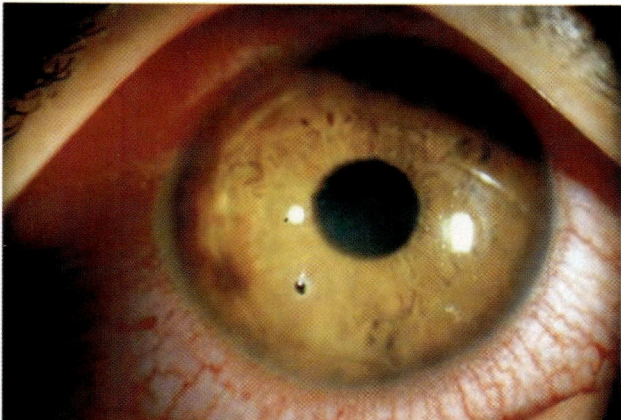

Figure 47.7 Corneal foreign body before removal

(Figure 47.7). Broad spectrum antibiotics and artificial tears are instilled after removing the foreign body from the cornea. The eye should be bandaged for 24 hours to facilitate healing of the corneal epithelium.

Corneal abrasions are a common reason for visit to the emergency department. They may be caused by small foreign bodies or by direct trauma due to finger nails, makeup brushes, toys, paper or twigs. The child usually complains of pain, foreign body sensation, tearing, and photophobia. Fluorescein staining and cobalt blue light helps in defining the extent of epithelial denudation. A careful search for foreign bodies should be made, especially when multiple linear corneal abrasions are present. Treatment is aimed at relieving the pain and promoting healing. Short acting cycloplegic agents such as tropicamide or cyclopentolate help reduce ciliary spasm and secondary iritis. Topical antibiotic instillation followed by a 24 hour patch is usually adequate for such cases. A follow-up

examination is required after 24 to 48 hours and if the abrasion has not healed, an ophthalmic referral should be sought. Do not patch if the mechanism of injury involves vegetable matter or the child is a contact lens user due to risk of development of corneal ulcer. Topical antibiotics (tobramycin, ofloxacin) should be instilled every 2-4 hours and the abrasion should be monitored daily till it heals.

Traumatic optic neuropathy can be diagnosed by the presence of a relative afferent pupillary defect in a recently traumatized eye that cannot be accounted for by any other ocular pathology. High dose intravenous steroids (~1 mg/kg/day dexamethasone or methylprednisolone in a loading dose of 30 mg/kg, followed by 5.0 mg/kg q 6 hr for 48 hours) should be given as soon as possible but definitely within 48-72 hours after the injury. An immediate ophthalmic consultation should be sought.

Fractures of the orbit (Blowout fractures) generally result from blunt injury such as a blow from a cricket ball or fist. The bones of the orbital rim usually remain intact, but there is a fracture of the floor of the orbit (sometimes the medial wall) with herniation of the orbital contents into the blowout site. This is suspected if there is diplopia in any direction of gaze or limitation of ocular movements, particularly upward gaze (Figure 47.8). Theses fractures are not always seen on X-ray orbit (tear drop sign) and CT scan is usually required (Figure 47.9). The child should be referred to an ophthalmologist who may consider surgical treatment in non-regressing and debilitating blowout fracture.

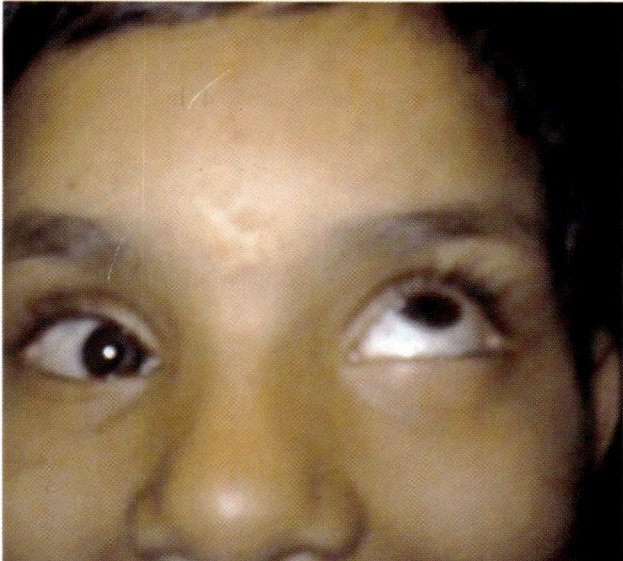

Figure 47.8 Right orbital floor fracture. Note the limitation in upward movement of right globe.

Section 4

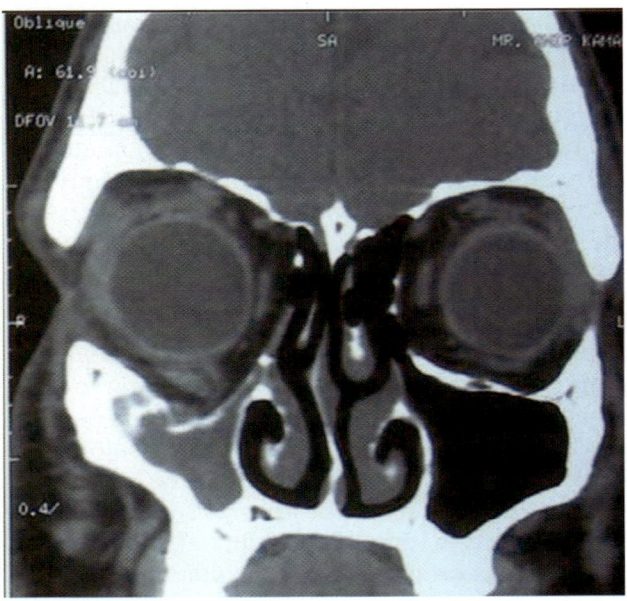

Figure 47.9 CT scan showing a right orbital floor fracture (blowout fracture)

Open Globe Injury

Open globe injuries include penetrating injuries (entry wound but no exit wound), perforations (entry and exit wounds) and globe ruptures (disorganized open globe with no well defined entry/exit site). They may be associated with a retained intraocular foreign body. Arrows, slingshots, pellets, pencils and hypodermic needles can produce this type of injury (Figures 47.10 to 47.12). Once a diagnosis of an open globe injury has been made, further examination should not be performed as this often entails pressure on the globe, with potential risk of extrusion of intraocular contents. All open globe injuries require surgery. The child should be kept fasting and the time since

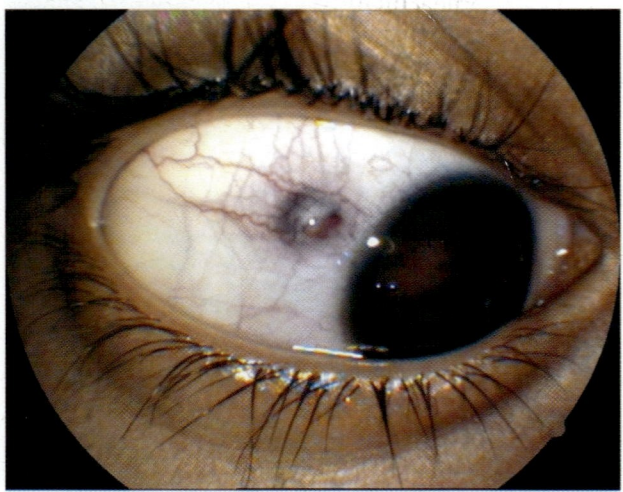

Figure 47.10 Needle stick injury to the globe with scleral perforation and uveal prolapse

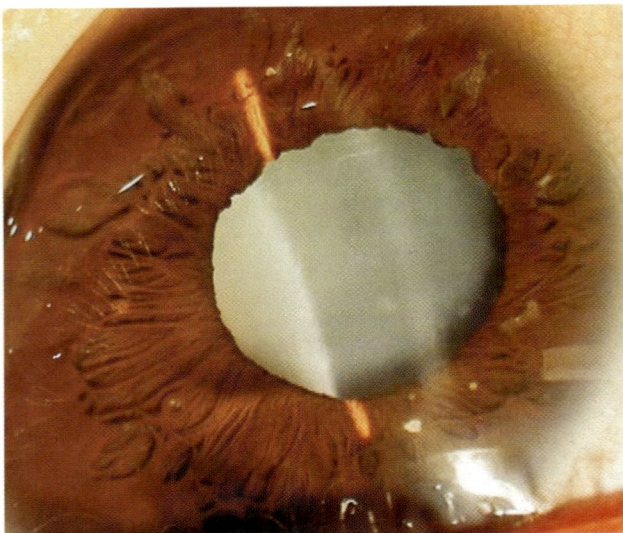

Figure 47.11 Traumatic cataract

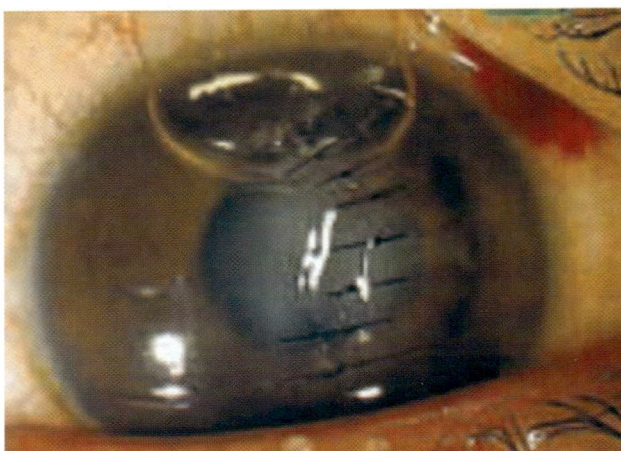

Figure 47.12 Repaired corneal perforation using a 10-0 monofilament nylon suture

last intake of food or drink noted. An eye shield should be placed on the affected eye, systemic antibiotics (cefazolin and gentamicin or ciprofloxacin) and antiemetics administered before referring the child for surgery under general anesthesia.[10, 11]

It is important to remember that in every case with a penetrating injury (especially in the region of the ciliary body or with prolapse of uveal tissue) one should watch the other eye for sympathetic ophthalmia. During follow up, the near vision of the fellow eye should be recorded on a daily basis and if possible retrolental flare should be ruled out (in consultation with an ophthalmologist) as these are the earliest symptoms and signs of sympathetic ophthalmitis.

Intraocular foreign bodies. Intraocular foreign bodies are serious open globe injuries that may not be suspected on initial examination. They carry the potential of causing blinding sequelae such as endophthalmitis, siderosis, chalcosis etc. Examination may show a perforating wound of the cornea, a hole in the iris, an irregular or peaked pupil, and an opaque lens. Ultrasonography and X-rays of the eye may be necessary to rule out the possibility of intraocular foreign body (Figure 47.13). Children with suspected intraocular foreign bodies should be referred immediately to an ophthalmologist.

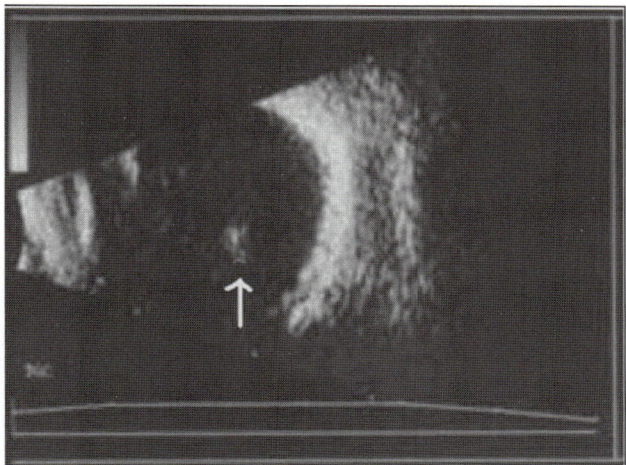

Figure 47.13 Intraocular foreign body seen on an ocular ultrasonogram image (white arrow)

CHEMICAL TRAUMA

Chemical injuries constitute an ocular emergency in which any delay in the initiation of treatment can lead to serious ocular damage.[12, 13] (Figures 47.14 and 47.15) These include injuries caused by alkali (lye, cement, plaster), acids, solvents, detergents, and other irritants e.g. mace. Alkali injury due to lime during whitewashing of houses and slaked lime (calcium hydroxide) in *chuna* packets are a common mode of injury.[14]

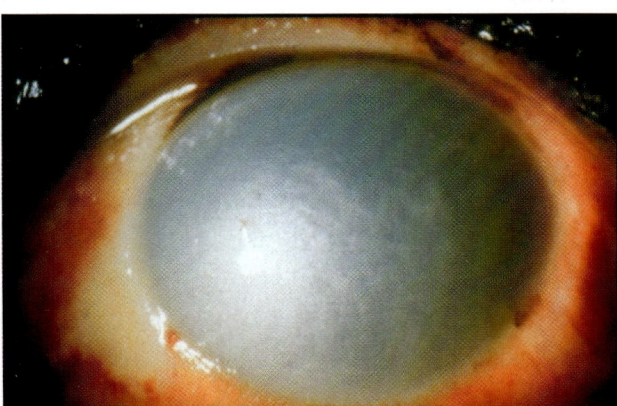

Figure 47.14 Alkali burn during acute stage

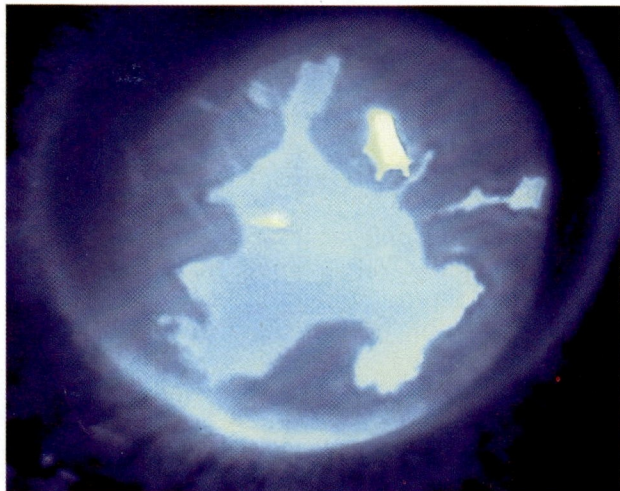

Figure 47.15 Post alkali burn epithelial defect stained with fluorescein

Alkalis such as ammonia or lime are far more destructive than acid burns because alkalis react with fats to form soaps, which damage cell membranes and allow further penetration of the alkali into the eye, while acids coagulate tissue proteins to form an eschar that limits further penetration of the acid. Such acid/alkali injuries are also common in laboratories at schools and industrial areas. It is not uncommon to see chemical and foreign body injuries to the eyes due to powdered colors during the festival of *Holi*.

All chemical injuries require immediate, copious and prolonged irrigation for at least 30 minutes. Fresh tap water is adequate for this purpose. One can also use normal saline or ringer lactate solution and use the drip set for irrigating the eye. It is helpful to place a topical anesthetic (proparacaine or xylocaine) and an eyelid speculum (provided corneal melting is not total) before starting the irrigation. After irrigating for half an hour, one should wait for 5-10 minutes to allow equilibration and then test the pH by touching the inferior conjunctival sac with litmus paper. Irrigation should be continued until a neutral pH (7.0) is achieved. A moistened cotton tipped applicator should be swept in the conjunctival fornices to remove any retained particles. This should be avoided if there is evidence of corneal melting or thinning. An analgesic should be given, topical antibiotic ointment and 1% atropine ointment should be applied and the eye should be patched before referring the patient to an ophthalmologist. While topical steroids are safe in the first week of injury, their unregulated use carries the risk of corneal melting and secondary infection and should preferably be left to the ophthalmologist. Use of alkalis to neutralize acids and *vice versa*

Section 4

should be avoided as they may produce a thermal reaction and exacerbate tissue damage. In lime burns the lid needs to be everted to examine and remove any foreign bodies.

THERMAL TRAUMA

Thermal injuries can occur when hot ashes, lighted matches or boiling liquids make contact with the eye before reflex blinking.[15] Most injuries are minor, involving the corneal epithelium and superficial stroma and are treated with topical antibiotic ointment, patching of the eye and analgesics. Thermal burn injuries to the eyelids and periorbital tissues are common. It should be remembered that the laser pointer which is in common use, can lead to a macular burn and children must be cautioned not to shine the laser pointer light directly into the eye.

Fireworks during *Diwali* and other festive occasions can cause direct mechanical injury and thermal burns. Serious damage to the eyes may be produced by explosive injuries. Ocular fireworks injuries are much more severe and dangerous in children than in adults. Prevention is of greater value. Children should wear protective eye gear and should be allowed to burst crackers only under adult supervision. Dangerous crackers like rockets should be avoided.[15]

Colors used in *Holi* can also cause chemical injury. Dada et al in a study of 40 patients reported chemical conjunctivitis in 95% of patients, corneal epithelial abrasion in 37.5% and superficial punctuate keratitis in 75%.[13] Treatment involves copious irrigation of the conjunctival sac with administration of broadspectrum antibiotics and cycloplegics. Topical steroids should be avoided until the epithelial defect has healed.

Prevention of Ocular Injuries

Health education on the preventive aspects of ocular injuries in schools as well as through mass media can help reduce the morbidity due to ocular injuries. The teachers should be well informed to teach preventive and promotive aspects of eye health care to the students. There should be awareness on the part of parents to the potential dangers of toys, airguns, fire crackers etc. The use of protective eye wear such as CR-39 plastic glasses and polycarbonate sport goggles during contact sports should be made mandatory for all children[14-18].

Table 47.2 Differential diagnosis of redness of eyes in children				
Features	**Acute conjunctivitis**	**Corneal abrasion**	**Acute iritis**	**Acute glaucoma**
Incidence	Very common	Fairly common	Uncommon	Rare
Etiology	Usually bacterial	Foreign body; abrasion	Usually unknown; may be associated with JRA	Developmental defects or obstruction of aqueous drainage channels
Redness	Diffuse injection of conjunctiva, more towards fornices	Diffuse injection of conjunctiva	Purple-red; circumcorneal congestion	Often diffuse injection of bulbar conjunctiva
Discharge	Moderate to heavy; mucoid or mucopurulent	Watery	None	None; tearing may occur
Visual acuity	Normal	Decreased	Decreased	Decreased
Corneal transparency	Clear	Variable haze; positive fluorescein stain	Clear or some haze	Hazy; cornea enlarged in congenital form
Anterior chamber depth	Normal	Normal	Normal; cloudy	Shallow; deep in congenital glaucoma
Pupil size	Normal	Normal	Constricted	Dilated
Intraocular pressure	Normal	Normal	Usually normal; may be low or elevated	Elevated
Conjunctival smear results	Causative organism identified	Normal	Normal	Normal

(Adapted from Ellis P. Eye.Current Pediatric Diagnosis and Treatment. Hay W *et al* Ed. 1991 Appleton and Lange, Connecticut.)

Section 4

NON-TRAUMATIC EMERGENCIES

The Red Eye

The red eye is one of the most common ophthalmic problems seen in clinical practice and may demand simple topical therapy and reassurance or an urgent referral to an ophthalmologist.[19, 20] The common causes of red eye are conjunctivitis (infectious, allergic and blepharoconjunctivitis), trauma, drugs, toxins or chemical reactions, corneal ulcer, iridocyclitis, glaucoma and episcleritis or scleritis and conjunctival foreign body (Table 47.2).

INFECTIONS

Conjunctivitis

The majority of cases of acute conjunctivitis are bacterial in etiology. It typically presents with a red eye, burning, stinging, foreign body sensation, ocular discharge and matting of the eyelids. Symptoms and signs may present unilaterally or bilaterally. Bacterial infections present with purulent discharge, while mucopurulent discharge is seen in viral and chlamydial infections. Viral infections and allergic reactions usually have a serous discharge.

Pneumococcus, *Haemophilus influenzae species* and Moraxella are the most common bacterial pathogens. Conjunctival swabs and cultures are usually not needed as the disease is self-limiting and resolves without treatment in a few weeks. A topical broad spectrum antibiotic like sulphacetamide, tobramycin or fluoroquinolones shortens the course to a few days. However, if the conjunctivitis is severe and the discharge copious, calcium alginate swabs of the conjunctival surface may be taken to rule out virulent organisms like gonococcus and meningococcus.

Viral conjunctivitis may be caused by adenovirus (most common), infectious mononucleosis, influenza virus, mumps virus, rubeola and varicella. Treatment is primarily symptomatic. Topical steroids should be avoided. Parinaud oculoglandular syndrome is caused by *Bartonella henselae*, and presents with unilateral granulomatous conjunctivitis with preauricular and submandibular adenopathy.

Conjunctivitis occurring in the first four weeks of life is called as ophthalmia neonatorum. The disease may be bacterial, viral, and chemical in etiology. The infection is usually contracted during passage through the birth canal. Prolonged rupture of membranes at the time of delivery greatly increases the risk of infection.

Effective prophylaxis has greatly reduced the incidence in developed countries. The Crede's method of instilling 2% silver nitrate has now become obsolete and has been replaced by topical administration erythromycin and tetracycline ointments to cover for chlamydiae.

Gonococcal conjunctivitis is caused by *Neisseria gonococci* and is by far the most serious. Typically it presents in the first 3-4 days, but may appear as late as 3 weeks. Marked chemosis with copious discharge is characteristic. The organism is capable of penetrating intact corneal epithelium and therefore corneal ulceration and globe perforation is always a risk. Systemic infection in the form of sepsis and meningitis may be associated. Gram staining of the conjunctival discharge usually shows the Gram-negative rods. Systemic therapy is mandatory. Increasing incidence of bacterial resistance has made penicillin and erythromycin therapy unreliable. Ceftriaxone given intramuscularly once a day for a week is highly effective. Topical irrigation of the eyes effectively washes and debrides the conjunctival discharge but topical antibiotics provide little advantage in the absence of corneal ulceration.

Chlamydial conjunctivitis has replaced gonococcus as the most common organism in developed countries. The organism may be acquired during passage through the birth canal, but unlike other agents it commonly ascends up to the uterus and may infect infants delivered by cesarean section. The conjunctivitis occurs later around one week of age (earlier if there has been premature rupture of membranes). Usually there is mild swelling, hyperemia, a papillary reaction with minimal discharge. A follicular reaction may be seen after 4 weeks of age. Diagnosis is made by indirect fluorescent antibody test, ELISA and culture of conjunctival scrapings. Chlamydial conjunctivitis may be associated with systemic infection viz, pneumonia and gastrointestinal infection which makes systemic treatment mandatory. Erythromycin is highly effective and tetracyclines are contraindicated in young children.

Rarely, *Herpes simplex* virus may cause ophthalmia neonatorum. The conjunctivitis presents late usually in the second week. Chemical conjunctivitis has become rare with the discontinuation of silver nitrate prophylaxis. It usually presents in the first 24 hours of life and is self-limiting improving spontaneously on the second day.

Nasolacrimal duct obstruction occurs in about 5% of newborns.[21] The majority present by a month of age with epiphora (watering from affected eye), sticky mucoid or mucopurulent discharge that accumulates and causes matting of eyelashes. Pressure on the lacrimal sac region often causes regurgitation of turbid fluid through the punctum. Children with nasolacrimal duct obstruction may develop an inflammation of the lacrimal sac (acute dacrocystitis) and present to the emergency with a red tender swelling below the medial canthus of the eye. This requires the administration of topical tobramycin drops and a short course of oral antibiotics. An ophthalmology consultation should be sought for further management.

Management is usually conservative in this age group and consists of regular sac massage by the mother with administration of broad spectrum antibiotics. The sac should be compressed after massaging or milking the canaliculi. The parent should be instructed to place the little finger over the medical canthus and press the lacrimal sac several times and massage the ducts by sliding the finger downwards along the side of the nose (Criggler's massage). This is repeated several times followed by administration of antibiotics. This procedure facilitates the opening of the nasolacrimal duct and discourages bacterial growth by emptying the sac. In cases not responding to massage within 6 months or developing acute episodes of dacrocystitis, surgery may be required.

Corneal ulcer

Infectious keratitis may be caused by bacterial, viral, fungal or protozoal infections[22] (Figure 47.16). Keratitis may occur as a primary event or may supervene when ocular surface is compromised by malnutrition, abrasion, use of topical steroids or wearing contact lenses. Pain, redness, watering, photophobia, discharge and a decrease in the visual acuity are the prominent symptoms. Localised white areas of corneal infiltration are characteristic.

It is a sight-threatening condition and immediate attention and urgent referral are warranted. *Topical steroids are permissible only after good control of infection and should never be used by the pediatrician.* If possible, the discharge and the scrapings from the base and the leading edge of the infiltrate should be sent for culture and sensitivity and smears stained with Gram stain and broad spectrum topical antibiotics started. One can initiate therapy with hourly fortified cephazolin (5%) and fortified tobramycin (1.3%) eye drops, given round the clock. As tobramycin is

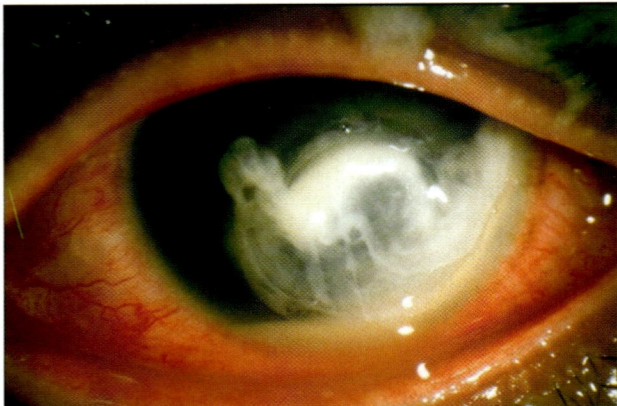

Figure 47.16 Extensive damage to anterior chamber of the eye secondary to bacterial keratitis

relatively toxic to the corneal epithelium, gatifloxacin is preferred by many ophthalmologists. Monotherapy with a fluoroquinolone antibiotic (0.3% ciprofloxacin or ofloxacin) is another option but it is not widely used these days. Cycloplegics such as homatropine, artificial tears, antiglaucoma medications (if the digital IOP is high), analgesics and vitamin A can be given as a supportive therapy. Antifungal drops are indicated only if fungal infection is documented by culture or smear (5% natamycin eye drops, 1 hourly at day time and 2 hourly at night). Eyes with a perforated ulcer, scleral extension of the infection, gonococcal or *Haemophilus influenzae* infection and one eyed patients, should be given systemic antibiotics. The follow up of a patient with corneal ulcer should be done by an ophthalmologist.

Ocular allergy

It is characterized by bilateral involvement, seasonal exacerbations, marked itching and absence of purulent discharge[23, 24]. Seasonal allergic conjunctivitis has its peak in spring and fall. It is triggered by specific airborne allergens e.g. pollen. The discharge is watery with boggy-appearing conjunctiva and the patient complains of itchy eyes. Perennial allergy is milder with little variations in seasons because it is related to more ubiquitous household allergens like dust mites and animal dander.

Vernal keratoconjunctivitis occurs in two distinct forms i.e. palpebral and limbal. Both are characterized by intense itching and a mucoid ropy discharge worse in spring and fall. The palpebral variant predominantly involves the upper eye lids and is characterized by a milky conjunctiva with cobblestone papillae in well developed cases. The limbal variety presents with gelatinous nodules at the limbus with a white central dot called as Horner-Trantas dot. The cornea is infrequently involved with punctate epithelial erosions and shield ulcer.

Atopic keratoconjunctivitis is rare in children with predominant involvement of the lower lid with papillae and scarring. Atopic dermatitis and bronchial asthma may be associated.

Treatment of ocular allergy is primarily symptomatic. The offending antigen should be avoided if possible. Oral antihistamines are not very effective. Topical medications like azelastine and levocabastine are preferred. Cold compresses are also effective in relieving symptoms. Mast cell stabilizers like cromolyn sodium, ketotifen fumarate, lodoxamide, nedocromil sodium and olapatadine are also effective. Topical nonsteroidal anti-inflammatory drops like ketorolac tromethamine may be tried. *It is important to use topical steroids judiciously due to potential risk of producing glaucoma.* Their use should be restricted to 3-4 days and the patient should be monitored for rise in intraocular tension.

Inflammation

Episcleritis/scleritis is characterised by a sectoral or diffuse redness of eyes due to engorgement of episcleral/scleral vessels (2.5% epinephrine blanches episcleral vessels but does not effect scleral vessels). It may be diffuse or nodular. It is important to rule out connective tissue disorders, herpes simplex, and tuberculosis. Topical and systemic NSAIDs are used as initial therapy and steroids are added if there is no response. Scleromalacia perforans and necrotizing scleritis are serious variants often seen with rheumatoid arthritis. They may require systemic immunosuppressive therapy with a scleral patch graft and should be managed by an ophthalmologist.

Uveitis in children is relatively uncommon and may present in the ER as a red eye. While the detailed management of uveitis is strictly in the domain of ophthalmology, it is necessary for the physician to be aware of certain general principles.[25] Children may not have any symptoms unless the disease is well advanced. Due to prolonged therapy, the compliance is poor and it is associated with increased incidence of side effects in children like cataract, steroid induced glaucoma, and band keratopathy.

An anatomic classification (anterior, intermediate and posterior) is quite useful. A specific cause is found in only 50-65% of cases. Juvenile rheumatoid arthritis (JRA) is the most commonly identified cause of uveitis in children. Toxoplasmosis is the most common cause of posterior uveitis. Children may present in a number of ways. Pain, redness and photophobia are common in acute anterior uveitis, but chronic uveitis may be asymptomatic or may present with diminished vision at a later stage. Anterior uveitis has an identifiable cause in only 50% of cases, and therefore a detailed diagnostic workup may be deferred unless the uveitis tends to become recurrent or chronic. In JRA, uveitis is chronic and most commonly occurs in the pauciarticular variety. Therapy is indicated only if there is 2+ or more cells and not merely for flare alone. Anterior uveitis occurs in 90% of cases with sarcoidosis. While older children present with multisystem involvement like adults, children less than 4 years may present with skin rash, uveitis and arthritis and may be confused with JRA. HLA B27 associated uveitis is rare. It is important for the pediatrician to be aware of sympathetic ophthalmia, which presents as a bilateral granulomatous panuveitis, that occurs after injury or surgery in one eye followed by development of uveitis in the fellow eye after a variable latent period.

Intermediate uveitis in children is usually idiopathic and presents as a chronic inflammation. Toxoplasmosis is the most commonly identified cause of posterior uveitis. Other causes include histoplasmosis, toxocariasis, Vogt Koyanagi Harada syndrome, Behcet syndrome and Masquerade syndrome. Many of these are serious diseases wherein early diagnosis is crucial for survival of the child e.g, retinoblastoma, leukemia, lymphoma, malignant melanoma. As a general principle uveitis in the pediatric age group should include assessment of the patient by a pediatrician, and should include testing for rheumatic and gastrointestinal disorders, tuberculin skin testing, FTA-ABS, serum protein electrophoresis, chest and sacroiliac radiography (when indicated). An ocular ultrasound and imaging should be done to rule out malignancy and foreign body. Topical and systemic corticosteroids form the mainstay of therapy. It is important to be aware of the numerous side effects of topical steroids which include glaucoma and cataract.

ACUTE PROPTOSIS

Preseptal and Orbital Cellulitis

Preseptal cellulitis is an inflammatory process involving the tissues anterior to the orbital septum. The common causes are listed below:

- Penetrating injury to the periorbital skin. *Staphylococcus aureus* and *Streptococcus pyogenes* are the most common pathogens.

- Severe conjunctivitis, skin infection such as impetigo and herpes zoster
- Secondary to respiratory or sinus disease
- Insect bite (Figure 47.17)
- Idiopathic

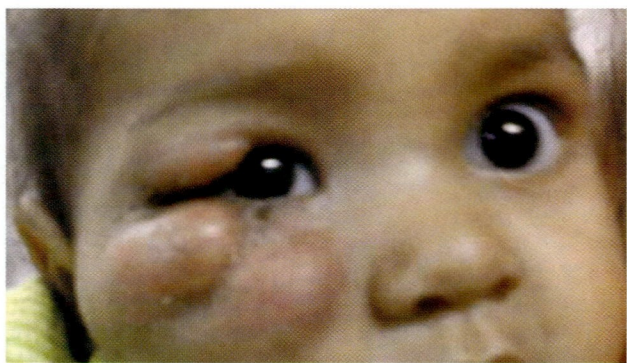

Figure 47.17 Pre septal cellulitis secondary to insect bite

The eyelid becomes taut and inflamed. Inflammation may extend to the eyebrow and forehead and the fellow eyelid may become edematous. There is no proptosis and the ocular movements are normal which serves to distinguish it from orbital cellulitis.

Children with mild infections and without any systemic features may be treated on an outpatient basis with oral cephalosporins or amoxicillin-clavulanic acid. Children below one year especially with systemic features should be treated with intravenous antibiotics.

Orbital cellulitis is an infection of the orbital tissues posterior to the orbital septum. Periorbital swelling, erythema, proptosis and ophthalmoplegia are common manifestations (Figures 47.18, 47.19). Two-thirds of the cases are due to an extension of a sinus infection. Other causes include orbital trauma, orbital and paranasal sinus surgery, local extension of a facial cellulitis and seeding from systemic bacteremia. A retained intraorbital foreign body can cause orbital cellulitis months later.

Children below 9 years of age are usually infected with isolated aerobic organisms. While those older than 9 years may have multiple pathogens both aerobic and anerobic. *S. aureus* and Gram-negative rods predominate in the neonates. Gram-negative infections are common in the immunosuppressed children.

Orbital cellulitis needs to be distinguished from orbital pseudotumor and orbital tumors like rhabdomyosarcoma. CT scanning is indicated in patients with orbital cellulitis to confirm orbital

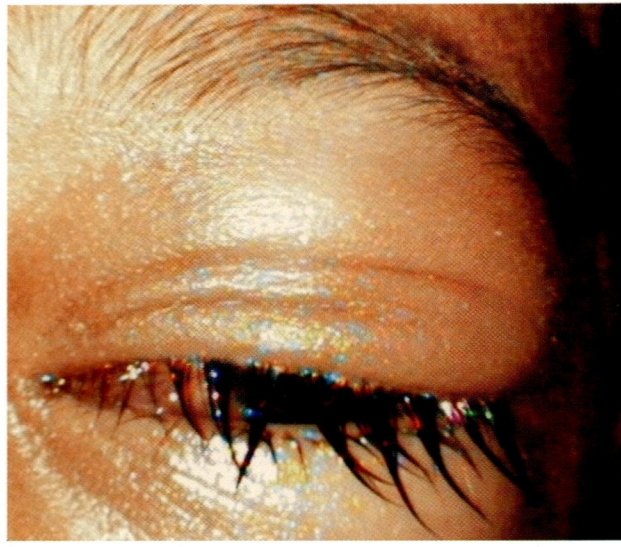

Figure 47.18 Marked chemosis and swelling due to orbital cellulitis

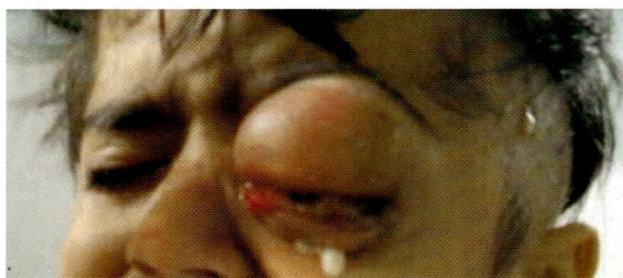

Figure 47.19 Marked proptosis due to orbital cellulitis. Note the purulent discharge from the eye

involvement, to document the presence of sinusitis and subperiosteal abscess and to rule out a foreign body in a patient with a history of trauma.

Orbital cellulitis is a serious infection and may lead to a variety of complications like cavernous sinus thrombosis, intracranial extension (subdural or brain abscess, meningitis, periosteal abscess), corneal exposure with secondary ulcerative keratitis, secondary glaucoma, septic uveitis, retinitis, exudative retinal detachment, optic nerve edema, inflammatory neuritis, infectious neuritis, CRAO and panophthalmitis. The diagnosis of cavernous sinus thrombosis is difficult during early stages. Paralysis of eye movements out of proportion to the degree of proptosis, decreased sensation along the maxillary division of the trigeminal nerve, and bilateral involvement constitutes a diagnostic triad.

Orbital cellulitis in children is a serious disease which requires hospitalization and treatment with broad spectrum antibiotics. Empirically cefuroxime or cefotaxime along with a penicillinase-resistant penicillin like naficillin or cloxacillin may be used until results from blood, nasal, nasopharyngeal cultures are available. Vancomycin and chloramphenicol may be used in children allergic or resistant to penicillin. Associated sinusitis should be treated in consultation with an otolaryngologist. Subperiosteal abscess mandates drainage if it compromises optic nerve function (reduced vision, RAPD), and if it is enlarging or is non responsive.

Other causes of acute proptosis in children include malignant tumors like rhabdomyosarcoma, metastatic neuroblastoma, leukemic infiltration, traumatic hematoma and foreign body.

Malignant tumors

Rhabdomyosarcoma is the most common primary orbital malignancy in children.[26, 27] The average age of presentation is around 5-7 years. Proptosis is the most common presenting sign and often develops acutely which leads to a diagnostic confusion with orbital cellulitis, but fever and systemic symptoms are absent. Supranasal quadrant is the most common site of involvement. A CT scan or MRI readily confirms the presence of a well circumscribed mass. A biopsy is needed for confirmation of diagnosis. Chemotherapy and radiotherapy form the mainstay of treatment.

A metastatic neuroblastoma presents with unilateral or bilateral proptosis with ecchymosis of lid. Sometimes ocular involvement is the presenting feature of the tumor. The primary malignancy is located in the adrenal gland or the sympathetic chain of the retroperitoneum. Horner's syndrome may be caused by a thoracic tumor. Opsoclonus or ocular bobbing is a paraneoplastic syndrome unrelated to orbital involvement and is characterized by rapid, multidirectional saccadic eye movements. It signifies a relatively good prognosis. Other features include hypertension due to compression of renal artery, abdominal fullness and pain, edema due to venous obstruction and bone pain. Treatment is done with radiation and chemotherapy but prognosis is dismal.

Leukemia is the most common malignancy of childhood. Ocular involvement includes retinal hemorrhage, orbital infiltration (causing proptosis, eyelid swelling, and ecchymosis), optic nerve infiltration (optic disc edema and loss of vision) and retinal deposits.

MISCELLANEOUS CONDITIONS

Lid swelling may be a caused by allergy to topical medications, insect bites, and infection (stye). The treatment is conservative. Allergic lid edema usually responds well to cold compresses and corticosteroid ointment. Stye (hordeolum externum) is a painful tender erythematous infection of the hair follicle of eye lashes. Most styes either resolve spontaneously or discharge anteriorly close to the lash roots. Resolution may be promoted by epilation of the eyelash associated with the infected follicle followed by hot compresses and application of antibiotic ointment. Systemic antibiotics may be necessary if preseptal cellulitis is present.

Stevens-Johnson syndrome is an acute inflammatory polymorphic disease affecting skin and mucous membranes and carries a mortality rate of 5-15%. Ocular involvement is seen in 50% of patients and ranges from mild mucopurulent conjunctivitis to severe perforating corneal ulcers. Blindness can occur from ulceration, perforation and vascularization.

The syndrome has been associated with various bacterial, viral, mycotic and protozoal infections, vaccines, collagen diseases and allergic reaction to many drugs. A prodrome of chills develops with pharyngitis, and tachypnea. This is followed by bullous mucous lesions especially in the oropharynx that heal without scarring. Ocular involvement begins with edema and encrustation of the eyelids. A conjunctivitis develops with serous discharge. Bullae develop in the palpebral conjunctiva that heal with scarring leading to symblepharon. Primary corneal involvement is rare but has been reported. Ocular morbidity is caused by the late complications like ectropion, trichiasis, symblepharon and a severe dry eye syndrome that is caused by multiple factors like scarring of the lacrimal duct orifices and destruction of the goblet cells of the conjunctiva.

Treatment involves close coordination between the pediatrician, dermatologist, otolaryngologist and the ophthalmologist. Systemic steroids do not have a proven role. Liberal use of preservative-free ocular lubricants and prevention of symblepharon by lysis with a glass rod smeared in antibiotic ointment or a symblepharon ring is recommended. Prompt recognition and treatment of microbial infections is of paramount importance.

CONCLUSION

The above mentioned list of ocular emergencies is meant only as a guide and is not exhaustive. Much is gained by experience and managing cases in liaison with an ophthalmologist. Ocular signs should be looked for while managing

Section 4

patients with systemic illness e.g. raised intracranial pressure and collagen vascular disorders. The pediatrician should be able to provide primary care where speed is crucial in management e.g. conjunctivitis, chemical burns and orbital cellulitis. Appropriate and early referral to an ophthalmologist is mandatory to preserve vision and improve the outcome.

REFERENCES

1. Levin, A. Eye emergencies: acute management in the pediatric ambulatory care setting. *Pediatric Emergency Care* 1991, 7(6): 367-377.

2. Day S. History, examination and further investigation. In: *Pediatric Ophthalmology*. Taylor D (ed). 2nd edition. Cambridge, MA; Blackwell; 1996

3. McKeown CA. The pediatric eye examination. In: *Principles and Practice of Ophthalmology*. Albert DM, Jakobiec FA, (eds). 2nd edition. Philadelphia; Saunders;1991

4. Juang PSC, Rosen P. Ocular examination techniques for the emergency department. *J Emerg Med* 1997; 15(6):793-810.

5. Hamid, R, Newfield, P. Pediatric eye emergencies. *Anesthesiol Clin North Amer* 2001, 19(2), 257-264.

6. Preferred Practice Patterns Committee. *Pediatric Ophthalmology Panel. Pediatric Eye Evaluations*. San Francisco; American Academy of Ophthalmology; 1997

7. Mason I, Stevens S. Instilling eye drops and ointment in a baby or young child. *Community Eye Hlth J* 2010, 23;72:15.

8. Bremner MH. Childhood eye injuries, 1983-1998. *Med J Aust* 1999; 170(12):618-619.

9. Childhood blindness. *Souvenir of Annual General Assembly of NSPB*, March 25, 2000

10. Linden JA, Renner GS. Trauma to the globe. *Emerg Med Clin North Amer* 1995; 13(3):581-605.

11. MacEwen CJ, Baines PS, Desai P. Eye injuries in children: the current picture. *Brit J Ophthalmol* 1999; 83:933-936.

12. Burns FR, Paterson CA. Prompt irrigation of chemical eye injuries may avert severe damage. *Occup Health Safety* 1989; 58(4):33-36.

13. Dada T, Sharma N, Kumar A. Chemical injury due to colors used at the festival of Holi. *Natl Med J India* 1997; 10(5):256.

14. Agarwal T, Vajpayee RB. A warning about the dangers of *chuna* packets. *Lancet* 2003 Jun 28; 361(9376):2247.

15. Dhir SP, Shishko MN, Krewi A, Maburka S. Ocular fireworks injuries in children. *J Pediatr Ophthalmol* 1991; 28:354-355.

16. Meiler WF. Trauma section XIX. In: *Principles and Practice of Ophthalmology*. Albert DM, Jakobiec FA (eds.), 2nd edition, WB Saunders Company, Pennsylvania, 2000; pp 5177-5326.

17. Garcia GE. Management of ocular emergencies and urgent eye problems. *Am Fam Physician*. 1996; 53(2):565-574.

18. Gothwal VK, Adolph S, Jalali S, Naduvilath TJ. Demography and prognostic factors of ocular injuries in South India. *Aust NZ J Ophthalmol* 1999; 27(5): 318-325.

19. O'Hara MA. Ophthalmia neonatorum. *Pediatr Clin North Amer* 1993; 40:715-725.

20. Baum J, Barza M. The evolution of antibiotic therapy for bacterial conjunctivitis and keratitis. 1970-2000. *Cornea* 2000; 19:659-672.

21. Kushner BJ. The management of nasolacrimal duct obstruction in children between 18 months and 4 years old. *JAAPOS* 1998; 2:57-60.

22. Mets MB, Noffke AS. Ocular infections of the external eye and cornea in children. In: *Focal Points: Clinical Modules for Ophthalmologists*. San Francisco; American Academy of Ophthalmology; 2002

23. Dinowitz M, Rescigno R, Bielory L. Ocular allergic diseases: Differential diagnosis, examination techniques and testing. *Clin Allergy Immunol* 2000; 15:127-50.

24. Heidemann DG. Atopic and vernal keratoconjunctivitis. In: *Focal points: Clinical Modules for Ophthalmologists*. San Francisco, American Academy of Ophthalmology; 2001

25. Dunn JP. Uveitis in children. In: *Focal Points: Clinical Modules for Ophthalmologists*. San Francisco: American Academy of Ophthalmology; 1995

26. Shields JA, Shields CL. Rhabdomyosarcoma: Review for the ophthalmologist. *Surv Ophthal* 2003; 48(1): 39-57.

27. Shields JA. In: Diagnosis and Management of Orbital Tumors. *Philadelphia; Saunders; 1989.*

Section 4

5

Accidents and Poisonings

Foreign Bodies in the Aero-digestive Tract

V Bhatnagar and M Srinivas

Children are notoriously fond of inserting objects into various orifices, either due to their innocence or as a result of the oral phase of psychological development. Objects inserted into the nose, ears, anus and vagina are usually easy to manage but foreign bodies in the mouth can find their way into the aero-digestive tract and can be hazardous and often life-threatening. Such accidents are fairly common and underscore the need for vigilance on the part of parents and child care providers. The majority of foreign body aspirations occur in children younger than 3 years of age. A high index of suspicion is necessary to make an early diagnosis since small children and even older ones with neurological, cognitive, or psychiatric disorders may not be able to provide a proper history of foreign body aspiration.

Foreign body aspiration accounts for approximately 5% of all unintentional deaths among less than 5 years old children in most developed countries accounting for the fifth leading cause of accidental deaths. A few studies on this subject have been reported from India[1-6]. However, the true incidence, morbidity and mortality related to foreign body aspiration in India is not known. The presentation and management of foreign bodies that are inhaled into the respiratory tract is quite different from those in the alimentary tract although the portal of entry through the mouth is common to both. This chapter, therefore, discusses the two types of foreign bodies separately.

FOREIGN BODIES IN THE RESPIRATORY TRACT

Aspiration of foreign bodies into the respiratory passages is encountered quite commonly in children and present as a surgical emergency with features of acute airway obstruction[7-8].

Anatomical Considerations

The larynx is relatively narrower than the trachea. Hence, only those foreign bodies which can go across the vocal cords and larynx can enter the trachea and bronchus. The larger ones either get entrapped at the level of the vocal cords or slip down into the esophagus. Less commonly, an aspirated foreign body may lodge at or near the glottis. A foreign body obstructing the glottis may present with acute airway obstruction, hoarseness and stridor. Partial glottic obstruction by smaller impacted objects, rarely may go unnoticed for a few days. Asphyxiation due to an impacted obstructing laryngeal foreign body carries a high mortality rate. Survivors of such near fatal events may end up with hypoxic encephalopathy.

The trachea bifurcates into the right and left main bronchi at the carina. In neonates the angle of bifurcation is almost equal. However, with growth the bronchi bifurcate at unequal angles and the configuration becomes similar to that in adults by 10-12 years, i.e. the right main bronchus is almost in line with the trachea and the left main bronchus takes off at a more acute angle. Thus in younger children foreign bodies may be found with equal frequency in the right and left bronchi but in older children the foreign bodies find their way into the right main bronchus more easily.

Pathological Considerations

Metallic, plastic and other inert foreign bodies do not cause any significant inflammatory reaction but may obstruct the lumen due to their size. Glass beads, which have a central hole, may allow the passage of air and near normal ventilation may continue despite the foreign body. Plastic whistles may produce audible expiratory sounds. Sharp and pointed foreign bodies may perforate the airway leading to catastrophic results.

Some organic foreign bodies may swell up in the airway and lead to delayed obstruction. Seeds, nuts and other vegetable foreign bodies e.g., peanuts, sunflower seeds, water melon seeds, castor seeds, pieces of treated betel nut etc. cause a severe inflammatory reaction because of various chemical components of the vegetable matter (Table 48.1). The resultant edema further compromises the lumen and the mucosa bleeds easily on touch. With a long standing foreign body exuberant granulation tissue develops around it leading to complete obstruction, collapse and bronchiectasis. Bronchoscopic identification and removal may become difficult due to bleeding from manipulation of the foreign body.

Table 48.1 Types of foreign bodies in the airways

Seeds, nuts and other vegetable matter (> 75%)
Peanut, almond, other dry fruits are most common. Betel nut, seeds, gram, peas, millet, pine nuts, pop corn, bone, etc. are less common.

Inert material (< 25%)
Metallic objects, pen caps, beads, whistle, pins, nails, screws and dislodgeable parts of toys etc.

Nowadays children are increasingly exposed to electronic gadgets containing button batteries. These are usually ingested but may be inhaled at times and they need urgent attention. More often foreign bodies cause partial obstruction with a ball-valve like mechanism leading to air trapping and obstructive emphysema. Pneumomediastinum and pneumothorax secondary to obstructive emphysema may be rarely seen. Mediastinitis, tracheoesophageal fistula and rarely catastrophic bleeding from major vessels may result due to foreign bodies.

The larger foreign bodies may lodge in the trachea; causing choking and suffocation. Smaller foreign bodies lodge in a main bronchus; these may subsequently change position or migrate distally. Atelectasis, pneumonia, lung abscess or bronchiectasis may result from long standing foreign bodies in the respiratory tract. Even if the foreign body is removed, the inflammatory changes may not be completely reversible. Once irreversible bronchiectasis develops then open surgical intervention may become necessary. In India, arecanut poses serious problems due to arecoline an alkaloid found in them. It is a partial agonist of muscarinic acetylcholine receptors and hence some of these children may present with intense bronchospasm posing diagnostic difficulty.

Clinical Features

Inhalation of foreign bodies is most commonly seen in children between 1-3 years of age and the incidence falls as the age advances. There is a 3:1 male preponderance[9]. The incidence is somewhat higher in the winter months and this seems to correlate with the availability of peanuts. In recent

years, an increase in the inhalation of small dislodgeable parts of toys has been reported[10].

A definite history of foreign body inhalation is not available in most patients. The most common presentation is with a history of sudden choking and coughing while playing or during feeding followed by wheezing, paroxysmal coughing with or without fever and respiratory distress. The most common clinical manifestation is the triad of cough, wheeze and unilateral restriction of air entry. Inspiratory and expiratory rhonchi are also heard in most patients. Often, a foreign body in the respiratory tract presents as atypical asthma which does not respond to bronchodilators. Complications of long standing foreign bodies in the respiratory tract viz. repeated pneumonia, lung abscess, atelectasis and bronchiectasis is a less common mode of presentation. The exact clinical picture may vary with the site of enlodgement of the foreign body.

Larynx. The onset is dramatic. There is sudden choking, aphonia and stridor or violent inspiratory efforts. Death follows rapidly if impaction is complete.

Trachea. Foreign bodies between the larynx and carina give rise to spasmodic paroxysmal coughing and wheezing. A characteristic thud can be appreciated on auscultation with a freely mobile foreign body. Hoarseness, hemoptysis, cyanosis and dyspnea may be present. Sometimes after the initial acute discomfort the child presents with a laryngotracheobronchitis or a bronchiolitis type of clinical picture[9].

Bronchus. The large majority of inhaled foreign bodies find their way into one of the bronchi. There is a variable degree of tachypnea, cough and wheezing. Auscultation reveals restriction of air entry on the side of foreign body enlodgement. Prolonged impaction may lead to pneumonitis and bronchiectasis.

Table 48.2 Clinical symptoms of inhaled foreign bodies

- Choking
- Respiratory distress
- Stridor
- Cyanosis
- Tachypnea
- Spasmodic cough
- Wheezing
- Recurrent episodes of pneumonitis with fever

Investigations (Figures 48.1 to 48.4)

The suspicion of foreign body inhalation is based on clinical grounds, sometimes even in the absence of clinical or radiological findings. The investigations are done for the localisation of the foreign body and to evaluate its effects on the respiratory tract. A plain antero-posterior X-ray of the chest including the neck and diaphragm usually suffices; a lateral film may be required if the foreign body is suspected to be in the larynx. Radio-opaque foreign bodies are easily visible. Collapse, consolidation, pneumonic patches, pneumo-mediastinum and pneumothorax are easy to discern. Bronchiectatic changes may develop with long

standing foreign bodies. However, indirect inferences and clinical correlations are more often required to determine the site of the foreign body. For example, bilateral hyperinflated lungs would indicate a tracheal foreign body, whereas bronchial foreign bodies are indicated by unilateral pathology on the X-ray. A unilateral hyperinflated lung with ipsilateral restriction of air entry would indicate a foreign body on the same side, the hyperinflation resulting from air trapping due to a ball valve mechanism. But, if the air entry is restricted on the contralateral side then the foreign body will be on that side and the hyperinflation will occur as a compensatory response due to loss of volume on the side of the foreign body. Skiagrams of chest taken during expiration demonstrate air trapping while fluoroscopy is useful for evaluation of diaphragmatic movements[11].

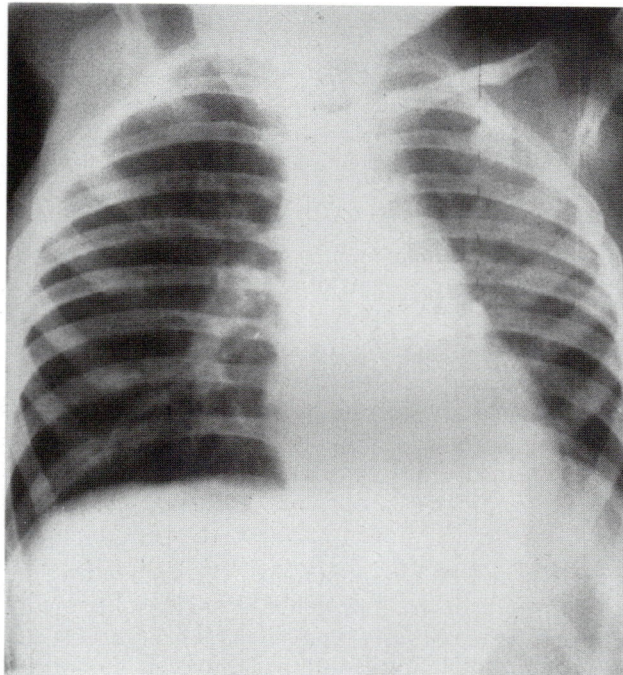

Figure 48.1a Radiolucent foreign body in the right main bronchus causing hyperinflation of the ipsilateral lung

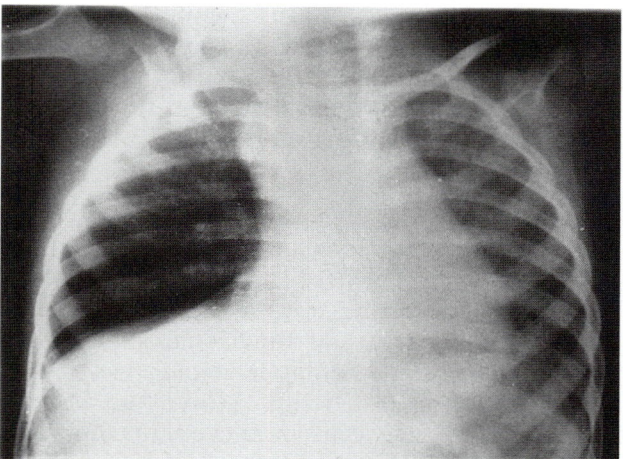

Figure 48.2a Radiolucent foreign body on the right side causing collapse of the lobe and hyperinflation of remaining ipsilateral lung

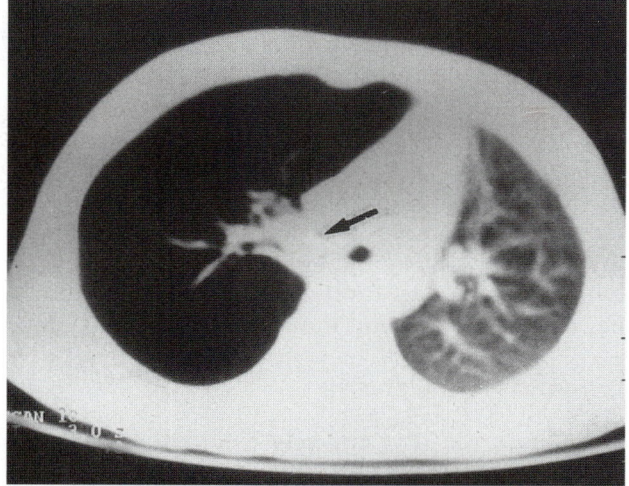

Figure 48.1b The foreign body, a peanut, in Figure 48.1a. seen on CT scan (arrow). It should be emphasized that CT scans are not necessary for diagnosis

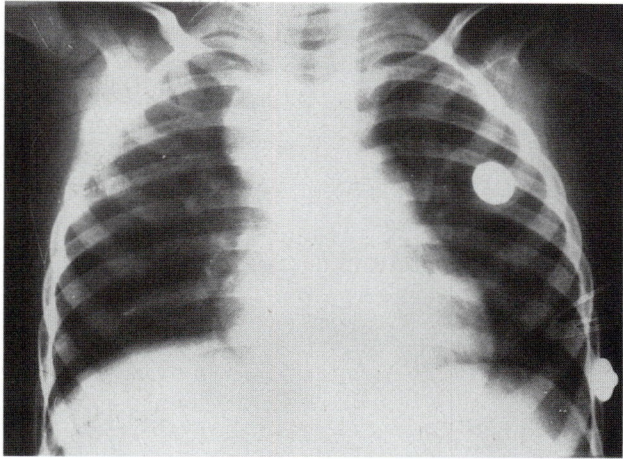

Figure 48.2b X-ray of the chest following bronchoscopic extraction of the foreign body followed by normal bilateral aeration of the lungs

Section 5

Chatterji and Chatterji[12] have summarised the various X-ray findings into four types of pictures in foreign body aspiration: (i) Bypass valve obstruction. This type results in a bypass valve that partially obstructs on both phases of respiration. The chest X-ray is normal because there is some aeration (albeit diminished) beyond the obstruction. Objects such as organic foreign bodies or small, flat items may not have any abnormalities on radiography. (ii) Check valve obstruction. Here the air is inhaled but cannot be expelled during expiration. Both lung fields fill up with air on inspiration, but hyperinflation of the ipsilateral lung occurs. (iii) Ball valve obstruction. This is caused by a partial obstruction from an object that intermittently prolapses and obstructs the affected bronchus. In this situation, mediastinal shift occurs toward the involved side and there is decreased air entry leading to early atelectasis and collapse. (iv) Stop valve obstruction. This denotes a complete bronchial obstruction where air passage is blocked both during inspiration and expiration. Such a condition results in consolidation of the involved bronchopulmonary segment with subsequent collapse.

CT scans and ventilation/perfusion scintigraphy are not required in the emergency evaluation of inhaled foreign bodies. They may have a role in the evaluation of long standing foreign bodies to assess the physical and functional state of the underlying lung. Virtual bronchoscopy has no role in an emergency setting. However, it may occasionally be useful in the evaluation of a suspected long standing foreign body[13]. Similarly, the role of MRI is very limited in the diagnostic work up of the child with suspected foreign body.

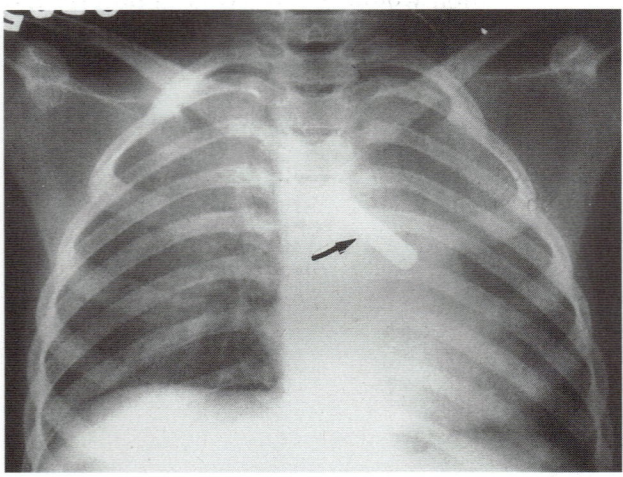

Figure 48.3 Radio-opaque foreign body in the left main bronchus. The compensatory hyperinflation on the right side is due to collapse of the left lung

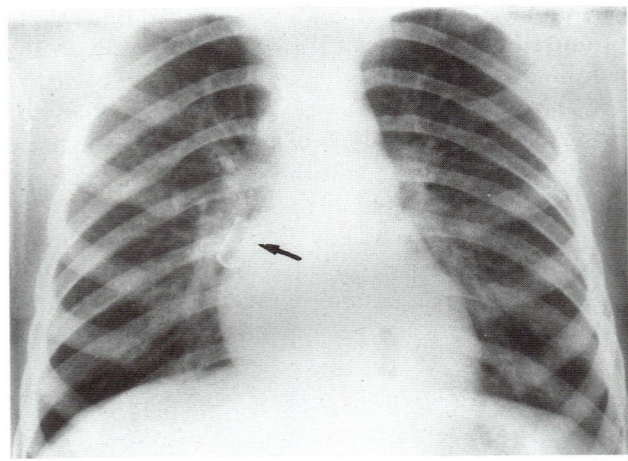

Figure 48.4 Radio-opaque foreign body in the right main bronchus. Both lungs appear equally aerated because the main central hole in the foreign body allowed normal ventilation to continue despite impaction

In life threatening situations, if clinical suspicion is strong and physical signs indicate the presence of an inhaled foreign body, the patient may have to be rushed to the operation theatre for a diagnostic cum therapeutic bronchoscopy even without an X-ray of the chest.

Management

Emergency management

Home first aid maneuvers like suspending the child up side down, thumping the back, groping with fingers in the pharynx, backblows, chest thrusts etc. may produce sustained pressure to facilitate expulsion of the foreign body but are fraught with danger because such maneuvers may cause impaction of foreign body. However, a large air flow and increased intrathoracic pressure may be produced to expel the foreign body by either subdiaphragmatic pressure or by encircling the patient in the prone position from behind with clasped hands while pushing and kneading the abdominal contents sharply up into the epigastrium towards the chest (Heimlich maneuver[11,14]). All these maneuvers are generally not recommended in children with foreign body aspiration. The child with a suspicion of foreign body inhalation should be rushed to a hospital immediately.

Hospital management

Once the diagnosis is established or even strongly suspected, a bronchoscopy should be done as soon as possible. Unnecessary delay may worsen the lung condition or run the risk of dislodgement and impaction of the foreign body at the larynx to cause immediate death. If the child is cyanosed and requires endotracheal intubation for ventilation in the emergency ward, arterial blood gas analysis is useful for judging the adequacy of the respiratory support. Pulse oximetry is the sheet anchor in monitoring of these children. In an intubated child, end tidal carbon dioxide levels are also useful for providing respiratory support.

Bronchoscopy is performed under general inhalation anesthesia preferrably with controlled ventilation and muscle relaxants, although successful extractions have been reported without muscle relaxation. A local anesthetic spray over the larynx greatly helps in reducing post-bronchoscopy laryngospasm[15-17]. A rigid ventilating bronchoscope of appropriate size with a fiberoptic light is currently the instrument of choice. Flexible bronchoscopes have also been successfully used[18] but always require a standby rigid brochoscope in case of failure. A variety of foreign body forceps are available for ease of extraction. After negotiating the larynx the endoscope should be advanced under vision so as to avoid pushing the foreign body into the smaller bronchi. After sighting the foreign body, it should be grasped with a suitable forceps and withdrawn along with the scope as a single unit. Following the extraction the endoscope should be reintroduced to ensure that there is no residual foreign body and also to clear the air passages of secretions under direct vision. Some advances have been made in the instrumentation e.g. an optical grasping forceps that helps in the extraction of foreign body. Good instruments and video imaging offers a clear magnified view that leads to higher success rates of retrieval and reduce the risk of residual foreign body[19-23].

Some specific foreign bodies may require special instruments like Fogarty catheter, floppy forceps, magnetic grasping forceps, etc. If possible, it is always useful to get the prototype of the foreign body inhaled by the child. This aids the surgeon to contemplate the exact method of grasping for extraction of the foreign body. Smooth beads may be difficult to hold and if they have the central hole, a Fogarty catheter or floppy forceps may be introduced into the central hole for retrieval of the foreign body. Sharp objects facing vocal cords need meticulous removal. In such situations a tracheostomy set should be kept as stand by in the operation theater. Tiny bits and pieces of foreign bodies inhaled by the child while chewing nuts and seeds may lodge in the segmental bronchi. All these small foreign bodies also need to be thoroughly extracted or sucked out meticulously. If this is not done, the child may go home with apparent recovery but will present later with recurrent chest infections and bronchiectasis requiring thoracotomy and lobectomy at a later date.

When the foreign body is visualized, the rigid bronchoscope is positioned proximally with just enough space to open the jaws of the optical forceps. The procedure should permit the ventilation via the side-ports of the bronchoscope sheath. Gentle suctioning is required if thick or purulent secretions are present and these should be sent for the culture and sensitivity. The foreign body is delicately grasped and every attempt is made to extract it in one piece and avoid damage to the surrounding mucosa of the trachea/bronchus. If the foreign body is larger than the lumen of the bronchoscope, it is grasped tightly with the optical forceps, brought to the tip of the bronchoscope, and then the bronchoscope, forceps and foreign body are removed as a single unit. It is important not to dislodge or push the foreign body distally during the procedure. If the foreign body dislodges during this maneuver, it is re-grasped and retrieved successfully. Rarely during extraction the foreign body may obstruct completely the main airway compromising the ventilation. In such a situation, the foreign body is pushed distally into a bronchus to allow ventilation through the healthy lung. If the foreign body is smaller than the diameter of the bronchoscope sheath, then the the optical forceps with the grasped foreign body is taken out. At times, the vegetable foreign body may swell up and may not be easily retrievable between the vocal cords. In such a rare situation, tracheotomy may be required. Long standing foreign bodies with a lot of granulation tissue may remain obscured. In such a rare situation thoracotomy may be needed to retrieve the foreign body. During thoracotomy one lung ventilation would be preferred to prevent the purulent material flooding the contralateral lung[24,25].

After the bronochoscopy some children may continue to have mild to moderate paroxysmal cough which can be effectively treated with humidification. A short course of antibiotics and chest physiotherapy is necessary. Postoperatively, an X-ray of the chest is always done to ensure that there is no pneumothorax and that the lung fields are equally ventilated. The child can be discharged after 24 hours of the bronchoscopy if there are no other contraindications. Algorithm for management of inhaled foreign body is shown in Figure 48.5.

Prevention

Parents should pay attention to the size and texture of the toys they buy for the children. Toys

Section 5

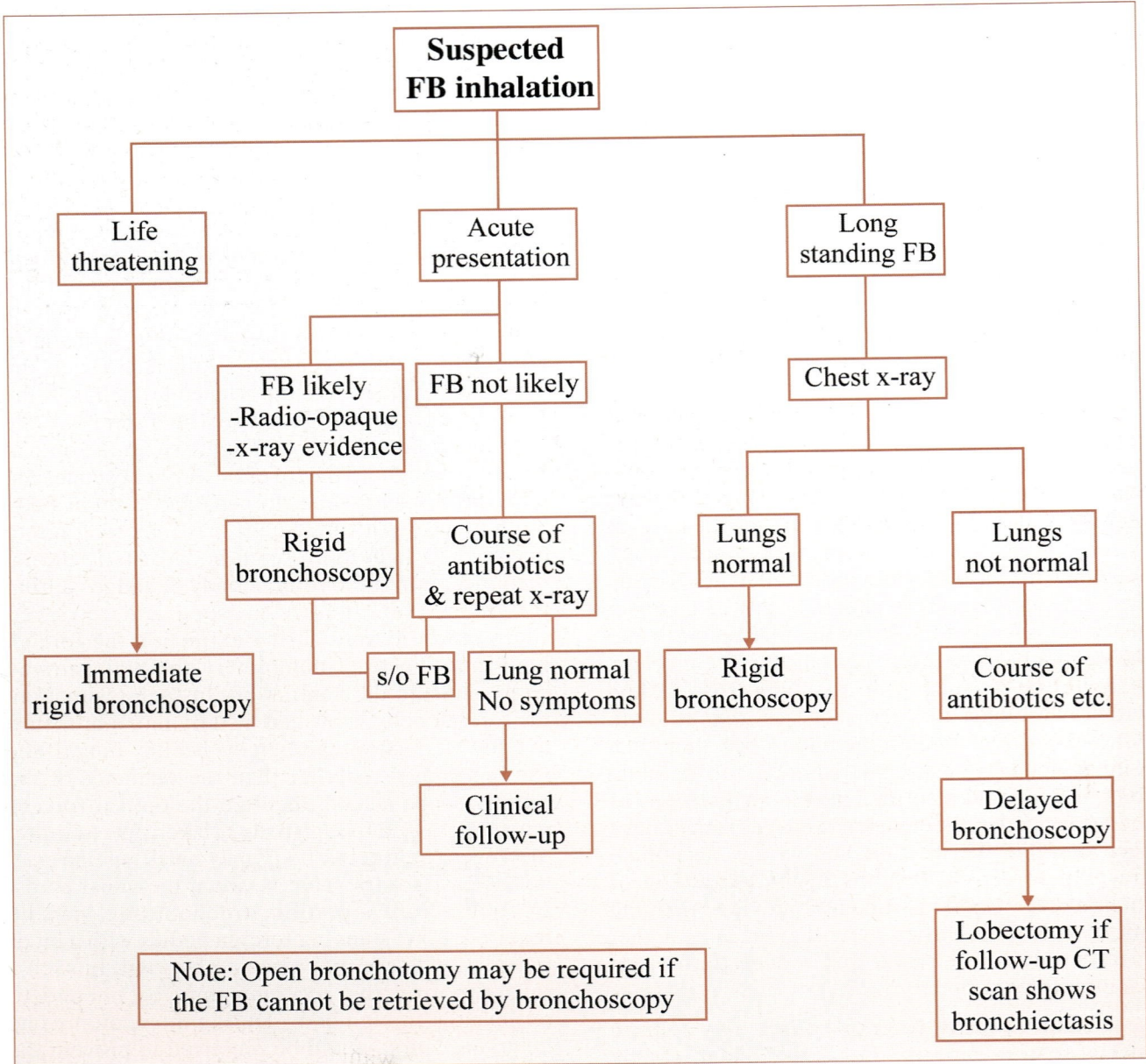

Figure 48.5 Algorithm for the management of an inhaled foreign body

with dislodgeable small parts should not be given to toddlers. It is important to educate the children regarding the hazards of putting the objects in mouth. Children less than 3 years of age should not be offered seeds and nuts which can be readily inhaled.

Complications

Almost all cases of foreign body inhalation can be discharged within 24 hours of successful foreign body retrieval by rigid bronchoscopy and do not get any complications. The complications of foreign body aspiration and its retrieval depends mainly on the delay in the diagnosis and delay in performing the bronchoscopy. The size, organic nature, shape, composition, location, and orientation of the aspirated object have a bearing on retrieval and complications. Cough, dyspnea, wheeze, hemoptysis, obstructive emphysema, atelectasis, tracheoesophageal fistula, bronchial stricture, pneumonia, polyp formation, bronchiectasis, lung abscess, bronchopleural fistula and pseudo tumor are listed as recognized complications. Bleeding from granulation tissue is usually mild. Long-standing bronchial obstruction can result in soiling of the contralateral bronchial tree as well. All these need extensive investigations by X-ray chest and

CT scan. Some of these complications will need appropriate open surgical procedures for management.

Prognosis

Almost all foreign bodies can be removed from the tracheobronchial tree using rigid bronchoscopy and carry excellent prognosis. The complication rate increases with delay in the diagnosis and delay in their retrieval.

FOREIGN BODIES IN THE ALIMENTARY TRACT

Ingestion of foreign bodies, like inhalation accidents, is also fairly common. The majority of ingested foreign bodies are spontaneously passed in the stool. However, those that do not do so may need endoscopic or operative removal[26].

Anatomical Considerations

The digestive tract has many naturally occurring areas of narrowing where foreign bodies can get lodged. At least three such sites are found in the esophagus; (i) at or just below the cricopharyngeus, where the vast majority of the swallowed objects are found; (ii) at the level of the aortic arch and (iii) at the cardioesophageal junction. The other areas which can restrict the passage of a foreign body are found in the stomach (pylorus), duodenojejunal junction and the ileocecal valve. Sometimes a foreign body may get lodged in the ampulla of rectum.

Pathological Considerations

An ingested foreign body, which is usually an inert metallic (e.g. coin) or plastic (e.g. small parts of toys) object, may get impacted at any of the physiological areas of constriction but it may also bring to light a pathological stricture by obstructing the lumen at the site of stricture (Table 48.3). In the alimentary tract, impaction of a foreign body may result in ulceration and pressure necrosis. Sharp objects may perforate any part of the gut. Depending on the site of impaction it may result in retropharyngeal abscess, empyema, a fistula (esophagotracheal/bronchial or esophagovascular) and if the perforation and/or impaction occurs in the abdomen then peritonitis can develop[2, 27].

The advent of 'button' cells or batteries has added to the long list of ingested foreign bodies. These are small mercury or alkaline cells and the large majority of ingested batteries are passed out in the stool uneventfully but following impaction their chemical components may leak out and cause focal liquefaction necrosis with resultant mediastinitis/peritonitis or the absorption of toxic material e.g. mercury may give rise to poisoning after absorption. Batteries impacted in the esophagus have also been reported to cause tracheo-esophageal fistula[28-30]. The management of button battery ingestion has been discussed in greater detail below. Psychological aberrations may result in a child eating non-edible objects (pica). Plucking one's own hair and eating them (trichotilomania) can lead to trichobezoar. Elder sibs have been known to 'feed' the younger ones with objects which can get impacted.

Clinical Features

The initial episode of foreign body ingestion may resemble that of foreign body inhalation but the coughing is not severe and there is minimal choking and gagging. This is usually followed by dysphagia, drooling of saliva and retrosternal/epigastric discomfort if the foreign body gets impacted in the esophagus. However, foreign bodies which go beyond the esophagus are usually asymptomatic and are passed out in the stool spontaneously within 4-5 days. Impaction in the alimentary tract will present with features of intestinal obstruction. Perforation of the gut, depending on the site, will lead to mediastinitis, empyema or peritonitis. The common symptoms of foreign body in the esophagus are listed in Table 48.4.

Table 48.3 Types of foreign bodies in the alimentary tract
Blunt objects (80%) Coins (>50%) Others – button battery, beads, key, pencil sharpener, suction catheter, trichobezoar etc.
Sharp objects (20%) Pins, nails, ear rings, ornaments, dislodgeable parts of toys
Multiple objects (rarely)

Table 48.4 Clinical symptoms of foreign body in the esophagus
• Drooling of saliva
• Dysphagia/odynophagia
• Foreign body sensation in throat
• Cough
• Fever
• Recurrent aspiration pneumonia
• Failure to thrive

Section 5

Investigations (Figures 48.6a and b)

Most of the ingested foreign bodies are radio-opaque. Hence, if the foreign body is suspected to be impacted in the esophagus, a plain antero-posterior and lateral X-ray of the neck and chest is all that is necessary in the emergency management. The abdomen should be included in the antero-posterior chest X-ray if the foreign body is suspected to have passed into the stomach or beyond. The progress of an ingested foreign body should be monitored by fluoroscopy or repeated plain skiagrams every 24-48 hours. Perforation by the foreign body can also be diagnosed on the plain X-ray by the findings of pneumothorax or free air under the diaphragm. But if an empyema has resulted from the perforation then a CT scan is required to assess the condition of the underlying lung.

Since the contrast studies, with either barium or water soluble contrast, carry a risk of aspiration it is better to perform diagnostic endoscopy which can also be therapeutic. CT scans, ultrasonography, and magnetic resonance imaging have been used to identify radiolucent foreign bodies.

If a large bolus of food matter gets impacted as a foreign body then esophageal stricture should be ruled out with the help of esophagoscopy and/or contrast studies. Foreign bodies like bezoars do not present as an emergency and various imaging modalities e.g. ultrasonography, barium studies and CT scans may be necessary for the diagnosis.

The hand held metal detector has been used for the localisation of ingested metallic foreign bodies[31].

Management

Impaction of an ingested foreign body rarely threatens life. Eating food which provides bulk eg. mashed potatoes or bananas may help in the passage of a foreign body down the esophagus into the stomach or if it has already passed down the esophagus then its further progress through the gastrointestinal tract is facilitated. Fishing for a foreign body in the pharynx with one's finger is not a good idea because even small children can bite hard! Children with impacted or symptomatic foreign bodies should be referred to a well equipped center for endoscopy. Algorithm for the management of an ingested foreign body is shown in Figure 48.7.

It is important to determine whether the foreign body is in the esophagus, stomach or beyond. The following prerequisites are desirable for management of an ingested foreign body:

(i) Intra-operative C-arm or digital X-ray facility, if available, should be utilized. (ii) Consent for neck exploration or thoracotomy in cases with

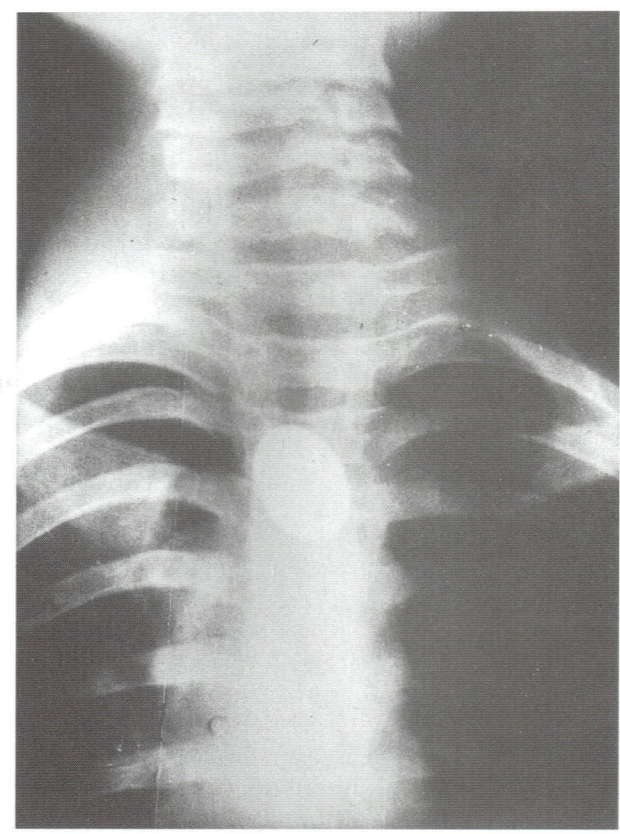

Figure 48.6a Coin impacted in the upper esophagus

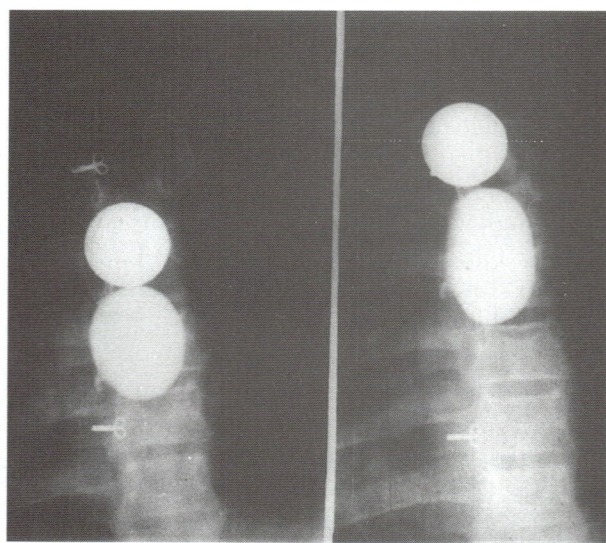

Figure 48.6b X-ray showing extraction using Foley's balloon catheter. The catheter has been passed beyond the coin and the balloon inflated with radio-opaque contrast. Gentle pull on the catheter disimpacts the coin and brings it up into the mouth from where it can be retrieved

long standing impacted foreign body. (iii) Stand by bronchoscopy in long standing anteriorly impacted foreign bodies. (iv) In long standing impacted foreign bodies, major vascular breach or injury should be kept in mind.

An X-ray of the neck, chest and abdomen should be repeated just before endoscopy to confirm the exact site of the impaction and monitor progression of the foreign body if any. Parenteral ketamine-midazolam or fentanyl-midazolam have been used during the extraction of esophageal foreign bodies but there is a risk of transient hypoxemia. Hence, esophagoscopy in children should always be performed under general anesthesia to avoid compromise of the respiratory tract during the procedure[32,33]. Endoscopy may be avoided for the extraction of foreign bodies impacted in the upper esophagus. However, the endoscope should be kept ready in the operation theater because the foreign body may move down. Magill's forceps can be effectively used for such impactions[34, 35]. For foreign bodies impacted lower down in the esophagus, endoscopy is required. The foreign body is visualised and preferrably extracted; it may be pushed down into the stomach if it cannot be gripped adequately with a foreign body forceps. If retrieval of a button cell through an endoscope is unsatisfactory because of inability to grasp it

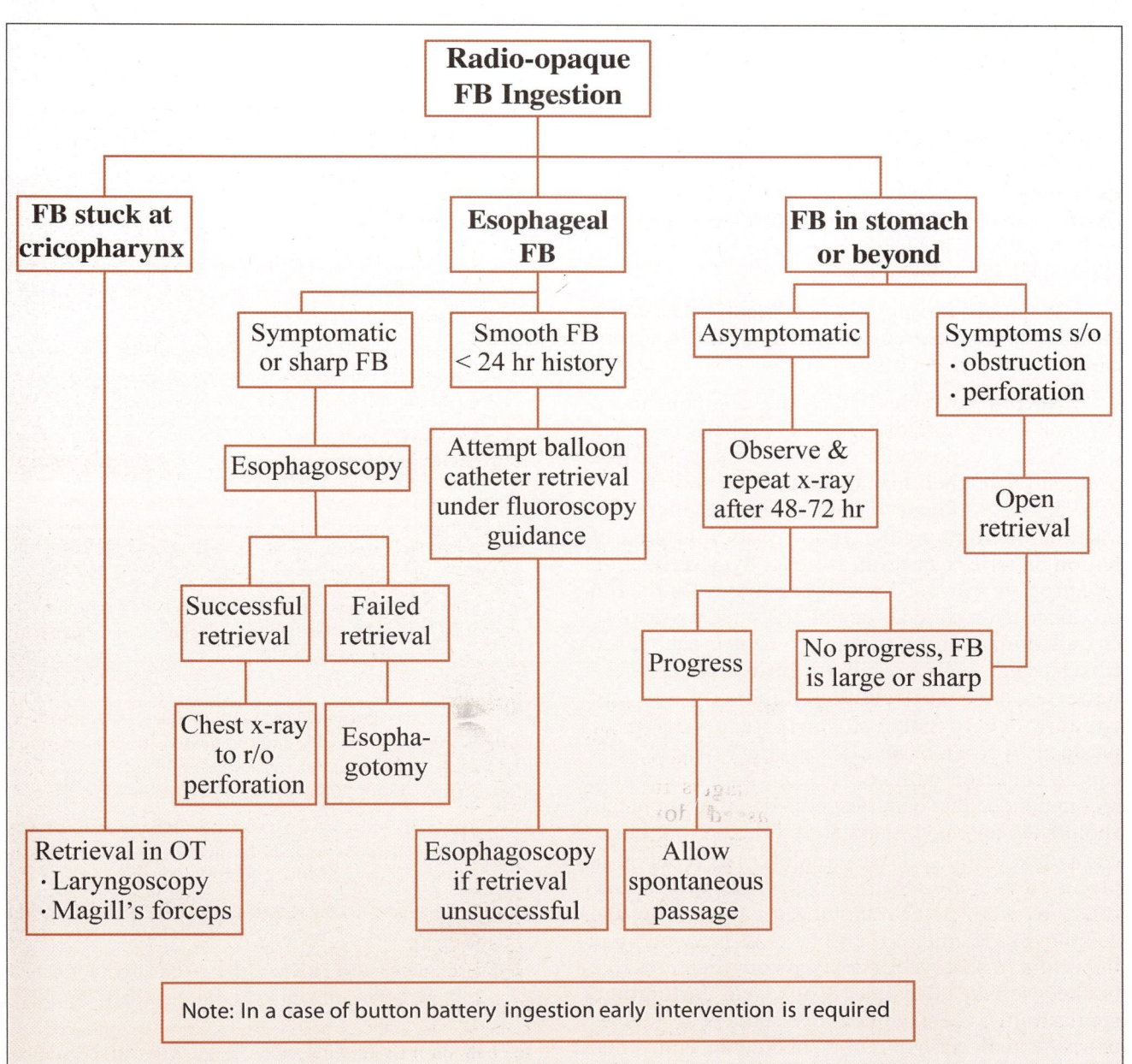

Figure 48.7 Algorithm for the management of an ingested foreign body

properly then open surgical removal should be considered[29, 33].

Smooth surfaced foreign bodies can be extracted by the Foley or Fogarty balloon catheter. The catheter is passed beyond the foreign body, the balloon is inflated so as to block the lumen of the esophagus and it is then gently pulled up. The foreign body is then spat out or it can be retrieved from the mouth of the patient. Care should be taken to avoid re-swallowing of the foreign body. This is a simple, safe and inexpensive method which does not require X-ray or fluoroscopic control and can be performed even in peripheral centers where facilities for endoscopy may not exist. This procedure is ideally suited for removal of coins from the esophagus. However, objects with irregular or sharp edges cannot be removed by this method[36].

The foreign bodies that have reached the stomach may be removed with an endoscope if it is large in size (> 2.0 cm diameter), long in length (> 10 cm) or sharp (open safety pin), if it is causing obstruction or perforation and when a coin or blunt object fails to leave the stomach in 3-4 weeks (Figure 48.6).

Trichobezoars present insidiously and require gastrotomy for their removal although small bezoars can be removed endoscopically[37].

Button batteries which are components of toys and games for children, if not properly disposed off, these are now increasingly being ingested accidently and their management strategies are still not clear[38-40]. These batteries can be mercury, alkaline or lithium cells. Injury from ingestion of button batteries can result from (i) hydroxylization (electrolytic current hydrolyzes tissue fluids and produces hydroxide at the battery's negative pole), (ii) alkalinization or (iii) pressure necrosis. Used (discharged) cells are also injurious since these batteries have sufficient residual voltage and capacitance to generate an external current, produce hydroxide, and cause injury. These cells can be confused with coins on an X-ray. It is now recommended that batteries lodged in the esophagus should be removed immediately since serious burns can occur within 2 hours. Endoscopic removal is preferred as it allows direct visualization of tissue injury as well. After removing a battery from the esophagus, if mucosal injury was present, it is important to observe for delayed complications like tracheoesophageal fistula, esophageal perforation, mediastinitis, vocal cord paralysis, tracheal stenosis or tracheomalacia, aspiration pneumonia, empyema, lung abscess, pneumothorax, spondylodiscitis, or exsanguination from perforation into a large vessel.

Prevention

Accidents due to foreign bodies are common in infants and toddlers due to their natural curiosity to explore the environment and due to carelessness and lack of awareness on the part of the attendants. Children must be constantly supervised and watched[41]. Nuts and seeds should not be offered to infants and young children. Objects like safety pins, buttons, glass beads, coins, tablets and toys with removeable small parts or those with sharp edges should be kept away from toddlers and young children. Preschool children with food in their mouths should not be triggered to laugh or cry as they can readily get choked. A foreign body in the airway and sometimes in the alimentary tract can be a life-threatening emergency requiring immediate treatment. It is, therefore, important that the public and primary health care workers should be educated in the first aid methods of dealing with such exigencies.

REFERENCES

1. Shivakumar AM, Naik AS, Prashanth KB, Shetty KD, Praveen DS. Tracheobronchial foreign bodies. *Indian J Pediatr* 2003 Oct;70(10):793-797.

2. Shivakumar AM, Naik AS, Prashanth KB, Yogesh BS, Hongal GF. Foreign body in upper digestive tract. *Indian J Pediatr* 2004 Aug;71(8):689-693.

3. Yadav SP, Singh J, Aggarwal N, Goel A. Airway foreign bodies in children: experience of 132 cases. *Singapore Med J* 2007 Sep;48(9):850-853.

4. Mathur NN, Pradhan T. Rigid pediatric bronchoscopy for bronchial foreign bodies with and without Hopkins telescope. *Indian Pediatr* 2003 Aug;40(8):761-765.

5. Singh JK, Vasudevan V, Bharadwaj N, Narasimhan KL. Role of tracheostomy in the management of foreign body airway obstruction in children. *Singapore Med J* 2009 Sep;50(9):871-874.

6. Kamath P, Bhojwani KM, Prasannaraj T, Abhijith K. Foreign bodies in the aerodigestive tract—a clinical study of cases in the coastal belt of South India. *Amer J Otolaryngol* 2006 Nov-Dec;27(6):373-377.

7. Sisenda TM, Khwa-Otsyula BO, Wambani JO. Management of tracheo-bronchial foreign bodies in children. *East Afr Med J* 2002; 79:580-583.

8. Bhatnagar V, Bazaz R, Mitra DK. Foreign bodies in the pediatric airway. *Indian J Pediatr* 1983; 50:519-523.

9. Esclamoda RM, Richardson MA. Laryngotracheal foreign bodies in children. *Amer J Dis Child* 1987; 141:259-262.

10. White DR, Zdanski CJ, Drake AF. Comparison of pediatric aieway foreign bodies over fifty years. *South Afr Med J* 2004; 97:434-436.

11. Gordon AS, Belton AK, Ridolpho TF. Emergency management of foreign body airway obstruction. In: Advances in Cardiopulmonary Resuscitation. Safer PU, Elam JO (eds). *Springer-Verlag, New York,* 1977, pp 39-50.

12. Chatterji S, Chatterji P. The management of foreign bodies in air passages. *Anaesthesia* 1972; 27: 390-395.

13. Cevizci N, Dokucu AI, Baskin D, Karadað CA, Sever N, Yalçin M, Bahadir E, Baºak M. Virtual bronchoscopy as a dynamic modality in the diagnosis and treatment of suspected foreign body aspiration. *Eur J Pediatr Surg* 2008 Dec;18(6):398-401.

14. Heimlich HL. A life saving maneuver to prevent food choking. *JAMA* 1975; 234:398-399.

15. Koloske AM. Bronchoscopic extraction of aspirated foreign bodies in children. *Amer J Dis Child* 1982; 136:924-929.

16. Pasaoglu I, Dogan R, Demericin M, *et al.* Bronchoscopic removal of foreign bodies in children: retrospective analysis of 822 cases. *Thorac Cardiovasc Surg* 1991; 39:95-98.

17. Soodan A, Pawar D, Subramanium R. Anesthesia for removal of inhaled foreign bodies in children. *Paediatr Anaesth* 2004; 14:947-952.

18. Swanson KL, Prakash UB, Midthun DE, Edell ES, Utz JP, McDougall JC, Brutinel WM. Flexible bronchoscopic management of airway foreign bodies in children. *Chest* 2002 May;121(5):1695-700.

19. Hilmi OJ, White PS, Oluwole M, Dunkley MP, McGurty DW. A randomised control trial of surgical task performance in rigid bronchoscopy: foreign body extraction with optical versus non-optical forceps. *Clin Otolaryngol Allied Sci* 1999; 24:499-501.

20. Martinot A, Deschildre A, Brichet A, Leclerc F. Indications of bronchial endoscopy in suspected tracheo-bronchial foreign body in children. *Rev Mal Respir* 1999; 16:673-678.

21. Sehgal A, Singh V, Chandra J, Mathur NN. Foreign body aspiration. *Indian Pediatr* 2002; 39:1006-1010.

22. Swanson KL, Prakash UB, Midthun DE, Edell DS, Utz JP, McDougall JC, Brutinel WM. Flexible bronchoscopic management of airway foreign bodies in children. *Chest* 2002; 121:1695-1700.

23. Yang CC, Lee KS. Comparison of direct vision and video imaging during bronchoscopy for pediatric airway foreign bodies. *Ear Nose Throat J* 2003; 82:129-133.

24. Bhatnagar V, Mitra DK. Surgical removal of tracheo-bronchial foreign bodies. *Indian J Pediatr* 1985; 52: 651-654.

25. Bhatnagar V, Mitra DK. Inhaled glass beads: problems in removal. *Indian Pediatr* 1985; 22:540-543.

26. Bhatnagar V, Mitra DK. Management of ingested foreign bodies. *Indian Pediatr* 1985; 22:519-522.

27. Antao B, Foxall G, Guzik I, Vaughan R, Roberts JP. Foreign body ingestion causing gastric and diaphragmatic perforation in a child. *Pediatr Surg Int* 2005; 21:326-328.

28. Alkan M, Buyukayavuz I, Dogru D, Yalcin E, Karnak I. Tracheoesophageal fistula due to disc battery ingestion. *Eur J Pediatr Surg* 2004; 14:279-282.

29. Chang YJ, Chao HC, Kong MS, Lai MW. Clinical analysis of disc battery ingestion in children. *Chang Gun Med J* 2004; 27:673-677.

30. Litovitz TL. Button battery ingestion. *JAMA* 1983; 2495-2497.

31. Schalamon J, Haxhija EQ, Ainoedhofer H, Gossler A, Schleef J. The use of a hand held metal detector for localisation of ingested metallic foreign bodies – a critical investigation. *Eur J Pediatr Surg* 2004; 163:257-259.

32. Hostetler MA, Barnard JA. Removal of esophageal foreign bodies in the pediatric ED: is ketamine an option? *Amer J Emerg Med* 2002; 20:96-98.

33. Stringer MD, Capps SNJ. Rationalizing the management of swallowed coins in children. *Brit Med J* 1991; 302:1321-1322.

34. Karaman A, Cavusoglu YH, Karaman I, Erdogan D, Aslan MK, Cakmak O. Magill forceps technique for removal of safety pins in upper esophagus: a preliminary report. *Int J Pediatr Otorhinolaryngol* 2004; 68:1189-1191.

35. Baral BK, Joshi RR, Bhattarai BK, Sewal RB. Removal of coin from upper esophageal tract in children with Magill's forceps under propofol sedation. *Nepal Med Coll J* 2010 Mar;12(1):38-41.

36. Agarwala S, Bhatnagar V, Mitra DK. Coins can be safely removed from the esophagus in children by Foley's catheter without fluoroscopic control. *Indian Pediatr* 1996; 33:109-111.

37. Bhatnagar V, Mitra DK. Childhood trichobezoars. *Indian J Pediatr* 1984; 51:489-492.

38. Amanatidou V, Sofidiotou V, Fountas K, Kalostou A, Tsamadou A, Papathanassiou V, Neou P. Button battery ingestion: the Greek experience and review of the literature. *Pediatr Emerg Care* 2011 Mar;27(3):186-188.

39. Litovitz T, Whitaker N, Clark L, White NC, Marsolek M. Emerging battery-ingestion hazard: clinical implications. *Pediatrics* 2010 Jun;125(6):1168-1177.

40. Litovitz T, Whitaker N, Clark L. Preventing battery ingestions: an analysis of 8648 cases. *Pediatrics* 2010 Jun;125(6):1178-1183.

41. Saki N, Nikakhlagh S, Rahim F, Abshirini H. Foreign body aspirations in infancy: a 20-year experience. *Int J Med Sci* 2009 Oct 14;6(6):322-328.

Section 5

49

Drowning

Pankaj Hari

Drowning is a leading cause of accidental deaths in children and results in substantial morbidity in the survivors. It is one of the greatest tragedies for the family and is largely preventable. In the past, terminologies used to describe drowning have been confusing. The World Congress on Drowning and the World Health Organization have put forth uniform definitions related to drowning[1]. Drowning is defined as a process resulting in primary respiratory impairment from submersion/immersion in a liquid medium. The term drowning is used regardless of the outcome. In addition it is recommended that terms such as near-drowning, secondary drowning, active drowning, passive drowning, silent drowning, wet drowning and dry drowning be abandoned.

Drowning has been an age-old problem and continues to occur worldwide. According to WHO drowning is the leading cause of injury related mortality in males aged 5-14 years[2]. There is less information on drowning related morbidity. It is estimated that for each drowning death there are 1-4 non fatal hospitalizations due to drowning. Most pediatric drowning victims are toddlers. The drowning rates peak at 0–4 years and again at 16-18 years of age[3].The adolescent peak is observed only in boys. Drowning accidents are about 10 times more common in adolescent boys than girls. Swimming in prohibited areas of ocean, boating, river rafting, scuba diving, daredevil behavior, intentional hyperventilation, use of alcohol and drugs are frequent antecedents of drowning in adolescents. Children with epilepsy and those with long QT syndrome are at increased risk of drowning. The patterns of drowning deaths are highly dependent upon the geographic factors. Majority of drowning deaths happen during swimming. Drowning events may assume epidemic proportions during floods.

Most drowning events in toddlers in rural areas occur in wells, ponds and large buckets. Children of affluent society may drown in swimming pool, inflatable pool, bathtub, commode, and washing machine. Bathtubs are a particular threat to infants who are unable to become upright if submerged. Momentary lapse of supervision, usually less than 5 minutes, is responsible for drowning of toddlers. However, bathtub submersions, particularly in children with evidences of physical abuse are likely to be inflicted rather than accidental or spontaneous[4].

PATHOPHYSIOLOGY

Sequence of Events

Following submersion, older children may panic, hold breath and struggle violently with automatic swimming movements. On the other hand, younger children may sink to the bottom without any noises, shrieks, physical movements or resistance. Voluntary breath holding continues until a break point is reached and the victim is forced to breathe under water, leading to aspiration of water. The 'breakpoint' is determined by the degree of hypercarbia and hypoxemia. The duration of breath holding is prolonged if it is preceded by hyper-ventilation.

Within minutes of first submerged breath, the victim develops secondary apnea. This is followed by involuntary gasping, resulting in aspiration of water. Finally, respiratory arrest ensues leading to further hypoxia. Prolonged hypoxia results in cardiac arrhythmia, cardiac arrest and brain death. In 10 percent of cases of drowning aspiration of small amount of water may trigger severe laryngospasm and the victim may succumb to hypoxia without significant aspiration of water.

During a drowning episode, exposure of face to cold water stimulates the trigeminal nerve, which transmits the afferent impulses to the medullary centers in the brain. This results in bradycardia, systemic hypertension and shunting of blood from cutaneous and splanchnic vessels to the heart and the brain. This is called diving reflex. Though relatively weak in children, this reflex is believed to offer some neuroprotection during a drowning episode[5]. Diving reflex may be absent in infants who are taught to swim or "water-proofed" at an early age. Table 49.1 provides a list of complications associated with drowning.

Table 49.1 Complications of drowning
☐ Hypothermia
☐ Regurgitation and aspiration
☐ Pulmonary edema
☐ Pneumonia
☐ Hypoxic encephalopathy
☐ Electrolyte abnormalities
☐ Rhabdomyolysis
☐ Renal dysfunction
☐ Cardiac arrhythmia
☐ Trauma
☐ Decompression illness in scuba divers

Hypothermia

Hypothermia develops rapidly after submersion in cold water. Cooling is faster in children as compared to adults due to larger surface area and decreased insulation by fat. The heat loss is also aided by ingestion of cold water. Rapid cooling (<30°C) results in decreased cerebral oxygen consumption and cardiac standstill much before decreased oxygen delivery results in cell death. Rapid onset of hypothermia allows the brain to tolerate longer periods of hypoxia and may be associated with improved neurologic outcome. Young children may survive submersion for up to 20 minutes or longer if the water temperature is below 10°C. Severe hypothermia also results in bradycardia, cardiac arrhythmia, central respiratory depression, deep coma and fixed dilated pupils. Other adverse consequences include pulmonary edema, hyperglycemia, disseminated intravascular coagulation and sepsis.

Pulmonary Effects

The most remarkable lung abnormality in drowning is pulmonary edema, although most victims do not aspirate enough water to result in serious alteration in blood volume[5]. The sequence of events resulting in pulmonary edema has been shown in Figure 49.1.

The respiratory disturbances depends less on the water composition and more on the amount of water aspirated. The pulmonary changes begin with laryngospasm or aspiration of small amounts of water. Aspiration of small amount of water can cause reflex pulmonary vasoconstriction leading to pulmonary hypertension. Loss or inactivation of surfactant leads to alveolar collapse and decreased lung compliance. Perfusion of nonventilated alveoli

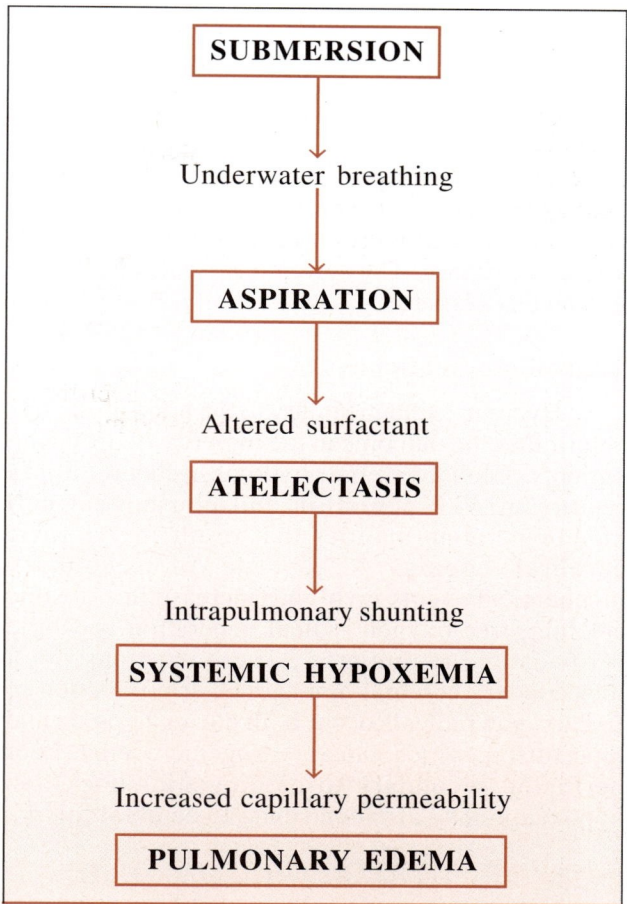

Figure 49.1 Respiratory pathophysiology in drowning

results in ventilation perfusion mismatch, which may increase up to 6-8 times of normal[5]. The ventilation perfusion mismatch may persist for several days even when the victim is clinically normal. Severe ventilation perfusion mismatch results in worsening of hypoxia. Persistent hypoxia and acidosis result in pulmonary edema. Significant airway obstruction may occur due to aspiration of stomach contents, foreign bodies and bronchospasm, which contribute to hypoxemia. Lung injury from fresh water and sea water drowning does not differ substantially as was believed earlier.

Less than 5 percent survivors of drowning may initially respond well to resuscitation but later develop respiratory deterioration. It may be seen during 3 to 72 hours after rescue and is most likely due to alterations in the composition or loss of surfactant.

Cardiovascular Consequences

Cardiac function in children is more tolerant to hypoxic insult than in adults. Cardiac abnormalities usually follow respiratory arrest and mainly include bradycardia and asystole[5]. However, ventricular fibrillation may also occur and is most likely due to hypothermia and hypoxia rather than hyperkalemia. Cardiac resuscitation is possible in most children with prolonged hypoxia[2]. However, cardiogenic shock due to myocardial contractility is common following resuscitation in severely affected children. The systemic vascular resistance is typically elevated.

Neurologic Sequelae

Hypoxic-ischemic injury to the brain ultimately determines the outcome in the majority of drowning patients. Global cerebral hypoxic-ischemic injury results in ATP depletion and consequent cell membrane abnormalities that result in cytotoxic cerebral edema. A cascade of secondary biochemical events involving increase in cytosolic calcium, free oxygen radical generation and lipid peroxidation are initiated[6]. These reactions result in secondary cerebral damage. Over production of free oxygen radicals occur both during hypoxia and reperfusion, which causes vasogenic edema. Poor perfusion secondary to cardiogenic shock and hypoxemia may also contribute to cerebral injury.

Fluids, Electrolytes and Hematological Alterations

In humans both fresh and seawater drowning do not result in significant alterations in blood volume and electrolytes. This may be because a majority of human drowning victims aspirate small amounts (<2.2 ml/kg) of water[5]. Nevertheless, hyponatremia and hypernatremia can occur with fresh and salt water drowning respectively.

Usually near-drowning is associated with hypovolemic shock. The hypovolemia is due to increase in capillary permeability and third space loss, secondary to hypoxia. Hyperglycemia may occur in drowning cases. This is secondary to catecholamine release due to stress. Hyperglycemia (blood glucose >250 mg/dl) may aggravate ischemic brain damage and result in poor neurological outcome. Disseminated intravascular coagulopathy may supervene.

Multi-organ Dysfunction

Several other organs including liver, kidneys and gastrointestinal tract may be affected because of hypoxia in drowning victims. Renal ischemia usually results in hematuria and albuminuria. Severe ischemic injury can lead to acute renal failure secondary to acute tubular necrosis. Drowned scuba diver may suffer from decompression sickness which is often difficult to recognize.

CLINICAL FEATURES

The clinical features are predominantly related to respiratory and nervous system and are determined by the submersion time. Central nervous system features vary from mild impairment in sensorium to deep coma, convulsions and even neurological deficits. A classification by Conn and Barker[7] based on Glasgow Coma Scale is a useful guide to the management of drowning victims. Children with normal or blunted sensorium generally have good outcome, whereas those who are comatose, apneic and pulseless have poor outcome.

Respiratory distress is present in a majority of near-drowning cases and pulmonary edema is frequently seen in severely affected children. Clinical examination may reveal cyanosis, crepitations and other features of congestive heart failure. The clinical picture may be complicated by cardiogenic shock, acute renal failure and disseminated intravascular coagulation.

Head and cervical spine injury should be ruled out in all drowning victims. Drowning can sometime be inflicted by the caretaker and younger children should be examined for evidences of abuse or inflicted injuries.

LABORATORY INVESTIGATIONS

Radiological. The chest X-ray may show various types of patchy opacities during the course of illness. The skiagram may reveal pulmonary edema, bronchopneumonia, pulmonary abscess and even empyema. The X-rays of skull, cervical spine and sometimes skeletal survey may be required to exclude fractures due to fall or abuse.

Biochemical and hematological changes. Low $paCO_2$, variable paO_2, metabolic acidosis, increased lactic dehydrogenase are common in patients with significant submersion injury. Occasionally, azotemia may be present. Electrolyte abnormalities such as hyponatremia, hypernatremia and hyperkalemia are uncommon. Hematological findings include hemoconcentration, leukocytosis, hemolysis and abnormal coagulation profile due to disseminated intravascular coagulopathy. The initial blood glucose may influence the eventual outcome and should be obtained in all cases.

Pulmonary function tests may reveal decreased forced expiratory volume (FEV-1), vital capacity and lung compliance. Ventilation perfusion scan may reveal ventilation-perfusion mismatch.

Renal and hepatic functions should also be assessed in cases with prolonged submersion time.

Electrocardiogram should be taken to exclude arrhythmia and ischemic changes, which may appear on rewarming.

Tracheal and throat swabs should be taken to identify any pathogenic organisms, which may be seen in drowning in excessively contaminated water such as sewers. Children suspected of poisoning or drug abuse should undergo toxicological screening.

MANAGEMENT

The most important goal of management is to improve tissue oxygen delivery as soon as possible in order to minimize cerebral hypoxic damage. The management of drowning has been summarized in a flow chart (Figure 49.2).

Resuscitation at site

The most important determinants of neurologically normal survival are prompt rescue from the water and immediate institution of basic life support[8]. Some bystander resuscitation is better than none. Cardiopulmonary resuscitation (CPR) should be initiated promptly to shorten the "no-flow" stage of cardiac arrest. Rescue breathing should be started without wasting much time in clearing aspirated water from the airways along with effective chest compressions. A combination of rescue breathing and chest compressions is superior to either of them instituted alone. Single rescuer should provide two rescue breaths before each cycle of 30 chest compressions. Rescue breathing rates much higher than 20 breaths per minute should be avoided to prevent impediment to venous return. During CPR, the primary determinant of stroke volume is the force of chest compressions. Adequate chest compression is provided by pressing the lower half of sternum to a relative depth of one third to one half of the anterior-posterior diameter of the chest. The rate of chest compression should be approximately 100 compressions per minute. Appropriately performed chest compressions can deliver 15-20% of the normal cardiac output that would suffice for successful resuscitation.

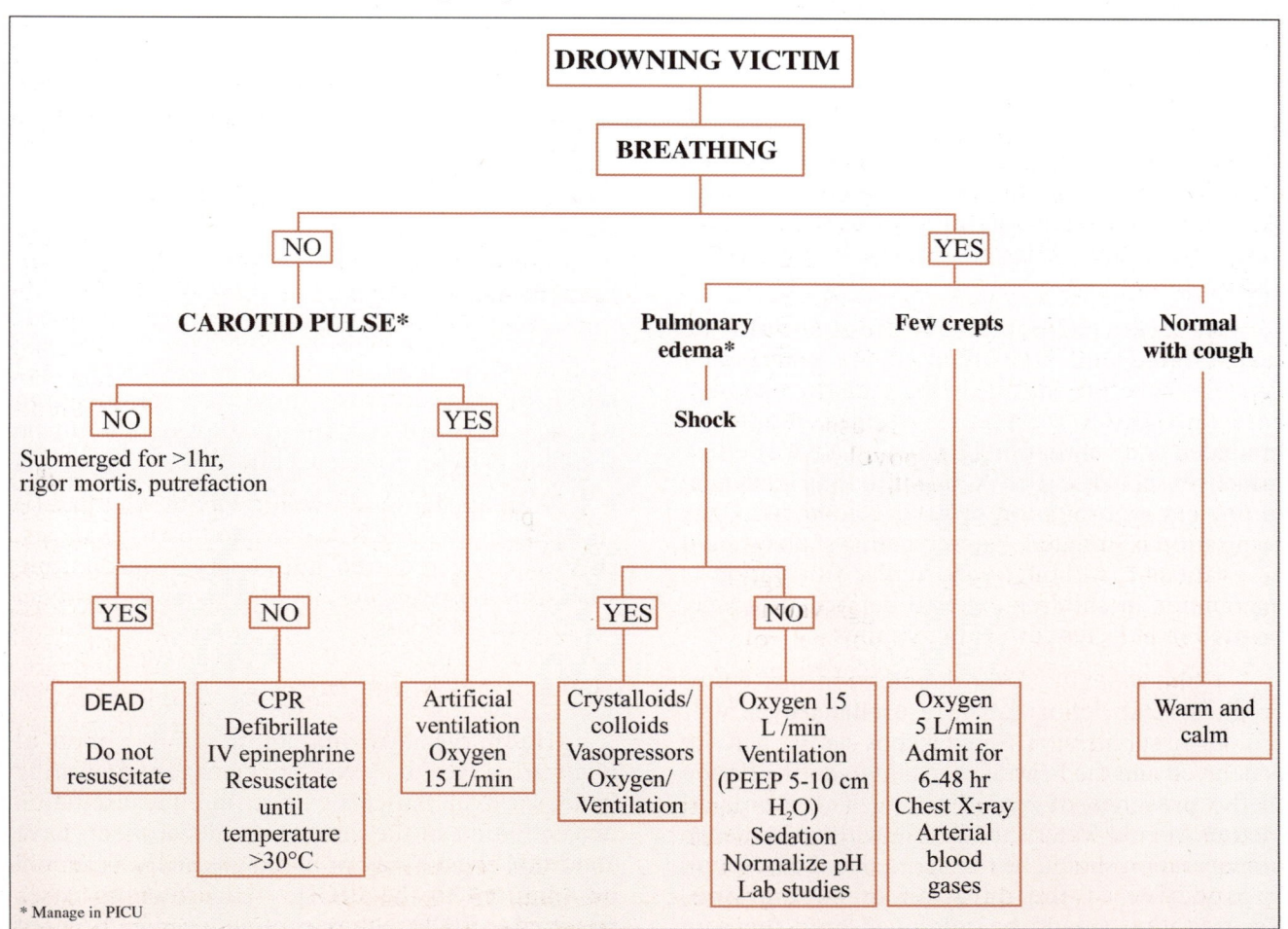

Figure 49.2 Algorithm for management of a drowning victim

Interruptions in chest compressions should be minimized to avoid absence of blood flow to the brain or heart. The victim should be immediately transported to a medical facility while continuing resuscitation during the transport. Oxygen at the highest concentration should be administered to the patient.

Hemlich's maneuver should not be performed except in cases when repeated attempts to open the airway and ventilate the victim have failed and an obstructed airway is suspected[2]. Chest compressions to clear the obstructed airway are preferable to abdominal thrusts because abdominal distension is common in drowning victims and it predisposes them to vomiting and aspiration. Spontaneously breathing drowning victim should be transported in right lateral decubitus position with the head lower than the trunk to minimize the risk of aspiration if vomiting occurs. Venous or intraossseous access is preferred for administration of life support drugs. The endotracheal route may be unreliable due to copious pulmonary edema fluid.

MANAGEMENT IN THE HOSPITAL

Emergency Department

All children with submersion should receive supplemental oxygen until investigations reveal that it is no longer needed. Children with short duration of submersion, who are alert and appear normal, should be monitored carefully for at least 6 to 12 hours to detect delayed onset of respiratory dysfunction.

Severely affected children should be resuscitated and stabilized in the emergency department before shifting to the pediatric intensive care unit (PICU). Apneic children should be intubated and ventilation begun with a bag. Sellick maneuver should be used if possible during intubation to prevent regurgitation of gastric contents. Once respiration is initiated, hemodynamic status should be evaluated. Although ventricular fibrillation is uncommon in children external defibrillation may be tried in pulseless drowning victims.

Cold water (< 5°C) submersion has better prognosis and victims can be resuscitated even after prolonged submersion. Spontaneous cardiac activity is delayed and the heart is resistant to defibrillation in the presence of hypothermia. Therefore, all victims of cold water submersion without evidence of maceration should be transported to the hospital, irrespective of the duration of submersion. Resuscitation should be continued until the core temperature is higher than 30°C. These patients should be aggressively rewarmed and repeat defibrillation attempted once the temperature is more than 30°C[9].

In contrast, warm water submersion has a poorer prognosis. In such cases, if the cardiopulmonary resuscitation is ineffective for 35-40 minutes, it may be discontinued at the rescue site or in the emergency room. Discontinuity of blood columns in the retinal vessels and 'swimming' appearance of retina are ominous signs and when present indicate that resuscitation is unlikely to be successful[10].

Drowning cases may not respond well to increasing FiO_2 alone due to significant intrapulmonary shunts and require positive end expiratory pressure (PEEP). PEEP improves oxygenation and ventilation by recruiting more alveoli and thereby increasing functional residual capacity of lungs. Comatose patients may vomit and aspirate stomach contents. Therefore, patients with significant submersion injury should have their stomach contents aspirated through a nasogastric tube.

Poor perfusion is evidenced by poor pulses, cold extremities, mottled appearance of skin and prolonged capillary refill time. Isotonic intravenous fluids should be administered to correct hypovolemia. Optimizing cerebral perfusion is more important and fluid administration should not be withheld in view of worsening cerebral edema. Ionotropic agents should be considered if perfusion does not improve after intravascular volume has been adequately expanded.

Blood sugar should be monitored in all patients with near drowning. In case of hypoglycemia, 1-2 ml/kg of 50% dextrose should be administered whereas dextrose containing solution should be withheld in hyperglycemic children.

Well appearing drowning victim who had (i) submersion for more than one minute, (ii) cyanosis, (iii) apnea or required pulmonary resuscitation, should be observed in the emergency department for at least 24 hours

Management in the PICU

Intensive care management is aimed at minimizing secondary cerebral damage and ensuring intact survival. Patients who required resuscitation or ventilation in the emergency department, have abnormal chest X-ray or blood gas analysis should be admitted to the PICU. All drowning cases admitted to PICU require continuous monitoring of pulse, temperature, respiration, blood pressure and electrocardiogram. Central venous pressure should preferably be monitored in all hemodynamically unstable patients. Frequent blood gas estimations is required in severely affected children.

Rewarming

Hypothermia can delay response to cardiopulmonary resuscitation besides causing several other complications. Rewarming should be started in a hypothermic child as soon as possible. Wet clothes should be removed. Surface rewarming should be started with radiant warmers and hot water bottles in patients with a core temperature of more than 30°C.

External rewarming in a markedly hypothermic child (< 30°C) may be ineffective. It can also result in severe localized burns at the rewarming sites. Additionally, rewarming of peripheral circulation first increases the risk of cardiac collapse in severely hypothermic children. Therefore, internal rewarming is needed in patients with a core temperature of less than 30°C. The gold standard for warming patients with cardiac arrest or shock is active internal warming with cardiopulmonary bypass or extracorporeal life support. Other methods include intravenous infusion of prewarmed (37°C-40°C) fluids, gastric, rectal or peritoneal lavage with warm fluids and administration of warm humidified oxygen.

Respiratory Management

Most near-drowning victims who survive the accident are likely to develop pulmonary edema. They have significant oxygenation defect and require ventilatory support[11]. Oxygen therapy with or without ventilation is the frontline therapy for drowning victims. Even awake and alert patients may remain hypoxic despite supplemental oxygen due to ventilation perfusion mismatch. A patient with paO_2/FiO_2 ratio of 300 or less usually requires continuous positive airway pressure (CPAP) in addition to oxygen[2]. CPAP is optimally provided by a nasotracheal or orotracheal tube. Patients on mechanical ventilation should be initially put on PEEP of 4-5 cm of H_2O, which may be increased to 10-15 cm of H_2O depending upon the status of oxygenation. However, high PEEP can cause pneumothorax and impair cardiac output by decreasing venous return to the heart. Therefore, normal intravascular volume should be maintained in patients receiving high levels of PEEP. Once the patient improves, the FiO_2 should be decreased to 0.5 or less to avoid adding oxygen toxicity to the pulmonary injury. Pulmonary dysfunction in

drowning cases tends to resolve due to regeneration of surfactant and PEEP can be tapered after 3-4 days. Furosemide should not be used to treat pulmonary edema as drowning victims may be hypovolemic. In severe cases, high-frequency oscillation and extracorporeal membrane oxygenation (ECMO) may be tried when conventional ventilation fails to alleviate hypoxemia[5].

Pulmonary air leaks, pneumonitis and acute respiratory distress syndrome (ARDS) should be considered in cases showing worsening of pulmonary function. The diagnostic triad of ARDS is non cardiogenic pulmonary edema, impaired oxygenation and bilateral pulmonary infiltrates. Secondary bacterial infections due to aspiration or because of assisted ventilation are common complications[12]. Tracheal aspirates and bronchoalveolar lavage specimens should be cultured for rational management of super added bacterial infection. Prophylactic antibiotics should be administered in cases of drowning in contaminated water. *Aeromonas* can cause a severe pneumonia that develops rapidly after drowning. Aspirated foreign body and sand may preclude effective ventilation and should be removed by fiberoptic bronchoscopy.

Prophylactic use of corticosteroids for pulmonary complications has not been shown to be beneficial. There are anecdotal reports of improvement in respiratory function following use of artificial surfactant, in cases of fresh water drowning[13].

Neurologic Management

The most significant and important complication of drowning accidents is anoxic-ischemic cerebral insult. Every effort should be made to prevent further damage by providing adequate oxygenation and perfusion. Patients with Glasgow coma scale (GCS) of less than 8 with raised intracranial pressure (ICP) can be hyperventilated to bring $paCO_2$ value between 25 and 30 mm Hg. Other therapies to reduce cerebral edema include head elevation to 30 degrees, fluid restriction and use of osmotic agents such as mannitol.

The role of aggressive ICP monitoring and therapies such as barbiturate coma, hypothermia and steroids for neuroprotection is controversial[5]. Studies evaluating therapies directed at controlling intracranial pressure and monitoring cerebral perfusion pressure have failed to demonstrate improvement in outcomes of drowning patients[2]. Seizures should be treated with benzodiazepines,

Section 5

which should be followed by administration of a loading dose of phenytoin. Pancuronium may be useful in agitated patients. Alternatively, morphine sulphate and benzodiazepines can be used for sedation. However, sedation may interfere with regular neurological examination, which is a useful predictor of outcome.

Correction of acid-base, electrolyte and blood glucose abnormalities is important to prevent secondary cerebral damage. Hyperthermia should be avoided as it can increase cerebral metabolism and lower seizure threshold. Occasionally, invasive cerebral mycosis due to *Aspergillus* and *Pseudallescheria* may occur in an immuno-compromised near-drowning victim and requires antifungal therapy.

Newer drugs that modulate reperfusion excitotoxic injury, free radical scavengers and moderate hypothermia are potential neuroprotective strategies that need to be evaluated in future.

Cardiovascular Management

Adequate intravascular volume should be ensured to facilitate perfusion to vital organs. Persistent cardiac dysfunction may occur due to hypoxia. Use of ionotropic agents such as dopamine and dobutamine may augment cardiac output in these cases. Pulmonary wedge pressure may be monitored in cases with severe cardiorespiratory dysfunction requiring high levels of PEEP.

PROGNOSIS

Drowning is associated with high case fatality and sequelae rates[14]. Early and accurate prognostication is essential to identify those children who are likely to die or have poor neurologic outcome. Children have relatively better outcome than adults particularly in ice-water submersion. Several predictors of outcome have been identified[2, 15, 16]. The predictors of outcome in the emergency department are listed in Table 49.2.

However, none of these variables either alone or in various combinations can predict the outcome with certainty. Serial neurologic examination during the first 24 –72 hours is probably the best predictor of outcome[18]. Usually one-third victims of warm water submersion who require CPR at the accident scene are likely to survive. However, most of the survivors are either neurologically intact or have minimal deficits.[9] Patients requiring prolonged resuscitation after warm water submersion generally do not survive or do so with profound neurologic impairment.

Despite all odds, a small proportion of children do make miraculous recoveries. Hence, each child should be treated on an individual basis. Aggressive resuscitation should be attempted in all children with unknown submersion time particularly in those who are drowned in cold water.

In patients reaching PICU after a submersion injury, 50-80 percent have intact neurologic survival. 25-30 percent cases die and 5-10 percent survive with neurologic impairment, which includes motor disability and mental retardation[19].

Futility and withdrawal of aggressive life-support therapy should be considered for severely affected victims who are likely to die or suffer profound neurologic impairment. Such decisions should, however, be made in consultation with the family. In general, studies indicate that 90% of children who survive submersion accidents and 68% of patients receiving CPR have good outcomes[20].

PREVENTION

The best hope for drowning victims lies in prevention. Parents, teachers and children should be educated and made aware of the risk and implications of submersion. Swimming pools should be equipped with safety measures and training in CPR and rescue techniques should be advocated among the swimming pool staff. Table 49.3 summarizes specific targeted messages that the

Table 49.2 Prognostic factors upon arrival in the emergency department	
Good prognosis	**Poor prognosis**
▫ Short submersion time	▫ Submersion duration >25 min
▫ Spontaneous respiration and heart beats are present	▫ Resuscitation time >25 min
▫ Glasgow coma scale >5	▫ Cardiac arrhythmia
▫ PRISM score of less than 25 and hemodynamic stability at admission in the emergency room[17]	▫ Fixed and dilated pupils on initial examination, GCS < 5
	▫ Severe acidosis (arterial pH < 7)
	▫ Apnea with no arterial pulse

pediatricians can provide to parents besides general water-safety advice[21].

Table 49.3 Targeted messages for prevention of drowning

- ☐ Small children should never be left alone or in the care of another young child even for a moment while in bath-tubs, water bucket, inflatable pool, fish tank.
- ☐ "Touch supervision" by an adult with swimming skills is advised when infants or toddlers are in the pool.
- ☐ Swimming lessons are not advised for children younger than 4 years.
- ☐ Parents sending children for swimming in pools should check for adequate fencing of pool and availability of life-guard at all times.
- ☐ Do not use inflatable arm band in place of life jackets.
- ☐ Showers are preferable to pool baths for children of any age with history of seizures.
- ☐ Provide CPR training to parents, care givers and pool owners.

The effectiveness of prevention in case of young children would depend upon the educational and socioeconomic status of the parents and the degree of supervision that they could provide. Many children can be saved if preventive strategies against drowning are implemented effectively.

REFERENCES

1. Idris AH, Berg RA, Bierens J, *et al.* Recommended guidelines for uniform reporting of data from drowning: the "Utstein style." *Resuscitation* 2003; 59: 45–50.

2. Orlowski JP, Szpilman D. Drowning. *Pediatr Clin North Amer* 2001; 48: 627-646.

3. Spyker DA. Submersion injury. Epidemiology, prevention and management. *Pediatr Clin N Amer* 1985; 32:113.

4. Gillenwater JM, Quan L, Feldman KW. Inflicted submersion in childhood. *Arch Pediatr Adolesc Med* 1996; 150:298-303.

5. Levin DL, Morriss FC, Toro LO, Brink LW, Turner GR. Drowning and near-drowning. *Pediatr Clin N Amer* 1993; 40:321.

6. Shaw KN, Briede CA. Submersion injuries: drowning and near drowning. *Emerg Med Clin North Amer* 1989; 7:355.

7. Conn AW, Barker GA. Fresh water drowning and near drowning an update. *Canad Anaesth Soc J* 1984; S31:S38.

8. Marchant J, Cheng NG, Lam LT, *et al.* Bystander basic life support: an important link in the chain of survival for children suffering a drowning or near-drowning episode. *Med J Aust* 2008; 188: 484-485.

9. Emergency Cardiac Care Committee and Subcommittee AHA. Guidelines for cardiopulmonary resuscitation and emergency cardiac care in special resuscitation situations. *JAMA* 1992; 268:2244.

10. Wilson RG. Resuscitation of children who nearly drown. *Brit Med J* 1991; 302:1404.

11. Lee KH. A retrospective study of near drowning victims admitted to intensive care unit. *Ann Acad Med Singapore* 1998; 27:344.

12. Van Berkel M, Bierens JJ, Lie RL, *et al.* Pulmonary edema, pneumonia and mortality in submersion victims; a retrospective study in 125 patients. *Intensive Care Med* 1996; 22:101-107.

13. Suzuki H, Ohta T, Iwata K, Yamaguchi K, Sato T. Surfactant therapy for respiratory failure due to near-drowning. *Eur J Pediatr* 1996; 153:383.

14. Joseph M, King WD. Epidemiology for hospitalization for near- drowning. *South Med J* 1998; 91:253.

15. Bayeda DH. Childhood submersion injuries. *J Emerg Nurs* 1998; 24:140.

16. Zuckerman GB, Gregory PM, Santos-Damiani SM. Predictors of death and neurologic impairment in pediatric submersion injuries. *Arch Pediatr Adolesc Med* 1998; 152:134.

17. Spack L, Gediet R, Splaingard M, Havens PL. Failure of aggressive therapy to alter the outcome in pediatric near-drowning. *Pediatr Emerg Care* 1997; 13:98-102.

18. Ibsen LM, Koch T. Submersion and asphyxial injury. *Crit Care Med* 2002; 30 (Suppl):S402-S408.

19. Seisjo B. Mechanism of ischemic brain injury. *Crit Care Med* 1988; 16: 954.

20. Sachdeva RC. Near drowning. *Crit Care Clin* 1999; 15:281-296.

21. American Academy of Pediatrics Committee on Injury, Violence, and Poison Prevention. Prevention of drowning. *Pediatrics* 2010; 126(1):178-185.

Section 5

Burns

R P Narayan

50

Human civilization only began after discovery of fire by prehistoric man. Fire is an immense source of energy and power. It has been man's endeavor to utilise it for useful purposes. Whenever he fails in this pursuit burns accidents occur. A curious child in his innocense to experience the miracle of fire often becomes a victim himself. Pediatric burns account for 25 percent of total admissions at our Center. Burns is largely a preventable disease. A remarkable decrease in incidence of burns has been observed in developed countries by enforcing legislation and education regarding preventable measures[1]. Inflammable clothes, unguarded heating equipment, hot water and liquids, loose flowing clothes etc. have been blamed as major causes leading to accidents. In our country there are no safety regulations. Fire is worshipped in our country. No celebration or ritual is complete without invocation of '*Agni Devta*'. Unsafe practices like using crackers, open *diya, agarbatti, havans,* erecting *shamianas* for marriages etc. are deep rooted in our culture. The functions and festivals are celebrated without any consideration for safety precautions. The effect has been compounded by our tendency to save money at the cost of safety. An imperfectly made lighting instrument in the form of a bottle containing kerosene oil with a wick coming out, without bothering for the stability of the bottle, putting candle at any place without proper candle stand or working with fire or hot liquids with a small baby in the lap or a toddler moving around are common examples of negligence.

Burns injury during infancy and childhood causes prolonged effect on the growing child. It leads not only to scars but also hampers the growth of the musculoskeletal system. Therefore, it is of utmost importance that all out efforts should be made at the time of managing these cases to ensure that the future outcome leads to minimum functional disability. One must also remember that burn is a serious trauma and it destroys many hopes and dreams forever. There is no computer in the world, which can compute the pain, misery and the shattered dreams of a burnt child. In the following paragraphs we will describe a practical and effective way of managing burns, with special emphasis on early detection and effective management of complications.

EPIDEMIOLOGY

Before the development of burns units, the incidence of burn injuries was thought to be very low. An average pediatric surgical ward looked after one or two burnt children at a time. With the creation of burns units, all cases of burns started pooling at one particular point and one was amazed to see the enormity of the problem[2]. Though burns is not a notifiable disease and no national data is available, one can get an idea of the incidence from the available data of Safdarjung Hospital, New Delhi which has the biggest burns unit in the country. In the year 2004 out of the 3455 burns patients, 680 were male and 321 were female pediatric patients. Therefore, it would appear that our population of children is at a slightly higher risk of thermal injuries as compared to the west.

Scalds account for less than 10% of the burns in the adult age group while in the pediatric age group 40% of total burn admissions are due to scalds and 60% are due to flame or other burns. However, it must be remembered that even in the pediatric age group in India, the incidence of flame burns is higher than the scalds though the number of scalds in pediatric age group is far higher than adults. In contrast, pediatric burns are mainly scalds with a very low percentage of flame burns in the west.

There is increased incidence of burns during festival seasons like Diwali and during marriage seasons. The various modes of thermal injuries include child falling into a frying vessel (*Kadhai*), sustaining burns from the flames of earthen lamp or *diya,* clothes catching fire from crackers or fire of *havan, holi* or *lohri.* There are some peculiar type of burns which are noticed during infancy when the cot catches fire by falling of an earthen lamp or a lantern and the hapless infant is not in a condition to protect himself and thus sustains quite extensive burns. Similarly falling of a hot object on the baby's leg or keeping convector heater close to leg and feet may lead to deep burns in the lower extremity. Hot water bottles should not be used to keep the babies warm and they should never come in direct contact with the baby due to potential risk of causing serious injury due to burns.

It is not uncommon in India, even in the rich community for the mother to sip hot tea or coffee with the child in the lap and a sudden movement of the infant may lead to extensive scalds on the chest and abdomen. Similarly an inquisitive toddler may pull the hanging wires of electric kettle and boiling water or milk may spill on the baby. Sometime a tablecloth on top of which hot teapot or milk pot has been kept may be pulled by an infant leading to extensive scalds. In the winter season it is not uncommon in many homes to prepare hot water in the kitchen and take it to the bathroom for the child's bath. During the movement of this hot water, the inquisitive child may topple the bucket leading to extensive scalds. Burns may also occur due to electrocution, lightning or by chemicals like acids and caustics but they are relatively uncommon causes. All these are preventable causes of burns and little thought and care will go a long way in preventing very painful and life-threatening burns. The pediatrician can play an important role in repeatedly passing on the safety information to the young parents about the precautions needed to protect the child against scalds and burns.

PATHOPHYSIOLOGY

Burns is basically a disease of skin which is the largest organ of the body. Injury to the skin results in loss of function which is in direct proportion to the area burnt. The important functions of the skin include barrier against micro-organisms, prevention of loss of body fluids and thermoregulation by preventing body heat loss. Dermis of the skin is very important layer for epithelialisation of wound and providing strength. Major burns produce widespread changes in body unlike minor burns where changes are localized. Important patho-physiologic changes in the body after severe burns are discussed below:

Circulatory Changes

Thermal injury causes increase in capillary permeability at burnt sites leading to loss of plasma into interstitial space. It occurs in all burn wounds regardless of size and depth. In burns above 25% of body surface area, increased capillary permeability is found all over the body. Membrane dysfunction of cells allows sodium to enter inside and potassium to leak out of the cells. The vascular integrity starts returning after 18-36 hours. The end result is progressive fall in plasma volume till capillary integrity is restored. Break down of skin barrier increases evaporative losses by 4-20 times during early stages of burns.

Major effect of the burns is because of hemodynamic changes due to excessive loss of fluid from intravascular compartment to extravascular compartment due to increased permeability of the capillaries. This loss is directly proportional to the extent of thermal energy. Even a small burn may have serious consequences in a child because of greater risk of hypovolemic shock. Following burns of moderate extent and severity, twice the normal plasma pool contained in the body may be lost. Swelling and edema of burns occurs due to loss of fluid from intravascular compartment to extravascular compartment. Release of local and systemic inflammatory mediators also contributes to the severity of edema.

Damage to the Cellular Elements of Blood

The heat energy may damage the cellular elements of blood. The red blood cells are destroyed immediately and some are permanently affected by the heat. The life span of red blood cells is reduced by 30 percent leading to slow protracted hemolysis. This effect on the cellular elements is directly proportional to the third dimension of injury i.e. depth of burns. The damage to red blood cells can be noticed in the form of hemoglobinuria which is seen in cases of full thickness burns. The damage to red cell structure is evident in the form of rigidity of cells and alterations in cellular shape seen in the peripheral blood smear. The red cells more fragile leading to long term changes in the form of shift to the left as new cells start forming in the body. However, this shift to the left may not be seen in many cases because of depressive effect of by-products of heat damaged skin on the bone marrow. There is initial rise in leukocytes but leukotaxis and phagocytosis are impaired. Plasma proteins including immunoglobulins show a rapid and persistent drop followed by a slow rise. There is increased vulnerability to infections due to break in the integrity of skin barrier and compromised immunocompetence and nutritional status. Platelet count falls but their adhesiveness increases with increased viscosity of blood which is resistant to the effects of heparin. The initial fall in fibrinogen level is followed by gradual recovery within 3-6 months. Fibrin degradation products are elevated immediately after the injury and remains so for 8-10 days. Hepatic transaminases show a prompt elevation soon after burns reaching a plateau within 2-3 days but elevated levels persist for several weeks.

Cardiac Changes

In extensive burns exceeding 50 percent, cardiac output falls by 30 percent of pre-burn values within 30 minutes of injury. Cardiac alterations, originally thought to be a response to hemodynamic changes, are now known to precede them. When the patient is lucky to survive without fluid therapy, cardiac output returns to normal level within 36 hours. However, with fluid therapy, cardiac output increases to supernormal level and remains so for a long period. Excessive cardiac strain is caused by development of progressive anemia, fluid mobilization, inadequate nutrition and electrolyte imbalance.

Pulmonary Changes

Thermal damage to airways may lead to edema of glottis, trachea, bronchi and bronchioles with decreased ventilation and trapping of secretions and inflammatory exudates. Pulmonary complications occur because of direct damage to the pulmonary tree and upper respiratory tract by the heat. The normal air contains 21% oxygen but during fire the surrounding hot air no longer contains 21% oxygen since it is utilised in the process of combustion. Thus the child trapped in fire may be continuously breathing air in which partial pressure of oxygen has fallen leading to severe hypoxia. The entry of hot air in the air passages leads to damage to the mucosa of pharynx and larynx and to the cilia lining the respiratory tract. This causes decrease in the ability of the pulmonary tree to throw out the secretions leading to congestion and hypostatic pneumonia. If these changes are not promptly corrected, they may have prolonged damaging effect leading to bronchopneumonia and respiratory failure[3, 4].

Renal Effects

Inadequate cardiac output due to cardiac damage and hypovolemia leads to diminished renal perfusion and reduced glomerular filtration rate. In children with extensive burns, acute tubular necrosis and renal shut down may occur. Hemoglobinuria due to destruction of red blood cells may also contribute to renal shut down[5].

Water Evaporation

Evaporation of water from burn wound is caused by loss of plasma exudates from skin surface during first 48 hours following burn. The evaporative losses from the skin may be as high as 6-8 liters per day in tropical conditions.

Metabolic Changes

Burn imposes hypermetabolic state in the body. Following moderate to severe burns there is negative nitrogen balance. In addition there is loss of proteins from the site of burns, which accounts for 20-25 percent of total nitrogen loss from the body. The tissue catabolism is enhanced by release of alpha adrenergic agents, cortisol and catecholamines. The aminoacids released from the muscle bed are transported to the liver and converted to glucose (neoglucogenesis). This provides a constant flow of readily available fuel to maintain essential functions of glucose-dependent tissues. Renin, angiotensin, ACTH and cortisol are elevated soon after thermal stress for a variable period. Free fatty acids and triglycerides are elevated while cholesterol and phospholipids are depressed in direct proportion to the severity and extent of burns. The burn patient should be nursed at higher room temperature for comfort compared to normal individual. The room temperature should be maintained between 28°C to 30°C to ensure elevated core body temperature between 37.5°C to 38.5°C. Higher ambient environment temperature decreases the basal metabolic rate of the patient.

While treating a child with burns, the following physiologic handicaps should always be kept in mind:

(i) The child has increased water and electrolyte losses, and caloric expenditure due to a larger body surface relative to weight.

(ii) Temperature regulating center under six months of age is immature and is maintained by non-shivering metabolic thermogenesis. Therefore, higher room temperature is needed to decrease the evaporative water loss and cooling.

(iii) Impairment of pulmonary function may necessitate early institution of ventilatory assistance to the child, as compensatory pulmonary mechanisms are easily overcome by stress.

(iv) Immature renal functions due to poor concentrating capacity and inefficient capacity to handle water load may readily precipitate osmotic imbalance and renal failure.

Assessment of extent of Burns

Morbidity and mortality of burn cases depends upon a large number of factors such as nature of burns (fire, hot liquids, chemical, electrical) and associated injuries and inhalation of smoke, extent of body surface involved; depth of burn; age of the patient; concomitant diseases such as pre-existing nutritional, renal, cardio-pulmonary, and metabolic diseases.

Burn area. The extent of burn is expressed as the size of surface area burnt in relation to total body area. "Rule of 5" is a convenient, easy and quick method for estimation of surface are in pediatric burns (Figure 50.1). "Rule of 9" is applicable only in children above 10 years of age. It has been modified for anthropomorphic differences of infancy and childhood (Figure 50.2). Accurate estimation of burn area can be made by using Lund and Browder chart[6] and can be used for all ages (Figure 50.3). Small areas of damage can be calculated using the palmar surface of the patient's own hand (from wrist to finger crease) which represents approximately 1% of the body surface.

Depth of burn. The depth of burn is dependent on the temperature of the burning agent and the duration of contact. Burns are classified as first, second and third degree, depending upon the amount of tissue destroyed (Figure 50.4). First degree burn is characterised by erythema, edema and blister formation of the skin and involves only the epidermis and portion of dermis and is very

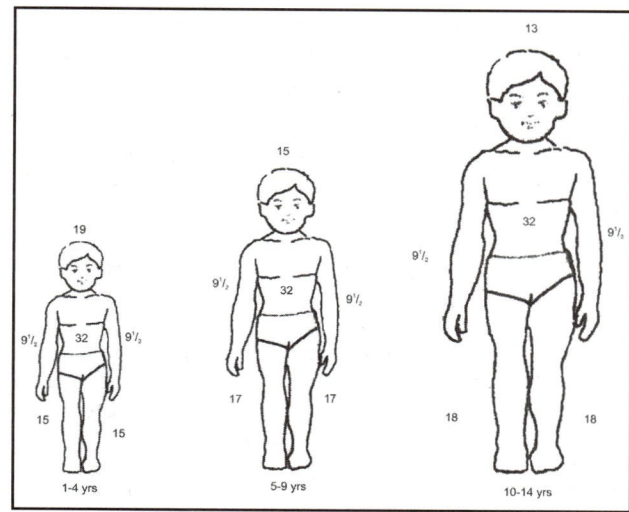

Figure 50.2 Modified "Rule of nines" for pediatric burns (Wallace's rule of nine)

painful (Figure 50.5). Second degree (deep dermal) burn is characterised by mottled pink and white appearance of skin which is not very sensitive to pain. It involves the epidermis and a three fourth portion of the dermis including the dermal papillae but leaves the sweat glands and hair follicles. First and second degree burns are included in partial thickness wound. Third degree burn destroys the full thickness of skin and often involves the underlying tissues as well. The area is depressed, dark and leathery in appearance without any sensations (Figure 50.6). Laser Doppler imaging is useful to assess the depth of burns.

The burns which are confined to superficial layers of dermis are called superficial partial thickness burns and they normally heal in less than two weeks time. The burns that have gone beyond papillary dermis are termed as deep dermal burns and they normally take more then two weeks for healing. It is important to remember that embryologically the skin is made up of two germinal layers that is ectoderm and mesoderm. Epidermis is derived from ectoderm and dermis is derived from mesoderm. Dermis is invaded by epidermis in the papillary dermis layer and therefore this layer has regenerative elements coming from epithelial tissues while the burns going into reticular dermis have practically no regenerative elements in the form of epithelial cells. These ultimately end up as deep scars and deformities due to contractures or leave behind ulcers which require skin grafting.

It must be remembered that burns are not homogenous in nature and there may be different areas with different thickness of burns. Therefore, it is necessary that each area should be assessed

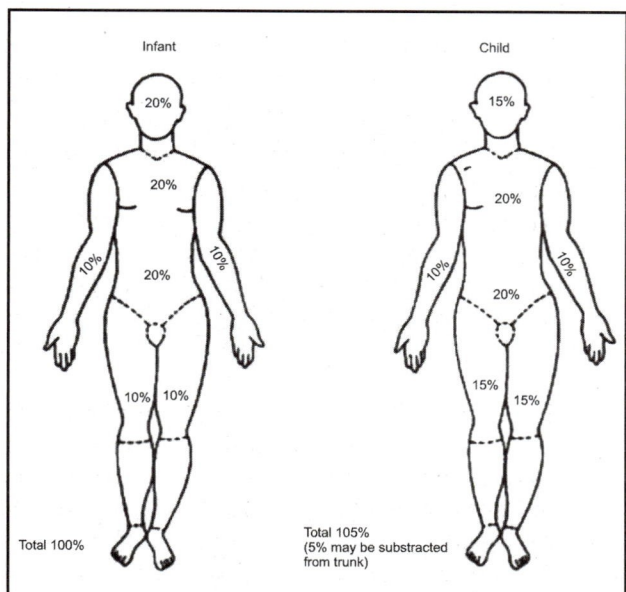

Figure 50.1 Estimation of burn area by "Rule of fives" (Lynch and Blocker 1963)

Relative Percentage of Areas Affected by Growth							
आयु (वर्षों में) -	Age in Years	0	1	5	10	15	Adult
सिरका आधा -	A-$^1/_2$ of head	$9^1/_2$	$8^1/_2$	$6^1/_2$	$5^1/_2$	$4^1/_2$	$4^1/_2$
जाधे का आधा -	B$^1/_2$ of one thigh	$2^1/_2$	$3^1/_2$	4	$4^1/_2$	$4^1/_2$	$4^1/_2$
निम्न पैरका आधा -	C$^1/_2$ of one leg	$2^1/_2$	$2^1/_2$	$2^1/_2$	3	$3^1/_2$	$3^1/_2$

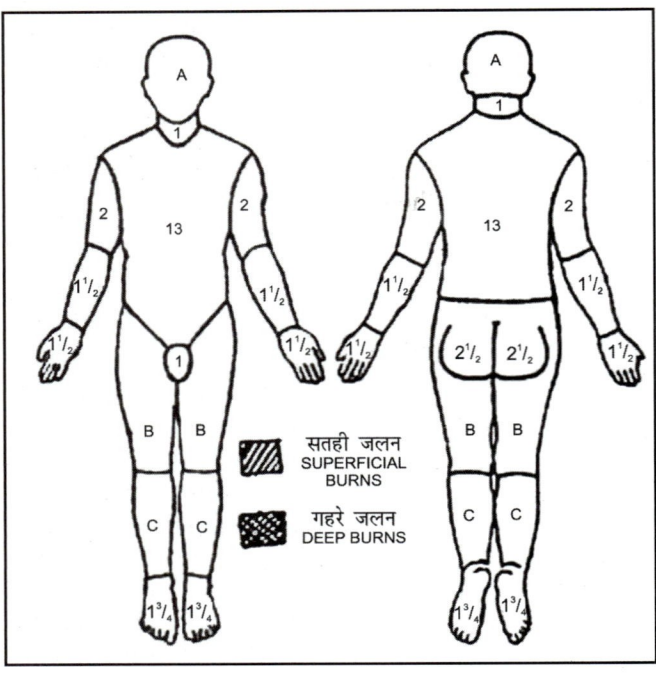

जलन विस्तार की गणना
Calculate Extent of Burn
पूर्ण अंकों में
Round to nearest whole number:

सिर/गला Head/Neck	
उपरी बाजू Upper Arms	-%
अग्र बाजू Forearms	-%
हाथ Hands	-%
पड Trunk	-%
नितम्ब Buttocks	-%
हाथ Hands	-%
जननांग Perineum	-%
जांघ Thighs	-%
निम्न पैर Lower Legs	-%
पंजा Feet	-%
योग TOTAL	-%

सतही जलन
SUPERFICIAL BURNS

गहरे जलन
DEEP BURNS

Figure 50.3 Lund and Browder chart for estimating the burn surface area

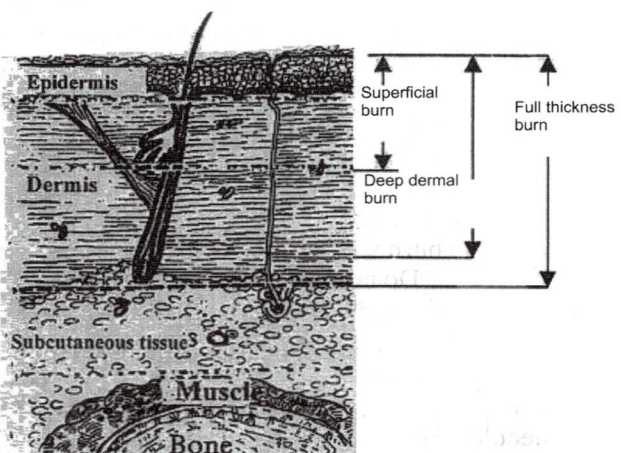

Figure 50.4 Section of skin showing depth of burn

independently and completely, properly marked and documented for management. Full thickness burns should be quickly subjected to surgical intervention while partial thickness burns should be treated by dressings.

Age. Extremes of life are poor risk patients. Patients less than 4 year of age have a higher mortality as compared to other age groups with

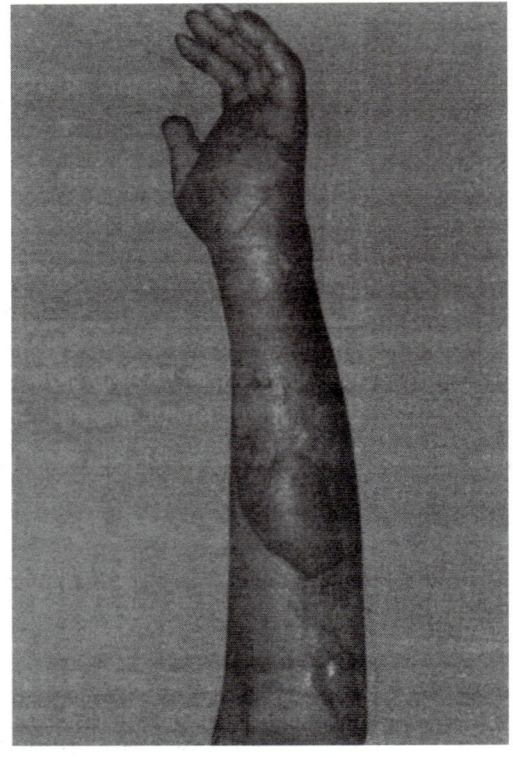

Figure 50.5 Superficial burn of upper limb

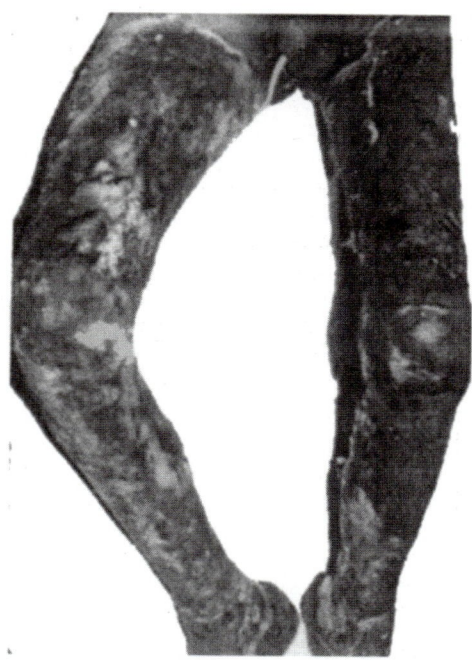

Figure 50.6 Full thickness burn of lower limbs

similar injury. Their body response to stress is not as good as in the older children and the smaller body mass provides less stores of protein and fat to cope with hypermetabolism.

Site of burns and associated injury. Burns of head, neck and chest lead to increased incidence of pulmonary complications. Burns of perineum are prone to early infection. Circumferential burns over chest and extremity are also associated with increased risk of complications. Skull fracture, head injury, abdominal injury and compound fractures associated with burns increase the risk of mortality by several folds[7].

Triage in Burns

Minor burns are usually treated on an ambulatory basis. These cases can be safely managed by a family physician and a pediatrician. They merely require local asepsis and management of the burn wound. Moderate burn requires treatment in a hospital and can be managed at a district hospital. The services of a plastic surgeon may be required when skin grafting is mandatory. Children with major burns should be provided first aid near the site of accident and transferred to a Burn Center when their general condition has stabilised.

TREATMENT

First Aid. The initial treatment provided at the scene of the burn accident is extremely important in minimizing the extent of the burn injury and in reducing complication. It is important to educate the public in first aid practices.

1. Eliminate the cause

   Flame burn. Fire should be extinguished by pouring water. Victim should not be allowed to run but should roll on the ground or should be wrapped with rugs or blankets to put off the fire.

   Electric burn. The local or main switch of electricity should be put off, before touching the victim.

   Chemical burn. The part should be thoroughly washed under running tap water for 30-45 minutes till pain and burning sensation disappears.

2. All the tight clothing should be loosened and free air movement should be ensured for breathing.

3. Pouring of excessive cold water over large burn areas in children may lead to hypothermia and severe hyponatremia due to absorption of water. Application of ice packs/cold water is advisable only to the localised area of burns like face/hands, which will relieve pain/burning sensation and edema. For that purpose ice should be sealed in a plastic bag for application rather than immersion of patient or extremity in ice-cold water which should be avoided. Direct contact with ice can cause more damage. Avoid undue contamination of the burn wound and position the patient in comfort. Drape the victim in clean, washed sheets. Avoid application of gention violet/ink/mercurochrome or other household material over the burn which is commonly done by the lay public. Do not use absorbent cotton directly on burn wounds as it may become adherent and difficult to remove. Blisters should not be peeled off, rather they should be made to collapse after puncturing them with a sterile needle. The first aid should be directed in cooling down the part as rapidly as possible to minimize further damage to skin and underlying structures.

4. Sleep-inducing painkillers should be avoided in children with head injury and respiratory burns.

5. If there are other associated injuries like head injury, fracture of bones, burns involving respiratory tract (inhaled hot air) patient should be shifted under medical supervision to the

Section 5

nearest hospital at the earliest. If transportation of the patient is delayed for more than half an hour, he should be offered oral drinks in small quantities at frequent intervals. Bulk intake of fluids should be avoided which may lead to vomiting and abdominal distension. Sips of oral rehydration solution (ORS), coconut water, glucose water, *sherbat,* milk, fruit juice, etc. can be offered.

Transportation. In ordinary circumstances a patient with isolated burns injury can be transported safely to a Burns Center within an hour or so of sustaining the injury. But if one has to transport a patient with other associated injuries, as mentioned above, an emergency medical services evacuation van, having well equipped resuscitation facilities is required. The Hi-tech evacuation vans should be staffed with well trained emergency medical technicians and nurses. Patients with large burns usually tolerate transfer/ transportation well for first 12 hours provided that initial resuscitative and stabilization measures have been adequate under the care of trained personnel before and during the period of transportation. After 24-48 hours, when edema is usually maximum, it is wise to defer the transfer of the patient for 5-6 days after burns. During this period the general condition of the patient will usually get stabilised

and he can be safely shifted to Burns Center subsequently for specialised care.

Hospital Management

Children with first and second-degree burns of less than 10% body surface area (BSA) may be treated on outpatient basis. The following children with burns should be admitted to the hospital for further management[7]:

1. Partial thickness burns of greater than 10 percent of the total body surface area.
2. Any full thickness burns likely to cause cosmetic or functional disability on recovery.
3. Burns of face, neck, hands, feet and perineum.
4. Burns associated with visceral and skeletal injuries.
5. Burns associated with suffocation and damage to respiratory system.
6. Burns associated with pre-existing serious disease.
7. Electrocution, lightning and chemical burns.

Initial Assessment

Management of ABC of trauma is very important[8]. Maintenance of airway is the first priority. Oral secretions should be sucked out. Child should be turned to one side and watched for adequacy of breathing. If there is difficulty in

Table 50.1 Classification and management of pediatric burns				
Extent	Depth	Severity	Place of treatment	Management
<10%	Superficial	Minor	Outpatient	• Conservative • Tetanus prophylaxis • Local wound care
<10%	Superficial + deep < 2%	Minor	Outpatient usually. Inpatient if hand or face is involved	• Conservative for superficial burns • Surgery for full-thickness burns
10%-30%	Superficial + deep dermal	Moderate	Inpatient	• Intravenous fluids • Conservative for superficial burns • Tangential excision for deep dermal burns
10%-30%	Full thickness	Major	Inpatient	• Intravenous fluids • Full thickness excision and skin graft
> 30%	Full thickness/ partial thickness	Major	Inpatient	• ICU care • Respiratory support • Dietary support • Conservative for superficial burns • Excision or delayed grafting for deep burns

breathing after clearing the airway, mouth-to-mouth respiration may be given. The initial assessment includes the general condition of the patient, estimation of the surface area burnt as well as the depth of burns and the presence of any associated injuries. The presence of associated injury should be carefully looked for especially in situations where there was explosion, vehicular accident or electrical injury and thus a complete physical examination including a neurological examination should be done. The presence of respiratory tract damage due to inhalation burns should be carefully looked for. Table 50.1 outlines the classification and basic principles of management of pediatric burns. All the extremities should be examined for pulses and in cases of circumferential burns, escharotomy may have to be done. Escharotomy is also essential in circumferential chest burns causing restriction of respiratory movements.

Fluid Resuscitation

Children with moderate to severe burns involving 15% or more BSA require intravenous fluid resuscitation to maintain adequate tissue perfusion. All inhalation injuries and high-tension electrical injuries, regardless of severity of burns, require venous access for administration of fluids. A wide bore cannula should be inserted in the vein as soon as possible, either by venesection or percutaneously. In case of difficulty, intraosseous route can be used for infusion.

As a guideline to fluid resuscitation in the first 24 hours, many formulae are available. They include administration of various crystalloids, colloids or both. The aim of resuscitating fluid is the restoration of body homeostasis. This is achieved by replacing the fluid sequestered as a result of thermal injury. Parkland formula is commonly used for calculation of fluids (Table 50.2). The total fluids given are 4 ml/kg/% of burn surface area, with half of the fluids given in the first eight hours and rest of the half in next sixteen hours. The time of administration is calculated from the time of accident instead of the time the patient reporting to the Burn Center. Ringer's lactate is the fluid of choice during first 24 hours. In infants and younger children, who are prone to hypernatremia, the fluid used is 0.33% sodium chloride instead of Ringer's lactate[9].

However, it must be kept in mind that the resuscitation formulas are only a rough guide to the fluid therapy and frequent clinical and laboratory assessment is necessary as a guide to hydration. The clinical assessment includes general appearance and sensorium, vital signs, capillary

Table 50.2 Plan for fluid resuscitation		
Formula	**Amount**	**Other measures**
Ringer's lactate	4 ml/kg/% of burn in first 24 hours 50% in 1st 8 hrs and 50% in next 16 hrs 2 ml/kg/% of burn in next 24 hrs	▪ Oral fluids ▪ Maintenance of urine output ▪ Cardiac support if required
Colloid formula	One plasma volume (5% of body weight) for every 15% burn + normal daily requirements	

filling time and urine output. Urinary output, by and large, is the best guide of tissue perfusion. Urine output of at least 0.5 ml/kg/hr is suggestive of adequate renal perfusion. It is important to avoid underhydration as well as overhydration. The laboratory tests include estimation of hematocrit, serum electrolytes, urinary osmolality and estimation of arterial blood gases.

The use of invasive monitoring like central venous pressure and pulmonary wedge pressure are not necessary in burnt children and are best avoided due to risk to sepsis. However, they may be required in patients with cardiac illness, severe anemia and metabolic problems like inappropriate secretion of ADH. Unless the child is in severe shock, oral fluids are started during the first 24 hours and one-fourth of the normal daily requirement may be given orally. Subsequently, the oral intake is increased and intravenous fluids are gradually reduced. However, intravenous fluids are stopped only when the child is taking and tolerating the calculated amount of daily requirement orally. During early phase, evaporative losses predominate. The burn wound may lead to loss of tremendous amount of fluids since the protective barrier of skin is lost. The following formula can be used to calculate the evaporative fluid loss in a burnt child:

Evaporative loss = Normal evaporative loss × 20 × % of burnt surface/100

After 24 hours, colloids may be given if serum proteins fall below 4 g/dl. However, in the case of respiratory burns, colloids like plasma are usually given in the initial phase of resuscitation to avoid pulmonary edema due to leakage of crystalloid solutions. In patients who have become acutely anemic because of large amount of red cell destruction, blood transfusion may be given after 24 hours. It is recommended that restrictive (Hb < 7.0 g/dl) blood transfusion policy is associated with

Section 5

reduced risk of complications and cost-savings[10,11]. Attention must also be paid to the potassium balance. After 24 hours usually potassium supplements are needed. This can be achieved by administration of potassium containing fluids or by adding potassium chloride in the infusate. Later on, potassium rich foods or oral supplements are usually adequate.

Airway Management

A large number of children with thermal burns have associated inhalation injury. Many children may have signs and symptoms of inhalation burns like hoarseness, stridor and carbonaceous sputum. In others the attention to the inhalation injury is drawn by clinical features like facial burns, singeing of nasal hair, and history of being burnt in a confined space[3].

A thorough assessment of the respiratory system should be made when inhalation burn is suspected. Chest radiographs, electrocardiogram and arterial blood gases are mandatory in these cases. When carbon monoxide poisoning is suspected, level of carboxyhemoglobin (HbCo) should be assessed. In many cases of full-thickness burns, unyielding eschar around the neck and chest may cause mechanical restriction to breathing and escharotomy should be done immediately.

Many of the patients with inhalation injury may be managed by simple supportive measures like humidified oxygen, chest physiotherapy, early ambulation, suction and pharmacological agents like bronchodilators. However, frequent clinical monitoring is required during the initial phase to detect the onset of complications like respiratory failure. Direct laryngoscopy and bronchoscopy may also be done for objective evaluation of inhalation injury. Bronchosocopic suctioning may help in clearing the airways[12].

In cases with critical injury to the airways, immediate active intervention may have to be done. The small aperture of the pediatric trachea predisposes to its obstruction. Bronchospasm, retained secretions and mucosal shedding may cause further complications. Endotracheal intubation and IPPV may be required in some cases especially if paO$_2$ is <80 mm Hg. IPPV is continued till blood gases and lung compliance have returned to within normal limits. Tracheostomy is generally avoided since it is associated with increased mortality because of infective complications. In case of suspected carbonmonoxide poisoning, administration of hyperbaric oxygen therapy may be beneficial.

In case of hydrogen cyanide toxicity, intravenous administration of sodium thiosulfate (125-250 mg/kg) and hydroxyl cobalamin are useful.

Tetanus Prophylaxis

The possibility of tetanus is always there in the presence of necrotic tissue. Nowadays most of children are well immunised against tetanus. Active immunisation with tetanus toxoid 0.5 ml SC is given at the time of accident. When the status of immunisation is unknown and there is gross contamination, passive immunisation with tetanus human immunoglobulins is indicated.

Sedation and Pain Control

It is important to provide adequate analgesia, anxiolytics and psychological support to reduce metabolic stress and achieve early stabilization. Superficial and partial thickness burns cause pain which is intensified by child's fear and anxiety. The application of ointments and dressings relieves the pain to some extent but analgesics are usually needed. Reassurance and support from parents and nurses also helps in calming the child. Intramuscular administration should be avoided during the initial phase of shock as there is erratic absorption. Commonly morphine sulfate is given intramuscularly or intravenously in a dose of 0.1-0.2 mg/kg. After the initial bolus injection, sedation and analgesia may be maintained in older children by patient-controlled analgesia pump. Otherwise morphine may be repeated every 4 hours. Once the shock phase is over, oral analgesics like paracetamol can be given. Paracetamol suppositories are invaluable for pain control when oral intake is contraindicated. Fentanyl lollipops are not available in our country. Often the problem is of apprehension rather than pain and drugs like chloral hydrate, promethazine and benzodiazepines are also useful.

For change of dressings, intravenous or inhalational agents may be used. Ketamine in analgesic doses (0.2-0.3 mg/kg) is useful in children for change of dressings. At some centers a mixture of air and nitrous oxide (Entonox) is used to relieve anxiety and pain during manipulations.

Nutritional Support

The burn injury produces a hyperketabolic state characterized by both protein and fat catabolism. Apart from increased nutritional demands of burn trauma and healing, there is additional requirement for rapid growth in pediatric patients. Children usually have less body fat and smaller muscle mass. The requirement of calories and nitrogen is very high during burns. Protein requirement is increased due to demand for wound healing and nitrogen loss through wound exudates and urine. Children are fussy and often refuse to eat during anxiety and distress. Malnutrition causes impaired wound healing, decreased resistance to infection and leads to cellular dysfunction. Enteral feeding as early as 3-6 hours post burn period should be encouraged as it decreases bacterial translocation from gut and reduces mucosal atrophy of the gut. In children under three years, maintenance of nutritional support is even more challenging because of immaturity of the gastrointestinal tract, small gastric volume and limited body stores of protein and other nutrients.

Various formulae are available for the calculations of caloric and protein needs in children of various age groups[13, 14] (Table 50.3). However, such a large intake of calories is difficult to achieve by oral feeding alone since the appetite is adversely affected due to pain, anxiety, fever and repeated wound dressings. In such cases, enteral tube feeding should be used. Enteral tube feeding has the advantage of preserving gastrointestinal integrity and decreasing the incidence of bacterial transmigration across the gut. Feeding tube should be properly fixed and sutures may be used to secure the tube in position. Enteral feeding through transpyloric route can be continued even during the periods of gastric ileus. Tube feeding is initially started at one fourth of the desired volume and increased at the rate of 5 ml per hour. Enteral feeding is often complicated by vomiting and diarrhea if sudden bolus feeds are given. Therefore, increase in enteral feeding should be gradual so as to prevent hyperosmolar diarrhea[15, 16]. The monitoring includes measurement of serum electrolytes, liver function tests, blood glucose and urinary urea and creatinine. Enteral milk is best tolerated by children. Hyperosmolar solutions should be avoided due to risk of development of diarrhea.

Parenteral nutrition should be used as a last resort in cases where enteral feeding is not possible because of prolonged alimentary tract dysfunction[17]. Complications associated with total parenteral nutrition include metabolic abnormalities, sepsis and immuno-suppression. Whatever the method of nutritional support used, particular care must be taken to provide supplements of vitamins especially vitamins B complex, vitamin A and vitamin C along with minerals like zinc and magnesium.

Table 50.3 Energy and protein requirements of burn patients

Energy needs of pediatric burn patients

After Hildreth et al[13, 14]

Age	Calories
0-12 months	2100 kcal/m² + 1000 kcal/m² burn area
1-11 years	1800 kcal/m² + 1300 kcal/m² burn area
12 years + above	1500 kcal/m² + 1500 kcal/m² burn area

Age	Calories
0-1 year	RDA+ 15 kcal /% burns
1-3 years	RDA + 25 kcal /% burns
4-15 years	RDA + 40 kcal /% burns

RDA of calories

Age	Calories per kg body weight
First 6 months	150 kcal
6 months-3 years	105 kcal
4-10 years	85 kcal
11-14 years (male)	60 kcal
11-14 years (female)	40 kcal

Protein requirement in pediatric burn patients

After Hildreth et al[13, 14]

Age	Proteins
Birth – 0.5 year	4.5 g/kg
0.5 – 2 years	4.0 g/kg
>2 years	3.5 g/kg
Davies and Liljedah	
13 gm/kg + 1 gm × % of burns	

Systemic Chemotherapy

No antibiotic cover is required during early post burn phase unless wounds are grossly contaminated though sepsis remains a common cause of death in burn patients. Use of prophylactic antibiotics may lead to the development of resistant strains of bacteria. The burn wound is initially sterile. After 24 hours and then regularly subsequently wound swabs for culture and sensitivity should be sent. Surface colonization does not warrant use of antibiotics unless signs of invasive sepsis are present. Blood culture should be obtained periodically. Nosocomial infections with methicillin-resistant *S. aureus* and *P. aeruginosa* are common. Systemic antibiotics depending upon the culture report are started if there are clinical evidences of sepsis like hectic rise in temperature, toxemia,

Section 5

altered sensorium, diarrhea, persistent vomiting or changes in the wound like neo-eschar formation. Wherever available, quantitative culture should be obtained by taking the burn wound biopsy. A count of $>10^5$ organisms/gm of tissue indicates sepsis[18]. To prevent spread of nosocomial infection, barrier nursing should be practiced. Patient already infected with resistant organisms should preferably be isolated.

Wound Care

After the initial assessment and resuscitation, attention should be paid to the local wound care[19]. Tight clothing and constricting ornaments like rings, bracelets and bangles should be removed immediately since they would be difficult to remove after the onset of edema. The wounds should be cleaned with copious amount of saline and any loose or dead skin should be removed. Whirlpool wash and pulsed lavage are useful to remove bacteria and loose debris. Swelling of the arms and legs can be reduced with a mechanical pump by using vasopneumatic compression. Blisters should not be excised but should be punctured and drained. During this period particular care should be taken to keep the environmental temperature comfortable since temperature regulation is disturbed following extensive burns. In small children and infants the room temperature is usually maintained on a higher side (28°C-30°C) to prevent hypothermia. If initial dressing and debridement is done gently, only mild sedation and analgesia may be needed. General anesthesia is rarely required during the initial dressing and debridement.

Circumferential, trunk and limb wounds should be dressed and burns over the face and perineum are left open. Thick layer topical ointment or cream is applied on the wound, followed by sterile vaseline gauze, cotton pads and bandages. The main role of the dressing is to absorb drainage, to provide protection and isolation of a wound from the environment and relief of pain. Following topical agents are commonly used. Advanced dressing techniques are available including VAC dressing which uses a closed system of suction to increase healing tissue.

Silver sulfadiazine

1% silver sulfadiazine cream is the most popular topical antimicrobial agent[20]. It has a broad-spectrum antimicrobial action. It is painless on application and does not stain clothes. The cream should be applied in a thick layer and since its anti-bacterial action lasts for about 24 hours, the dressing should be changed daily. Disadvantages include poor penetration into eschar and transient leucopenia. When used on second degree burns, a yellowish pseudo-eschar may form. Recently, zinc sulfadiazine and cerium sulfadiazine have become available but clinical experience has not shown their superiority over silver sulfadiazine.

Mafenide acetate cream

It is also known as sulphamylon. It has very good eschar penetration. However, it is a carbonic acid inhibitor and can cause acid base disturbances. It is not available in our country.

Silver nitrate

It is used as 0.5% solution. It was widely used before the availability of silver sulfadiazine cream. However, it causes staining of clothes and dressings and electrolyte disturbances due to excessive loss of sodium and potassium.

Many other antimicrobial creams and ointments like neomycin, polymyxin and bacitracin, povidone-iodine or framycetin can be used as topical agents for small areas of burns[21]. It must be remembered that absorption of these agents may lead to systemic toxicity especially in large burns. Therefore, before starting any agent its absorption pattern and toxicity should be ascertained. Thus creams and ointments containing gentamicin, framycetin, neomycin and povidone-iodine should be avoided in extensive burns because of systemic toxicity. Early and effective local management of burn wounds is summarized in Figure 50.7.

Surgical Management

The classical surgical management of full thickness or deep dermal burns is to wait for the eschar to separate and then apply split-thickness grafts over the granulating areas. This entailed a long period of wait for many weeks before wound closure could be achieved exposing the patient to septic and metabolic complications. Early surgical excision of the burn wound is one of the major advances which has lead to decreased morbidity and mortality in pediatric burns[22]. It is usually done between third to fifth post-burn day.

Excision and grafting

It is required in third degree burns involving less then 15 percent of body surface area and for burns over the hands. Surgical excision of burn is done followed by immediate skin autograft or

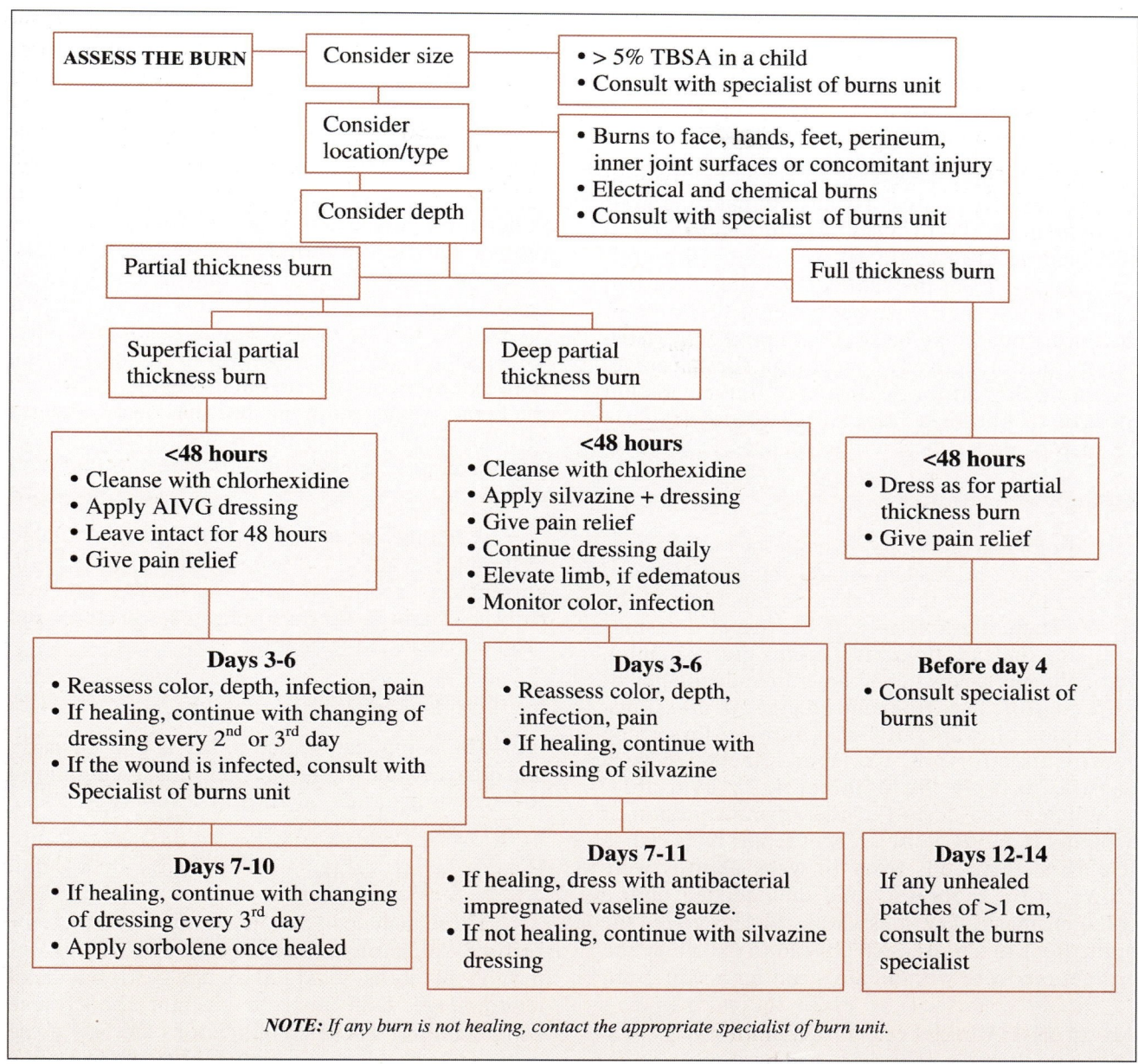

Figure 50.7 Algorithm for local management of burns

delayed auto-grafting after 24 to 48 hours to obtain homeostasis. In second and third degree burns of hands, excision and grafting must be done immediately to avoid formation of hypertrophic scars, which can lead to contractures and deformities.

Tangential excision. It is practiced in deep dermal burns between 2 to 5 days after the accident when the necrotic tissue is removed with the help of skin dermatome by cutting repeated superficial slices of eschar until a punctate bleeding surface of potentially viable dermis appears which is immediately grafted. The application of graft is essential following tangential excision and by this technique small degree dermal burns may completely heal within 7 to 10 days.

Skin grafting. Third degree burns are grafted when the necrotic tissue has been removed completely and the wound is covered with healthy granulation tissue. Wound swab cultures must be taken before skin grafting. The presence of *Streptococcus pyogenes* is an absolute contraindication to grafting. When wound culture is positive, a five day course of erythromycin is usually effective to eradicate streptococci. It is mandatory to obtain negative cultures of the wound before grafting the raw areas. The general condition of patient must be improved optimally before grafting by supportive measures to improve nutrition, fluid and electrolyte balance, hemoglobin and serum proteins.

A thin split thickness graft is commonly used to cover extensive areas because thinner the graft the more likely it is to "take" and the donor site will also heal rapidly within 10 days. A further graft can be taken from the same donor site about two weeks later. In an occasional patient, the extent of the burn wound may be so great that the available donor sites are grossly inadequate for coverage. Use of mesh graft for expansion of limited amount of skin to obtain a larger area of coverage is mandatory under these circumstances.

Biological dressings

Biological dressings are temporary skin covers derived from various human and animal tissues and they try to restore few of the lost functions of the skin[23]. There are a variety of biological dressings available such as allografts, porcine grafts, amnion and collagen sheets. They have the advantages of pain control, less frequent change of dressings, prevention of evaporative and nitrogen losses and control of infection. Collagen sheets are very popular as they are commercially available, economical and devoid of risk of transmission of hepatitis B and HIV. In a recent report by Swedish scientists, fetal cells from 14-week abortus were grown in the laboratory and then seeded onto a collagen mesh. The mesh was used to cover the burnt areas in children which lead to excellent and prompt recovery without any need for a skin graft.

Alternative wound cover

These include a number of dressing materials like biobrane, duoderm and hydrocolloid dressings. These are synthetic dressings, like biologic dressings and are useful for management of partial thickness burns. They are easy to apply and are devoid of any risk of spread of infections like HIV and hepatitis B.

Artificial skin

A number of synthetic materials have been devised as replacement of dermis and they basically help in preventing evaporative losses. A number of synthetic skin substitutes like Integra, Epigard, Biobrane, Hydron, Opsite, etc. are available in the market. These materials are more useful after excisional surgery where autografts are not available. However, at present they are not freely available in our country. The exorbitant cost restricts their use in extensive burns. Their main advantage is "off the shelf" availability.

Skin culture

In cases with extensive burns and paucity of donor sites, human keratinocytes from a small skin biopsy sample are cultured. After three weeks, sheets of epidermal cells are obtained and can be used for covering extensive raw areas (Figure 50.8). This facility is now available at our Center. This technology is very helpful in saving patients with extensive burns who otherwise die. However, the keratinocytes cultured sheet has disadvantages of delayed availability of 3-4 weeks after biopsy, poor take, unsatisfactory cosmetic results and high cost.

A number of newer modalities are available to promote healing. Ultrasound waves and electric current are credited to promote healing process. Cold UV light is useful to eliminate bacteria and promote new skin formation.

COMPLICATIONS

The complication due to burns may be early and delayed. The victim must be closely monitored to prevent and promptly manage these complications.

Early complications

These include hypovolemic shock, respiratory failure, pulmonary and systemic infection, thrombophlebitis, renal failure and gastroduodenal hemorrhage. One must be vigilant about these complications. These complications are less if the initial shock phase is properly managed. The gastroduodenal hemorrhage usually occurs after 7-10 days and is also known as Curling's ulcer. It should be managed by measures like gastric lavage, H^2 blockers and blood transfusion. Acute renal failure should be dealt by peritoneal dialysis initially followed by hemodialysis. All these complications should be promptly identified and managed adequately because of high risk of mortality.

Late complications

An awareness of late complications is very essential because many of them can be prevented by proper initial management. Most of the late complications are because of scarring which leads to disfigurement, contractures and slow growth[24]. Hypertrophic scars and pigment abnormalities

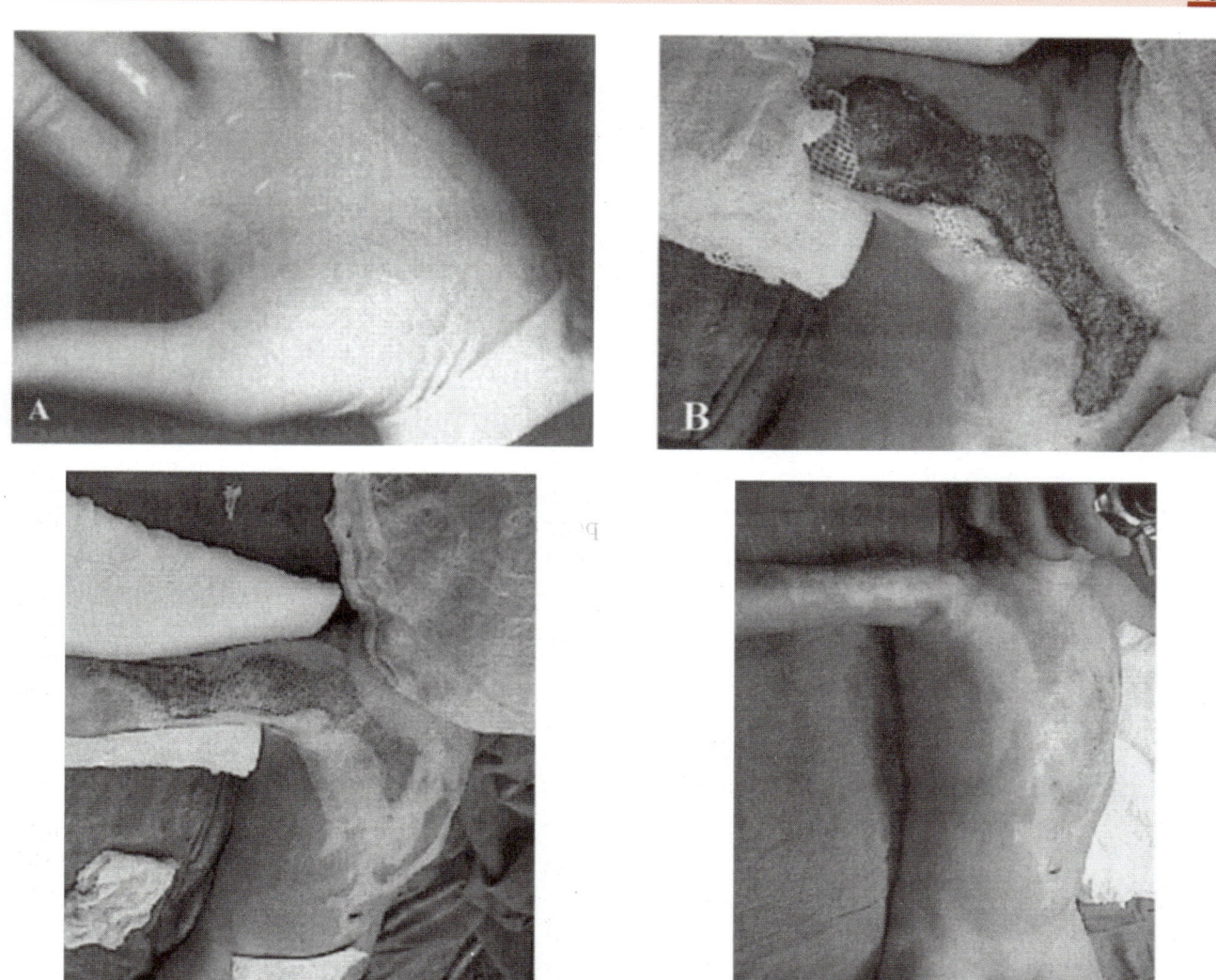

Figure 50.8 Burn wound coverage by cultured keratinocytes: (A) Cultured keratinocytes sheet; (B) Full thickness burn wound over right upper arm, shoulder and upper chest; (C) Wound covered with cultured keratinocytes sheet; (D) Healed wound after 21 days of application

(Figure 50.9A) cause lot of distress to the child and parents. Scarring can be minimised by early excision and grafting of areas that are likely to form hypertrophic scars.

Contractures occur because of delayed healing of deep burns across flexor surfaces and cause functional loss and deformities (Figure 50.9B and C). In order to prevent contractures, burn wounds should be excised or grafted early. Those areas that are likely to form contractures should be kept extended by use of proper splints. Splinting and physiotherapy should be started from the first day itself and the child should be ambulated as early as possible.

In cases where contracture and scarring has occurred inspite of best efforts, reconstructive surgery has to be done. Contractures should be released early in critical areas like eyelids and lips without waiting for scar maturation. One should be prepared to do repeated release surgeries to prevent growth disturbances. The possibility of the patient developing Marjolin's ulcer (carcinoma in a burn scar) must always be kept in mind especially where there is a long-standing scar (Figure 50.9D). It is important to remember that electrical and chemical burns are predisposed to develop a number of early and late complications.

ELECTRICAL BURNS

Electrical burns have high morbidity and mortality. These accidents are becoming very common due to rapid rural electrification, use of substandard electrical fittings and appliances, lack

Section 5

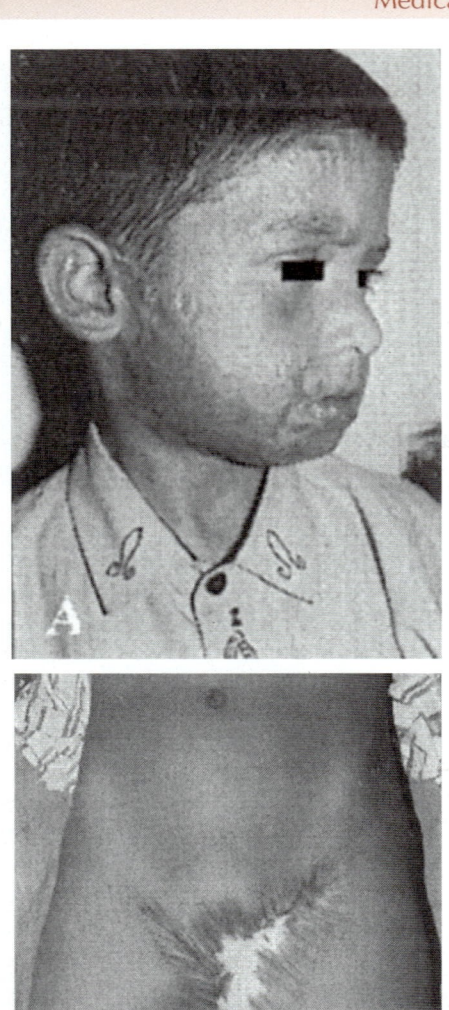
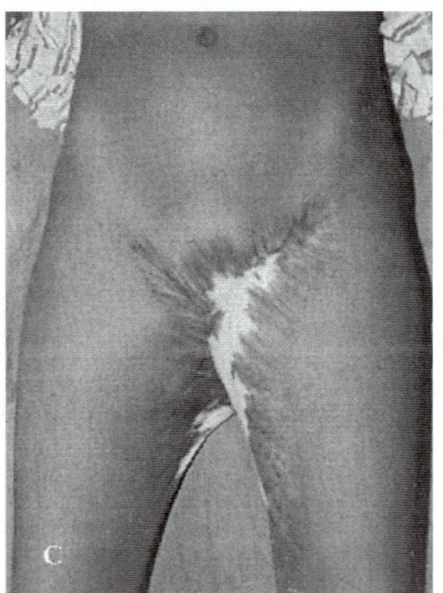
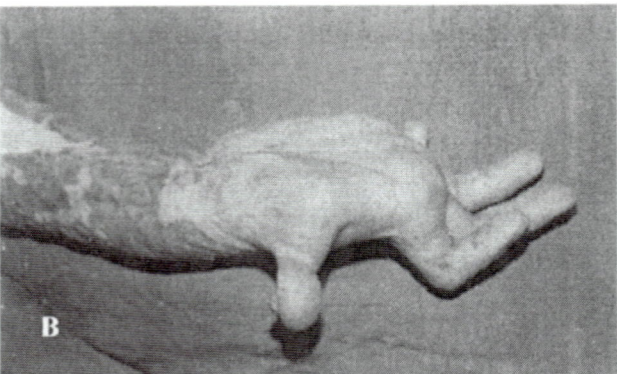
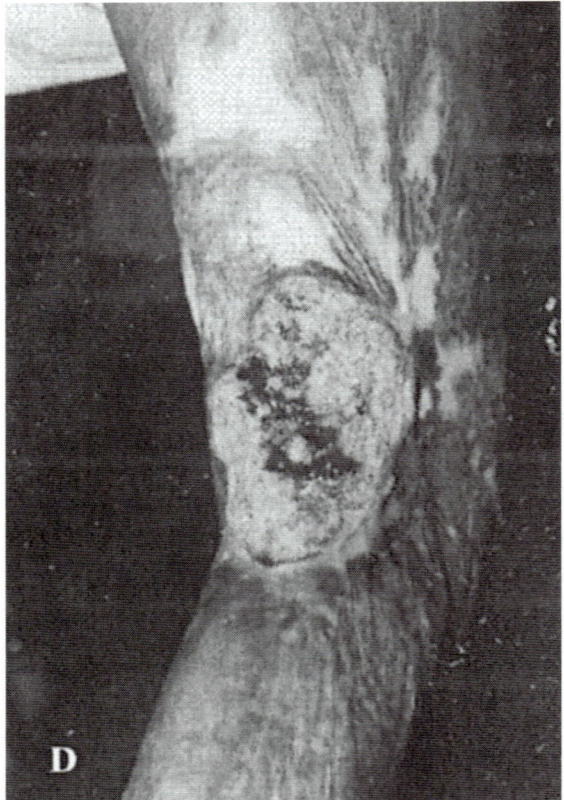

Figure 50.9 Complications of burn: (A) Hypertrophic scar of face; (B) Contracture of hand; (C) Perineum contracture; (D) Squamous cell carcinoma following burn ulcer

of safety norms and ignorance. Burns occur due to passage of electric current in the body which acts as resistance and conversion of electrical energy into heat. An inquisitive child putting an electrical wire into the angle of mouth is not an uncommon event in the west although it is rarely seen in our country.

Most of the pediatric electrical burns in India occur due to high tension electrical injuries. These commonly occur while children are flying kites with fine metallic strings or they try to catch hold of kites entangled in electrical poles thus sustaining major burns. However, in children below five years,

usually low tension injury is seen because of contact with plugs and sockets at home. In case of electric shock, the feeding electric switch or the main switch of electricity supply should be put off before touching the victim.

The electrical current flows through the body from the entry point to the exit point, which are usually depressed due to explosion of tissues due to current. The current flows preferentially through the tissues which are better conductors. Electric burns are very deceptive to look at. There may be a small area of burn on the skin but there is greater damage to muscles, nerves and blood vessels. This leads to extensive damage to the deeper tissues and almost all cases of high tension injuries (voltage of electricity above 1000 volts) to limbs require fasciotomies, serial debridements and reconstructive procedures. In many cases early amputation has to be done. Therefore, all such patients must be evaluated by a surgeon as soon as possible. The systemic effects of electrical burns may be quite serious and include cardiac rhythm abnormalities especially ventricular fibrillations and brain damage. These should be appropriately managed. Nervous tissue is highly susceptible to electrical injury because of its low resistance. There is loss of recent memory but neuromotor sequelae may be delayed for several months. These children also require greater amount of intravenous fluids because of deep tissue damage and massive edema. High infusion rates and administration of mannitol are recommended when there is hemoglobinuria and/ or myoglobinuria.

CHEMICAL BURNS

In children chemical burns usually occur at home. These may be accidental or homicidal. Although many types of chemicals are implicated, commonly acid and alkali burns are seen. To understand the effect of chemical burns one must keep in mind the basic structure of the cell. Cell wall is made up of protein interphase with lipid molecules. Acids react with the protein moiety leading to denaturation of proteins. This forms a dry eschar which prevents further absorption of the chemical. Therefore, systemic effects are not seen in majority of acid burns. However, there are exceptions in case of phenol and hydrofluoric acid burns. In the case of alkaline burns, the alkali dissolves the lipids and this causes further entry of alkali into the cells. Destruction of cells releases lysozomes causing liquefaction necrosis which is progressive in nature.

The first step in management is to wash the burnt area thoroughly with water. Buffered solutions like monobasic and dibasic phosphate may also be used. Since chemical burns are usually deep, early excision and grafting should be done to prevent long term sequelae.

PHYSICAL AND PSYCHOSOCIAL REHABILITATION

Physical rehabilitation involves optimal body and limb positioning, splinting, exercises (active and passive movements), assistance with activities of daily living and gradual ambulation. The child should return to school as soon as possible and his teachers and classmates should be motivated and encouraged to accept him and provide him emotional support. Psychosocial rehabilitation of the child is an important component of management of burns since profound psychosocial disturbances commonly occur[25, 26]. Injury, illness and hospitalization produces regressive behavior in children. When child is admitted to the hospital, the trauma of isolation and seclusion is minimised if the child has full visibility of other children, visitors and nurses. During the later phase a close cooperation is required between parents, teachers and attending physician to help the child gain better self esteem and social integration. The psychosocial rehabilitation should aim at making the child emerge as a hero out of the tragedy rather than a victim worthy of pity.

The onus of burn care does not rest on the shoulders of the burn specialists alone. Family doctors, pediatricians, general surgeons are also called upon to provide care to burn patients in the emergency department. Effective and holistic management of burn patients demands a close cooperation between a large number of specialists like specialized and dedicated nurses, plastic surgeon, physical therapist, occupational therapist, neuropsychologist, recreational therapist and respiratory therapist. Most of the burn victims are shunned by medical community as hopeless cases. Thorough knowledge of latest advances in management of burns reduces the morbidity and mortality of unfortunate victims. Dabhwali (Haryana) and Kumbhkonam (Tamil Nadu) fire disasters highlight greater awareness and the importance of prevention and provision of timely and effective burn care to the fire victims in our country.

REFERENCES

1. Chapman JC, Sarhadi NS, Watson AC. Declining incidence of paediatric burns in Scotland – A review of 1114 children treated as outpatients and inpatients in a regional center. *Burns* 1994; 20:106-10.

2. Mercier C, Blond MH. Epidemiological survey of childhood burn injuries in France. *Burns* 1996; 22: 29-34.

3. Almeida MA. Inhalation lesions in the burn patient. *Acta Med Port* 1998; 11:171-5.

4. Hunt JL, Agee RN, Pruitt BA Jr. Fibreoptic bronchoscopy in acute inhalation injury. *J Trauma* 1975; 15:641-9.

5. Jeschke MG, Barrow RE, Wolf SE, Herndon DN. Mortality in burned children with acute renal failure. *Arch Surg* 1998; 133:752-6.

6. Lund C L, Browder N C. The estimation of areas of burns. *Surg Gynecol Obstet* 1944; 79:352.

7. Herndon DN. (ed). In: *Total Burn Care*. WB Saunders Company Ltd. Philadelphia, 1996.

8. Sheridan R, Ramensnyder J, Prelack K, Petras L, Lyndon M. Treatment of seriously burned infant. *J Burn Care Rehabil* 1998; 19:115-8.

9. Carvajal FH. A physiologic approach to fluid therapy in severely burned children. *Surg Gynecol Obstet* 1980; 150:379-84.

10. Jeschke MG, Herndon DN. Blood transfusion in burns: Benefit or risk. *Crit Care Med* 2006, 34: 1882-1883.

11. Palmieri TL, Lee T, O'Mara MS, Greenhaigh DG. Effects of a restrictive blood transfusion policy on outcomes in children with burn injury. *J Burn Care and Res* 2007, 28(1): 65-70.

12. Fidkowsky KW, Fusaylov G, Sheridan RL, Kote CJ. Inhalation burn injury in children. *Pediatr Anaesth* 2009, 19 (suppl 1): 147-154.

13. Hildreth M A, Cverjal H F. Caloric requirements in burn children: a simple formula to calculate daily caloric requirement. *J Burn Care Rehabil* 1982; 3:78-80.

14. Hildreth M A, Herndon D N, Desai M H, Duke M A. Caloric needs of adolescent patients with burns. *J. Burn Care Rehabil* 1989; 10:523-6.

15. Trocki O, Michelini JA, Robbins ST, Eichelberger MR. Evaluation of early enteral feeding in children less than three years old with smaller burns (8 – Weber 25 percent TBSA). *Burns* 1995; 21:17-23.

16. Guenter PA, Settler R G, Permutter S, Marino D L, Desimone G A, Rolendii RH. Tube feeding related diarrhea in acutely ill patients. *J Parenter Enteral Nutr* 1991; 15:277-80.

17. Derganc M. Parenteral nutrition in severely burned children. *Scand J Plast Reconstr Surg* 1979; 13:195-200.

18. Weber JM, Seridan RL, Pasternack MS, Tompkins RG. Nosocomial infections in paediatric patients with burns. *Am J Infect Control* 1997; 25:195-201.

19. Hess A, Ofori Kuma FK, Tandoh JF. Are closed dressings of burns in children effective? *West Afr J Med* 1996; 15:117-22.

20. Fox CL. Silver sulfadiazine – A new topical therapy for pseudomonas in burns. *Arch Surg* 1968; 96:184-8.

21. Monafo WW, Fredman B. Topical therapy for burns. *Surg Clin North Am* 1987; 67:133-45.

22. Tompkins RG, Remensnyder JP, Burke JF *et al*. Significant reduction in mortality for children with burn injuries through the use of prompt eschar excision. *Ann Surg* 1988; 208:577-85.

23. Hull BE, Finley RK, Miller SF. Coverage of full-thickness burns with bilayered skin equivalents: A preliminary clinical trial. *Surgery* 1990; 107:496-502.

24. Rutan RL, Herndon DN. Growth delay in postburn pediatric patients. *Arch Surg* 1990; 125:392-5.

25. Blakeney P, Meyer W, Moore P *et al*. Social competence and behavior problems of pediatric survivors of burns. *J Burn Care Rehabil* 1993; 14:65-72.

26. Gordon MD. Burn Care Protocols: Paediatric recreational therapy after thermal injury. *J Burn Care Rehabil* 1987; 8:336.

51

Electrocution and Lightning

Daljit Singh and Hitesh Dhawan

INTRODUCTION

Electricity, lightning and radiation are physical agents that can result in injuries and death. These are clubbed under "environmental emergencies". Electrical injury is a relatively common, complex and potentially devastating form of physical trauma with a unique pathophysiology carrying high morbidity and mortality. It encompasses a wide spectrum and includes lightning injury, high-voltage injury, and low-voltage injury[1-3]. Clinical manifestations range from transient unpleasant sensations without apparent injury to massive tissue damage with both occult and delayed complications[4]. Some electrocutions are instantly fatal. Unlike thermal burns, electric injuries commonly involve multiple body systems and pose great challenge with regards to accurate assessment and management. Familiarity with the mechanisms of injury and the principles of therapy improves the outcome of the victim[5].

Over the last century, records for environmental injuries and mortality indicate that lightning has consistently been one of the top 3 environment-related causes of death and the second most common storm-related cause of death, exceeded only by floods. In typical years, deaths from lightning surpass deaths from tornados, tsunamis, hurricanes, and earthquakes. Extreme ambient temperatures, including extreme winter and summer heat, are generally the most common environmental killers[6].

EPIDEMIOLOGY

Any form of energy, when not properly controlled or harnessed, can result in serious danger to those who come in its contact. The dangers inherent with electricity can generally be divided into two categories: direct and indirect. The direct danger is the damage that the electricity itself can cause to the human body, such as cessation of breathing or regular heart beats, or burns. The indirect dangers include the damage that can result

from consequences such as a fall, an explosion, or a fire. The widespread use of electricity and the application of electrically powered machinery have caused an increase in the number of electrical injuries[7]. Approximately 20% of all electrical injuries occur in children, with a bimodal peak incidence being highest in toddlers and adolescents. Most electrical injuries that occur in children are at home, with extension cords (60-70%) and wall outlets (10-15%) being by far the most common sources in this age group[8]. Electrical burns account for 2-3% of all burns in children that require emergency room care. In modern society electrocution can occur when a mobile camera or digital flash camera is used near high voltage electrical lines. The current can pass through the flash light or the camera and electrocute the operator. In kite flying season the thread may get entangled with high voltage wires thus posing a risk of electrocution.

Electrical injuries are one of the most severe forms of injury in civilians in an industrialized society resulting in an estimated 1000 deaths per year and about 3000 admissions to specialized burn centers per year. Up to 40% of serious electrical injuries are fatal.[2-4] According to the National Crime Record Bureau of India, 1507 persons died from lightning in India during the year 2001, about 1% of all deaths due to natural and other accidental causes. In Orissa state alone, about 300 persons were killed by lightning in 2004. Studies have shown that the chances of being struck increased by wearing or carrying a metal object or by simply being wet.

Ninety percent of lightning strikes from cloud to cloud; only about 10% of lightning strikes are from cloud to ground (CG). Any object under or near the thundercloud will have an opposite charge induced in it, be it a television tower, a tree, a person, or a blade of grass. Multiple upward waves of current rise from these objects. Most of them do not contact the main lightning channel but may have sufficient energy to cause injury. Eventually, the downward wave may come is contact with one or more of the upward streamers to complete the lightning circuit. At that point, a return stroke fills all of the branches and the lightning strikes.[5]

PATHOPHYSIOLOGY

Electricity is classified as either direct current or alternating current. Direct current (DC) flows in a constant direction e.g. batteries. High-voltage direct current is used as a means for the bulk transmission of electrical power. Alternating current (AC) is an electric flow that regularly reverses its direction. Each forward-backward motion interval is called a cycle. Electric current in India alternates with a frequency of 50 Hz and normal residential voltage supply is 220-240 volts. The usual waveform of an AC power circuit is a sine wave, because this results in the most efficient transmission of energy, but at the same time, it is also more dangerous than DC. This is because of "hold on" effect it imparts making the muscles undergo a tetanoid spasm which prevents the victim from releasing the live conductor. According to Ohm's law, the flow of current is directly related to the voltage difference and inversely proportional to the electrical resistance between two points in a circuit: I = V/R wherein I is the current that flows through the body (amperes), V is the voltage difference between two points (volts) and R is the resistance between the two points in the closed circuit (ohms). A decrease in the resistance, therefore, causes an increase in the current, while the voltage remains constant.

The three major mechanisms of electricity-induced injury are as follows: [6,10,11]

1. Electrical energy causing direct tissue damage, altering cell membrane resting potential, and eliciting muscle tetany.
2. Conversion of electrical energy into thermal energy, causing massive tissue destruction and coagulative necrosis.
3. Mechanical injury with direct trauma resulting from fall or violent muscle contractions.

Clinical Features

The degree of electric injury is determined by the magnitude of energy delivered, resistance encountered, type of current, pathway of current, and duration of contact (Table 51.1). Systemic effects and tissue damage are directly proportional to the magnitude of current delivered to the victim. Electrical shock is classified as high voltage (>1000 volts) or low voltage (< 1000 volts). As a general rule, high voltage is associated with greater morbidity and mortality, although fatal injury can occur with the usual household current (220 volts).

Table 51.1 Physiologic effects of different electrical currents[12]	
Effect (1 second contact)	**Current (milliamperes)**
Tingling sensation/perception	1-4
Let go current ➤ Children ➤ Women ➤ Men	 3-4 6-8 7-9
Skeletal muscle tetany (Freezing to circuit)	16-20
Respiratory muscle paralysis	20-50
Ventricular fibrillation	50-120

Current travels down the path of least resistance. Nerve and muscle tissues have lower resistance than skin tissue. The current pathway determines which tissues are at increased risk and what type of injury is likely to occur. High-voltage injuries tend to cause deep internal injuries, myoglobinuria, renal failure, shock and massive loss of tissues and function. Electrical current that passes through the head or thorax is more likely to produce fatal injury. Transthoracic currents can cause fatal arrhythmia, direct cardiac damage, or respiratory arrest.[13] Transcranial currents can cause direct brain injury, seizures, respiratory arrest, and paralysis. Electrothermal tissue injury results in tissue edema; therefore, the development of a compartment syndrome can occur in any compartment of the body (Figure 51.1). The leg is the most commonly involved site. An injured extremity may not show external signs of injury but

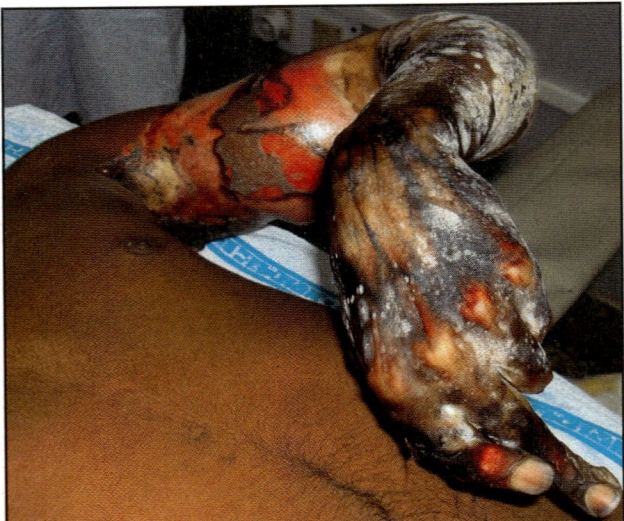

Figure 51.1 High voltage electric burns of left upper extremity
(*Courtesy* : DMCH Burns Unit Archives)

at times there may be exogenous thermal burns due to sparking or endogenous thermal burns known as Joule or electric burn.

Lightning cannot be classified as either direct current or alternating current. The physics of lightning is incredibly complex and substantially different from the physics of generated electricity. Lightning may injure an individual in six ways. [5,14,15]

(i)   Direct strike (3-5% of injuries).

(ii)   Side splash from another object (30%).

(iii)   Contact voltage from touching an object that is struck (1-2%).

(iv)   Ground current effect as the energy spreads out across the surface of the earth when lightning hits a distance away from the person (40-50%).

(v)   Upward leader that does not connect with the downward leader to complete a lightning channel (20-25%).

(vi)   Blunt trauma if a person is thrown away and barotrauma from being close enough to experience the explosive force of lightning.

Because lightning injuries are so infrequently reported compared with fatalities, a rule of thumb developed from many studies suggest that injuries occur about 10 times more often than fatalities. Although most injuries occur outdoors, many people are injured indoors every year, for example people getting landline telephone-mediated strikes. [16,17] Use of cell phones, iPods, and other portable electronic devices do not increase the risk of injury except distracting the individual from paying attention to warning signs such as storm clouds and thunder. Injuries range from tiny static electricity exposure to massive cardiac arrest. [13, 18-21] Lightning strike can send the heart into asystole. Blunt force injuries from falling, being thrown by muscle contractions, or barotrauma from the explosive force of a nearby lightning strike may occur. [13] External injuries are usually superficial and appear as filigree burns or "Lichtenberg figures" (linear arborescent pattern of contusions and lacerations). Other common complications of lightning injuries include tympanic membrane rupture and cataract. Lightning strikes are primarily a neurologic injury that affects all 3 components of the nervous system; central, autonomic, and peripheral. Hypothermia should also be considered when victim is soaked with rainwater. Lightning injuries tend to cause few external or internal burns and rarely cause myoglobinuria. On the other hand, cardiac and respiratory arrest, vascular spasm, neurologic damage, and autonomic instability play a great role. [22] There is usually little tissue loss although there may be permanent functional impairment. Therefore, the treatment of lightning victims rarely requires massive fluid resuscitation, fasciotomies for compartment syndromes, mannitol and furosemide as diuretics, alkalinization of the urine, amputations or large repeated debridements.

Laboratory Investigations

The laboratory evaluation of the patient sustaining an electrical injury depends on the extent of injury. All patients with evidences of conductive injury or significant surface burns should have the following laboratory tests: CBC, electrolyte level, serum myoglobin, blood urea nitrogen, creatinine level and urinalysis with special attention to myoglobinuria. In patients with severe electrical injury or suspected intra-abdominal injury, amylase aspartate, alanine transaminases, alkaline phosphatase and clotting indexes should also be obtained. Sending blood for type and cross-match should be considered, particularly if major debridement is necessary. Arterial blood gas determinations are indicated if the patient needs ventilatory support or alkali therapy.

All patients should be evaluated for myoglobinuria, a common complication of electrical injury. A patient in whom an ortho-toluidine dipstick examination of the urine is positive for blood, but no red blood cells are seen on microscopic examination, should be presumed to have myoglobinuria and treated accordingly.

Creatine kinase (CK) levels should be determined and isoenzyme analysis performed. Peak CK levels have been shown to predict the extent of muscle injury, risk of amputation, and ultimate hospital stay. However, the clinical value of a single CK estimation in the acute setting has not been established. Cardiac enzyme levels should be interpreted with care in diagnosing myocardial infarction in the setting of electrical injury. The peak CK level is not indicative of myocardial damage in electrical injury because of the associated injury to muscles.

Rescue and First aid

The victim must be promptly separated from the source of electric current but the rescuer must not touch the victim until main power supply has been put off. Flames must be extinguished otherwise the current will continue to flow through the tissues. The rescuer must stand on a dry, non-conducting surface like folded newspaper, flattened card board carton or a rubber mat and use a non-conductive object such as wooden rod or broomstick to push

Section 5

the victim away from the source of current. Never use a damp or metallic object to touch the victim. Provide comfort, cuddling, emotional support and cardio-pulmonary resuscitation when needed. In a case of lightning victim, aggressive and prolonged CPR is mandatory even if appreciable time has elapsed after the strike. *All victims of electric shock and lightning must be immediately taken to the hospital irrespective of the severity of injury at the entry point.*

MANAGEMENT

Patients with electrical injury should be initially evaluated as a burn and trauma patient.[23,24] Airway, breathing, circulation, and immobilization of the spine should be performed as a part of primary care. A high index of suspicion must be maintained and victim should be evaluated for hidden injuries. Intravenous access, cardiac monitoring, and measurement of oxygen saturation should be started during the primary survey. Fluid replacement is the most important aspect of the initial resuscitation.[24] As with conventional thermal injury, electrical injuries cause massive fluid shifts with extensive tissue damage and acidosis; therefore, monitoring patient's hemodynamics is important. A Foley's catheter is helpful in monitoring urine output and tissue perfusion.

Medical Therapy

Initial fluid resuscitation should aim for urine output of greater than 0.5 ml/kg/hr if no signs of myoglobinuria are present and preferably greater than 1 ml/kg/hr if myoglobinuria is present. Since lightning burns are usually superficial, using a standard formula, such as the Parkland formula, may be helpful.

Parkland Formula
4 ml/kg/ % of burnt surface
1. Half of the fluids given in 1st 8 hours and the remaining half in 16 hrs
2. For next 24 hrs administer 2 ml/kg/% of burnt surface
3. Time of administration is calculated from the time of incident and not from the time of admission.

Because of the iceberg effect of the cutaneous injury, coupled with the extensive destruction of the underlying structures, the fluid requirements are much greater than in a comparable thermal burn. Based on the Parkland formula, fluid replacement should be increased by 2-3 times, depending on the total surface area potentially involved. For example, an increase by 3 is required if the surface area is 20% and by 2 (or less) according to an increased percentage of burned skin. These formulae estimate necessary initial resuscitation volume over the first 24 hours from the time of the burn. An isotonic balanced saline solution (eg, Ringer's lactate solution) is used for fluid resuscitation. Urinary output as an indicator of hemodynamic status and kidney functions should be closely monitored. Constant adjustments based on hourly urine output are required. Decrease or increase of fluid rates may be necessary to maintain urine output of 0.5-1 ml/kg/hr.

An indwelling urinary catheter insertion is mandatory. Hematuria or dark urine prompts the need for more aggressive therapy to prevent myoglobin-induced tubular necrosis. This is treated with rapid administration of fluids and bicarbonate. Sodium bicarbonate is given at 1-2 mEq/kg. With extensive injuries, acidosis and myoglobinuria is expected and bicarbonate needs to be administered with the initial fluid bolus. Mannitol 1.0 g/kg body weight should be administered to promote osmotic diuresis. The target urine output should be 2-3 ml/kg/hr, with a urine pH greater than 6.5. Bicarbonate treats the underlying acidosis and alkalinizes the urine, making myoglobin more soluble. Additional diuretics may be administered. Acetazolamide is the drug of choice because it also alkalinizes the urine. However, diuresis must be promoted with extreme caution to avoid hyperosmotic hypoalbuminemia. Nonsteroidal anti-inflammatory drugs (NSAIDs) for the first few days are used as a prophylaxis to prevent long-term neurologic damage and to treat chronic pain syndromes that may develop from sympathetic nervous system injuries caused by lightning. Use of long-term ibuprofen, vitamin C (1 g/d), and vitamin E (400 U/d) have been shown to decrease long-term effects of injury and scarring with electrical damage. A nasogastric tube should be placed in the seriously injured patient because of the risk of adynamic ileus and stress ulceration. Ulcer prophylaxis with H-2 blockers or sucralfate is advocated. The steps in the management of electrocution are shown in Figure 51.2.

Surgical Therapy

The affected extremities should be splinted in a functional position to minimize edema and contracture formation. The hand should be splinted in 35-45 degrees extension at the wrist, 80-100 degrees flexion at the metacarpophalangeals and almost full extension at the proximal interphalangeal and distal interphalangeal joints to minimize the space available for edema formation. During the

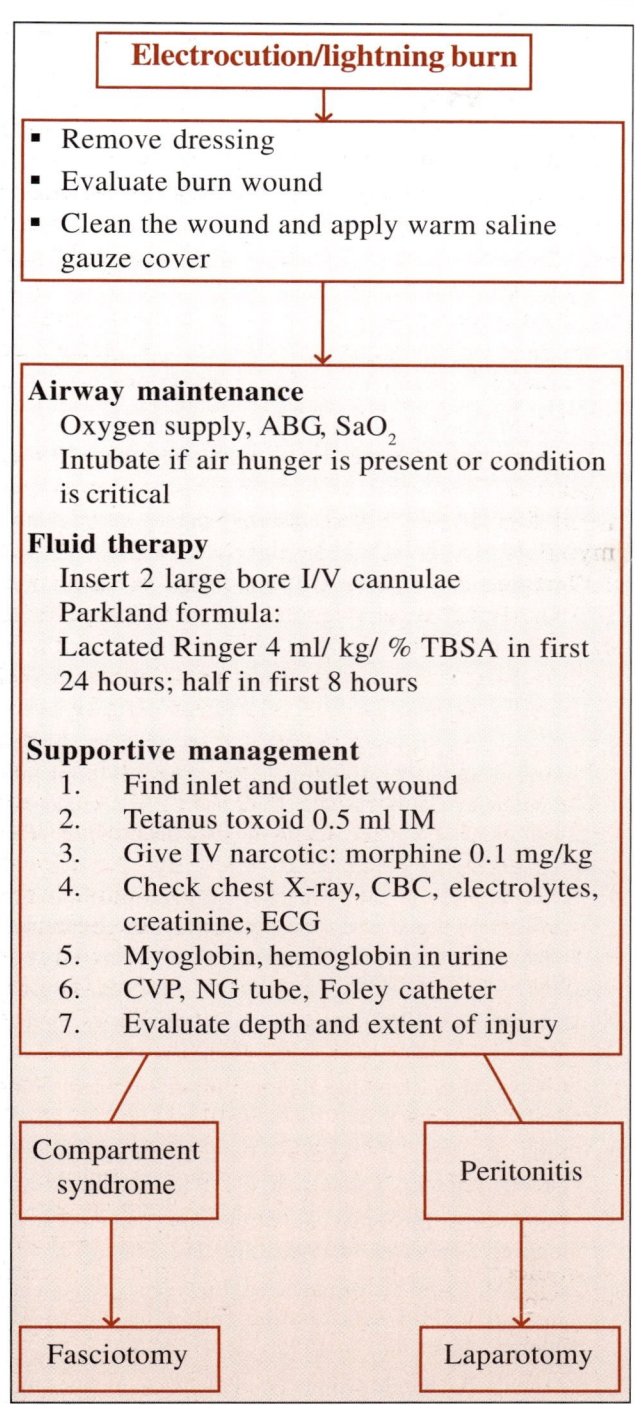

Figure 51.2 Flow chart for management of electric burns

first several days of hospitalization frequent monitoring of the neurovascular status of all extremities is essential.

Functional outcome of an electrical burn wound is inversely proportional to the time elapsed before the start of the reconstructive procedure(s).[23, 24] As part of the nature of the electrical trauma, tissue damage leads to vascular thrombosis and necrosis of skin and muscles. This leads to gross limitation for manipulation of local tissues for reconstruction. The optimal management of these wounds has evolved through various stages like initial debridement, decompression (fasciotomy), aggressive planned debridement and early skin grafting with the goal of preserving vital structures.[23, 24]

Fasciotomy serves a dual role of a therapeutic and a diagnostic tool in the treatment of electrical injuries. The fact that a burn with a relatively small surface area may hide massive underlying tissue destruction cannot be overemphasized. Therefore, any swelling or signs of impaired circulation must be aggressively evaluated and managed.

Sometimes it is impossible to resuscitate a patient with a large amount of dead muscle, and an emergency operation to amputate the injured extremity or remove the destroyed tissues may be necessary. Amputation rates reported in the literature vary from 10 to 68%.[25]

Complications

The most common causes of deaths include pneumonia, sepsis, and multiple organ failure because of the complexity of the injury. Compartment syndromes are common and should be identified early and managed promptly. Other complications include local infection (as with any burn injury), neurologic injury from the initial insult, and complex regional pain syndrome (CRPS). The associated injuries carry their own risk of complications.[26] Neurologic complications such as loss of consciousness, disorders of memory and concentration, peripheral nerve damage, and delayed spinal cord syndrome may occur. Damage to the brain may result in a permanent seizure disorder.[27,28] Long-term psychiatric sequelae in children may continue into adulthood.

Outcome and Prognosis

The location and extent of injury, the development of complications, and the functional damage determine the outcome and prognosis. Recent advances in ICU care, resuscitation, nutritional support, and surgical techniques, along with availability of skin substitutes, have significantly improved outcomes. Early physical and occupational therapy can reduce the severity of long-term sequelae.

Prevention

Most electrical injuries are preventable. All household electric sockets should be covered with plastic or rubber safety caps, so that children cannot insert their fingers or metal objects in the socket. The damaged appliances, extension, cords, plugs and ungrounded outlets should be repaired or replaced. Children should be kept away from electric appliances and should be taught about the dangers of electricity when they are old enough to understand. Children should be refrained from climbing any electrical system like a pole or electrical transformer. They should not be allowed to switch on and off the switches or electrical gadgets. Electrical toys should not be given to young children. The electrical appliances should never be switched on or off with wet hands or while standing in water. The location of fuse boxes and circuit breakers in home, school and place of work should be clearly identified.

Lightning fatalities are becoming less common with agriculture becoming less labor intensive and most homes and work places are provided with indoor plumbing and wiring that creates a "Faraday cage effect" with some grounding in most buildings. During thunderstorm children should be kept indoors and one should avoid the use of telephone, computer and hair dryer because these can act as conduits for lightning. If lightning strikes when you are outdoors, one should keep away from any metallic objects and should preferably sit or lie down on the ground. You can take shelter in a car while keeping the radio and mobile in off mode. Cyclists and motor cyclists should dismount and move some distance away from their bikes until the storm has passed.

REFERENCES

1. Browne BJ, Gaasch WR. Electrical injuries and lightning. *Emerg Med Clin North Amer* 1992; 10(2): 211-229.

2. Fontanarosa PB. Electrical shock and lightning strike. *Ann Emerg Med* 1993; 22(2 Pt 2):378-387.

3. Martinez JA, Nguyen T. Electrical injuries. *South Med J* 2000; 93(12):1165-1168.

4. Dega S, Gnaneswar SG, Rao PR, Ramani P, Krishna DM. Electrical burn injuries. Some unusual clinical situations and management. *Burns* 2007; 33(5): 653-665.

5. Cooper MA, Andrews CJ, Holle RL. Lightning injury. In: Wilderness Emergencies. Auerbach (Ed). *CV Mosby;* 2006:chapter 3.

6. Lopez RE, Holle RL, Heitkamp TA. Lightning casualties and property damage in Colorado from 1950 to 1991 based on storm data. *Weather and Forecasting* 1992, 10:114-126.

7. Leibovici D, Shemer J, Shapira SC. Electrical injuries: current concepts. *Injury* 1995; 26(9):623-627.

8. Baker MD, Chiaviello C. Household electrical injuries in children. Epidemiology and identification of avoidable hazards. *Amer J Dis Child* 1989; 143(1):59-62.

9. Lee RC, Zhang D, Hannig J. Biophysical injury mechanisms in electrical shock trauma. *Annual Rev Biomed Eng* 2000; 2:477-509.

10. Carleton SC. Cardiac problems associated with electrical injury. *Cardiol Clin* 1995;13(2):263-266.

11. Cooper AM. Emergent care of lightning and electrical injuries. *Semin Neurol* 1995,15(3): 268-278.

12. Arnoldo B, Klein M, Gibran NS. Practice guidelines for the management of electrical injuries. *J Burn Care Res* 2006; 27(4):439-447.

13. Fish R. Electric shock, Part II: Nature and mechanisms of injury. *J Emerg Med* 1993; 11(4):457-462.

14. Bier M, Chen W, Bodnar E, Lee RC. Biophysical injury mechanisms associated with lightning injury. *Neuro Rehabilitation* 2005; 20(1):53-62.

15. Cooper MA. A fifth mechanism of lightning injury. *Acad Emerg Med* 2002; 9(2):172-174.

16. Andrews CJ, Cooper MA, Darveniza M. Lightning Injuries: Electrical Medical, and Legal Aspects, Boca Raton FL (Ed), *CRC Press* 1992.

17. Cooper MA. Emergent care of lightning and electrical injuries. *Semin Neurol* 1995; 15(3):268-278

18. Cooper MA, Holle R, Andrews C. Field J. Electrical current and lightning Injury. In: The Textbook of Emergency Cardiovascular Care and CPR. *Lippincott, Williams & Wilkins;* ACLS for the Experienced Provider, AHA/ACEP; 2009: 498-511.

19. Cooper MA, Johnson SA. Cardiopulmonary resuscitation and early management of the lightning strike victim. In: Cardiopulmonary Resuscitation. *Humana Press;* 2005.

20. Cooper, MA. Electrical and lightning injuries. *Emer Med Clin N Amer* 1984, 2 (3): 489-501.

21. Cooper MA. Lightning injuries: prognostic signs for death. *Ann Emerg Med* 1980; 9(3):134-138.

22. Fish R. Electric shock, Part I: Physics and pathophysiology. *J Emerg Med* 1993;11(3):309-312.

23. Cooper MA. Emergent care of lightning and electrical injuries. *Semin Neurol* 1995; 15(3):268-278

24. Colic M, Ristic L, Jovanovic M. Emergency treatment and early fluid resuscitation following electrical injuries. *Acta Chir Plast* 1996; 38(4):137-141.

25. Arnoldo B,Klein M,Gibran NS. Practice guidelines for the management of electrical injuries.*J Burn Care Res* 2006; 27:439-447.

26. Cherington M. Neurorehabilitation of the multifaceted and complicated neurologic problems associated with lightning and electrical injuries. *Neuro Rehabilitation* 2005; 20(1):1-2.

27. Critchley M. Neurological effects of lightning and electricity. *Lancet* 1934; 1:68-75.

28. Kelley KM, Pliskin N. Meyer C, Lee RC. Neuropsychiatric aspects of electrical injury: the nature of psychiatric disturbance. *Ann N Y Acad Sci* 1994; 720:213-218.

S Mahadevan and Vinod K Paul

52 Animal and Insect Bites

Children commonly fall prey to bites of animals and insects because of their innate curiosity and innocence. The problem is more common and serious in developing countries due to several reasons. The underdeveloped rural habitat is commonly infested with potentially dangerous species of animals and insects. Underprivileged children may lack simple means of protection like shoes and adequate clothing to cover the body. Medical expertise is often not available in the close proximity and valuable time may be lost in transporting the patient. Recourse to unscientific folk remedies may further compromise the prognosis. Among the more important conditions resulting from animal and insect bites are rabies and snake envenomation. These can present as serious life-threatening emergencies necessitating expeditious and specialized management.

RABIES

Rabies is one of the most feared of all human diseases. Rabies has plagued mankind since ancient times. The disease was described as early as 3000 BC. Rabies is characterised by long incubation period, striking clinical presentation of hydrophobia and an almost invariably fatal outcome[1]. The etiologic agent is a bullet-shaped virus containing single-ribonucleic acid (RNA) and belonging to the Mononegavirales order, Rhabdoviridae family and Lyssavirus genus.

The disease is primarily a zoonosis, an infection of carnivores which occasionally spills into human hosts. Rabies is endemic in most parts of the world except Australia, Taiwan, Japan and some parts of Europe. In South-East Asia, the Indian subcontinent and Africa, rabies is a major public health problem. Although exact figures are not available, it is estimated that over 25,000 persons die due to rabies every year in India and 500,000 undergo antirabies immunisation[2]. A survey of 41 medical colleges revealed that rabies accounted for one out of every 2000 admissions[2]. As per the latest national survey conducted in 2003 about 20,000 people die of rabies every year in India and in more than 95 percent cases the transmitting vectors are dogs. In the majority of endemic regions including India, dogs are the principal vectors of rabies, stray dogs in the rural and urban localities perpetuate the cycle of infection by dog-to-dog transmission. Cats, monkeys, mongoose, jackals and cattle are occasionally responsible for this disease in our country. Bat rabies has not been reported from India although it is a major problem in Latin America. Foxes, wolves and skunks are other vectors. In India, common rodents viz. rats, mice, bandicoots and squirrels have not so far been shown to transmit rabies. However, mongoose in India is known to suffer from rabies and the possibility of transmission of disease from infected mongoose to other rodents and human beings cannot be ruled out. Hence rodent bites which show a tendency to be unusually aggressive must be viewed with suspicion and treated as per the merit of the individual case[2]. A carrier state of rabies has been recently described, epidemiologic importance of which is not understood as yet[3].

Pathogenesis

Rabies virus entry occurs through wounds or direct contact with mucosal surfaces. The virus cannot penetrate intact skin. Inhalation of rabies virus can also produce the disease, a mechanism that appears to operate in bat rabies. Human beings have developed rabies after visiting the caves infested by insectivorous bats even in the absence of any bite from the bats. Inhalation of aerosol of live virus in the laboratory has also resulted in rabies. Human-to-human transmission through infected secretions is theoretically possible. However, the only cases of human-to-human spread of rabies occurred through corneal grafts, the donors had died of ascending paralysis simulating Landry-Guillain-Barré syndrome. Transplacental infection can occur among the animals but it has not been reported in humans. Interesting reports of delivery of healthy babies following cesarean section of mothers with rabies are available.

Initial viral replication takes place within the striated muscles at the site of inoculation. Recent experimental evidence suggests that acetyl cholinesterase receptors may also serve as receptors for the rabies virus[4]. Other receptors for rabies virus include neural cell adhesion molecules (NCAM) and nerve growth factor receptors. Its binding to these receptors, which are present in high density at the neuromuscular junction, thus provides a mechanism whereby the virus gets concentrated at local sites in the vicinity of the peripheral nerves. The virus then spreads centripetally to the central nervous axoplasm. Viremia, although demonstrated, is probably unimportant in the pathogenesis of rabies. Involvement of the brain starts in the limbic system. This explains the characteristic manifestations of behavioural changes during early stages of the disease. Following extensive multiplication in the cerebral grey matter, virus spreads centrifugally along autonomic nerves to reach the peripheral tissues including salivary glands, skin, cornea, skeletal muscles, lungs, liver and kidneys. Infected saliva serves as a vehicle for further transmission of the virus.

Pathology

The picture is essentially that of viral encephalitis. The eosinophilic cytoplasmic inclusions, the Negri bodies, are pathognomonic of rabies. They are distributed throughout the brain particularly in Ammon's horn, cerebral cortex, brain stem, Purkinje cells of cerebellum and dorsal spinal ganglia. Absence of Negri bodies, however, does not rule out the diagnosis of rabies.

Clinical Features

The incubation period of rabies ranges between 20 to 90 days in 90 percent of cases, although it may vary from 10 days to over a year. Incubation period of bites on the face averages around 5 weeks and that for bites on the limbs around 7 weeks. Only about 50 percent of those bitten by rabid animals actually develop clinical rabies because of the variable quantum of virus in the saliva[5].

During the initial 1 to 4 days, the patient suffers from prodromal symptoms consisting of fever, myalgia, headache, easy fatiguability, sore throat and changes in the mood. *Paresthesias or fasciculations at the site of bite at this stage are highly suggestive of impending rabies*. This manifestation occurs in 50 to 80 percent of patients. Prodrome is followed by manifestations of encephalitis akin to other viral encephalitides. Alterations in behaviour, sensorium and thought; excessive motor activity; muscle spasms and upper motor neuron paralysis; and features of autonomic distrubances such as hypotension, perspiration, pyrexia, excessive lacrimation and salivation form the constellation of manifestations at this stage. Meningismus, opisthotonos and seizures may also be present. Most patients exhibit phases of agitation, hallucinations and confusion alternating with lucid state.

This phase is followed by florid disease dominated by profound involvement of the brainstem. Multiple cranial nerve involvement leads to diplopia, facial palsy, difficulty in swallowing, frothing and paralysis of laryngeal muscles. The most characteristic finding is hydrophobia. It refers to violent spasms of the muscles of deglutition, diaphragm and accessory respiratory muscles on attempted swallowing of liquids. In its severe form, hydrophobic spasms may be precipitated even by mere sight, sound or mention of water. A draught of air over the face may also trigger the reflex spasm (aerophobia).

Some cases of rabies present with ascending paralysis resembling Landry-Guillain-Barré syndrome. This form of paralytic rabies is seen particularly in patients bitten by vampire bats. Phobic spasms occur in only 50 percent of these patients. During the early stages of paralytic rabies, notable signs include piloerection and myoedema. The latter occurs at percussion sites; usually over the chest, deltoid muscles and thighs. Patients with a full blown picture of rabies do not survive for more than a week. Late stages of rabies are associated with asphyxia, aspiration, cardiac dysrhythmias and myocarditis. Death occurs due to respiratory failure.

Rabies in Animals

Dog. The incubation period is usually 14 to 60 days. The infection occurs through the bite of another rabid animal. Rabies in dogs takes two forms, namely the furious and the dumb rabies[3, 6]. In both types a distinct change in temperament is characteristic. In the commoner furious rabies, dog manifests restlessness and tendency to bite any object without provocation; biting animals, human beings and inanimate objects like twigs, stones, tins, sticks and rags. The dog shows a tendency to wander away from home and run amok often covering many miles before returning. The paralysis of larynx often leads to inability to bark. Pharyngeal paralysis results in characteristic drooling at the mouth due to swallowing difficulty. Over the next few days, the stage of irritability subsides and the animal seeks a secluded place and dies of rapidly progressive paralysis: The dog with dumb rabies appears depressed and withdraws itself. It does not bite and lapses into sleep followed by coma and rapid death. Once the dog manifests clinical signs of rabies, it generally dies within a week.

Cat. The manifestations of rabies in cats resemble furious rabies of dogs. Cats hide in isolated corners and attack unprovoked anyone coming near them. The cat may strike forepaws in air as if it were catching imaginary mice.

Diagnosis

The diagnosis of rabies can be made with reasonable accuracy on the basis of history of dog bite, the presence of paresthesias at the site of bite and hydrophobia[1]. At times, it may be difficult to clinically differentiate rabies from encephalitis due to arboviruses, enteroviruses or herpes simplex virus. Early involvement of the brainstem points to the diagnosis of rabies. The clinical picture of rabies may at times resemble Landry-Guillain-Barré syndrome, poliomyelitis, post-vaccinal (rabies) encephalomyelitis and heat stroke. Careful history, physical examination and cerebrospinal fluid examination will usually exclude these conditions. Rabies can be differentiated from tetanus by the

presence of trismus in the latter and hydrophobia in the former. Botulism, unlike rabies, does not manifest with sensory symptoms. Hysteria in an individual exposed to rabid animal and the fear of rabies may be difficult to rule out. However, hydrophobia and characteristic behavioral changes are not easy to imitate. Confirmatory diagnosis of rabies can be made on post-mortem as well as antemortem by a variety of tests[6-8].

Postmortem Diagnosis of Rabies in Animals and Humans

The postmortem diagnosis of rabies utilizes the brain tissues for antigen detection, viral isolation or histopathologic examination (Table 52.1). Flourescent antibody (FA) technique for antigen detection is a rapid and sensitive method. Using bilateral impressions (or smears) of tissue samples of hippocampus and brain stem further enhances the sensitivity of the test. The enzyme linked imunosorbent assay, called rapid rabies enzyme immuno diagnosis (RREID) detects virus nucleocapsid antigen in brain tissue. Since, it does not need a microscope, it can be done in the field and is suitable for epidemiological work. Virus can be isolated by intracerebral inoculation of brain tissue into mice. The suckling (less than 3 days old) mice are more suitable than the weanling or adult mice. The mice are killed and brain is examined for Negri bodies on histopathology or FA test is done on the brain tissue. The histopathological technique takes 20 days whereas the use of FA can reduce it

Table 52.1 Laboratory diagnosis of rabies		
Diagnostic test	**Postmortem diagnosis in animals or humans**	**Antemortem diagnosis in humans**
Antigen detection • Flourescent antibody (FA) • Rapid rabies enzyme immunodiagnosis (RREID)	 Brain tissue Brain tissue	 Corneal impression Skin biopsy, saliva
Virus isolation • Murine neuroblastoma cell culture • Intracerebral mouse inoculation	 Brain tissue Brain tissue	 Saliva Cerebrospinal fluid, saliva
Histologic examination	Brain tissue	Not applicable
Antibody titers • Mouse serum neutralization test (MNT) • Rapid flourescent focus inhibition test (RFFIT) • Enzyme linked immuno-sorbent assay (ELISA)	Not applicable	 Serum, CSF Serum, CSF Serum, CSF

Section 5

to 3 to 4 days. Rabies virus can also be cultured on murine neuroblastoma cell line giving results in just 2 days. Direct histopathologic examination of animal/human brain is done by the Seller's staining, the sensitivity of which is 75 percent[6]. It is a rapid and cheap test. The results are available within 2 hours: If histopathology is equivocal or negative, flourescent antibody test can be performed by fixing the smears in acetone for 18 hours.In India the major institutions providing diagnostic services for rabies are the Central Research Institute, Kasauli (HP); the National Institute of Communicable Diseases (22 Sham Nath Marg, Post Box 1492, Delhi –110 054), Pasteur Institute of India, Conoor - 643103 (Nilgiris) and Indian Veterinary Research Institute, Izatnagar-243 122, Bareilly (UP).

Antemortem Diagnosis of Rabies in Humans

In recent years antemortem diagnosis of rabies has become feasible (Table 52.1). The choice of technique for diagnosis varies according to the stage of the disease. Antigen detection is generally sensitive during the first few days, while virus neutralizing antibodies in cerebrospinal fluid and serum usually tend to appear after 7-10 days of illness.

Antigen detection by the FA technique can be done using corneal impression, skin biopsy, or saliva. The sensitivity of the FA test on the corneal impression (taken by lightly touching the cornea with a microscope slide) is only 30-35 percent[2]. FA testing on corneal impressions is rarely reliable in most clinical settings and is, therefore, not recommended.

Skin biopsy should be taken from back of the neck including the hair follicles and a peripheral nerve. Sensitivity of skin biopsy is better than that of corneal specimens. Examination of at least 20 sections is required to detect rabies nucleocapsid inclusions around the base of hair follicles. Patient's saliva can be used for making smear for FA staining or for isolation of virus.

Rabies virus isolation can be performed using neuroblastoma cells or the intracranial inoculation of mice. Virus isolation is preferably performed on saliva samples or other biological fluids such as tears and cerebrospinal fluid. The success rate depends upon the antibody status (more positive results are obtained in antibody-negative patients) and on the intermittence of viral shedding.

Neutralizing antibodies in the serum or cerebrospinal fluid of non-vaccinated patients can be measured using a virus neutralization test such as the rapid fluorescent focus inhibition test (RFFIT) or the fluorescent antibody virus neutralization (FAVN) test. Virus-neutralizing antibodies in serum tend to appear on an average 8 days after the clinical symptoms appear.

Magnetic resonance imaging can be helpful in diagnosis. Abnormal, ill defined, mildly hypersignal T2 images involving the brainstem, hippocampus, hypothalamus, deep and subcortical white matter, and deep and cortical grey matter are indicative of rabies. Computerized tomography of the brain is of no diagnostic value.

Anti-rabies Treatment

Antirabies treatment consists of two equally important aspects, namely, the management of the wound and the rabies prophylaxis.

Management of the Wound

Local treatment of the wound is of utmost importance. The aim is to cleanse the wound and neutralise as much virus load as possible. The guidelines are shown in Table 52.2.Wound management must be accomplished at the earliest. When wound management is done properly; this

Table 52.2 Management of the dog bite wound		
Do's		
1.	Cleansing	Wash thoroughly with soap and running water for 5 minutes
2.	Chemical treatment	Apply alcohol or tincture iodine or aqueous solution of iodine or quarternary ammonium compounds (like cetavalon or savlon)
3.	Antirabies serum (ARS)	When ARS is indicated and the bite is less than 24 hours old, most or all of ARS should be infiltrated around the wounds.
4.	Other measures	Tetanus toxoid should be given if otherwise indicated. Antibiotics may be administered if wound appears unhealthy
Don'ts		
1.	No cauterization of the wound	
2.	No stitching of the wound. If stitching is unavoidable, infiltrate the ARS around the wound and then apply minimum of stitches	
3.	Wounds are best closed by secondary suture after proper cleansing and daily wound care for a week. Infection is much less of a problem when this is practised, and cosmetic end results are better.	
4.	No application of turmeric, chilly powder or oil over the wound	

by itself, can reduce the risk of infection from 60 percent to nearly 20 percent[6].

Rabies Prophylaxis

It consists of rabies vaccine with and without antirabies serum. Rabies prophylaxis in a given case is planned keeping in mind the type and site of bite, the condition and immunization status of the biting animal and whether the animal is available for observation for 10 days or not. Antirabies prophylaxis is indicated when the animal shows signs of rabies, when the animal is not available for observation, when laboratory tests of the brain of the biting animal have confirmed the diagnosis of rabies and when the patient is bitten unprovoked by a wild animal (Table 52.3). Prophylactic regimen once initiated may be discontinued if the biting animal remains healthy for 10 days during the period of observation. In case of doubt, it is advisable to give the prophylaxis rather than withhold it especially by using the safe tissue culture vaccines, which are being used even for pre-exposure immunisation.

Anti-rabies Serum

Passive immunization with anti-rabies serum combined with local treatment of wound and active immunization provides best protection to the exposed individual. Rabies immunoglobulin (RIG) should be given for all category III exposures, within 7 days of exposure[8]. It should be given in a single dose of 20 IU per kg of body weight for human RIG, and 40 IU per kg of body weight (maximum 3000 IU) for heterologous equine RIG, at the same time as the first dose of vaccine. The RIG should be infiltrated around and into the wound, even if the lesion has begun to heal. Care is needed when injecting into tissue compartment for example into the finger. Any remaining RIG should be injected intramuscularly at a site distant from the site of vaccine. If RIG is unobtainable when the first dose of vaccine is given, it may be given upto day 7 of bite[8]. The total recommended dose of RIG if insufficient to infiltrate in all the wounds, may be diluted with sterile saline 2 or 3 fold to permit thorough infiltration.

Serum sickness occurs in 1-6% of patients usually 7 to 10 days after injection of equine RIG. This complication has not been reported after treatment with human RIG. Skin testing may detect the rare case of IgE-mediated (Type 1) hypersensitivity to equine serum protein. However, the majority of reactions to equine RIG resulting from complement activation are not IgE mediated,

Table 52.3 Guidelines for rabies prophylaxis advocated by the WHO			
Category	**Type of contact with a suspected or confirmed rabid domestic or wild[a] animal, or animal unavailable for observation**	**Recommended treatment**	**Remarks**
I	Touching or feeding of animals and licks on intact skin	None, if reliable case history is available	Stop treatment if animal remains healthy throughout the
II	Nibbling of uncovered skin. Minor scratches or abrasions without bleeding. Licks over broken skin	Administer vaccine immediately[b]	observation period[c] of 10 days or if animal is killed humanely and found to be negative for rabies by appropriate laboratory techniques
III	Single or multiple transdermal bites or scratches with oozing of blood. Contamination of mucous membrane with saliva (i.e. licks)	Administer the anti-rabies serum as well as the vaccine immediately[b]	Stop treatment if animal remains healthy throughout the observation period[c] of 10 days or if animal is killed humanely and found to be negative for rabies by appropriate laboratory techniques

a.	Exposure to rodents, rabbits and hares seldom, if ever, require specific anti-rabies treatment.
b.	If an apparently healthy dog or cat from a low-risk area is placed under observation, the situation may warrant delaying initiation of treatment.
c.	This observation period applies only to dogs and cats. Except in the case of threatened or endangered species, other domestic and wild animals suspected as rabid should be killed humanely and their tissues examined using appropriate laboratory techniques. Treatment should be started as early as possible after exposure, but in no case should it be denied to exposed persons whatever time interval might have elapsed.

and cannot be predicted by skin testing[9]. A negative skin test does not rule out the occurrence of anaphylactic reaction. If the skin test is positive, treatment with human RIG should proceed. If the latter is not available special precautions should be taken while using the equine RIG (e.g. pretreatment with intramuscular adrenaline and antihistamine) and the patient should be observed for at least one hour after the injection[10].

Rabies Vaccine

The long incubation period of rabies provides a unique opportunity to give protection by active immunisation even after exposure to the infection. The currently available vaccines belong to two classes namely, the nervous tissue vaccines and the tissue culture vaccines. The avian embryo (duck/chicken) vaccines are out of vogue.

Nervous Tissue Vaccines

Nervous tissues vaccines are obtained from artificially infected brains of the sheep (sheep brain vaccine) or of the suckling mice (suckling mouse vaccine). In India, only the sheep brain vaccine is manufactured. This is a 5 percent emulsion of the infected sheep brain, the virus being inactivated by beta-propiolactone (BPL). The vaccine needs to be stored between 4°C to 10°C.

The Central Institute of Research, Kasauli and the Pasteur Institute, Conoor are the manufacturers of BPL-inactivated nervous tissue antirabies vaccines in India. The dose schedule recommended by these institutes are based on classification of exposure (Table 52.4). The vaccine is given subcutaneously into the abdominal wall using a long (37 mm) needle.

The vaccines prepared from the brain tissues of animals contain neuroparalytic factors like myelin. Neuroparalytic complications are common and occur in 1 in 4000 to 1 in 11,000 vaccinees. Children are less susceptible to these ill effects. Manifestations appear between 7 to 14 days after the first dose and are a consequence of acute demyelinating encephalomyelitis. Different clinical neurological syndromes may occur and they include

Table 52.4 Classification of bite and dose schedules of nervous tissue vaccines manufactured at Kasauli and Conoor

I	Classification of rabies exposure for deciding dose of nervous tissue vaccines
Class	**Characteristics**
I.	Slight or negligible exposure i.e. minimum risk and includes all cases of licks (except those on fresh cuts and abrasions with oozing of blood which may be considered as class II)
II.	Moderate exposure i.e. definite but moderate risk. All bites except those on the head, neck, face, palms and fingers and less than five wounds in number. Licks on fresh cuts and scratches with oozing of blood.
III.	Severe exposure i.e. definite and grave risk. Licks on mucosa, all bites on neck or above, palm and fingers. Lacerated wound/wounds anywhere on the body and multiple bites (5 or more wounds). Wolf, jackal and other wild animal bites. Class II exposure but delay of 14 days or more in seeking treatment.

II.	Dose schedules of nervous tissue rabies vaccines				
Vaccine and nature of exposure	**Adult dose**	**Pediatric dose (body wt <30 kg)**	**Route**	**Schedule**	**Booster(s)**
1. BPL Inactivated Vaccine (Central Research Institute, Kasauli)					
Class I	2 ml	2 ml	SC*	7 daily doses	Nil
Class II	5 ml	2 ml	SC*	14 daily doses	One dose 3 weeks or later after the 14th injection
Class III	5 ml	2 ml	SC*	14 daily doses	One dose 7 days after 14th dose. Second booster 2 weeks or later after the first booster.
2. BPL Inactivated Vaccine (Pasteur Institute, Conoor)					
Class I	2 ml	1 ml	SC*	7 daily doses	
Class II	3 ml	3 ml	SC*	10 daily doses	
Class III	5 ml	3 ml	SC*	10 daily doses	
* Subcutaneous in the anterior abdominal wall.					

mononeuritis multiplex, dorsolumbar transverse myelitis, ascending paralysis akin to Landry-Guillain-Barre syndrome, and acute meningo-encephalitis.

With the appearance of first manifestations of neuroparalytic reactions, the offending vaccine should be discontinued. If the risk of rabies warrants further vaccination, tissue culture vaccine may be given instead. Steroids are recommended for the management of neurotoxic manifestations. Mortality due to adverse reactions is 15 to 20 percent. Recovery usually takes 2-3 weeks but some survivors may have permanent neurological sequelae.

Tissue Culture Vaccines

Vaccines prepared in cell culture are highly immunogenic and virtually free of side effects. Three such vaccines are now widely available, namely, the human diploid cell strain vaccine (HDCs), purified chick embryo cell (PCEC) vaccine and purified vero cell vaccine (PVRV). They all have a potency of over 2.5 iu. per dose. In India PCEC is marketed as Rabipur (cost Rs.280/- per dose), PVRV as Verorab (cost Rs. 296/- per dose) and HDCs as MIRV [Merieux Inactivated Rabies Vaccine] (cost Rs. 995/- per dose).

The recommended dose schedule for post exposure prophylaxis is given in Table 52.5. The standard (Essen Protocol) schedule consists of five doses given by intramuscular route, on days 0, 3, 7, 14 and 30. The first dose must be given as soon as possible. The sixth dose, on day 90, is recommended in following victims:

(i) Those given passive immunization with RIG (category III bite)

(ii) Immunosuppressed due to any chemical, physical, pathological or physiological (old age) causes.

Injection should be given in the deltoid or in anterolateral part of the thigh (in children). The dosage schedule remains same for all age groups including neonates. *Gluteal region must not be used for administering the vaccine as the abundant fat in this region slows the absorption and delays the immune response.*

Two alternative schedules have also been found effective[8]. In the abbreviated multisite intramuscular schedule, the so called 2-1-1 regimen (or Zagreb protocol), one dose each of the tissue culture vaccine is given in the right and left deltoid muscle simultaneously (day 0), followed by one dose on day 7 and day 21. This schedule induces an early antibody response and is especially useful when the treatment does not include administration of antirabies serum. A low cost intradermal schedule (Thai Red cross group) is also reported to be effective. One dose (0.1ml) each of the vaccine is given at two sites (either forearm or upper arm), on days 0, 3 and 7. This is followed by a single intradermal dose at one site only on days 30 and 90. Separate syringe and needle should be used for each dose. Intradermal injection must, however, be given by the staff who are well trained in this technique. *If vaccine is inadvertently given into the subcutaneous tissue, it is likely to be ineffective.* The reconstituted vial should be stored at 4°C to 8°C and used as soon as possible.

Tissue culture vaccines have hardly any side effects. Local swelling, pain, erythema or induration may be encountered some times. Mild fever, myalgia, lymphadenopathy and allergic skin reactions are reported occasionally.

	Vaccine	Each dose*	Route+	Schedule**
Table 52.5 Post-exposure dosage schedule for tissue culture vaccines				
1.	Human Diploid Cell Vaccine (HDCV, MIRV)	1 ml	Intramuscular	Days 0, 3, 7, 14 and 30
2.	Purified Chick Embryo Cell Vaccine (PCEC, Rabipur)	1 ml	Intramuscular	Days 0, 3, 7, 14 and 30
3.	Purified Vero Cell Vaccine (PVRV, Verorab)	0.5 ml	Intramuscular	Days 0, 3, 7, 14 and 30

* All age groups
+ In the deltoid or anterolateral thigh (children). Never use the gluteal region and subcutaneous sites.
**Day 0 refers to the day on which the vaccination is started and not the day of exposure. An additional 6th dose on day 90 is considered optional.

Section 5

In case the vaccination is started with the nervous tissue vaccine in a patient, it is possible to shift to a tissue culture vaccine. However, full course of the latter needs to be given. Previously, ACIP recommended a 5-dose rabies vaccination regimen with human diploid cell vaccine (HDCV) or purified chick embryo cell vaccine (PCECV). The new recommendations reduce the number of vaccine doses to four. The reduction in doses recommended for PEP was based in part on evidence from rabies virus pathogenesis data, experimental animal work, clinical studies, and epidemiologic surveillance. These studies indicated that 4 vaccine doses in combination with rabies immune globulin (RIG) elicited adequate immune responses and that a fifth dose of vaccine did not contribute to more favorable outcomes. For persons previously unvaccinated with rabies vaccine, the reduced regimen of 4 doses of 1.0 ml HDCV or PCECV should be administered intramuscularly. The first dose of the 4-dose course should be administered as soon as possible after exposure (day 0). Additional doses should be administered on days 3, 7, and 14 after the first vaccination. ACIP recommendations for the use of RIG remain unchanged. For persons who previously received a complete vaccination series (pre- or postexposure prophylaxis) with a cell-culture vaccine or who previously had a documented adequate rabies virus-neutralizing antibody titer following vaccination with a noncell-culture vaccine, the recommendation for a 2-dose PEP vaccination series has not changed. Similarly, the number of doses recommended for persons with altered immunocompetence has not changed; for such persons, PEP should continue to comprise a 5-dose vaccination regimen with 1 dose of RIG. The immunosuppressive agents should be stopped during rabies PEP unless unavoidable. In these children serum should be examined for seroconversion rapid flourescent focus inhibition test (RFFJT) 1-2 weeks after completing PEP. Recommendations for pre-exposure prophylaxis also remain unchanged, with 3 doses of vaccine administered on days 0, 7, and 21 or 28. Prompt rabies PEP along with effective wound care, infiltration of RIG into and around the wound, and multiple doses of rabies cell-culture vaccine continue to be highly effective in preventing human rabies.

Post-exposure prophylaxis in a previously vaccinated person

Previously vaccinated persons include those individuals who have received 3-dose preexposure or postexposure series of HDCV or PLEV, within 2 years with a documented history of seroconversion. These individuals are administered two doses of vaccine on day 0 and day 3. There is no need to administer human rabies immune globulins (HRIG).

Important Considerations

Some important considerations regarding antirabies immuno-prophylaxis are listed below:

(i) Post-exposure prophylaxis is also indicated in bites due to cats, monkeys and mangoose.

(ii) It may be appropriate to double the first dose of vaccine (whatever schedule is used) in the following situations[10].

  (a) In patients who seek treatment after a delay of 48 hours or more.

  (b) In patients where RIG is indicated, but is unavailable.

  (c) In patients with underlying chronic disease (e.g. liver cirrhosis);

  (d) In patients who are congenitally immuno-deficient or suffering from Acquired Immuno Deficiency Syndrome (AIDS).

  (e) In patients taking immunosuppressive drugs (including corticosteroids and anti-malarials).

  (f) In the severely malnourished.

  (g) In case of patients at a particularly high risk of rabies (multiple wounds on and above neck and on other parts of the body supplied with many nerves)

(iii) The tissue culture vaccines can be safely given to pregnant/lactating women as well as to infants and children.

(iv) Antirabies vaccines are stored at 4°C to 8°C, and should not be stored in the freezer compartment.

(v) There have been 14 reported cases of rabies despite post-exposure vaccine treatment with cell culture vaccine. The "failures" are attributed to delay in starting prophylaxis (>72 hours), lack of anti-rabies serum therapy when it was indicated, injections at the gluteal site and poor host defences.

Pre-exposure Prophylaxis

Veterinarians, laboratory workers, animal handlers, wildlife officers, postmen, health personnel etc. are at a high risk of contracting rabies. They should be actively immunized with a tissue culture vaccine. The dosage schedule is given in Table 52.6. Two schedules have been recommended by WHO.

Vaccine	Dose	Route	Dose Schedule	
			Primary	Booster*
o Human diploid Cell vaccine (MIRV)	1 ml	Intramuscular	Days 0, 7 and 28	Every 1-3 years
o Purified chick-embryo cell vaccine (Rabipur)	1 ml	Intramuscular	Days 0, 7 and 28	Every 1-3 years
o Purified vero cell vaccine (Verorab)	0.5 ml	Intramuscular	Days 0, 7 and 28	Every 1-3 years

Table 52.6 Dose schedule for pre-exposure rabies prophylaxis[8]

* Serum sample should be tested for rabies virus-neutralizing antibodies every 6 months to 1 year. A booster should be administered when the titer falls below 0.5 iu/ml.

Three doses on day 0, 7 and 28 or on day 0, 28 and 56 followed by one booster after one year make up the schedule. The titer of neutralizing antibodies should be checked to assess the immune response after completion of the course. A titer of over 0.5 i.u. per ml should be maintained.

Immunisation of Animals

Pre-exposure immunisation of dogs, cats and domestic animals is mandatory. Dogs below 3 months and cats below 6 months do not mount an effective immune response. The vaccination should be delayed upto the appropriate age.

Veterinary antirabies vaccine

This is a 20 percent sheep brain suspension infected with modified rabies virus. The single primary vaccine is followed by boosters at 6 months and every year. The dose is 5 ml for dogs and 3 ml for cats[3].

Modified live virus vaccine

This is based on 33 percent chick embryo suspension infected with modified virus. A dose of 3 ml is given as a single injection with boosters every 3 years. Parenteral vaccine employing tissue culture lines and oral vaccine using monoclonal antibody technique have been tried recently[8].

Key Facts

o Rabies occurs in more than 150 countries and territories.

o Worldwide, more than 55,000 people die of rabies every year.

o 40% of people who are bitten by suspect rabid animals are children under 15 years of age.

o Dogs are the source of 99% of human rabies deaths.

o According to some estimates, approximately 5,00,000 people in India receive every year the post-exposure vaccination treatment that consists of 5 vaccine doses and costs Rs. 1500 (excluding the cost of general wound care, hospitalization and time away from work). According to MK Sudarshan's survey (2007) the full cost of post-exposure treatment of humans that have been bitten in India is $25 million.

o Wound cleansing and immunization within a few hours after contact with a suspect rabid animal can prevent the onset of rabies and death.

o Every year, more than 15 million people worldwide receive a post-exposure preventive regimen to avert the disease which is estimated to prevent 3,27,000 rabies deaths annually.

o Two forms of the disease can follow. People with furious rabies exhibit signs of hyperactivity, excited behaviour, hydrophobia and sometimes aerophobia. After a few days, death occurs by cardio-respiratory arrest.

o Paralytic rabies accounts for about 30% of the total number of human cases. This form of rabies runs a less dramatic and usually a prolonged course than the furious form. The muscles gradually become paralyzed, starting at the site of the bite or scratch. Coma slowly develops, and eventually death occurs. The paralytic form of rabies is often misdiagnosed, contributing to the under-reporting of the disease.

o Transmission can also occur when infectious material (usually saliva) comes into direct contact with human mucosa or fresh skin wounds. Human-to-human transmission by bite is theoretically possible but has never been confirmed.

Section 5

Treatment of Rabies[8]

Although rabies in humans almost inevitably ends in death, a few instances of recovery have been recorded. All these patients had received immediate post-exposure treatment. The diagnosis in these patients was based upon the demonstration of high levels of rabies virus- neutralizing antibodies in serum and spinal fluid but no rabies antigen was detected.

The following therapeutic measures have been tried in clinical rabies, but without any evidence of effectiveness. Administration of vidarabine; multisite intradermal vaccination with cell-culture vaccine, administration of alpha-interferon and rabies immunoglobulin by intravenous as well as intrathecal routes, administration of anti-thymocyte globulin, high doses of steroids, inosine pranobex, ribavirin and the antibody-binding fragments of rabies immunoglobulin G. Intensive medical care and assisted ventilation may prolong life by few days[11].

The clinical course of the disease, with either excitation or paralysis as the predominant symptom, is of short duration and entails much suffering. Patients remain conscious, often aware of the nature of their illness, and are usually extremely agitated, particularly when excitation is predominant. This is compounded by the fact that they become isolated because of the perceived risk of transmission of the disease to contacts. Although rabies transmission from person-to-person has never been documented it is theoretically possible because secretions may contain the virus. Nursing staff should, therefore, be informed of the potential risk of contamination (especially during intensive care) and should wear goggles, mask and gloves. Those with cuts or abrasions on skin should not be permitted to come in contact with the patient. Hand washing should be practiced. Attendants must avoid direct contact of their skin and mucous membranes with the saliva of the patient. The patient's clothes and utensils should be disinfected. Rabies prophylaxis is recommended to doctors, nurses and attendants who may have unwittingly come in contact with the secretions of a patient with rabies. It may, however, be mentioned that no authentic case of direct human-to-human transmission of rabies has been reported. If contamination does occur through the skin or mucous membranes, the nursing staff should receive post-exposure treatment. *However, there is a risk of transmission of rabies through corneal transplants. Therefore, organs of patients with any neurological disease should not be used for transplantation.*

Prevention

Stray animals are a public health problem in India and needs to be controlled by municipal health authorities and animal lovers. Pets should be looked after with utmost care and concern and effectively protected with vaccines. Children should be sensitized to develop a humane and compassionate attitude towards animals and provided with following basic safety tips to safeguard against bites by domestic and stray animals.

- Do not disturb any animal that is sleeping, eating or feeding her puppies.
- Do not approach or touch an unfamiliar animal.
- When an unfamiliar animal approaches, never run but be stoic and still.
- Never stare and run seeing a stray dog, instead look away and ignore him.
- Always allow the pet dog to see and sniff you before touching it.

SNAKEBITE

India and the South Asian countries constitute the majority of world snakebite deaths. Some of these countries have taken active interest by developing locally relevant protocols to overcome dependency on western textbooks for management of snake envenomation. All doctors should be aware of the best methods of treating snakebite in local settings. The national protocol for snakebite management, developed and approved by Government of India, has guidelines that are need based and do not blindly follow a foreign model. The international experts had a great role in developing this protocol. Emergency care for children in India with snake envenomation should not suffer due to misguided notions or policies on anti-snake venom (ASV). Ensuring availability of ASV and allocating resources in a sustainable manner to meet the wide spread demand are indeed important. With an acceptable standard of quality care and better evidence-based outcomes, wider dissemination and implementation of the national protocol is our immediate need[12].

Magnitude of the Problem

According to the 2008 Global Snakebite report, co-authored by Indian workers and WHO, the annual mortality due to snake bite is 5.6-12.6 per 100,000 population. According to a recent report by the American Society of Tropical Medicine and

Hygiene, more than 2.5 lakh cases of snake bites occur in India leading to 46,000 deaths every year. The statistics are shocking because India is neither home to the largest number of snakes in the world nor there is a shortage of anti-venom (AV). A 28-member National Protocol Development Group (NPDG) was created by Ministry of Health and Family Welfare, Government of India to provide national guidelines for rational management of snake bites. The national snake bite management protocol was approved and published by MOH and ICMR in 2006. It is important to understand that almost 70% of snake bites are caused by non-venomous species. And even when a bite is caused by a poisonous snake, in almost half the cases it is a ''dry bite'' i.e. no venom is injected. Many a deaths due to snake bites can be prevented by following the correct first aid method of ''Do it Right'' and following the treatment guidelines provided in the national protocol[13-16].

Types of Snakes and their Venom

The symptomatology due to snake bite is termed as ophitoxemia. In India, venomous snakes fall into two categories, defined by their venom action and the symptoms manifested by the bite.

Neurotoxic: Cobra and Kraits, whose venom acts on the central nervous system.

Anti-hemostatic: Vipers and Pit vipers, where the venom attacks the blood and circulatory systems.

India is rich in snake fauna and it is impossible for other than an experienced herpetologist to recognize and identify all possible snakes. Snake taxonomy is a complex process and color is the least reliable means of identification as most species have a wide color range. In India almost two-third of bites are by Saw-scaled viper, about one-fourth by Russel's viper and smaller proportions by cobra and kraits.

Mechanism of Action of Neurotoxic Venom

Normally, when the brain signals a muscle to contract, an impulse passes down the nerve to the neuromuscular junction where acetylcholine is released which crosses the synaptic gap, attaches to the receptor cells, allowing the signal to continue to the muscle to enable it to contract. Neurotoxic venom interferes with this process by two mechanisms.

All Indian cobra venoms produce alpha-bungarotoxin which acts post synaptically. This means that the venom attaches to the receptors at

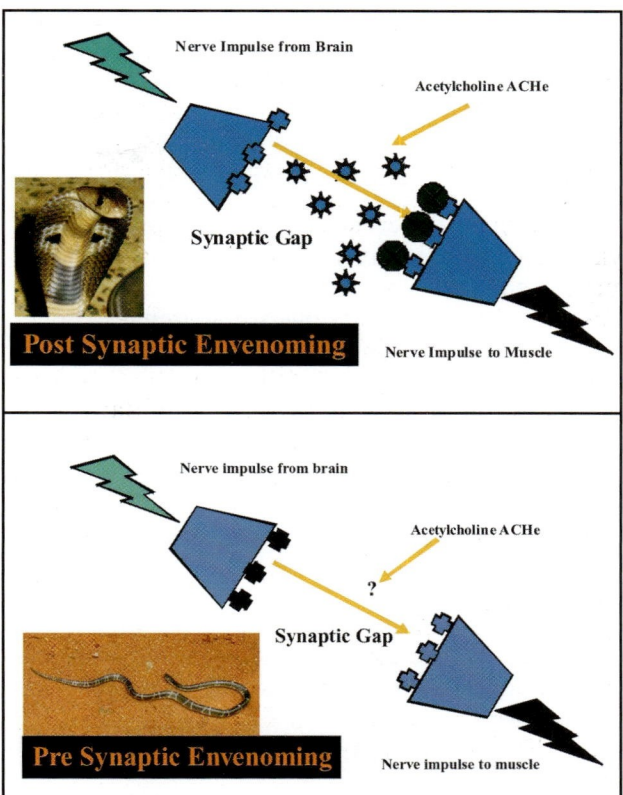

Figure 52.1 Post- and pre-synaptic neurotoxic envenoming due to cobra and krait bites

the muscle side of the neuromuscular junction, thus blocking them so that the acetylcholine cannot attach thus preventing the signal from the brain reaching the muscle (Figure 52.1). Krait species produce a venom containing beta-bungarotoxin which is pre-synaptic in its action and destroys the synaptic vesicles on the brain side of the junction which are responsible for the production of acetylcholine.

In both cases, the toxic effect is the same, leading to descending paralysis, starting with the facial muscles and descending to involve the diaphragm, the main muscle which controls breathing. It is important to remember that respiratory arrest rarely follows instantly after a bite as the venom takes time to circulate and bind. Also there may be insufficient venom to block or destroy all the cells. However, once drooping of eyelids is observed (ptosis), consideration must be given to the possibility of imminent respiratory arrest and arrangements made for assisted ventilation. In krait envenomation pupils may be dilated, fixed and non-reactive simulating brainstem death.

A neurotoxic victim may be completely paralysed and appear dead but it is crucial to remember that if neurotoxic victim can be kept alive by assisted ventilation, the body will eventually

Section 5

unblock or lead to recovery of the affected cells spontaneously. Anti-snake venom (ASV) will neutralize the venom in the blood stream and neostigmine can prolong the half life of acetycholine molecules so that they have a greater chance of finding and binding to the receptor cells.

The main difference between a post and pre-synaptic neurotoxic envenomation is significant only during recovery. In cobra victims, recovery of consciousness can be very quick upto minutes, hours or days, depending on how much venom has been injected and how quickly the neostigmine was administered after the bite. In krait victims, recovery may take several days, or weeks as the body has to repair the damaged synaptic vesicles before the paralysis ceases and the victim could breathe without support.

Neostigmine Test

In case of neurotoxic envenomation, the 'Neostigmine Test' should be administered.[17-20] This test involves administration of neostigmine (0.04 mg/kg) IM, along with intravenous atropine (0.05 mg/kg).

The patient should be closely observed for one hour to assess the effect of neostigmine. The following observations are useful for objective assessment.

1. Single breath count.
2. Severity of ptosis (mm of iris uncovered by the eyelid).
3. Inter-incisor distance (Distance between the upper and lower incisors).
4. Length of time that the upward gaze can be maintained
5. FEV 1 or FVC (If available).

The aforementioned parameters should be assessed every 10 minutes. The beneficial effects of neostigmine are likely to be evident within 20-30 minutes. If the victim responds to the neostigmine test, it should be continued in a dose of 0.5 mg of neostigmine IM every half hourly along with 0.6 mg of atropine IV every 8 hour by continuous infusion. If there is no improvement in the neurological symptoms after one hour, the neostigmine should be stopped.

Some authors have suggested that it may be possible to treat patients with anticholinesterase drugs alone, in the case of elapid bites. However, this approach ignores the value of neutralizing the free flowing venom by anti-snake venom before it can attach and cause the damage.

Mechanism of Action of Anti-hemostatic Venom

Anti-hemostatic venoms also act in two ways both of which are likely to occur in viper bites. The venom neutralizes the clotting factors in the blood so that it becomes thin and watery (incoagulable) and profuse bleeding occurs through blood vessels which are damaged by other constituents of the venom (Figure 52.2).

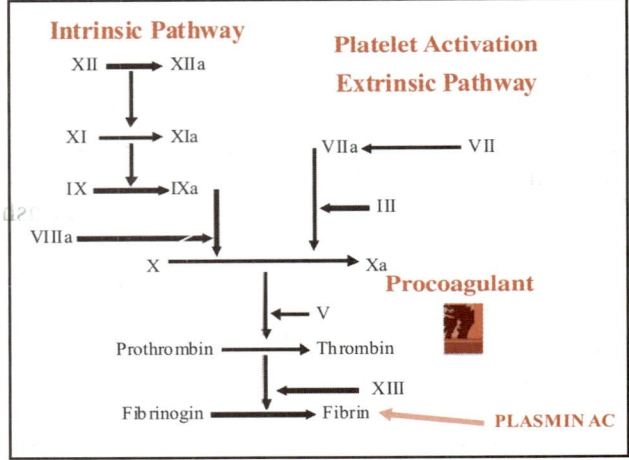

Figure 52.2 Clotting abnormalities due to viper bite

The venom travels through the blood and the lymphatic system and can cause bleeding and bruising away from the bite site. Bleeding is normally first observed from the gums and this is a clear sign that the victim has actually been envenomed. Bleeding can also be observed from the nose and previous wounds or bite site.

Life-threatening internal bleeding may occur. Stomach ache, hematemesis, blood in the urine or stools are all potential signs of serious internal bleeding. Intracranial bleeding is suspected by evidences of raised intracranial pressure, alteration in consciousness, limb paralyses or changes in the size of pupils and their inequality. Severe bleeding may cause hypotension, reduced renal perfusion and acute renal failure as evidenced by back ache, reduced urine output or anuria. The victims of viper bites (Russell's viper and Humped nose Pit viper) can die of shock and its consequences due to intractable bleeding[18-20].

A 20-minute whole bleed clotting test (20 WBCT) is done to assess whether victim has been envenomed and therefore needs ASV. The test must be done in a new clean and dry glass container, and take only 20 minutes as the name suggests. Anti-snake venom (ASV) neutralizes circulating venom in the blood but cannot reverse the necrosis or swelling at the site of bite. After administration of

ASV when all the venom has been neutralized, the body is likely to take about 6 hours to restore synthesis of clotting factors in the liver.

Reassure the Victim

It is important to keep the victim of snake bite as calm and relaxed as possible because panic may lead to neurogenic shock and tachycardia and rise in blood pressure may facilitate spread of venom through blood stream. The victim should be told that majority of snake bites occur by non-venomous species and even if a bite is caused by a venomous snake, it is likely to be a "dry bite" in almost one-half the cases. The common practice of cutting or enlarging the bite wound or sucking the venom is condemned. It is not effective and may cause super-added bacterial infection. There is no need to wash or dress the bite wound or apply any ointment or home made paste.

The bitten limb should be kept immobilized or splinted (like a fracture) to delay the absorption or venom. The victim should be carried and not allowed to walk. *The common practice of applying a tight bandage or a tourniquet above the site of bite is no longer recommended.* It may aggravate tissue damage at the bite site and ischemic damage to the limb or digits (even gangrene) if bandage is too tight or it is not released intermittently. At times when tourniquet is suddenly released at the hospital, it may cause excessive bleeding from the bite wound or lead to sudden surge of venom into blood stream with adverse effects.

Take the victim to the hospital

The victim must be taken to the nearest hospital as soon as possible. *No time should be wasted in giving folk remedies because they have no proven benefit.* The outcome of snake bite depends on how soon the supportive therapy and specific anti-snake venom (ASV) is given to the victim. A delay of few hours may prove fatal.

Supportive Care

Assess the vital signs, adequacy of breathing, circulation and CNS status. Pain, worry and anxiety should be allayed by administration of an appropriate opioid analgesic and sedative.

ABC approach is crucial to support Airway, Breathing and Circulation.

Intravenous Ringers' lactate or normal saline should be started to maintain circulation. Excessive bleeding should be managed by administration of fresh blood transfusion. Tetanus toxoid should be administered if indicated. Superadded bacterial infection should be treated by appropriate antibiotics by covering both Gram-positive and Gram-negative pathogens.

Anti-snake venom (ASV) Therapy

Anti-snake venom should be administered as soon as envenomation is established. Early administration of ASV is life saving because it promptly neutralizes the venom in the blood stream[19-24]. There are a number of misconceptions about ASV which are clarified below.

1. ASV neutralizes circulating venom in the blood stream. It cannot unlock the venom which is tagged to the receptors or tissues. Earlier the ASV is given, better are the chances of recovery. It may be difficult to save the snake bite victim if it reports to the hospital after 2-3 days.

2. Most cases of snake bite in India need 8-10 vials of ASV[12]. Large doses of ASV in excess of 30 vials (anti-hemostatic viper bites) and 20 vials in neurotoxic bites (cobra and krait) are unnecessary. The snakes can inject only a certain amount of venom to the victims, therefore, the dose of ASV is identical whether the victim is a neonate, child or an adult.

3. ASV should be administered only when envenomation has been clearly established either by presence of neurotoxic symptoms or abnormalities in the 20 WBCT[19-22]. ASV should be used judiciously because it is not only scarce but it may cause severe allergic reactions. After administration of ASV, the victim should be closely watched for 30 minutes. The allergic manifestations can be treated by temporarily withholding ASV and by administration of adrenaline 0.01 mg/kg IM.

4. ASV is available as freeze dried powder and is reconstituted with 10 ml normal saline or dextrose. It is given as IV infusion at 20 ml/kg per hour which is gradually slowed down.

5. ASV is species specific and it is more effective in snake bites in the southern parts because bulk of ASV in India is produced from the venom of snakes "milked" in Tamil Nadu.

6. In case of poor response to ASV, the same dose can be repeated after one hour in

neurotoxic and after six hours in hemotoxic envenomation.

Tell-tale Signs

It is crucial for the treating doctor to know what time the victim was bitten and which snake was responsible for the bite. The victim or observers should kill or catch the snake and take it to the hospital in a secure box / bag just in case it is not dead! It is important to note the time of onset of symptoms by watching the victim carefully.

1. Check for drooping eyelids, difficulty in speaking and swallowing or dribbling.
2. Double vision or diplopia.
3. Difficulty in breathing.
4. The taste of blood in the mouth.
5. Bruising or bleeding away from the bite site.
6. The rate of progress of any swelling mark by noting its time of onset and extent on the skin with a pen every 10 minutes.
7. In particular, watch for any evidence when the victim cannot hold up his / her head, as this can be a sign of imminent respiratory failure and you may have to give artificial respiration during the journey if the victim is to reach the hospital alive.

Assisted Ventilation

Most snake bite deaths due to cobra or krait can be prevented by providing artificial breathing till victim reaches the hospital. Airway should be kept patent and free from any secretions. Mouth-to-mouth resuscitation or assisted breathing with an Ambu bag can be provided at the site of bite or during transport to the hospital. All attempts should be made to keep the victim alive till he/she is transported to the nearest health care facility. Refer to Chapter 57 for technical details for providing mouth-to-mouth resuscitation and assisted ventilation with a bag and mask. Every Sub-center and Primary Health Center in the country must be equipped with functional first aid equipment for assisted ventilation and health care professionals should be adequately trained to provide effective artificial breathing.

Complications

Apart from venom-related neurotoxic (cobra, krait) and hemostatic manifestations (Russel's viper, Saw scaled viper), the victims are likely to have a large number of complications as listed below.

(i) Panic, anxiety and neurogenic shock.

(ii) Marked edema and bleeding at the site of bite (viper).
(iii) Respiratory paralysis.
(iv) Hypotension, shock and cardiac arrest.
(v) Bleeding manifestations due to hemotoxins and disseminated intravascular coagulation (DIC).
(vi) Acute kidney injury (AKI).
(vii) Acute respiratory distress syndrome (ARDS).
(viii) Superadded bacterial infection at the site of bite, tetanus and septicemia.

OTHER ANIMAL AND INSECT BITES

SCORPION STING

Scorpion stings are a major public health problem in many tropical and subtropical countries like Africa, South India, the Middle East, Mexico, and South Latin America. Out of 1.2 million stings per year, 3250 people die (0.27%)[25]. Number of deaths from scorpion sting are 10 times greater compared to the poisonous snake bite deaths. About 30-50% fatality due to acute pulmonary edema with scorpion sting has been reported from India before the use of prazosin. Hence the proper and early management of a child with scorpion sting is imperative in the emergency department which can help us to save precious lives.

Pathogenesis

The most important clinical effects of envenomation are neuromuscular, neuroautonomic, or local tissue effects caused by potent neurotoxin. The primary targets of scorpion venom are voltage-dependent ion channels, of which sodium channels are the best studied[26]. Venom toxins alter these channels, leading to prolonged neuronal activity. Many end-organ effects are secondary to this excessive excitation. Autonomic excitation leads to severe cardiopulmonary effects[27-28]. Somatic and cranial nerve hyperactivity results from neuromuscular overstimulation. Children exhibit severe reactions because of larger ratio of venom to the body weight.

History and Examination

Ask for the time of the sting, nature of the event (number of stings, site), local symptoms and systemic manifestations. The duration of progress to systemic symptoms ranges from 5 minutes to 4 hours after the sting. The symptoms generally persist for 10-48 hours. The following features are commonly seen.

1. Local tissue effects like edema, redness, tenderness, ascending hyperesthesia (appears by first 4 hours).

2. Signs of parasympathetic dysfunction include hypotension, bradycardia, excessive sweating, salivation, lacrimation, urination, defecation, priapism[27], and gastric emptying. Sweating and salivation persists for 6-13 hours[29].

3. Signs of sympathetic dysfunction include tachycardia, S_3 gallop, arrhythmias, hypertension, hyperthermia, features of pulmonary edema, cool extremities (inotropic phase → hypovolemic phase) which persists for 24 to 72 hours. Pulmonary edema can develop within ½ to 3 hours after the sting due to myocardial dysfunction.

4. Cranial nerve effects such as difficulty in swallowing, nystagmus, blurring of vision and fasciculations.

5. Restlessness and involuntary jerky movements, seizures, altered consciousness, cerebral thrombosis, thalamus induced systemic paresthesia, hemiplegia and aphasia.

During recovery stage (48-72 hr) hypotension can be seen; but the extremities will be warm with good volume pulse and child will be otherwise well[29]. This state, due to an exhausted catecholamine stores awaiting replenishment, requires no intervention with dopamine agonists.

Investigations

(a) Blood sugar (to look for hyperglycemia) and electrolytes if there is excessive salivation, sweating, vomiting and diarrhea are present.

(b) ECG to look for sinus tachycardia, ST segment elevation in V1, tall T waves in V2 to V6, prolonged QTc, left ventricular hypertrophy (by voltage criterion S-wave in V1 plus R-wave in V5 > 35 mm), ventricular repolarisation abnormalities and bundle branch block.

(c) X-ray chest if features of pulmonary edema are present.

(d) Creatine kinase and urine analysis to look for rhabdomyolysis.

(e) 2D ECHO to look for diffuse global biventricular hypokinesis with a decreased left and right ventricular ejection fraction. This dysfunction can appear just a few hours after the sting and usually normalizes within 4-8 days. ECHO is not required in the emergency management of scorpion bite.

Management of Scorpion Sting

General Measures

1. Maintain airway, assess breathing and circulation. Keep the child in propped up position, and administer oxygen if needed. Intubation and ventilator support should be given to deliver required PEEP if severe features of pulmonary edema are present.

2. Local treatment for pain by using ice packs, local anesthetics like xylocaine 2%, oral diazepam 0.1-0.3 mg/kg/dose, NSAIDs like paracetamol or ibuprofen. Morphine should be avoided as narcotics worsen arrhythmias. Those with severe local pain have less cardiovascular manifestations.

3. Monitor heart rate, respiratory rate, blood pressure, look for S_3 gallop, basal crepts every ½ hourly for first 3 hours, every hourly for next 4 hours and then every 4 hourly till improvement is seen.

4. Ensure administration of adequate oral fluids to the child. Give maintenance intravenous fluids (N/5) if needed to prevent hypovolemia due to vomiting, diarrhea, sweating, hyper-salivation, and insensible water loss.

Specific pharmacotherapy

Prazosin

In children with features of autonomic storm, Prazosin is the main stay of treatment which is a competitive alpha-1 adrenoreceptor antagonist.[30,31] It should always be available in the emergency department and should be given as early as possible to reduce the gap between the sting and first dose of prazosin which determines the outcome. Prazosin suppresses sympathetic outflow and activates venom-inhibited potassium channels. It decreases the preload, afterload and blood pressure without increasing the heart rate. Prazosin counters vasoconstriction induced by endothelins through accumulation of cyclic GMP (cGMP). It also inhibits phosphodiesterase enzyme.

Prazosin is available as 1 mg tablets and the dose is 30 µg/kg/dose oral. Whenever there is evidence of autonomic hyperactivity, it should be given immediately. If the child vomits, then it can be given through a nasogastric tube and intake of plenty of oral fluids should be encouraged. Sudden standing or lifting the child abruptly should be avoided to prevent first dose phenomenon[29]. Dose should be repeated after 3 hours and then every 6 hourly

Section 5

till signs of improvement are seen like warm extremities and reduced tachycardia.

If the child is restless, oral or intravenous diazepam 0.1-0.3 mg/kg can be given. It also alleviates the toxin's ability to stimulate specific ion channel.

Management of pulmonary edema

For severe cardiovascular changes like pulmonary edema with or without hypotension, aim is to reduce the afterload without affecting the preload. Intravenous furosemide 1-3 mg/kg can be given if the child is not hypovolemic. Start on inotropic support like dobutamine 6-20 µg/kg/min with afterload reducing agent like nitroglycerine (0.5-5 µg/kg/min) if there is decompensated shock[32] or sodium nitroprusside infusion (0.3-5 µg/kg/min) if there is normal blood pressure or hypertension or compensated shock. When the child is on infusion with nitroprusside or nitroglycerine, proper monitoring for the signs of improvement or worsening should be looked for like oxygenation, BP, work of breathing, heart rate and hepatomegaly. Infusion rates should be titrated with the clinical response. Administer prazosin 1 hour before stopping the infusion.

Scorpion antivenin

Mono specific F(ab)2 antivenom serum prepared by immunizing horses is available for clinical use from Haffkine Biopharma Mumbai, since 2002[33]. Mesobuthus tamulus is common in the Western Maharashtra, Saurashtra, Kerala, Andhra Pradesh, Tamil Nadu, and Karnataka states of India. Two randomised controlled trials have shown that it is useful in critically ill children with neurotoxicity[34] and fast recovery occurs when given along with prazosin[33]. More clinical trial results are awaited. The common Do's and Don'ts in the management of scorpion sting are given in the Box.

SPIDER BITES

Most spiders are not particularly dangerous to humans, lacking either potent venom or fangs capable of penetrating human skin. Arachnidism is the envenomation caused by a spider bite. The venomus spider species found in India are Loxosceles and Latrodectus.

Widow spider (Latrodectus species)

Female of this species have a body that measures 1.5 cm in length and a leg span around 4-5 cm. Males of this species are approximately 30%

Common do's and don'ts in the management of scorpion sting	
Do's	**Don'ts**
❖ Administer prazosin as soon as possible in autonomic storm.	❖ Do not give morphine to alleviate pain.
❖ Monitor vital signs and oxygenation.	❖ Do not use atropine and steroids.
❖ In pulmonary edema use dobutamine with SNP infusion.	❖ Do not give ACE inhibitors.
❖ In decompensated shock try nitro-glycerine infusion.	❖ Do not administer antivenin without skin testing

the size of female and pose no threat to humans because their fangs are too short to penetrate the skin. A bite by female spider is known as latrodectism. Latrodectus mactans commonly found in North America and Europe is not found in India. However, other Latrodectus species do occur which have more or less similar clinical effects. The poisoning is due to neurotoxic venom (alpha latrotoxin) that leads to continuous release of acetylcholine and norepinephrine at the presynaptic junction.

Clinical manifestations. The bite is like a pin prick and has characteristic twin red-spots with slight swelling. Local pain gradually becomes severe. In about 30 minutes the venom exerts powerful toxic effects. The manifestations include sweating, vomiting, tachypnea, tachycardia and hypertension. The hallmark is the appearance of repetitive muscular spasms, especially of the abdominal musculature. The abdomen is characteristically board like mimicking an acute abdomen. Severe envenomation leads to shock, delirium, coma and death in 4 to 5 percent cases. Children tend to manifest more severe effects.

Treatment. The mainstay of management is the maintenance of airway, breathing and circulation. Wound debridement and tetanus prophylaxis are essential. Cold packs and analgesics help in relieving pain. In more severe cases opioids can be used. Muscle relaxants such as methocarbamol and diazepam have been used. Calcium gluconate 10%, 0.1 to 0.2 ml/kg IV have traditionally been used for the relief of muscle spasms. It has been found relatively ineffective when compared with intravenous opioids and benzodiazpines. Antihypertensive medications should be given if hypertension does not respond to pain relief and muscle relaxation. Latrodectus antivenin is rapidly effective and curative but it is not available in India.

Brown Recluse spider (Loxosceles species, voilin or brown fiddle black spider)

This is a nocturnal hunter who can live for months without food and water. It is typically non-aggressive except when attacked or trapped. The female is more dangerous than the male. The venom is a complex mixture of cytotoxins of which sphingomylinase-D seems to be the most important.

Clinical manifestations. The clinical course after a bite is fairly predictable. The bite may be moderately painful but often goes unnoticed. Within 30-60 minutes after the bite, there is burning and pruritus at the local site. After becoming erythematous, indurated and painful, a hemorrhagic blister is formed within hours of the bite. As the blister sloughs, it leaves a necrotic enlarging ulcer, which is especially prominent when skin overlying areas of high fat content, such as the thighs and buttocks is affected. Systemic symptoms include fever, chills, nausea, vomiting, a generalized scarlatiniform rash, and arthralgias. Hemolysis, disseminated intravascular coagulation and renal failure may complicate the clinical course and may be life-threatening especially in small children.

Treatment. Accepted mainstay of treatment includes appropriate tetanus prophylaxis and frequent cleansing and dressing of the wound. Diphenhydramine 5 mg/kg/day orally with a maximum dose of 25-30 mg every 6 hours is effective in relieving pruritus. To reduce necrosis, dapsone[35] or colchicine[36], have been recommended. The victims should be tested for G6PD deficiency prior to dapsone therapy. The use of steroids and excision of the bite is controversial. An antivenin is under development.

HYMENOPTERA STINGS

Hymenopterous insects include bees, wasps, hornets, ants, etc.

BEES AND WASPS

Of all the bees, the worker honey bees and the bumble bee sting in defence. Commonly it is the swarm of bees which attack together. Honey bees sting only once, since the inserted stings get stuck to the wound, whereas bumble bee stings repeatedly. Several allergens found in bee venom include dopamine, histamine, phospholipase A_2, hyaluronidase, apamin (neurotoxin), acid phosphatase, allergen c and adolapin. Meletin account for 50% of the venom and cause tissue damage, pain, hemolysis and rhabdomyolsis. Histamine is present in concentrations as high as 1.5%.

Wasps in India belong to two species, Vespa species which are large and red or yellow in color, and Polistes which are small and honey yellow in color. The wasp venom is different from bee venom. In addition to phospholipase A_2, hyaluronidase and acid phosphatase, it is also known to contain antigen 5, mast cell degranulating peptide and kinin. The non-allergic direct effects of hymenopteran stings usually consists of severe pain, itching, local wheal and intense induration. The manifestations of hypersensitivity reaction may be alarming. Even a single sting may produce urticaria, laryngeal edema, bronchospasm and anaphylactic shock in a hypersensitive individual. Rarely, Bell's palsy, optic neuritis, polyneuropathy and myasthenia gravis may follow a sting. Massive honey bee envenomation may lead to life-threatening rhabdomyolysis, renal insufficiency and multi-organ dysfunction[37].

Treatment. The sting, if visible should be removed with a pointed needle or knife blade, taking care not to press the sting releasing more venom. Removal of sting is beneficial if done immediately after the sting because venom is absorbed into the circulation within one minute of sting. Non-allergic manifestations can be satisfactorily treated with local cooling, application of soothing lotions (calamine) or an anesthetic cream. Oral analgesic and antihistamine may be given for relief of pain and itching. Anaphylactic manifestations demand immediate administration of adrenaline (0.01 ml/kg of 1: 1000 solution intramuscularly) which can be repeated after 20-30 minutes. Pharyngeal edema may occur due to stings of swallowed honey bees. Occasionally, steroids, endotracheal intubation, assisted ventilation, parenteral fluids and vasopressors may be needed as life-saving measures. Diphenhydramine, prednisolone and aminophylline may be necessary.

Skin testing and hyposensitization is indicated in victims of hypersensitivity due to hymenopteran stings. A delayed reaction may appear 1-2 weeks after the sting characterised by fever, malaise, headache, polyarthritis and lymphadenopathy.

Section 5

Children with more than one sting per kg body weight should be kept under extended observation upto 24 hours after envenomation.

ANTS

A large variety of distinct groups of ants exist, each with different toxins and allergens. The majority of the ant stings are only slightly painful and just pruritic. However, the fire ant's bite can result both in localized and systemic reactions. Fire ants are named for the burning pain inflicted by their sting. They vary in color from dark red to brown or black. Although the mandibles are used for grasping (biting), the venom is introduced with a 0.5 to 1.0 mm stinger extruded from the abdomen. Unlike bees and wasps, fire ants sting slowly, injecting their venom over seconds to minutes. Fire ant stings are usually not immediately painful[38]. They have a necrotizing toxin, solenamine, which is neurotoxic and hemolytic in nature.

Clinical Manifestations[38]

Local. Pain is followed by appearance of pruritic wheal and flare. A characteristic pustule develops within 24 hours. Large local reactions are defined as painful, pruritic swelling at least 5 cm in diameter and are contiguous with the sting bite.

Systemic manifestations include hypotension, respiratory difficulty, upper airway edema, angioedema, urticaria, gastrointestinal distress, stridor, syncope and pruritus. Life-threatening systemic reactions usually involve cardiovascular and/or respiratory systems.

Treatment. Application of cold compresses may help to relieve the swelling and discomfort. The risk of secondary infection can be reduced by cleansing sting sites with soap and water and applying local antiseptics. Oral or topical antihistamines may relieve pruritus and reduce edema. Large local reactions may be treated with oral corticosteroids, oral H_2 antagonists, and analgesics. Cutaneous and systemic reactions can be managed with oral or injectable antihistamines. More severe reactions necessitate immediate intramuscular injection of 0.3 to 0.5 ml of 1:1000 solution of epinephrine, repeated at 10-minute intervals if necessary. Anaphylactic manifestations are treated as in case of bee envenomation.

BEETLES

These are non-biting insects causing local irritation through their secretions (body fluids). The blister beetle (the commonest being Spanish fly,

Lytta vescicatoria) contains the toxic principle cantharidin, concentrated mostly in the genitalia. Body contact with this produces the typical blistering dermatitis. The Rover beetle toxin contains pederin and its derivatives which produces the typical whiplash dermatitis.

Clinical features. Both the toxins are dermal irritants and vesicants. Ocular exposure may cause conjunctivitis, keratitis, iritis and edema. Ingestion may cause severe irritation, excoriation of the mucosa, blistering and necrosis of the upper GI tract. Nausea, vomiting, diarrhea, salivation, abdominal pain, tenesmus and GI hemorrhage may occur. Strangury and hematuria may occur. In severe cases hypotension, ventricular arrhythmias, respiratory depression and kidney damage may occur.

Treatment is mainly supportive. No specific antidote is available. Emesis should not be induced. Severe cases may need respiratory and cardiovascular support. For local treatment, application of antihistamine or corticosteroid ointment is recommended for a few days.

LIZARD BITE

There are two venomous species of lizards (the Gila monster, Heloderma suspectum and the Mexican beaded lizard, Heloderma horridum). Bites by them are infrequent and usually occur following attempts to capture or handle them. These are not found in India. No specific treatment is required for lizard bites.

CATERPILLAR

Caterpillars are larval stage of butterflies and moths. More than 50 species possess specialized hairs containing venom. These get scattered by wind and on dermal contact leads to localized dermatitis of urticarial type, manifested by severe pain, erythema and papular eruptions. Ocular contact causes conjunctivitis and inhalation leads to respiratory disturbances. Other features are nausea, vomiting, shock and convulsions. Treatment, apart from local decontamination with water and removal of hair, includes local application of antihistaminic. Occasionally parenteral antihistaminics and calcium gluconate are required for systemic manifestations.

CENTIPEDE BITES

Centipede bites are seldom serious. Venom produces local pain and swelling. Symptomatic treatment is all that is necessary. Centipedes are known to traverse narrow body passages especially ear canal, posing serious difficulty in their extraction.

RAT BITE FEVER

Two organisms, namely *Spirillum minor* and *Streptobacillus moniliformis*, introduced through the bite of an infected rat may produce an acute illness. Clinical manifestations include maculopapular skin rash, relapsing fever, arthritis and lymphadenitis. Infection with *S. minor* causes fever, induration, swelling, ulceration at the site of bite, lymphadenopathy and skin rash occurring days to weeks after the primary wound has healed (Sodoku). Penicillin is the drug of choice. Tetracycline can be given if patient is allergic to penicillin. There is no need for anti-rabies prophylaxis following rat bite.

CAT SCRATCH DISEASE

It is a benign, non bacterial suppurative lymphadenitis following a lick or scratch by a kitten or cat. The causative agent is possibly a Chlamydiae-like organism *B. henselae*. The disease affects children and young adults. A primary painless, non-pruritic skin lesion develops at scratch site after 3-5 days. In 2 week's time regional lymph nodes enlarge and caseate. These may persist for several months but eventually show resolution. Rarely, fever, malaise, anorexia and weight loss may occur. A positive skin test (Hanger-Rose test) helps in the diagnosis. Specific serological tests are also available. The disease is self-limited. An occasional case may need aspiration of lymph nodes and oral azithromycin or parenteral gentamicin therapy.

PAPULAR URTICARIA

This is a manifestation of bites due to several insects and is peculiar to the first decade of life. It represents as a delayed hypersensitivity reaction. The lesions are localized to the trunk and extensor surfaces of the extremities. They consist of hyperpigmented papulo-nodular eruptions which begin as a wheal with a central punctum. Pruritis is intense. The appearance of new lesions is associated with flaring up of the apparently quiescent lesions. An attempt should be made to identify the offending insect (usually fleas, mosquitoes, mites etc.) and adequate precautions taken to protect the child against them. Treatment is symptomatic, consisting of antipruritic agents, soothing lotions and topical steroid ointment in patients with intense lesions.

REFERENCES

1. Ahuja S, Misra CN, Saxena SN. Rabies and its control. *Indian Pediatr* 1984; 21:105-111.

2. Sehgal S, Bhatia R. Rabies: Epidemiology, Prinicples of Control and Treatment. *National Institute of Communicable Diseases, Delhi,* 1992.

3. Park JE, Park K. Rabies. In: Textbook of Preventive and Social Medicine, *Jabalpur, Bhanot Publishers* 1997; 207-214.

4. Lentz TL, Burrage TG, Smith AL, Crick J, Tignor GH. Is acetylcholine receptor a rabies virus receptor? *Science* 1982; 215:182-184.

5. Sayre MP, Lucid EJ. Viral infections in the emergency department. In: Principles and Practice of Emergency Medicine. Schwartz GR, Cayton CG, Manglesen MA, Mayer TA, Hanke BK (eds.). *Lea and Febiger; Philadelphia,* 1992; pp 1857-1872.

6. Sehgal S, Bhatia R. Rabies. *Gonway Printers Bombay;* July 1992.

7. Koch FJ, Sagartz JW , Davidson DE, *et al.* Diagnosis of human rabies by cornea test. *Amer J Clin Pathol* 1975; 63:509-515.

8. Use of a reduced (4-dose) vaccine schedule for post exposure prophylaxis to prevent human rabies. MMWR Recommndations and reports 2010:59-RR2.

9. Wilde H, Sirikawin S, Sabcharoen A, *et al.* Rabies post exposure treatment failures in canine rabies in endemic Asian countries. *Clin Infect Dis* 1996; 22:228-232.

10. Gode GR, Jayalakshmi RS, Rajiv AV, *et al.* Intensive care in rabies therapy: clinical observations. *Lancet* 1976; 2:6-8.

11. National Snakebite Management Protocol (India), 2008 *Indian J Emerg Pediatr* 2009:1 (2) 63-84.

12. Lim BL. Venomous land snakes of Malaysia. In: Snakes of Medical Importance - Asia-Pacific Region. Chou LM, Gopalkrishnakone P, (Eds.) *National of University of Singapore;* 1990:387-417.

13. Looareesuwan S, Viravan C, Warrell DA. Factors contributing to fatal snake bite in the rural tropics: analysis of 46 cases in Thailand. *Trans R Soc Trop Med Hyg* 1988; 82(6):930-934.

14. Warrell DA. Clinical toxicology of snakebite in Africa and the Middle East and Asia. In: Clinical Toxicology of Animal Venoms and Poisons. *CRC Press;* 1995: 433-594.

15. Banerjee RN, Sahni AL, Chacko KA, Vijay K. Neostigmine in the treatment of Elapidae bites. *J Assoc Phys India* 1972; 20: 503 – 509.

16. Gold BS. Neostigmine for the treatment of neurotoxicity following envenomation by the Asiatic cobra. *Ann Emerg Med* Jul 1996;28:87-89.

Section 5

17. Thomas PP, Jacob J. Randomized trial of antivenom in snake envenomation with prolonged clotting time. B*rit Med J* 1985: 291: 177-178.

18. Kakrani AL. Rationale of anti-snake venom therapy: Randomized controlled trials. *J Assoc Phys India* 1999: 47: 367 – 368.

19. Tariang DD, Philip PJ, Alexander G, *et al.* Randomized controlled trial on the effective dose of anti-snake venom in cases of snake bite with systemic envenomation. *J Assoc Phys India* 1999; 47: 369 – 371.

20. Vijeth SR, Dutta TK, Shahapurkar J, Sahai A., *et al.* Dose and frequency of anti-snake venom injection in the treatment of Echis carinatus (saw scaled viper) bite. *J Assoc Phys India* 2000; 48: 187-191.

21. Srimannarayana, *et al.* Randomised controlled trial on the effective dose of anti-snake venom in case of snake bite with systemic envenomation. *J Assoc Phys India* 2000; 48: 458 – 459

22. Seth AK, Verma PP, Pakhetra R., *et al.* Randomised controlled trial on the effective dose of anti-snake venom in case of snake bite with systemic envenomation. *J Assoc Phys India* 2000; 48: 756.

23. Srimannarayana J, Dutta TK, Sahai A., *et al.* Rational use of anti snake venom (ASV): Trial of various regimens in hematoxic snake envenomation. *J. Assoc Phys India* 2004; 52:788 - 793.

24. Chippaux J.P, Goyffon M. Epidemiology of scorpionism: a global appraisal. *Acta Trop* 2008;107: 71-79.

25. Ismail M. The scorpion envenoming syndrome. *Toxicon* 1995; 33:825-858.

26. Bawaskar HS. Diagnostic cardiac premonitory signs and symptoms of red scorpion sting. *Lancet* 1982;1: 552-554.

27. Freire-Maia L, Pinto GI, Franco I. Mechanism of the cardiovascular effects produced by purified scorpion toxin in the rat. *J Pharmacol Exp Ther* 1974;188: 207-213.

28. Mahadevan S. Scorpion sting. *Indian Pediatr* 2000; 37:504-514.

29. Bawaskar HS, Bawaskar PH. Clinical profile of severe scorpion envenomation in children at rural setting. *Indian Pediatr* 2003; 40: 1072-1075.

30. Bawaskar HS, Bawaskar PH. Management of scorpion sting. *Heart* 1999; 82:253 -254.

31. Narayanan P, Mahadevan S, Serane VT. Nitroglycerine in scorpion sting with decompensated shock. *Indian Pediatr* 2006; 43: 613-617.

32. Bawaskar HS, Bawaskar PH. Efficacy and safety of scorpion antivenom plus prazosin compared with prazosin alone for venomous scorpion (Mesobuthus tamulus) sting: randomised open label clinical trial. *BMJ* 2011;342:c7136.

33. Boyer LV, Theodorou AA, Berg RA, Mallie J, Chavez-Mendez A, Garcia-Ubbelohde W, *et al.* Antivenom for critically ill children with neurotoxicity from scorpion stings. *N Engl J Med* 2009; 360:2090-2098.

35. Ress RS, Altenbern DP, Lynch JB, *et al.* Brown recluse spider bites. A comparison of early surgical excision. *Ann surg* 1985; 202:659-663.

36. Russel FE. Venomous animal injuries. *Curr Prob Pediatr* 1973; 3:1-47.

37. Belten DP, Richardson WH, Tong TC, Clark RF. Massive honey bee envenomation-induced rhabdomyolysis in an adolescent. *Pediatric*s 2006; 117:231-235.

38. Stafford CT, Hoffman DR, Rhoades RB. Allergy to imported fire ants. *South Afr Med J* 1989; 82:1520-1527.

53

The Child with Polytrauma

Gayatri Munghati and M Bajpai

INTRODUCTION

The term polytrauma lacks a universally accepted definition[1]. It can be defined as simultaneous insult to a number of body regions, the combined result of which is life-threatening[2]. Trauma is the leading cause of death among children aged less than 14 years in US; 15000-25000 deaths in this age group annually can be attributed to trauma alone. It is also the leading cause of disability (3-10 times the mortality). Twenty five percent of pediatric emergency visits are due to trauma. Blunt trauma tops the list of mode of injury with falls and vehicular accidents being the most common cause. Boys by virtue of their outgoing bold nature are affected more often than girls[3-5].

The precise number of deaths and injuries due to specific causes or any scientific estimates of trauma deaths in India are not available from any single source. However, population based studies and hospital based studies as also the various data collecting bodies show vehicular accidents as the leading cause of injury. Mortality in age group of less than 14 years due to trauma is 9-11.2% of total mortality. The ratio of deaths to severe injuries needing hospitalization and to minor injuries is 1:20:50. One third of the disabilities are due to injuries[6]. The deaths and disabilities are expected to increase in future due to rapid motorization of India combined with lack of safety environment. Prevention, acute and long-term care and rehabilitation are the major challenges faced today.

Not only the pattern of injury but also the physiological response of a child differs from that of an adult. This puts a great onus on the part of the pediatric trauma care team to possess the necessary expertise in the management of these cases.

BASIC DIFFERENCES BETWEEN A CHILD AND AN ADULT

General

1. Lesser protective fat and connective tissue.

2. The force of impact is dissipated over a small surface area. Energy transmitted during injury delivers greater force per unit body volume.

3. Large surface area to body weight ratio resulting in greater heat loss with increased risk of hypothermia.

4. Increased requirements of maintenance fluids, trace elements and minerals.

Skeleton

1. Bones are immature, porous with incomplete calcification.

2. Greenstick fractures are seen only in children.

3. Injuries to growing bones and their epiphyses are attended with unique problems of growth disturbances, overgrowth, angular deformation and shortening.

Thorax

1. Compliant and compressible chest wall allows transfer of energy underneath without fracture of ribs.

2. Hidden injuries are common. Rib fractures in a child is likely to be associated with serious visceral injuries.

3. Different spectrum of injuries as compared to adults e.g.
   (a) Pulmonary contusions
   (b) Traumatic asphyxia
   (c) Commotio cordis

4. Mobile mediastinum resulting in displacement and kinking of vessels and compression of heart resulting in shock and airway obstruction.

Abdomen

1. Poor protection due to uderdeveloped rib cage.
2. Less cushioning by intra-abdominal and peri-renal fat.
3. Less protection by muscles of flank and abdomen.
4. Relatively large intra-abdominal solid organs.

5. The increased mobility of kidneys result in unique disruption of PUJ seen only in pediatric age group.

6. Presence of pre-existing abnormalities of solid organs e.g. Pelviureteric junction obstruction (PUJO), ectopic kidneys, presence of fetal lobulations in kidneys and spleen.

Head and Neck

1. Greater head size relative to body weight.
2. Neck muscles are not fully developed.
3. Excessive intracranial fluid makes the brain more susceptible to wave like forces.
4. Lesser myelination of neurons and nerve fibers.
5. Thinner and softer cranial bones.

Other characteristics

1. Profound psychological effects of trauma.
2. Long term effects of bone injury and splenectomy.
3. Lifelong impacts of disability due to spinal injury.

Therefore, pediatric trauma as an entity has distinctive features in children compared to adults. Those who treat injured children should recognize and understand these important distinctions and address the special needs of the child during resuscitation and further management.

Assessment of Severity of Trauma

The severity of trauma and its outcome can be assessed on the basis of vital signs, Glasgow Coma Score and severity of trauma. Two commonly used scores are pediatric trauma score and revised trauma score (Tables 53.1 and 53.2). Higher trauma scores are associated with better chances of survival.

Trimodal Distribution of Trauma Deaths

The pattern of distribution of trauma deaths was described by Donald Trunkey 20 years back[7]. In case of children it requires revision. In classic description of major trauma the peak incidence of deaths occurs within minutes after injury and accounts for 45% of deaths. Majority of these

Table 53.1 Pediatric trauma score (PTS)			
Patient characteristics	**Score**		
	+ 2	**+ 1**	**-1**
❑ Weight (kg)	> 20	10-20	< 10
❑ Airway	Normal	Maintainable	Not maintainable
❑ Systolic blood pressure (mm Hg)	> 90	50-90	< 50
❑ CNS	Awake	Obtunded	Comatose
❑ Open wound	None	Minor	Major
❑ Skeletal fracture	None	Closed fracture	Open fracture

The child should be referred to Trauma Center when PTS is 8 or less

Table 53.2 Revised trauma score (RTS)			
Glasgow coma score	**Systolic BP (mm Hg)**	**Respiratory rate (per minute)**	**Score**
13-15	> 89	10-29	4
9-12	76-89	> 29	3
6-8	50-75	6-9	2
4-5	1-49	1-5	1
≤ 3	0	0	0

The child should be referred to Trauma Center when RTS score is 12 or less
Adapted from *J Trauma* 1989, 29: 623-629

deaths are due to head or cardiovascular injuries. Prevention is the only effective measure against this early peak of deaths. Second peak occur within one to four hours after injury and is responsible for 34% of deaths. The majority of these deaths occur due to CNS bleeds, solid organ and thoracic injuries. This peak can be prevented by early resuscitation. Pediatric resuscitation focuses on this 'golden hour'. However, the period of initial stability decreases as age decreases. The third peak of late deaths is ascribed to sepsis, SIRS is seen less frequently in children. Recent studies have shown the absence of third peak which may be the result of improved medical care. However, the first peak remains the same, indicating the need to focus on preventive measures[8,9].

Basic Trauma Life Support

It is usually defined as prehospital emergency service using non-invasive life-saving procedures including cardiopulmonary resuscitation, bleeding control, splinting of broken bones, artificial ventilation, basic airway management and administration of oral or rectal medications. It is instituted by either untrained personnel or paramedics[10].

In emergency setting, two alternative strategies have generally been adopted[11]:

1. *Scoop and run.* The patient is transported to a higher level hospital as quickly as possible, with minimal prehospital treatment.

2. *Stay and play.* The patient is stabilized on site before transportation.

The tactic of choice is determined by the nature of the emergency, the available services, and the possibilities of starting the treatment at the site or the nearby hospital.

Advanced Trauma Life Support

The priorities in resuscitation of a child with polytrauma remain the same as those of an adult. These have been effectively promoted by the Advanced Trauma Life Support Group (ATLS). The ATLS philosophy is to "Treat the lethal injury first, then reassess and treat again". The systematic approach comprises of primary survey, resuscitation and management of potentially life-threatening injuries and a definite secondary survey[10].

Primary Survey

This structured management strategy, the ABCDE approach focuses on recognition and management of immediate life threatening injuries. **A**ssess and stabilize **A**irway, **B**reathing, **C**irculation, **D**isability (evaluate neurological condition), **E**xposure of the patent and **E**nvironment control.

Airway with Cervical Spine Control

Rapid assessment and maintenance of the airway is the first step in resuscitation. Hypoxia due to failure to maintain a patent airway is a common cause of cardio-respiratory arrest. Following points should be considered.

(i) Ability of the child to cry, speak normally and breathe spontaneously.

(ii) Inspection of oral cavity for presence of vomitus, secretions, dislodged teeth or other foreign bodies.

(iii) Presence of stridor, wheeze, nasal flaring and sternal retractions.

(iv) Presence of maxillo-facial injuries and cyanosis.

There are certain important anatomical differences in the airway of children that require special consideration during opening and maintaining the airway. The short neck and large head results in passive neck flexion and airway obstruction if the child is placed supine. Therefore, a pediatric back board should have a torso mattress or occiput recess to prevent potentially dangerous neck flexion[12]. The soft floor of the oropharynx is easily compressed by inexperienced fingers attempting to lift the jaw. The large tongue and small mandible make the upper airway narrow and easily occluded. Small reductions in the diameter of airway from swelling, blood or foreign bodies may impair air flow severely. The mass of adenoid tissue makes placement of nasopharyngeal airway difficult. The larynx is large and placed anteriorly making visualisation difficult. The epiglottis is horse-shoe shaped and projects posteriorly making intubation difficult. The cricoid ring is the narrowest part. All these factors favour the use of straight blade laryngoscope to place an uncuffed endotracheal tube in a child less than 8 years of age. Cuffed tubes are not recommended in infants and children less than 8 years as it may lead to pressure necrosis of cricoid cartilage[13].

The various measures to be undertaken for airway management are summarized below.

(i) *Suction.* The finger sweep method advocated in adults should be avoided in children as it may impact the foreign body or induce laryngeal spasm. Instead gentle suction should be used to dislodge the foreign body[14].

(ii) *Jaw thrust.* It should be achieved by lifting the mandible and care should be taken not to compress the floor of the mouth.

(iii) *Head tilt and chin lift.*

(iv) *Oral airway.* Nasopharyngeal airway should be avoided.

(v) *Cervical spine immobilization.* In children with significant trauma or when history is unavailable, cervical spine injury should be assumed and immobilization measures instituted (Figure 53.1). Measures should be taken off only after ruling out spinal injury by thorough clinical and radiological examination.

(vi) *Bag and mask ventilation.* When short term ventilatory support is required.

(vii) *Orotracheal intubation.* Size of the tube is dictated by the age of the child and is given in Table 53.3. Indications for endotracheal intubation are listed below.

- Respiratory arrest or failure (hypoventilation, arterial hypoxemia despite supplemental oxygen therapy or severe respiratory acidosis)
- Actual or potential airway obstruction
- Coma or significant alteration in mental status (GCS or modified pediatric GCS of 8 or less)
- To facilitate hyperventilation when appropriate (e.g. transtentorial herniation)
- Anticipated need for prolonged ventilatory support (e.g. thoracic injuries)
- Decompensated shock

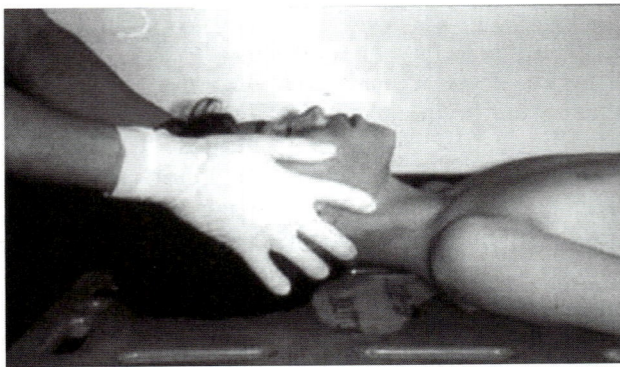

Figure 53.1 Cervical spine should be immobilized before further assessment of the child

(viii) *Surgical cricothyroidotomy.* In cases when intubation is not possible because of maxillofacial injuries or congenital anomalies, cricothyroidotomy should be undertaken. Following stabilization it should be converted to formal tracheostomy.

The flow chart summarises the various steps for the maintenance of an adequate airway (Figure 53.2).

BREATHING AND VENTILATION

In a child with polytrauma difficulty in breathing and inadequate ventilation can usually be attributed to either head injury (impaired respiratory drive) or thoracic injury (impaired lung expansion). Hypoventilation and hypoxia are common causes of cardiac arrest in children. Assess the following parameters in the emergency room.

- ○ *Breathing*
  - Rate
  - Depth
  - Effectiveness of respiration

Age (years)	Endotracheal tube internal diameter (mm)	Length of trachea (cm)	Depth of insertion (cm from lips)	Size and blade
Newborn	3.0 uncuffed	3.0	10	1, straight
1	3.5-4.0 uncuffed	4.3	11	2, straight
3	4.0-4.5 uncuffed	5.3	13	2, straight
5	4.5-5.0 uncuffed	5.7	16	3, straight
7-10	6.0-6.5 uncuffed	7.0	20	3, straight
Adult	7.0-8.0 uncuffed or cuffed	10.0+	22+	curved
General	Diameter of child's little finger 16 +age (yrs)/4	--	Age in years + 10	Straight/curved

Table 53.3 Guidelines for size of endotracheal tube in various age groups

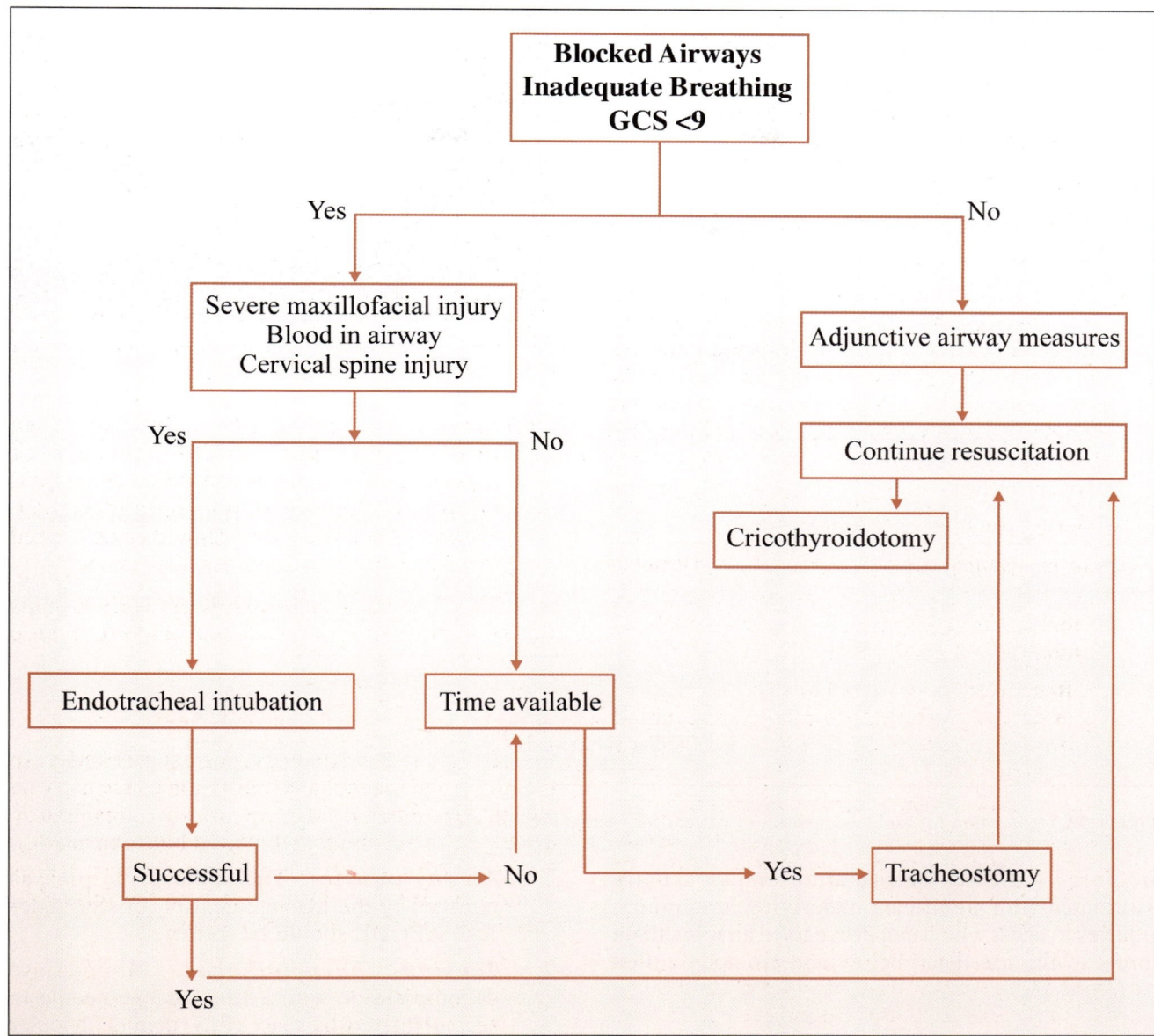

Figure 53.2 Algorithm for maintenance of adequate airway

- ○ *Chest wall movements*
  - • Bilaterally decreased
  - • Unilaterally decreased
  - • Paradoxical movements
- ○ *Mediastinal shift*
  - • Tracheal deviation
  - • Displacement of point of maximal cardiac impulse
  - • Distended neck veins
  - • Asymmetric air entry
- ○ *Percussion note*
  - • Dull
  - • Resonant
- ○ *Oxygen saturation*

Approximately 11-48% of pediatric head injuries are severe[15,16]. When child is not able to maintain respiration due to head injury immediate endotracheal intubation should be undertaken. After intubation, 100% oxygen should be delivered with tidal volume of 10-12 ml/kg. PaO_2 of more than 80 mmHg and a $PaCO_2$ 30-35 mm Hg should be maintained. PEEP should not exceed 5 cm H_2O pressure. The goal is to prevent secondary brain injury by optimising oxygenation and cerebral perfusion by minimising intracranial pressure. Head injury is best managed by moderate hyperventilation and hypocapnia ($PaCO_2$ between 30-35 mm Hg) to reduce intracranial pressure[17].

Injury to thoracic organs can be severe even in the absence of rib fractures. Presence of rib

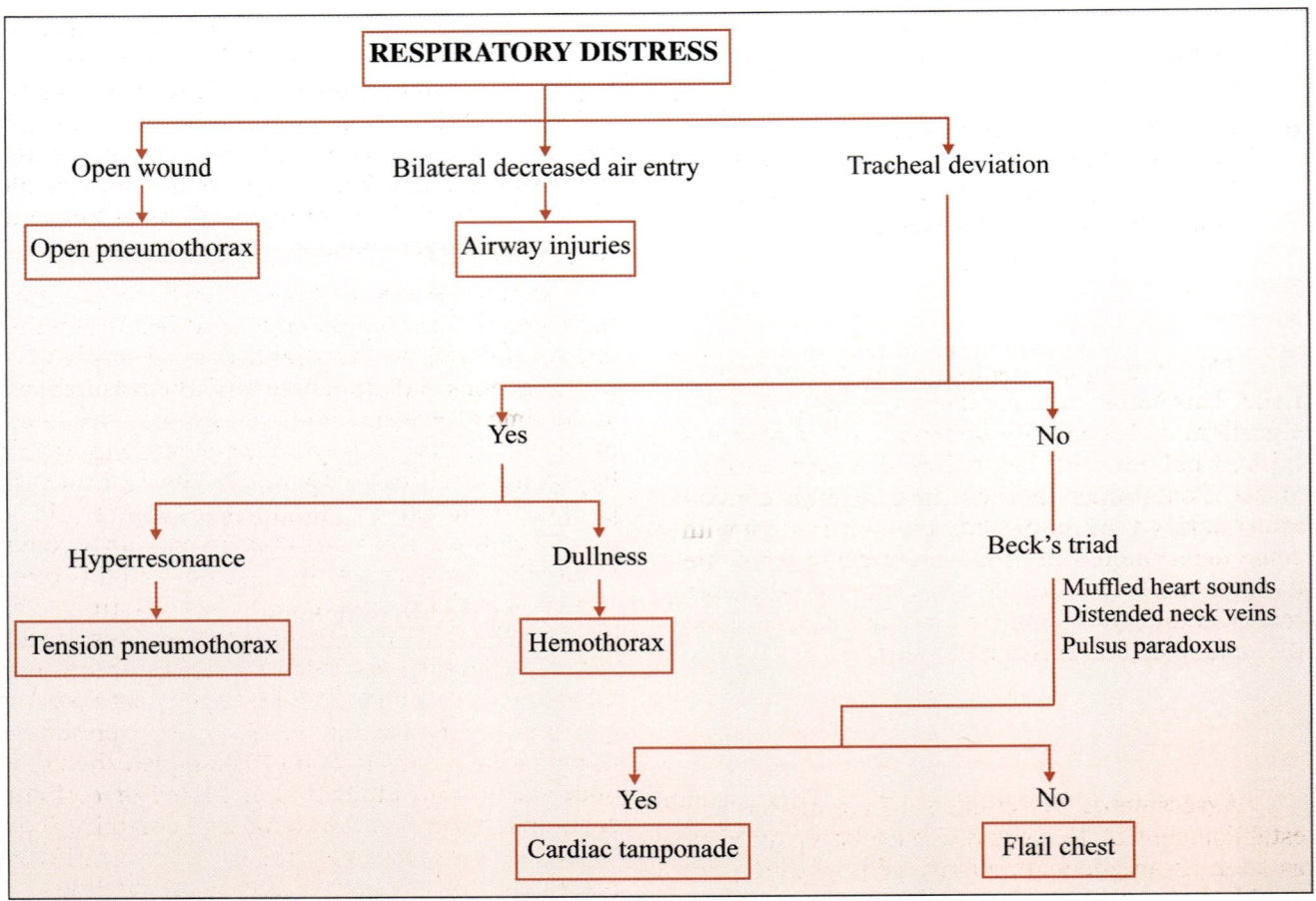

Figure 53.3 Algorithm for rapid assessment of patient for "lethal six" injuries

fractures indicates deformation and is usually associated with significant underlying lung injury. Injuries to chest which can prove to be an immediate threat to life are listed below and are aptly called as *lethal six*.

LETHAL SIX

1. Airway injuries
2. Open pneumothorax
3. Tension pneumothorax
4. Hemothorax
5. Flail chest
6. Cardiac tamponade

The diagnosis of above conditions should be established rapidly followed by quick intervention. Diagnosis is usually based on clinical examination and X-ray chest may be done if patient's condition is stable enough to permit the same. Figure 53.3 summarizes stepwise assessment of "lethal six".

The management of these conditions is outlined as follows.

1. *Airway injuries*. The same principles as outlined in the management of airway under A of ABCDE should be followed.

2. *Tension pneumothorax*. Immediate decompression with a 12-14 gauge needle in second intercostal space (ICS) in midclavicular line or in the fifth ICS in anterior axillary line. This maneuver should be followed by tube thoracostomy in 5th ICS and connected to underwater seal bag.

3. *Open pneumothorax.* The wound should be immediately sealed on the three sides. Alternatively an occlusive dressing should be applied along with a tube thoracostomy in 5th ICS.

4. *Hemothorax.* Immediate tube thoracostomy is life saving. Thoracostomy may be required if blood loss is more than 20% of blood volume or the rate of blood loss through thoracostomy is more than 1-2 ml/kg/hour.

5. *Flail chest.* Endotracheal intubation with elective ventilation is recommended. Prophylactic tube thoracostomy may be

needed for associated pneumothorax or hemothorax. Adequate pain management is of utmost importance.

6. ***Cardiac tamponade***. Pericardiocentesis through subxiphoid approach should be done. Thoracotomy may be required for open drainage and repair if pericardiocentesis fails.

Role of emergency room or on-site thoracotomy

This is a highly controversial and debatable issue. This heroic measure interrupts the diagnostic algorithm and is usually undertaken in a severely injured patient who has suffered a near cardiac arrest. Penetrating thoracic trauma with cardiac arrest during transfer or blunt thoracic trauma with acute deterioration of vitals and cardiac arrest are the indications for on-site thoracotomy. Although recent studies show some improvement in survival, the outcomes are universally poor[18-20].

CIRCULATION AND CONTROL OF HEMORRHAGE

Assessment. Assessment of circulation and establishment of IV access should be undertaken as soon as an adequate airway and breathing are established. Children possess the unique ability to maintain blood pressure even in the face of a significant fluid and blood loss. Blood pressure, therefore, cannot be considered as a reliable indicator of hypovolemia[20]. Tachycardia precedes hypotension and is a more reliable indicator of hypovolemic shock. However, pulse rate can be altered in certain conditions like associated brain injury where one may encounter bradycardia. Bradycardia is also a feature of severe hypoxia. On the other hand an anxious child may have tachycardia without hypovolemia.

Urine output is a reliable indicator of end organ perfusion and is monitored for assessment of hypovolemia and adequacy of fluid resuscitation. Urine output should be maintained between 1-2 ml/kg/hour in a child more than one year of age and more than 2 ml/kg/hour in less than one year old child. Table 53.4 summarises the signs and symptoms of hypovolemia.

Intravenous access. Two large bore intravenous lines should be established preferably above and below the diaphragm. Samples for investigations and cross matching should be drawn at the time of placement of venous line. Placement of IV access can prove to be quite challenging in a hypotensive child. If two attempts to establish peripheral line fails, an intraosseous line should be established in a child less than 6 years. In a young child bone marrow is quite vascular and this route can be used effectively for resuscitation. The preferred site for intraosseous access is the anteromedial surface of tibia 2-3 cm below the tibial tuberosity. In an older child a venous cut down of great saphenous vein above the ankle is preferred. Central vein catheterization if attempted should be undertaken with utmost care. Failed or difficult cannulation can result in significant complications. Femoral route is the preferred route for central line placement due to relative ease of cannulation.

Fluid resuscitation. Resuscitation should begin with rapid infusion of isotonic solution such as Ringer's lactate or normal saline 20 ml/kg over a period of 15-20 min. The bolus can be repeated twice during fluid resuscitation. If hypotension persists in spite of administration of 40 ml/kg of RL or NS, transfusion of cross matched or O-negative packed RBCs should be administered. Adequacy of resuscitation can be judged by improvement in color of skin, dermal circulation, skin temperature, increase in blood pressure, decrease in pulse rate,

System	<25% blood loss	25-45% blood loss	>45% blood loss
Table 53.4 Signs and symptoms of hypovolemia in children			
Cardiac	Weak pulse, tachycardia	Marked tachycardia, thready pulse, systolic BP < 70 mm Hg	Severe tachycardia, absent pulses or BP < 50 mm Hg.
Central nervous system	Lethargic, irritable, confused	Altered sensorium, dulled response to pain	Comatose or obtunded
Skin	Cool clammy, capillary refill > 2 sec.	Decreased capillary filling, cold extremities, capillary refill > 3 sec.	Pale, cold, mottled skin, cyanosis, capillary refill > 5 sec.
Kidneys	Slight decrease in urine output, increased specific gravity	Marked oliguria with increased BUN	No urine output

Section 5

etc. The most reliable indicator of adequate fluid resuscitation and euvolemia remains the urine output as it indicates end organ perfusion. If child responds to resuscitation and perfusion is established, fluid infusion is gradually decreased to maintenance levels.

If stabilization does not occur it indicates ongoing blood loss. Hemorrhage from external sites is usually obvious e.g. open wounds, and compound fractures. In the absence of an external injury blood loss from cavities like abdomen, pelvis and thoracic cavity should be suspected. Other causes of persistent hypotension include cardiac tamponade, unrecognised myocardial injury and missed spinal injury.

The concept of 'hypotensive fluid resuscitation' is increasingly being studied in ongoing uncontrolled hemorrhage. This entails that patient does not receive aggressive fluid resuscitation till the hemorrhage is controlled. Increase in blood pressure may dislodge soft clots and can lead to further aggravation of bleeding which may be difficult to control. Moreover, dilution of blood decreases oxygen carrying capacity and dilution of clotting factors hinders formation of clot[22].

ASSESSMENT OF DISABILITY AND CONSCIOUSNESS

A rapid neurological assessment should be undertaken for identification of serious injuries that may have a bearing on airway maintenance. A useful tool for rapid assessment of gross neurologic dysfunction is AVPU scale.

A - Alert
V - Verbal response
P - Pain response
U - Unresponsive

Glasgow Coma Scale (GCS) is a commonly used and easily reproducible tool for assessment of neurologic injury[23]. Pediatric GCS is especially useful for children 5 years of age or younger[24]. (Table 53.5).

Exposure and Prevention of Hypothermia

Once the basic tenets of ABCD have been followed, the child should now be exposed completely to assess the injuries in detail. Particular attention should be given to areas where injuries are more likely to be missed such as axillae, buttocks, rectum etc. Children have large surface area to body weight ratio and heat loss is greater. Every precaution should be taken to avoid hypothermia. The emergency room should be air conditioned and kept warm in winter. Overhead warmers or radiant warmers are useful to create warm micro-environment. Also the fluids used for resuscitation should be warmed to body temperature before infusion.

SECONDARY SURVEY

Secondary survey is undertaken once the child is stabilized. The goal of secondary survey is to identify conditions which are potentially life threatening and to institute measures to correct them. It comprises of detailed clinical examination accompanied with laboratory and radiological investigations leading to planning of an appropriate management strategy.

Clinical Assessment

'SAMPLE' history is obtained.
S – Symptoms
A – Allergies
M – Medications
P – Past illnesses
L – Last meal
E – Events and environment

Vital parameters such as pulse rate, blood pressure, respiratory rate and temperature are monitored. Pallor, hydration and cyanosis are looked for. Log rolling of the patient is done for a detailed head to toe examination. All external injuries are carefully examined and note is made regarding their extent and depth. Head is examined to look for signs of brain injury and facio-mandibular fractures. Ear and nose are examined for any evidences of bleeding or bruising. Bony skeleton is examined for crepitus, tenderness, and deformation. Chest is carefully examined for evidences of internal injuries, flail chest, fracture of ribs and pneumothorax and hemothorax. Abdomen is examined for tenderness, bruises, lap belt sign and periumbilical darkening or pigmentation of skin due to intraperitoneal hemorrhage (Cullen's sign) or acute hemorrhagic pancreatitis (Grey Turner's sign). One must not forget to examine axillae, buttocks, groins and perineum as injuries to these sites can be missed if not specifically looked for. Foley's catheterization is done if there are no overt signs of urethral trauma. Gastric decompression should be done by placing nasogastric (NG) tube. Placement of NG tube is contraindicated if basal fracture of skull is suspected. In this case an orogastric tube will be more appropriate.

Table 53.5 Pediatric Glasgow Coma Scale			
Eye opening			
Greater than 1 year old	**Less than 1 year old**		**score**
Spontaneously	Spontaneously		4
To verbal command	To shout		3
To pain	To pain		2
No response	No response		1
Motor response			
Greater than 1 year old	**Less than 1 year old**		**score**
Obeys commands	Spontaneous movements		6
Localises pain	Localises pain		5
Flexion withdrawal	Flexion withdrawal		4
Flexion abnormal (decorticate rigidity)	Flexion abnormal (decorticate rigidity)		3
Extension (decerebrate rigidity)	Extension (decerebrate rigidity)		2
No response	No response		1
Verbal response			
>5 years	**2-5 years**	**< 2 years**	**score**
Oriented	Appropriate words/phrases	Smiles/coos appropriately	5
Confused	Inappropriate words	Cries but consolable	4
Inappropriate words	Persistent cries and screams	Persistent inappropriate crying and/or screaming	3
Incomprehensible sounds	Grunts	Grunts, agitated and restless	2
No response	No response	No response	1

The PGCS score is graded as minor 13-15, moderate 9-12 and severe 3-8. Lower the score, worse is the outcome.

LABORATORY INVESTIGATIONS

A baseline hemoglobin and hematocrit should be checked. This is repeated every hour for four hours to look for ongoing hemorrhage as evidenced by hemodilution. Serum electrolytes, urea, creatinine and coagulation profile should be done. Urine should be examined for blood with dipstick if there is no gross hematuria. If positive, microscopy should be done to quantify the microscopic hematuria[25]. Insignificant microscopic hematuria (less than 50 RBCs /hpf) usually clears in 72 hours. Persistent or rising hematuria should be investigated for genitourinary trauma.

Radiological Investigations

Skiagrams. The clinical examination should be followed by X-rays of the injured extremities and chest. The usefulness of skiagrams for detection of fractures is limited in children as the pattern of fractures is different. The growing ends of bones can be mistaken for fractures. Significant trauma can occur in the absence of fractures. The only useful X-ray is that of chest which may show presence of pleural collection, mediastinal shift and condition of lungs. Diaphragmatic ruptures may also be picked by X-ray chest[26]. In addition it helps to confirm the position of intercostal and endotracheal tubes.

Ultrasound examination (USG). Ultrasonography has an important role in the evaluation of pediatric trauma victims. Focused abdominal sonography for trauma (FAST) has sensitivity of 63-99% and specificity of 79-97% for the diagnosis of hemoperitoneum[27-33]. Among hemodynamically stable patients who are not taken immediately to the operating room, FAST serves as a useful screening tool to assess the need for further investigations. A negative FAST may be helpful in avoiding unnecessary CT scan[34]. FAST cannot, however, reliably exclude intestinal injury. USG is also useful for post injury monitoring if serial follow-up imaging is required[35].

Contrast enhanced CT (CECT) scan. It is the most common and effective means of correctly categorizing the patients into surgical or non surgical management group. It should be done in all stable patients when intrabdominal injury is suspected. Suspicion of intraabdominal injury is suggested by the magnitude of the trauma, presence of clinical signs or a positive FAST. CT accurately identifies the site of bleeding, organs injured and the extent of injury[36]. Identification of the site of ongoing hemorrhage can lead to endovascular or surgical intervention. CT is the diagnostic procedure of choice for assessment of retroperitoneal injuries, as neither FAST nor DPL adequately assesses the retroperitoneum[37]. CT, however, is relatively insensitive for the diagnosis of acute pancreatic injuries[38,39]. Definite diagnosis and staging would require endoscopy, magnetic resonance cholangio-pancreatography (MRCP) or intraoperative assessment.

Magnetic resonance imaging (MRI). It is a useful tool for evaluation of brain and spinal cord injury. In children injuries to spinal cord can occur in the absence of spinal fractures. In the SCIWORA (spinal cord injury without radiographic abnormality) syndrome, MRI is valuable in delineating the site and extent of spinal cord injury. Early diagnosis of spinal cord injury is essential because high dose intravenous methylprednisolone within 8 hours of injury is associated with improved motor outcome at one year. In a child with a bloody knee effusion without an apparent fracture, MRI evaluation may demonstrate a significant ligament or cartilage injury. It is also useful for evaluation of suspected pancreatic injuries[40].

Radionuclide scan. A technetium 99m bone scan is desirable in a child with multiple fractures. It is useful to identify areas of unsuspected skeletal injuries in an abused child. The sites with increased tracer uptake can be further studied in detail by obtaining radiographs.

Intravenous urography (IVU). Although once a modality of choice for evaluation of genitourinary trauma, it has been replaced by CECT. The only role of IVU is when an unstable patient is taken directly to operating room without imaging.

In this situation on table IVU can be done with 2 ml/kg of contrast. It is helpful to determine the presence of two functioning kidneys, extravasation of contrast and renal pedicle injuries[41].

DEFINITIVE MANAGEMENT

Treatment is planned on the basis of clinical assessment and reports of investigations and patient is directed to the appropriate destination for definitive management of the injuries. The steps for management of a child with polytrauma are summarized in Table 53.6.

Despite primary and secondary survey some injuries can still be missed, hence the concept of

Table 53.6 Steps for management of a child with polytrauma
❑ Notify a trauma surgeon with pediatric expertise.
❑ Immobilize the neck with a semirigid collar or head immobilizer.
❑ Clear the oropharyxn with a rigid suction device if indicated. Insert orogastric tube.
❑ Assess vital signs, Airway, Breathing, Circulation, Disability (CNS assessment) and Exposure (Body temperature).
❑ Administer 100% oxygen with a non-breathing mask if the child is awake and breathing spontaneously.
❑ Ventilate with 100% oxygen using a bag and mask if the child has significant respiratory distress or altered mental status.
❑ Provide advanced life support with assisted ventilation if spontaneous breathing efforts are poor or labored and there is respiratory failure. Provide hyperventilation for 15-30 minutes if you suspect increased intracranial pressure with impending brain herniation.
❑ Assess circulation while maintaining airway and breathing. Initiate chest compressions and control external bleeding with pressure if indicated.
❑ Treat tension pneumothorax and hemothorax by needle aspiration and thoracostomy.
❑ Establish vascular access, obtain blood samples for base line parameters, blood type and cross match studies.
❑ If signs of inadequate perfusion are present, rapidly infuse 20 ml/kg of isotonic saline or Ringer's lactate. Infuse a second or even third crystalloid bolus if signs of shock persist. Consider transfusion of blood products as and when necessary for treatment of major hemorrhage and blood loss.
❑ Provide holistic management by active and close cooperation with a pediatric surgeon, orthopedic surgeon, neurosurgeon, chest therapist, occupation and rehabilitation expert, psychologist and medical social worker.

tertiary survey has developed. The incidence of missed injuries is between 2-50% and have the potential to be a clinically significant factor for patient's morbidity[42]. Factors which delay the identification of injuries during the initial evaluation in the emergency department include an altered level of consciousness from a closed head injury, use of sedation and paralytic agents for intubation, and hemodynamic instability.

The *tertiary survey* is defined as a patient evaluation that identifies all injuries after the initial resuscitation and operative intervention.[43] The timing of this survey is variable, but typically occurs within 24 hours after admission and is repeated when the patient is awake, responsive, and able to communicate. It is a comprehensive review of the medical record with emphasis on the mechanism of injury and pertinent co-morbid factors. It includes the repetition of the primary and secondary surveys, a review of all laboratory data including radiographic studies[44]. Any new physical findings require further studies to rule out missed injuries.

Nutrition often gets neglected in an injured child. Malnutrition is associated with immune depression, increased risk of sepsis, poor wound healing and increased surgical morbidity and mortality. Children with trauma are more susceptible to iatrogenic malnutrition as they have relatively higher metabolic rate and low endogenous energy reserves. Following the initial shock phase of the metabolic response to trauma, daily protein and energy requirements may be approximately double that of uninjured state. The child may be unwilling or unable to to take nutritious food. Early enteral feeding should be instituted through gastric or jejunal route. Parenteral route is used when enteral feeding is contraindicated[45].

PREVENTION

The majority of injuries in adults and children can be prevented. Simple precautions can be taken to avoid injury to self and others. More than half of trauma is because of motor vehicle accidents. Seat belts are useful to prevent serious automobile injuries. Placing children in proper safety restraints (car seats, booster seats, etc.) and in the back seat are also useful to prevent or reduce the magnitude of vehicular injuries. Education of children emphasising safety aspects and education of motorist as also of pedestrians should be promoted. Government should ensure strong legislation regarding the road safety rules and use of safety restraints.

REFERENCES

1. Nerida, Zsolt JB. The definition of polytrauma: the need for international consensus. *Injury* (Suppl 4), November 2009;40:S12-S22

2. Ott R, Kramer R, Martus P, Bussenius-Kammerer M, Carbon R, Rupprecht H. Prognostic value of trauma scores in pediatric patients with multiple injuries. *J Trauma* 2000; 49: 729–736.

3. Bajpai M, Mitra DK. Recent advances in the management of pediatric trauma. In: Trauma. Misra MC (Ed.) *Interprint publishers* 1993.

4. A survey of pediatric injuries seen at AIIMS: National workshop on trauma held at PGIMER, Chandigarh, Nov. 30 – Dec. 1, 1991

5. Stafford PW, Blinman TA, Nance ML. Practical points in evaluation and resuscitation of the injured child. *Surg Clin North Am* 2002 Apr;82(2):273-301.

6. NCMH background papers. Burden of Disease in India (New Delhi, India), September 2005: 325-347

7. Trunkey DD. Trauma. *Lancet* 1983;249:25–35.

8. Demetriades D, Murray J, Charalambides K, *et al.* Trauma fatalities: time and location of hospital deaths. *J Am Coll Surg* 2004;198:20–26.

9. Demetrios Demetriades, Brian Kimbrell, Ali Salim, *et al.* Trauma deaths in a mature urban trauma system: Is "Trimodal" distribution a valid concept? *J Am Coll Surg* 2005; 201:343–348.

10. Liberman M, Roudsari BS. Prehospital trauma care: what do we really know? *Curr Opin Crit Care* 2007, 13:691-696.

11. Gold CR. Prehospital advanced life support vs "scoop and run" in trauma management. *Ann Emerg Med* 1987, 16:797-801.

12. Herzenberg JE, Hensinger RN, Dedrick DK, *et al.* Emergency transport and positioning of young children who have an injury of the cervical spine: The standard backboard may be hazardous. *Bone Joint Surg Am* 1989;71:75.

13. Tollefsen WW, Chapman J, Frakes M, Gallagher M, Shear M, Thomas SH. Endotracheal tube cuff pressures in pediatric patients intubated before aeromedical transport. *Pediatr Emerg Care* 2010 May; 26(5): 361-363.

14. Cashman J. P. and Bellw M.J. The multiply injured child. *Current Orthopedics* 2002, 16, 442-450.

15. Beauchamp MH, Ditchfield M, Babl FE, Kean M, Catroppa C, Yeates KO, Anderson V. Detecting traumatic brain lesions in children: CT versus MRI versus susceptibility weighted imaging (SWI). *J Neurotrauma* 2011 June; 28(6):915-27. Epub 2011 June 9.

16. Mabrouk Bahloul, Hedi Chelly, Anis Chaari, Imen Chabchoub, *et al. J Emerg Trauma Shock* 2011 Jan-Mar; 4(1): 29–36.

Section 5

17. Stafford PW, Blineman TA, Nance ML. Practical points in evaluation and resuscitation of the injured child. *Surg Clin North Am* 2002; R2:273-302.

18. Hofbauer M, Hüpfl M, Figl M, Höchtl-Lee L, Kdolsky R. Retrospective analysis of emergency room thoracotomy in pediatric severe trauma patients. *Resuscitation* 2011 Feb; 82(2):185-9. Epub 2010 Nov 20.

19. Gomez G, Fecher A, Joy T, Pardo I, Jacobson L, Kemp H. Optimizing outcomes in emergency room thoracotomy: a 20-year experience in an urban Level I trauma center. *Am Surg* 2010 Apr;76(4):406-410.

20. Lögters T, Lefering R, Schneppendahl J, Alldinger I, Witte I, Windolf J, Flohé S; Interruption of the diagnostic algorithm and immediate surgical intervention after major trauma—incidence and clinical relevance. Analysis of the trauma register of the German society for trauma surgery. *Unfallchirurg* 2010 Oct; 113(10):832-838.

21. Quinlan DM, Gearhart JP. Blunt renal trauma in childhood: Features indicating severe injury. *Brit J Urol* 1990; 66:526.

22. Wigginton JG, Poppolo LP, Pepe PE. Advances in resuscitative trauma care. *Minerva Anaesthesiol* 2011; 77; 1-10.

23. Teasdale G., Jennett B., Assessment of coma and impared consciousness. A practical scale. *Lancet* 1974; Jul 13, 2 (7872): 81-83.

24. James HE. Neurologic evaluation and support in the child with an acute brain insult. *Pediatric Ann* 1986; 15:16–22.

25 Perez-Brayfield MR, Gatti JM, Smith EA, Broecker B, Massad C, Scherz H, Kirsch AJ. Blunt traumatic hematuria in children. Is a simplified algorithm justified? *J Urol* 2002 June;167(6):2543-46.

26. Iochum S, Ludig T, Walter F, *et al.* Imaging of diaphragmatic injury: a diagnostic challenge? *Radiographics* 22 (Spec No.):S103-S116.

27. Rozycki GS, Ochsner MG, Schmidt JA, *et al.* A prospective study of surgeon-performed ultrasound as the primary adjuvant modality for injured patient assessment. *J Trauma* 1995;39:492-500.

28. Fernandez L, McKenney MG, McKenney KL, *et al.* Ultrasound in blunt abdominal trauma. *J Trauma* 1998; 45:841-848.

29. McKenney MG, Martin L, Lentz K, et al. 1,000 consecutive ultrasounds for blunt abdominal trauma. *J Trauma* 1996;40:607-612.

30. Soudack M, Epelman M, Maor R, *et al.* Experience with focused abdominal sonography for trauma (FAST) in 313 pediatric patients. *J Clin Ultrasound* 2004; 32: 53-61.

31. Richards JR, Knopf NA, Wang L, *et al.* Blunt abdominal trauma in children: evaluation with emergency US. *Radiology* 2002; 222:749-754.

32. Benya EC, Lim-Dunham JE, Landrum O, *et al.* Abdominal sonography in examination of children with blunt abdominal trauma. *Am J Radiol* 2000;174:1613-1616.

33. Holmes JF, Brant WE, Bond WF, *et al.* Emergency department ultrasonography in the evaluation of hypotensive and normotensive children with blunt abdominal trauma. *J Pediatr Surg* 2001;36:968-973.

34. Bode PJ, Edwards MJ, Kruit MC, *et al.* Sonography in a clinical algorithm for early evaluation of 1671 patients with blunt abdominal trauma. *Am J Roentgenol* 1999, 172:905-911.

35. Luks FI, Lemire A, St-Vil D, *et al.* Blunt abdominal trauma in children: the practical value of ultrasonography. *J Trauma* 1993, 34:607-610.

36. Shanmuganathan K. Multi-detector row CT imaging of blunt abdominal trauma. *Semin Ultrasound CT MR* 2004, 25:180-204.

37. Al-Salamah SM, Mirza SM, Ahmad SN, *et al.* Role of ultrasonography, computed tomography and diagnostic peritoneal lavage in abdominal blunt trauma. *Saudi Med J* 2002, 23:1350-1355.

38. Bigattini D, Boverie JH, Dondelinger RF. CT of blunt trauma of the pancreas in adults. *Eur Radiol* 1999, 9:244-249.

39. Coppola V, Vallone G, Verrengia D, *et al.* Pancreatic fractures: the role of CT and the indications for endoscopic retrograde pancreatography. *Radiol Med* (Torino) 1997, 94:335-340.

40. Fulcher AS, Turner MA, Yelon JA, *et al.* Magnetic resonance cholangiopancreatography (MRCP) in the assessment of pancreatic duct trauma and its sequelae: preliminary findings. *J Trauma* 2000, 48:1001-1007.

41. Mercader VP, Gatenby RA, Curtis BR. Radiographic assessment of genitourinary trauma. *Trauma* 1996; 13:129.

42. Janjua, KJ, Sugrue, M, and Deane, SA. Prospective evaluation of early missed injuries and the role of tertiary trauma survey. *J Trauma, Injury, Infection, and Critical Care* 1998, 44, 1000-1007.

43. Grossman, MD and Born, C. Tertiary survey of the trauma patient in the intensive care unit. *Surgical Clin N Amer* 2000, 80(3), 805-824.

44. Janjua, KJ, Sugrue, M and Deane, SA. Prospective evaluation of early missed injuries and the role of tertiary trauma survey. *J Trauma, Injury, Infection, Critical Care,* 1998, 44, 1000-1007.

45. Anthony H. In: Care of the Critically ill Child. Macnab AJ, Macrae DJ, Henning R (eds.). *Edinburgh: Churchill Livingstone,* 2001, pp. 447–456.

Section 5

Head Injury

Deepak Kumar Gupta, Pankaj Ailawadhi and AK Mahapatra

54

It is almost 30 years ago that McLaurin, a famous pediatric neurosurgeon said "child is not a small adult". He emphasized that the protocol being followed for the management of head injuries in adults cannot be used in under-5 children. The total number of head injuries in a year in India is over one million accounting for 300,000 pediatric cases. In USA, brain injuries are responsible for 7000 deaths per year which is more than any other single cause of mortality, and at least 29,000 children suffer from permanent post-traumatic neurological sequelae each year[1]. The mechanism of injury, type of pathology, management modalities and specific problems in children with head injuries are different than adult population[2-4].

MECHANISM OF INJURY

The pediatric population can be subdivided into 4 groups (a) infants below 1 year which includes neonates, (b) pre-school children between 1-5 years, (c) school going children up to 10 years and (d) children and adolescents above the age of 10 years. Head injury in neonates occurs due to birth trauma. The common correlates of birth trauma are cephalopelvic disproportion, prolonged labor and difficult delivery. Injury can also be due to the use of forceps or vacuum extraction for delivery. The above mentioned causes lead to brain injury during head engagement. During the moulding of fetal head, there is overriding of parietal bones over each other and frontal and occipital bones override the parietal bones. This normal process gets exaggerated during an obstructed labor leading to various types of intracranial hemorrhages and brain edema. The above situation can be made worse due to the application of forceps and vacuum extraction. The aforementioned traumatic complications in the neonates can be avoided by timely cesarean section.

Head injuries in toddlers below 5 years of age are more frequently due to fall from a height, or an object falling on the head of a child. Falls account for over 80 percent of injuries in this group. But when all the pediatric age groups are considered together, falls contribute to head injuries in over 55 percent cases[5]. Low height falls at home e.g. fall from bed rarely cause significant neurological morbidity. Fall from a height greater than 4 feet and falls from stairs are sometimes associated with more severe injuries such as contusions, subarachnoid hemorrhage and depressed skull fracture. Older children more often get involved in automobile and road accidents or fall from roof tops while flying kites. Recently, school bus accidents have significantly contributed to pediatric head injury. Severity of head injury is related with the velocity of the vehicle and impact of accident. Diffuse axonal injury, acute subdural hematoma and multiple contusions are associated with high speed. Concussions and focal contusions are common when collision involves two low speed vehicles. Children also get injured while crossing the road. Head injury may occur in children during recreation and sports activities especially while playing football.[6, 7]

Accidental penetrating injuries and crush injuries can occur at home. The most common mechanism of accidental penetrating injuries in children involves a fall onto a sharp object such as pencil or a stick. The orbital roof is the commonest site of entry. Crush injuries occur as a result of fall of heavy objects on the head due to pranks of the child at home. Very rarely, children can get involved in a blast injury or a missile injury as a part of global involvement during terrorist attack.

PATHOLOGY

Pathology of head injury in children is similar to those in adults. However, a large number of factors significantly modify the ultimate changes in the brain. These factors include thickness of the skull, presence of open fontanels, type of sutures and developing brain. Pathological changes in brain may be primary or secondary. Primary injury includes all types of hematomas, cerebral contusion and laceration while secondary changes mostly consist of cerebral edema, hypoxic and ischemic injury, as a part of perfusion defect in the brain, as the developing brain is specially susceptible to ischemic damage (Table 54.1).

Table 54.1 Common pathology in brain in children with head injuries
Neonates
• Cephalhematoma
• Ping pong skull fracture
• Ischemic-hypoxic injury
• Acute subdural hematoma
• Intracerebral hematoma
• Brain swelling
Toddlers
• Depressed and comminuted fracture
• Concussion
• Extradural and subdural hematoma
• Contusion
• Laceration
• Brain swelling
• Combinations
Older children
• Extradural hematoma
• Subdural hematoma
• Cerebral contusion/laceration
• Intracerebral hemorrhage
• Ischemic-hypoxic injury
• Brain swelling

SPECIFIC INJURIES

NEONATES

Hematoma of Scalp and Skull Fracture

Some degree of birth trauma occurs to every newborn baby during moulding, leading to edema and hematoma of scalp. However, these conditions are often treated by the pediatrician and are not referred to the neurosurgeon. The edema of the scalp is well known as caput succedaneum. Occasionally, large cephalhematoma can give rise to hypovolemic shock needing blood transfusion. The fracture of skull in a neonate is rare. However, due to elasticity of skull bones a typical fracture called as "ping pong" fracture may develop. The fracture could be a fissured fracture or a depressed fracture. The linear fracture is the commonest type. As the dura is densely adherent to the bone, when it gets torn it leads to a growing skull fracture. This occurs in children less than 5 years of age. Due to non-pneumatised paranasal sinuses the fracture through anterior cranial fossa is also common in children which can lead to leakage of CSF through the nose.

Intracranial Hemorrhage

An exaggerated moulding of skull bones during labor, or careless use of forceps may lead to intracranial hemorrhage in neonates. Extradural hematomas are rare in neonates, because dura is densely adherent to the skull bone. Rupture of delicate surface veins lead to acute subdural hematoma, which is not rare in newborn babies. Sometimes subdural hematoma may occur in the posterior fossa. Rarely, a serious intracerebral hematoma may result; leading to neonatal death. Hematoma can be formed even in the absence of skull fracture[4, 8-10]. About 20-25 percent of neonatal deaths are due to intracranial hemorrhage though most of them are non-traumatic and limited to sick preterm babies[11].

TODDLERS AND OLDER CHILDREN

Children between 5-15 years are commonly involved in accidents at home, school and roadside. One of the common causes of fall from the rooftop is during the season of kite flying. Another type of common injury in children occurs due to automobile accidents and is called as "Baby dash board syndrome". When toddlers are allowed to travel while standing or sitting on the front seat, and car is suddenly brought to a halt by a head-on collision, the head may be squashed between the mother and the dashboard. In such a situation the total kinetic energy brakes against the hard dashboard leading to serious head injury.

Concussion of the Brain

Concussion generally means a reversible neurological dysfunction. This can follow trivial injuries with transient loss of consciousness. The memory loss is a part of the concussion leading to both retrograde and post-traumatic amnesia (PTA). Small children may be "stunned" for a short time and may not give classical history of unconsciousness. There may be confusion, transient disturbances of vision and equilibrium, and headache. The etiology of concussion is believed to be an injury at the occipital area and shearing strain at the brainstem level. Loss of consciousness may also be due to kinking of posterior cerebral arteries. The children usually recover promptly from concussion. CT scan usually does not show any abnormality. However, in experimental animals, concussion is associated with diffuse damage to axons, both in cerebral cortex and brainstem.

Contusion of the Brain

A cerebral contusion i.e. bruising of the brain parenchyma(Fig 54.1) may present as focal symptoms at the site of injury (coup) or on the area of brain opposite to the injury (countercoup).

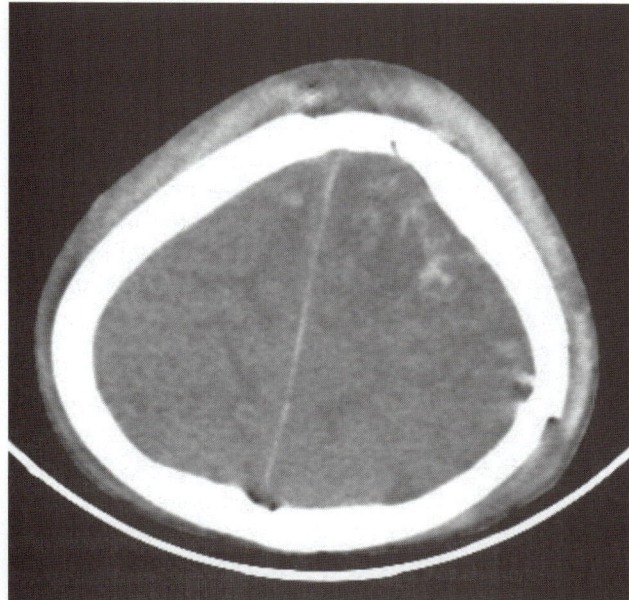

Figure 54.1 Showing left frontal contusions with surrounding edema

Fracture of the Skull

The fractures are usually linear and most commonly parietal in location. Fractures may cross the suture lines and vascular grooves. In younger children skull is pliable and depressed fracture may look like a "dimple" on a gutta-percha doll's head. Children falling from a greater height may have a comminuted fracture (Figure 54.2). These fractures lead to dural tear and laceration of brain leading to compound injury. Over 50-60 percent children with fracture have associated brain damage. Fracture can also involve anterior or middle fossa giving rise to CSF rhinorrhea or CSF otorrhea. Fracture of anterior cranial fossa may involve orbit and give rise to orbital hematoma and black eyes. Fracture going through the orbit (Figure 54.3) rarely can give rise to traumatic blindness (optic nerve injury)[12, 13-16]. When fracture line involves the petrous bone, the skin overlying the mastoid process is discolored and is popularly called as "Battle sign". Petrous bone fracture may be associated with bleeding from the ear, CSF otorrhea and facial palsy[17-18].

Growing Skull Fractures/Leptomeningeal Cyst

Growing skull fracture or "craniocerebral erosion" is a rare complication of skull fractures seen mainly in infancy and early childhood[12]. It is characterised by progressive enlargement of the fracture line. This late complication is also known as a "Leptomeningeal cyst"[19] because of its frequent association with a cystic mass filled with CSF (Figure 54.4). Growing skull fractures usually occur after severe head trauma during the first three years of life (particularly in infancy) and almost never after the age of 8 years. Incidence reported is only 0.05% to 0.1% of all skull fractures in childhood. During this stage, the brain volume is increasing rapidly, which in part is responsible for its development. Though the pathogenesis of growing skull fractures is multifactorial, the predominant factor in their causation is the presence

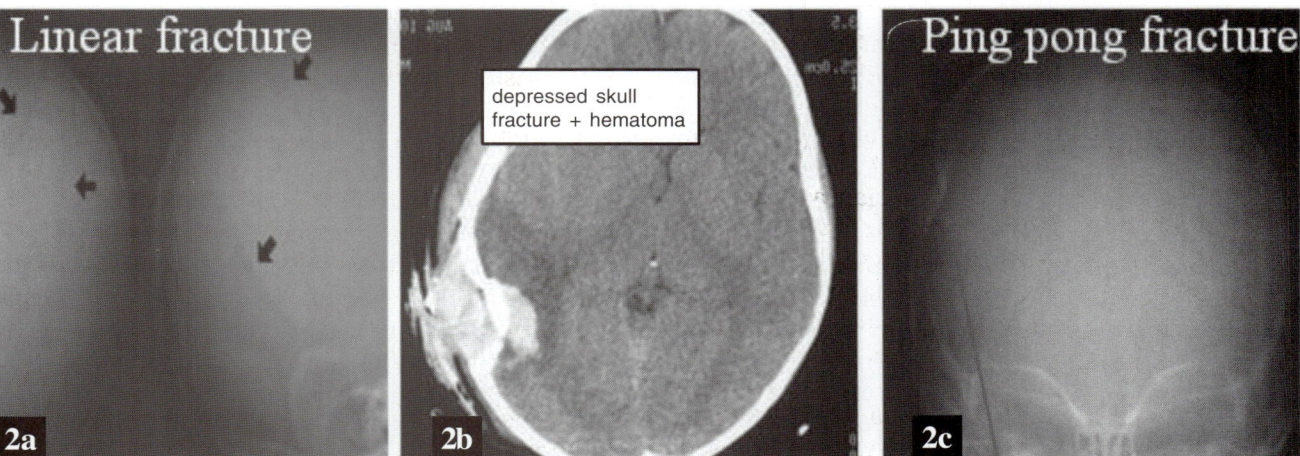

Figure 54.2 CT scan showing skull fracture (from left to right: linear skull fracture (54.2a), depressed skull fracture with underlying contusion (54.2b) and ping pong fracture (54.2c)

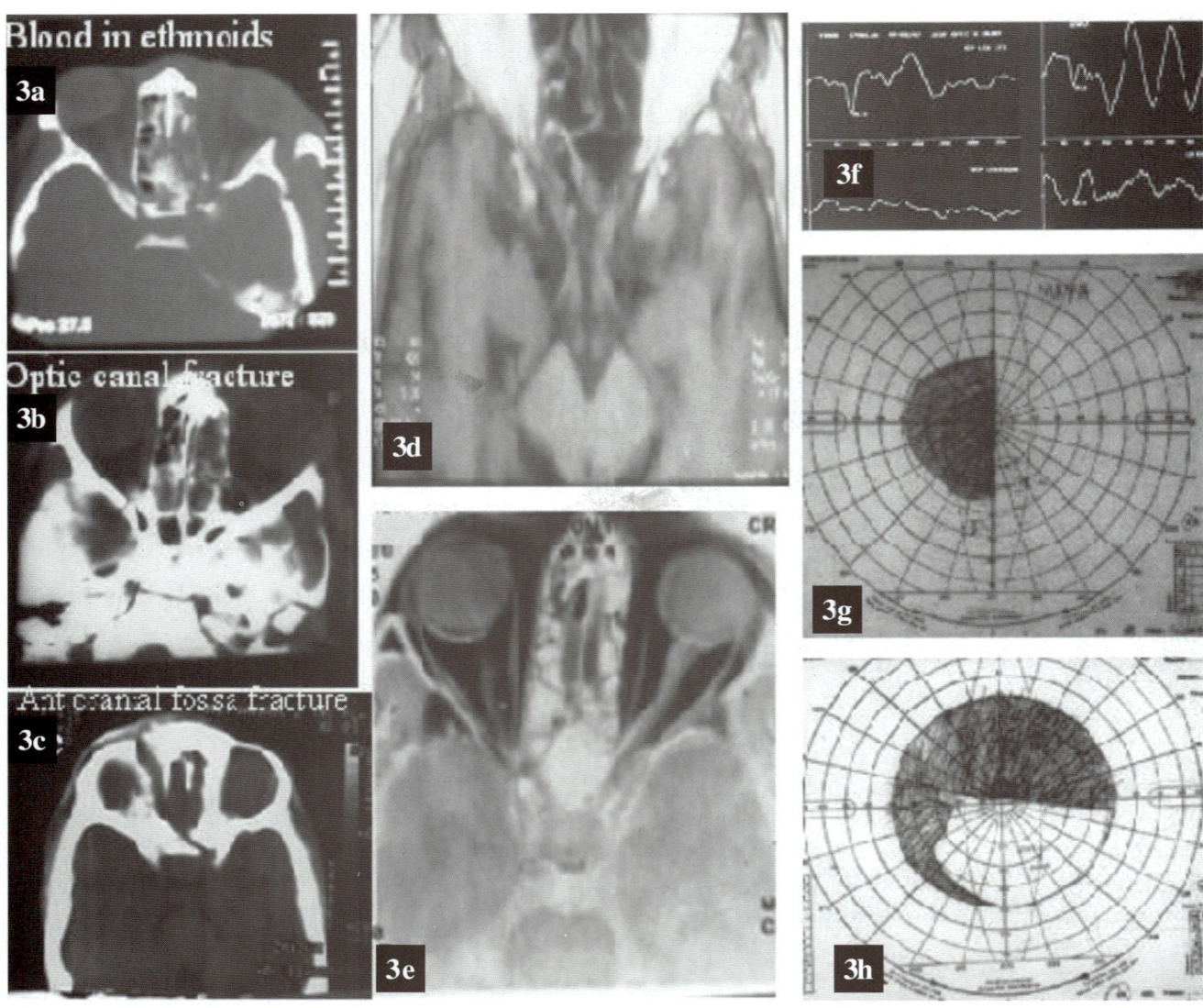

Figure 54.3 NCCT head with orbital cuts showing optic nerve injury 54.3a Anterior cranial fossa fracture with blood in ethmoids, 54.3b: Optic canal fracture right side, 54.3c: Anterior cranial fossa fracture, 54.3d and 54.3e: MRI showing optic nerve injury, 54.3f: VEP study tracings in a patient with optic nerve injury, 54.3g and 41.3h: Visual field charting in a patient of head injury showing field defects

of lacerated dura mater. The pulsatile force of the brain during its maximum growth will cause cerebral or subarachnoid herniation through the lacerated dura, which causes the fracture in the thin skull to enlarge. This interposition of tissue prevents osteoblasts from migration and inhibits fracture healing. The resorption of the adjacent bone by the continuous pressure from tissue herniation through the bone gap adds to the progression of the fracture line. The brain extrusion may be present shortly after diastatic linear fracture in neonates and young infants resulting in focal dilatation of the lateral ventricle near the growing fracture. This focal dilatation is reversible and may normalize after surgical repair. The cranial defects never increase if the underlying dura is intact and also craniotomy

performed without watertight closure of dura does not cause a growing fracture. Therefore, for growing fractures to develop a dural laceration is a must along with a fracture line. Another risk factor is severity of the underlying trauma. A linear fracture associated with hemorrhagic contusion of underlying brain suggests a trauma significant enough to cause dural laceration. The brain at the growing fracture site shows a cerebromeningeal cicatrix formation. Cystic changes at the site of region of growing fracture may occur due to cystic encephalomalacia. Post-traumatic aneurysms and subdural hematomas have also been reported to accompany growing skull fractures[10, 20]. Though most patients show damage to underlying brain, this finding is not a prerequisite for the development of

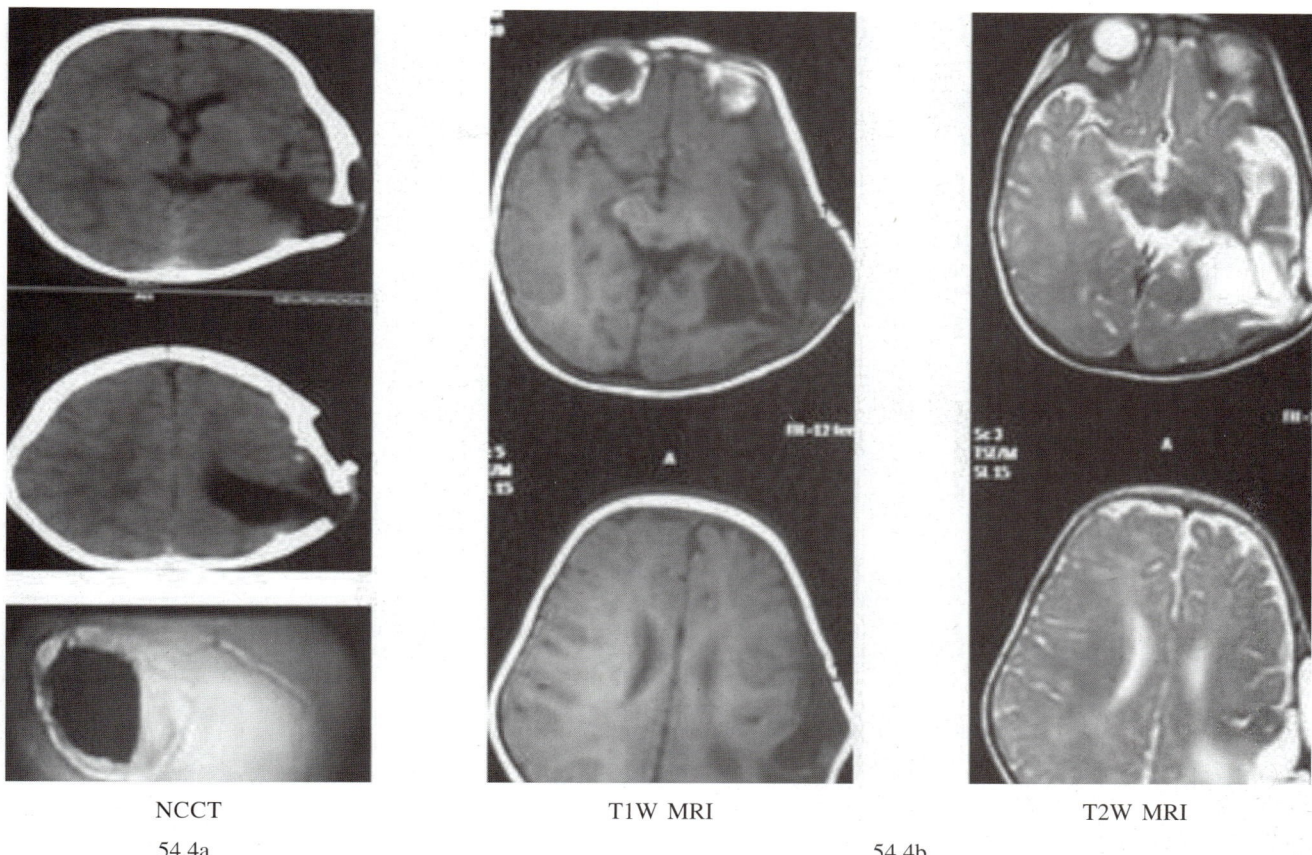

NCCT   T1W MRI   T2W MRI

54.4a   54.4b

Figure 54.4a NCCT with 3 D reconstruction showing left parietal growing skull fracture, 54.4b: MRI showing growing skull fracture with associated intradiploeic cyst

growing skull fractures. The growing skull fractures after reaching to maximum extent will cease to grow and remain stable throughout adulthood. Depressed fracture usually does not become a growing fracture but a linear fracture extending from a depressed one can start growing. A fracture with a diastasis of more than 4 mm may be considered at risk of developing a growing skull fracture[5, 21, 22]. The most common site is the parietal region[23]. Growing fractures can be seen even in older individuals usually in linear fractures in thin areas of skull base associated with dural laceration of orbital roof, ethmoid plate, and frontal sinus[12]. These fractures commonly present as a progressive, often pulsatile, scalp mass that appears sometime after head trauma sustained during infancy. They may be associated with seizures, hemiparesis, psychomotor retardation, but an asymptomatic palpable mass may be the sole sign. A growing fracture at the skull base may present with ocular proptosis or CSF rhinorrhea or otorrhea.

A plain radiograph may show a fracture line that crosses a coronal or lambdoid suture but it is usually limited to a parietal bone. On CT, a hypodense lesion is seen near the fracture site (Figure 54.4). Intracranial hypodense area may be due to encephalomalacia, arachnoid loculation or cortical atrophy[19].

Owing to the risk of progressive neurological deterioration and development of a seizure disorder, surgical correction of growing fractures, which involves removal of gliosed brain, duraplasty and cranioplasty, is recommended.

Extradural Hematoma

In younger children extradural hematomas are rare as the dura is adherent to skull bone in this age group. Hematomas may be of arterial or venous in origin depending on the type of fracture and vessel involved by the fracture (Figure 54.5). Blood may also get collected as a result of bleeding from fracture line and usually form a thin layer of clot. Mostly hematomas are temporal or frontal in location. Rarely, posterior fossa extradural hematomas are also observed[24, 25]. Ammarati and

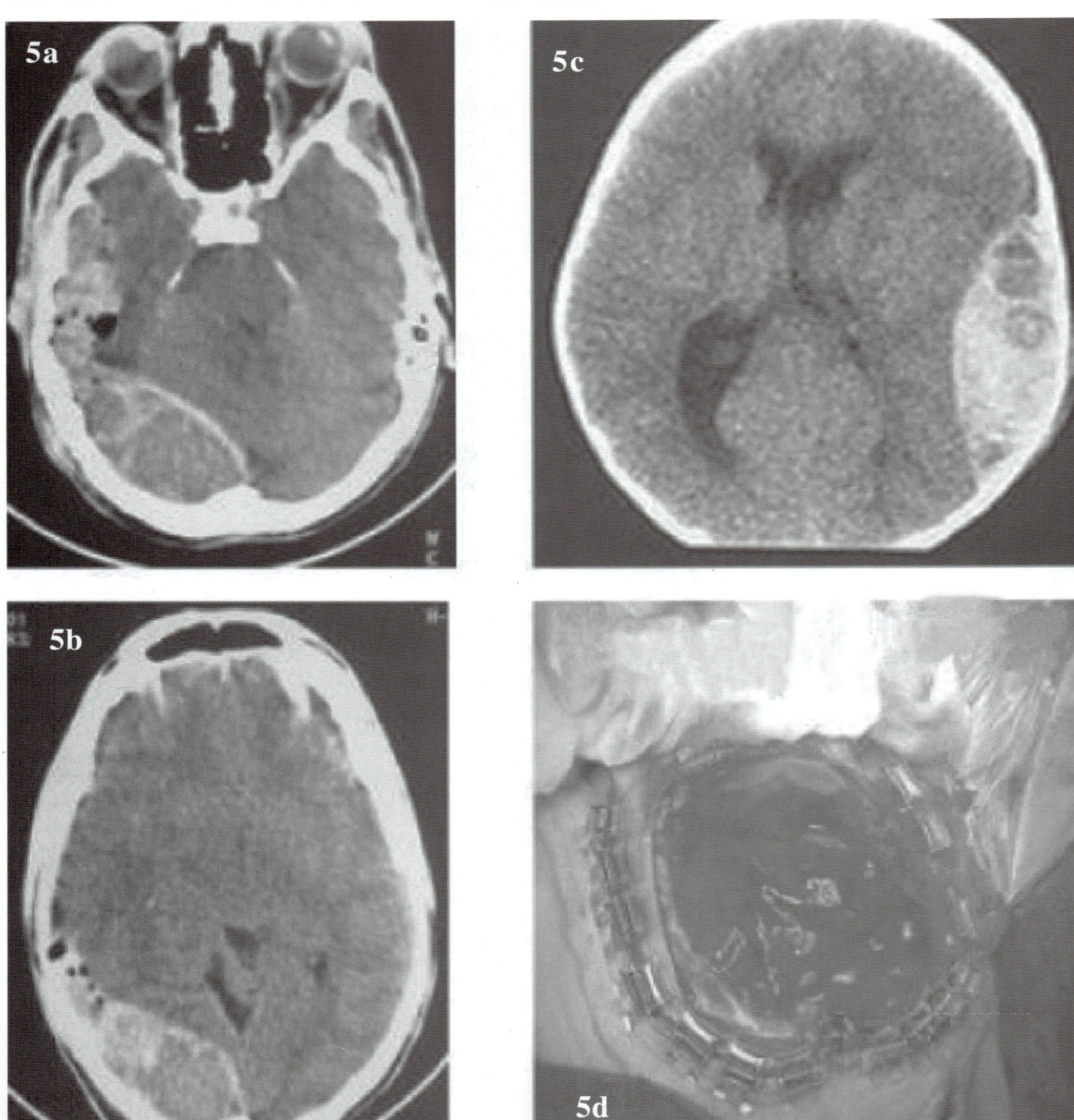

Figures 54.5 CT scan appearance of extradural hematoma. 54.5a and b Large biconvex extradural hematoma in posterior fossa with right temporal extension with significant mass effect, 54.5c Left parietal EDH, 54.5d: Intraoperative view showing EDH

Tomita[18] reviewed 36 cases of acute posterior fossa extradural hematomas in children. These hematomas can also extend above the tentorium cerebri in significant number of cases[25, 26].

Acute Subdural Hematoma

Acute subdural hematomas (SDH) are common in children. There are two peaks, one in infancy and the second among older children. Acute SDH is usually a result of severe injury; rarely it may follow a minor injury in children with a bleeding disorder[10, 27, 28]. Frequent falls and injury to the head accounts for a higher incidence of SDH. When the sutures are not fused, the hematoma can grow slowly and is termed as "growing subdural hematoma". The hematoma may remain silent for some time because the cranium can expand to

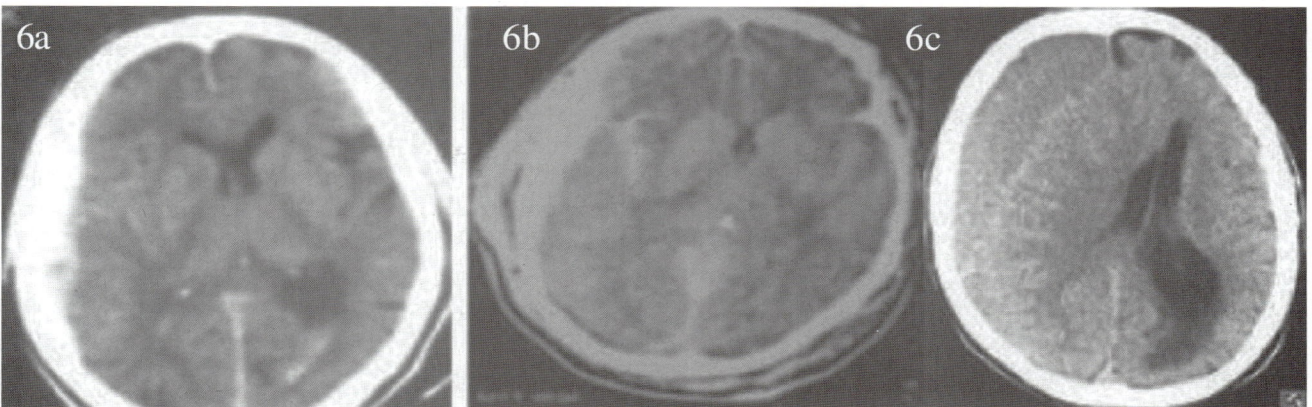

Figure 54.6 CT appearance of subdural hematoma. 54.6a and b Acute subdural hematoma, 54.6c: Subacute subdural hematoma

accommodate the SDH. In children with open fontanels, raised ICP is indicated by a tense anterior fontanel, which may be wrongly diagnosed as hydrocephalus by the treating doctor. Rarely, acute subdural hematoma can be located in the posterior fossa (Fig. 54.6a-c).

Chronic Subdural Hematoma

A subdural hematoma is a collection of blood in the space between the outer layer (dura) and middle layers of the covering of the brain (the meninges) (Figure 54.7). Only a slight hit on the head or even a minor fall without hitting the head may be enough to tear veins in the brain, often without fracturing the skull. There may be no external evidence of bruising on the surface of the brain. The chronic form of subdural hematoma is less risky, as pressure of the veins against the skull lessens the bleeding[29]. Prompt medical care can reduce the probability of permanent brain damage. Infrequently, chronic subdural hematoma in brain may calcify (also called "armour brain") which requires a major operation[30]. In childhood, hematomas are a common complication of falls. A subdural hematoma also may be an indication of child abuse, as evidenced by the shaken baby syndrome[31, 32].

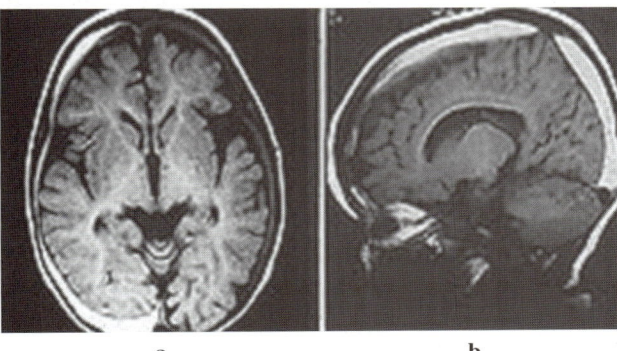

a   b
Figure 54.7a and b Chronic subdural hematoma seen on MRI

Clinical features

The common symptoms of chronic SDH include headache, episodes of confusion and drowsiness, and one-sided weakness or paralysis. There may be convulsions, drowsiness or loss of consciousness and coma after head injury. Pupils may be dilated or asymmetric. In infants, symptoms may include increased intracranial pressure (ICP), growing head size, bulging fontanel, vomiting, irritability, lethargy, and seizures. In cases of child abuse, there may be fractures of the skull or other bones.

Diagnosis

A chronic subdural hematoma may be missed, but a slow loss of consciousness after a head injury is assumed to be due to a hematoma unless proved otherwise.

Treatment

Small hematomas that do not cause any symptoms may resolve spontaneously. A large subdural hematoma with raised ICP should be surgically evacuated. Liquid blood can be drained through burr holes, drilled into the skull. Limited craniotomy/craniectomy may be required to remove a large hematoma or to coagulate the bleeding vein. Corticosteroids and diuretics can be given to control brain swelling[23]. After surgery, anticonvulsant drugs (such as phenytoin) may help controlling or preventing the seizures, which can begin as late as two years after the head injury.

Prognosis

If treatment is provided early, recovery is usually complete. Headache, amnesia, attention problems, anxiety, and giddiness may continue for some time after surgery. Children tend to recover much faster.

Child Abuse and Battered Baby Syndrome

Child abuse presents in many forms[31-33]. It is best defined as a purposeful infliction of physical or emotional harm, sexual exploitation, and/or neglect of basic needs (nutrition, education, and medical care). Caffey[32] in 1946 reported a series of patients with multiple fractures and a chronic subdural hematoma, which fit the profile of what today is defined as the shaken baby syndrome (SBS)[33-35]. Kempe et al[34] coined the term battered child syndrome. Battered child syndrome refers to children who have undergone physical abuse that has left them with both physical and psychological trauma.

In the west males are affected more commonly than females. The perpetrator is usually alone with the victim. Males are the abusers in 90% of the cases. The abuser is usually the biological father or in some cases the mother's boyfriend. The most common female attacker is a baby-sitter. The typical abused child is younger than 6 months. More than half of the patients that present to the emergency department (ED) or a physician's office have no history of prior abuse. One-fourth have a history of minor trauma. A small percentage present with a seizure[35], with varying levels of consciousness (e.g., coma, and apnea, respiratory arrest)[30]. Other symptoms include failure to thrive, poor feeding, and other vague symptoms[31, 33]. Common historical accounts that suggest abuse include injury inflicted by sibling, a fall down the steps, suddenly turned blue and stopped breathing, left alone for a few minutes, and fell from a low height. Only after obtaining a computed tomography (CT) scan and finding evidence of intracranial pathology is the true nature of the problem discovered.

Pathology

The most common intracranial lesion is the subdural hemorrhage. The symptoms are related to signs of increased intracranial pressure (ICP), but some patients may not have any evidence of ICP. Other findings include cerebral edema, subarachnoid hemorrhage, and even intra-parenchymal hemorrhage[31]. Skull fractures are seen in as many as 95% of patients with serious intracranial injury[36]. The fracture is usually in the occipital or parietal bones. Abuse should be considered if the patient has bilateral depressed fractures or multiple fractures, especially if they cross suture lines. Retinal hemorrhage is a characteristic and diagnostic feature of SBS. It can be detected even before intracranial hemorrhages are seen. Several types of retinal hemorrhages have been described[31].

The standard diagnostic triad of "Shaken Baby Syndrome" (SBS) include subdural hematoma, retinal hemorrhages, and lack of history of a motor vehicle accident or a fall from an appreciable height. Some have referred to this as the "Shaken Baby Triad."[35].

Physical signs

Ludwig[31] has emphasized the following presenting physical findings of SBS:

- An enlarged head circumference was seen in slightly more than half of cases as well as a bulging anterior fontanel.

- Non-specific bruising was noted in one-third of the cases.

- Neurologic involvement is seen in fewer than 50% of cases.

- The key to diagnosis is the presence of retinal hemorrhages, which are seen in 80% of the patients[37, 38].

Investigations

Laboratory studies for SBS are non-specific and are not diagnostic. Leucocytosis is seen in approximately 50% of patients. Serum chemistry findings are usually normal but these may reveal evidence of acidosis. The cerebrospinal spinal fluid may be bloody, possibly indicating the presence of a subarachnoid hemorrhage.

The key diagnostic test for SBS is neuroimaging (Figure 54.8). CT scan of the brain is sufficient to diagnose subdural hemorrhage, cerebral edema, and/or subarachnoid hemorrhage. Magnetic resonance imaging (MRI) as a follow-up study can determine the extent of the neurologic injury. It may be helpful for continued management and prognosis. As long, as the anterior fontanel is still open; ultrasound can identify an intracranial hemorrhage. A negative head ultrasound, however, does not rule out intracranial pathology.

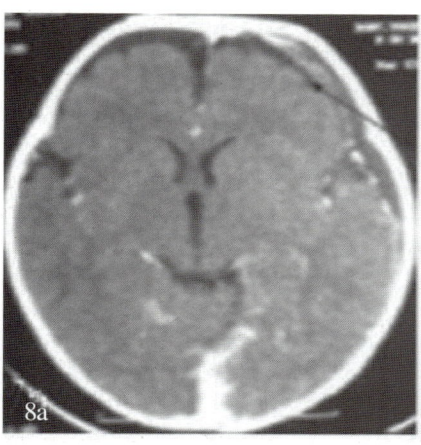 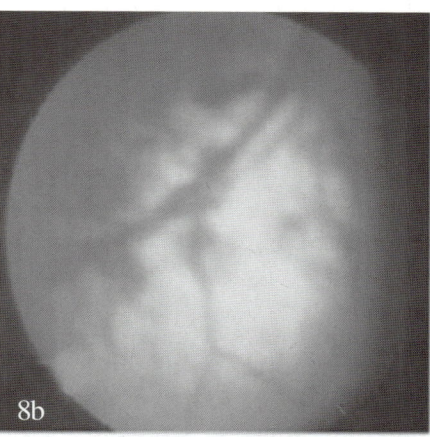 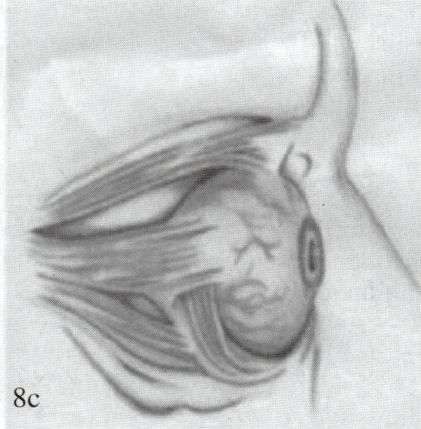

Figure 54.8a Showing subdural hematoma, 54.8b Fundoscopy picture of retinal hemorrhages. 54.8c Ocular hemorrhages due to child abuse

An ophthalmologic evaluation is extremely important and helpful in diagnosis. A dilated eye examination is preferable, but in the ED, all patients (regardless of the presenting complaint) should have a retinal examination with a direct ophthalmoscope. Papilledema indicates the presence of increased ICP, and retinal hemorrhage strongly points to the diagnosis of SBS. All patients who are suspected of abuse must have a long-bone skeletal survey to check for new or healing fractures, which also helps in the diagnosis. Serum alkaline phosphatase is elevated if there are multiple fractures.

Management

Medical care. Supportive care is the mainstay of treatment in child abuse. Blood pressure and vital signs should be supported and maintained. Provide mechanical ventilation as needed. Treat increased ICP, if present.

Surgical care. Intracranial monitoring may be necessary, especially when raised ICP is a problem. In the presence of subdural hematoma, surgical evacuation may be necessary. Obtain an ophthalmic evaluation by an ophthalmologist who is well versed in identifying eye findings in abused children. The ophthalmologist is required for the initial evaluation and possibly for the follow-up as well. Referral to a physician who specializes in abuse cases can be helpful but is not mandatory.

Following recovery from the neurologic injury, physical therapy and occupational therapy are helpful. For patients in whom speech/language may be affected, speech therapy is advised. The reasons for child abuse should be sought and remedial measures should be instituted to prevent recurrence.

Mild Traumatic Brain Injury and Concussion

Its been realized that in spite of an apparently normal CT head, there might be subtle organic brain damage, which may be associated with distressing neuropsychological sequelae in these patients[39, 40]. A typical review of head injured patients admitted to a neurosurgical service found that 5% were severe (GCS score ≤ 8), 11% were moderate (GCS score 9 to 12), and 84% were minor (GCS score 13 to 15)[34]. In spite of these figures, however, patients with minor head injuries can be offered little except reassurance.

Diagnostic criteria. The most widely used definition of minor head injury is a set of criteria published by the members of the Mild Traumatic Brain Injury Interdisciplinary Special Interest Group (BISIG) of the American Congress of Rehabilitation Medicine (Handbook 16th)[41] which states that:

1. Loss of consciousness should not exceed 30 minutes.
2. After 30 minutes the initial GCS score should be between 13 and 15.
3. Post-traumatic amnesia does not exceed 24 hours.

Following minor head injury, a syndrome called as 'post-concussion syndrome' has been reported to occur in upto 80% of the patients[42]. This syndrome includes symptoms such as headache, irritability, poor concentration, memory disturbances, dizziness, anxiety and depression. Persistent postconcussion syndrome, defined as persistence of symptoms of postconcussion syndrome beyond three months, is seen in more than 30% of the patients, and upto 15% may have persistent, disabling symptoms beyond six months.

Section 5

Pathophysiology. The hippocampus is especially vulnerable to mechanically induced head injury and to other types of insults such as ischemia, hypoxia, and seizures. The extent of hippocampal damage may be correlated with severity of memory impairment. Newer investigative modalities such as SPECT and PET due to their high sensitivity appear as an attractive proposition for studying structural damage in such patients (Figure 54.9). In a study conducted at AIIMS using SPECT in children with persistent postconcussion syndrome and abnormal SPECT brain[43], all children showed medial temporal (86%) or frontal (13%) hypoperfusion and no patient showed any hyperperfusion. This finding of areas of hypoperfusion in minor head injury has been described previously[44] and may result from vasospasm, direct vascular injury[45] and perfusion changes due to alterations in remote neuronal activity (diaschisis). There is evidence to show that brain is more vulnerable to ischemic injury after minor head injury and it has been hypothesized that SPECT findings representing hypoperfusion may in fact lead to secondary ischemic injury[45].

Imaging studies. In the recent years, with its widespread availability, the use of CT for minor head injury has become increasingly common. Various modalities ranging from neuropsychological testing[46], evoked potential testing, to newer radiological techniques such as PET, SPECT and MRI have been investigated as tools to correlate cerebral dysfunction with symptoms in cases of minor head injuries. Umile et al[40] found that 90% of patients of minor head injury and postconcussion syndrome had abnormal findings on PET or SPECT imaging. Though PET is slightly superior to SPECT in terms of spatial resolution, SPECT is much more affordable and widely available making it attractive as a cost-effective investigative and diagnostic tool in post-concussion syndrome. In a study by Agarwal et al[37] SPECT showed a sensitivity of 80% which is excellent when compared to abysmally poor sensitivities of 9% for CT and 46% for MRI scan recorded by others.

Treatment

Management of minor head injury revolves around two broad issues; firstly, the use of investigative procedures such as SPECT, PET and neuropsychological testing as a means of prognostication and secondly, treatment strategies for postconcussion syndrome. Investigative tools such as SPECT, PET and neuropsychological assessment help in prognostication, especially in pre-school children (less than five years of age) as there is good evidence to suggest that even minor head injury, if occurring at an early age that is critical for the development of certain skills, may cause persistent psychoneurological deficits. Most neurosurgeons can do little except giving reassurance and prescribing analgesics and anti-vertigo medications to children with minor head injuries. Recently, a nootropic agent, piracetam has been tried in such patients. Piracetam has a unique mode of action which is not entirely clear, may be explained by its neuroprotective properties, mediated through effects on the cell membrane. Piracetam improves membrane bound cell functions including ATP production and secondary messenger activity[49, 50]. It has also been shown that piracetam has beneficial effects on the cerebral blood flow, by decreasing the adhesivity, aggregation, and deformability of erythrocytes along with flow thrust

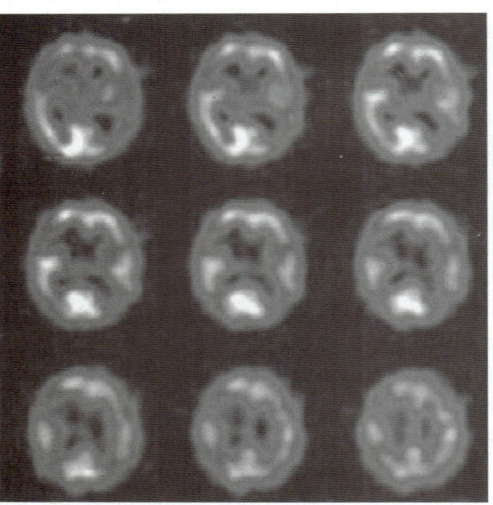
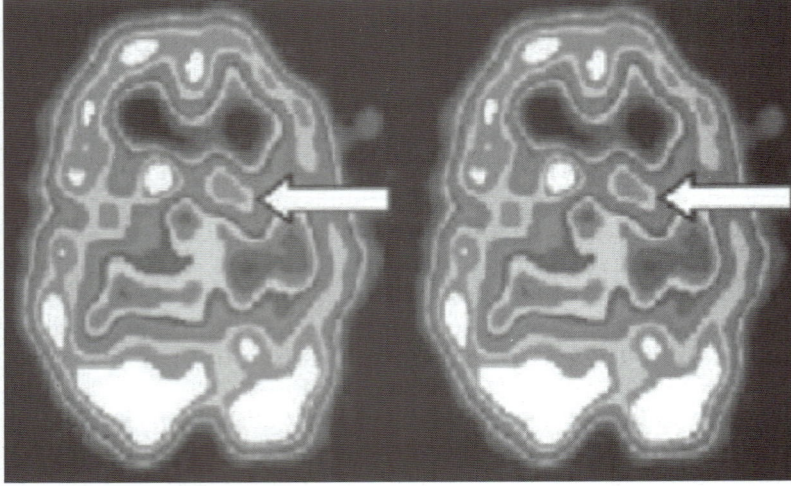

Figure 54.9a SPECT scan in a case of severe head injury, 54.9b SPECT scan in a case of minor head injury showing localized left temporal hypoperfusion (pointed arrow)

tension of the blood. We conducted a randomised-controlled trial and found that low dose piracetam successfully reversed cerebral perfusion deficits and resulted in accelerated symptomatic improvement in patients with post-concussion syndrome[37]. Results show that cerebral perfusion defects occur in majority of the cases of post-concussion syndrome following mild traumatic brain injury. These perfusion defects *per se* may be responsible for the clinical manifestations of post-concussion syndrome and this is further borne out by the improvement in regional blood flow and the reversal of perfusion abnormalities on SPECT, along with alleviation of clinical symptoms of post-concussion syndrome. In children with minor head injury, medial temporal lobe (hippocampus and other associated structures) is particularly vulnerable to direct mechanical trauma as well as indirect injury secondary to hypoperfusion, which on SPECT imaging appears as medial temporal lobe hypoperfusion, and these children may be more likely to develop features of persistent postconcussive syndrome. Serial SPECT studies may, therefore, also serve as a platform for testing the efficacy of various neurobehavioral and pharmacological interventions.

Post-traumatic Dural Sinus Thrombosis

Post-traumatic dural sinus thrombosis (DST) in children has rarely been described in the literature[51]. Steifel *et al*[51] treated 131 children with minor or severe head injury requiring a cranial computed tomography (CT) scan, observed DST in eight patients (6.1%), five with mild and three with severe cranial trauma. Diagnosis is suspected either because of a skull fracture crossing over a dural sinus or because of a hyperdensity at a dural sinus. Enhanced CT scan is used to confirm the diagnosis of DST. No specific symptoms related to DST are observed. DST is usually managed conservatively in most patients and recovery is usually uneventful. Recanalization of the sinus is documented to occur within three weeks to six months. Neither surgical nor any medical intervention is indicated in post-traumatic DST in children.

BRAIN EDEMA

Cerebral contusion consists of heterogeneous areas of hemorrhagic brain necrosis and infarction. Contusions developing at the site of impact are coup contusions and those opposite the cranial impact are contracoup contusions. Coup contusions are due to direct injury to the brain tissue and its surface

vessels by fracture fragments. Contracoup contusions results from tangential or angular head motion. Angular head motion produces high tensile strains throughout the brain. These tensile strains are concentrated adjacent to the irregular bony surface e.g. frontal and temporal areas. In clinical practice contusions of frontal and temporal lobes are common (Figure 54.10a, 54.10b).

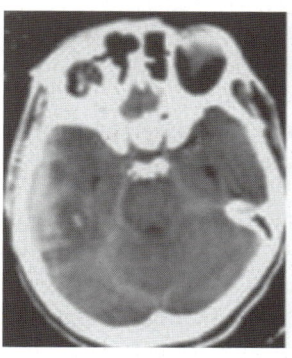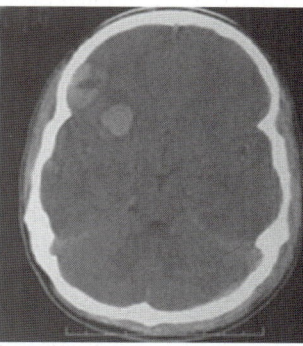

Figures 54.10a and 10b CT scan showing right temporal and right frontal contusions

There are certain differences the way child's brain responds to an injury, as compared to an adult. In adults cerebral edema is more often due to increase in water content which is called as vasogenic edema. In children the swelling is intractable and the brain volume increases rapidly. The condition is termed as "malignant brain edema"[8, 52]. This is by and large due to venous congestion or stasis. Brain injury leads to a cascade of events leading to release of neurotransmitters[53, 54]. These substances disturb the autoregulation leading to break down of blood brain barrier (BBB). The break in blood brain barrier gives rise to loosening of tight junction in the capillary walls and there is leakage of fluid into the extravascular spaces giving rise to brain edema which can be focal or generalised[53].

Recently, brain swelling is increasingly being recognised in association with head injury. This is basically due to vascular congestion. In the past a term called as "luxury perfusion" was described in angiography, which suggested an increased blood circulation in an infarcted area. Sometimes children may suddenly die due to generalised brain swelling. Lobato[53] described acute hemispheric brain swelling in children with cerebral trauma. Pathophysiological mechanism of brain swelling, however, is poorly understood. Post-mortem usually reveals venous congestion. In contusion or intracerebral hematoma, the focal brain swelling occurs due to release of neurotransmitter[55]. However, formation of diffuse edema or swelling in the absence of focal brain lesion is difficult to explain. Cerebral edema may occur due to hypoxia in an unconscious child due to obstruction of airways or aspiration. It is sometimes difficult to understand, whether the vasocongestion is due to neurogenic vasoparalysis or is caused by hypoxic autoregulation failure; leading to vasodilatation and increased blood flow. Recently transcranial Doppler studies have shown significant abnormalities of flow velocity and pulsatility index in head injured patients[56].

Traumatic Ischemic Brain Damage

Over the last two decades, it has been clearly established that the ischemic brain damage is an important pathological finding in the brain following the head injury (Figure 54.11). The studies conducted by Graham *et al* and others have shown that the incidence of ischemic damage is 85-90% in case of severe head injuries[16, 56, 57]. Ischemia may be focal or diffuse due to microcirculatory failure. The hypoxic ischemic damage is probably the most frequent secondary brain damage following head injury. Ischemic damage is not uncommon in children with head injuries. The delicate vasculature in children and sludging effect of blood in capillaries due to increased viscosity may lead to microcirculatory failure. The potent cause of ischemia is hypotension and raised ICP. Fall in cerebral perfusion pressure (CPP) below 60-70 mm of Hg may lead to cerebral hypoperfusion and

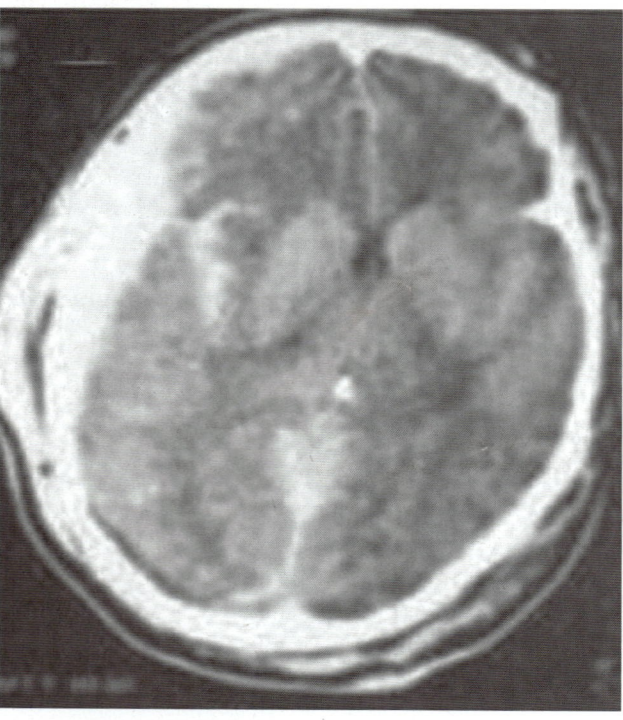

Figure 54.11 CT appearance of diffuse cerebral edema. Note small chinky lateral ventricles

ischemia leading to anerobic glucose metabolism and accumulation of lactic acid and glutamate. Accumulation of oxygen free radicals lead to opening up of calcium channels with influx of calcium into the neurons. The ischemic damage is more common in hippocampus and basal ganglia[57, 58].

MANAGEMENT OF PEDIATRIC HEAD INJURIES

It has been observed that head injured patients fare better when treated early at a trauma center. Two studies have looked specifically at pediatric head injury patients and have found increased survival in those who were transferred to a trauma center with special qualifications to treat children. Brain trauma foundation pre-hospital guidelines of 2007 also recommend that pediatric patients with suspected severe TBI should be transported directly to a facility with specific qualification to treat pediatric patients[59] . However, life saving measures should be started at the site of the accident .The following are the aims of first aid maneuvers:

(i) Resuscitation; (ii) prevention of a second accident and (iii) safe transport of the injured patient under optimum conditions

The "**ABC**" **approach** (A= airways, B= breathing, C= circulation) is aimed at rapid assessment, provision of life support measures followed by more detailed clinical assessment and specific treatment. Until the patient arrives at hospital, care must be taken to ensure that the airways remain clear. Clearing of the upper airways of vomitus, blood and secretions is crucial for intact survival.

Emergency Room Care

The child should be examined carefully but quickly. The airway patency and blood pressure should be checked. The respiratory obstruction and hypotension are the two most important factors causing mortality, followed by intracranial hematoma. Intracranial hematoma takes time to develop and requires CT scan to establish the diagnosis as opposed to respiratory obstruction which can cause rapid clinical deterioration in the neurological status of the patient. If patient's airway cannot be maintained with simple oral airway or a nasopharyngeal tube, the child should be intubated. If due to any reason, intubation is not possible or delayed, an immediate tracheostomy is an accepted alternative in patients having respiratory obstruction.

Neonates and children can develop shock due to scalp hematoma or bleeding from a lacerated wound. A simple long bone fracture may lead to 70-100 ml blood loss, which can result in shock in a child with a weight of 10 kg. The systemic arterial blood pressure should be monitored and kept within normal range to maintain cerebral perfusion pressure. Crystalloid solution (Normal saline or Ringer's lactate) should be infused through a reliable intravenous line. Hypotonic solutions should not be used as they can induce or aggravate already existing brain edema by lowering serum osmolality. In all children with a head injury the source of internal bleeding, must be looked for. In an unconscious patient with hypotension, hemopneumothorax, abdominal trauma and pelvic fracture should be carefully ruled out. Miller[34] found additional systemic injuries in 49 percent cases of severe head injuries, the most common being fracture of limb/s. In their study, fracture of a long bone, chest injury, abdominal injury and spinal injury were observed in 30%, 29%, 29% and 6% cases respectively.

Neurological Assessment

Information regarding precise time of injury and mechanism of injury should be obtained. Acceleration injury as a result of vehicular accidents and falls is associated with a serious and diffuse brain injury and polar contusion. History of the child's neurological status at the scene of the accident and during transport should be sought from police, relatives or any witness. A detailed report from a referring hospital regarding the patient's condition helps in proper assessment. Neurological assessment is crucial to determine the extent of the damage to the brain. However, assessment in children under 2 years of age is much more difficult while children above 10 years of age do not pose any difficulty in examination. The examination of level of consciousness and presence of focal neurological deficit is the two most important aspects. Glasgow coma scale (GCS) designed for the adults has been modified for infants[5, 9, 28] and is called as children coma scale (CCS) and modified GCS[7, 60]. Their comparison is given in Table 54.2. Another scale called pediatric coma score has been developed which takes into consideration size of the patient, respiratory status, systolic blood pressure, CNS status, open wound and fractures (Table 54.3).

For rapid evaluation some pediatric neurosurgeons have modified Glasgow coma score and a mnemonic is used to depict it with AVPU. **A** stands for alert and conscious, **V** signifies response to verbal command; **P** denotes that the patient

Table 54.2 Modified coma scales for infants[7,50]		
Glasgow Coma Scale (GCS)	**Children coma scale (CCS)**	**Modified GCS (MGCS)**
Eye opening		
4 Spontaneous	4 (same)	4 (same)
3 To speech	3	3
3 To pain	2	2
1 None	1	1
Motor		
6 Obeys	6 (same)	6 (reaches)
5 Localizes	5	5
4 Withdraws	4	4
3 Abnormal flexion	3	3
3 Abnormal extension	2	2
1 None	1	1
Verbal		
5 Oriented	5 Smiles, interacts	5 Babbles/gestures
4 Confused	4 Cries, interacts	4 Cries for needs
3 Inappropriate words	3 Consolable, moans	3 Cries, non-specific
2 Sounds	2 Restless, irritable	2 Sounds
1 None	1 None	1 None

Table 54.3 Pediatric coma score

Abnormality	Score*		
	+2	+1	-1
Size of the body frame	Normal or mild abnormality i.e. normal weight-for-age	Major abnormality i.e. under/over weight	Severe or life-threatening abnormality i.e. overtly malnourished/ obese
Respiratory status	Normal breathing	Mild abnormality	Severe distress/ life-threatening obstruction
Systolic BP	Normal	Mild hypotension	Shock
CNS status	Normal	Drowsy or focal deficit	Coma
Open wound	None	Multiple small punctures	Single or multiple lacerated wounds
Fractures	Nil	Small bones like clavicle, Colle's, phalanges etc.	Large bones, pelvis, femur, vertebrae, etc.

*Score +12 outcome excellent, +6 outcome in-between, -6 poor outcome, vegetative state, or death

responds to pain, while **U** symbolises unresponsiveness.

By and large 25 percent children are admitted with a history of loss of consciousness and another 25 percent may be drowsy and irritable[11]. Drowsy or lethargic state in a child should be taken seriously as a large number of these children may have intracranial hematoma and they can deteriorate rapidly.

Focal Neurological Deficit

Presence of hemiparesis, monoparesis or hemiplegia is indicative of focal brain damage. Examination of cranial nerves is important; 3rd nerve palsy is considered as the most significant finding in a patient with head injury. Presence of unilateral or bilateral dilated fixed pupils is not uncommon depending upon severity of injury and transtentorial herniation. Bilateral fixed dilated pupils usually indicate a severe injury and signify a poor outcome. Rarely a child can be conscious and have a fixed dilated pupil, with a positive consensual light reflex. This is indicative of an optic nerve injury[61]. Seventh nerve involvement may be of upper motor type, as a part of hemiparesis. Lower motor neuron facial palsy can occur due to fracture of petrous temporal bone. These children manifest with a bruise over the mastoid process and bleeding through the ipsilateral ear. Hearing loss and CSF otorrhea may also be associated with facial palsy.

Cerebellar signs are rarely observed in children with head injury. When present it is always indicative of a posterior fossa lesion such as extradural or subdural hematoma and cerebellar contusion[24, 25, 62—64]. Acute subdural hematomas can occur in neonates due to birth trauma and till 1997 less than 100 cases have been reported in the world literature[62]. Irritability hypotonia, lethargy, tense anterior fontanel and rarely opisthotonic posture are the characteristic findings in these neonates. Drowsiness and fine horizontal nystagmus are useful correlates of extradural hematoma[24, 25].

Investigations

Following the availability of CT scan, the role of plain X-ray skull has been a subject of controversy. There is little doubt about the medicolegal significance of X-ray skull. The presence of fracture in a case of minor head injury provides a useful clue to the possibility of intracranial hematoma. It is difficult to get a good quality X-ray skull in children unless child is properly restrained. In unconscious patients and children, compound head injury with brain matter coming out, CT scan is the investigation of choice.

A CT scan of brain is indicated immediately in all patients with moderate and severe head injury to rule out any intracranial mass lesion. The primary approach to a large extradural hematoma or subdural hematoma with significant midline shift is surgical drainage. In contrast, patients with diffuse head injury and compressed cisterns should be treated in an ICU with proper monitoring and management of respiratory, cardiovascular and metabolic parameters.

In the absence of CT scan facility, burr hole exploration is recommended. Most extra-axial intracranial lesions can be localised and the possibility of false negative results after six-hole exploration appears to be negligible. Subsequently, a CT scan of abdomen should be planned when abdominal injury is strongly suspected. X-ray chest and pelvis are useful to exclude pneumohemothorax and fracture of pelvis respectively. An abdominal paracentesis is useful for diagnosing hemoperitoneum, but a negative tap does not necessarily exclude the diagnosis. Diagnostic peritoneal lavage may be required for diagnosing hemoperitoneum. Cervical injury may also lead to hypotension. A failure to detect these injuries in an unconscious patient may lead to drastic consequences.

Emergency Management

The following steps should be taken when a child with severe head injury reports to the emergency department:

1. Maintenance of airways
   - Nasopharyngeal tube or oral airway
   - Intubation
   - Tracheostomy

2. Establish breathing (ventilation)
   - Position
   - Bag and mask ventilation
   - Assisted ventilation

3. Sustain circulation
   - Maintenance of systemic BP
   - Good intravenous line
   - CVP line
   - Crystalloid infusion
   - Blood transfusion if required

4. Foley's catheterization and nasogastric intubation

5. Neurological assessment
   - GCS score
   - Pupillary size and reaction to light

6. Associated injuries

7. Investigations
   - X-ray skull AP/translateral
   - X-ray chest
   - X-ray cervical spine AP/translateral
   - Non contrast CT scan head

If required X-ray pelvis, X-ray abdomen, or CT abdomen and arterial blood gases (ABG) should be checked.

Management in the Intensive Care Unit

The intensive care management of both surgically treated and medically managed cases of head injury are similar. The potentially treatable factors such as hypoxia, hypercapnia, hypotension and intracranial hypertension should be identified and treated accordingly. The outcome from severe head injury to a large extent depends on recognition and early treatment of the preventable secondary damage.

The following parameters should be monitored:

1. Neurological status

2. Intracranial pressure

3. Cerebral perfusion pressure

4. Vital signs and physiological parameters: Heart rate, breathing rate, blood pressure, temperature, fluid intake and output

These parameters would guide in providing proper medical and surgical management.

Neurological monitoring

Neurological assessment will help in detecting early deterioration, improvement or static clinical condition of the patient during therapy. No investigation can serve as a substitute for good neurological assessment and observation.

Intracranial pressure monitoring

Studies in pediatric patients have demonstrated improved outcomes for those patients who undergo aggressive monitoring and management of ICP. The outcome is poor when ICP is persistently elevated above 20 mm Hg[65].

Normally, the resting ICP is between 0 to 15 mm of Hg. Transient elevation of ICP occurs during straining, coughing or in Trendelenburg position. A sustained ICP of greater than 20 mm Hg is clearly abnormal. An ICP between 20 and 40 mm Hg is considered as moderate intracranial hypertension. If the ICP is greater than 40 mm Hg, head injury is likely to be severe and it is usually considered as a life-threatening intracranial hypertension. Increased ICP occurs in 50%-70% of the patients even after evacuation of intracranial hematoma. The incidence of intracranial hypertension is greater after evacuation of an intracerebral hematoma, 71% compared with 39% after evacuation of a subdural or epidural hematoma.

The association between the severity of intracranial hypertension and a poor outcome after severe head injury is well recognised. Miller[34] reported that the mortality rate increased from 18% to 92% and the frequency of good outcomes decreased from 74% to 3% in patients who had severe intracranial hypertension that could not be lowered below 20 mm Hg. Though there are no specific guidelines for ICP monitoring in pediatric patients, a threshold for placing a monitor at a GCS of 8 or less is generally accepted[65].

Indications for monitoring of ICP in patients with head injury[66]

1. Patients with GCS score of less than 8 in whom the decision to surgically evacuate the hematoma is equivocal.

2. Inability to monitor serial neurologic examination in a patient undergoing elective ventilation for traumatic brain swelling.

3. Patients with multiple small intracranial hematomas not meriting surgical evacuation.

4. Patients with good coma scale with hematoma diagnosed on CT scan.

5. Patients with multiple hematomas of which only the largest one was evacuated.

6. Postoperative patients who are paralysed and being electively ventilated.

Methods for ICP monitoring

Two types of ICP monitoring devices are available, fluid-coupled and non-fluid coupled. The fluid-coupled devices are placed in the ventricles, subarachnoid space or the subdural spaces and are connected to a pressure transducer through a fluid filled line. The ventriculostomy catheter remains the standard against which all of the newer monitors are compared. Ventricular catheter also allows cerebrospinal fluid drainage for therapeutic purposes. It can be placed easily and quickly in most patients with head trauma, even those who are having a mass effect. Disadvantages of ventricular catheter include infection rate of 8% to 10% and a small risk of intracranial hemorrhage[67]. Subdural bolt (Richmond screws) which is placed in the subdural space is less invasive. Subdural and epidural devices are comparatively less reliable and are associated with a higher rate of blockage.

Non-fluid coupled system such as the Camino intraparenchymal monitor is placed within the parenchyma of the brain[66]. It is not associated with any variations in pressure transmission, which is seen with devices placed in the subarachnoid or dural layers, and it is not prone to clogging. This system, however, is expensive but the risks involved are similar to the fluid-coupled systems.

Management of raised ICP

Treatment of raised ICP should be started after removal of all remediable factors e.g. any intracranial hematoma significant enough for surgical evacuation. Most investigators report improved outcome with treatment if ICP is maintained between 15 to 20 mm Hg[68]. Intracranial pressure of more than 20 mm Hg should be treated because of potential risk of transtentorial herniation.

The *"Monro-Kelli"* doctrine states that the total intracranial volume will remain essentially constant by virtue of displacement if any one of the primary intracranial components i.e. brain parenchyma, blood, or CSF is increased (e.g. cerebral edema or tumor). If there is development of intracranial hematoma, one of the primary intracranial components must be displaced otherwise the ICP would increase.

Therefore, reducing cerebral blood volume (head-up positioning, hyperventilation and barbiturates); reducing CSF volume (CSF drainage); and reducing brain tissue volume (osmotic diuretics and glucocorticoids) can control ICP. Ventriculostomy and CSF drainage are most effective for treatment of refractory hypertension[69]. Other conventional treatments, such as neuromuscular blockage, sedation and analgesia exert less specific effects.

Position of the patient's head. Ventilated head injured patients should be nursed with their head maintained in a neutral position at 15 to 30 degrees above horizontal. This enhances cerebral venous drainage. This is an effective method to decrease ICP and may also decrease the likelihood of subsequent ICP spikes. Care should be taken to note the level of the external auditory meatus, which is the zero reference point for the calibration of ICP monitors.

Hyperventilation. Hyperventilation to maintain an arterial $paCO_2$ between 25 to 30 mm Hg will reduce ICP by promoting cerebral vasoconstriction and subsequent reduction of cerebral blood flow (CBF). The onset of action is within 30 seconds and peaks within 8 minutes after $paCO_2$ drops to the desired level[14]. In case the patient does not rapidly respond the prognosis for survival is generally poor. Prolonged hyperventilation loses its effectiveness and therefore is of limited value beyond acute phase. The partial pressure of carbon dioxide should not fall below 25 mm Hg because this may lead to profound vasoconstriction and ischemia in normal and injured areas of brain. The major difficulty with managing hyperventilation is the difficulty in assessing its effect on CBF. One useful approach to resolve this problem is the use of jugular venous saturation monitoring. Gopinath[15] found that the hypocapnia ($paCO_2$ <30 mm Hg) increased the incidence of cerebral desaturation [decreased jugular bulb oxygen stauration ($SjvO_2$)]. According to 2003 guidelines, prophylactic hyperventilation ($paCO_2$<35 mm Hg) should be avoided but mild hyperventilation ($PaCO_2$ of 30-35 mm Hg) can be considered for elevated ICP that is refractory to other treatments[69].

Osmotic agents. As per 2003 guidelines , both mannitol and hypertonic saline are considered acceptable for use as hyperosmolar therapy after brain injury[70]. When there is deepening coma, pupillary inequality or other deterioration of the neurologic signs, mannitol may be life saving. Mannitol (0.25 to 1.0 gm/kg) can effectively reduce cerebral edema by producing an osmotic gradient that draws intraneuronal and interstitial water into the vascular space and reduces brain volume.

The effect of mannitol depends on the dose, rate of infusion, serum osmolality and patient's state of hydration. The osmotic effects of mannitol occur within minutes of its administration and peak at about 60 minutes after the bolus has been administered. The ICP-lowering effects of a single bolus of mannitol may last for 6 to 8 hours. Mannitol has neuroprotective effect and reduces the concentration of oxygen free radicals that may promote cell membrane lipid peroxidation. Mannitol also promotes cerebral blood flow by reducing blood viscosity and microcirculatory resistance. It reduces RBC deformability and, therefore, improves oxygen carrying capacity.

Mannitol can induce hypovolemic hypotension. Repeated doses of mannitol increases serum osmolality. This reduces the effectiveness of mannitol and may cause dilutional hyponatremia and precipitate acute renal failure. Also repeated episodes of diuresis may wash out the renal medullary concentration gradient and thereby interfere with the ability of the kidneys to concentrate the urine. As mannitol enters areas of damaged blood brain barrier (BBB), mannitol may concentrate within brain tissue, producing reversed osmotic effect. By reducing brain volume, tamponade effect of extraaxial hematoma may be decreased or lost, allowing more bleeding to occur into the traumatic site. It has been found that mannitol in a dose of 0.25 g/kg appears to be as effective as 1 gm/kg in terms of beneficial effect on ICP. Serum osmolality should not be allowed to increase beyond 320 mOsm/l.

Furosemide is a loop diuretic often used in patients with head injury. Evidence suggests that furosemide works synergistically with mannitol in lowering ICP. It may lead to significant dehydration and hypokalemia. *There is no role of corticosteroids for the treatment of raised ICP following head injury.*

Sedation. Sedation is often indicated in agitated and restless patients. Restlessness and irritability may be because of pain, which interferes with diagnostic and therapeutic procedures and results in increased ICP. A variety of different sedating agents commonly used to facilitate ventilation are diazepam, midazolam, opiates and more recently propofol.

Barbiturates are effective in lowering ICP. Second tier therapy with barbiturates is required in selected patients with refractory intracranial hypertension. Barbiturates have a potent depressant effect on cerebral electrical activity and metabolism of brain. They also cause vasoconstriction, which leads to decreased cerebral blood flow (CBF) and ICP. In patients with intracranial hypertension, barbiturates cause maximal reduction in ICP in those patients whose initial ICP was abnormally high. This decrease in ICP is often associated with an increase in cerebral perfusion pressure (CPP).

Thiopental, a short acting barbiturate, is most commonly used to control intracranial hypertension. Thiopental should be given to patients admitted to an intensive care unit who are provided with intensive neurosurgical care. Barbiturate therapy should be accomplished with an intravenous loading dose of 10 mg/kg of thiopental given during 30 minutes. During administration of loading dose, if the patient's blood pressure decreases, the intravascular volume should be increased and dopamine infusion should be started. This dose should be followed by a constant infusion of thiopental at a rate of 5 mg/kg/hr during the next 3 hours. The maintenance dose should be restricted to 1 mg/kg/hr.

Propofol is a relatively new sedative-hypnotic with a very rapid onset and short duration of action. As an intravenous anesthetic agent, propofol has many advantages in treating raised ICP. It reduces cerebral metabolic rate of oxygen ($CMRO_2$) and cerebral blood flow (CBF). It also lowers systemic blood pressure and usually results in net decrease in cerebral perfusion pressure (CPP)[11, 68, 69].

Decompressive craniectomy

Although decompressive craniectomy can reduce ICP, its effect on outcome has been less clearly established. The 2003 guidelines offer decompressive craniectomy (Figure 54.12a & b) as an option as a weakest level of recommendation, in patients who meet all or some of the following criteria: (i) diffuse cerebral swelling on imaging, less than 48 hours after injury, (ii) no episodes of sustained ICP higher than 40 mm Hg before surgery, (iii) GCS score higher than 3 at some point after injury, and (iv) secondary clinical deterioration or clinical evidence of herniation.[71]

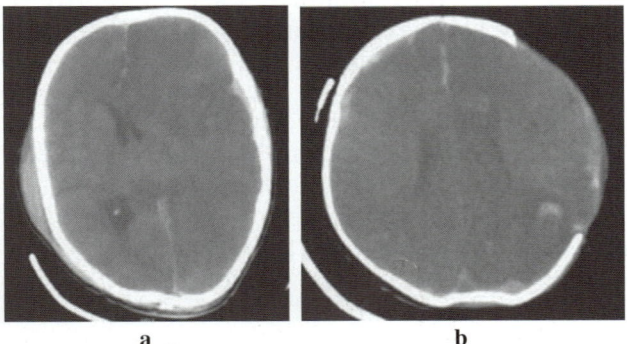

a   b

Figure 54.12 (a) showing frontoparietal acute subdural hematoma with mass effect/ midline shift and brain infarction and (b) post decompressive craniectomy

Seizure Prophylaxis

Upto 9 percent of all patients who sustain blunt head trauma suffer from early post-traumatic seizures[72]. The incidence of early post-traumatic seizures approaches 42 percent in patients who have sustained penetrating head trauma[73]. Although the occurrence of seizures in the immediate post-trauma period has no predictive value for future epilepsy, early seizures can cause hypoxia, hypercarbia, and release of excitatory neurotransmitters and increased ICP, which can worsen secondary brain injury. Therefore, all paralysed head injured patients should have prophylactic anticonvulsant therapy during the acute phase. If patient is having convulsions, benzodiazepines are effective in rapidly controlling seizures. Diazepam is given intravenously in a dose of 0.1 mg/kg (upto 5 mg) IV every 5 minutes upto a maximum total dose of 20 mg. For long term anticonvulsant therapy, phenytoin is given in a loading dose of 15 mg/kg IV at a rate of 50 mg/minute. The maintenance dose is 5 mg/kg IV every day[74-76].

Indications for anticonvulsant therapy

Incidence of early seizures in patients with closed head injury ranges from 2-5%. The presence of risk factors will further increase the incidence of early post traumatic epilepsy. Young et al[75] randomized 204 patients into two groups. One group received phenytoin within 24 hours of admission and plasma concentration of at least 10 ug/ml was achieved. No significant reduction in the incidence of early or late post traumatic seizures was found between the treated and placebo group. Tempkine et al[76] randomized 404 patients with severe head trauma and observed that phenytoin was effective in preventing seizures during the first week after cerebral injury (3.6% among treated versus 14.2% control) but was no better than placebo in exerting a protective effect during the remainder of the study period. It was, therefore, concluded that phenytoin should be given to patients at risk of post traumatic seizures during the first week after trauma and then discontinued unless further seizures occur. Compilation of the available data supports prophylactic administration of phenytoin for prevention of early seizures but it was not found to be useful in preventing late post-traumatic seizures. Other antiepileptic drugs such as sodium valproate, and phenobarbitone have not been adequately evaluated for their use as prophylactic anticonvulsant agents in head injury patients.

Acute post-traumatic seizures should be treated aggressively with benzodiazepines and a loading dose of phenytoin. Inadequate control of early post-traumatic seizures results in severe hypoxic and secondary metabolic damage of the already injured brain. Current pediatric guidelines recommend a 7-day course of prophylactic antiepileptics after head injury to decrease the risk for early seizures[77].

SEQUELAE

Previously it was thought that infants are at a lower risk of long term sequelae, but recent studies have shown that infants may have slow development of intelligence than older children after similar head injuries. Similarly, children younger than 6 years had more difficulty in executive control and had higher risk of memory loss after head injuries than did older children. In addition, 40% of children have a persistent change in personality after severe head injury. It has also been seen that the incidence of behavioral problems correlates with severity of head injury (36% in those with severe injury and 22% in those with moderate injury).

In 2008 , around 2000 patients requiring neurosurgical care showed up at level 1 trauma center facility of our institute. Out of these, 183 (9.15%) were pediatric patients i.e. <18 years of age. 129 (70.4%) patients sustained the injuries as a result of fall from height whereas 50 (27.3%) patients had suffered road traffic accidents. The remaining 4 (2.1%) patients had history of physical assault. Male patients outnumbered the females and constituted 66.1% (121/183) of all patients. 75 (40.9%) patients were admitted with minor head injuries whereas severe head injuries were seen in 65 (35.5%) patients. Moderate head injuries were seen in 23.4% patients. 141 (77%) patients were managed conservatively whereas 42 (23%) patients required surgery. Mortality rate was 20.2% (37 out of 183 patients). 50.7% mortality (33/65) was seen in severely head injured patients whereas mortality rate in moderately head injured patients was 9.3% (4/43). No mortality was seen in minor head injury patients.[78-81]

CONCLUSIONS

Children pose difficulties in the assessment of the severity of head injury and early neurosurgical consultation is indicated. Patient must be stabilized and intubated if indicated before transfer to the neurosurgical department. Overhydration must be avoided. When emergency surgery is warranted it must be undertaken as per the guidelines mentioned earlier. Blood loss and hypotension are common features in children and add to the mortality and morbidity. Early blood transfusion should be given to replace blood loss and maintain adequate oxygenation. Because of the differences in the pathaphysiological responses of the brain, intracranial mass lesions are less frequent, diffuse brain swelling sets in very easily following even minor injuries. In general outcome of severe head injury in childhood is considerably better than those of adults owing to the greater neuronal plasticity, provided they are managed appropriately. The common neuromotor sequelae following head injury in children include seizures, attention deficit hyperactivity disorder (ADHD), behaviour disorders and learning disability.

REFERENCES

1. Kraus JF, Rock, Hemyari P. Brain injuries among infants, children, adolescents and young adults. *Am J Dis Child* 1990 (144): 684-691.

2. King DR. Trauma in infancy and childhood: Initial evaluation and management. *Pediatr Clin N Am* 1985 32: 1299-1309.

3. Moront ML. The injured child. An approach to care. *Pediatr Clin N Am* 1994, 41: 1201-1226.

4. Sambasivan M. Epidemiology: Pediatric head injuries. *Neurology India (Supplement)* 1995, 43: 57-58.

5. Walia BS. Severe pediatric head injury. An analysis of 109 patients. MCh *Thesis submitted to AIIMS,* 1996.

6. Baker DP, Flower C, Li G, Laine M. Head injuries incurred by children and young adults during informal recreation. *Am J Publ Health* 1994, 84: 649-652.

7. Ewing-Cobbs L Miner ME, Fletcher JM, *et al.* Intellectual motor and language sequelae following closed head injury in infants and pre-schoolers. *J Pediatr Psychol* 1989, 14: 531-547.

8. Bruce DA, Alavi A, Bilaniuk L, *et al.* Diffuse cerebral swelling following head injuries in children: The syndrome of "Malignant brain edema". *J Neurosurg* 1981, 54: 170-178.

9. Bruce DA, Scheet C, Ware JD, Sutton L.N. Outcome following severe head injury in children. *J Neurosurg* 1978, 48: 679-688.

10. Chidambaram B. Head injuries: Special problems in children. *Neurology India (Supplement)* 1995, 43: 68-73.

11. Farling PA, Johnston JR, *et al.* Propofol infusion for sedation of patients with head injury in intensive care: a preliminary report. *Anaesthesia* 1989, 44: 222-226.

12. Suri A, Mahapatra AK. Growing fractures of the orbital roof. A report of two cases and a review. *Pediatr Neurosurg* 2002, 36(2): 96-100.

13. Mahapatra AK, Tandon PN. Post-traumatic intradiploic pseudomeningocele in children. *Acta Neurochir (Wien)* 1989, 100(3-4): 120-126.

14. Chan KH, Miller JD, Dearden NH, *et al.* The effects of changes in cerebral perfusion pressure upon middle cerebral artery blood flow velocity and jugular bulb

venous oxygen saturation after severe brain injury. *J Neurosurg* 1992 77: 55-61.

15. Gopinath SP, Robertson CS, Contant CF, *et al.* Jugular venous desaturation and outcome after head injury. *J Neurol Neurosurg Psychiatry* 1994, 57: 717-723.

16. Graham DI. Pathology of hypoxic damage in brain, hypoxia and ischemia. *J Clin Path (supplement)* 1977, 11: 170-180.

17. Paul C Francel, John Honey C. Mild brain injury in children including skull fracture and growing skull fracture. In: Youmans Neurological Surgery, H Richard winn (Ed.), *Saunders Co* 5th edn, 2004, pp 3461-3472.

18. Ammarati M, Tomita T. Posterior fossa extradural hematoma in childhood. *Neurosurgery* 1985, 14: 541-544.

19. Mahaptra AK. Posterior fossa extradural hematoma. *Indian Pediatr* 1990, 27: 989-992.

20. Gupta PK, Mahapatra AK, Lad SD. Posterior fossa extradural haematoma (PFEDH). The Oman experience. *Pan Arab Neurosurgery* 2001, 5: 1-7.

21. Bagchi AK. Head injury in neonates. In: An Introduction to Head Injury. AK Bagchi (Ed.), *Oxford University Press, Calcutta* 1980, p 77-80.

22. Zuccarello M, Facco E, Zampieri P, Zanardi L, Andrioli GC. Severe head injury in children. Early diagnosis and outcome. *Child Nerv Syst* 1985, 1: 158-162.

23. Edon MR, Doppen Berg, John D Ward. In: Youmans Neurological surgery, H Richard Winn (Ed.), *Saunders Co* 5th edn 2004, pp 3473-3480.

24. Sharma RR, Mahapatra AK, Pawar SJ, Sousa J. Symptomatic calcified subdural hematoma *Pediatr Neurosurg* 1999, 31: 151-154.

25. Duhaime AC, Christian CW, Rorke LB, *et al.* Nonaccidental head injury in infants- the "shaken baby syndrome". *N Engl J Med* 1998, 338:1822-1829.

26. Caffey J. The whiplash shaken infant syndrome. Manual shaking by the extremities with whiplash induced intracranial and intraocular bleedings, linked with residual permanent brain damage and mental retardation. *Pediatrics* 1974, 54:396-403.

27. Billmire ME, Myers PA. Serious head injury in infants: Accident or abuse? *Pediatrics* 1985, 75: 340-342.

28. Kempe CH, Silverman FN, Steele BF, *et al.* The battered child syndrome. *JAMA* 1962, 181:105-112.

29. Duhaime AC, Sutton LN. Delayed sequelae of pediatric head injury. In: Complications and Sequelae of Head Injury. Barrow D (Ed.) Park Ridge III, *American Association of Neurological surgeons,* 1992, pp 169-186.

30. Meservy CJ, Towbin R, Mc Laurin RL, *et al.* Radiographic characteristics of skull fractures resulting from child abuse. *Am J Radiol* 1987, 149:173-175.

31. Ludwig S. Child abuse. In: Textbook of Pediatric Emergency Medicine, Fleischer GR, Ludwig S (Eds). *Baltimore, Williams and Wilkins,* 2nd Edn 1988, pp 1127-1163.

32. Harcourt B, Hopkins D. Ophthalmic manifestations of the battered baby syndrome. *BMJ* 1971, 3: 398-401.

33. Watson MR, Fenton GW, McClelland RJ, Lumsden J, Headley M, Rutherford WH. The post-concussion state: Neurophysiological aspects. *Br J Psychiatry* 1995; 167:514-521.

34. Miller JD. Minor, moderate and severe head injury. *Neurosurg Rev* 1986; 9:135-139.

35. Mild Head Injury Interdisciplinary Special Interest Group of the American Congress of Rehabilitation Medicine. Definition of mild traumatic brain injury. *J Head Trauma Rehabil* 1993; 8:86-88.

36. Hugenholtz H, Stuss DT, Stethem BA, Richard MT. How long does it take to recover from a mild concussion? *Neurosurgery* 1998; 22:853-858.

37. Agarwal D., Naveen K., Bal CS, Mahapatra AK. Post concussion vertigo. Is the cause central? Correlation with SPECT and CT. *Neurosciences Today* 2003, 7: 33-36.

38. Jacobs A, Put E, Ingels M, Bossuyt A. One-year follow up of technicium-99m-HMPAO SPECT in mild head injury. *J Nucl Med* 1996; 37:1605-1609.

39. Hoffman PAM, Stapert SZ, van Kroonenburgh MJPG, Jolles J, de Kruijk Jelle, Welmink JT. MR imaging, single-photon emission CT, and neurocognitive performance after mild traumatic brain injury. *AJNR* 2001, 22:441-449.

40. Umile EM, Sandel E, Alavi A, Terry CM, Plotkin RC. Dynamic imaging in mild traumatic brain injury: support for the theory of medial temporal vulnerability. *Arch Phys Med rehabil* 2002, 83:1506-1513.

41. Peuvot J, Schanck A, Deleers M, *et al.* Piracetam-induced changes to membrane physical properties: a combined approach by 31P nuclear magnetic resonance and conformational analysis. *Biochem Pharmacol* 1995, 50:1129-1134.

42. Benzi G, Pastoris O, Villa RF, *et al.* Influence of ageing and exogenous substances on cerebral energy metabolism in post hypoglycemic recovery. *Biochem Pharmacol* 1985, 34: 1477-1483.

43. Stiefel D, Eich G, Sacher P. Posttraumatic dural sinus thrombosis in children. *Eur J Pediatr Surg* 2000 Feb, 10 (1): 41-44.

44. Cock MW, Levin I A, Joseph MP, *et al*. Traumatic optic neuropathy: A meta-analysis. *Arch Otolaryngol Head Neck Surg* 1996, 122:389-392.

45. Mahapatra AK, Tandon DA, Bhatia R, Bannerji AK. Optic nerve injury in children. A study of 35 cases. *Child's Nerv System* 1991, 7 (5): 287.

46. Mahapatra AK. Indirect optic nerve injury in children. A study of 35 patients. *J Neurosurg Sci* 1992, 36: 79-84.

47. Mahapatra AK. Optic nerve injury - A study of 530 patients. *Clinical Neurology Neurosurgery* 1997, Vol. 99 Suppl: S201 (Abstract)

48. Healy GB. Hearing loss and vertigo secondary to head injury. *N Eng J Med* 1982, 306: 1029-1031.

49. Luerssen TG. Skull fractures after closed head injury. In: Principles and Practice of Pediatric Neurosurgery, Al-bright L, Pollack I, Adelson PD (eds.). *New York, Thieme Medical* 1999, pp 813-829.

50. Lang DA, Teasdale GM, *et al*. Diffuse brain swelling after head injury, more often malignant in children than adults. *J Neurosurg* 1991, 80: 675-680.

51. Long DM. Traumatic brain edema. *Clinical Neurosurg* 1982, 29: 174-202.

52. Mohanty S, Dey PK, Sharma HS, *et al*. Role of histamine in traumatic brain edema. An experimental study in rats. *J Neurol Sciences* 1989, 90: 87-97.

53. Labato RD. Post-traumatic brain swelling. In: Advances and Technical Standards in Neurosurgery. L. Symon (Ed.) 1993. *Springer Verlag, (Wien) New York* vol. 21, pp 3-38.

54. Yang BO, Feng Z, Zhang Z, Sun H. A transcranial Doppler study of drainage of cerebrospinal fluid and intracranial haematoma. In: Modern Trends in Management of Neurotrauma. P.S. Ramani, A. Sharma (Eds.), *Lavanya Print Pvt. Ltd., Bombay,* 1994, p 36.

55. Dharker SR, Mitta RS, Bhargav N. Ischemic lesion in basal ganglia in children after minor head injury. *Neurology India (Suppl)*, 1995 43-47.

56. Graham DI, Adama JH. Doyle D. Ischemic brain damage in brain in fatal non missile head injuries. *J Neurol Sciences* 1978, 39: 213-234.

57. Hahn YS, Chyung C, Martha JB, *et al*. Head injuries in children under 36 months of age. *Child's Nerv Syst* 1988 4: 34-49.

58. Mahapatra AK, Tandon DA. Traumatic optic neuropathy in children. A prospective study of 50 patients. *Pediatr Neurosurg* 1993 19: 34-39.

59. Guidelines for the management of severe traumatic brain injury. *J Neurotrauma* 2007; 24 (suppl 1): S1-S106.

60. Gupta DK, Subodh Raju, Mahapatra AK. Predictors of outcome in acute subdural hematoma in severe head injury patients. *Indian Neurotrauma* 2004, 1:37-44.

61. Sousa J, Sharma RR, Pawar SJ, Mahapatra AK, Lad SD. Bilateral dilated unreactive pupils in pediatric patients following severe head injury. Long term outcome. *Pan Arab Neurosurg* 2002, 6: 39-46.

62. Pervin RG, Rutka JT, Drake JM, *et al*. Management and outcome of posterior fossa subdural hematomas in neonates. *Neurosurg* 1997, 40: 1190-1200.

63. Mendelsohn D, Levin HS, Bruce D, Lilly M. MRI after head injury: relationship to clinical features and outcome. *Child's Nerv Syst* 1992, 8: 445-452.

64. Aguas J, Begue R, Di Ez J. Brainstem injury diagnosed by MRI. An epidemiological and prognostic reappraisal. *Neurocirugia (Astur)*. 2005, 16(1): 14-20.

65. Adelson PD, Bratton SL, Carney NA, *et al*. Guidelines for the acute management of severe traumatic brain injury in infants, children, adolescents. Indications for intracranial pressure monitoring in pediatric patients with severe traumatic brain injury. *Pediatr Crit Care Med* 2003; 4:S19-S24.

66. Lundberg N, Troupp H, Lorin H, *et al*. Continuous recording of the ventricular fluid pressure in patients with severe acute traumatic brain damage. *J Neurosurg* 1965, 22: 581-590.

67. Luerssen T, Chestnut R. Post traumatic cerebrospinal fluid infections in the Traumatic Coma Data Bank: The influence of type and management of ICP monitors. In: Intracranial Pressure VIII. Avezaat C, Van Eyndhoven J, Mass A, *et al*. (Eds.) *Berlin: Springer-Verlag,* 1993 157-163.

68. Marik PE. Propofol: therapeutic indications and side effects. *Curr Pharma Des* 2004; 10(29): 3639-49.

69. Adelson PD, Bratton SL, Carney NA, *et al*. Guidelines for the acute management of severe traumatic brain injury in infants, children, adolescents. The role of cerebrospinal fluid drainage in the treatment of severe pediatric traumatic brain injury. *Pediatr Crit Care Med* 2003; 4:S38-S39.

70. Adelson PD, Bratton SL, Carney NA, *et al* : Guidelines for the acute management of severe traumatic brain injury in infants, children, adolescents. Use of hyperosmolar therapy in the management of severe pediatric traumatic brain injury. *Pediatr Crit Care Med* 2003; 4:S40-S44.

71. Adelson PD, Bratton SL, Carney NA, et al . Guidelines for the acute management of severe traumatic brain injury in infants, children, adolescents. Surgical treatment of pediatric intracranial hypertension. *Pediatr Crit Care Med* 2003; 4:S56-S59.

72. Kennedy CR, Freeman JM. Post traumatic seizures and post-traumatic epilepsy in children. *J Head Trauma Rehab* 1986, 1 (4): 66.

Section 5

73. Tempkin NR, Dikmen SS, Winn HR. Post-traumatic seizures. *Neurosurg Clin North Am* 1991, 2: 425-435.

74. Hahn YS, Fuch S, *et al*. Factors influencing post-traumatic seizures in children. *Neurosurgery* 1988, 22: 864-867.

75. Young B, Rapp, RP, *et al*. Failure of prophylactic administered phyenytoin to prevent late post-traumatic seizures. *J Neurosurg* 1986, 58: 236-241.

76. Tempkin NR, Dikman SS, *et al*. A randomised, double blind study of phenytoin for the prevention of post-traumatic seizures. *N Eng J Med* 1990, 323, 498-502.

77. Adelson PD, Bratton SL, Carney NA, *et al*. Guidelines for the acute management of severe traumatic brain injury in infants, children, adolescents. The role of antiseizure prophylaxis following severe pediatric traumatic brain injury. *Pediatr Crit Care Med* 2003; 4:S72-S75.

78. Ewing Cobbs L, Prasad MR, landry SH, *et al*. Executive functions following traumatic brain injury in young children. A preliminary analysis. *Dev Neuropsychol* 2004; 26:487-512.

79. Keenan HT, Bratton SL: Epidemiology and outcomes of pediatric traumatic brain injury. *Dev Neuropsychol* 2004; 26:256-263.

80. Max JE, Koele SL, Castillo CC, *et al*. Personality change disorder in children and adolescents following traumatic brain injury. *J Int Neuropsychol Soc* 2000; 6:279-289.

81. Schwartz L, Taylor HG, Drotar D, *et al*. Long term behavior problems following pediatric traumatic brain injury: prevalence, predictors and correlates. *J Pediatr Psychol* 2003:28:251-263.

Section 5

55

Poisoning in Children

P Ramesh Menon and Rakesh Lodha

INTRODUCTION

A poison is an agent of injury (disturbance to internal milieu) to human beings, usually by chemical reaction, when a sufficient quantity is absorbed through epithelial linings such as the skin or gut. A poison is often distinguished from a toxin and venom. Toxins are poisons produced via a biological process in nature, and venoms are usually toxins that are injected by a bite or sting of an insect or animal to cause their effect.

Poisoning is a common medical emergency in childhood. Most exposures involve oral ingestion (three-quarters), occur at home (>90 percent), and are unintentional (> 80 percent). Suicide attempts or gestures are more common in older children and adolescents. There are very few community-based data in India regarding incidence of poisoning. This is due to several reasons including a lack of standardized case definition[1].

Reports available in literature are based on hospital studies. Figures from these reports indicate that poisoning is the cause for 0.64-11.6 percent of total pediatric admissions and is responsible for 0.6 percent of all deaths during childhood. There is regional variability largely influenced by the life style, socioeconomic and cultural habits of people and functioning of regulatory and surveillance systems[2].

Toddlers are at an increased risk of accidental poisoning because of their spontaneous activity, curiosity, innocence, mouthing of objects and imitation of adults. Poisoning may result from pica, thirst or hunger. It may be a manifestation of insecurity, self-injury due to guilt feelings or attention seeking behaviour. Toxicity due to pharmaceutical agents may occur due to self administration by parents for minor ailments, prescription of drugs by quacks and due to ignorance of doctors.

In developing countries due to rapid industrialization and change in living habits, without proportionate increase in education and awareness, the incidence of poisoning is increasing especially due to medications, industrial chemicals, pesticides and insecticides.

CAUSES OF POISONING

In our country, majority of episodes still involve household substances. Recent trends show increase in incidence of toxicity related to medicines and chemicals used in agriculture[3, 4]. Common causes of poisoning in India are given in Table 55.1.

Table 55.1 Important causes of childhood poisoning in India	
Toxic substance	**Incidence (%)**
• *Kerosene and other hydrocarbons*	8-55
• *Household products:* Insecticides, rodenticides, phenol, alkalies (caustic soda, unslaked lime), acids, turpentine, eucalyptus oil, camphor, naphthalene, "neem" oil, alcohol, copper sulfate.	14-30
• *Pharmaceutical products:* Phenothiazines, opiates, tincture opii, diphenoxylate, iron salts, barbiturates, aspirin, piperazine, antiseptics, anticonvulsants, antihypertensives, etc.	16-30
• *Plants and plant products:* Dhatura (datura fastuosa), yellow oleander (*Thevetia nerifolia*), white oleander (*Nerium odorum*), castor seeds (*Ricinus communis*), Chandrajyoti seeds (*Jatropha curcas*).	6-32
• *Food poisoning*	7-15
• *Environmental poisoning:* Elapidae (cobra, krait), viperdae (Russell's viper, saw-scaled viper) bites, scorpion /bee / wasp stings, insect bites.	7-11

EPIDEMIOLOGY

Most of the common pediatric poisonings in the developed world are innocuous and most of the pediatric patients are discharged after a brief period of observation in the emergency room[4-6]. Data available from National Poison Information Center, New Delhi suggests a high incidence of poisoning in children (36.5%)[7]. Accidental mode (79.7%) as well as intentional attempts (20.2%) were reported. Recent review from a single centre by Kohli et al[8] reported 96.9% of accidental exposure in children. The most vulnerable age group was between 1-6 years. Household products (47%), drugs (21.8%), agricultural pesticides (9.1%), industrial chemicals (7.9%), bites and stings (3.2%) and plants (1.5%) are the common poisons reported in the national database. Five percent (5.3%) were classified as miscellaneous and 4% as unknown. Common household products included kerosene, pyrethroids, thermometer mercury, rodenticides, phenyl, detergents and corrosives. Drugs included anticonvulsants, thyroid hormones, benzodiazepines, analgesics and oral contraceptives. Agricultural pesticides included aluminum phosphide, organochlorines and organophosphates.

A majority of substances do not cause any significant problems, when ingested in a small quantity. A representative list of innocuous poisons is given in Table 55.2.

Table 55.2 Non toxic common household agents
• Cosmetics, hair dye, hair oil, cream emulsions, mascara, lipstick.
• Shampoos, toothpaste, shaving cream, toilet soaps.
• Lead pencils, matches, cigarettes, candles, chalk, clay, water colors, newspaper, adhesives, ballpoint pen ink, fountain pen ink (blue, black), toy pistol "caps".
• Antacids, antibiotics, oral contraceptives, mercury of thermometers.
• House lizards discovered in food.
• Fertilizers (non-nitrate containing).
• Nail polish and its remover (acetone), depilators, skin lighteners (hydroquinone), after-shave lotions (alcohol) are moderately toxic. Talcum powder may be inhaled by infants with serious consequences.

GENERAL APPROACH TO MANAGEMENT

Initial Assessment and Life Support

Irrespective of the substance ingested, initial management of these children is identical. Most of the children are brought to hospital due to fear of expected untoward effects. Each poisoned child should be assessed immediately for requirement of support of airway; ventilation and circulation for basic life support and these measures should be immediately instituted regardless of the responsible toxin. *Do not try to discover or remember a specific antidote when the child is not breathing*

or is in shock. Observe the rate and depth of respiration and pooling of secretions in throat. In an obtunded comatose patient, the neck should be slightly extended, and secretions in the throat should be sucked. If respiration is depressed, cyanosis, SpO_2 and ABG should be looked for because hypoxia/hypercarbia may be responsible for obtunded sensorium. Circulatory status can be gauged by assessing heart rate, quality of pulse, blood pressure, skin color, temperature and capillary refill time. Any sick child with symptoms of intoxication should have an intravenous line quickly. In critically ill children central venous line may be necessary.

History

In most situations clinical suspicion of poisoning is raised as the symptom complex does not fit in a known pattern or there is a classical pattern of symptomatology (Toxidromes) mimicking known clinical conditions, with a dramatic onset[9]. For example, acute liver failure due to paracetamol poisoning, hyperglycemia with ketosis and CNS depression by acetone or theophylline intoxication (mimic diabetic ketoacidosis) and hyperthermia and tachypnea of salicylate poisoning (simulate acute lower respiratory tract infection).

After initial assessment and stabilization, the identification and quantification of the poison should be sought. Following relevant information should be obtained[10].

1. What was ingested? The name or class of agent and whether formulation was liquid or solid.

2. Time since ingestion, because clinical signs and symptoms need to be interpreted accordingly (*progression versus improvement*) and treatment modalities already offered in relation to the time of ingestion (*pretoxic, toxic and resolution phase*).

3. The total amount of poison or toxic material ingested is assessed by seeing the residual amount in the container or remaining number of tablets.

4. Route of exposure i.e. oral, topical, ocular, respiratory.

5. The presence of co-existent disease, such as G6PD deficiency, myocardial dysfunction and mental subnormality.

6. Whether the patient is receiving other medications, which may interact with the poison?

A careful screening of family members for medications and potentially toxic products, including a social history and information regarding family background should not be forgotten.

Certain drugs may cause fatality even if consumed in small amounts by young children e.g. Tricyclic antidepressants, antipsychotics, quinine derivatives, calcium channel blockers (including sustained release tablet), opioids and oral hypoglycemics[11].

Physical Examination

Patient should be examined for evidences of local irritative effects on the oropharynx and gastrointestinal system. Specific focus should be placed on neurological and cardiorespiratory findings. Further clues are often obtained by careful evaluation of eyes (pupillary size, nystagmus, and lacrimation), skin changes, and unusual breath odor. It is possible to recognize certain syndromes specific or characteristic for a toxin (Toxidromes i.e. constellation of signs and symptoms that help to classify a patient into a category for toxin identification) which are given in Tables 55.3 and 55.4.

Identification of the Poison

Once basic life support and initial diagnostic efforts are instituted, specimens of blood, urine and

Table 55.3 Symptoms and signs of common poisonings	
Symptomatology	**Important causes**
1. Odor	Kerosene, arsenic, phosphorus, organophosphates (garlic odor), camphor, chloral hydrate, alcohol, cyanide (bitter almonds).
2. Sweating	Organophosphates, salicylates, acetaminophen (increased); atropine (decreased)
3. Fever	Salicylates, anticholinergics, kerosene, camphor
4. Hypothermia	Opiates, barbiturates
5. Coma	Barbiturates, opiates, diazepam, salicylates, organophosphates, carbon monoxide, kerosene, antihistamines, organochlorines
6. Delirium	*Dhatura*, salicylates, antihistamines, barbiturates
7. Ataxia	Piperazine, kerosene, anticholinergics, phenothiazines, antihistamines, organochlorines
8. Abnormal movements	Phenothiazines
9. Convulsions	Organophosphates, organochlorines, phenothiazines, phenol, camphor, amphetamines, isoniazid, kerosene, antihistamines, aminophylline, benzylbenozoate, salicylates, strychnine, lead.

10. Pupils
    Meiosis
    Mydriasis
	
	Opiates, organophosphates, chloral hydrate, early stages of barbiturates
	Atropine, oleander, antihistamines, sympathomimetic agents

11. Burns of mouth	Corrosives, tincture iodine
12. Cardiac arrhythmias	Aluminium phosphide, digitalis, phenol, cisapride, phenothiazines, theophylline, kerosene, carbon monoxide, tricyclic antidepressants, oleader
13. Tachycardia	Atropine, theophylline
14. Bradycardia	Digitalis, beta blockers, quinidine
15. Gastrointestinal	Plant products (castor, *Chandrajyoti* seeds), iron, camphor, oleander, naphthalene, acetaminophen, salicylates, food poisoning; hemorrhagic gastroenteritis (iron, salicylates, phenol, arsenic); flruoescent vomitus (phosphorus).
16. Paralytic ileus	Opiates, anticholinergics
17. Respiratory changes	Salicylates, atropine, oleander (hyperventilation) ; barbiturates, opiates (depression); kerosene (distress)
18. Metabolic acidosis	Phenol, iron, salicylates (usually with high anion gap).
19. Hemoglobinuria	Naphthalene, viper bite
20. Methemoglobinemia	Aniline dyes, nitrites, phenacetin, sulfones
21. Hypotension	Iron, barbiturates, anticholinergics, phenothiazines, opiates, phosphorus, aluminum phosphide
22. Anemia	Iron, naphthalene, lead, snake venom
23. Jaundice	Arsenic, iron, naphthalene, phosphorus, acetaminophen.

		Table 55.4 Common toxidromes		
Findings	**Adrenergic**	**Anti-cholinergic**	**Anti-cholinesterase**	**Opioid**
Heart rate	Increased	Increased	Decreased	Decreased
Temperature	Increased	Increased	No change	No change
Pupils	Dilated	Dilated	Constricted	Constricted
Mucosa	Wet	Dry	Wet	No change
Skin	Diaphoresis	Dry	Diaphoresis	Normal

gastric fluid should be obtained for appropriate toxicological analysis and screening. Urine is useful for many qualitative screens. Blood is necessary for quantitative determinations. If nature of poison is not known or a possibility of poisoning is considered as one of the differential diagnosis, following investigations are helpful[12].

1. *Bedside screening.* Certain poisons can be identified by simple bedside tests. Ferric chloride test is performed on patient's urine. 5-10 drops of freshly prepared 10% ferric chloride solution is added to 10 ml of boiled and acidified urine. Presence of salicylates in urine is indicated by burgundy red color, purple green color suggest phenothiazine, while violet color indicates presence of phenol derivatives[13]. Microscopic examination of urine may show characteristic oxalate crystals in ethylene glycol poisoning. The arterial blood is chocolate colored in methemoglobinemia without any change in color on exposure to air but it turns to pink on addition of few crystals of KCN.

2. *Toxic screen.* Examination of blood and urine by qualitative spot chromatography or thin layer chromatography is useful for identification or confirmation of a suspected poison. For unknown substances a screening test may be performed for commonly encountered toxins/ poisons. All these require a good toxicology laboratory support and are not very cost effective[14, 15].

3. *Osmolality.* Certain volatile poisons change the osmolality of blood. These include methanol, ethanol, acetone, isopropanol and ethylene glycol. The osmolar gap (difference between calculated and measured osmolality) is increased in poisoning due to these substances[16].

4. *Anion gap.* Anion gap is increased in poisoning due to paraldehyde, methanol, iron, isoniazid, ethylene glycol and salicylates. It is decreased in poisoning due to bromides and lithium[17].

5. *Radiology.* Plain X-ray film of abdomen or chest may be able to detect presence of radio opaque poisons. The radio opaque poisons are chloral hydrate, heavy metals, iodine, iron, phenothiazine, potassium compounds, and enteric-coated formulations[17].

6. *Diagnostic trial.* If the diagnosis of poisoning is in doubt inspite of strong clinical suspicion; administration of antidote for the most likely poison not only assist in diagnosis but also helps in early initiation of treatment. The commonly used antidotes are flumazenil (for benzodiazepines), deferoxamine (for iron), naloxone (for opiates), atropine (for organophosphates), diphenhydramine (for acute intoxication due to phenothiazines) and pyridoxine (for isoniazid toxicity)[13].

MANAGEMENT

Following basic first-aid measures at the site may prove life saving[18].

Ingested poison

- Wash the mouth thoroughly with water.
- Do not induce vomiting unless in hospital.
- Do not give salt water, raw eggs, mustard, vinegar etc. orally.
- Do not attempt neutralization in case of corrosives.
- Withhold food and drinks.

Eye contact

- Irrigate eyes with tepid water for at least 15 minutes making sure that the eye lids are open.

Inhalation damage

- Move the patient from exposure site to fresh air.

- Wear protective equipment in case you need to enter the area.
- Ensure clear airway.

Dermal contact

- Remove contaminated clothing.
- Wash skin thoroughly with soap and water for at least 15 min.
- Do not apply any medications or ointments on the affected area unless advised.

Once the child is in the hospital, the aim is to (i) prevent further absorption of poison, (ii) enhance elimination of poison, (iii) administer antidote and prevent re-exposure.

Prevention of further Absorption

Dilution

Simple dilution is indicated when the toxin exerts a local irritatant or caustic effect on oral, esophageal or gastric mucosa. These substances include acids, alkalis, and household cleansing agents. Both water and milk are acceptable as diluting agents. If suspected poison is medicinal toxin, simple dilution is contraindicated because it may increase dissolution rate of tablets or capsules and promote rapid transit into the lower intestinal tract. However, administration of fluids during induction of emesis is appropriate.

GI decontamination

According to recent recommendation there is no place for routine gastric lavage, emesis or activated charcoal[9]. For inhalational, dermal and ocular exposures first aid measures (vide supra) may be instituted.

Most liquid products get absorbed within 30 minutes and solids within 1-2 hours. It is recommended that gastric evacuation should be considered seriously only in patients who present early to the hospital; the ingested poison is poorly adsorbed by the activated charcoal and in critically sick patients[19-21]. Gastric evacuation may be of value up to 24 hours post ingestion, but is most effective if done within 1-2 hours. If the ingested material is non toxic, its amount is small and child is asymptomatic, no evacuation is required.

The procedure of choice for GI decontamination, if needed, is administration of activated charcoal, with whole bowel irrigation (WBI) in a few situations. The practice of universal evacuation by gastric lavage or emesis is no longer recommended. A controlled trial in adult patients has shown no added benefit of gastric evacuation in addition to administration of activated charcoal[22]. Orogastric lavage may be considered for certain uncommon situations.

Emesis may occur spontaneously following ingestion of many substances. The use of emetics including ipecac syrup has declined in the recent past[23]. It has been abandoned except as a home remedy when delay is anticipated to transport the victim to an appropriate medical facility. A dose of 30 ml for adolescents, 15 ml for children and 10 ml for infants under one year of age given with at least 8 ounces of water or other liquids has been shown to induce vomiting in nearly 100 percent of patients[19,20]. Other emetics like mechanical stimulation of the pharynx, table salt, copper sulfate, tartar emetics, and zinc sulfate, apomorphine, detergent, raw egg, dry mustard powder have been used to induce vomiting. Three tablespoons of detergent with 8 ounces of water is able to induce vomiting in children within few minutes with no side effects. This is a useful alternative when syrup ipecac is not available[6,22]. Induction of emesis is contraindicated in cases of hydrocarbon ingestion.

Gastric lavage is a commonly used procedure for evacuation of stomach but its use in pediatric patients remains controversial. It should be tried in critically sick patients with altered sensorium. The child is placed in left lateral position with head end low. A large orogastric tube with multiple lateral holes at the distal end and a funnel at the proximal end is preferable to a narrow nasogastric tube. Normal saline 15 ml/kg (maximum of 200-400 ml/cycle) is poured into the raised funnel, which is then lowered to allow drainage by gravity into a bucket. The procedure is repeated till the affluent is clear. In comatose (impaired gag reflex) children, gastric lavage should be done after intubation with cuffed endotracheal tube. Use of tap water or hypertonic saline may cause electrolyte imbalance[19-21].

Binding Agents

Activated charcoal. It is prepared by the pyrolysis of organic material such as wood pulp. It is activated by an oxidizing gas flow at high temperature to produce a fine network of pores. It adsorbs a wide variety of organic materials in the gastrointestinal tract thus minimizing absorption of the toxin. *Its use should be considered in all cases of poisoning except iron, cyanide and when orally administered antidotes are used.* It is most effective if given during first few hours after ingestion. It is given in a dose of 1 gm/kg/ dose mixed in sufficient amount of water (slurry) or sweet drinks orally or through nasogastric tube. It can be repeated every four hours for at least four doses or until charcoal is seen in the stools. Some people recommend repeated doses of charcoal without preceding emesis. A saline cathartic or sorbitol is usually administered with each dose[25]. Repeated doses of activated charcoal are useful in poisoning due to carbamazepine, barbiturates, dapsone, quinine, theophylline, salicylates, digoxin and phenytoin[26]. Activated charcoal has been shown to be effective in poisoning due to phenobarbitone, theophylline, digitoxin and nortriptyline even when the drug was taken parenterally. It is contraindicated in victims with paralytic ileus, intestinal perforation and where it interferes with oral antidote (N-acetyl cysteine)[21]. The suggested mechanism of action is removal of sequestrated toxin in the bowel wall by dialysis and reduction of enterohepatic circulation of toxin. Burnt toast (universal antidote) does not possess the adsorptive properties of activated charcoal. Recently a superactivated charcoal has been introduced with a surface area three times that of activated charcoal and it adsorbs 2.5 to 2.8 times more toxins.

Other binders. Clays such as attapulgite, bentonite, Fuller's earth, kaolin, and pectin have been studied besides cholestyramine. These are less effective than activated charcoal. Carbonized resin and modified silicagel were found to be as effective as activated charcoal in adsorbing methanol, ethylene glycol, kerosene and turpentine in-vitro[6].

Cathartics

Cathartics are seldom used. Sodium sulphate is contraindicated if there is congestive cardiac failure and magnesium sulphate is contraindicated in patients with renal failure.

Whole Bowel Irrigation[6,19,20,27,28]

Whole bowel irrigation (WBI) is a recent addition to the emergency treatment of poisoning. It removes the unabsorbed drug from the entire gut and possibly removes absorbed poison from the gut mucosa. It is a useful procedure for decontamination of gut. The indications for WBI include poor binding of ingested poison to activated charcoal, massive ingestion, late presentation, sustained release formulation of poison and ingestion of toxic solid material (e.g. disc battery). It is contraindicated in the presence of intestinal obstruction due to mechanical cause or ileus, intestinal perforation or hemorrhage.

Isotonic balanced electrolyte solution containing propylene glycol is administered in doses of 30 ml/kg/hr in children (2 liters/hour in adolescents) by nasogastric tube or through oral route. The infusion rate can be modified according to the tolerability of the patient. It is continued till the effluent fluid from the rectum is clear. It may require up to 4–6 hours. WBI is useful in iron poisoning and intoxication with sustained release or enteric coated preparations.

Enhancing Excretion

The methods for enhancing the elimination of absorbed poison include diuresis, dialysis and hemoperfusion. Because of some potential risk in their use, these measures are indicated only in patients where the recovery would be otherwise unlikely or where a specific significant benefit is expected[29,30].

Diuresis

Diuresis may be useful in cases of poisoning with agents that are excreted primarily through the renal route. Osmotic diuretics are preferred agents as these also prevent reabsorption of toxins by the renal tubules. Alkalization or acidification of urine enhances excretion of drugs and thus increase efficacy of diuretics. Weak acidic drugs are excreted better when urinary pH is alkaline while weak alkalis are excreted better with acidic urine pH. The important prerequisites for initiating diuresis are listed below:

1. The drug should be well excreted through the renal route.
2. The systolic blood pressure should be more than 90 mm of Hg.
3. There is no evidence of cardiac failure or respiratory insufficiency.
4. Renal functions are normal.
5. Blood levels of drug, if available, are in potentially toxic range.

The diuresis can be induced with 20 percent mannitol in initial doses of 0.5 gm/kg and then repeated to ensure a urinary output of 6-9 ml/kg/hour. Osmotic diuresis is continued until the blood levels of drug are in the pharmacological range or the patient is stable.

Urinary alkalization can be achieved by use of sodium bicarbonate (1-2 mEq/kg) intravenously as infusion, over a period of 1-2 hours and continued thereafter (target urine pH $\geq$ 8.0). It is useful in salicylates and barbiturate intoxication.

Acidification of urine is usually initiated with ammonium chloride in a dose of 75 mg/kg/dose

(22.75 mEq/kg/dose) orally or through nasogastric tube every 6 hours to keep the urine pH 5 or less. As an adjunct to this therapy, ascorbic acid in a dosage range of 0.5–2.0 gm in 500 ml of fluid can be administered intravenously at a maintenance infusion rate every 6 hours. Acidification is useful for weak bases like amphetamine, quinine and strychnine. A forced diuresis can be achieved by increasing the rate of intravenous fluid infusion with intermittent injections of furosemide.

Dialysis

Dialysis is particularly useful if electrolyte or acid base abnormalities exist. Dialysis is effective if the toxin is of low molecular weight, highly water soluble, has small volume of distribution and poorly bound to protein[9]. Indications of dialysis can be divided into patient-related and drug-related[29,30].

Patient-related indications of dialysis

(i)   Anticipated prolonged coma with high likelihood of complications.
(ii) Development of renal failure or impairment of normal excretory pathways
(iii) Progressive clinical deterioration.

Drug-related indications of dialysis

(i)   Satisfactory membrane permeability.
(ii) A good correlation between plasma drug concentration and drug toxicity of the agent.
(iii) Plasma levels in the potentially fatal range or presence of a significant quantity of an agent which is normally metabolized to toxic substances.
(iv) Significant enhancement of clearance of drug with dialysis.

Hemodialysis is the most effective means of dialysis, but it is technically demanding. Peritoneal dialysis is considerably less effective but is more readily available, simple and safe. However, substances that are highly protein bound are dialyzable only if protein is added to the dialysis fluid. If indicated 5% albumin can be added to dialysis fluids in first few cycles.

Hemodialysis is useful for poisoning with salicylates, acetaminophen, chloroquine, chloramphenicol, camphor, propranolol, ethylene glycol, vancomycin, and snake bite. Peritoneal dialysis may be useful in salicylate poisoning.

Hemoperfusion and Hemofiltration

Hemoperfusion is the process of passing blood through an extracorporeal circuit containing an adsorbent. The detoxified blood is returned to the patient. It is also effective in removal of toxic drugs. Although there are some reservations regarding the extent to which hemoperfusion can be utilized, it appears to be as effective as or even more effective than hemodialysis for a number of agents. Indications for its use are similar to those for hemodialysis[29,30]. Hemoperfusion is useful for toxins with low water solubility and with high affinity for the adsorbent e.g. carbamezepine, barbiturates, theophylline[31]. Hemofiltration can remove compounds with high molecular weight and is of use in poisoning due to amnioglycosides, theophylline, iron and lithium.

Pharmacological Antidotes

In a number of toxins, drugs and poisons a specific antidote is available. Antidotes, where indicated, should be immediately administred in some poison like sodium nitrate/sodium thiosulphate (cyanide), atropine (cholineesterase inhibitors), methylene blue (methemoglobinemic agents), oxygen (carbon monoxide), and naloxone (narcotic respiratory arrest). Other antidotes usually do not require such urgent administration and may be given subsequent to initiation of other management modalities. When available, antidotes do not diminish the need for supportive care or other therapy. Table 55.5 lists the commonly used antidotes with their doses. It is desirable that all pediatric emergency rooms should prominently display charts of specific antidotes with their doses and mode of administration[12,13].

Unknown Poison/Suspected Poisoning

Children who are poisoned do not always have a clear history of exposure. General features that suggest the possibility of poisoning include acute onset, age between 1-5 years, substantial environmental stress, multiple organ system involvement, altered consciousness, and a puzzling clinical picture. Physical examination may give important clues (Tables 55.3, 55.4 and 55.6). All such children should be hospitalized and samples of blood, urine, gastric lavage should be collected for analysis. They should be managed by gastrointestinal decontamination; enhancement of excretion and other supportive measures outlined *vide supra*.

Unconventional poisons

Unconventional poisons/toxins include herbal products, inhalational agents, polychlorinated biphenyls (PCBs), polycyclic aromatic hydrocarbons

Table 55.5 Specific antidotes

	Poison	Antidote
1.	Acetaminophen (paracetamol) Toxic dose: 150 mg/kg	N-acetyl cysteine 140 mg/kg followed by 70 mg/kg every 4 hours for 68 hours (17 doses) as oral (preferred) solution mixed with fruit juice.
2.	Amphetamines Toxic dose: 50 mg	Chlorpromazine 1 mg/kg IM or IV
3.	Atropine	Pilocarpine 2-4 mg orally or 0.25 – 0.5 mg IM. Physostigmine 1-2 mg IM every 30 min
4.	Belladonna (*dhatura*)	Physostigmine 0.5–2.0 mg IM every 30 min. Neostigmine is ineffective because it does not enter the CNS
5.	Benzodiazepines	Flumazenil IV in incremental doses of 0.1, 0.2, 0.3, 0.5 mg at 1-min intervals until desired effect is achieved.
6.	Carbon monoxide	100 % oxygen inhalation or hyperbaric oxygen therapy.
7.	Cyanide Fatal dose : 200 – 300 mg	i. Amyl nitrite (vaporal) 0.3 ml inhalation for 15-30 sec after every min. ii. Sodium nitrate 3% solution, 0.33 ml/kg (max10 ml) slowly IV. iii. Sodium thiosulphate 1.65 ml/kg 25% solution (max 50 ml) at a rate of 2.5 – 5.0 ml per min IV.
8.	Ethylene glycol	Ethanol 10 ml/kg 10% solution IV or 1ml/kg of 95% by mouth. Maintenance dose is 1.5ml/kg/hr 10% solution IV or 3 ml/kg/hr 10% solution IV during hemodialysis.
9.	Heavy metals I. Mercury i, iii II. Arsenic i III. Lead i, ii, iii, iv	i. British anti-lewisite (BAL) 12-24 mg/kg/day in 6 divided doses IM (BAL or dimercaprol 100 mg/ml ; 3 ml amp) ii. EDTA (calcium disodium ethylene diamine tetra acetic acid) 50-75 mg/kg/day in 4 div doses IM or IV as 0.2 – 0.4% solution (200 mg/ml ampoule) iii. D-penicillamine 20-40 mg/kg per day orally for 5 days. iv. Oral thiamine and dimercapto succinic acid (DMSA) is useful.
10.	Heparin	1.0 mg protamine sulfate for 100 units heparin as 1% solution IV (10 mg/ml ampoule).
11.	Iron Toxic dose : 35 mg/kg	Deferoxamine 15 mg/kg/hr IV infusion. Therapy needed for 12-36 hours till urine color becomes normal (desferal 500 mg/vial).
12.	Isoniazid	Pyridoxine 1.0 mg IV for every 1.0 mg of isoniazid upto a maximum of 500 mg if amount of isoniazid ingested is unknown.
13.	Methemoglobinemia	Methylene blue 1-2 mg/kg/hr IV 1% solution. May be repeated after 4 hours (10 mg/ml ampoule). Maximum dose is 7 mg/kg.
14.	Methyl alcohol	Ethyl alcohol (ethanol) 0.75-1.0 ml/kg IV followed by 0.5 ml/kg every hourly IV as 5% solution in sodium bicarbonate. Alternatively it can be given as 3-4 ounces of whisky (45% alcohol) every 4 hourly for 1-3 days in adults (Inj ethanol 2 ml ampoule).
15.	Morphine, other opiates, semi and synthetic narcotics (heroin), meperidine, lomotil (diphenoxylate hydrochloride), and pentazocin	Naloxone 0.1 mg/kg IV (max 2 mg). Repeat every 2-3 min till the reversal of toxic effects or a cummulative dose of 10 mg is reached (Inj narcan 0.4 mg/ml).
16.	Organophosphorous poisoning (insecticides which are cholinesterase inhibitors)	i. Atropine 0.02 – 0.05mg/kg/dose IV every 15-30 min till signs of atropinization develop. For continuous infusion 0.02-0.08 mg/kg/hour after the initial bolus. ii. PAM or pralidoxime (2-Pyridine aldozime methiodide) 25-50 mg/kg IM or IV as 5% solution over 15-30 minutes. The dose may be repeated after 1-2 hours and then at 10-12 hours intervals if cholinergic signs recur. For continuous infusion 9-19 mg/kg/hour after the initial bolus of 25-50 mg/kg.
17.	Phenothiazine and metoclopramide (extra-pyramidal reactions)	Diphenhydramine 1-2 mg/kg/IV every 30 min. (benadryl cap 25 mg; 50 mg; elixir 12.5 mg/5 ml; amp 50 mg/ml; vials 10 mg/ml).
18.	Propranolol (beta-blockers)	Atropine 0.01-0.02 mg/kg per dose SC every 5-10 min to achieve full atropinisation. Glucagon 0.25 – 1.0 mg IM or IV. (Glucagon amp 1 mg/ml).
19.	Warfarin, dicumarol	Vitamin K 5-10 mg IM or IV (Inj kapilin 10 mg/ml)

Source: Singh M and Deorari AK. Drug Dosages in Children. *CBS Publishers & Distributors, Pvt Ltd, New Delhi,* 9th edition 2015; pp 186-192.

(PAH) to which infants and children are getting more and more exposed in the current scenario. A discussion of these and a slow yet definite "*thought*" poisoning, e.g. violence in media/addictions/alcoholism/cartoons; competition instead of cooperation among children; exploitation of natural resources creating ecological imbalance etc. is beyond the scope of the chapter.

INDIVIDUAL POISONINGS

The clinical picture and brief treatment of common poisons is summarized in Table 55.6.

	Poison	Symptoms and signs	Supportive management*
	Table 55.6 Symptomatology and supportive management of various poisons		
1.	Arsenic (Rat poison)	Abdominal pain, vomiting, bloody diarrhea, cardiovascular collapse	BAL (dimercaprol) 3-5 mg/kg/dose IM every 4 hours for 2 days, every 6 hours for additional 2 days and every 12 hours for upto 7 additional days.
2.	Phenol	Local burns, nausea, vomiting, bloody diarrhea, convulsions, pulmonary edema, cardio-respiratory depression	Dilution with water or milk, then give activated charcoal and olive oil 30 ml stat and 10 ml every hourly
3.	Camphor	Nausea, vomiting, epigastric pain, muscular irritability, seizures	Hemoperfusion
4.	Naphthalene	Nausea, vomiting, hemoglobinuria, pain, jaundice, acute tubular necrosis	Forced alkaline diuresis, blood transfusion.
5.	Copper sulphate	Burning pain in mouth and throat, vomiting, watery or bloody diarrhea, hemolysis, anuria, jaundice, collapse and convulsions	Water, milk, egg white per oral, BAL (see doses given in arsenic poisoning) or d-penicillamine 100 mg/kg/day (max 1 gm) PO divided doses for upto 5 days. For long term use the dose should not exceed 40 mg/kg/day.
6.	Castor seeds, *Chandrajyoti seeds*	Violent vomitings, abdominal pain, bloody diarrhea	IV fluids, blood transfusion if required.
7.	Yellow and white oleander seeds	Dysphagia, burning in throat, vomiting, abdominal pain, diarrhea, varying degree of heart block, muscular twitchings, tetanic seizures, drownsiness, lock jaw with white seeds.	Treatment for heart block, IV fluids.
8.	*Dhatura* (Belladona alkaloids)	Muscarinic blockage, tachycardia, hot dry skin, fever, dilated pupils, urinary and bowel retention, initial hypertension followed by hypotension, confusion, disorientation, ataxia, picking or grasping movements, seizures, psychomotor hallucinations, coma	Activated charcoal, physostigmine 0.5 mg IV/IM/SC may repeat every 15 minutes until desired effect is achieved. Subsequently can be repeated every 2-3 hours.
9.	Acetaminophen	Stage I (12-24 hours): Nausea Stage II (24-48 hours): Clinical recovery Stage III (72-96 hours): Peak hepatotoxicity Stage IV (7-8 days): Recovery. *See text*	Avoid activated charcoal if N-acetyl cysteine is to be given. N-acetyl crysteine is specific antidote (*vide supra*).
10.	Salicylates	Tinnitus, fever, sweating, hyperventilation, nausea, vomiting, respiratory alkalosis and metabolic acidosis, restlessness, dehydration, fluid retention, gastric hemorrhage, pulmonary edema, hepatitis.	Forced alkaline diuresis, hemodialysis or hemoperfusion, vitamin K.
11.	Barbiturates	Respiratory depression, hypotension, hypothermia, cerebral edema, acute renal failure, and coma. Isoelectric EEG tracings can occur.	Cardio-respiratory support, forced alkaline diuresis, hemodialysis/hemoperfusion.

(Contd.)

Section 5

	Poison	Symptoms and signs	Supportive management*
Table 55.6 Symptomatology and supportive management of various poisons (Contd.)			
12.	Lead	Anorexia, abdominal pain, vomiting, constipation, anemia, abnormal behaviour, paresis of muscles, convulsions, coma, intellectual deterioration	Laxatives and enema. Mild cases : d-penicillamine 10 mg/kg twice daily orally. Severe cases : Calcium EDTA. Mannitol for cerebral edema.
13.	Benzyl benzoate	Convulsions, excitement and incoordination	Admit*
14.	Piperazine citrate	Dizziness, disorientation, ataxia, drowsiness, seizures	Admit*
15.	Tincture iodine	Oral burns, gastric irritation	Gastric lavage with soluble starch solution. Leave 1-5% sodium thiosulfate solution in stomach.
16.	Food poisoning	Incubation period for staphylococcus 1-6 hours, salmonella 12-18 hours. Nausea, profuse vomiting, abdominal pain and diarrhea followed by recovery within 24 hours.	Maintenance of hydration with IV fluids. Antibiotics are not required.
17.	Botulism	Bulbar paralysis, weakness, postural hypotension, dryness of mucosa and respiratory paralysis. Incubation period is 12-36 hours.	Cardiorespiratory support, pencillin and specific antitoxin if available.
18.	Tricyclic antidepressants	Drowsiness, lethargy, coma, seizures, tachycardia, hypotension, flutter, fibrillation other arrythmias, hypoventilation, respiratory arrest.	Sodium bicarbonate, lidocaine.
19.	Calcium channel blockers	Bradycardia, AV block, hypotension, confusion, lethargy, coma, hyperglycemia	WBI (if sustained release preparation), atropine, pacemaker, fluids vasopressors, IV calcium, glucagon.
20.	Ethylene glycol	1-12 hours: GI symptoms, CNS manifestations, 12-24 hours: Arrythmias, muscle pains, tetany > 24 hours: Cardiac failure, cerebral edema	Gastric decontamination and activated charcoal not useful, correction of acidosis, antidotes like ethanol, fomepizole and dialysis.

* Supportive care and gut decontamination for all unless specifically contraindicated.

Selected poisonings are described below in detail.

CORROSIVE INGESTION

Common substances involved in accidental ingestion are washing soda, unslaked lime, powerful detergent granules, toilet and drain cleaners, button alkali cells and acids.

Toxicology

Acids produce coagulation necrosis, which causes superficial damage, while alkalis cause a deep and penetrating liquefaction necrosis often with severe consequences. Acid ingestion may cause gastric perforation and peritonitis, while with alkalis severe damage is more common in the esophagus and it is associated with mediastinitis and pneumonia in severe cases.

Clinical Picture

Children may have protean manifestations. Common symptoms and signs are vomiting, dysphagia, drooling, epigastric abdominal pain and refusal to drink liquids. Respiratory distress with stridor (due to glottic edema), signs of shock, esophageal perforation with mediastinitis, gastric perforation with peritonitis are present in severe cases. Sometimes there may be history of ingestion of corrosives but examination of the mouth and pharynx may be normal. Absence of oral burns and lack of symptoms do not rule out involvement of esophagus. Presence of two or more symptoms namely vomiting, drooling, stridor or oropharyngeal burns correlates well with esophageal and laryngeal injury. Upper GI endoscopy should be performed within 24-48 hours and after 2-3 weeks by an experienced person to determine the extent of injury[29].

Treatment

Detailed history may help in the identification and the amount of corrosive ingested. Gut decontamination procedures are contraindicated. Neutralization of offending agent by acid/alkali is also not recommended. The child may be given a very small amount of water or milk to wash away any residual caustic from the oral mucosa. This amount should be small so as not to overload the stomach and induce vomiting. Milk of magnesia and antacids may be used to neutralize strong acids. If skin or eyes are exposed; a thorough and prolonged irrigation with water is necessary. Eye injuries due to alkali is an ophthalmic emergency.

To prevent secondary injury from reflux of gastric acid into esophagus, proton pump inhibitor (PPI), H-2 blockers or therapeutic doses of antacids should be given. Acid suppression should be continued for 6-8 weeks in these children. Use of steroids for prevention of esophageal stricture formation is controversial. Recent data indicates that the esophageal stricture formation depends on severity of injury and it is not altered by administration of corticosteroids[33-36]. As soon as the child is able to swallow; liquids are offered by mouth. Drinking is a form of self-dilatation and may decrease the likelihood of esophageal stricture formation. Antibiotics should be used if infection is suspected. Drooling and dysphagia persisting beyond 12-24 hours have been reported to be good predictors of scar formation and should prompt upper GI endoscopy[37].

Recently other methods have been investigated to prevent stricture formation. One mechanical method is the placement of a rubber tube in the esophageal lumen, which allows the esophagus to scar down leaving a functional lumen. Other pharmacological agents used in animal studies for prevention of esophageal stricture include beta aminoproprionitrite and penicillamine[32].

KEROSENE AND OTHER HYDROCARBONS

Petroleum distillate hydrocarbons are present in many household products. These compounds may be divided into two groups based on their volatility (vapor pressure related), viscosity (sheer force related), surface tension and their respiratory manifestations.

(i) *High volatility.* Kerosene, petroleum, ether, gasoline and paint thinner.

(ii) *Low volatility.* Furniture polish, lubricating oil, paraffin wax, mineral and sea oil.

Toxicology

Petroleum distillate hydrocarbons are not absorbed from gastrointestinal tract. The systemic toxicity generally results from absorption via the lungs following aspiration; important exceptions are the non-petroleum distillate hydrocarbons (benzene, carbon tetrachloride, chloroform, turpentine, xylene, and toluene) which are absorbed from the gastrointestinal tract. Due to its low surface tension, kerosene tends to get aspirated into the lungs during ingestion, vomiting and inhalation of vapors. Kerosene toxicity may occur in neonates if it is applied over skin, indicating that transdermal absorption can also result in toxic effects. Ingestion of 30 ml may prove lethal. Intravenous kerosene injections have been reported among IV drug abusing teenagers, causing major injury to the pulmonary capillaries.

Clinical Features

Symptoms and signs of ingestion include the following:

Topical effects. Irritation of oral, esophageal and gastric mucosa.

Pulmonary effects. Fever, tachycardia, tachypnea, cough, cyanosis and rarely pulmonary edema may occur. These findings of chemical pneumonitis result from aspiration and may develop over 1-24 hours after aspiration of high and low volatility substances. Kerosene and other lighter liquids produce severe pneumonitis early in the course.

Respiratory symptomatology sometime ensues within minutes of the ingestion. It almost always begins within first six hours (including chest roentgenogram abnormalities). Children who are asymptomatic for 6 hours are unlikely to develop pneumonia later. Distress generally worsens over next 24 to 48 hours. Most victims recover by 3 to 8 days.

The skiagram of chest may show fine punctate mottled densities in the perihilar region and mid lung fields followed by ill defined patchy densities, which may coalesce to form large areas of consolidation. Pneumonitis is usually bilateral and involves multiple lobes. Lower lobes are more severely affected. Localized areas of atelectasis are often present. Pleural effusion, pneumatoceles, pneumothorax, pneumomediastinum and subcutaneous emphysema are found infrequently. Radiological abnormalities

Section 5

may be present in the absence of clinical pneumonia. Pneumatoceles may appear 2-3 weeks after clinical resolution

CNS effects. Euphoria, headache, restlessness, weakness, muscle twitchings, in-coordination, confusion, drowsiness, lethargy, stupor, coma and convulsions may occur. These effects are secondary to hypoxia, acidosis or absorption of low volatility, high viscosity substances that sometimes get absorbed from the intestine.

Other features. Liver damage, renal tubular damage, bone marrow suppression and myocardial toxicity have also been reported[38].

Treatment

Evacuation of stomach by emesis or lavage does not benefit the child; rather they increase the risk of aspiration and are thus contraindicated. Dilution with (palm) oil or milk, commonly used as a household remedy for hydrocarbon exposure results in detrimental effects, due to changes in volatility, viscosity and miscibility. This should not be done. When hydrocarbons are mixed with pesticides, heavy metals or other toxic substances or in case of ingestion of hydrocarbons such as benzene, carbon tetrachloride, then gastric lavage or emptying is indicated. One of the indications for gastric lavage is when the amount of hydrocarbon ingested exceeds 1 ml/kg. In unconscious patients, gastric lavage after intubation with a cuffed endotracheal tube is the method of choice.

Supportive treatment includes correction of hypoxia by administration of oxygen and maintenance of fluid and electrolyte balance. For wheezing, selective beta-2 agonists are preferred over epinephrine as latter may cause arrhythmias. Antibiotics are required if secondary bacterial infection is suspected. Steroid therapy has no role.

Children who are asymptomatic and X-ray of chest does not show any abnormality, can be sent home after 24 hours of observation. Children who are asymptomatic at 6 hours but show some lesions on X-ray chest, though they are less likely to develop any problems later but it is preferable to admit these children for observation unless one is certain that the child can be closely followed-up on ambulatory basis[38,39].

ORGANOPHOSPHATE POISONING

Organophosphate compounds are commonly used as insecticides in household (1-2% weight/volume solution) and agriculture (40-50% w/v solution). The compounds used in household are less toxic. The solvents used for these products are hydrocarbons. The commonly used compounds are methyl parathion (Agrolex), dichlorovos (Agrovan, Vapox), fenthion (Bytex, Fenthiosul), malathion (Finit), diazinon (Agrozinon), fenitrothion (Tik 20), and tetra ethyl pyrophosphate etc.

Toxicology

The toxicity may occur due to accidental or intentional ingestion or following absorption through skin. Organophosphate compounds act by phosphorylating the active or esteritic site of acetylcholine esterase leading to an irreversible inhibition of the cholinesterase resulting in excessive accumulation of acetylcholine at receptor sites.

Clinical Features

Most childhood poisonings occur by ingestion. These compounds are well absorbed from all the routes; sometimes symptoms may be localized to the site of exposure. A small amount spilled on the skin may cause localized excessive sweating or muscle twitchings, while inhalation of dust or vapor may cause nasal irritation, rhinorrhea, broncho-constriction, wheezing and increased bronchial or salivary secretions. To a certain extent, the severity of intoxication can be related to the type of receptor activity that dominates the clinical presentation. Various clinical features according to type of receptor involved are given in Table 55.7. At low doses of organophosphates, muscarinic symptoms may be most prominent. In more severe intoxication, nicotinic and central muscarinic activity may predominate. Thus tachycardia and hypertension

---

Table 55.7 Signs and symptoms of poisoning due to cholinesterase-inhibitors

Muscarinic (mnemonic SLUDGE)
Salivation, **l**acrimation, **u**rination, **d**efecation/diarrhea, bronchoconstriction, wheezing, increased pulmonary secretions, bradycardia, nausea, emesis, **GI** (abdominal) cramps, intestinal hypermotility, **e**xcessive sweating and constriction of pupils.

Nicotinic
Muscle fatigue, twitchings, fasciculations, paralysis of respiratory muscles with diminished respiratory effort, tachycardia, hypertension, pallor, hyperglycemia

Central nervous system
Anxiety, restlessness, confusion, headache, emotional lability, slurred speech, ataxia, generalized seizures, hypotension, Cheyne-Stokes respiration, central respiratory paralysis, depression of cardiovascular center and coma.

can be important signs of severe poisoning and should not delay therapy or confuse the unfamiliar clinician that expects the patient to have bradycardia[40,41].

Fatalities caused by organophsophate poisoning are due to respiratory arrest and are attributable to all three types of receptor over-stimulation. Death can occur within minutes of exposure to large amounts.

Diagnosis

A clinical diagnosis of acute organophsophate poisoning is made by history, physical examination, presence of cholinergic signs and response to antidote administration. *A clinical classification for severity based on organ system involvement has been proposed as given in Table 55.8.* The definitive diagnosis can be made by estimation of red cell cholinesterase activity. The treatment should not be delayed pending reports of cholinesterase activity. The sample for cholinesterase activity estimation should be drawn before administration of cholinesterase reactivator. In advanced laboratories, sensitive methods for estimation of urinary metabolites of several organophosphates such as malathion and parathion are also available[37]. However, cholinesterase levels

Organ system	Severity of symptoms		
	Severe	**Moderate**	**Mild**
GI system	Massive haemorrhage, gut perforation, 2nd or 3rd degree burns, severe dysphagia	Diarrhea, vomiting, bloody stools, jaundice	Abdominal cramping, loss of appetite, nausea, oral irritation, constipation
Respiratory system	Cyanosis and respiratory depression, pulmonary edema, respiratory arrest	Diffuse radiographic abnormalities, pleuritic chest pain, respiratory depression, bronchospasm, dyspnea	Cough, airway irritation, rhinitis, sneezing
Nervous system	Coma, paralysis, seizure, stupor, widespread neurologic impairment	Confusion, hallucination, blurred vision, ataxia, slurred speech, syncope, hearing loss, localized neuropathy/ paresthesias	Hyperactivity, headache, profuse sweating, dizziness, tremor, tinnitus, drowsiness
Cardiovascular system	Bradycardia: HR <60 in children, <80 neonates. Tachycardia: HR > 190 children, >200 neonates. Cardiac arrest /MI, shock	Bradycardia: HR 60–80 in children, 80–90 neonates. Tachycardia: HR 160–190 children, 160–200 neonates. Chest pain, dysrhythmia hyper/hypotension	Isolated extrasystoles, mild transient hypertension
Metabolic	Acid/base disturbance (pH <7.15 or >7.7), severe electrolyte imbalance	Elevated anion gap, acidosis (pH 7.15–7.30), alkalosis (pH 7.60–7.69)	Fever of short duration. mild hyperglycemia
Renal	Anuria, renal failure	Hematuria, oliguria, proteinuria	Polyuria
Muscular	Muscle rigidity and rhabdomyolysis, compartment syndrome	Fasciculations, rigidity, weakness	Muscle weakness, muscle pain
Dermatologic	Burns: 2nd degree >50% total BSA, Burns: 3rd degree >2% BSA	Bullae, burns: 2nd degree <50% BSA Burns: 3rd degree of <2% BSA	Edema, swelling, erythema, irritation, urticaria
Ocular	Corneal ulcer corneal perforation, loss of vision	Corneal abrasion ocular burn, visual changes	Lacrimation, mydriasis miosis, pain/ conjunctivitis
Others	–	–	Fatigue, malaise

Table 55.8 Grading of severity of signs and symptoms of poisoning due to pesticides[1]

do not correlate with severity of organophosphate poisoning.

Treatment

General supportive measures are instituted immediately. Anticholinergic therapy is initiated in all suspected organophosphate poisoning. Atropine is given until cholinergic signs are reversed or patient is atropinized. Signs of atropinization include dry mouth, warm, dry and flushed skin, dilated pupils, decreased pulmonary secretions, and increasing heart rate (if bradycardia was an earlier sign). The doses of atropine (see Table 55.5) can be repeated to maintain reversal of cholinergic signs at least for 24 hours. The interval for administration of atropine can be titrated to the patient's physical signs. In an intubated child, control of bronchial secretions is a useful sign for monitoring frequency of dosing and adequacy of response to atropine. Some cases may require prolonged treatment with an infusion of atropine.

Pralidoxime is a specific antidote for organophosphates (see Table 55.5). Pralidoxime does not reverse the CNS effects and atropine does not have any effect on respiratory impairment due to muscle weakness. Both the drugs should be used together in severely poisoned children. In severe poisoning more frequent dosing of pralidoxime is required. In such cases, after the initial bolus dose, continuous intravenous infusion in doses of 9-19 mg/kg/hour has also been tried. Preliminary studies suggest benefit from blood alkalinisation with sodium bicarbonate in organophsophate poisoning, but there is insufficient evidence to support its routine clinical use[42].

Certain drugs are contraindicated in patients poisoned with anti-cholinesterases; these include morphine, theophylline, caffeine, furosemide and ethacrynic acid. The child should be observed at least for 24-48 hours even after recovery to ensure that cholinergic signs do not recur as the effect of atropine and pralidoxime wane off.

Obidoxime chloride may be administered in a dose of 4-8 mg/kg/dose, as an alternative, for children with organophosphate poisoning. Other oximes include diacetyl monoxime (DAM), H-series of oximes (eg. H16 and HLO7). They have better CNS penetration. Human BuChE-based bioscavengers are also used for prophylaxis and treatment of intoxications/poisoning by these compounds. Also, BuChE has been integrated in biosensors for prevention of biological terrorism/warfare. Intravenous magnesium can be given for control of tachyarrhythmias.

Other chronic effects of organophosphate poisoning

A demyelinating polyneuropathy in organophosphate poisoning is well documented. Several compounds have been implicated including triorthocresylphosphate (TOCP), merphos, mipatox, trichlorton, methamidophos and possibly laptophos. The symptom complex of the illness consists of ascending paralysis which begins after 2 weeks of recovery from intoxication or following chronic exposure. Sensory disturbances, weakness, diminished tendon reflexes; muscle fasciculations and tenderness are initial manifestations. During subsequent weeks to months, flaccid paralysis and muscle wasting may occur. Recovery may take up to two years and may be incomplete with residual spastic diplegia[38].

CARBAMATE POISONING

Carbamate insecticides are reversible cholinesterase inhibitors. They differ from organophosphates in several aspects. The signs of intoxication are of shorter duration and they do not penetrate CNS; therefore no neurological manifestations are seen. They are more readily absorbed from skin and gastrointestinal tract . The common carbamate compounds are propoxur (Baygon), propoxure (Protox bait), carboryl (Agrovin), methomyl (Lannate), carbofuran (Agrofuran), akdcarub (Temik), etc.

Treatment consists of general measures with atropine administration intravenously (refer to details given in the section on organophosphate poisoning). Pralidoxime should not be used because of spontaneous recovery of cholinesterase and may enhance lethality of some carbamates such as carboryl. However, if the source of cholinergic poisonings is not precisely known, a trial of pralidoxime is warranted [40,41].

ORGANOCHLORINE INSECTICIDE POISONING

These are lipid soluble low molecular weight compounds with a wide range of toxicity. The commonly available compounds are DDT, gamma benzene hexachloride (Gamascab, scarab, scarlex), aldrin (Aldrin 30), kethane and methoxychlor. Toxicity of gamma benzene hexachloride, a compound used for scabies and lice infestation does not occur if applied in therapeutic doses but overzealous application or accidental ingestion may cause toxicity.

These compounds alter electrophysiologic and enzymatic properties of membranes. Acute poisoning is the result of abnormal nerve transmission. In CNS it results in generalized seizures. Clinical features of intoxication are variable. They include nausea, vomiting and CNS stimulation. CNS symptoms include apprehension, excitability, ataxia, disorientation, dizziness or generalized seizures. Treatment is supportive and directed at specific signs. Seizures are controlled with anticonvulsants. The half-life of gamma benzene hexachloride is 21 hours, thus supportive care needs to be given for more than 24 hours[41].

PARACETAMOL (ACETAMINOPHEN) POISONING

Paracetamol is a safe analgesic antipyretic agent in therapeutic doses. Hepatic damage after paracetamol overdose occurs due to increased formation of highly reactive intermediate (N-acetyl-p-benzoquinonimine) which is produced by its metabolism through P-450 cytochrome oxidase system. N-acetyl-p-benzoquinonimine is normally detoxified by endogenous glutathione, but the increased production induced by paracetamol overdose may deplete glutathione stores allowing the intermediate metabolite to react with and destroy hepatocytes. Hypatotoxicity may occur when a dose of more than 150 mg/kg is ingested. Few cases of life-threatening hepatotoxicity have occured due to therapeutic misadventures but most cases of fatal liver damage occur due to intake of paracetamol for suicidal intentions. Death may occur within 2-7 days of ingestion.

Clinical Manifestations

The clinical features of paracetamol toxicity are divided into 4 stages.

Stage 1 (6-24 hr). There is anorexia, nausea, vomiting, pallor and excessive sweating with cold skin.

Stage 2 (24-48 hr). The clinical evidences of hepatic dysfunction supervene. There is jaundice, enlarged tender liver and deranged liver functions with elevated liver enzymes and prolonged prothrombin time. Renal dysfunction is manifest by oliguria and elevation of blood urea and creatinine.

Stage 3 (48-96 hr). The symptoms of stage 1 reappear and hepatic coma supervenes with gross evidences of hepatic dysfunction.

Stage 4 (4 days–2 weeks). After optimal supportive and specific therapy recovery may occur gradually during 1-2 weeks period. It may take 3 months for liver histology to return back to normal.

Management

The blood level of paracetamol should be monitored after 4 hours of ingestion and serially thereafter. If serum paracetamol level is >200 ug/ml at 4 hr, >100 ug/ml at 8 hr and >50 ug/ml at 16 hr there is a high risk of hepato-toxicity. Elevation of hepatic transaminases >1000 units/l is associated with serious hepatic damage[3]. The supportive management includes induction of emesis or gastric lavage followed by activated charcoal to adsorb unabsorbed paracetamol. Supportive treatment includes correction of hypoglycemia, maintenance of hydration, electrolyte balance, treatment of coagulopathy, hemodialysis for acute renal failure and management of fulminant hepatic failure. N-acetyl cysteine (NAC) is a specific antidote and should be started ideally within 8 hours but preferably within 16 hours of ingestion. NAC acts as an antidote by enhancing glutathione stores, providing a glutathione substitute and facilitating nontoxic sulfate conjugation of paracetamol in the liver. Oral NAC protocol is as effective as intravenous therapy which is popular in Great Britain and Canada. Activated charcoal is contraindicated when oral NAC protocol is followed. Side effects include nausea, vomiting and epigastric discomfort. Any dose that is vomited within one hour of administration should be replaced. The standard principles of management of hepatic coma should be followed. Recovery is heralded by return of consciousness and improvement in the hepatic function tests.

An alternative drug, though less effective, is oral methionine 2.5 g stat followed by 2.5 g 4 hourly up to a total of 10 g over 12 hours. Activated charcoal may provide additional hepatoprotective effect although it entails intravenous NAC administration. Once hepatic failure occurs, NAC is contraindicated.

Forced alkaline diuresis is of no value. Frequent monitoring of the liver function tests are needed. Most patients (99%) will recover within a week. The following are poor prognostic factors in established hepatic failure due to paracetamol i.e. pH <7.3, PT > 100 sec, grade III or more of hepatic encephalopathy, elevated serum bilirubin > 4 mg/dl, SGOT > 1000 iu/l. Factor VIII: Factor V ratio of > 30 indicates the worst outcome.

Section 5

PHENOTHIAZINE INTOXICATION

Phenothiazines are commonly used drugs for a variety of clinical problems. The onset of toxic manifestations may be delayed for 6-24 hours after the ingestion and they may be intermittent in nature. The various systems affected by toxic manifestations include central nervous system, cardiovascular system, cutaneous, hepatic, ocular and hematological systems[43].

Clinical Manifestations

Three major clinical categories are indentified.

Acute overdose. If a child ingests a large dose, the presenting manifestations may be meiosis, hypotension, dysrhythmias and coma. Disturbance of temperature homeostasis is also common. Respiratory depression is unusual.

Extrapyramidal symptoms. Younger children are more prone to extrapyramidal signs and have generalized manifestations. In adolescents and adults, the signs are localized. The patient is usually alert and awake; there may be torsion of head and neck, dystonia, choreiform movements, oculogyric crises and tremors.

Neuroleptic malignant syndrome. It is an uncommon but potentially life-threatening effect of phenothiazine (fluphenazine) and other antipsychotic (butyrophenon) drugs. The characteristic features of this syndrome include fluctuating mental status progressing to coma and extrapyramidal symptoms especially rigidity, fever, diaphoresis, tachycardia and hypo or hypertension. Laboratory findings include elevated white blood count, CPK and transaminases. It is more common in children who have relatives with idiopathic Parkinson's disease. The clinical features evolve over 24 to 72 hours. There is no relationship between dose and duration of drugs administered and neuroleptic malignant syndrome[45].

Treatment

Treatment of phenothiazine poisoning consists of supportive care to stabilize vital organs. For extrapyramidal manifestations; benztropine mesylate 0.5 mg/kg or diphenhydramine 2 mg/kg is given intravenously slowly over 2-5 minutes. If parenteral preparations are not available; same doses can be given orally. Phenothiazines have a long half-life and therefore to avoid recurrence of symptoms, same dose can be repeated every 6-8 hours for 24-36 hours. Diazepam has also been used successfully in acute dystonia secondary to phenothiazine toxicity. For ventricular dysrhythmias, phenytoin or lidocaine is the drug of choice. In serious poisonings where dysrythmias and convulsions do not respond to routine management, physostigmine can be used with due precautions[44].

The treatment of neuroleptic malignant syndrome consists of temperature reduction by hydrotherapy, ventilatory and cardiovascular support. Dantrolene in doses of 0.5 mg/kg orally every 12 hours has shown to be useful in reducing muscle rigidity and oxygen consumption in a few patients[45].

IRON POISONING

Iron poisoning is one of the most common potentially fatal intoxication in children. Widespread availability of iron tablets particularly during pregnancy and post-natal period and ignorance of general public about its potential lethality contribute to the high incidence of iron poisoning.

Toxicology and Clinical Manifestations

Toxicity of iron is due to its direct effect on the gastrointestinal mucosa and the presence of free iron in circulation. The effects are divided into five stages (i) Gastrointestinal; (ii) Relative stability; (iii) Shock; (iv) Hepatic necrosis and (v) Gastric scarring.

(1) *Gastrointestinal toxicity.* This is primarily due to direct mucosal injury, especially on gastric and small intestinal mucosa by producing coagulation necrosis and platelet aggregation. Clinical manifestations in this stage are vomiting, diarrhea, colicky abdominal pain, hematemesis and melena. This stage lasts for about 2 to 12 hours.

(2) *Stage of relative stability.* This poorly described second stage of iron intoxication begins as early as 3 to 4 hours after ingestion and lasts as long as 48 hours. During this phase patient appears better, while absorbed iron accumulates in the mitochondria and various body organs.

(3) *Stage of circulatory collapse.* Acute circulatory failure, acidosis, and hypoglycemia characterize this phase. The various contributory factors for shock include hypovolemia due to external losses and third space loss due to increased capillary permeability, acidosis and decreased cardiac output.

(4) *Stage of hepatic necrosis.* This is a rare clinical manifestation of iron intoxication. After apparent recovery, 2-4 days after ingestion of iron,

severe hepatic necrosis with elevation of trans-aminases and bilirubin may occur.

(5) *Stage of gastric scarring.* Following an acute corrosive insult to the gastrointestinal tract, the healing process may result in area of stenosis in both the stomach outlet and small intestine. These late consequences of iron poisoning rarely occur and may present as late as 2 to 6 weeks after the initial event.

Laboratory Investigations

Determination of the estimated dose taken is the first step. If ingestion is less than 20 mg/kg of elemental iron, there is generally little risk of toxicity and no specific treatment is indicated. When 20-60 mg/kg elemental iron had been ingested, supportive management and follow up is required. If the amount of elemental iron taken is more than 60 mg/kg, it is an indication for detailed evaluation.[46] Adolescent and adult overdoses should be considered as intentional and require careful evaluation regardless of the alleged dose taken. In addition, clinical condition of the child is an important indicator for initiation of the treatment even if the estimated dose is low. The value of serum iron and total iron binding capacity determination for estimation of intoxication is controversial. Serum iron values of more than 350 ug/ dl is taken as a risk for serious intoxication and values of more than 1000 ug/dl is associated with a steep rise in morbidity and mortality[46]. X- ray abdomen may show radio-opaque shadows giving rough indication for the amount ingested and need for their removal by endoscopy.

Additional baseline laboratory tests include white blood cell count and blood glucose determination. An arterial blood gas and bicarbonate determination is important to monitor the development of metabolic acidosis. Serum calcium and coagulation studies are also indicated in severe intoxication. Determination of serum electrolytes is useful in the overall fluid management of the patient. Liver function tests may be abnormal after 24 hours of ingestion.

Treatment

The general measures for management of iron intoxication include early gastric evacuation by emesis with syrup of ipecac or gastric lavage. Antacids may be useful for complexing iron in the stomach and decreasing corrosive effect of acid upon denuded gastric mucosa. Use of activated charcoal, intragastric deferoxamine and phosphate solutions as complexing agents are of no therapeutic value.

In all cases of serious iron intoxication, chelation therapy with intravenous infusion of deferoxamine should be started During deferoxamine infusion careful monitoring of blood pressure is required. The chelation therapy should be continued till serum iron falls below 300 ug/dl. If laboratory monitoring is not possible it is recommended to continue the infusion of deferoxamine for 24 hours after the urine color has become clear[46,47].

Apart from gastric decontamination and chelation, supportive care by ensuring fluid and electrolyte balance forms an important part of management. In severe intoxication, exchange blood transfusion and hemodialysis may be used in addition to other therapeutic measures[46]. In selected patients whole bowel irrigation may be helpful.

ISONIAZID POISONING

The toxic dose varies between 5-10 gm. The symptoms appear within 30-60 minutes of ingestion. Gastrointestinal irritation, CNS manifestations (lethargy, confusion, seizures and coma) and respiratory depression may occur. The blood INH level of > 50 mg/dl is toxic. Besides supportive measures (prompt gastric lavage, administration of activated charcoal and correction of metabolic acidosis with sodium bicarbonate) pyridoxine is a specific antidote and is given intravenously in a dose of 1.0 mg for every mg of INH ingested. When the amount of INH ingested is unknown, administer 500 mg of pyridoxine IV and repeat every 5-20 min if needed.

CARBON MONOXIDE POISONING

Carbon monoxide (CO) is an odorless, colorless, non-irritating gas present in atmosphere in concentration of less than 0.001%. Excessive CO may be produced due to incomplete combustion of carbon containing substances. CO poisoning occurs following accidental fire in a close area, and use of coal or kerosene stove for keeping rooms warm during winter.

Clinical Features

CO binds with hemoglobin and produce caboxy hemoglobin (COHB) resulting in hypoxia. The signs and symptoms depends on the proportion of COHB. With COHB less than 10% there may be shortness of breath and dilatation of cutaneous vessels. Levels of COHB of 20% may produce headache and tightness in frontal region. COHB level of 20–50% may produce irritability, nausea, vomiting, weakness, dizziness, diminished vision, confusion, and fainting on exertion. As the COHB crosses 50% level, loss of consciousness and convulsions may occur. A level of COHB between 60–80% may be fatal.

Treatment

Treatment of CO poisoning consists of 100% oxygen inhalation. Hyperbaric oxygen may relieve hypoxia early as it also provides oxygen to tissues by dissolved oxygen in the plasma. Patient with hypercarbia and respiratory failure may require ventilatory support. Cerebral edema may occur. Mild acidosis should not be corrected as it may help to reduce hypoxia by shifting the oxygen dissociation curve to the right[48-51].

ALUMINIUM PHOSPHIDE POISONING

Aluminum phosphide is a grain preservative. It is available as tablets (Celphos, Alphos, Quickphos, Phosphotek and Phostoxin). It releases phosphene, carbon monoxide and ammonia gases. Toxic effects are produced due to disturbance in activities of various body enzymes. In adolescents it may be ingested with an intention to commit suicide. Fatal dose for an adult is 150-500 mg.

Clinical Manifestations

In moderate to severe poisoning almost all systems are involved. Gastrointestinal symptoms include nausea, vomiting, burning epigastric pain, diarrhea and excessive thirst. Clinical manifestations related to cardiovascular system are hypotension, cardiac arrhythmia, myocardial ischemia, myocarditis, pericarditis and congestive cardiac failure. The respiratory manifestations vary from cough and dyspnea to adult respiratory distress syndrome. There may be hepatomegaly, increased transaminases and occasionally clinically evident jaundice. Both oliguric and non oliguric renal failure may occur. The patient may be anxious and restless. With increasing severity there may be convulsions and terminally coma. The diagnosis of aluminum phosphide poisoning is based on history of ingestion. Presence of hypotension, arrhythmia, foul or decaying fish like smell and metabolic acidosis strongly suggest its possibility. Confirmatory test include analysis of blood or gastric fluid for phosphine gas.

Treatment

Treatment is supportive. There is no specific antidote. For decreasing the absorption of poison gastric lavage with $KMnO_4$ may be carried out but at the same time other supportive care should be started immediately. If it is likely to take a long time to transport the patient to the hospital or patient comes late; gastric lavage may be deferred. Activated charcoal is administered. Cathartics can be used for evacuation of gut. For decreasing organ toxicity intravenous administration of magnesium sulphate has been advocated in adults. The doses for adults are 1 gram of magnesium sulphate stat followed by 1 gram over next 2 hours and finally 1.0–1.5 grams every 4–6 hours for 3–5 days. The role of magnesium sulphate in children is not well established. In one series a dose of 200 mg/kg every 4-6 hours demonstrated benefit to the patients[52]. Hypoxia, shock, metabolic acidosis and ARDS should be treated appropriately[53]. Arrhythmia if present may not respond to conventional drugs and sometime may show good response to magnesium sulphate.

Prognosis

Mortality is very high and depends on dose of aluminum phosphide consumed, and the lag period between ingestion and reporting to hospital. Most of the fatalities result within 1 to 90 hours (mean 28 hours) of ingestion of poison. Cause of death in majority of patients is peripheral circulatory failure due to cardiac toxicity[52, 53].

OPIOID POISONING

Opioids include broad spectrum of compounds including natural alkaloids (morphine, codeine), semisynthetic derivatives (heroin, hydromorphine, and oxycodon), and synthetic derivatives (butorphenol, fentanyl, levorphenol, meperidine, methadone, propoxyphen, and pentazocin). Intoxication due to various opioids may occur due to accidental ingestion or due to therapeutic mishap. In adolescence it may occur due to drug abuse.

Clinical Features

The triad of respiratory depression, meiosis and impaired conciousness is characteristic of opioid poisoning. Cardiovascular manifestations include hypotension, bradycardia and arrhythmia (intraventricular conduction defects, heart block, bigemini and nonspecific ST-T wave changes). Non cardiogenic pulmonary edema manifesting as hypoxemia, cyanosis, respiratory distress, tachypnea, crepitations and respiratory and metabolic acidosis may be present. Seizures may occur due to hypoxia or due to primary toxic effect of meperidine and propoxyphene. Intoxication due to antidiarrheal agents containing diphenoxylate and atropine combination may present with a mixed clinical picture of opioids and anticholinergic effects.

Treatment

Management of opioid poisoning consists of initial stabilization and providing life support, administration of specific antidote naloxone, gut decontamination and symptomatic treatment. If the patient is in respiratory failure, assisted ventilation should be provided. Naloxone is a specific antidote and its administration helps in confirmation of diagnosis and early reversal of toxic effects. American Academy of Pediatrics has recommended initial dose of 0.1 mg/kg in children weighing less than 20 kg including newborns. In children weighing more than 20 kg the minimum initial dose of 2 mg is recommended. The doses are repeated every 2-3 minutes till the toxic effects are reversed or a maximum cumulative dose of 10 mg is reached. After initial reversal of toxic effects further doses can be administered if there is recurrence of respiratory or CNS depression[54]. Intoxications due to methadone, propoxyphene, pentazocin, diphenoxylate and codeine require higher doses of naloxone for reversal of toxic effects[55].

THEOPHYLLINE POISONING

Theophylline is a commonly used drug for asthma by oral or parenteral routes. Because of its narrow therapeutic window, toxicity may result due to accidental ingestion or therapeutic mishap.

Clinical Features

Theophylline toxicity produces symptoms related to gastrointestinal tract (GIT), cardiovascular system and central nervous system (CNS). The GIT manifestations include nausea, vomiting, epigastric pain and hematemesis. Cardiac toxicity may manifest as hypotension and arrhythmia (premature ventricular beats, bigemini, ventricular tachycardia and fibrillations). CNS toxicity include anxiety, restlessness and seizures. There may be varying degree of hypokalemia, hypophosphatemia, hyperglycemia, leukocytosis and metabolic acidosis. The blood levels of theophylline are in toxic range. The levels are repeated every 2-4 hours in severe poisoning till they are below 20 ug/ml[13].

Treatment

Gastrointestinal decontamination remains the important mode of treatment in theophylline toxicity.

Administration of activated charcoal is an essential component. Repeated doses of charcoal help in rapid decrease in the blood theophylline levels possibly by gut dialysis. Whole bowel irrigation may be considered if the patient has ingested enteric-coated tablets and/or the blood levels are increasing despite charcoal administration. If facility exists, charcoal hemoperfusion is another modality to reduce the blood levels of theophylline rapidly.

Seizures are controlled with benzodiazepines and barbiturates. Phenytoin may not be very effective. Seizures may be refractory and may require general anesthesia. Supportive care for GI symptoms include antacids and H-2 receptor blocking agents. Hypotension and cadiac arrhythmia should be treated appropriately[13].

PREVENTION OF POISONINGS

Every episode of poisoning should be probed in detail to identify the circumstances that lead to the accident. The opportunity should be taken to allay guilt feelings and impart proper advice to the parents to avoid recurrence of misadventure. There is a need to create public awareness and impart health education through mass media to prevent accidental poisonings. Practitioners need to consider a community's ecology and social context of risk as it pertains to "wicked" problems. The term "wicked" is used to characterize problems that are multifactorial, dynamic in nature, and resistant to resolution. There are several characteristics of "wicked" problems that can apply to environmental health issues. For example, there are multiple stakeholders who define the problem differently and who possess uncoordinated solutions. In addition, the feasibility of numerous solutions may be viewed differently due to the varied perspectives and interests of many stakeholders. Remedial measures should focus on how to best manage them.

The well baby clinics should not lay emphasis merely on vaccine preventable diseases but should provide information to the parents in the art of child care, provision of nutrition and prevention of accidents and poisonings. Most poisoning accidents occur at home especially in the kitchen. Kerosene, detergents, soap solutions, cleaning liquids etc. should not be stored in the open containers and left on the floor. They should be kept in proper containers having child-proof screw caps and stocked in cupboards. The toxic nonconsumable liquids should never be stored in the conventional soft drink bottles, which is a common cause of accident. The thirsty toddler is a common victim of such a tragedy. Insecticides should never be stored in the kitchen and always kept in firmly sealed containers. The drugs should be prescribed in limited supplies and dispensed in child proof foils and bottles. They should be kept in cupboards away from the reach of inquisitive children. Children are great imitators and one should avoid taking medicines in their presence. Unused surplus medicines should be disposed off properly or flushed in the toilet. The dressing table should not be decorated with cosmetics if the family has under-five children.

REFERENCES

1. Thundiyil JG, Stober J, Besbelli N, Pronczuk J. Acute pesticide poisoning: a proposed classification tool . *Bull World Health Organ* 2008; 86: 205–209.

2. Dutta AK, Seth A, Goyal PK, *et al*. Poisoning in children: Indian scenario. *Indian J Pediatr* 1998; 65: 365-370.

3. Gupta S, Govil YC, Misra PK, Nath R, Srivastava KL. Trends in poisoning in children: experience at a large referral teaching hospital. *Natl Med J India* 1998; 11: 166-168.

4. Jesslin J, Adepu R, Churi S. Assessment of prevalence and mortality incidences due to poisoning in a south Indian tertiary care teaching hospital. *Indian J Pharm Sci* 2010 ;72:587-91.

5. Lamireau T, Llanas B, Kennedy A, Fayon M, Penouil F, Favarell-Garrigues JC, *et al*. Epidemiology of poisoning in children: a 7-year survey in a pediatric emergency care unit. *Eur J Emerg Med* 2002; 9: 9-14.

6. Fine JS, Goldframe LP. Update in Medical Toxicology. *Pediatr Clin North Am* 1992; 39:1031-1051.

7. Srivastava A, Peshin SS, Kaleekal T, Gupta SK. An Epidemiological study of poisoning cases reported to the National Poisons Information Center, All India Institute of Medical Sciences, New Delhi. *Hum Exp Toxicol* 2005; 24(6):279 – 285.

8. Kohli U, Kuttiat VS, Lodha R, Kabra SK. Profile of childhood poisoning at a tertiary care centre in North India. *Indian J Pediatr* 2008 ;75:791-4.

9. Riordan M, Rylance G, Berry K. Poisoning in children 1: General management. *Arch Dis Child* 2002; 87(5): 392-96.

10. Kisoon N, Vidyasagar D. Poisoning. *Indian J Pediatr* 1991; 58:431-438.

11. Bar-Oz B, Levichek Z, Koren G. Medications that can be fatal for a toddler with one tablet or teaspoonful: a 2004 update. *Paediatr Drugs* 2004; 6(2):123- 126.

12. Seikel K, Keyes DC. Poisoning: principles of management. In: Essentials of Pediatric Intensive Care. II edition, Levine DC, Morriss FC (Eds) New York 1997 pp 853-868.

13. Wolf AD, Berkowitz ID, Liebelt E, Rogers MC. Poisoning and critically ill child. In: Text Book of Pediatric Intensive Care, Roger M C (Ed.), 3rd edition. *Williams and Wilkins, Baltimore,* 1996; pp 1315-1392.

14. Belson MG, Simon HK. Utility of comprehensive toxicologic screening in children. *Am J Emerg Med* 1999; 17:221-224.

15. Helper B, Sutheimer C, Sushine I. Role of the toxicology laboratory in suspected ingestion. *Pediatr Clin North Am* 1986; 33:245-256.

16. Chabali R. Diagnostic use of anion and osmolar gap in pediatric emergency care. *Ped Emerg Care* 1997; 13:204-210.

17. Savitt DL, Howkins HH, Roberts JR. The radio opacity of orally ingested medications. *Ann Emerg Med* 1981; 16:331-333.

18. National Poisons Information Center. Accessed from http://www.aiims.edu/aiims/departments/pharmacology/NPIC/home.htm on July 18, 2011.

19. Bond GR. The poisoned child; evolving concept in care. *Emerg Med Clin North Am* 1995; 13:343-355.

20. Fleisher GR, Keanrey TE, Herretig F, *et al*. Gastric decontamination in the poisoned patients. *Pediatr Emerg Care* 1991; 7:378-381.

21. Phillips S, Gomez H, Brent T. Pediatric gastrointestinal decontamination in acute toxic ingestion. *J Clin Pharmacol* 1993; 33:497-507.

22. Ponds SM, Lewis-Driver DJ, Williams GM, Green AC, Stevenson NW. Gastric emptying in acute overdose, a prospective randomized control trial. *Med J Aust* 1995; 163:345-349.

23. Manoguerra AS, Cobaugh DJ. Guidelines for the management of poisoning. Guideline on the use of ipecac syrup in the out-of-hospital management of ingested poisons. *Clin Toxicol* (Phila) 2005; 43(1): 1 – 10.

24. Rodgers GC Jr, Fort P. Use of dish soap as an emetic in out patient management of accidental poisonings. *Pediatr Res* 1984; 18:232.

25. Jones J, Mc Mullen MJ, Dougherty J, *et al*. Repetitive doses of activated charcoal in treatment of poisoning. *Am J Emerg Med* 1987; 5:305-307.

26. Vale JA , Krenzelok EP, Barceloux GD. Position statement and practice guidelines on the use of multidose activated charcoal in the treatment of acute poisoning. American Academy of Clinical Toxicology; European Association of Poisons Centers and Clinical Toxicologists. *J Toxicol Clin Toxicol* 1999; 37:731-751.

27. Tenebein M. Whole bowel irrigation as a gastrointestinal decontamination procedure after acute poisoning. *Med Toxicol* 1988; 3: 77-84.

28. Tenenbein M. Position statement: Whole bowel irrigation. American Academy of Clinical Toxicology; European Association of Poisons Centers and

Clinical Toxicologists. *J Toxicol Clin Toxicol* 1997; 35:753-762.

29. Peterson RG, Peterson LN. Cleansing the blood-hemodialysis, peritoneal dialysis, charcoal hemoperfusion, forced diuresis, and exchange transfusion. *Pediatr Clin North Am* 1986; 33:675-686.

30. Ponds SM. Diuresis, dialysis and hemoperfusion. *Emerg Med Clin North Am* 1984; 2:29- 37.

31. Pond SM. Diuresis, dialysis,and hemoperfusion. Indications and benefits. *Emerg Med Clin North Am* 1984; 2:29-45.

32. Rothstein FC. Caustic injuries to the esophagus in children. *Pediatr Clin N Am* 1986; 33:665-673.

33. Anderson FD, Rousetin P, Randolph GJ. A controlled trial of steroids in children with corrosive injury of esophagus. *N Eng J Med* 1990; 323: 637-642.

34. Karnak I, Tanyel FC, Buyukpamukcu N, Hicsonnee A. Combined use of steroids, antibiotics, and early bougienage against stricture formation following caustic esophageal burns. *J Cardiovas Surg* 1999; 40:307-310.

35. Ulman I, Mulof O. A critique of systemic steroids in the management of caustic esophageal burns in children. *Eur J Ped Surg* 1998; 8:71-74.

36. G. Stiff, A. Alwafi, B. I. Rees, J. Lari. Corrosive injuries of the esophagus and stomach: experience in management at a regional pediatric centre. *Ann R Coll Surg Engl* 1996 ; 78: 119–123.

37. Nuutinen M, Uhari M, Karvali T, *et al*. Consequences of caustic ingestions in children. *Acta Paediatr* 1994; 83:1200-1205.

38. Klein BL, Simon JE. Hydrocarbon poisoning. *Pediatr Clin North Am* 1986; 33:411-419.

39. Anas N, Namosonthi V, Ginsburg CM. Criteria for hospitalizing children who have ingested products containing hydrocarbons. *JAMA* 1981; 246: 840-844.

40. Lifsitz M, Shahak E, Sofer S. Carbamate and organophosphate poisoning in young children. *Pediatr Emerg Care* 1999; 15:102- 103.

41. Mortensen ML. Management of acute childhood poisonings caused by selected insecticides and herbicides. *Pediatr Clin North Am* 1986; 33: 421-445.

42. Roberts DM, Buckley N. Alkalinisation for organophosphorus pesticide poisoning. Cochrane Database of Systematic Reviews 2005, Issue 1. Art. No.: CD004897. DOI: 10.1002/14651858. CD004897. pub 2.

43. Senanayak N, Johnson MK. Acute polyneuropathy after poisoning by a new organophosphate insecticide. *N Eng J Med* 1982; 306:155-157.

44. Knight ME, Roberts RJ. Phenothiazine and butyrophenon intoxication in children. *Pediatr Clin North Am* 1986; 33: 299-309.

45. Smego RA, Durack DT. The neuroleptic malignant syndrome. *Arch Intern Med* 1982; 142:1183-1185.

46. Banner WJ, Tong TG. lron poisoning. *Pediatr Clin North Am* 1986; 33: 393-410.

47. Henertig FM, Karl SR, Wentraub WH. Management of severe iron poisoning with enteral and intravenous deferoxamine. *Ann Emerg Med* 1983; 12:306-309.

48. Dolan MN. Carbon monoxide poisoning. *Canad Med Assoc J* 1985; 133: 392-398.

49. Liebelt EL. Hyperbaric oxygen therapy in childhood carbon monoxide poisoning. *Curr Opin Pediatr* 1999; 11:259-264.

50. Myers RA, Linberg SE, Cowley RA. Carbon monoxide poisoning. The injury and its treatment. *J Am Coll Emerg Phys* 1979; 8:479-488.

51. Waisman D, Shupak A, Weis ZG, Melamid Y. Hyperbaric oxygen therapy in pediatric patients: the experience of the Israel Naval Medical Institute. *Pediatrics* 1998; 102:653-658.

52. Singh UK, Chakroborty B, Prasad R. Aluminum phosphide poisoning a growing concern in pediatric population. *Indian Pediatr* 1997; 34:650-651.

53. Chug SN. Aluminum phosphide poisoning, present status and management. *J Assoc Phys India* 1992; 40:401-405.

54. American Academy of Pediatrics Committee on Drugs. Naloxone doses and route of administration for infants, children: addendum to emergency drug doses for infants and children. *Pediatrics* 1990; 86:484-485.

55. Kunkel DB. Narcotic antagonist update. *Emerg Med* 1987; 19:97-108.

Emergency Procedures and Medications

Pain Relief and Sedation

56

Meharban Singh

> *People are more scared of pain than death. And most people will do anything to avoid pain but not so much for gaining pleasure.*

Pain is the most common signal or symptom of disease and often coexists with fever in most inflammatory conditions. Pain indeed is a protective mechanism on the part of body to limit tissue injury. Pain in young children is less often recognized and under treated compared to older children and adults[1]. Many children present to the emergency department with musculo-skeletal pains and abdominal colic. Pain may occur due to physical trauma following day-to-day activities, sports injuries and road-side accidents. Children are prone to accidental burns, chemical injuries and electrocution. Pain and anxiety are caused in children by various diagnostic and therapeutic procedures. Apart from fear and pain in the child, the procedures also cause lot of anxiety and concern to parents and attendants.

MECHANISM OF PAIN

Pain is perceived through spinal and central nervous system pathways which are triggered by a cascade of biochemical mediators. Tissue damage or inflammation releases a number of inflammatory mediators like bradykinin, prostaglandins, leukotrienes and potassium. These mediators eleborate a polypeptide called as "substance-P" which aggravates local inflammatory signs by further release of bradykinin, histamine and serotinin (Figure 56.1)[2].

ASSESSMENT OF SEVERITY OF PAIN

Pain is subjective with both physical and emotional components like anxiety, fear and terror. Threshold of pain is different in different individuals. Pain is difficult to recognize in children and is often under recognised and undertreated. Infants cannot vocalize and localize pain and they merely cry. There is a need to have a device like algometer or

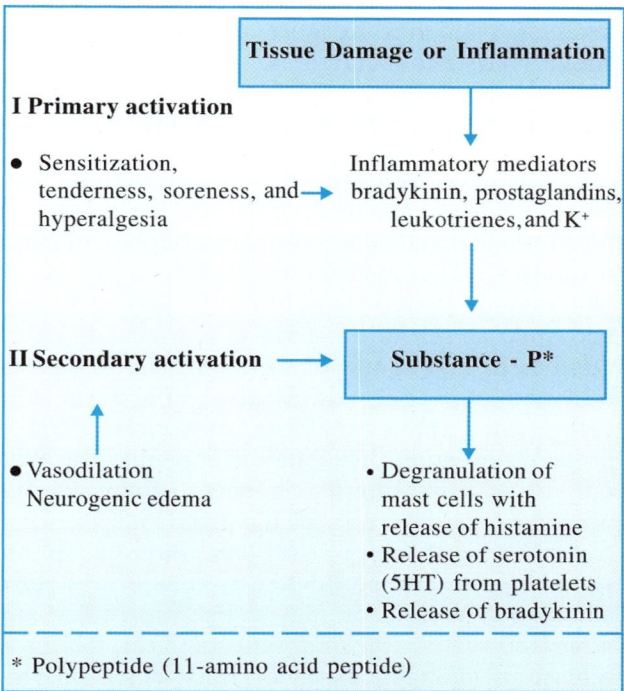

Figure 56.1 Biochemical mediators of pain

nocimeter to assess the severity of pain. Changes in facial expression (facial action coding system), nature of cry, motor activity and autonomic responses can be used for assessment of severity of pain in infants and young children. In school going children, numerical rating scale, visual analogue scale and McGill pain questionnaire can be used to assess the severity[3]. The location, severity, quality, duration, radiation and other characteristics of pain provide useful diagnostic clues.

MYTHS REGARDING PAIN

Till recently it was believed that newborn babies feel less pain due to lack of myelination of CNS and poor development of the cortex. There is enough neuro anatomic evidence to suggest that pain pathways are well developed as early as 24-25 weeks of gestation as evidenced by the presence of nocioceptive nerve endings in the skin,

823

arborization of dendritic processes in the neocortex, and synaptic genesis of thalamocortical fibers. Therefore, neonates and young infants do feel pain and its adverse physiological consequences. There is a mistaken belief that children have higher tolerance for pain. Infact young children are more delicate and less stoic, and they are likely to feel more anxiety, discomfort and pain. There is a wrong perception that children have little or no memory for a painful experience. In the absence of any scientific evidence, it is wrongly believed that children are more likely to have side effects of analgesics and they are more vulnerable to develop addiction to opioid narcotics.

BIOLOGICAL CORRELATES OF PAIN

Pain is associated with at least four components i.e. physical, emotional, autonomic or physiological and neuro-endocrine or biochemical responses[4]. The common emotional correlates of pain include anxiety, fear, terror, nausea, sickening and sinking sensation. Pain is associated with a number of autonomic or physiological responses because of vagal stimulation. They include tachycardia, rapid breathing, elevation of blood pressure, sweating and dilatation of pupils. The child may make struggling movements of limbs (during procedure) or there may be localized muscle spasm over the site of injury or inflammation i.e. sprain, psoas abscess and peritonitis. A number of neuro-endocrine responses may cause morbidity and adversely affect the outcome of pain. There is release of endogenous endorphins which provide comfort and sense of wellbeing. The release of stress hormones like cortisol and catecholamines is associated with various physiological responses. Pain is usually associated with hyperglycemia due to release of cortisol and glucagon, and suppression of insulin. Severe pain may cause elevation of pulmonary artery pressure with right-to-left shunting of blood, hypoxia, hypercarbia and elevation of serum pyuvate and lactate levels. Pain may adversely affect body defences and immune mechanisms of the body thus adversely affecting recuperative and healing capabilities of the patient.

CHOICE OF ANALGESICS

The basic role of physician is to relieve human suffering and pain. Pain and discomfort must be relieved to provide comfort and improve the quality of life. Early and effective treatment of pain is associated with reduced morbidity and enhanced survival by reversing neuroendocrine responses which are associated with pain. Figure 56.2

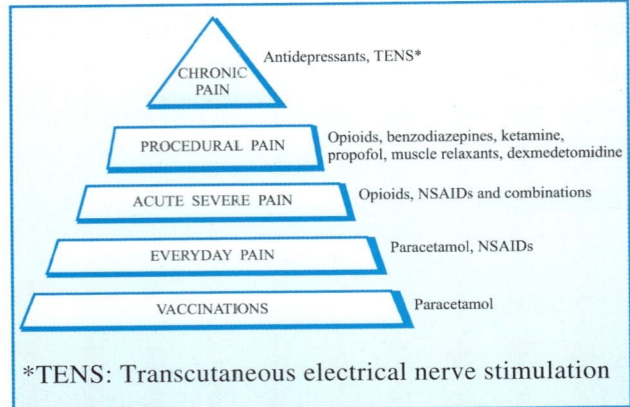

Figure 56.2 Pyramid of pain

summarizes the choice of analgesics and sedatives for various painful conditions and situations in children[4].

Indications for use of Analgesics

Analgesics and sedatives must be prescribed in children to relieve pain and anxiety. Emotional support, comfort of mother's lap, cuddling and caressing are useful to provide comfort and relieve fear and anxiety due to pain.

Newborn Babies

Pain in neonates is often unrecognized and undertreated. There is no doubt that neonates do feel pain and analgesics should be routinely prescribed during their medical care. Sucrose (0.5-2.0 ml of 20% solution) or sucking at breast or dummy nipple provides comfort during minor procedures like venipuncture or heel stick by virtue of distraction and possibly due to its pharmacological effect.[5] Surface anesthetic should be used before heel stick and venipuncture and baby comforted by skin-to-skin contact, cuddling and caressing after the procedure.[6]

Paracetamol is the drug of first choice for relief of pain due to traumatic delivery, congenital fracture, cellulitis, abscess, osteomyelitis and arthritis. Non-steroidal antiinflammatory drugs (NSAIDs) are not recommended for use in newborn babies as an analgesic.

Children

The indications for giving analgesics to children are listed in Table 56.1. Paracetamol is the drug of first choice for treatment of discomfort due to vaccinations and minor every day pains. When pain is more severe and is due to serious injury, infection or auto immune disorder, it is best treated with a non-steroidal antiinflammatory drug (NSAID). In case of severe pain due to polytrauma

Table 56.1 Indications for administration of analgesics

- ❑ Vaccinations
- ❑ Teething
- ❑ Viral and bacterial infections
- ❑ Non-inflammatory conditions
  Headache or migraine, tooth ache, dysmenorrhea, sprains and serious injuries
- ❑ Inflammatory conditions
  Infections
  Cellulitis, facio-myositis, arthritis, osteomyelitis, abscess
  Auto-immune or collagen vascular or connective tissue disorders
- ❑ Procedures
  Diagnostic and therapeutic
- ❑ Post-surgical pain

or malignancy, a combination of opioids and NSAIDs is used. The management of pain and anxiety should be given priority in the emergency department. Intractable pain due to terminal cancer and burns can be managed by patient-controlled analgesia (PCA) with the help of a device that delivers a pre-designed dose of an opioid drug when the patient pushes a button. The device can be programmed to restrict the upper limit of the total hourly dose so that over dosing is impossible. The adolescent patient can self titrate the dose to serve the optimal needs for pain relief. Children with chronic intractable pain due to neurogenic disorders are managed with antidepresants and transcutaneous electrical nerve stimulation (TENS)[7]. Table 56.2 gives the dosages and adverse effects of commonly used analgesics.

Visceral Pain

Colicky abdominal pain due to intestinal colic, renal colic and biliary colic is managed by a combination of analgesic with an antispasmodic and activated dimethicone (intestinal colic). Simple home remedies which are effective for treatment of 'wind' and infantile colic include prone positioning, hot fomentation, application of asfoetida (*hing*) around the navel and administration of concoction of fennel seeds (*sonf*), carom seeds (*ajwain*), dil or fennel oil. Dicyclomine hydrochloride 5-10 mg q 8 hr and drotaverine hydrochloride 20-40 mg q 8 hr are useful oral antispasmodic agents. They can be administered in combination with paracetamol or mefenamic acid. Hyoscine butylbromide 10-20 mg q 8 hr can be administered per oral, rectal, IM or IV in cases of severe colic.

Non-pharmacologic Strategies

The alternative non-drug therapies for pain control include emotional and psychological support to the patient. Physiotherapy, massage and active and passive movements are useful for management of musculoskeletal disorders due to trauma, connective tissue diseases and neurological sequelae. Accupunture and accupressure by experts in the field can produce amazing relief from chronic pain. Transcutaneous electrical nerve stimulation (TENS) has been exploited effectively for treatment of chronic intractable pain. Surgical excision of localized malignancy followed by radiotherapy is curative for cancer. Other alternative therapies which are credited to relieve pain include yoga, physiotherapy, acupressure or acupuncture, meditation, music and laughter therapy.

Pain Modulation

There is an in-built mechanism based on a brain circuit involving frontal cotex and hypothalamus which can modify response to painful stimuli by release of endogenous opioids, enkephalins and beta-endorphins. The pain can be tolerated by will power, poise, suggestions and distraction. The proper handling and behavior of the doctor and parents can modify child's response to pain. Distraction, praise, reassurance, information and explanation by the parents or the physician can have a positive effect on the response of the child towards a painful event like physical examination, injection or a procedure[8]. On the other hand sympathizing, admonishing and criticizing the child has a negative effect leading to more discomfort and pain to the child. Atheletes and soldiers are known to suffer from serious accident and injuries during sports and war with relatively minor perception of pain because they are "focussed and distracted" for a supreme cause. At times, mere expectation of pain (injection or procedure) can produce a "fright and fear reaction" even before the noxious event.

SEDATION FOR PROCEDURES

Procedural sedation is defined as the administration of sedatives or dissociative agents, with or without analgesics, to induce a state that allows the patient to tolerate unpleasant procedure while maintaining cardiorespiratory stability.

Children do not cooperate during various procedures because fear and anxiety are out of proportion to the actual pain. Young children have high vagal tone and they are more reactive, fussy, easily frustrated and readily cry. Depending upon the age, child should be given relevant information

Section 6

	Analgesic	Dose	Side effects
❑	Paracetamol	15 mg/kg q 4-6 hr oral or rectal	Nephropathy, hepatic damage
NSAIDs			
❑	Acetyl salicylic acid	15 mg /kg q 4-6 hr oral	Bleeding, peptic ulcer, hepatic and renal damage, tinnitus, Reye syndrome
❑	Ibuprofen	10 mg/kg q 4-6 hr oral	Peptic ulcer, GI bleeding, skin rash
❑	Naproxen	5-10 mg/kg q 12 hr oral	Peptic ulcer, renal dysfunction
❑	Mefenamic acid	5-8 mg/kg q 6-8 hr oral	Cotitis, seizures, bleeding, renal dysfunction, skin rash
❑	Diclofenac sodium	1.5 mg/kg q 12 hr oral	Peptic ulcer, GI bleeding
❑	Indomethacin	1.0 mg/kg q 8 hr oral	Peptic ulcer, GI bleeding, renal damage
❑	Ketorolac	0.5 mg/kg q 6 hr oral, IM or IV	Renal and hepatic dysfunction
Opioids			
❑	Morphine sulfate	0.1-0.2 mg/kg q 8-12 hr IV or IM	Apnea, seizures, bronchospasm, rise in intracranial tension, seizures, and hepatic dysfunction
❑	Pethidine hydrochloride (Meperidine)	1-2 mg/kg 8-12 hr IV or IM	
❑	Codeine phosphate	1.0 mg/kg q 6-8 hr oral	Respiratory depression, bronchospasm, seizures, rise in intracranial pressure, liver dysfunction, and constipation
❑	Oxycodone	0.05-0.15 mg/kg q 4-6 hr oral	Renal and hepatic dysfunction.
Mild sedatives			
❑	Triclofos sodium	10-20 mg/kg oral	Cumulative toxicity with prolonged use
❑	Promethazine hydrochloride	0.5-1.5 mg/kg oral	Dry mouth, nasal stuffiness, and blurred vision

Table 56.2 Dosages and side-effects of commonly used analgesics

regarding the procedure. The child must be given the comfort and confidence of parental presence during the procedure. Infant should preferably be kept in the mothers' lap which provides security and confidence to the child. Parental humor, distraction, praise and reassurance provide comfort and emotional support to the child during the procedure. The commonly performed diagnostic and therapeutic procedures in children are listed in (Table 56.3). A topical anesthetic and/or systemic analgesic-sedative must be given whenever an invasive procedure is performed (Table 56.4). Procedural sedation and analgesia enhances the cooperation of the child and allays the anxiety and fear of the child as well as the parents.

Levels of Sedation

American Society of Anesthesiologists (ASA) has proposed a clinical classification of levels of sedation which has been adopted by American Academy of Pediatrics (Table 56.5)[9]. Children with mild to moderate sedation are considered to have "conscious sedation" which is safe and without any risks. When deep sedation or general anesthesia is planned, fasting, pre-sedation assessment, monitoring during sedation and after the procedure are manda-

tory to prevent any complications and mishaps. The common life-threatening adverse events during deep sedation include vomiting, excessive oral and lung secretions, apnea, desaturation, airway obstruction, cardiac arrhythmia and hypotension.

Pre-sedation Assessment

A detailed pre-sedation assessment of the patient is mandatory if deep sedation is planned[10]. Baseline parameters like age, sex, weight, vital signs presence of any systemic disease, allergy to drugs, current medications, previous sedation etc. should be recorded. Airway is assessed by the neumonic HEENT i.e. head, ears, eyes, nose and throat for any anatomical variations and tonsillar hypertrophy. The risk category of the patient can be assigned as shown in Table 56.6.

Informed Consent

The parents should be explained about the nature of procedure, drug/s to be used for sedation, likely side effects and complications. After explaining risks, benefits and potential side effects of sedation and procedure, a written consent must be obtained from the parents or attendant.

Table 56.3 Indications for procedural sedation and analgesia

Diagnostic procedures

- ❑ Lumbar puncture
- ❑ Bone marrow and tissue biopsies
- ❑ Arthrocentesis
- ❑ Endoscopies
- ❑ Sexual assault examination
- ❑ Radiologic and neuroimaging studies (CT, MRI)

Therapeutic procedures

- ❑ Endotracheal intubation
- ❑ Suturing
- ❑ Wound care and dressing
- ❑ Incision and drainage of abscess
- ❑ Reduction of fracture and dislocation
- ❑ Aspiration of fluid from serosal cavities
- ❑ Removal of foreign body
- ❑ Debridement of wound and burns
- ❑ Tube thoracostomy
- ❑ Central intravenous line placement
- ❑ Urethral catheterization or bladder puncture
- ❑ Peritoneal dialysis
- ❑ Any other painful procedure

Table 56.4 Types of analgesic-sedatives used during various procedures

- ❑ Heel stick
  Skin-to-skin contact, cuddling, caressing, glucose solution, breast feeding or dummy nipple, surface anesthetic like EMLA* (eutectic mixture of local anesthetic lignocaine and prilocaine) and EMLAP*
- ❑ Emergency room suturing, dressings, burn debridement, fracture reduction, drainage of abscess
  Opioids, diazepam or midazolam
- ❑ Radio-imaging studies
  Triclofos sodium, promethazine, propofol, midazolam, and dexmedetomidine
- ❑ GI endoscopies and bronchoscopy
  Midazolam + ketamine
- ❑ Biopsies and invasive diagnostic or therapeutic procedures
  Surface anesthetic, midazolam with or without ketamine
- ❑ Neurophysiology studies
  Triclofos sodium, promethazine and midazolam
- ❑ Intubation
  Morphine with or without muscle relaxant

* May cause methemoglobinemia in preterm babies

Table 56.5 Levels of sedation as proposed by American Society of Anesthesiology (ASA)

Physiological effects	Minimal sedation	Moderate sedation	Deep sedation	General anesthesia
Responsiveness	Normal response to verbal commands	Purposeful response to verbal or tactile stimulation	Purposeful response following repeated or painful stimulation	Not arousable even on painful stimulation
Airway	Unaffected	No intervention is required	Intervention may be required	Intervention is often required
Spontaneous ventilation	Unaffected	Adequate	May be inadequate	Usually inadequate
Cardiovascular functions	Unaffected	Usually maintained	Usually maintained	May be impaired

Table 56.6 Classification of the patient on the basis of physical status (ASA)

Class	Criteria
Class 1	A normally healthy subject
Class 2	A patient with a local or mild systemic disease
Class 3	A patient with a severe systemic disease
Class 4	A patient with a life-threatening disease
Class 5	A moribund patient who is not expected to survive without the procedure or operation

Fasting

No fasting or dietary restrictions are required for mild to moderate or "conscious sedation". In case of deep sedation, about 4 hours fasting is adequate in infants while in older children fasting (non-clear fluids like formula, milk, soup and solid food) for 6-8 hours reduces the risk of vomiting, airway complications and aspiration[11]. NPO for clear fluids is recommended for 2 hours before the procedure. When procedure is life saving and mandatory but patient is not fasting, it is advised to perform the procedure under "conscious sedation".

Section 6

Personnel and Equipment

At least two well trained pediatricians should be available for giving sedation and undertaking the procedure. When deep sedation is contemplated, pediatric intensivist or anesthesiologist should be available for giving sedation/anesthesia, monitoring during and after the procedure[11]. Expertise and facilities should be available at hand for providing advanced pediatric life support. A large number of emergency drugs, disposables and monitoring equipments like multi-channel vital sign monitor, EKG machine, pulse oximeter, end tidal carbondioxide monitor ($EtCO_2$) and defibrillator should be available as discussed in Chapter 1.

The child should be closely monitored during procedural sedation. The basic equipments and supplies required during the procedure can be remembered by the acronym SOAPME[12] as follows:

S (Suction) : Suction catheters and suction apparatus

O (Oxygen) : Adequate oxygen supply and flow meters

A (Airway) : Oropharyngeal or nasopharyngeal airways, laryngoscope blades, endotracheal tubes, face masks, bag-valve-mask or equivalent device

P (Pharmacy) : Emergency drugs and antagonists

M (Monitors) : Vital sign monitor, non-invasive blood pressure monitor, pulse oximeter, end-tidal carbondioxide monitor, ECG machine

E (Equipment) : Procedure light, disposables and supplies for conducting the procedure

Monitoring during the Procedure

A time-based record should be maintained during procedural sedation which should include vital signs, level of sedation, drugs used and any complications encountered. During deep sedation it is desirable to attach the patient to a vital sign monitor. Any adverse drug reactions and their management should be documented. In advanced centers, when facilities are available, pulse oximetery, capnography ($EtCO_2$) can be used for early detection of hypoventilation while bispectral index monitoring is useful to assess the depth of sedation with encephalographic signals[12]. There are a variety of quantitative sedation scores available which can be used to measure the level of sedation and guide administration of sedative drugs or need for antognists.

Post Procedure Care

The patient should be closely monitored after the procedure till full consciousness is achieved. There is increased risk of complications immediately after the procedure because cardio-respiratory depressant effects of sedative drugs may become more pronounced when pain of procedure is no longer present. The patient should be fully oriented, should have stable vital signs and be able to accept oral feeds before the discharge. When a patient had no adverse events during procedural sedation, he can be usually discharged after 30 minutes of the procedure[13]. Recovery from ketamine sedation may be associated with ataxia for 12–24 hours and child's activities should be restricted during this period.

SEDATIVE DRUGS AND THEIR DOSAGES

A single drug or a combination of drugs may be used depending upon the procedure to be performed. After the initial appropriate dose, the subsequent doses are given at an interval of 3-5 minutes to achieve full sedation. The following groups of drugs are commonly used for procedural sedation.

OPIOIDS

Opioids are often used in combination with benzodiazepines as they produce analgesia and sedation without causing loss of memory. The common side effects include respiratory depression, hypotension, bronchospasm, emesis, urinary retention and ileus[14]. The adverse effects can be reversed by administration of naloxone.

Morphine

It is a naturally occurring prototypical opioid agonist which produces analgesia, euphoria and sedation. It is given intravenously in a dose of 0.1-0.2 mg/kg followed by infusion at a rate of 20-60 µg/kg/hr. Onset of action occurs after 10-15 minutes with a half life of about 2-3 hours. It can also be given through subcutaneous, intramuscular and oral route. Excretion of active metabolite of morphine occurs by the kidneys, which is slow in neonates and infants making them more susceptible to morphine induced respiratory depression. Its long duration of action is useful for relief of post procedural pain but it may prolong somnolence in the patient. Morphine may lead to histamine release which is characterized by bronchospasm, vasodilation, hypotension and itching. Pethidine or meperidine is no long popular due to less predictable sedation and serious side effects.

Fentanyl

It is a semisynthetic opioid agonist with a wide therapeutic window, rapid onset and short duration of action. Fentanyl is 75–200 times more potent than morphine[15]. It does not release histamine, has no adverse effects on myocardium and does not cause any cardiovascular instability even with large doses. Respiratory depression is a major concern with fentanyl and it may cause chest wall rigidity in neonates and infants especially when rapidly infused. It is not suitable for procedures involving the face as it may cause intense facial pruritis. It is administered intravenously in a dose of 0.3-1.5 µg/kg in children below 6 years and 1-5 µg/kg in children above 6 years followed by constant infusion at a rate of 1-10 µg/kg per hour.

Remifentanil

It has highly predictable onset of action with a short duration of sedation because of half life of 5 minutes. It is safe in children with hepatic and renal dysfunction but is associated with greater risk of apnea and respiratory depression and should preferably be administered by an anesthetist[16]. It may be given as an intravenous infusion at a rate of 0.025-0.05 µg/kg/min alone or with low doses of benzodiazepines.

BARBITURATES

Barbiturates produce sedation by depressing reticular activating system. They relieve anxiety and cause amnesia but have no analgesic effects. They are useful in patients with raised intracranial pressure because they cause cerebral vaso-constriction. The common side effects include apnea, hypoventilation and hypotension. They are contraindicated in patients with documented hypersensitivity and porphyria. Benzodiazepines are preferred over long acting barbiturates because of availability of flumazenil as a specific antidote.

Pentobarbital

It is a short acting barbiturate which has sedative, hypnotic and anticonvulsant effects. It is given in a dose fo 2-5 mg/kg IV, IM, orally or through rectal route. Onset of action occurs in 1-5 minutes after intravenous administration and effect lasts for 15-45 minutes. Rapid bolus administration may cause apnea, respiratory depression, laryngospasm and vasodilation. In susceptible children it may produce paradoxical excitement instead of sedation[17].

Methohexital

It is an ultrashort acting barbiturate with immediate onset of action. It is rapidly metabolised in the liver leading to rapid recovery compared to other barbiturates. Methohexital is given intravenously in a dose of 0.75-1.0 mg/kg stat, followed by 0.5 mg/kg/dose every 2-3 minutes for maintenance. Common adverse effects include myoclonus, excessive nasopharyngeal secretions, transient upper airway obstruction, stridor and emergence phenomenon[18].

Thiopental

It is a useful induction agent for endotracheal intubation. The onset of action occurs within 30-40 seconds with a half-life of 3-8 hours. Induction dose is 2-5 mg/kg IV. Children can tolerate higher doses per unit body weight compared to adults.

BENZODIAZEPINES

They are most useful for procedural sedation because of their anxiolytic, amnesic, hypnotic and muscle relaxant effects. The loss of short-term memory and availability of a specific antidote (flumazenil) are other advantages but they lack analgesic effect. Long-term use of benzodiazepines may be associated with dependency and withdrawal symptoms such as rebound agitation and even seizures in some patients.

Diazepam

It modulates post synaptic effects of GABA-A transmission, resulting in an increase in pre-synaptic inhibition in the limbic system, thalamus and hypothalamus. The negative attributes of diazepam include risk of apnea, long half-life, erratic absorption and lack of dosing schedule below the age of 30 days. It is administered in a dose of 0.25 mg/kg IM or IV slow bolus over 3 minutes to avoid respiratory depression. Rectal dosing schedule depends upon the age of the child, i.e. 2–5 years; 0.5 mg/kg; 6–11 years; 0.3 mg/kg, >12 years; 0.2 mg/kg. Excessive sedation and respiratory depression can be reversed by adminstration of flumazenil 0.01–0.02 mg/kg IV, which can be repeated every minute upto maximum cummulative dose of 1.0 mg.

Midazolam

Midazolam is preferred over diazepam and may be used alone or in combination with opioids and ketamine. It has a rapid onset, short duration of action and fewer side effects[19]. It is water soluble and can be given through various routes including parenteral, oral, nasal and per rectal. The dose of midazolam is 0.05-0.15 mg/kg by parenteral route, 0.05-0.75 mg/kg by oral or rectal route and 0.25-0.5 mg/kg by intranasal route. About 25% of initial dose may be given as repeat doses to maintain desired level of sedation. Over dosage of midazolam may cause somnolence, confusion, impaired coordination, diminished reflexes and hypotension. Flumazenil can be used to reverse excessive sedation due to midazolam.

DISSOCIATIVE SEDATIVES

Ketamine

It is a dissociative anesthetic with an excellent profile for conducting painful emergency procedures by virtue of its analgesic, amnesic and sedative properties without causing loss of protective reflexes[20]. Patients given ketamine often look as if they are in a cataleptic state. Side effects of ketamine include excessive salivary and bronchial secretions with risk of laryngospasm which can be prevented by concomitant administration of atropine. Unusual adverse effects, due to emergence phenomenon is less common in children, and include disturbing dreams and hallucinations. The emergence phenomenon can be prevented by administration of midazolam 5 minutes before ketamine[21]. Life-threatening arrhythmia may occur following bolus administration of ketamine. It is contraindicated in patients with raised intracranial or intraocular pressure, pulmonary disorders, hyperthyroidism and uncontrolled hypertension[22]. It is administered in an intravenous dose of 1-2 mg/kg or intramuscular dose of 3-4 mg/kg.

HYPNOTICS

Etomidate

It is a carboxylated imidazole sedative or hypnotic agent without any analgesic properties. It has a short duration of action with fewer side effects compared to pentobarbital. It can block cortisol production which is a serious drawback of etomidate which limits its long term use. It produces transient reduction in cerebral blood flow with benefits of modulation of intracranial and intraocular pressures. Etomidate has a better respiratory and hemodynamic safety profile. It has a rapid onset (within 1 min) and short duration of action (5-15 min). It is administered in a dose of 0.1-0.4 mg/kg intravenously[23].

Propofol

It is an ultrashort acting hypnotic which is commonly used for procedural sedation. It has a useful antiemetic effect and is credited to lower intracranial pressure but lacks in analgesic properties. It is a useful agent for use in children undergoing imaging studies. It can be coadministered with ketamine.[24] Side effects include hypoventilation, hypotension, tachycardia, myoclonus, and excessive sedation[25]. The usual dose is 0.5-1.0 mg/kg intravenously followed by 100-200 ug/kg/min as a constant infusion. Fentanyl may be coadministered to provide analgesia for painful procedures.

Triclofos sodium

It is an excellent hypnotic and sedative agent but lacks analgesic and amnestic effects. Onset of action is slow and lasts for 6-8 hours. Paradoxical agitation may occur especially in association with pain. It is administered in a dose of 20 mg/kg in infants, 250-500 mg in 1-5 years and 500-1000 mg in 6-12 years orally. It is commonly used for sedation during radio-imaging studies. It is contraindicated in patients with renal or hepatic impairment.

Nitrous Oxide

Nitrous oxide is a sweet-smelling gas which produces anxiolysis, amnesia and mild to moderate analgesia. It is used as a mixture of 30-50% of nitrous oxide (maximum upto 70%) and oxygen[26,27]. The onset of action occurs within 1-2 minutes of inhalation followed by recovery within 5 minutes after stoppage of inhalation. It has minimal effect on cardiovascular and respiratory systems and airway reflexes. Vomiting is the common side effect occurring in 10-20% cases. Diffusion hypoxia may occur when nitrous oxide concentration is more than 50%. It can be relieved by administration of 100% oxygen for 5 minutes after the procedure. Nitrous oxide is contraindicated in children with pneumothorax, eye injury, abdominal distension due to intestinal obstruction and altered sensorium.

Dexmedetomidine

It is a newer selective alpha-2 receptor agonist. Dexmedetomidine is credited to have sedative, analgesic and sympatholytic properties. It has a wide safety profile and wide range of dosages can be given without any cardiovascular and respiratory adverse effects. The common side effects include hypertension or hypotension and bradycardia. It is mainly used in radiological procedures, sedation in mechanically ventilated children, invasive procedures like awake craniotomy and cardiac catheterization[28,29]. It is given intravenously in a loading dose of 1-2 µg/kg followed by a continuous infusion at a rate of 0.1-0.2 µg/kg/hour. It can be coadministered with opioids and benzodiazepines.

Combination Formulations

A number of analgesic-sedative drugs are used in combination for their additive and synergic effects. The commonly used combinations for procedural sedation include morphine-midazolam and midazolam-ketamine. When an opioid and benzodiazepine combination is used, the dose of opioid should be titrated first, followed by administration of benzodiazepine for further sedation because opioid poses greater risk of respiratory depression.

The Child-friendly Hospital Ambience

In order to reduce the anxiety and fear of children towards pediatricians and hospitals, there is a need to create child-friendly ethos and ambience. There should be plenty of soft musical toys and culture-specific cartoon characters to gain the confidence of children. Pediatricians should be gentle, caring, campassionate and friendly in their approach towards children. They should handle children as children (play-like informal or unstructured approach) and not patients! The child should be encouraged to have hands-on experience with the gadgets of the doctor. *Children should never be given threats of injections and doctors to modify their behavior.* During clinical examination, minor procedures or administration of vaccines, preschool child should be provided with the comfort and security of the mother's lap. There is hardly any indication for administration of medications through parenteral route in ambulatory pediatric practice except for giving vaccines and treatment of anaphylaxis with epinephrine. In view of ever increasing number of vaccines, there is a need to develop "multiple antigens" vaccines, and painless transcutaneous, nasal or oral vaccines.

REFERENCES

1. Alexander J, Manno M. Under use of analgesia in very young pediatric patients with isolated pain injuries. *Ann Emerg Med* 2003, 41: 617-622.

2. Fields HL, Martin JB. Pain: pathophysiology and management. In: Harrison's Principles of Internal Madicine. Fauci AS, Braunwald E, Kasper DL, *et al.* (Eds). *Mc Graw Hill, New York,* 17th Edition, 2008, pp. 81-87.

3. Gilbert CA, Lilley CM, Craig KD, *et al.* Post operative pain expression in preschool children: Validation of the the child facial coding system. *Clin J Pain* 1999, 15(3): 192-200.

4. Singh M. Pain in children: practical issues and concerns. *Indian J Pract Pediatr* 2001, 3:146-149.

5. Stevens B, Yamada L, Lee GY, et al. Sucrose for analgesia in newborn infants undergoing painful procedures. *Cochrane Database Syst Rev* 2013, Jan 31, 1: CD001069. doi: 10.1002/14651858; CD 001069. Pub 4.

6. Singh M. The need for analgesia and sedation in newborn babies. *Perinatology* 2001, 3: 240-242.

7. Merkel SI, Gutstein HB, Malviya S. Use of transcutaneous electrical nerve stimulation in a young child with pain from open perineal lesions. *J Pain Symptom Management* 1999, 18(5): 376-381.

8. Sweet SD, McGrath PJ, Symons D. The roles of child reactivity and parenting context in infant pain response. *Pain* 1999, 80: 655-661.

9. Comprehensive Accreditation Manual for Hospitals, Oakbrook Terrace, Il. *Joint Commission on Accreditation of Healthcare organization,* 2005.

10. American Academy of Pediatrics, American Academy of Pediatric Dentistry. Charles J Cotes, Stephen Wilson. The Work Group on Sedation Guidelines for Monitoring and Management of Pediatric Patients during and after Sedation for Diagnostic and Therapeutic Procedures: An Update. *Pediatrics* 2006, 118: 2587-2602.

11. American College of Emergency Physicians. Clinical Policies Subcommittee on Clinical Policy. Procedural sedation and analgesia in the emergency department. *Ann Emerg Med* 2005, 45: 177-196.

12. Bell JK, Laasch HU, Wibraham L, England RE, Morris JA, Martin DF. Bispectral index monitoring for conscious sedation in intervention. Better, safer, faster. *Clin Radiol* 2004, 59: 1106-1113.

13. Newman DH, Azer MM, Pitetti RD, Singh S. When is a patient safe for discharge after procedural sedation? The timing of adverse effect events in 1,367 pediatric procedural sedations. *Ann Emerg Med* 2003; 42:627-635.

14. Lewis K P, Stanley GD. Pharmacology. *Int Anesthesiol Clin* 1999, 37: 73-86.

15. Chudnofsky CR, Wright SW, Dronen SC, Borron SW, Wright MB. The safety of fentanyl use in the emergency department. *Ann Emerg Med* 1989, 18: 635-639.

16. Rosow CE. An overview of remifentanil. *Anesth Analg* 1999, 89 (Suppl): S1-S3.

17. Malviya S, Voepel-Lewis T, Tait AR, *et al.* Pentobarbitol vs chloral hydrate for sedation of children undergoing MRI: Efficacy of recovery characteristics. *Pediatr Anesthesiol* 2004, 14: 589-595.

18. David R, Freyer AE, Schwanda DJS, Richard MH, *et al.* Intravenous methohexital for brief sedation of pediatric oncology out patients: physiologic and behavioral responses. *Pediatrics* 1997, 99(5): 8-15.

19. Wright SW, Chudnofsky CR, Dronen CR, Wright MB, Borron SW. Midazolam use in the emergency department. *Am J Emerg Med* 1990; 8: 97-100.

20. Chudnofsky CR, Weber JE, Stoyanoff PJ, *et al.* A combination of midazolam and ketamine for procedural sedation and analgesia in adult emergency department patients. *Acad Emerg Med* 2000; 7: 228-235.

21. Green SM, Krauss B. Clinical Practice Guidelines for Emergency Department: ketamine dissociative sedation in children. *Ann Emerg Med* 2004, 44: 460-471.

22. Mason KP, Padua H, Fontaine PJ, Zurakowski D. Radiologist supervised ketamine sedation for solid organ biopsies in children and adolescents. *AJR Am J Roentgenol* 2009, 192 (5): 1261-1265.

23. Rothermal LK. Newer pharmacological agents for procedural sedation of children in the emergency department: etomidate and propofol. *Curr Opin Pediatr* 2003, 15: 200-203.

24. Scheier E, Gadot C, Leiha R, Shavit I. Sedation with the combination of ketamine and propofol in a pediatric ED: A retrospective case series analysis. *Amer J Emerg Med* 2015, 33(6): 815-817.

25. Bassett KE, Anderson JL, Pribble CG, Guenther E. Propofol for procedural sedation in children in the emergency department. *Ann Emerg Med* 2003; 42: 773-782.

26. Burnweit C, Diana-Zerpa JA, Nahmad MH, *et al.* Nitrous oxide analgesia for minor pediatric surgical procedures: An effective alternative to conscious sedation? *J Pediatr Surg* 2004; 39: 495-499.

27. Tobias JD. Applications of nitrous oxide in the pediatric population. *Pediatr Emerg Care* 2013, 29(2): 245-265.

28. Phan H, Nahata MC. Clinical uses of dexmedetomidine in pediatric patients. *Pediatr Drugs* 2008, 10(1): 49-69.

29. Buck ML. Dexmedetomidine use in pediatric intensive care and procedural sedation. *J Pediatr Pharmacol Ther* 2010, 15(1): 17-29.

Section 6

57 Assisted Ventilation

Sindhu Sivanandan and Rakesh Lodha

57.1 Introduction

Mechanical ventilation was first introduced during the polio epidemics in 1950. Bjørn Ibsen, an anesthetist recommended positive pressure ventilation via tracheostomies, thereby reducing the mortality from 84% at the start of the polio outbreak to 26%[1]. During the 1880s, positive pressure ventilation was delivered by using a simple foot operated bellow to pump air into the trachea[2]. Mechanical ventilators can be of two categories, negative pressure ventilators or 'iron lungs' where negative pressure is applied to the surface of the thorax (rarely used now) and positive pressure ventilators where positive pressure is applied to the airway opening. Mechanical ventilation can be instituted with an endotracheal tube or tracheostomy (invasive positive pressure ventilation), or with a mask (non-invasive positive pressure ventilation). The last three decades has seen tremendous technological advances with the development of high frequency ventilators, microprocessor operated ventilators and newer modes of ventilation. Despite the advances in technology, conventional assisted ventilation remains the mainstay of treatment. At the same time there has been a better understanding of factors responsible for ventilator induced lung injury (VILI). Gentle ventilation with low tidal volumes and 'open-lung' strategy of using positive end-expiratory pressure (PEEP) are employed in order to minimize VILI. There has been a growing interest in non invasive respiratory support (either by nasal continuous positive airway pressure (nCPAP) or nasal positive pressure ventilation (nPPV) especially in neonates to avoid the risks and side effects of endotracheal intubation, ventilator associated pneumonia and lung injury.

57.2 Indications for Mechanical Ventilation

The most common indications for initiating mechanical ventilation are listed below[3].

1. **Reversal of hypoxemia**. Hypoxemic respiratory failure is characterized by failure of the lungs to maintain oxygenation. Blood gas analysis shows a PaO2 $\leq$ 60 mmHg (SaO2 < 90%). Hypoxemia can usually be treated with oxygen and non invasive methods like continuous positive airway pressure (CPAP).

However, if the fraction of inspired oxygen (FiO_2) requirement is greater than 60% to maintain $SaO_2 > 90\%$ or if hypoxemia is associated with ventilatory failure causing carbon dioxide retention, mechanical ventilation may be required.

2. **Reversal of acute respiratory acidosis**. Carbon dioxide retention and respiratory acidosis occurs when ventilatory pump mechanism fails. Pump failure can occur when either the respiratory muscles (diaphragm / chest wall muscles) or their neural control fails. Acute respiratory acidosis ($PaCO_2 > 50\text{-}55$ mmHg) with pH < 7.25 is an indication for mechanical ventilation. Frequently respiratory failure is a result of both hypoxemic and hypercapnic failure (failure of oxygenation and ventilation).

3. **Apnea.** The treatment of apnea depends on the underlying cause. Apnea can be central (absence of respiratory efforts), obstructive (absence of airflow in spite of respiratory efforts) or mixed. Infants or children with obstructive apnea respond to CPAP delivered through nasal prongs and nasal canulae but those with central apnea require mechanical ventilation until spontaneous respiratory efforts are established. In children with obstructive sleep apnea syndrome, CPAP therapy has shown to improve sleep architecture, day time sleepiness, neuro cognitive function and quality of life[4].

4. **In the delivery room.** Intubation and mechanical ventilation should be considered in the following situations; (a) failure to establish adequate spontaneous respiration despite positive pressure ventilation by bag and mask, (b) to administer prophylactic or early rescue surfactant in extremely preterm infants and (c) neonates with congenital diaphragmatic hernia.

Other short-term indications for mechanical ventilation

5. **To relieve respiratory distress**. Mechanical ventilation can be employed temporarily to perform the respiratory functions thereby decreasing the work of breathing, oxygen consumption and relieve patient discomfort while the primary disease process improves.

6. **Anesthesia.** Cardiac, abdominal, neurosurgery and other surgical procedures which might require neuromuscular blockade and control of air way.

7. **To secure an airway**. In patients with depressed sensorium, head injury, poor airway reflexes and in those recovering from anesthesia and during transport of a sick patient.

8. **To decrease systemic or myocardial oxygen consumption**. Examples include septic and cardiogenic shock.

9. **To reduce intracranial pressure (ICP)**. To lower elevated ICP through controlled hyperventilation.

10. **To stabilize the chest wall** in children with flail chest

While assessing a patient for respiratory support, one must try to evaluate following parameters[5]:

1. The nature of the problem (failure of oxygenation (PaO_2) or ventilation ($PaCO_2$), or both)
2. The underlying pathophysiology (hypoventilation, lung disease like pneumonia, meconium aspiration, asthma, respiratory distress syndrome etc) and
3. Formulate a goal i.e. target oxygen saturations and $PaCO_2$ that are acceptable for the patient. An otherwise healthy child intubated for surgery should have a goal of pH = 7.40, $PaCO_2$ = 40 mm Hg, PaO_2 = 60 mm Hg. In a patient with chronic lung disease $PaCO_2$ of 60-65 mm Hg and SaO_2 >88% may be acceptable.

Although mechanical ventilation is life saving, it is associated with a number of complications[6]. Ventilator associated lung injury can be produced by *barotrauma* (lung damage attributable to the application of high airway pressure), *volutrauma* (due to high inspired tidal volume), *biotrauma* (un physiological stress/strain promote the release of pro-inflammatory cytokines leading to lung inflammation) and *atelecto trauma* (lung injury secondary to repeated opening and closing of lung units)[7].

57.3 Pulmonary Physiology

57.3.1 Anatomy

Lung is a dichotomously branching airway system. According to Weibel's model[8], the first 16 generations make up the conducting airways ending in the terminal bronchioles. The next three generations constitute the respiratory bronchioles. This is the transitional zone. Finally, there are three genera-tions of alveolar ducts and one generation of alveolar sacs. These last four generations constitute the true respiratory zone which participates in gas exchange. Beyond the 16th generation the cross sectional area of lung dramatically increases. The mode of gas flow in the conductive airways is convective or 'bulk' flow and that in the respiratory zone is by molecular diffusion. The conducting airways do not participate in gas exchange and constitute the anatomic dead space. In adults this "dead space" is approximately 2.2 ml/kg[9] or 30% of the tidal volume. In early infancy this volume may be > 3 ml/kg largely because of the higher extra thoracic component (naso-oropharynegeal volume[10]). The normal dead space / tidal volume (V_D/V_T) ratio is 0.3. In other words dead space occupies about 1/3 of total tidal volume.

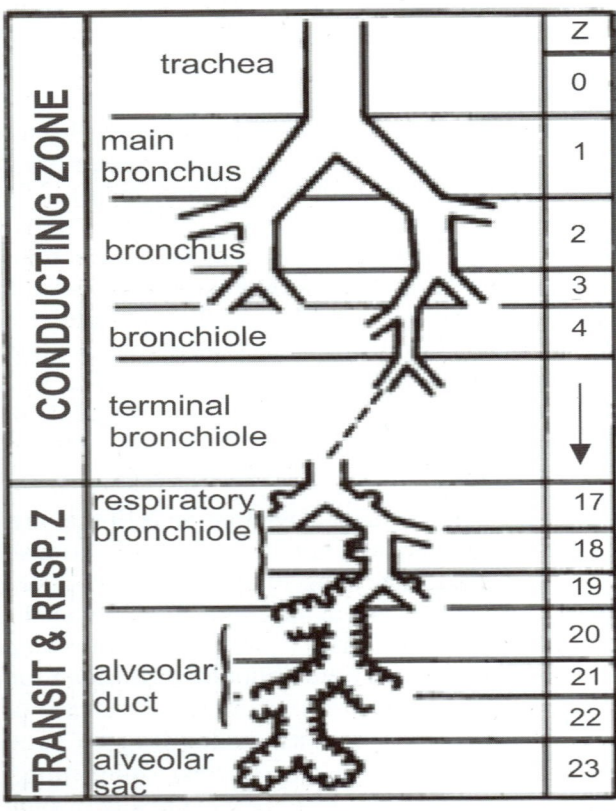

Figure 57.1 Weibel model (8) of airways with its 23 generations. Conduction zone: transport; transition zone: transport and gas exchange; the respiratory zone (alveoli) gas exchange

57.3.2 Gas exchange

Alveolar ventilation

Minute ventilation is the product of tidal volume and respiratory rate (VT × RR) where VT is the tidal volume and RR is the respiratory rate. Since dead space air does not participate in gas exchange, CO_2 elimination depends on alveolar ventilation which is (VT–DS) × RR, where, DS is the anatomical dead-space volume. Normal $PaCO_2$ is 35-45 mmHg. Factors that increase anatomic dead space are breathing thorough a mouth piece and a valve or the interposition of Y connector in the ventilatory circuit. This is called the apparatus dead space. Endotracheal tube and tracheostomy decrease the anatomical dead space by 50%. In health, the alveolar dead space is negligible. In lung disease the increase in alveolar dead space can be due to ventilation of under-perfused alveoli (e.g. pulmonary embolism or poor ventilation of perfused alveoli) or bronchoconstriction or obstruction as in asthma, bronchitis, and chronic obstructive airway disease. In disease states the alveolar dead space can contribute to as high as 80-90% of tidal volume. In addition a right to left shunt at the ductal or atrial level can cause deoxygenation of systemic circulation and is called shunt dead space. The sum of anatomical, alveolar and shunt dead space is called physiological dead space. The result is ventilation perfusion mismatch and this can lead to both hypoxemia and hypercarbia.

Alveolar ventilation can be increased by increasing tidal volume or respiratory rate. Assume a 10 kg child ventilated at a rate of 30/min with V_T 4 ml/kg. Dead space volume = 2 ml/kg. Alveolar ventilation= $(V_T - V_D) \times RR$ = 600 ml. If VT is increased to 5 ml/kg, the rest remaining the same, alveolar ventilation = 900 ml. If RR is increased to 40/min, the rest remaining the same, alveolar ventilation = 800 ml. However, it should be noted that indiscriminate increase in tidal volume to wash out CO_2 can lead to volutrauma, hyperinflation, V/Q mismatch and undesirable CO_2 retention.

Oxygenation

Oxygenation occurs by diffusion of oxygen across the alveolar capillary membrane. Normal PaO_2 is 80-100 mm Hg when breathing room air at sea level. Ventilation perfusion mismatch is the most common and hence the most important cause of hypoxemia. Other causes include decreased FiO_2, right to left shunt and impaired diffusion. The prime determinants of oxygenation are FiO_2 and the mean airway pressure (MAP). MAP is modified by changes in peak inspiratory airway pressure (PIP), positive end-expiratory pressure (PEEP) and the I: E (Inspiratory : Expiratory time) ratio (Table 57.1).

$$MAP = \frac{k (Ti \times PIP) + (Te \times PEEP)}{Ti + Te}$$

(k= constant, which is dependent on the shape of the pressure waveform)

MAP can be increased by increasing the PIP, PEEP, Ti, RR and flow.

Table 57.1 Determinants of oxygenation and ventilation and the ventilator parameters	

Oxygenation	❑ FiO_2
	❑ Mean airway pressure
	  • PIP
	  • PEEP
	  • I:E ratio
	  • Flow

Ventilation	❑ Minute ventilation= Tidal volume × rate
	❑ Tidal volume
	  • Compliance and resistance of lung
	  • Delta P = PIP-PEEP Rate
	❑ Rate
	  • Ti ,Te and I:E ratio

Alveolar gas equation

The PAO_2 is calculated using the alveolar gas equation. It relates the alveolar concentration of oxygen PAO_2 to three variables: FiO_2, $PaCO_2$ and the respiratory quotient (R) (Box).

$$PAO_2 = FiO_2 \times (P_{atm} - P_{H20}) - \frac{(PaCO_2)}{R}$$

FiO_2	=	fraction of inspired O_2 (21% at room air)
Patm	=	atmospheric pressure (760 mm Hg at sea level)
PH_2O	=	partial pressure of saturated vapor (47 mm Hg at 37°C)
$PaCO_2$	=	partial pressure of carbon dioxide in the arterial blood (assumed to be equal to the partial pressure of CO_2 in the alveoli [$PACO_2$] given the high diffusion coefficient of CO_2)
R	=	respiratory quotient (~0.8)

Parameters used to monitor oxygenation are listed below:

- Alveolar-arterial PO_2 difference (A-a) PO_2. The problem with the use of (A-a) PO_2 is its tendency to change as FiO_2 changes. This gradient is normally less than 10 mm Hg when breathing room air but increases to 30-60 mm Hg when breathing 100% O_2.

- PaO_2/FiO_2 ratio is a more commonly used measure of oxygenation and is easier to calculate. The normal value ranges between 300 and 500. PaO_2/FiO_2 of < 200 indicates acute respiratory distress syndrome and a PaO_2/FiO_2 between 200-300 acute lung injury.

- Oxygenation index (OI), is calculated using the following equation:

$$OI = \frac{Mean\ airway\ pressure \times FiO_2 \times 100}{PaO_2}$$

Increasing values of OI indicate a worsening of oxygenation. The OI could be considered a more robust index than the PaO_2/FiO_2 ratio, because it takes into con-sideration the mean airway pressure, thus providing a better pathophysiologic assessment of impaired lung function.

Mechanics of respiration[11]

The respiratory system can be thought of as a single tube (representing the airways) attached to a single bag representing the lung and chest wall (Figure 57.2).

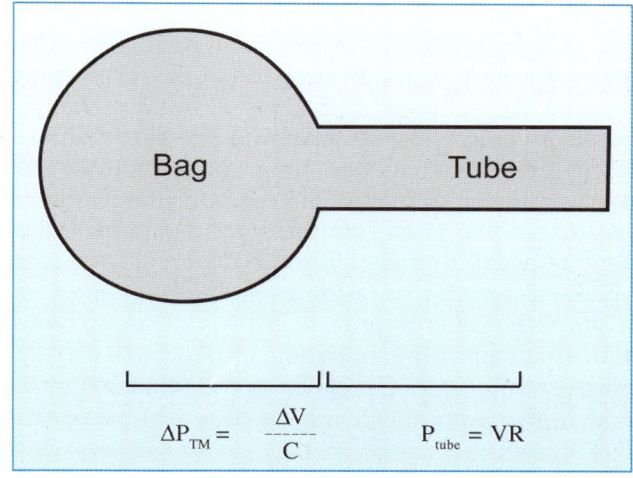

$$\Delta P_{TM} = \frac{\Delta V}{C} \qquad P_{tube} = VR$$

Figure 57.2 Bag and tube analogy of the respiratory system

Resistance: The air flowing into the lungs has to overcome the airway resistance and the elastic and frictional resistance of the lungs and chest wall. The airways contribute to 80% of the total resistance. The resistance to the flow of air through a long narrow tube is proportional to the length of the tube and inversely proportional to the 4th power of radius. The resistance (R) to airflow can be expressed by dividing the driving force by the flow across the airways: R= Pressure difference (cm H_2O) / Flow (Liter/second). Nasal airway resistance contributes to two-thirds of total upper airway resistance, the glottis and larynx less than 10% and the trachea and the first five

Table 57.2 Factors affecting resistance in mechanical ventilation	
Type of flow	Resistance is higher when flow is turbulent as compared to laminar flow
Flow rate	Flow rates exceeding 3 L/min through 2.5 mm ETT and 7.5 L/min through 3 mm ETT produce turbulence
Length of endotracheal tube (ETT)	Resistance is linearly proportional to ETT tube length. Cutting the tube length to half decreases the resistance by 50%
Diameter of the ETT	Resistance is inversely proportional to the 4th power of radius. A small diameter ETT or mild narrowing of bronchi produce exponential increase in resistance
Density of the gas	Heliox mixture (helium 80% and oxygen 20%) is 60% less dense than air and decreases the airway resistance by one third when used in patients with obstructive airway disorders

generations contribute to the remainder Table 57.2[12].

Compliance. Compliance describes the elastic properties of various parts of the respiratory system. Compliance represents a volume change per unit change in pressure. The pressure volume (P-V) curve for isolated lung shows that as the trans-pulmonary pressure increases the lung volume increases. The graph obtained is a hysteresis; the compliance during inspiration is different from that obtained during expiration as additional energy is required during inspiration to inflate and recruit more alveoli. The slope between two points on the pressure volume loop is called as compliance. Lungs with higher compliance have a steeper slope on the P-V curve.

The difference between static and dynamic compliance is that static compliance is measured at zero air flow and dynamic compliance is measured during air flow through the lungs. Since dynamic compliance is measured during airflow, it reflects not only the lung and chest wall stiffness, but also the airway resistance. If static compliance and dynamic compliance are both decreasing, it means that the lung is becoming stiff, e.g. pulmonary edema, consolidation etc. If the dynamic compliance has decreased whereas the static compliance has remained relatively unaffected, it means that the airway is obstructed e.g. endotracheal tube obstruction or bronchospasm.

The static compliance curve can be used to select the ideal level of PEEP for a mechanically ventilated patient (Figure 57.3). At the lower

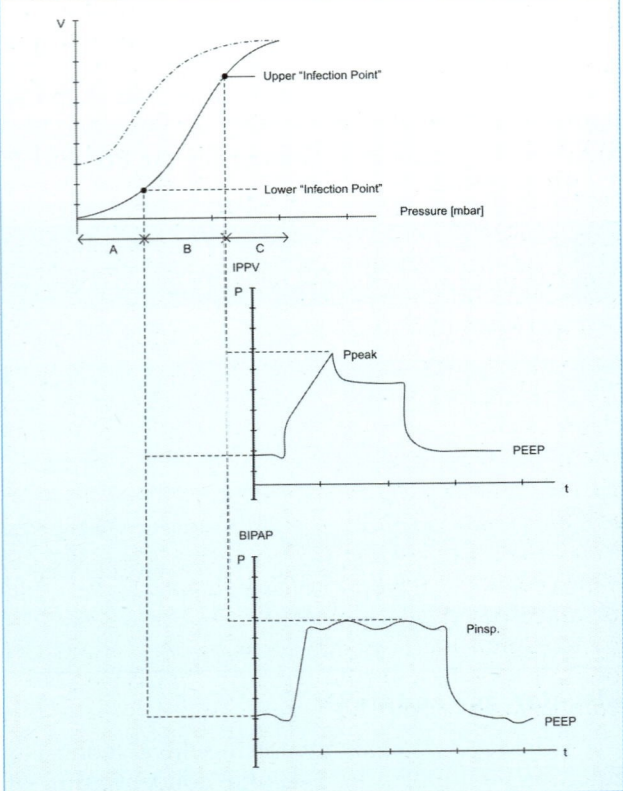

Figure 57.3 Pressure-volume loop or compliance curve

inflection point most of the collapsed alveoli will open and beyond the upper inflection point over distension of the alveoli will occur. It is generally accepted that ventilation should take place as far as possible within the linear compliance area. Near the lower inflection point there is a risk of atelecto trauma and near the upper inflection point there is a risk of over distension. The lower inflection point can be overcome by setting a PEEP. The tidal volume or peak inspiratory pressures must then be selected to ensure that the upper inflection point will not be exceeded.

Time constant

The rate of filling of an individual lung unit is referred to as its time constant. A time constant is the product of the resistance and compliance of a particular lung unit. It has been estimated that it takes the equivalent of five time constants for the lung to completely fill (or to empty) Figure 57.4 demonstrates the concept of time constant. Time constant (sec) = Resistance (cm H_2O/L/sec) × compliance (L/cm H_2O). For example, in a healthy infant with a resistance of 30 cm H_2O/L/sec and compliance of 0.004 L/cm H_2O, one time constant would be 0.12 second. For complete equilibration pressure (five time constants or 5 × 0.12 sec) an inspiratory or expiratory phase of 0.6 second will be necessary. This information is useful while setting a ventilator's inspiratory and expiratory time.

Lungs that have decreased compliance as in respiratory distress syndrome have a shorter time constant and lungs with increased airway resistance as in meconium aspiration syndrome have longer time constant. Table 57.3 shows the compliance (CL), resistance (R) and time constant (Kt) in normal and abnormal states in the newborn. The clinical application of the concept of time constant is that very short inspiratory times may lead to incomplete tidal volume delivery resulting in a decrease in peak inspiratory pressure (PIP) and mean airway pressure (MAP) (Figure 57.4). Insufficient expiratory time may cause an increase in functional residual capacity, gas trapping and build up of pressure in the alveoli and distal airways. This is called inadvertant PEEP or auto PEEP. This is manifested as increased work of breathing, hypercapnia that worsens or is poorly responsive to increase in ventilatory rate, cardiovascular compromise (cyanosis, hypotension and metabolic

acidosis) and as a hyper expanded lung with flattened diaphragm on a chest radiograph.

57.4. Basics of Mechanical Ventilation

Mechanical ventilators are designed to assist or replace the work of the respiratory muscles and the thorax to maintain the gas exchange function of the lungs. In order to use these effectively, one should understand the basics of these 'complex' machines[13]. We shall briefly discuss the set up of a positive pressure ventilator.

1. **Power input.** There can be two different ways of running a ventilator; electrical or pneumatic (using compressed gases).

2. **The pneumatic circuit.** Compressed air or oxygen is delivered to the ventilator at 50 psi pressure. In the mixing chamber, the pressure is reduced and the gases are blended to get the desired FiO_2. The inspiratory valve controls the flow and pressure of the inspired gases. The gases are filtered, warmed and humidified before delivery to patient circuit. During expiration gases flow out passively through the expiratory valve into the atmosphere. The expiratory valve closes during inspiration and is also responsible for maintaining the PEEP (Figure 57.5).

3. **The microprocessor.** ventilators have an electronic microprocessor that controls the inspiratory and expiratory valves, monitors the pressure, flow and volume of delivered gases and displays the alarms.

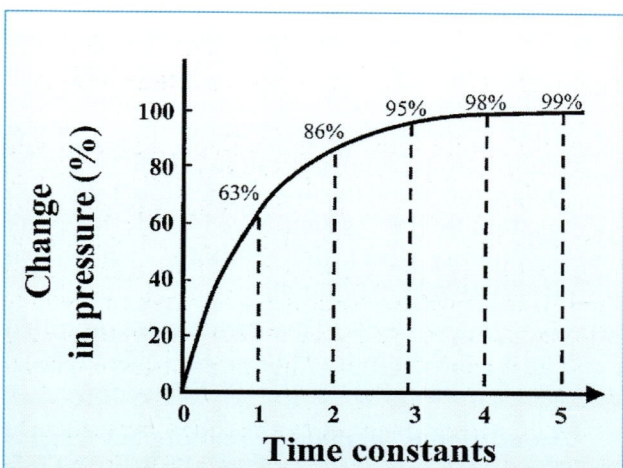

Figure 57.4 Concept of time constant. Percentage change in pressure in relation to the time (in time constants) allowed for equilibration

Table 57.3 Compliance (CL), resistance (R) and time constant (Kt) in normal and abnormal states in the newborn			
Condition	**CL (L/cm H$_2$O)**	**R (cm H$_2$O/ L/sec)**	**Kt (sec)**
Normal	0.005	20	0.10
HMD	0.001	20	0.02
MAS	0.003	100	0.30

HMD: Hyaline membrane disease, MAS: Meconium aspiration syndrome

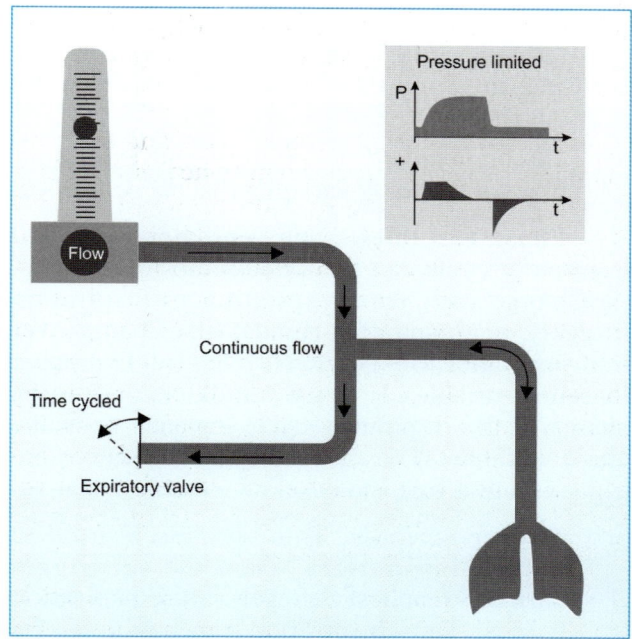

Figure 57.5 Design of a simple pressure controlled ventilator

57.4.1 Classification of mechanical ventilators[14]

A ventilator can be classified by describing the following variables

1. Control variable
   (a) Time
   (b) Pressure
   (c) Volume
   (d) Flow

2. Phase variables
   (a) Trigger
   (b) Limit
   (c) Cycle
   (d) Baseline variable

3. Conditional variables

Control variable. It is the variable that the ventilator controls to cause inspiration. There are 4 main variables that can be regulated by the ventilator i.e. pressure, volume, flow, and time. The first 3 are inter-related and time can influence all the three. The control variable remains constant as the ventilatory load changes.

(a) *Pressure controlled.* They control the *airway pressure* (positive pressure ventilators). The pressure wave form does not change with changes in compliance and resistance of the lung.

(b) *Volume controlled.* These ventilators deliver a *constant tidal volume* even if the resistance and/ or compliance of the respiratory system varies.

(c) *Flow controlled.* These have a *constant volume waveform, but the volume is not measured* or used as a feedback signal to alter the flow.

(d) *Time controlled.* Inspiratory and expiratory times are the only variables that are controlled.

Phase variables. Each ventilator-controlled respiratory cycle can be divided into four phases, (i) Change over from expiration to inspiration (trigger); (ii) Inspiration (limit); (iii) Change over from inspiration to expiration (cycle); (iv) Expiration (baseline variable). How the ventilator controls the phases of the respiratory cycle depends upon the phase variables. Thus the four phase variables are trigger, limit, cycle and baseline variable.

(a) *Trigger variable.* This variable is used to initiate inspiration. When the set trigger variable reaches a preset value inspiration begins. Thus inspiration can begin after a predefined time (Time trigger). For example

the ventilator initiates a breath every 1 second independent of patient effort if the rate is set at 60/min. Inspiration can be initiated by the patient (patient triggering). When ventilator detects a patient effort by changes in air way pressure or inspiratory flow (pressure or flow trigger) a breath is initiated. Flow triggering is more sensitive than pressure triggering. When the trigger is initiated by the patient, the ventilator tries to synchronize the breath with the patient's inspiratory effort.

(b) *Limit variable.* In any ventilator, the value of the limit variable cannot be exceeded at any time during inspiration. This limiting variable can be pressure, flow or volume. For example if pressure is the limiting variable, the set pressure cannot be exceeded during inspiration. The inspiration is not terminated when the limit is reached. The decision to end inspiration and to begin expiration is made by the cycle variable.

(c) *Cycle variable.* This variable is used to terminate inspiration, once a preset value is reached. The most commonly used cycle variable is time. The other cycle variables are pressure, flow and volume. For example in volume cycled ventilator the ventilator cycles from inspiration to expiration after a preset volume has been delivered. In flow cycle, when the flow during inspiration falls to a certain level (typically 25% of the peak inspiratory flow), the ventilator cycles from inspiration to expiration

(d) *Baseline variable.* This variable is controlled during the expiratory phase and is the positive end expiratory pressure (PEEP) setting.

Conditional variables. Conditional variables are those that are examined by the ventilator's control logic and invoke an action if a threshold is met. Examples include the synchronization of mandatory and spontaneous breaths (synchronized intermittent mandatory ventilation) and the delivery of sigh breaths.

Spontaneous versus mandatory breaths. A spontaneous breath is one for which inspiration is both started (triggered) and stopped (cycled) by the patient. If inspiration is either triggered or cycled by the machine, the breath is classified as mandatory. For a patient connected to the ventilator, spontaneous breaths may be assisted or unassisted, but mandatory breaths by definition are assisted. Depending on who or what is controlling the 3 phase variables (trigger, limit, cycle), 4 modes of different kinds of breaths can be defined (Table 57.4).

Table 57.4 Classification of available mechanical ventilator breaths			
Breath type	**Phase variable**		
	Trigger	**Cycle**	**Limit**
Mandatory	Machine	Machine	Machine
Assisted	Patient	Machine	Machine
Supported	Patient	Patient	Machine
Spontaneous	Patient	Patient	Patient

57.4.2 Modes of mechanical ventilation

There are four modes of ventilation, namely intermittent mandatory ventilation, synchronized intermittent mandatory ventilation, assist/ control ventilation and pressure support ventilation[15] (Figure 57.6).

(a) **Mandatory or controlled ventilation**. It is also called as continuous mandatory ventilation (CMV). Mandatory breaths are controlled entirely by the machine, i.e. all breaths are triggered, limited and cycled by the ventilator. The clinician sets a minimum rate per minute.

The patient can trigger the ventilator but all the delivered breaths are controlled by the ventilator including those breaths above the set rate. Modern microprocessor ventilators have the ability to sense the patient's efforts and to synchronize the ventilator breaths with the patient initiated breaths. This avoids patient-ventilator asynchrony. Depending on the control variable chosen CMV can be volume or pressure controlled

(b) **Synchronized intermittent mandatory ventilation (SIMV).** In SIMV, a set number of mandatory breaths per minute are synchronized with the patient initiated breaths. If the patient breathes above the set rate, the extra breaths are allowed but will not be supported by the ventilator unless one also adds the pressure support option to SIMV. The advantage of this mode is that it allows spontaneous breaths in between the mandatory breaths. As the patient's condition improves, there is a gradual increase in spontaneous breaths and simultaneous reduction in mandated breaths allowing a gradual transition towards extubation.

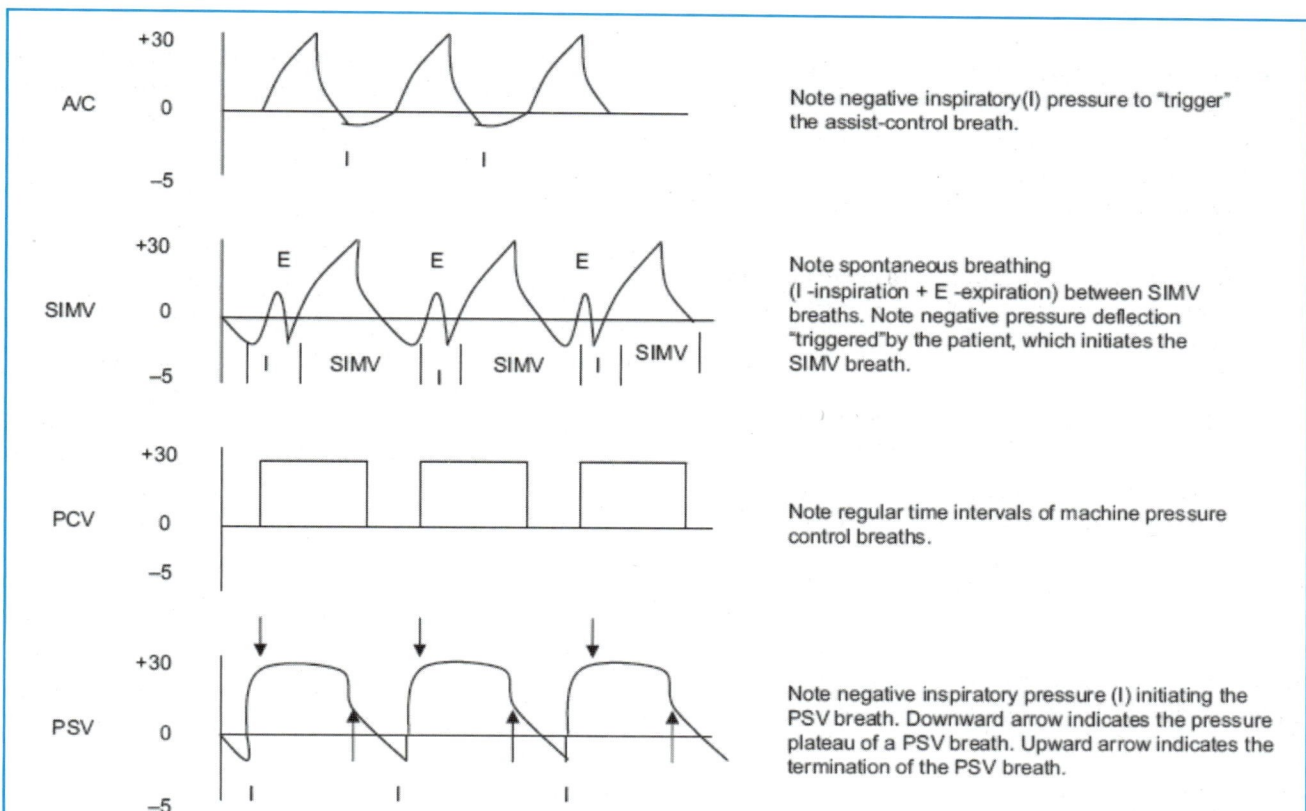

Figure 57.6 Pressure waveforms in the different modes of mechanical ventilation. A/C indicates assist-control ventilation; SIMV, synchronized intermittent mandatory ventilation; PCV, pressure control ventilation; PSV, pressure support ventilation. Intermittent mandatory ventilation is not shown

Depending on the control variable chosen SIMV can be volume or pressure controlled.

(c) **Assist/Control ventilation (A/C).** In this mode all spontaneous breaths that exceed the trigger sensitivity result in the delivery of a mechanical breath (assist) synchronous to the patient's inspiratory effort. If the patient fails to breathe or cannot trigger the ventilator, a control breath will be provided at the desired interval.

(d) **Continuous spontaneous ventilation.** Every breath is generated spontaneously by the patient. The patient determines the rate, inspiratory and expiratory times. The breaths are triggered and cycled by the patient but limited by the ventilator. CPAP (Continuous positive airway pressure) and PSV (Pressure support ventilation) are the most common modes of spontaneous ventilation. CPAP is discussed later in the section of non invasive ventilation.

Pressure Support Ventilation[16]. In a spontaneously breathing patient who is connected to the ventilator, the narrow high resistance ETT, the ventilatory circuit and its associated dead space and the demand flow valve provide additional work of breathing. These elements constitute the imposed work of breathing. PSV is a spontaneous ventilatory mode in which an inspiratory pressure boost is provided to overcome the imposed work of breathing or to provide additional support to a mechanically ventilated patient. PSV is a flow-cycled but time-limited mode that supports each spontaneous breath. The patient has control over the rate and the inspiratory time and the clinician has control over the inspiratory pressure and time limit. Typically, the pressure support level has been set at 30% to 50% of the difference between PIP and PEEP (partial support), or at a level to deliver an adequate tidal volume (full support). PSV is generally used in conjunction with SIMV, usually as a weaning strategy. In patient's with decreased effort or apnea, the SIMV provides a backup rate but in patients with reliable respiratory drive PSV can be used alone. Benefits of PSV include improvement in patient–ventilator synchrony, perceived improvement in patient comfort and reduced need for sedation.

The advantages and disadvantages of the different modes[17] are listed in Table 57.5.

Table 57.5 Advantages and disadvantages of various modes of mechanical ventilation		
Mode	**Advantages**	**Disadvantages**
Intermittent mandatory ventilation	• All breaths are mandatory • Unloads the respiratory muscles	• Patient ventilator asynchrony
Assist control	• The set tidal volume and minute ventilation are guaranteed • Allows the patient to initiate a breath but all breaths will be assisted • Breaths are delivered in synchrony with the patient's spontaneous effort • Unloads the respiratory muscles. Useful in acute phase of illness	• If the spontaneous respiratory rate (SRR) is high, all breaths would still be assisted and this can lead to hyperventilation and respiratory alkalosis. • When SRR is high patient ventilator asynchrony and air trapping can occur • If used for a long time, respiratory muscle wasting can occur
Synchronized intermittent mandatory ventilation	• Breaths are delivered in synchrony with the patient's spontaneous effort • Allows spontaneous breathing in between the mandatory breaths which are unsupported unless pressure support is added. • Allows patient comfort and at the same time keeps respiratory muscles active	• Work of breathing can be high if spontaneous breaths are not supported
Pressure support	• Patient controls the rate, inspiratory time and flow rate • Patient is comfortable with less need for sedation	• Cannot be used in patients with poor drive • Pressure support needs to be adjusted based on changing lung mechanics

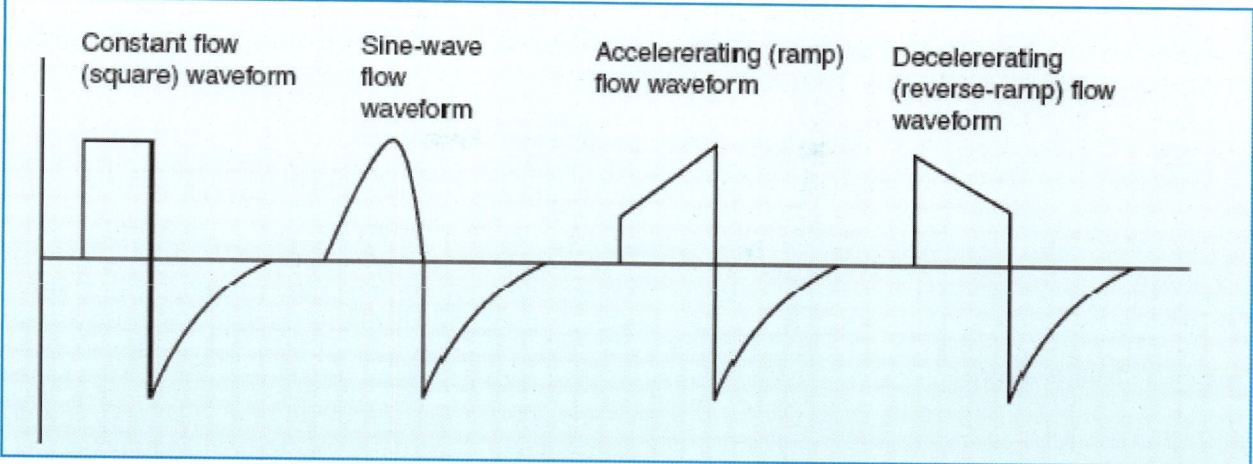

Figure 57.7 Different types of flow waveforms

For each control variable, following waveforms are possible (Figure 57.7).

(a) Rectangular (pressure and flow control)
(b) Sinusoidal (flow and volume control)
(c) Accelerating or decelerating (flow control).

57.4.3 Modalities of ventilation

Modality refers to the target or limit variable of the mechanical breath. Thus conventional mechanical ventilation is either pressure controlled or volume controlled (Table 57.6). Newer modes include volume guarantee ventilation, airway pressure release ventilation and Mandatory minute ventilation.

Pressure controlled ventilation. Traditional neonatal ventilators are continuous flow, time-cycled, pressure-limited ventilators (PLV). These ventilators deliver a positive pressure up to a predetermined pressure limit above PEEP during the selected Ti and at a set frequency. The tidal volume (V_T) delivered will depend on the difference between PIP and the baseline or positive end expiratory pressure (PEEP) and the mechanics of the respiratory system. VT delivered may not be consistent when compliance changes. For example, when lung compliance improves following the administration of surfactant, the delivered VT will be high if the PIP is not reduced. The following parameters are set in PLV ventilators; inspiratory and expiratory time (T_I, T_E, which together determine the RR), PIP, PEEP, inspiratory flow rate and FiO_2. The tidal volume delivered can now be measured in newer ventilators. Pressure-limited ventilators continue to be the primary mode of ventilation in newborns because of its relative simplicity, ability to ventilate effectively despite large ETT leak, improved intra pulmonary gas

distribution due to the decelerating gas flow pattern and the presumed benefit of directly controlling the PIP. The major disadvantage of pressure-limited ventilation is that the VT varies with changes in lung compliance and excessively large VT can lead to inadvertent hyperventilation and lung injury from volutrauma. The flow time curve in PLV shows a decelerating flow pattern (Figure 57.8).

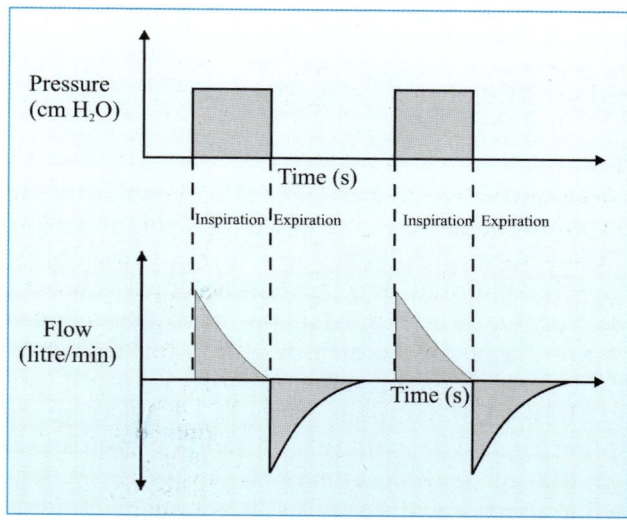

Figure 57.8 Pressure control ventilation. Note the rectangular pressure wave form and descending ramp (exponential) flow pattern. The peak pressure and tidal volume delivery occur early in the inspiratory phase 'front end loaded'

Volume controlled ventilation. Volume-targeted (VTV) or volume controlled ventilation aims to deliver a consistent tidal volume (V_T). The pressure required to deliver a set V_T depends on lung mechanics; if the compliance is low the ventilator will increase the pressure and conversely if compliance is low, the pressure is auto weaned (Figure 57.9). Volume targeted modes have been in use in pediatric and adult practice for many years.

Table 57.6 Pressure controlled versus volume controlled ventilation		
Parameter	Pressure controlled	Volume controlled
Tidal volume	Variable (depends on lung mechanics)	Constant
PIP	Constant	Variable (depends on lung mechanics)
Peak alveolar pressure	Constant	Variable
Flow pattern	Decelerating	Preset
Peak flow	Variable	Constant
Common to both modalities		
Inspiratory time (Ti)	Preset	Preset
Minimum rate	Preset	Preset
Modes	IMV, SIMV, A/C	IMV, SIMV, A/C
Advantages	• PIP remains constant throughout the cycle, hence less risk of barotrauma. • The decelerating flow pattern and the front ended breaths are more effective in treating stiff, atelectatic lungs	• Constant tidal volume delivery and hence less risk of volutrauma. • Back-end loaded breaths work better in high lung volume states and in heterogeneous disease states. • Auto weaning of pressures as compliance improves.
Disadvantages	• Variable tidal volume delivery. Risk of volutrauma if PIP is not decreased when compliance improves	• Risk of barotrauma in low compliance lungs if PIP is not monitored • Fixed inspiratory flow can lead to flow starvation if patient's demand flow is high. This could lead to increased work of breathing.

Modern microprocessor-controlled ventilators can measure and deliver even small tidal volumes using flow sensors placed at the Y piece between the ventilator circuit and the endotracheal tube. V_T delivery based on expired tidal volume measurement is more accurate because it is less influenced by ETT leak. Measurement of both inspired and expired tidal volumes allow ETT leaks to be quantified. The benefits of volume controlled ventilation include consistent V_T delivery, less volutrauma (avoiding high V_T), less atelectotrauma (avoiding low V_T) and more stable $PaCO_2$. A meta analysis of 12 RCTs[18] that compared volume controlled versus pressure controlled ventilators in the neonate found that the use of VTV modes resulted in a reduction in the combined outcome of death or bronchopulmonary dysplasia [typical RR 0.73 (95% CI 0.57 to 0.93)]. VTV modes also resulted in reduction in pneumothorax, days of ventilation, hypocarbia and the combined outcome of periventricular leukomalacia or grade 3-4 intraventricular hemorrhage.

Volume guarantee ventilation[19]. Volume guarantee (VG) is a new composite ventilatory modality that has the advantages of pressure-limited, time-cycled, continuous-flow ventilation as well as those of volume-controlled ventilation. The operator sets a target expired V_T and the ventilator adjusts

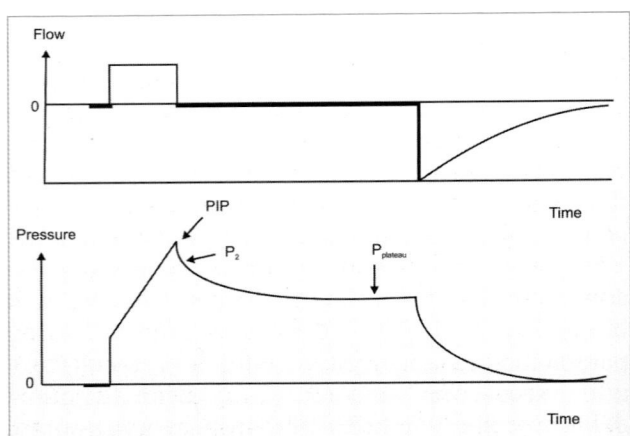

Figure 57.9 Volume controlled ventilation. Flow waveform can be set as constant flow pattern as shown in the figure or as descending ramp. With the constant flow pattern (square flow waveform), the airway pressure increases linearly throughout the inspiration and the peak pressure and volume are achieved at the end of inspiration (back end loaded)

the PIP for the next inflation based on the measurement of the expired V_T of the previous breath. Studies have reported that with VG, more than 60% of the breaths were delivered within the set target V_T[20]. VG can be used with SIMV or A/C or PSV modes. Target V_T is set based on the underlying disease condition. VT of 4-6 ml/kg is appropriate for infants with RDS, VT > 8 ml/kg can cause volutrauma and < 3 ml/kg can cause atelectatotrauma and ineffective ventilation. In VG, the operator sets the PIP max. This PIP limit is different from the delivered PIP because the ventilator adjusts the delivered PIP to achieve the target V_T. The PIP max should be set high enough to allow fluctuations around the working PIP. A low set PIP max may not allow the target VT to be delivered and produces alarms; conversely a very high set PIP max may not alert the operator of the rising working PIP and changes in lung mechanics. Klingenberg and colleagues[19] recommend starting VG with a PIP max of 25-30 cm H_2O. Thereafter, the PIP max can be adjusted 5-10 cm H_2O above the working PIP. The clinician should monitor the working PIP in VG ventilation. Increasing PIP or low VT alarms can be caused by ETT leak, patient-ventilator asynchrony, worsening lung conditions, ETT obstruction etc. If ETT leak is greater than 50%, VG mode becomes less efficient because measurement of expired V_T is inaccurate. VG ventilation automatically weans the PIP as the lung condition improves. Kingenberg and colleagues do not recommend weaning V_T below 3.5 ml/kg and suggest that extubation should be considered if the MAP is less than 8-10 cm H_2O, with the set VT 3.5-4.5 ml/kg and the blood gases are satisfactory (Figure 57.10).

Airway pressure release ventilation (APRV). APRV was developed as a lung protective mode, allowing recruitment while minimizing ventilator induced lung injury[21]. APRV is essentially a pressure control mode where the operator sets a high and a low pressure. The amount of time spent at the higher pressure (T high) is generally 80% to 95% of the cycle, and the amount of time at the lower pressure (T low) is 0.6 to 0.8 seconds. Since the T low is very short, a residual volume of air remains in the lung, creating intentional auto-PEEP. This auto-PEEP prevents lung derecruitment. APRV produces tidal ventilation by causing the release of airway pressure from an elevated baseline to simulate expiration. The elevated baseline facilitates oxygenation, and the timed releases aid in carbon dioxide removal. In addition, APRV allows unrestricted, spontaneous breathing throughout the entire breathing cycle. Advantages

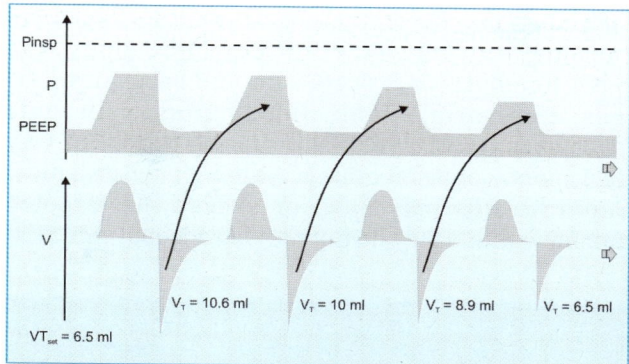

Figure 57.10 Principle of volume guarantee ventilation

of APRV include significantly lower mean airway pressures for a given tidal volume, the ability to allow spontaneous breathing throughout the breathing cycle, lesser lung injury and decreased need for sedation[22]. Figure 57.11 demonstrates airway pressure release ventilation. P high and P low are set by the operator and the optimal release time (the very short time in low pressure or T low) in APRV is also set based on the time constant of the expiratory flow.

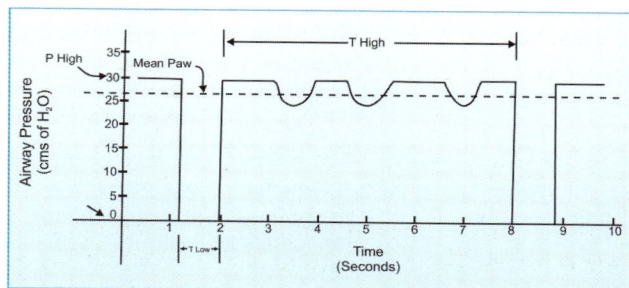

Airway pressure release ventilation terminology. P_{aw}= airway pressure; P high = 30 cm H_2O; P low = 0 cm H_2O. T high= 6 sec; T low = 0.8 sec

Figure 57.11 Principles of airway pressure release ventilation

Mandatory minute ventilation (MMV). MMV is a mode of ventilation that combines features of synchronized intermittent mandatory ventilation (SIMV) and pressure support ventilation (PSV)[23]. In MMV, the clinician chooses a minimum minute volume (the product of tidal volume and frequency) for the patient. If the patient's spontaneous breathing, which is augmented with PSV, meets or exceeds the minute volume, no mandatory ventilator breaths are provided. If, however, the patient's minute volume falls below the pre selected minimum, the ventilator will provide "catch up" breaths at a fixed frequency to ensure that the patient receives this preselected minute ventilation. In patients with reliable respiratory drive, MMV enables nominal ventilator support if they are able to generate the minimum minute ventilation. This allows expedient weaning with only the PEEP, pressure support, and FiO_2 to adjust, thus decreasing the need for blood gas monitoring. The disadvantages include decreased alveolar ventilation during periods of very fast spontaneous breathing. Although these shallow rapid breaths may meet or exceed the targeted minute volume they do not provide adequate alveolar minute ventilation and could lead to alveolar collapse.

57.4.4. Ventilatory parameters.

The various parameters that are set in a ventilator and their physiological roles are shown in the Table 57.7 The key settings that regulate the pressure-limited ventilators are; inspired oxygen

Parameter	Description	Role in ventilation	Side effects
Peak inspiratory pressure (PIP)	The highest pressure that occurs during the inspiratory phase of the cycle, usually seen at or near the end of inspiration. Higher PIP indicates increased airway resistance as in bronchospasm or decreased lung compliance	PIP affects tidal volume and minute ventilation and hence CO_2 removal. Higher PIP also increases mean airway pressure and improves oxygenation	Excessive PIP may cause barotrauma. High PIP alarm may occur due to airway secretions, kinked ET tube, pneumothorax or high airway resistance as in bronchial asthma
Positive end expiratory pressure (PEEP)	This is the positive airway pressure at the end of expiration. Opening of alveoli is done by joint effort of PEEP and opening pressures in response to the tidal volume. PEEP prevents the closure or collapse of the recruited alveoli during expiration.	PEEP increases the functional residual capacity, improves ventilation perfusion matching and oxygenation. It also increases the mean airway pressure. Since delta P= PIP-PEEP determines the tidal volume, an increase in PEEP can decrease the tidal volume and reduce CO_2 elimination.	Excessive PEEP can lead to overdistension of lung units, gas trapping and barotrauma. It impedes venous return, decreases cardiac output, decreases cerebral perfusion
Tidal volume	In volume controlled ventilator tidal volume is set instead of PIP	Regulates minute ventilation and therefore the CO_2 removal.	High tidal volumes lead to volutrauma.
Frequency (Rate)	Number of set breaths per minute	Minute ventilation is the product of VT and frequency. Hence increasing the rate helps in CO_2 elimination. Higher frequency facilitates better synchronization.	Use of high rates can compromise inspiratory and expiratory times. Low Ti can lead to low VT being delivered and low Te can lead to gas trapping
Inspiratory time, expiratory time and I:E ratio	An adequate Ti is 3-5 time constants. Expiratory time constant is slightly longer because airway resistance is higher during expiration	Infants with RDS have shorter time constants and Ti of 0.2-0.5 second is adequate, whereas infants with chronic lung disease have longer time constants and may benefit from a longer Ti of 0.6-0.8 seconds	Changes in Ti, Te and I:E ratio have only modest effects on gas exchange
FiO_2		Influences alveolar oxygen tension and increases PaO_2	High FiO_2 can cause oxygen toxicity
Flow	A minimum flow rate needed is 2.5-3 times the minute volume. The operating range in neonatal ventilators is 4-10 liters/min.	Flow pattern is square wave in volume controlled ventilation and descending ramp in pressure controlled ventilation. Other forms are ascending ramp and sinusoidal.	Inadequate flow may contribute to air hunger, asynchrony and increased work of breathing, whereas excessive breathing can contribute to turbulence, inefficient gas exchange and inadvertent PEEP

Table 57.7 Ventilator parameters and their physiological role

concentration (FiO_2), peak inspiratory pressure (PIP), respiratory rate (RR), positive end expiratory pressure (PEEP), inspiratory to expiratory ratio (1:E) and flow rate. Mean airway pressure (MAP) can be calculated as follows:

$$MAP = \frac{k\ (PIP \times Ti) + (PEEP \times Te)}{Ti + Te}$$

The MAP is the true measure of average pressure actually being perceived by the airways (depending upon the compliance of the lungs) and is altered by changes in a number of ventilator parameters (PIP, PEEP, inspiratory time, duration of cycle etc). It should be maintained between 8-12 cm H_2O.

Ventilator Variables

The ventilator variables in pressure-controlled and volume-controlled ventilators are shown in the box.

	Pressure controlled ventilation	Volume controlled ventilation
Variables set	1. PIP 2. Rate 3. Inspiratory time or I:E ratio 4. PEEP 5. Trigger sensitivity	1. Tidal volume 2. Rate 3. Inspiratory time (controls flow rate) 4. PEEP 5. Trigger sensitivity

Inspired oxygen concentration (FiO_2)

Higher inspired oxygen concentrations are potentially toxic especially in preterm infants. FiO_2 greater than 0.5 has been implicated in absorption atelectasis and tracheobronchitis[24]. In preterm infants oxygen toxicity is implicated in the development of retinopathy of prematurity, bronchopulmonary dysplasia and free radical injury of the developing brain. Although ventilation induced lung injury is more deleterious than oxygen toxicity, it is essential to use the lowest concentration of oxygen to achieve appropriate oxygenation goals. Although the optimal oxygen saturation for preterm infants is still not defined, a number of studies have indicated that a high saturation (>93-95%) is detrimental to these infants when compared with a lower saturations between 88–93%[25]. For ongoing management of preterm infants, SpO_2 targets of 85–93% seem to be most appropriate, with alarm limits set within 1 to 2% of these targets[26]. In term

and near term infants and older children who are mechanically ventilated it is acceptable to target SaO_2 between 90-95%. Oxygen causes pulmonary vasodilatation and one should target normal SaO_2 (92-95%) and PaO_2 (60-90 mm Hg) in babies with persistent pulmonary hypertension of the newborn (PPHN). In PPHN, the traditional practice of targeting a high PaO_2 (>100 mmHg) and low $PaCO_2$ to achieve pulmonary vasodilatation has been shown to be potentially harmful to the developing lung and cerebral perfusion[27]. In children with cyanotic congenital heart disease SaO_2 between 70-75% acceptable if tissue oxygenation is good. Increasing the FiO_2 has little effect in increasing PaO_2 in children with cyanotic congenital heart disease, because of the presence of fixed right-to-left shunt. Many clinicians use SaO_2 measurements using a pulse oximeter rather than PaO_2 by arterial blood gas analysis as it affords a cheap and continuous non-invasive method to monitor oxygen administration. Appropriate FiO_2 is delivered by blenders that mix oxygen and compressed air into precise concentrations. Unlike older models, many new ventilators have built-in blenders. These are generally accurate but periodic checks are necessary to confirm the accuracy of the oxygen concentration being delivered. Several portable oxygen analyzers or in-line sensing devices can be used to check the oxygen concentration being delivered to the patient. Although there is no single safe prescription of FiO_2, one should try to set an acceptable SaO_2 target that is appropriate to the patient and the lung condition. Hypoxemia is also equally harmful. The initial FiO_2 can be set at 0.5 and FiO_2 can be increased or decreased in steps of 0.05 based on the target SaO_2. Because both FiO_2 and mean air way pressure affect oxygenation, the parameter that is more effective and less toxic should be adjusted to achieve target SaO_2. When FiO_2 requirement is > 60%, increasing the MAP is preferred. When FiO_2 requirement is <30-40%, one should try to decrease the MAP.

Tidal volume

This is the primary parameter to be set in volume controlled ventilation. The initial set V_T depends on the age of the patient. It is 4-6 ml/kg in preterm infants, 6-8 ml/kg in term infants and in older children. An inappropriately low V_T (< 3 ml/kg) can lead to atelectasis, hypoxemia and hypercarbia and excessive V_T (> 8 ml/kg) can cause volutrauma in infants. High-volume lung injury occurs as a result of tidal ventilation above the upper inflection point of the pressure-volume curve. Low-volume lung injury results from ventilation beginning

Section 6

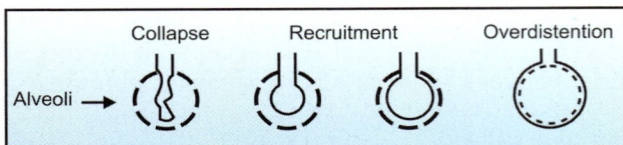

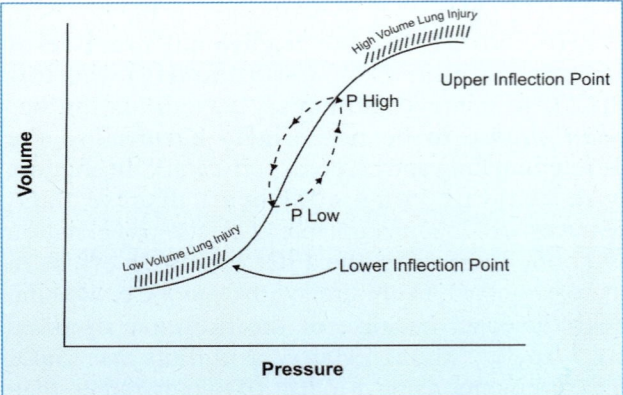

Figure 57.12 Pressure volume curve. Appropriate selection of tidal volume and pressures (PIP and PEEP) is essential to avoid lung injury

below the lower inflection point[28]. If the expired tidal volume measured by the ventilator is less than the set V_T, there can be an air leak (Endotracheal tube leak, circuit leak or broncho-pleural fistula). Peak pressure varies with each breath in VC ventilation depending on the lung compliance and resistance. Peak pressures can be used to monitor improvement (lower PIP) and worsening (higher PIP) lung condition.

Peak inspiratory pressure (PIP)

In pressure controlled ventilators, PIP is the primary modality that is selected and the difference in pressure (Delta P= PIP-PEEP) determines the tidal volume delivery. For a given PIP, the tidal volume delivered will vary depending on the lung compliance, airway resistance and the time constant. Depending upon the underlying disease condition, start with an appropriate level of PIP necessary to produce adequate chest excursion and breath sounds. If the ventilator has a V_T monitor, adjust the PIP in increments of 1-2 cm to achieve a desired V_T based on the patien's age; 4-6 ml/kg in preterm, 6-8 ml/kg for term neonates and 7-10 ml/kg in older children. PIP is the primary variable that determines tidal volume in a pressure-limited time-cycled ventilator. Increasing the PIP will not only increase the V_T but also increase the mean air way pressure. Thus, this parameter can be adjusted to improve both oxygenation and ventilation. Low PIPs may not be able to provide adequate tidal volume and can lead to hypoxia and hypercapnia, while high PIPs are associated with the risk of

pulmonary barotrauma in the form of air leaks and bronchopulmonary dysplasia (Figure 57.12). The increase in intra thoracic pressure may decrease venous return to the heart.

Positive end expiratory pressure (PEEP)

Adequate PEEP prevents alveolar collapse, maintains lung volume at the end expiration and improves ventilation-perfusion relationships. PEEP is the most effective parameter that increases MAP. Both extremely high and low PEEPs are associated with retention of carbon dioxide. It is important to remember that though both PIP and PEEP increase MAP and improve oxygenation, but PEEP has opposite effect on carbon dioxide. The normal physiologic PEEP is approximately 3 cm H_2O. The initial PEEP is usually kept at 4-5 cm H_2O. Then the PEEP is increased in steps of 1-2 cm until the optimum PEEP (above the lower inflection point) is achieved. An optimal PEEP is one where desired blood gases are achieved (PaO_2 >60 mm Hg or SaO_2 >90%) with an acceptable low FiO_2 (usually < 50%) without affecting hemodynamic stability. Excessive elevation of PEEP (above the higher inflection point) may cause over distension, baro trauma, gas trapping, hypercarbia and impair venous return to the right heart.

Respiratory rate (RR)

Usually, the initial RR is set based on the normal RR for that age, the underlying condition and patient's efforts at generating spontaneous respirations. The normal RR varies by age i.e. 40-60/min in the neonatal period, decreasing to 20-40/min in early childhood and 15-25/min in older children. The ventilator rate is based on the decision whether the ventilator is taking over the work of breathing completely or partially. In the early stages when the disease process is still evolving, it is logical to unload the respiratory muscles and decrease the patient's work of breathing. To achieve this, the ventilator rate is kept within the normal range or higher than the normal spontaneous respiratory frequency. Higher rates may also be set in restrictive lung disease eg. respiratory distress syndrome (RDS) and acute respiratory distress syndrome (ARDS) where the time constant is less allowing quick filling and emptying of lung units. Lower rates are set in patients with high airway resistance like chronic lung disease, meconium aspiration syndrome and asthma where it is necessary to allow adequate time for expiration and where permissive hypercapnia can be accepted. Since RR determines minute ventilation (minute ventilation = tidal volume × RR) higher respiratory rate is useful for carbon dioxide wash out and to increase minute ventilation. If rates are too high respiratory alkalosis, auto PEEP and barotrauma can occur and if rates are too low hypoxemia, hypoventilation and increased work of breathing can occur.

Inspiratory-expiratory ratio (I:E ratio)

The normal ratio of the inspiratory time to the expiratory time (I: E ratio) is approximately 1:2. Increasing the 'I' time increases the MAP and improves oxygenation. A shorter inspiratory time encourages lung emptying (by allowing more time for exhalation). When the inspiratory time is lengthened so that it is at least as long as the expiratory time (an I: E ratio of 1:1), the I: E ratio is said to have become inverted. Inverse ratio ventilation (IRV) is used in acute respiratory distress syndrome as it appears to improve V/Q matching and decrease shunting. Since this pattern of breathing is unphysiological, it can increase patient discomfort and may necessitate use of sedatives. By shortening the expiratory time, IRV can lead to air trapping. Prolonged expiratory time (I:E ratio 1:2, 1:3) is indicated in ventilation of infants with obstructive airway disease.

Inspiratory time

Inspiratory time that is set depends on the time constant of the lung condition. One should allow 3-5 time constants for adequate filling and emptying of lung units. In neonates with RDS, a Ti of 0.3-0.5 is adequate whereas neonates with chronic lung disease (longer time constant) may benefit from higher Ti of 0.6-0.8 seconds. In older children a Ti of 1 second is adequate.

Flow rate

In neonates, flow rate of oxygen-air mixture of 4-8 liters/ minute is usually sufficient to ensure adequate ventilation. Changes in flow rate have not been well studied in infants but they seem to have lesser impact as compared to adults. High flow rate above 10 l/min can lead to turbulence and gas trapping due to inadvertent PEEP. Only volume-targeted modes of ventilation offer a choice in terms of flow wave patterns. For a given VT and I: E ratio one can choose a square, accelerating, decelerating or sine wave form but the square wave form is the most common one. In pressure-targeted ventilation, to maintain the constancy of pressure, the inspiratory waveform is necessarily decelerating.

Trigger sensitivity

The purpose of trigger sensitivity is to coordinate the delivery of the inspiratory breath with patient's own inspiratory effort. The patient's spontaneous efforts produce a negative change in flow or pressure within the circuit that the ventilator detects. Thus the trigger could be a pressure or flow trigger. In general increased sensitivity is preferable so that the patient spends less energy in triggering the ventilator and there is better patient-ventilator synchrony. However, excessively high sensitivity may result in false or auto-triggering (ie spontaneous triggering of the ventilator by changes in airway like water droplets in the circuit and not by patient efforts).

57.4.5 How to adjust ventilator settings?

During acute stage of the disease, ventilator settings are always in a dynamic state and require frequent alterations. Judicious clinical monitoring along with pulse oximetry and periodic blood gas analyses are crucial for the success of ventilatory therapy. The parameters indicating the adequacy of ventilation are listed in Table 57.8.

Table 57.8 Clinical and laboratory indices of adequate ventilation
Clinical parameters
□ Adequate chest expansion □ Adequate air entry □ Absence of retractions □ Pink color □ Prompt capillary filling (within 2 -3 sec) □ Normal blood pressure
Pulse oximetry
Oxygen saturation 90-95% in term babies and children
Blood gases
• paO$_2$ 50-80 mm Hg • paCO$_2$ 40-50 mm Hg (In a chronic disease up to 60 mm Hg) • pH 7.35-7.45

Depending upon the clinical condition of the patient and status of blood gases, appropriate changes should be made in the ventilator settings (Table 57.9).

The changes in the ventilator settings must be made in short steps. PIP and PEEP should be altered only by 1.0 cm H$_2$O at a time, rate 2 breaths/ min, FiO$_2$ in steps of 0.05 (5%) and Ti in installments of 0.05 seconds. Blood gas estimation should be done after 20-30 minutes of each change.

Section 6

Table 50.9 Blood gas abnormalities and changes in the ventilator settings to correct them						
Blood gas abnormality	**Corrective measure**					**Comments**
	FiO$_2$	**Rate**	**PIP**	**PEEP**	**Ti**	
Hypercapnia sure that PEEP is not too high and (PaCO$_2$ >50 mm Hg)	-	↑	↑	-	-	Can also increase Te. Make sure there is no auto PEEP phenomenon.
Hypocapnia (PaCO$_2$ <35mm Hg)	–	↓	↓	-	-	-
Hyperoxia (PaO$_2$ >100 mm Hg)	↓	↓	↓	↓	↓	-
Hypoxia (PaO$_2$ <50 mm Hg)	↑	-	↑	↑	↑	If chest excursions are adequate, it is better to increase FiO$_2$
Total ventilatory failure (PaCO$_2$ too high and PaO$_2$ too low)	Depends upon the cause					Check that chest is moving with each ventilation and endo-tracheal tube is not blocked. Check for air leak and ventilator malfunction.

57.4.6 Monitoring the Ventilated Patient

Patient monitoring

Babies requiring mechanical ventilation require close monitoring to optimize the respiratory support and limit the potential complications of ventilator induced lung injury, oxygen toxicity, air leaks and nosocomial infections[29]. Although a number of electronic devices aid in monitoring a sick infant, clinical examination is very important.

Physical examination. Breathing rate, evidence of respiratory distress, ausculation for equal air entry and ventilator-patient synchrony should be observed. Rapid shallow breathing and the presence of subcostal or intercostal recessions in ventilated babies may suggest 'air hunger' or 'increased work of breathing' which can be corrected by adjusting the ventilatory settings. Cardiovascular parameters monitored include skin color, heart rate, perfusion (capillary refill), blood pressure and urine output.

Monitoring oxygenation. Arterial blood gas (ABG) analysis has remained the gold standard for monitoring the adequacy of gas exchange. It is preferable to have an indwelling arterial cannula if frequent ABGs are required. The ABG measures PaO$_2$ directly from blood, and uses values of temperature, pH, PaCO$_2$ and PaO$_2$ to calculate the percent oxyhemoglobin saturation. Capillary blood gases do not reliably predict arterial PaO$_2$. Pulse oximeter is a simple bed side non-invasive tool that allows accurate and continuous monitoring of arterial oxygen saturation (SaO$_2$). They are very accurate when oxyhemoglobin concentrations are greater than 60%. However, it fails to detect hyperoxia when SaO$_2$ is greater than 94% and often underestimate SaO$_2$ when perfusion to the extremity is compromised as in circulatory shock or local edema. They can also be inaccurate if other forms of hemoglobin (i.e methemoglobin or carboxy-hemoglobin) that absorb light at similar wavelengths as oxyhemoglobin or deoxyhemoglobin are present. As discussed earlier, for ongoing management of preterm infants, SaO$_2$ targets of 85–93% seem to be most appropriate, with alarm limits set within 1 to 2% of these targets[26]. In term and near term infants and older children who are mechanically ventilated it is acceptable to target SaO$_2$ between 90-95%. In children with PPHN target SaO$_2$ between 92-95% and in children with cyanotic congenital heart disease SaO$_2$ between 70-75% are acceptable if tissue oxygenation is good.

Ventilation. PaCO$_2$ determined from an ABG is a reliable measure of ventilation. A free flowing capillary sample is an acceptable alternative. Peripheral venous samples are inaccurate measures of systemic pH and PaCO$_2$. Capnography and transcutaneous CO$_2$ detectors provide non-invasive alternatives to monitor ventilation. In addition to detecting end-tidal CO$_2$ (EtCO$_2$), capnography provides information about respiratory rate and rhythm, dead space calculations, confirmation of endotracheal tube (ETT) placement, displacement or obstruction of the ETT and patient–ventilator asynchrony. The combination of very low EtCO$_2$ value and a high PaCO$_2$ could be due to ETT not in the airway or due to impaired pulmonary blood flow secondary to low cardiac output or pulmonary embolism. Transcutaneous carbon dioxide (TcPCO$_2$) measured by using skin electrodes are relatively independent of sensor site and skin thickness. It may be falsely high in severe shock.

Chest radiograph. Chest radiography is the most commonly used imaging modality in the intensive care unit for the diagnosis of complications during assisted ventilation. The findings to look for in a chest radiograph include position of the endotracheal tube, central lines and umbilical catheters. Optimal positioning for ETT is approximately 1–1.5 cm above the carina. Displacement of the tube into the esophagus is indicated by a low ETT position, a tracheal column distinct from the ETT, poor aeration of lungs and gaseous distension of the gastrointestinal tract. One should also pay attention to the volume of the lungs (atelectasis or over expansion) and the cardiac outline. Flattening of the diaphragm and lung expansion reaching the tenth rib suggests over expansion and increased risk of pulmonary air leaks and lung injury.

50.4.7 Monitoring pulmonary graphics

Pulmonary graphics monitoring has emerged as a valuable tool to assess patient ventilator interaction, study pulmonary mechanics, response to therapy, readiness to wean and to detect complications of ventilation at an early stage[30]. The basic parameters that are measured include the pressure (P) necessary to cause a flow (V''') of gas to enter the airway and increase the volume (V) of the lungs. From this compliance (C=DV/DP), resistance (R = flow × volume), time constant (compliance × resistance) and elastic work of breathing can be derived.

The flow sensor collects the air flow data and transmits them to the microprocessor that displays the graphics and the calculated values. If the air flow sensor is located close to the patient's airway the data is more accurate than if a flow sensor is located distally or back in the machine. There are two types of wave forms; scalars and loops. In a scalar waveform the control variables (pressure, volume and flow) are plotted on the Y axis and time (seconds) in the X axis. In the loop waveform, one control variable is plotted against another (volume plotted against pressure or flow against volume). The ventilator graphic display provides the following parameters:

1. Scalar waveforms

    (a) Pressure waveform
    (b) Flow waveform
    (c) Volume waveform

2. Loop waveform
    (a) Pressure volume loop
    (b) Flow volume loop

3. Calculated values
    (a) Compliance
    (b) Resistance

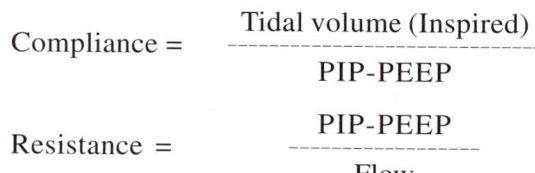

$$\text{Compliance} = \frac{\text{Tidal volume (Inspired)}}{\text{PIP-PEEP}}$$

$$\text{Resistance} = \frac{\text{PIP-PEEP}}{\text{Flow}}$$

Pressure waveform

(a) The shape of the curve represents the breath type eg pressure limited (square) and volume limited (triangular).

(b) The components of the pressure wave form curve: PIP is the maximum pressure point on the curve, PEEP is the baseline pressure, and mean airway pressure (MAP) is the area under the curve. Plateau pressure is measured during inspiratory hold or prolonged I time.

(c) Other information obtained

    (i) *Triggering.* It is indicated by the presence of a negative deflection immediately preceding inspiration (Figure 57.13).

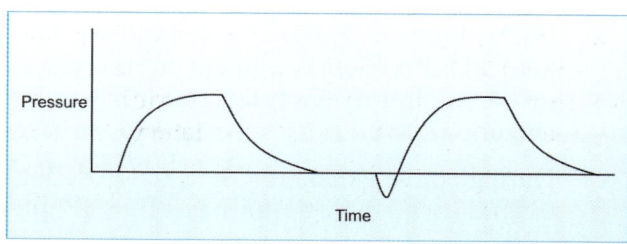

Figure 57.13 Patient-triggered breaths are indicated by negative deflection below the baseline

    (ii) *Airway obstruction* is indicated by disproportionate rise in peak airway pressure relative to the plateau pressure and decreased compliance is indicated by elevated both peak and plateau pressures (Figure 57.14). A decrease in PIP following administration of bronchodilator indicates a good response.

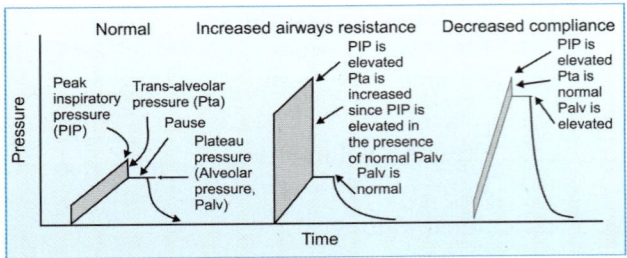

Figure 57.14 Pressure-time scalar in volume controlled constant flow ventilation

(iii) *Air trapping.* PEEP that fails to return to the baseline indicates air trapping.

Volume waveforms

(a) In a constant flow, volume limited ventilation, the upstroke is inspiration and down stroke is expiration and the corresponding peak volume on the Y axis is the tidal volume. Figure 57.15 demonstrates the volume-time scalar in a volume controlled ventilation.

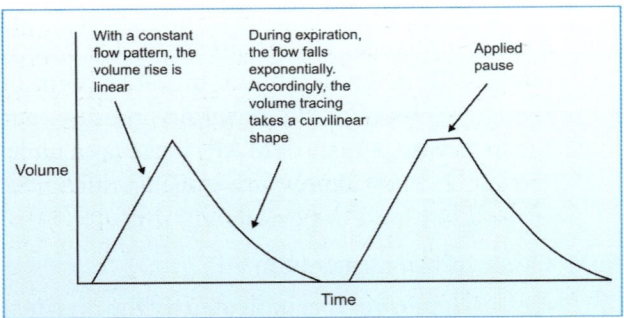

Figure 57.15 Volume-time scalar in a volume controlled ventilation

(b) Other information obtained include, endotracheal tube leak, bronchopleural fistula and auto PEEP which is evident by the failure of the expiratory limb to return to baseline (Figure 57.16).

(c) During active exhalation the expiratory limb extends well below the base line (Figure 57.17).

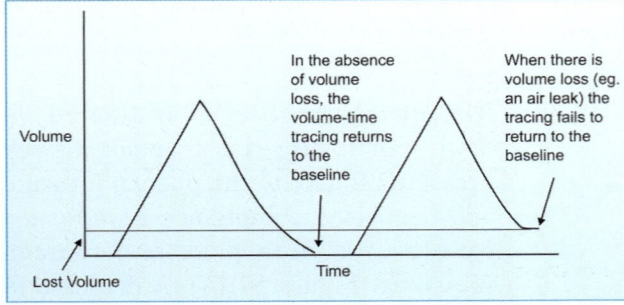

Figure 57.16 Volume time scalar indicating the presence of air leak

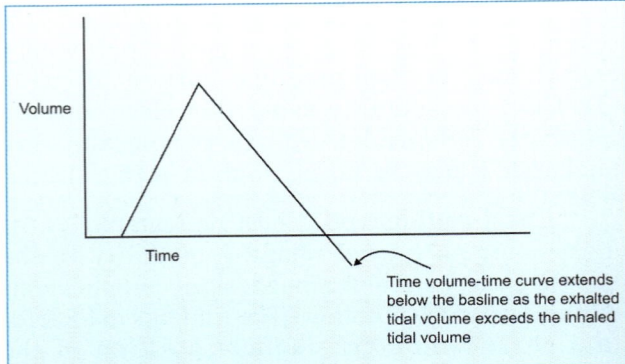

Figure 57.17 Volume time scalar indicating active exhalation

Flow waveforms

The shape of the flow waveform is square in volume ventilation and descending ramp in pressure ventilation (Figure 57.18).

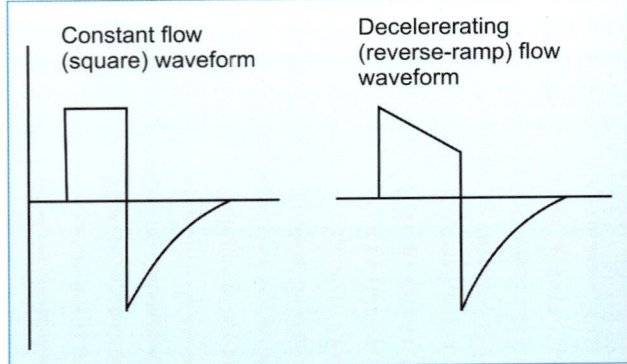

Figure 57.18 Flow time scalar in volume controlled (square) and pressure controlled ventilation (decelerating)

Inspiratory flow waveform is marked above the abcissa and the expiratory waveform below it. The peak flow during inspiration is peak inspiratory flow rate and that during expiration is peak expiratory flow rate. When the expiratory limb touches the base line, lung deflation is complete. Failure of the expiratory flow to return to zero indicates gas trapping and auto PEEP or air leak. If the expiratory flow limb is deeply curved and takes a longer time to return to the baseline, it indicates airway obstruction (Figure 57.19). Because of the extensive loss of lung parenchyma and the resultant loss of elastic recoil, the usual peaked configuration of the PEF is replaced by a more relaxed, rounded contour (Figure 57.20). A good response to inhaled bronchodilator is indicated by reversal of the above.

Graphic loops

Pressure-volume (P-V) loops. The pressure is plotted on the X axis and volume on the Y axis.

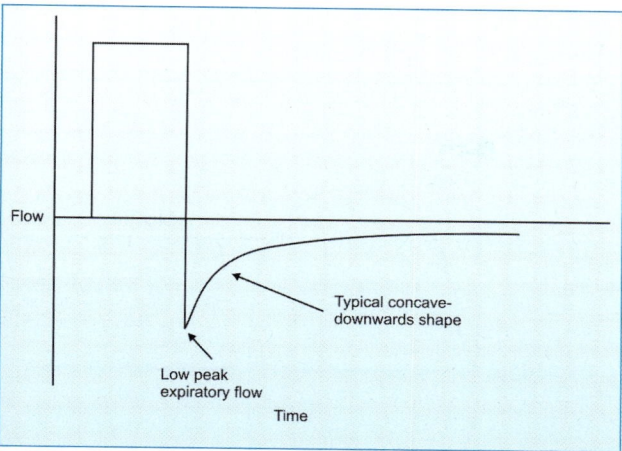

Figure 57.19 Prolongation of expiratory limb and low peak suggestive of increased airway resistance

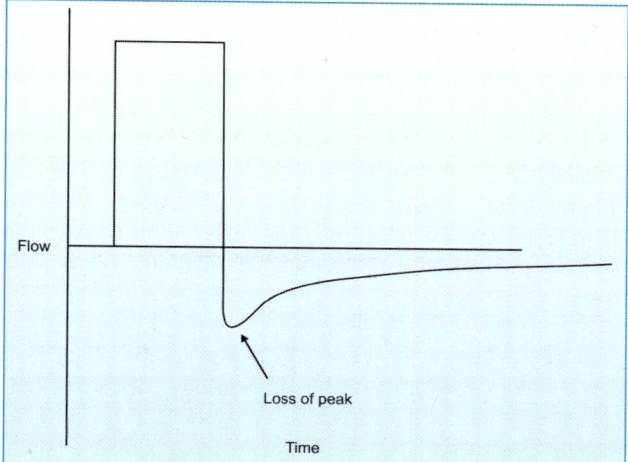

Figure 57.20 Rounded contour of expiratory limb is seen in emphysema

On the P-V loop, notable measurements on the X axis are PEEP and PIP, and on the Y axis is the inspired tidal volume. Since volume change in relation to pressure change defines compliance, the PV loop displays compliance of the respiratory system. Since the loops are plotted during airflow, it also provides useful information about airway resistance. A line drawn between each end points of the curve is the compliance line and the slope of the line indicates the compliance of the system. Normally the compliance line is 45 degrees from the horizontal. If this slope is more towards the vertical axis, compliance is improving, and conversely compliance is decreasing if this line moves nearer to the horizontal axis. Other uses of PV loop are listed below.

(a) The patient triggered breaths are indicated by a negative deflection at the beginning of the loop (Figure 57.21).

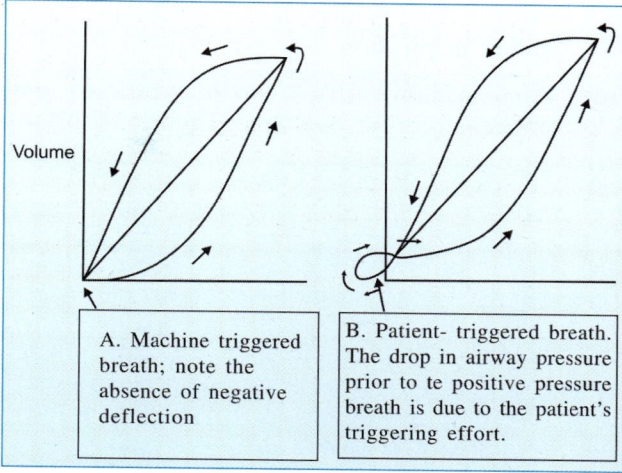

Figure 57.21 P-V loops demonstrating machine versus patient triggered breaths

(b) Choosing an appropriate inspiratory pressure. An over distended lung is less compliant and therefore there is less volume change towards the end of pressure inflated breath compared to the initial inflation. This leads to flattening of the terminal part of the inspiratory curve to give a characteristic beaked shape to the pressure–volume loop (Figure 57.22). The compliance of the last 20% of the curve is lower than the compliance of the entire loop. When this occurs evaluate the appropriateness of VT and PIP and try to lower one of these.

(c) Inadequate flow is indicated by inadequate hysteresis. There is little separation between the inspiratory and expiratory limbs. Air hunger

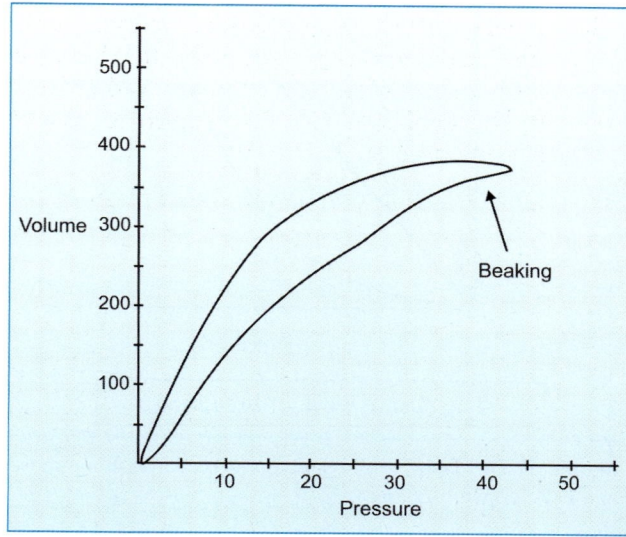

Figure 57.22 A P-V loop that flattens at the upper end producing a bird's beak appearance indicates hyperinflation and further increase in pressure result in little or no increase in volume

creates the "figure-eight" appearance at the end of inspiration.

(d)   Air leak is identified by the expiratory limb not reaching the base line (Figure 57.23).

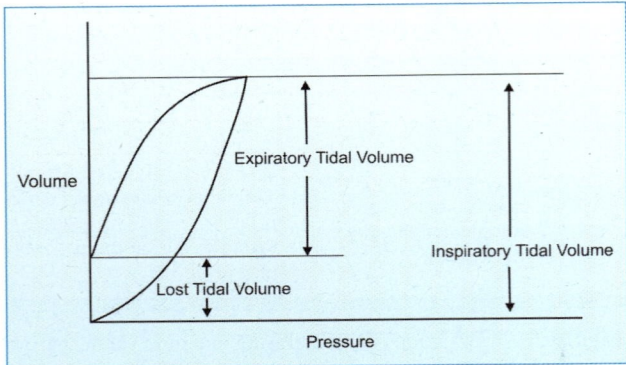

Figure 57.23 P-V loop demonstrating air leak. The expiratory limb fails to reach baseline

(e)   Elastic and resistive work of breathing. The area shaded in green represents the elastic work of breathing and that in yellow resistive work of breathing (Figure 57.24). Changes in the shape of P-V loop can indicate increased elastic work (when compliance decreases) and increased resistive work (when there is bronchospasm)

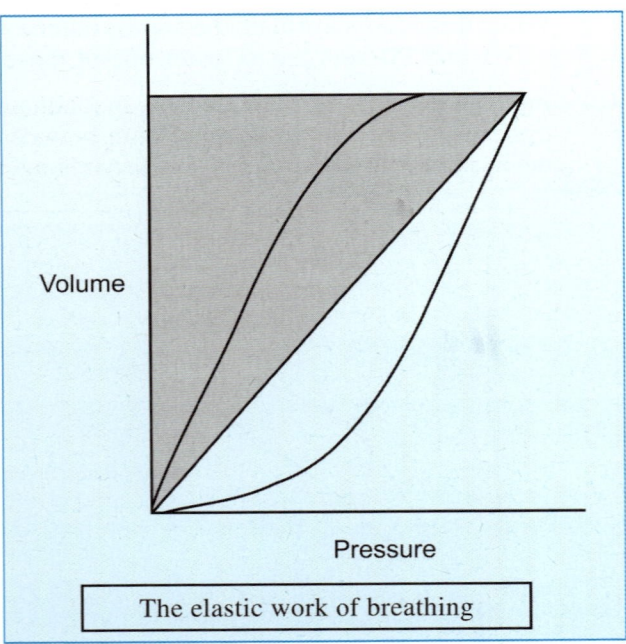

The elastic work of breathing

Figure 57.24 Elastic and resistive work of breathing shown in a P-V loop

Flow volume loops. Flow is plotted on the Y axis and volume on the X axis. Inspiration is above the abscissa and expiration below it. The shape of the inspiratory limb is square with volume breaths

and decelerating in the pressure controlled breaths (Figures 57.25 and 57.26).

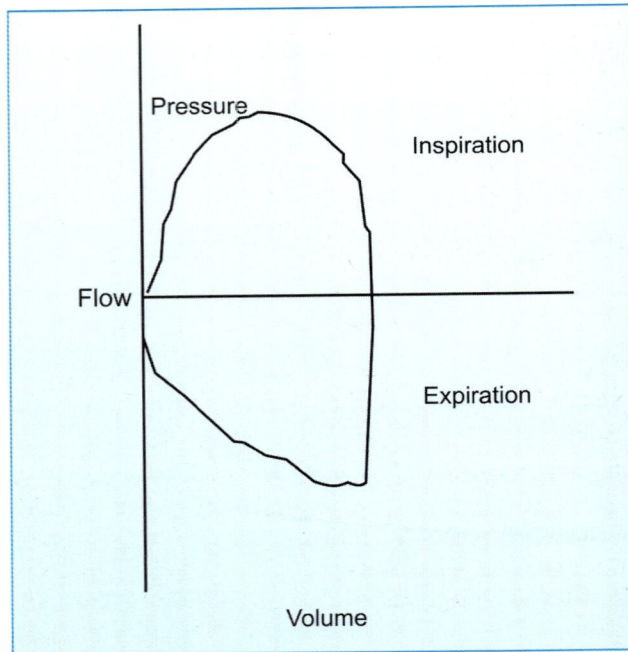

Figure 57.25 A normal flow volume loop should be circular or oval in appearance. The upper and lower limits representing peak inspiratory and expiratory flows should be nearly equal

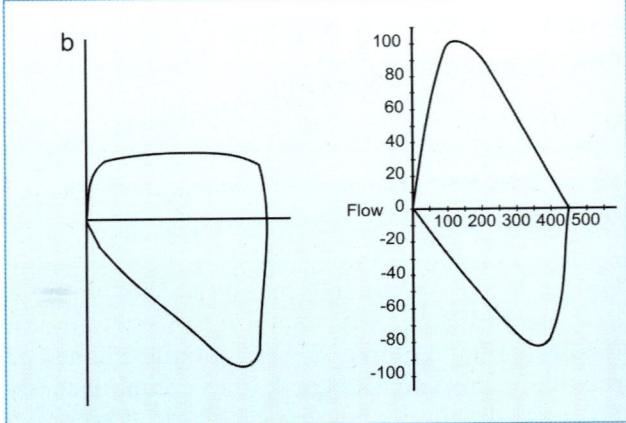

Figure 57.26 Flow volume loop in volume and pressure controlled ventilation

Other advantages of flow volume loop includes (i) increased airway resistance where in both the flow and tidal volume are reduced, (ii) Effectiveness of bronchodilators with marked improvement in inspiratory and expiratory flow rates, (iii) air leaks, and (iv) airway secretions.

57.5 High Frequency Ventilation

High-frequency (HF) ventilation is a general term that refers to a family of ventilator techniques that utilize ventilator rates greater than 60 breaths/

minute and tidal volumes that are usually less than or equal to the anatomical dead space of the airways[31]. They can be classified into four types: high-frequency positive pressure ventilator (HFPPV), high frequency flow interrupter (HFFI), high-frequency jet ventilator (HFJV), and high-frequency oscillatory ventilator (HFOV). The mechanisms involved in achieving gas exchange using tidal volumes smaller than dead space volume ($V_T < V_D$) remains controversial. The basic difference between HFV and conventional ventilation (CV) is that in CV the movement of gas from the airways to the alveoli is by bulk flow, whereas in HF multiple modes of gas transport occur including bulk convection, high frequency 'pendelluft', convective dispersion, taylor type dispersion and molecular diffusion[32]. During high frequency ventilation, minute ventilation and the CO_2 washout are proportional to the product of ventilator frequency and the square of the tidal volume ($V_T^2 \times RR$). This is unlike CV where minute ventilation is $V_T \times RR$. Airway pressures monitored in a HF ventilator is measured distally, inside the trachea, whereas the pressures displayed on the conventional ventilator is a proximal value. In most HF devices expiration is due to passive recoil of the patient's lung except in HFO in which the device actively sucks gas during expiration. The basic set up of HFO is shown in Figure 57.27.

High frequency ventilation is generally considered beneficial in severe pulmonary failure because it uses tidal volumes smaller than dead space (less volutrauma), it enables the safe application of higher PEEP and MAP to open collapsed alveoli and to keep them open (less barotrauma and atelecto trauma) and it improves ventilation/perfusion (V/Q) matching by ensuring uniform aeration of the lungs[33].

Since HFO and HFJV are the most commonly used HF devices in neonatal and pediatric patients the following discussion will focus on these modalities.

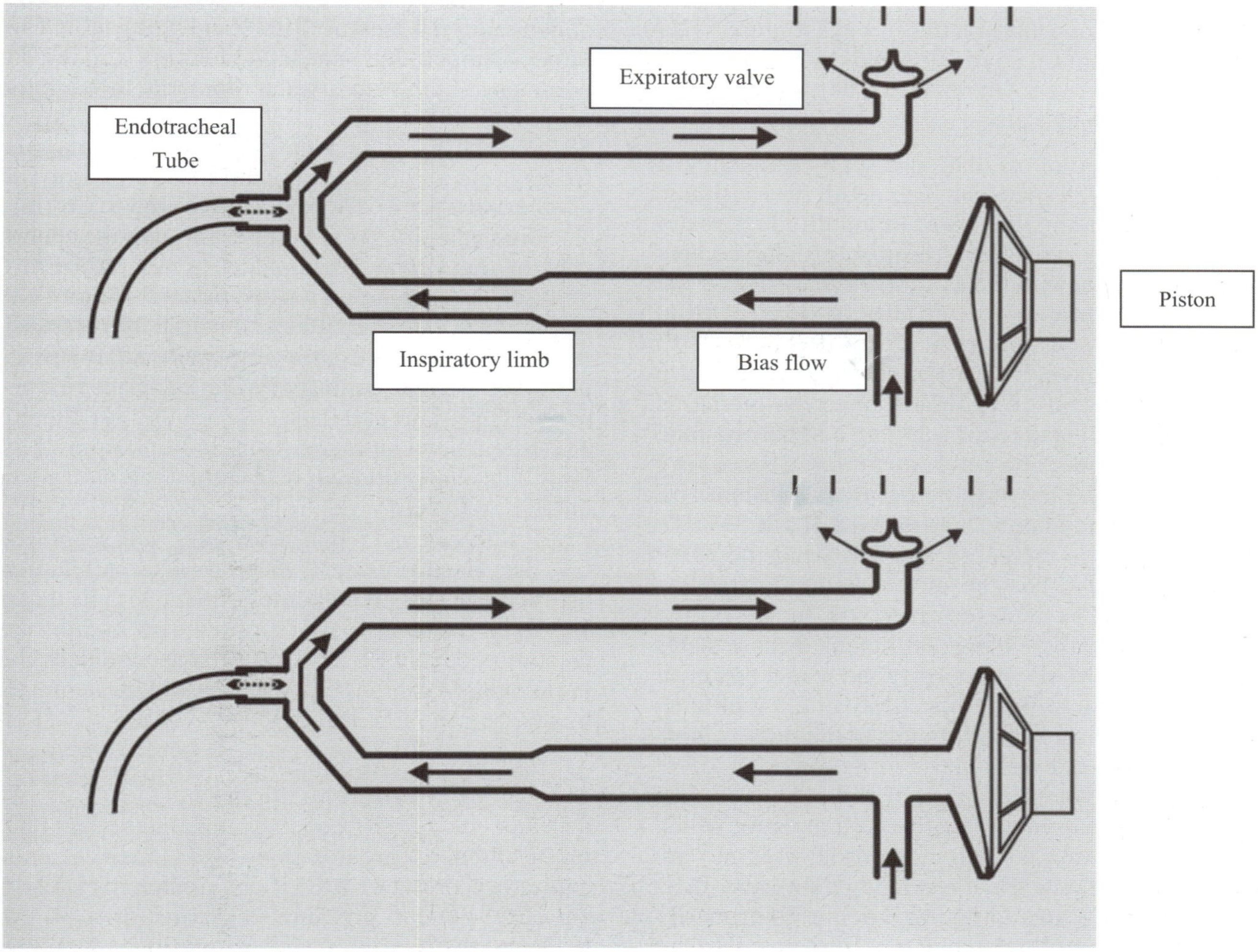

Figure 57.27 Basic set up of high frequency oscillator

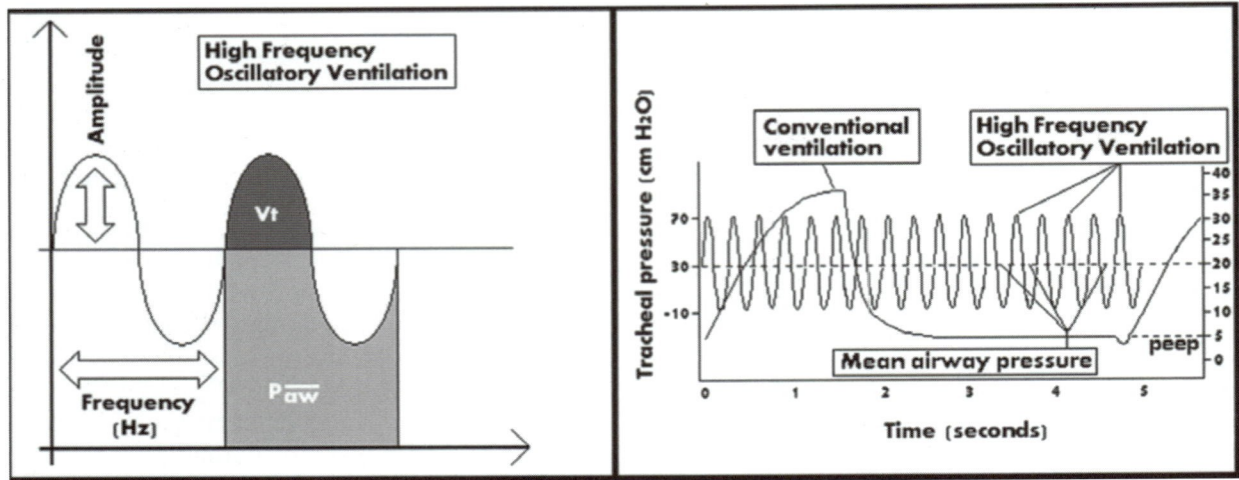

Figure 57.28 Sinusoidal waveform of high frequency oscillator. The horizontal line corresponds to the continuous distending pressure or MAP and height of the waveform from the horizontal represents the amplitude

High frequency oscillator[33]. HFO (Sensor Medics 3100A, Viasys Healthcare, Yorba Linda, CA) consists of a piston or diaphragm that moves back and forth at high frequencies. The to and fro movement oscillates a constant stream of gas, called the bias gas flow, through the airways. Figure 57.27 shows the basic set up of HFO and the Figure 57.28 shows the waveform in HFO as compared to conventional ventilator.

The speed of oscillation is set by frequency; 1 Hertz = 60 cycles/second. The depth of oscillation is set by adjusting the power or amplitude. Greater the amplitude, greater is the piston displacement and more tidal volume is delivered. In HFO, the inspiratory time is set initially at 33% of total respiratory cycle time (e.g. 22 milliseconds at 15 Hz, 41 milliseconds at 8 Hz, 55 milliseconds at 6 Hz). The percent of Ti should never be increased because it will lead to air trapping and barotrauma. Ti should only be increased by decreasing frequency, thus leaving the I:E ratio constant. I:E ratio is approximately 1:2 for 3-15 Hz at 33% Ti. Oxygenation is increased by increasing the MAP and FiO_2. MAP has the most profound effect on oxygenation as it determines the lung volume available for gas exchange. For many disease states the optimum MAP will correspond to 8-9 posterior ribs on an antero-posterior chest film. Amplitude, which most closely corresponds to the tidal volume delivered by conventional ventilation, can affect oxygenation when inflation of the patient's lungs by MAP is marginal. The three parameters which affect ventilation (CO_2 removal/tidal volume) are Amplitude (Delta-P), Frequency (Hz) and % I-Time. A change in ventilation is achieved primarily by altering amplitude and to a lesser extent by frequency while I:E ratio is not changed.

High frequency jet ventilation. HFJV (Life Pulse High-Frequency Ventilator; Bunnell Inc., Salt Lake City, Utah) is characterized by a (normally) fixed brief inspiratory time, passive expiration, and coupling with a conventional ventilator for provision of conventional breaths, PEEP, and bias flow[34]. Life Pulse, Bunnell Jet ventilator delivers small tidal volumes at high velocity at a rapid rate through the jet nozzle via a special ET tube adapter (Figure 57.29). The ET tube adapter has 2 side ports, one for gas injection via a conventional ventilator and another port for distal airway pressure monitoring. The high velocity gas penetrates through the central core of the airway and exhaled gases return in a counter-current helical flow pattern around the inspired gas. This facilitates mucociliary clearance in the airways. Pressure amplitude (PIP-PEEP) produces V_T and controls $PaCO_2$. The inspiratory time is kept short at 0.02 seconds and is not altered. The frequency can range from 240-660 bpm (4-11 Hz). The conventional ventilator that is used in tandem with HFJV controls the oxygenation. PIP, PEEP and rate (2-5 bpm) and FiO_2 are set in the CV. The back up rate (2-5 bpm) also called sigh breath facilitates alveolar recruitment with its larger V_T. Once the alveoli are recruited sigh breaths are discontinued and PEEP or MAP is used to keep the lungs open. Changes in oxygenation are achieved by altering the PEEP in CV[35].

Although the exact time to switch from conventional to HF ventilation is not clear, one can consider either high frequency modalities when FiO_2 requirement is greater than 60%, positive end-expiratory pressure (PEEP) is greater than 12-15 cm H_2O, plateau pressure is greater than 30 cm H_2O, and the arterial oxygen saturation is less than 90%[36].

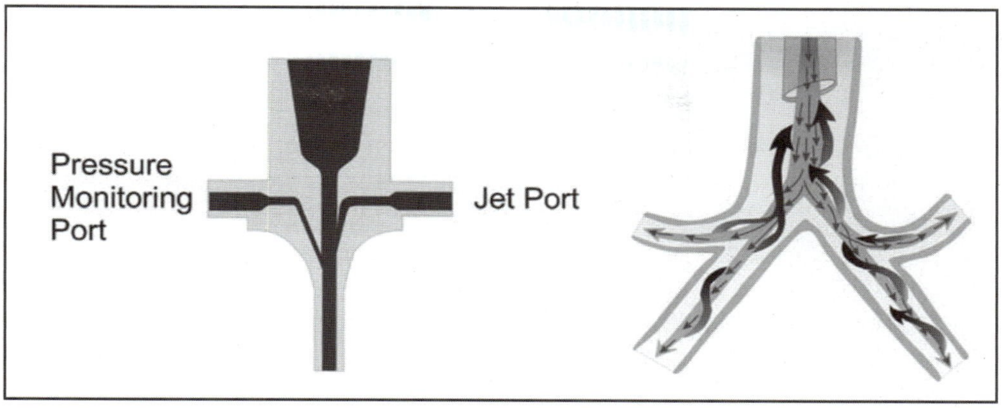

Figure 57.29 Special endotracheal adapter used with Bunnell Life pulse and the high velocity gas flow during inspiration and expiration in HFJV

HFJV is considered as an early or late rescue therapy in the treatment of severe respiratory failure unresponsive to CV. The role of HFJV as the initial therapy (prophylactic use) in lung conditions is not clear. HFJV is specifically considered in the following situations[37, 38].

1. Air leak syndrome due to tracheoesophageal fistula, bronchopleural fistula, pneumothorax, and pulmonary interstitial emphysema[38].

2. Pulmonary hypoplasia secondary to congenital diaphragmatic hernia, respiratory distress syndrome, selected cases of meconium aspiration syndrome, pneumonia and poor compliance secondary to abdominal distension.

The proposed benefits in these conditions stem from effective CO_2 elimination, rapid resolution of air leaks, ability to ventilate better in cases of airway disruption (tracheoesophageal fistula), ability to use high PEEP safely, less interference with venous return (better hemodynamics), mobilization of secretions and above all less lung injury.

The indications for HFO are similar to *vide supra* but the most dramatic effects are seen in conditions associated with poor lung inflation. However, HFO is not effective in patients with obstructive airway disease. The use of HFO is associated with gas trapping in these cases. In patients with shock, high MAP can further compromise venous return and decrease cardiac output. If decreasing the MAP adversely affects oxygenation, these patients would benefit by volume loading and inotropes.

Setting up the high frequency ventilator (Table 57.10)

(i) Choosing the right patient: One should know the underlying pathophysiology of the lung disease (air leak, pulmonary hypoplasia, non homogenous condition like meconium aspiration).

(ii) Choosing the right ventilator: HFJV in a case of air leak.

(iii) Choosing the right time: In cases with severe refractory respiratory failure unresponsive to conventional ventilation, the decision to start HF ventilation should be made early before onset of lung injury.

(iv) Choosing the appropriate settings

Patients on HF ventilator require diligent nursing care and clinical monitoring. Suctioning is performed only when indicated and closed in line suction catheters are preferred. Frequent disconnection from high frequency ventilator should be avoided to prevent atelectasis. Regular blood gases and chest radiographs should be obtained to monitor $PaCO_2$ levels and lung expansion. Both hypocarbia and lung over expansion are harmful.

Disadvantages and complications of HFV

High frequency ventilation is not the first line therapy for every patient with respiratory failure. However the benefits are incredible in certain lung conditions and in refractory respiratory failure. Incorrect patient choice and ventilator settings can cause complications. Mucosal damage to the trachea and bronchi reported in earlier studies was due to inadequate humidification. The increased incidence of intraventricular hemorrhage and periventricular leukomalacia reported in earlier studies is due to in advertent hyperventilation. This can be prevented by careful attention to $PaCO_2$ levels. The common limitations of HF include air trapping and inadvertent PEEP if an inappropriately high frequency of breaths is used. Cardio-circulatory compromise may occur because high

Table 57.10 Guidelines for settings and monitoring required during high frequency ventilation

Settings	HFO	HFJV	Monitoring
MAP	Start with 1-2 cm higher than the MAP in conventional ventilator. Increase MAP in increments of 1-2 cm. The goal is to maintain optimal lung inflation and the lowest level of FiO_2 necessary to maintain an oxygen saturation of 90-95%.	Start with a MAP 1-2 cm higher than that on CV. This is done by adjusting the PEEP in tandem with CV. Set the PIP as on the previous CV. Patients are then stabilized with sigh breath rate of 5 bpm and FiO_2 is adjusted to produce appropriate SaO_2. CMV is then switched to CPAP mode, and PEEP is increased until SaO_2 is restabilized. Thus, CMV breaths are only used intermittently.	An adequate MAP should produce good lung expansion (8th posterior ribs in AP chest radiograph). SaO_2 to be maintained >90-95% with a FiO_2 <30%. Higher MAP can interfere with venous return. Monitor for clinical signs of decreased systemic perfusion by noting capillary refill, blood pressure, central venous pressure, heart rate, and urine output.
Ventilation	Adjust *amplitude* in order to produce an adequate wiggle of chest and abdomen *Frequency* 10 Hz -15 Hz. Use higher frequency in smaller babies. 15 Hz in <1000 grams *Ti* 33% is maintained	*Pressure amplitude* (PIP-PEEP) determines CO_2 removal. Set the *rate* between 240-660 bpm. Use lower rates 240-360 bpm in larger patients and those with air leak/obstructive airway disease. *Ti* is kept constant at 0.02	Monitor on the basis of $PaCO_2$ targets. Hypercarbia can be corrected by increasing the amplitude or decreasing the frequency in HFO or by altering the PIP in Jet ventilator. Rates can be decreased as a secondary measure if there is air trapping. %Ti in HFO and Ti in Jet ventilator is not altered
Recruitment maneuvers	Use higher MAP transiently to open up collapsed alveoli.	Use back ground IMV or sigh breaths to recruit alveoli. Once oxygenation is stable, switch back to CPAP mode and use MAP to keep alveoli open.	
Weaning	Weaning should be a slow process. Wean the FiO_2 first followed by MAP when FiO_2 is < 30%	Wean FiO_2 first. Once < 30% wean the PEEP. PIP is lowered in response to CO_2 levels. Ventilator rate is not decreased as a weaning strategy. Infants can be weaned directly to CPAP or to CV when the PIP is <12-14 and PEEP is < 6 cm H_2O	

MAP can interfere with venous return. Fluid boluses and inotropes may be needed to support cardiac output if MAP cannot be decreased without compromising oxygenation.

57.6 Disease Specific Initial Ventilator Settings

Newborn Babies

Respiratory distress syndrome (RDS)

Respiratory distress syndrome is characterized by surfactant deficiency. High surface tension in the alveoli leads to alveolar collapse, atelectasis, V/Q mismatch. This is manifested by increased work of breathing, hypoxemia and hypercarbia. In preterm infants with RDS, early use of continuous positive air way pressure (CPAP) may decrease the need for mechanical ventilation. Mechanical ventilation and surfactant administration should be considered in babies with significant work of breathing, apnea, hypoxemia (PaO_2 < 50 mm Hg), FiO_2 requirement >40-50% and hypercarbia (PaO_2 > 60 mm Hg). In an early phase of RDS, accepting a $PaCO_2$ of 45 to 55 mm Hg with a pH between 7.20 to 7.25 allows gentle ventilation. Respiratory support in early RDS is shown in the box[39].

Ventilatory goals are to achieve adequate oxygenation and ventilation without causing lung

> **Initial ventilator settings for RDS**
>
> Early therapeutic CPAP
> Early surfactant
> Rapid rates 40-60/min
> Moderate PEEP 4-5 cm H_2O
> Low PIP 10-20 cm H_2O
> Short Ti 0.25-0.4 S
> Low tidal volume 3-6 ml/kg
> Early extubation to nasal CPAP

injury. Acceptable goals are; SaO_2 88-92%, pH 7.25-7.35, PaO_2 50-60 mm Hg, $PaCO_2$ 45-55 mm Hg . A recent systematic review and meta-analysis shows that volume-targeted ventilation (VTV) compared with pressure-limited ventilation (PLV) reduce death and bronchopulmonary dysplasia, pneumothorax, hypocarbia and severe cranial ultrasound abnormalities[18]. Since the risk of lung injury and the development of broncho-pulmonary dysplasia(BPD) is related to the duration of invasive mechanical ventilation, there has been a trend towards increasing use of noninvasive ventilation with nCPAP or noninvasive positive pressure ventilation (NIPPV) to protect the preterm infant's lungs[40]. In ventilated infants the following strategies can be employed to provide gentle ventilation[39].

1. *Permissive hypercapnia.* accepting $PaCO_2$ up to 60 mm Hg

2. *Permissive hypoxemia.* In the early phase of RDS, it is appropriate to maintain the oxygen saturation between 87% and 92% and the arterial oxygen tension between 40 and 60 mm Hg. If BPD is established, to avoid the development of cor pulmonale, it may be reasonable to maintain slightly higher targets (SpO_2 89-94% and minimum PaO_2 of 50 mm Hg.

3. *Minimal peak pressures, low V_T and rapid rates.* Studies have shown that a faster ventilator rate with a lower tidal volume produces less volutrauma compared to to a slower ventilator rate with a larger TV. When attempts are made to use small TV and low PIP, the MAP which is the key determinant of ventilation-perfusion matching may need to be maintained by the use of adequate PEEP. Based on these clinical data, recommended initial settings for conventional ventilation (CV) of neonates with RDS are a respiratory rate of 40 to 60 breaths per minute, a PIP at which minimal chest excursions during inspiration is noted (usually 10-20 cm H_2O), moderate PEEP (4-5 cm H_2O), and a relatively short Ti (0.25-0.4 sec).

4. *Ventilator adjustments.* CO_2 elimination is better achieved by increasing rate rather than by increasing the PIP, as an increase in PIP will increase TV and may induce volutrauma. Similarly, if there is hypocarbia, the PIP rather than ventilator rate should be first reduced if the chest rise is adequate. If atelectasis occurs, higher PIP may be transiently required, and following resolution of the atelectasis, it is important to reduce PIP rapidly. Maintaining an adequate MAP is essential to optimize FiO_2.

5. *Extubation.* can be attempted when there is adequate spontaneous respiratory effort and the infant is on low ventilator settings (rate 10-25/min, FiO_2 < 0.4, PIP low with good lung compliance). Extubabtion to NCPAP and loading with methyl xanthenes should be considered in preterm infants less than 28 weeks gestation to decrease the incidence of extubation failure and apneic episodes.

6. *Early therapeutic CPAP and early surfactant treatment* followed by rapid extubation to CPAP may help reduce mechanical ventilation-induced lung injury and possibly reduce BPD.

Chronic lung disease or bronchopulmonary dysplasia

A 2001 NICHD (National Institute of Child Health) consensus statement defines BPD as a requirement for supplemental oxygen for 21 of the first 28 days of life, and identifies 3 grades of severity of BPD (mild, moderate, severe) depending on the duration and level of supplemental oxygen and mechanical ventilatory support at 36 weeks postmenstrual age in preterm infants[41].The lung pathology in BPD is heterogeneous with areas of atelectasis alternating with air trapping. The compliance is reduced and the airway resistance is high. This produces higher time constants. The goals are to employ minimum ventilatory settings to achieve gas exchange[39]. One can accept higher

> **Ventilatory settings in BPD**
>
> Slower rates   20-40/min
> Moderate PEEP 4- 8 cm H_2O
> Lowest PIP required 20-30cm H_2O
> Longer Ti   0.4-0.7 sec
> VT 5-8 ml/kg or more

$PaCO_2$ levels if pH is > 7.25 (pH 7.25-7.30, PaO_2 50-70 mm Hg, and $PaCO_2$ up to 55 60 mm Hg). Infants with BPD tolerate higher PEEP (5-7 cm H20) and require lower rates (20-40/min) because of the higher time constant. Infants with cystic changes in chest radiograph are more prone to air trapping.

BPD is not a mere continuum of lung disease secondary to RDS and the effects of mechanical ventilation but involves injury and impaired development of alveoli and pulmonary capillaries. Hence a number of adjuvant therapies have been tried to prevent or treat inflammatory response in BPD. Of note is the use of methylxanthines, such as caffeine for the treatment of apnea in preterm babies. Results from the Caffeine for Apnea of Prematurity (CAP) trial showed that caffeine significantly reduced BPD at 36 weeks' corrected age[42].

Pulmonary interstitial emphysema (PIE) and air leaks

The main principles for ventilation of PIE are to further reduce barotrauma by decreasing the peak airway pressure, MAP and PEEP and by increasing the expiratory time to minimize further gas trapping. Permissive hypercapnea ($PaCO_2$ up to 60 mm Hg) and low arterial oxygenation (PaO_2 > 50 mmHg) may need to be accepted to avoid further air leaks. The following ventilator settings are recommended:

Ventilatory settings in PIE	
PIP	12-15 cm H_2O
PEEP	4-6 cm H_2O
Rate	Appropriate rate without compromising the expiratory time
I:E ratio	1:2 to 1:3

High frequency Jet ventilation allows better ventilation at lower peak and mean air way pressures resulting in resolution of PIE. A symptomatic pneumothorax that complicates the air leak syndrome may require needle aspiration or chest tube insertion.

Meconium aspiration syndrome

Respiratory distress in meconium aspiration syndrome is characterized by areas of atelectasis due to complete airway obstruction by particulate meconium and areas of air trapping (obstructive emphysema) due to ball valve effect and incomplete obstruction by meconium. Lung mechanics in MAS

includes increased airway resistance, prolonged time constant, increased FRC as well as decreased compliance. These infants are vulnerable to develop PPHN with perpetuation of hypoxia due to right-to-left shunting of blood through foramen ovale or the ductus arteriosus. The incidence of air leaks, either spontaneous or following ventilation is very high.

Most clinicians try to avoid the use of positive pressure support (CPAP or mechanical ventilation) in these infants for fear of air leaks and supplemental oxygen alone (eg. an oxygen hood) is tried first[43]. Adequate systemic oxygenation (PaO_2 between 60-80 mm Hg and SaO_2 between 92-97%) should be maintained to avoid PPHN, but PaO_2 beyond 80 mm Hg does not provide any benefit to decrease pulmonary artery pressures[44]. However, FiO_2 >80% may be harmful and some form of positive pressure is required. Mechanical ventilation should be considered in MAS if PaO_2 is < 50 mm Hg, $PaCO_2$ > 60 mm Hg or pH < 7.25 in an oxygen enriched environment with FiO_2 > 0.8[45]. The recommended ventilatory settings are given in the box[43]. Lower PIP, moderate PEEP, lower rates (40-60/min) and adequate expiratory time (0.5- 0.7 seconds) are used and permissive hypercapnia is tolerated to facilitate gentle ventilation. If lungs are hyperexpanded PEEP is reduced further and expiratory time is prolonged. Where MAS is complicated by PPHN, mild hyperventilation and higher FiO_2 can be considered. But the strategy of achieving hypocapnia and alkalosis by hyperventilation has adverse effects including lung injury, sensorineural deafness and poor neurological outcome[46]. In such situations other modalities like inhaled nitric oxide and high frequency ventilation should be considered early.

Ventilatory settings in meconium aspiration syndrome	
PIP	Use lower PIP (not exceeding 25 cm H_2O)
PEEP	4-6 cm H_2O
Rate	40-60/ min
I:E ratio	1:2 to 1:3

Congenital diaphragmatic hernia (CDH)

Management of a neonate with CDH requires a well-coordinated multidisciplinary team. Herniation of of abdominal contents in the thorax coincides with the period of pulmonary parenchymal and vascular development. Pulmonary hypoplasia results in decreased surface area for gas exchange (leading to hypoxemia, hypercarbia and acidosis) and increased pulmonary vascular resistance (PPHN). In most cases the diagnosis of CDH is established antenatally. Delivery room resuscitation should include avoidance of bag and mask ventilation and immediate endotracheal intubation. Any delay in obtaining an airway can intensify the resultant acidosis and hypoxia, which can increase the risk of pulmonary hypertension. A nasogastric tube is placed in the stomach and connected to continuous suction for decompression of the abdominal contents and expansion of lung tissue. Initial ventilator settings should aim to produce gentle ventilation and acceptable SaO_2 levels (pre ductal SaO_2 >85%), pH 7.25-7.35 and $PaCO_2$ 45-65 mm Hg. Metabolic acidosis and high lactate concentrations reflect poor tissue perfusion and cardiac compromise. These patients may respond to volume loading and inotropic support.

Ventilatory settings for CDH	
PIP	20-22 cm H_2O (< 25 cm)
PEEP	3-5cm H_2O
MAP	<12 cm H_2O
Rate	20 - 40/min
Ti	0.35 sec
FiO_2	50-100%

High frequency ventilation should be considered if high peak pressures >25 mm Hg are required or if there there is persistent hypercarbia >60 mm Hg or hypoxia (Preductal SaO_2 <85%) unresponsive to conventional ventilation. Adjunctive therapies include inhaled nitric oxide, prostaglandins and sildenafil for the management of PPHN. Surfactant therapy has not been shown to improve outcomes in infants with CDH[47]. Surgical correction should only be attempted after ensuring respiratory and cardiovascular stability.

Mechanical ventilation for non-pulmonary conditions

Birth asphyxia, apnea of prematurity and immediate post operative care are some of the

Ventilatory settings in non-pulmonary conditions	
PIP	12-14 cm H_2O
PEEP	3-4 cm H_2O
Rate	30 -40/min
Ti	0.3- 0.4 sec
I:E ratio	1:2

situations where mechanical ventilation is instituted until spontaneous efforts are established by the patient. In many of these conditions the lungs are either normal or has minimal underlying problem. These babies can be ventilated with minimal settings. Ventilatory goals are pH 7.35-7.45, $PaCO_2$ 35-45 mm Hg and SaO_2 between 92-95%. Post surgical patients can develop lung atelectasis and may require higher settings.

Mechanical ventilation in older children

Principles of mecahnical ventilaton in children beyond the neonatal period are not different from that in neonates. Certain lung conditions like asthma, bronchiolitis and acute respiratory distress syndrome are seen beyond neonatal period whereas pneumonia is common to both age groups.

Pneumonia

Although most children with pneumonia can be managed in the community, indications for admission include oxygen saturations less than 92%, respiratory rate greater than 70 breaths per minute for infants or 50 breaths per minute for children, apnea, dyspnea and grunting during breathing, poor feeding and signs of dehydration[48]. Indications for ventilatory support include FiO_2 > 60% to maintain SaO_2 > 92%, severe respiratory distress and apnea.

The main guiding principle is to titrate the FiO_2 and the PEEP depending on the severity of the underlying disease to achieve normal oxygen saturation. Use a tidal volume (V_T) of 8-10 ml/kg if using volume control ventilation. In pressure control ventilation PIP is decided by aiming at optimal chest rise and by monitoring the delivered tidal volume. The initial rates are kept according to the child's expected respiratory rate for age.

Ventilatory settings for pneumonia	
V_T	6- 8 ml/kg
PIP	20-25 cm H_2O
PEEP	4-5 cm H_2O
Rate	40 - 50/min (infants)
	30 - 40/min (older children)
I: E ratio	1:2

Acute severe asthma

Intubation of patients with severe asthma is recommended only in certain situations like acute impending ventilatory failure, severe hypoxia and rapid deterioration in the child's mental state because there are intrinsic difficulties in ventilating such patients and the increased risk of barotrauma. In severe asthma, the abnormally high airway resistance results in increased work of breathing. The inspiratory transpulmonary pressure may be as high as 50 cm H_2O, compared with 5 cm H_2O during normal tidal breathing[49]. Expiration becomes an active event in order to empty the lungs via markedly narrowed airways. Incomplete emptying leads to hyperinflation , air trapping and auto-PEEP (alveolar pressure fails to return to zero at the end of expiration and remains positive) (Figure 57.30). The pressure (in excess of the atmospheric pressure) within the airways and alveoli at the end of exhalation is referred to as auto (intrinsic) PEEP. The auto-PEEP leads to an added inspiratory load on the patient who has to generate extra flow to overcome the auto-PEEP to trigger the ventilator. The adverse cardiac effects of auto-PEEP include decreased cardiac output and hypotension. A hyperinflated lung is also less compliant because it is more expanded.

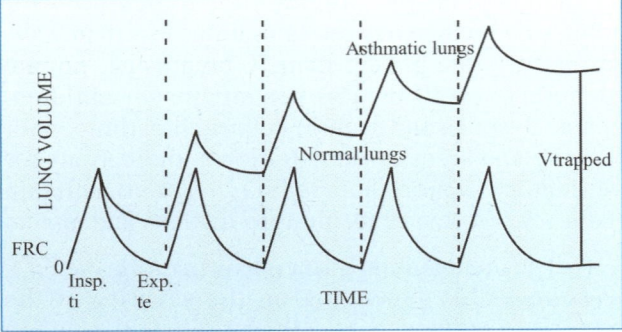

Figure 57.30 Mechanism of dynamic hyperinflation in the setting of severe airflow obstruction. The next inspiration begins before complete exhalation of the tidal breath; this leads to air trapping and increased end-expiratory lung volume.

Goals of ventilation in status asthmaticus are to maintain adequate oxygenation, permissive hypercapnia and adjusting minute ventilation (peak pressure, tidal volume, and rate) in order to maintain an arterial pH of >7.2, $PaCO_2$ between 50-55 mm Hg and SaO_2 > 95%. As opposed to disorders of static compliance with short time constants such as acute respiratory distress syndrome that can be managed with relatively faster respiratory rates, disorders of resistance such as asthma require relatively slow rates for adequate ventilation[50]. Typically slow ventilator rates with prolonged expiratory phase, minimal end-expiratory pressure, and short inspiratory time are used in order to minimize dynamic hyperinflation and air trapping.

For older children, one may begin with volume control (VC) mode using settings of V_T of 5–6 ml/kg, RR approximately half of the normal for age,

I:E ratio of 1:3 and PEEP of 2–3 cm of H_2O[51]. The use of PEEP in the asthmatic patient receiving mechanical ventilation is controversial. Due to the presence of auto-PEEP the patient fights the ventilator and exhibits tachypnea, tachycardia, discoordinate thoraco-abdominal movements[52]. In such cases counterbalancing the auto-PEEP by adding an appropriate level of extrinsic PEEP (approximately 85% of PEEP) decreases the work of breathing[53]. In infants, pressure controlled ventilation may be used with PIP adjusted to achieve adequate ventilation; the settings of rate, I:E ratio and PEEP are the same as above.

Although VC mode is traditionally used in acute asthma, there are concerns of unequal ventilation because relatively less obstructed airways with shorter time constants are likely to receive more volume throughout inspiration as compared with more obstructed airways with longer time constants. Advocates of PCV believe that constant inflation pressure, relatively less obstructed lung units with shorter time constants will achieve pressure equilibration during early inspiration and more obstructed areas with longer time constants will continue to receive additional volume in late inspiration. This will result in more even distribution of inspired gas and delivery of more tidal volume for the same inflation pressure[50]. However, with either mode, the principles are the same. Bronchodilator therapy and systemic corticosteroids are indispensible in the management of acute severe asthma.

Asthmatic patients on ventilator are at high risk of barotrauma and need monitoring of peak alveolar pressure, mean airway pressures, auto-PEEP and hemodynamic status as well as chest radiographs to assess lung expansion. As the lung condition improves, the exhaled VT increases and $PaCO_2$ begins to fall. The PIP should be reduced accordingly. In volume mode, the peak pressure required to deliver the set VT decreases and the patients can be weaned off the ventilator early.

Ventilatory settings in a child with status asthmaticus	
V_T	6- 8 ml/kg
PIP	20-25 cm H_2O
PEEP	3- 4 cm H_2O
Rate	20 - 30/min (infants)
	10- 20/min (1-5 years)
	8-12/min (6-12 years)
I:E ratio	1:3 to 1:4

Acute respiratory distress syndrome (ARDS)

ARDS is an acute and rapidly progressive pulmonary disease of a noncardiac nature, characterized by progressively diffuse, bilateral pulmonary infiltrates on the chest radiograph, and severe arterial hypoxemia resistant to oxygen therapy alone (PaO_2/FiO_2 ratio $\leq$ 200 for ARDS and $\leq$ 300 for ALI). ARDS is a heterogenous disorder with alveolar collapse, protein rich edema fluid in the alveoli in the acute phase (lasts 7-10 days) progressing to fibrosing alveolitis in chronic phase. Interspersed with atelectatic alveoli are normal areas resulting in markedly reduced volume of lung for ventilation in ARDS. Resolution of injury can occur during either phase. Low lung compliance and short time constants are hallmarks of the disorder.

The two strategies of ventilatory support in ARDS are listed below[54]:

1. *Open lung approach.* Low tidal volumes and plateau pressures, with PEEP sufficiently high to ensure that the alveoli open at end-expiration (open lung approach).

2. *ARDS net approach.* Small tidal volumes (< 6 ml/kg), low plateau pressures (< 35 cmH_2O), respiratory rate to control $PaCO_2$ and pH within as normal a range as possible, with PEEP titrated to achieve an acceptable oxygenation (PaO_2 between 80 and 100 mm Hg.).

The flow chart describes the ventilatory settings, target gases and weaning in either setting (Figure 57.15).

Open lung approach Pressure controlled ventilator Assist/control (acute phase) or SIMV	ARDS net approach Volume controlled-Pressure limited Assist/control (acute phase) or SIMV
1. Set PIP to achieve a VT 4-8 ml/kg 2. Ensure peak alveolar pressure < 25-30 cm H_2O 3. Ti 0.3- 1.0 (based on age). The I:E ratio may be increased to 1:1 or 2:1 (inverse ratio ventilation) to improve oxygenation. 4. Rate 20-40/min (based on age) 5. PEEP: Above lower inflection point if PV loop available, otherwise, use between 8 - 20 cm H_2O. PEEP should be progressively increased by 2–3 cm H_2O increments to maintain SaO_2 between 90 and 95% with FiO_2 <0.6.	1. Set VT < 6 ml/kg 2. Limit plateau pressure < 30 cm H_2O 3. Ti 0.3- 1.0 (based on age) The I:E ratio may be increased to 1:1 or 2:1 (inverse ratio ventilation) to improve oxygenation. 4. Rate 20-40/min (based on age) 5. PEEP: Above lower inflection point if PV loop available. Otherwise, use between 8 - 20 cm H_2O. PEEP should be progressively increased by 2–3 cm H_2O increments to maintain SaO_2 between 90 and 95% with FiO_2 <0.6.

Target gases
pH= 7.30-7.45
PaO_2 = 55-80 mm Hg, SaO_2 88-95%
$PaCO_2$ = 45 mm Hg
[Consider accepting pH> 7.25 and $PaCO_2$ >45 mm Hg if higher peak pressures are required]

Corrective actions
pH< 7.25

- Increase PIP if peak pressure < 30 cm H_2O
- Increase rate if peak pressure > 25-30 cm H_2O
- Consider accepting lower pH

Hypoxemia (SaO_2 < 90%)
- Increase PEEP
- Increase FiO2

Severe hypoxemia
- Prone positioning
- High frequency ventilation
- Inhaled nitric oxide

Weaning

pH >7.45/ $PaCO_2$<45 mm Hg
- Decrease PIP/ VT
- Decrease rate

SaO_2>95%
- Wean FiO_2< 60%
- Wean PEEP

Figure 57.31 Algorithm for ventilatory management of ARDS

Extubation is planned once the child's respiratory condition improves allowing decrease in ventilator settings to FiO$_2$ of less than 40%, PEEP of 4–5 cm H$_2$O, rate of 15/min or less, PIP of less than 15 cm H$_2$O; the child is hemodynamically stable and sensorium is normal/near normal with presence of protective reflexes[56].

Adjunctive therapies in ARDS

Prone position. Prone positioning can be considered in children who have significant hypoxemia in spite of usual ventilation strategies. Prone position has potential physiological benefits, including the recruitment of dorsal (nondependent) atelectatic lung units, improved respiratory mechanics, decreased ventilation perfusion mismatch, increased secretion drainage, reduced mechanical compression by heart[57]. A recent RCT in children with ARDS who were randomized to prone positioning for 20 hours a day for 7 days, showed no benefit in mortality or duration of ventilation despite a short term improvement in oxygenation[58].

Nitric oxide. Inhaled nitric oxide (iNO) is a potent pulmonary vasodilator and can be used in patients with hypoxemia. A meta-analysis of multiple studies in children and adults showed that iNO improved oxygenation without changing mortality[59].

High frequency ventilation. This modality can be considered in children with severe disease who require very high mean airway pressure on conventional ventilation (>20-25 cm H$_2$O) although studies have not shown a survival benefit despite improvement in oxygenation. Its use should be considered early in the management of children with large air leaks[60].

Surfactant therapy. Surfactant can be used as an adjunctive therapy in severe ARDS. A meta-analysis of six trials of surfactant therapy in children with acute respiratory failure including bronchiolitis and ALI showed decreased mortality, increased ventilator free days, and decreased duration of mechanical ventilation[61].

Children with normal lungs (shock, flaccid paralysis)

In these conditions, the aim is to mimic normal breathing pattern as far as possible (Box).

57.7 Weaning from the Ventilator

Weaning is a process of gradual transition from mechanical to spontaneous breathing by decreasing the support provided by the ventilator.

Ventilatory settings in children with normal lungs	
V$_T$	6-8 ml/kg
PEEP	3- 4 cm H$_2$O
Rate	40 /min (infants)
	20 - 30/min (older children)
I:E ratio	1:2-1:3

Because of the inherent risks associated with mechanical ventilation (injury to the airway and lungs, risk of ventilator associated pneumonia, patient immobility) it is advantageous to discontinue ventilatory support as soon as there is resolution of the underlying condition for which ventilation was instituted. Examples include resolution of pneumonia or RDS, reversal of anesthesia, establishment of spontaneous breathing in cases of apnea, head injury, resolution of septic shock etc. For the majority of patients (75%) weaning and extubation are established easily while it is prolonged and difficult in the rest[62]. Patients should be assessed for their readiness to wean by considering the following parameters.

(i)   Resolution of underlying condition causing respiratory failure.

(ii)   Adequate gas exchange with minimal settings; PaO$_2$ > 60 mm Hg with FiO$_2$ < 30- 40% and PEEP < 5 cm H$_2$O.

(iii) Adequate spontaneous breathing efforts.

(iv)   Hemodynamic stability (normal cardiac function with minimal or no inotropic support).

(v)   Absence of major organ dysfunction.

(vi)   Normal electrolytes, adequate nutrition and normal body temperature also facilitate successful weaning.

Patients on a ventilator need extra help to overcome the imposed work of breathing contributed by the ventilator tubing, demand valves and endotracheal tube. Hence support should be provided to over come this imposed work of breathing (a tidal volume of 4 ml/kg).

Strategies for weaning. There is evidence from literature to show a reduction in the duration of mechanical ventilation, weaning duration and stay in the intensive care unit with the use of standardized weaning protocols[63]. The general principles are to wean the potentially injuries parameters first, limit changes to one parameter at a time, avoid changes of large magnitude and to assess patient response after each change as shown in Figure 57.32[64].

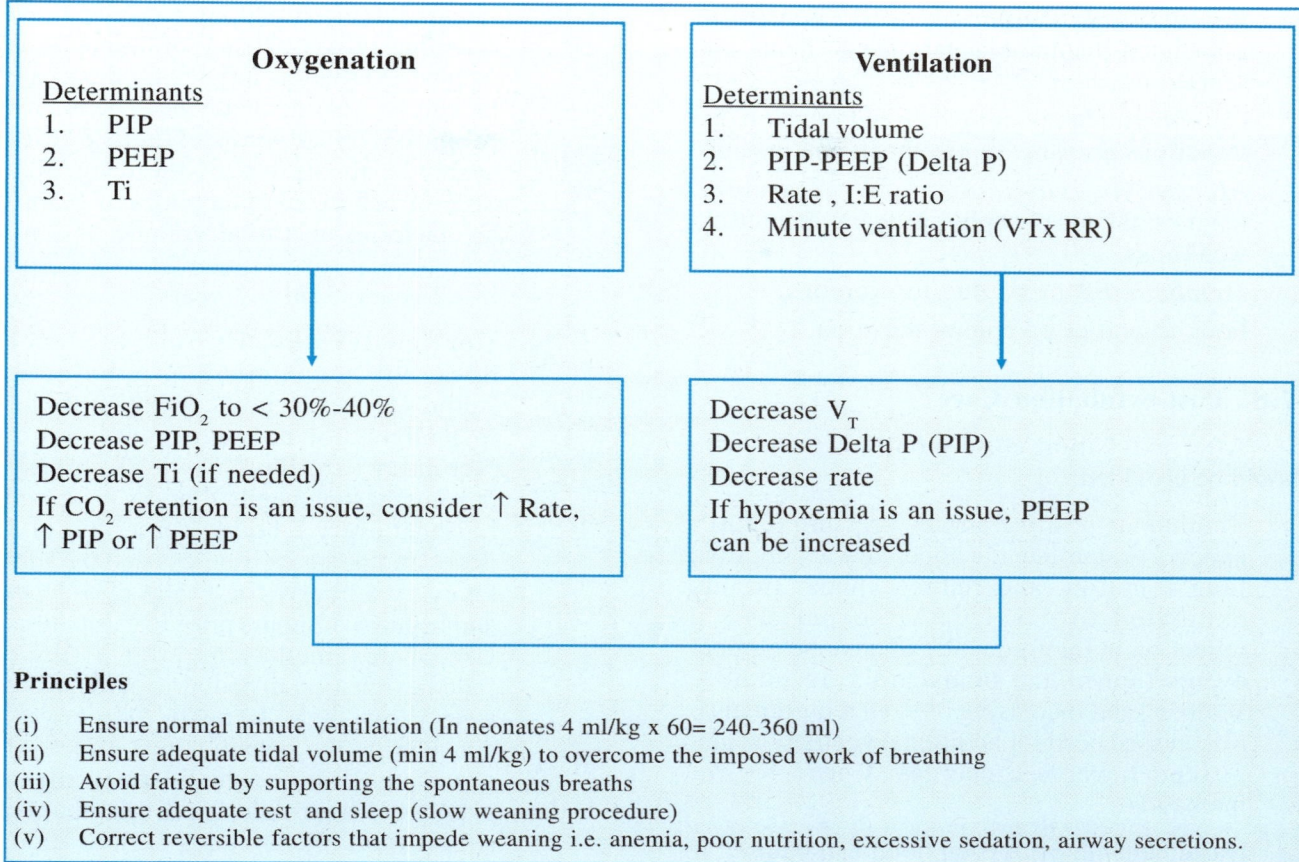

Oxygenation

Determinants
1. PIP
2. PEEP
3. Ti

Ventilation

Determinants
1. Tidal volume
2. PIP-PEEP (Delta P)
3. Rate , I:E ratio
4. Minute ventilation (VTx RR)

Decrease FiO_2 to < 30%-40%
Decrease PIP, PEEP
Decrease Ti (if needed)
If CO_2 retention is an issue, consider ↑ Rate,
↑ PIP or ↑ PEEP

Decrease V_T
Decrease Delta P (PIP)
Decrease rate
If hypoxemia is an issue, PEEP
can be increased

Principles

(i)   Ensure normal minute ventilation (In neonates 4 ml/kg x 60= 240-360 ml)
(ii)   Ensure adequate tidal volume (min 4 ml/kg) to overcome the imposed work of breathing
(iii) Avoid fatigue by supporting the spontaneous breaths
(iv)   Ensure adequate rest and sleep (slow weaning procedure)
(v)   Correct reversible factors that impede weaning i.e. anemia, poor nutrition, excessive sedation, airway secretions.

Figure 57.32 Step-wise weaning protocol

Weaning can either be accomplished by trials of spontaneous breathing on the endotracheal tube for progressively longer periods of time, or by gradually decreasing the level of support on IMV, SIMV+PS, or pressure support ventilation (PSV).

1. During a T-piece trial, the patient is disconnected from the ventilator, a T-piece is attached to the endotracheal tube, and an appropriate concentration of oxygen is administered through one limb of the T-piece. The patient is encouraged to breathe on his own through the endotracheal tube, initially for brief intervals of time. These periods of spontaneous breathing are progressively increased until the patient is capable of breathing on his own for a reasonable period of time without manifesting any signs of distress. In a CPAP trial patient is not disconnected from the ventilator but given a minimum CPAP pressure. Trials of spontaneous breathing should be terminated immediately at any stage should any signs of cardio-respiratory distress develop.

2. In assist or control modes, each spontaneous effort would result in the delivery of mandatory breath. So decreasing the rate has no effect as long as patient's RR is more than the set rate. Wean PIP but maintain a delta P to deliver adequate VT. One can also decrease the trigger sensitivity so that the patient has to make greater efforts to trigger the ventilator.

3. Weaning methods in SIMV are similar to IMV, i.e. weaning is achieved by decreasing the SIMV rate and PIP. However, one should avoid using a very low SIMV rate and try to maintain a tidal volume delivery of at least 4 ml/kg. If children require continuing minimal support through SIMV, an alternative approach is to use pressure support ventilation (PSV) in conjunction with SIMV.

Common causes of failure to wean

Some of the causes of extubation failure are given below. Many of these conditions are reversible or amenable to appropriate therapy. Hence one should try to correct these before labeling a patient as extubation failure.

1. *Neurological.* Sedation, apnea of prematurity and decreased respiratory drive.

2. *Respiratory.* Superimposed ventilator associated pneumonia, laryngeal edema and secretions.

3. *Cardiovascular.* poor myocardial function due to various reasons, septic shock and anemia.

4. *Electrolyte imbalance.* Low potassium, magnesium and phosphorus aggravate muscle weakness.

5. *Metabolic alkalosis* due to diuretics.

6. Poor enteral or parenteral nutrition.

57.8   Post-extubation Care

After extubation close monitoring and care should be provided.

1. Continuous positive airway pressure (CPAP) appears to stabilize the upper airway, improve lung function, and reduce apnea. Infants extubated to nasal CPAP, experience a reduction in the frequency of adverse clinical events (apnea and bradycardia, respiratory acidosis, and increasing oxygen requirement), a decreased need for additional ventilation, and a trend towards a decreased need for re-intubation.

2. Nasal cannula or oxygen hood can be used if there is oxygen requirement. Patients without pre existing lung condition do well on room air.

3. Preterm babies at risk of apnea of prematurity may benefit from caffeine loading at least 2 hours prior to extubation. Caffeine base is administered in a dose of 10 mg/kg loading dose followed by maintenance at 3-5 mg/kg/day 24 hours after the loading.

4. Other pharmacologic agents often used to facilitate the process of weaning but not routinely recommended are diuretics and bronchodilators in chronic lung disease.

5. Clinically relevant post-extubation laryngeal edema occurs in up to 30% of extubated patients, and 4% of patients need to be reintubated[65]. If stidor is severe with increased work of breathing consider re-intubation. The decision whether or not to treat laryngeal edema depends on the severity of symptoms. Ensure warm humidified air or oxygen for inhalation. The following medications can also be considered.

   (a) **Epinephrine.** Epinephrine acts through local stimulation of β-adrenergic receptors to cause vasoconstriction and reduce edema. Randomized controlled rials that prove efficacy of epinephrine in post-extubation laryngeal edema are lacking[66]. Also neonates may be at risk of potential adverse effects due to systemic absorption of the drug. The dose of nebulized epinephrine is 0.5ml/kg made up to a total volume of 3 ml with normal saline (maximum of 2.5 ml in <2 years; 5 ml > 2 years)[67].

   (b) **Corticosteroids.** Current evidence does not recommend prophylactic steroids to prevent post extubation stridor in pediatric or neonatal population[68]. Neonatal studies used 0.5mg/kg dexamethasone begun 4 hours prior and repeated every 8 hourly for a total of 3 doses and pediatric studies used 0.5 mg/kg every 6 hourly for a total of 6 doses and begun 6-12 hours prior to extubation. Use of dexamethasone after a single failed extubation in pediatric patients did not show any benefit. However, considering the potential side effects of dexamethasone, one should use it only in patients at high risk of post extubation stridor (multiple attempts at intubation, airway injury or instrumentation). Dexamethasone can be administered orally or parenterally.

57.9   Supportive Care during Ventilation

Nurses caring for mechanically ventilated children should have knowledge about the child's medical condition and the indications for mechanical ventilation. Proper assessment of vital signs supplemented by electronic monitoring of heart rate, oxygen saturation, blood pressure, end tidal or transcutaneous carbon dioxide measurements are essential. Hydration status, urine output and enteral and parenteral intake are also monitored. Physical examination should include monitoring for respiratory distress, chest symmetry, chest wiggle or vibrations in high frequency ventilator, air entry, presence of added sounds and cardiac murmur. Other important steps in nursing care pertaining to mechanically ventilated infants is summarized below.

1. **Thermal homeostasis**. The infant should be nursed in a thermoneutral environment by using servocontrolled warmers or incubators. Intravenous fluids should be pre-warmed and direct contact with cold X-ray plates should be avoided

2. **Endotracheal tube position**. The position of ET tube should be documented in the nursing flow sheet and checked during each assessment. Its position should also be checked on skiagrams. A properly placed tube should lie below the level of clavicles at T2 vertebral level above carina.

3. **Endotracheal tube suctioning**[69]. Suction is performed only as needed based on patient assessment. Indications for suctioning are given below.

   (a) Visible secretions in ETT.
   (b) Audible secretions or presence of rhonchi, coarse and/or decreased breath sounds.
   (c) Changes in respiratory rate and/or rhythm.
   (d) Oxygen desaturations or bradycardia.
   (e) Changes in blood gas values (increased $PaCO_2$ and/or decreased PaO_2).
   (f) Restlessness and agitation.
   (g) Increased proximal airway pressure on the ventilator.

   Procedure. A sterile closed suction system is preferred. Open endotracheal suctioning is used if closed system is unavailable or unsuccessful in removing secretions. Appropriate sized catheter is selected for the specific size of the airway used. A 6.0 French catheter is used for 2.5 ETT, while an 8.0 French catheter is used for a 3.0 or 3.5 ETT. Proper asepsis should be ensured throughout the procedure. FiO_2 is increased 5-10% above the existing oxygen requirements. Insert the catheter so that its tip ends at the tip of the ETT and does not touch the carina. Negative pressure should not exceed 100 mm Hg and not for more than 15 seconds and it should be applied only during withdrawal of the catheter. The number of catheter passes should not exceed 3 per suctioning procedure. Normal saline should *not* be instilled routinely. After suctioning, the patient is reconnected to the ventilator as soon as possible if the open technique is used. If the infant was pre-oxygenated, oxygen is weaned back to baseline requirement.

   Complications. The common complications of the the procedure include bradycardia, hypoxia, hypercarbia and tracheal mucosal damage. After the procedure, lung de-recruitment and atelectasis can occur if the ventilator was disconnected from the patient. This can lead to hypercarbia and increased oxygen requirements. When using the open method, the suction catheter should be changed after each patient use and when using the closed in line suction, catheter should be changed every 72 hours or when soiled.

4. **Prevention of ventilator associated pneumonia (VAP)**[70]. The Canadian Critical Care Trials Group has recommended the following guidelines for the prevention of ventilator associated pneumonia. Their recommendations include, orotracheal route of intubation rather than nasotracheal intubation, use of new ventilator circuits for each patient, and the circuits need to be changed only if they become soiled or damaged, change of humidifiers every 5 to 7 days or as clinically indicated and use of closed endotracheal suctioning system. They noted that use of bacterial filters and prophylactic inhaled or oral antibiotic therapy does not influence the incidence of VAP and hence are not recommended. Elevation of the head of the bed to 45° and the use of the oral antiseptic chlorhexidine may decrease the incidence of VAP.

5. **Chest physiotherapy**. Chest physiotherapy techniques include, manual percussion with proper cupping of hand or with a face mask, vibration of the chest wall, postural drainage using gravity and assisted coughing. The presumed benefits of these maneuvers include loosening and dislodgement of secretions and gravity assisted drainage from smaller to larger airways from where the secretions can be coughed up or suctioned. However, studies have shown that chest physiotherapy administered in pediatric patients is associated with (a) a higher rate of atelectasis and a longer hospital stay[71]; (b) a higher rate of gastroesophageal reflux[72] and (c) increase in intracranial pressure, cerebral blood flow and a higher rate of intracranial hemorrhage in mechanically ventilated newborn infants[73]. Hence, in mechanically ventilated children, chest physiotherapy should not be routinely performed until safety and efficacy of such therapy is established by further studies[74].

6. **Prone positioning**. Prone position during mechanical ventilation has been used to improve oxygenation in severe hypoxemic respiratory failure. The benefits appear to be due to recruitment of alveoli, redistribution of ventilation toward the dorsal regions resulting better ventilation/perfusion matching, and the elimination of compression of the lungs by the heart[75]. The potential adverse effects include facial edema, pressure ulcers, inadvertent

Section 6

extubation, loss or displacement of central vascular catheters and increased need for sedation. Although the majority of patients undergoing prone positioning experienced an improvement in their oxygenation studies have not demonstrated a survival benefit. Despite these limitations, Girard and Bernard[76] concluded that prone positioning may be considered a reasonable short-term therapy for patients with ARDS requiring high FIO_2 (> 0.6) or elevated plateau pressure (> 30 cm H_2O). Nursing implications include monitoring of vital signs, care of endotracheal tube, central lines and careful position change after an interval of at least 6-8 hours.

ADJUVANT THERAPY

Surfactant treatment. pulmonary surfactant is composed of phospholipids, neutral lipids and proteins synthesized and secreted by type 2 alveolar epithelial cells. Surfactant preparations for use are derived from minced lung preparation or lung lavage extracts of animals or made synthetically. Surfactant administration in preterm infants with respiratory distress syndrome (RDS) has brought about a 50% decrease in the odds of neonatal death and 30-50% reduction of pulmonary air leaks. Surfactant can be administered prophylactically in neonates <26 weeks gestation or as an early rescue therapy (within 2 hours) of onset of signs and symptoms of RDS. Supplemental oxygen requirement > 30-40% on nasal CPAP and need for mechanical ventilation for RDS are indications for early rescue therapy. Other uses of surfactant therapy in neonates include lung diseases where inactivation of natural surfactant can occur. These conditions include meconium aspiration syndrome (MAS), group B streptococcal pneumonia, pulmonary hemorrhage, persistent pulmonary hypertension with coexistent parenchymal damage and chronic lung disease (CLD). However, surfactant therapy does not seem to offer significant benefit in babies with congenital diaphragmatic hernia[77, 78]. Children with acute lung injury (ALI) and acute respiratory distress syndrome show qualitative and quantitative deficiency in pulmonary surfactant. The meta-analysis by Duffett et al.[61] showed that surfactant therapy in children with ARDS was associated with significantly lower mortality (relative risk 0.7, CI 0.4–0.97, p = 0.04) and increased ventilator free days, significantly shorter duration of MV, shortened duration of PICU stay, and lower use of rescue therapy. Other conditions where surfactant therapy has been tried in children with respiratory failure include viral pneumonia, hydrocarbon aspiration, near-drowning, severe inhalation injury and burns, idiopathic pulmonary hemorrhage, and aspiration pneumonia[78].

Inhaled nitric oxide[79]. Nitric oxide is a colorless odorless gas which causes potent and selective vasodilatation of the pulmonary vasculature by increasing the cyclic guanosine monophosphate in the vascular smooth muscle cells in the lungs. It can thus reduce pulmonary vascular resistance (PVR) and improve oxygenation in newborns with severe hypoxemic respiratory failure and persistent pulmonary hypertension. Unlike other vasodilator drugs nitric oxide does not cause systemic hypotension because it is inactivated by avid binding to hemoglobin. The supra-systemic PVR causes right-to-left shunting through the ductus arteriosus and/or the foramen ovale leading to hypoxemia and acidosis that further increase the PVR. This leads to a vicious cycle. PPHN can be primary or secondary to a variety of clinical conditions, including birth asphyxia, sepsis, pneumonia, polycythemia, meconium aspiration syndrome (MAS) and antenatal exposure to NSAIDs. The condition usually involves term/near-term neonates, but preterm neonates with hyaline membrane disease (HMD) also have an element of PPHN. PPHN is suspected when there is persistent hypoxemia that is poorly responsive to oxygen, a pre-ductal to post-ductal SaO_2 difference greater than 10% and confirmed by echocardiography that demonstrates the right-to-left shunt (ductal or foramen ovale level) with normal cardiac anatomy. Echocardiography also helps to rule out cardiac conditions with a ductal dependent systemic blood flow lesions like coarctation of aorta, interrupted aortic arch and hypoplastic heart syndrome where iNO use is contraindicated, and also to evaluate left ventricular function.

1. *Indications.* The approved indications for iNO therapy include term or near-term babies born at > 34 weeks gestation with hypoxemic respiratory failure (PaO_2 < 100 mm Hg on 100% FiO_2 and an oxygenation index of > 25 and evidence of PPHN. iNO does not benefit newborns with congenital diaphragmatic hernia and its role in neonates < 34 weeks gestation is still under investigation.

2. *Dose.* Starting dose is 20 ppm and the therapy is usually begun in the first week of life. Due to the rapid onset of action of iNO, a response (improvement in PaO_2 or oxygenation index), if present, can be seen quickly (within 1 hour). Because of lack of evidence, it is not

recommended to continue iNO in non responders. However, before discontinuing therapy one should ensure adequate alveolar recruitment by using sufficient MAP if infant is on a ventilator because an apparent lack of response could be secondary to sub-optimal lung inflation in infants with parenchymal lung disease.

3. *Delivery methods.* Currently the three FDA-approved commercially available delivery devices for the administration of iNO are the INOvent (Datex-Ohmeda), iNOmax DS (Ikaria), and AeroNOx (International Biomedical). iNO therapy can be administered to babies on conventional mechanical ventilator, high frequency ventilator as well as those on nCPAP.

4. *Weaning.* In responders, the initial dose of iNO should be weaned to the minimum dose that consistently produces a therapeutic response. Finer et al.[80] noted that iNO in a dose as low as 1–2 ppm was as efficacious as 10 or 20 ppm. The dose of iNO should be weaned to 1 ppm before an attempt is made to discontinue therapy. Increasing the FiO_2 by 20% prior to discontinuation can prevent the rebound hypoxemia usually seen with discontinuation.

5. *Duration of therapy.* The usual duration of therapy is about 5 days which equates with the clinical resolution of PPHN.

6. *Side effects.* These are rare. Methemoglobinemia rarely occurs at the usual therapeutic dose of 20 ppm but can be seen with a higher dose of 80 ppm. However, it is reasonable to monitor methemoglobin levels by co-oximetry.

7. *Outcome.* Cochrane meta-analysis of 14 RCTs that evaluated the efficacy and safety of iNO has shown that inhaled nitric oxide improves the outcome in hypoxemic term and near term infants by reducing the incidence of the combined endpoint of death or need for ECMO[81]. The reduction seems to be entirely due to reduction in need for ECMO; mortality is not reduced. Oxygenation improves in approximately 50% of infants receiving nitric oxide. Among long term neuro-developmental outcomes, there was no difference in the incidence of disability, deafness and development scores among children who received iNO and those that did not. In summary the Cochrane meta-analysis shows that it appears reasonable to use inhaled nitric oxide in an initial concentration of 20 ppm for term and near term infants with hypoxic respiratory failure who do not have a diaphragmatic hernia.

Aerosol therapy in mechanically ventilated patients[82, 83]

Inhaled aerosols commonly bronchodilators and corticosteroids are used in mechanically ventilated patients. Devices suitable for aerosol delivery during mechanical ventilation are small volume nebulizers and metered-dose inhalers (MDI). Aerosol delivery in intubated patients is significantly lower than in non intubated patients and is determined by various factors including the type of device, mode of ventilation, use of humdification etc. The presence of ETT is a significant barrier for effective aerosol therapy. Effective aerosol delivery can be achieved if appropriate techniques are adopted.

(i) Use of an holding chamber with MDI results in a four- to six-fold greater delivery of aerosol.

(ii) Placing a nebulizer at a distance of 30 cm from the ETT is more efficient than placing it between the patient Y and the endotracheal tube, because the ventilator tubing acts as a spacer.

(iii) Operating the nebulizer/ MDI during inspiration is more efficient.

Complications include (a) contamination of nebulizers which can lead to aerosolization of bacteria and increased risk of pneumonia, (b) disconnection of ventilator circuit during aerosol administration can lead to loss of PEEP and atelectasis. This is off set by the use of in line adapters attached to the inspiratory limb of the circuit.

Compared to nebulizers, MDIs are easy to administer, involve less personnel time, provide a reliable dose of the drug and are cost effective. A good response to bronchodilator use is indicated by decrease in peak airway pressure, plateau pressure and auto PEEP if present.

Physiological effects of mechanical ventilation

Unlike normal spontaneous breathing, a mechanical ventilator maintains a positive intra thoracic pressure which increases during inspiration to push in air into the lungs and decreases during expiration to allow elastic recoil of lungs. Venous return to the right heart is greatest when the intra-thoracic pressure becomes more negative during

Section 6

inspiration in spontaneous breathing. However, during mechanical ventilation, the venous return is greater during exhalation when the mean positive airway pressure decreases. Many of the benefits as well the deleterious effects of mechanical ventilation can be attributed to the positive mean airway pressure. Some of the physiological changes are listed below.

1. *Effects on upper airway.* Laryngeal edema, injury to trachea, bypassing the humidification of upper airway and palatal grooving due to prolonged ET tube placement.

2. *Effects on pulmonary system.* Positive MAP decreases the pulmonary shunt and ventilation perfusion mismatch. It opens up collapsed alveoli and maintains them in open state (alveolar recruitment). However, excessive mean airway pressure can over distend alveoli, increase pulmonary vascular resistance and lead to barotrauma. Volutrauma (excessive tidal volume), atelectotrauma (cyclical opening and closing of alveoli) and biotrauma are other mechanisms of ventilator induced lung injury. Excess of inspired oxygen can lead to oxygen toxicity. Prolonged mechanical ventilation also predisposes to ventilator associated pneumonia by promoting colonization of respiratory tract by bacteria originating from oropharynx or gastro intestinal tract.

3. *Cardiac effects.* Higher MAP interferes with venous return and right heart filling. The increased pulmonary vascular resistance can interfere with left ventricular filling. Both can decrease cardiac output and lead to hypotension necessitating the use of volume replacement and vasopressors.

4. *Renal effects.* Urine output may decrease secondary to decreased cardiac output or reduced atrial natriuretic hormone release.

5. *Gastrointestinal effects.* Gastric distension and stress ulcers can occur. Infants and children require nasogastric feeding or parenteral nutrition. Inadequate intake of proteins and calories lead to catabolism of respiratory muscles and excessive feeding with carbohydrates leads to increased CO_2 production. Maintaining gastric acidity is useful in preventing ventilator associated pneumonia.

6. In children with head injury or cerebral edema, the higher mean airway pressure can *raise intracranial pressure* by compromising cerebral venous return

7. *Patient ventilator asynchrony.* Lack of synchrony can result in patient fighting the ventilator due to inappropriate ventilator settings or choice of mode of ventilator.

57.10 Ventilator Emergencies

The common causes of sudden deterioration in the condition of a ventilated child can be remembered by the acronym DOPE.

D: Displacement of the tube
O: Obstruction of the tube
P: Pneumothorax
E: Equipment failure

Common problems that can be encountered during the course of mechanical ventilation are listed below[84].

(a) Acute respiratory distress
(b) Hypoxemia or sudden desaturation
(c) Acute hypercarbia
(d) Hypotension
(e) Pulmonary hemorrhage

1. **Acute respiratory distress.** This is manifested as tachypnea, increased work of breathing, chest retractions, use of accessory muscles of respiration, tachycardia and hypotension. Possible causes include equipment failure, endotracheal tube issues and disease-related causes. If patient shows improvement after being removed from the ventilator and on hand bagging, an equipment failure is likely. If there is no improvement after being bagged, check tube position. Displacement of the tube above the vocal cords or into the right main stem bronchus or obstruction of the tube by secretions are the common tube problems. Bronchospasm, pneumonia, pulmonary edema and air leak like pneumothorax can lead to dyspnea and patient discomfort. Clinical examination and chest X-ray can help in making a diagnosis. Appropriate interventions include use of bronchodilators, treatment of the underlying condition that leads to pulmonary edema like control of cardiac failure, fluid restriction, diuretics and needle aspiration or chest tube drainage in cases of symptomatic pneumothorax.

Another cause of increased work of breathing is dynamic hyperinflation (DH) or auto-PEEP. If the ventilator delivers a breath before the patient has exhaled fully, this will lead to air trapping and the lung cannot empty to the FRC. In normal circumstances the end expiratory pressure equals atmospheric pressure. In the presence of dynamic hyper inflation the alveolar pressure remains positive relative to atmospheric pressure. The DH may be the consequence of any factor that prevents adequate exhalation within the allotted time like, short expiratory time, higher respiratory rate or higher tidal volume. When DH exists, the work of breathing is high because the patient has to generate pressure equal to the level of auto-PEEP plus the negative inspiratory flow to trigger the ventilator. Strategies for decreasing DH include facilitating expiration by increasing the expiratory time, decreasing the rate and accepting a higher $PaCO_2$ (permissive hypercapnia). Finally, adding external PEEP (equal to 75%-85% of the auto-PEEP) can decrease work of breathing and patient distress.

Another important cause for a patient fighting a ventilator is inadequate pain relief or inadequate sedation. However, before using sedatives or muscle paralysis one should rule out potentially remediable and life threatening aforementioned causes.

2. **Hypoxemia and hypercarbia.** The approach is similar to a patient presenting with acute respiratory distress.

3. **Hypotension.** Common causes of hypotension include hypovolemia, myocardial dysfunction, and impairment of venous return due to higher mean airway pressure and sepsis/systemic inflammatory response syndrome. Medications like sedatives and muscle relaxants can also produce hypotension by decreasing the vascular tone. Treatment should be aimed at correcting the underlying cause. In cases where higher MAP is needed for adequate oxygenation, adequate volume loading and use of inotropes should be considered.

4. **Pulmonary hemorrhage.** The main causes include pulmonary edema, trauma to trachea due to repeated suctioning, necrotising pneumonia, tracheobronchitis, pulmonary embolism, bleeding disorders, pulmonary artery catheters etc. Treatment is based on the underlying cause. Conditions that lead to a decrease in lung compliance like pulmonary edema or pneumonia need a higher PEEP to maintain oxygenation.

Pneumothorax. Risk factors for the development of pneumothorax in mechanically ventilated patients include use of high MAP, prolonged Ti, patient ventilator asynchrony and the presence of an underlying lung condition like MAS, PIE, pulmonary hypoplasia etc. Occurrence of a pneumothorax in mechanically ventilated patients is manifest by an acute onset of respiratory distress, cyanosis, episodes of apnea or bradycardia, decreased air entry in the affected side, mediastinal shift and hypotension. Transillumination may reveal increased transmission of light in the affected side. However, identification of pneumothorax may be difficult in ventilated patients. With volume ventilation, the peak airway pressure progressively increases producing a high pressure alarm. With PCV, the delivered tidal volumes decrease progressively since peak aiway pressure is constant. Attention to the peak pressures and delivered VTs and appropriate setting up of alarms are essential to detect complications early. Iatrogenic pneumothoraces due to positive pressure mechanical ventilation may lead to the development of a bronchopleural fistula or a tension pneumothorax[85]. These patients require needle aspiration or chest tube insertion and simple observation is not adequate[86].

Needling of the chest is performed using a butterfly needle or intravenous cannula in the second intercostal space in the midclavicular line. The anterior axillary line between the 4th or 5th intercostal space (Buelau position) is safe for performing thoracostomy in preterm and term infants[87]. Appropriate sized chest tube is 10 Fr in small infants, 12 Fr and for bigger infants and larger size for children. Although single and two bottle patient drainage units are available, the commercial three compartments PDU offer more advantages. In this arrangement, one compartment acts as a fluid collection bottle, the second as a water seal that prevents aspiration of air back into the pleural space, and the third as a pressure-regulating chamber, all incorporated into one disposable plastic unit[88].

Patients requiring chest tube drainage on a mechanical ventilator require close monitoring. Bubbling should be constant in the pressure regulating chamber, otherwise the amount of suction applied to the system is unknown. Air should not bubble from the water seal chamber unless there is a persistent airleak (pneumothorax, broncho-pleural fistula).

Leaks in the chest tube system can also produce bubbling in the chamber in the absence of air leaks.

Patients on positive pressure ventilation are at a high risk of tension pneumothorax if the tube is clamped or obstructed. Hence clamping the chest tube should be done only under close monitoring prior to chest tube removal. If clamping does not result in accumulation of pneumothorax, the chest tube can be safely removed.

57.11 Non-invasive Ventilation

Non-invasive ventilation (NIV) is the delivery of ventilatory support without the need for an invasive artificial airway. The advantages of NIV include avoiding the complications of endotracheal intubation, lesser need for sedation and increased patient autonomy. Non invasive strategies include continuous positive airway pressure, Bi level positive airway pressure and nasal intermittent positive pressure ventilation.

57.11.1 Continuous positive airway pressure

In CPAP positive pressure is applied to the airways of a spontaneously breathing baby throughout the respiratory cycle. CPAP and positive end-expiratory pressure (PEEP) support the airways and prevent atelectasis by avoiding alveolar collapse to a level below functional residual capacity (FRC). CPAP splints the upper airway. It also alters the shape of the diaphragm and increases diaphragmatic activity. It improves lung compliance and decreases airway resistance, improves ventilation-perfusion mismatch and reduces oxygen requirements with subsequent reduction in the work of breathing. CPAP conserves surfactant on the alveolar surface. The indications for CPAP are listed below.

(i) In the delivery room, nCPAP is an acceptable alternative to endotracheal intubation and prophylactic surfactant therapy for preterm infants born between 25-28 weeks gestation.

(ii) Respiratory distress syndrome. Early CPAP therapy may decrease the need for intubation in infants with respiratory distress secondary to surfactant deficiency.

(iii) Post extubation period. Direct extubation to CPAP in infants decreases the need for reintubation by preventing atelectasis and decreasing apnea.

(iv) Obstructive sleep apnea. In older children CPAP can be used in OSA, to splint the upper airway. CPAP therapy has shown to improve sleep architecture, day time sleepiness, neuro-cognitive function and quality of life.

CPAP delivery devices

CPAP can be delivered through an endotracheal tube (not used because of increased resistance), long nasopharyngeal tube and single nasal prong and an ETT cut to a shorter length. The nasal mask and short binasal prongs are more commonly used in neonates because they can fit snugly to the nose and cause less trauma and better seal.

CPAP generating devices[89]

Bubble CPAP. Bubble-CPAP involves a source of gas flow (typically 6–8 L per minute in a neonate), an air-oxygen blender, humidifier, and a T-piece, the expiratory arm of which is inserted in a bottle of water[90]. The depth of immersion determines the CPAP pressure delivered. The loss of pressure due to a large leak around the prongs or prong dislodgement, is detectable by the disappearance of the bubbling. Bubble CPAP is characterized by wide, noisy variations in peak-to-peak intra-prong pressures and tubing submersion depth is a highly inaccurate and unreliable estimate of actual delivered B-NCPAP[91]. Although the system is inexpensive and easy to use, careful monitoring is essential to avoid adverse events like pneumothorax[92].

Ventilator CPAP. CPAP can be delivered by a ventilator using the PEEP control. Ventilators maintain the delivered CPAP pressure close to the set pressure by automatic adjustments at the expiratory valve[91].

Variable flow CPAP system. They include the infant flow driver and the Arabella system. The infant flow driver has a conventional flow source with a manometer. The desired CPAP pressure is controlled directly by adjusting the flow. Pressure in the system is generated at the level of the nasal device (Generator) via dual injector jets directed toward the nasal prongs. When the patient inspires, the Bernoulli effect of the jet injector converts the kinetic energy to pressure energy. During exhalation, the gases flip around through the expiratory limb due to Coanda effect. The constant gas flow maintains the CPAP pressure even during exhalation. More research is required to determine whether the IFD has clinically important benefits over less expensive bi-nasal systems[89].

Bilevel positive airway pressure. This non invasive mode differs from CPAP by a basic mechanism that during BiPAP, the patient breathes spontaneously at a high and low pressure levels[93]. BiPAP is delivered using a suitable nasal interface and a generator like infant flow advance and infant flow SIPAP. A high pressure (for SiPAP, max. 15 cm H_2O and IFD max. 11 cm H_2O), a low CPAP pressure (4-6 cm H_2O), rate (10-30/min) and Ti (0.5-1 second (the time that would be spent on high pressure level during each cycle) are the parameters that are set in the BiPAP. Compared to CPAP, BiPAP was shown to produce greater oxygen saturation and lower $PaCO_2$ in preterm babies. The improvement in oxygenation is due to the increased MAP during BiPAP and the improvement in ventilation might be attributed to the difference between the two pressure levels that produces two different FRCs. This alteration induces a small tidal volume[93].

57.11.2 Non-invasive positive pressure ventilation (NPPV)

There is a growing interest in NPPV in neonates because; about half of all infants started on CPAP for RDS may fail such a therapy and require intubation and surfactant therapy and about a third of these infants may fail extubation to CPAP[89].

NIPPV is accomplished by using a nasal interface like a tight-fitting mask or prongs and a positive pressure ventilator or specialized devices like infant flow advance. This technique is well established in adults and children where tight fitting masks and flow sensors can be used for synchronization. However, in neonates these interfaces do not achieve adequate seal and the use of flow sensors is not possible in the presence of air leak[94]. The exact mechanism of action of NIPPV is uncertain as there is little evidence that the delivered pressures result in chest rise.

The devices that have been used to provide NIPPV include conventional ventilators and special devices like the Infant Flow SiPAP and Infant Flow Advance. There are no recommended settings for NIPPV in infants. In one study[95] babies extubated to SNIPPV received synchronized IMV at the same rate as they were receiving before extubation, PIP was increased by 2 to 4 cm H_2O, whereas the PEEP was kept ≤ 5 cm H_2O. FiO_2 was adjusted to maintain oxygen saturations 90 to 96% on pulse oximetry. The flow rate was kept at 8 to 10 L/min. In these babies a nasogastric tube was placed open to the atmosphere to avoid gastric distension[95].

There is growing evidence that the use of NIPPV decreases the rate of extubation failure in preterm infants and can be considered as a primary mode of support to reduce the need for intubation in RDS[89]. It is also used in the treatment of obstructive sleep apnea in older children.

57.11.3 Nasal cannulae

Low flow rates (0.5-2 L/min) are generally used to deliver oxygen. The gases may or may not be humidified. Non humidified gases dry out the nasal mucosa, and cause obstruction and bleeding. High flows heated humidified nasal cannulae deliver flow greater than 2 L/min and are used to deliver some pressure in addition to oxygen. However, pressures delivered are highly variable and depend on the size of the infant's nose, the size of the cannula and the presence of leak. In preterm infants there is a possibility of high pressures being transmitted with flows exceeding 2 L/min. Until more data is available experts recommend using CPAP rather than high flows to deliver pressure[89, 96].

57.12 Ventilator Induced Lung Injury

Mechanical ventilation may lead to injury of the lungs or exacerbate the pre-existing condition that led to the need for mechanical ventilation. Ventilator-induced lung injury (VILI) involves alveolar structural damage, pulmonary edema, inflammation, and fibrosis and it is associated with surfactant dysfunction[97]. Recovery includes clearance of pulmonary edema and alveolar structural repair. The pathophysiology of ventilator induced lung injury is summarized in Table 57.11.

Table 57.11 Pathophysiology of VILI

- ❑ Lung injury
  - Cellular and structural damage
  - Alveolar edema
- ❑ Inflammation
- ❑ Fibrosis and recovery
- ❑ Edema clearance
- ❑ Repair
  - Removal of intra-alveolar debris
  - Restoration of the extracellular matrix
  - Re-epithelialization of the alveolar surface
  - Formation of new capillaries

Various predisposing factors for VILI include *Volutrauma* which refers to the damage caused by overdistension of the lung by delivery of too much gas, *Barotrauma*, or excessive pressure, which may damage airway epithelium and disrupt alveoli, *Atelectotrauma* which refers to the damage caused by the repeated opening and closing (the cycle of recruitment and subsequent de-recruitment) of lung units, *Biotrauma* which is a collective term to describe the injurious effects of infection and inflammation (and oxidative stress) on the developing lung and *Rheotrauma* which refers to injury caused by inappropriate airway flow. In the preterm lung, VILI may interfere with lung development that occurs after birth.

Adopting lung protective ventilator management strategies to avoid the "mechanical" elements of ventilator induced lung injury is specially important in ventilating premature lungs because they are more susceptible to lung injury. The ideal mode of ventilation should maintain adequate and consistent tidal volume and minute ventilation at low airway pressures. This can be accomplished by ventilating the lung close to the normal functional residual capacity. This occurs at the midportion of the inflation limb of the pressure-volume loop, where compliance is greatest and the zones of lung injury can be avoided.

Kraybill et al[98] in 1989 reported that infants with the highest levels of carbon dioxide had the lowest incidence of CLD . This led to the concept of permissive hypercapnia, its rationale as a protective lung strategy being that it may decrease volutrauma, decrease the duration of positive pressure ventilation, reduce alveolar ventilation, reduce complications associated with hypocapnia, and increase oxygen unloading from hemoglobin at the tissue level.

In mechanical ventilation, patient-ventilator asynchrony results in complications like inefficient gas exchange, gas trapping, air leaks and irregular cerebral blood flow velocity. The advent of miniature transducers and sophisticated microprocessor based mechanical ventilators ushered the era of patient triggered ventilation (PTV) with synchronous modes. Avoidance of asynchronous breathing may result in the need for less pressure, facilitate weaning by making pressure the primary weaning variable, and significantly reduce gas trapping and air leaks, all of which may help in reducing VILI.

REFERENCES

1. Trubuhovich RV. Further commentary on Denmark's 1952-53 poliomyelitis epidemic, especially regarding mortality; with a correction. *Acta Anaesthesiol Scand* 2004 Nov;48 (10):1310-1315.

2. Bone RC, Eubanks DH. The basis and basics of mechanical ventilation. *Dis Mon* 1991 Jun; 37(6): 321-406.

3. Slutsky AS. Consensus conference on mechanical ventilation—January 28-30, 1993 at Northbrook, Illinois, USA. Part I. European Society of Intensive Care Medicine, the ACCP and the SCCM. *Intensive Care Med* 1994; 20(1):64-79.

4. Freedman N. Treatment of obstructive sleep apnea syndrome. *Clin Chest Med* 2010 Jun; 31(2):187-201.

5. Lands LC. Applying physiology to conventional mechanical ventilation. *Pediatr Respir Rev* 2006; 7 Suppl 1:S33-S36.

6. Sandur S, Stoller JK. Pulmonary complications of mechanical ventilation. *Clin Chest Med* 1999 Jun; 20(2): 223-247.

7. Gattinoni L, Protti A, Caironi P, Carlesso E. Ventilator-induced lung injury: the anatomical and physiological framework. *Crit Care Med* 2010 Oct;38(10 Suppl): S539-S548.

8. Weibel ER. Morphometry of the human lung: the state of the art after two decades. *Bull Eur Physiopathol Respir* 1979 Sep-Oct;15(5):999-1013.

9. Nunn JF, Campbell EJ, Peckett BW. Anatomical subdivisions of the volume of respiratory dead space and effect of position of the jaw. *J Appl Physiol* 1959 Mar;14(2):174-176.

10. Numa AH, Newth CJ. Anatomic dead space in infants and children. *J Appl Physiol* 1996 May;80(5):1485-1489.

11. West JB, (ed.) Respiratory Physiology- The Essentials. 7th ed. *Philadelphia, USA: Lippincott Williams and Wilkins;* 2004.

12. Ferris BG, Jr., Mead J, Opie LH. Partitioning of respiratory flow resistance in man. *J Appl Physiol* 1964 Jul;19:653-658.

13. Chatburn RL. Understanding mechanical ventilators. *Expert Rev Respir Med* 2010 Dec;4(6):809-819.

14. Chatburn RL. Classification of mechanical ventilators. *Respir Care* 1992 Sep; 37(9):1009-25.

15. Donn SM. Neonatal ventilators: how do they differ? *J Perinatol* 2009 May;29 Suppl 2:S73-S78.

16. Sarkar S, Donn SM. In support of pressure support. *Clin Perinatol* 2007 Mar; 34(1):117-128.

17. Hasan A, (ed.) The Conventional Modes of Mechanical Ventilation: *Springer;* 2010.

18. Wheeler K, Klingenberg C, McCallion N, Morley CJ, Davis PG. Volume-targeted versus pressure-limited ventilation in the neonate. *Cochrane Database Syst Rev* 2010(11):CD003666.

19. Klingenberg C, Wheeler KI, Davis PG, Morley CJ. A practical guide to neonatal volume guarantee ventilation. *J Perinatol* 2011 Jul 14.

20. Keszler M, Abubakar K. Volume guarantee: stability of tidal volume and incidence of hypocarbia. *Pediatr Pulmonol* 2004 Sep;38(3):240-245.

21. Modrykamien A, Chatburn RL, Ashton RW. Airway pressure release ventilation: an alternative mode of mechanical ventilation in acute respiratory distress syndrome. *Cleve Clin J Med* 2011 Feb; 78(2):101-110.

22. Frawley PM, Habashi NM. Airway pressure release ventilation: theory and practice. *AACN Clin Issues* 2001 May; 12(2):234-246.

23. Guthrie SO, Lynn C, Lafleur BJ, Donn SM, Walsh WF. A crossover analysis of mandatory minute ventilation compared to synchronized intermittent mandatory ventilation in neonates. *J Perinatol* 2005 Oct; 25(10):643-646.

24. Carvalho CR, de Paula Pinto Schettino G, Maranhao B, Bethlem EP. Hyperoxia and lung disease. *Curr Opin Pulm Med* 1998 Sep; 4(5):300-304.

25. Maltepe E, Saugstad OD. Oxygen in health and disease: regulation of oxygen homeostasis: clinical implications. *Pediatr Res* 2009 Mar; 65(3):261-268.

26. Finer N, Leone T. Oxygen saturation monitoring for the preterm infant: the evidence basis for current practice. *Pediatr Res* 2009 Apr; 65(4):375-380.

27. Konduri GG, Kim UO. Advances in the diagnosis and management of persistent pulmonary hypertension of the newborn. *Pediatr Clin North Amer* 2009 June; 56(3):579-600.

28. Hickling KG. The pressure-volume curve is greatly modified by recruitment. A mathematical model of ARDS lungs. *Amer J Respir Crit Care Med* 1998 Jul; 158(1):194-202.

29. Jubran A, Tobin MJ. Monitoring during mechanical ventilation. *Clin Chest Med* 1996 Sep;17(3):453-473.

30. Becker MA, Donn SM. Real-time pulmonary graphic monitoring. *Clin Perinatol* 2007 Mar; 34(1):1-17.

31. Cronin JH. High frequency ventilator therapy for newborns. *J Intensive Care Med* 1994 Mar-Apr; 9(2):71-85.

32. Slutsky AS, Drazen JM. Ventilation with small tidal volumes. *N Engl J Med* 2002 Aug 29; 347(9):630-631.

33. Stawicki SP, Goyal M, Sarani B. High-frequency oscillatory ventilation (HFOV) and airway pressure release ventilation (APRV): a practical guide. *J Intensive Care Med* 2009 Jul-Aug; 24(4):215-229.

34. Musk GC, Polglase GR, Bunnell JB, McLean CJ, Nitsos I, Song Y, *et al.* High positive end-expiratory pressure during high-frequency jet ventilation improves oxygenation and ventilation in preterm lambs. *Pediatr Res* 2011 Apr; 69(4):319-324.

35. Friedlich P, Subramanian N, Sebald M, Noori S, Seri I. Use of high-frequency jet ventilation in neonates with hypoxemia refractory to high-frequency oscillatory ventilation. *J Matern Fetal Neonatal Med* 2003 June; 13(6):398-402.

36. Hemmila MR, Napolitano LM. Severe respiratory failure: advanced treatment options. *Crit Care Med* 2006 Sep; 34(9 Suppl): S278-S290.

37. Lampland A L MM (ed.). High Frequency Ventilation. 5th ed. *Missouri: Elsevier, Saunders;* 2011.

38. Keszler M, Donn SM, Bucciarelli RL, Alverson DC, Hart M, Lunyong V, *et al.* Multicenter controlled trial comparing high-frequency jet ventilation and conventional mechanical ventilation in newborn infants with pulmonary interstitial emphysema. *J Pediatr* 1991 Jul; 119(1 Pt 1):85-93.

39. Ambalavanan N, Carlo WA. Ventilatory strategies in the prevention and management of bronchopulmonary dysplasia. *Semin Perinatol* 2006 Aug; 30(4):192-199.

40. De Paoli AG, Morley C, Davis PG. Nasal CPAP for neonates: what do we know in 2003? *Arch Dis Child Fetal Neonatal Ed* 2003 May; 88(3):F168-F172.

41. Jobe AH, Bancalari E. Bronchopulmonary dysplasia. *Amer J Respir Crit Care Med* 2001 Jun;163(7):1723-1729.

42. Schmidt B, Roberts RS, Davis P, Doyle LW, Barrington KJ, Ohlsson A, *et al.* Caffeine therapy for apnea of prematurity. *N Engl J Med* 2006 May 18; 354 (20): 2112-2121.

43. Goldsmith JP. Continuous positive airway pressure and conventional mechanical ventilation in the treatment of meconium aspiration syndrome. *J Perinatol* 2008 Dec; 28 Suppl 3:S49-S55.

44. Mourani PM, Ivy DD, Gao D, Abman SH. Pulmonary vascular effects of inhaled nitric oxide and oxygen tension in bronchopulmonary dysplasia. *Amer J Respir Crit Care Med* 2004 Nov 1;170(9):1006-1013.

45. Ambalavanan N SR, Carlo W (Ed.) Ventilatory Strategies. 4th ed. *Philadelphia: WB Saunders;* 2003.

46. Walsh-Sukys MC, Tyson JE, Wright LL, Bauer CR, Korones SB, Stevenson DK, *et al.* Persistent pulmonary hypertension of the newborn in the era before nitric oxide: practice variation and outcomes. *Pediatrics* 2000 Jan;105(1 Pt 1):14-20.

47. Van Meurs K. Is surfactant therapy beneficial in the treatment of the term newborn infant with congenital diaphragmatic hernia? *J Pediatr* 2004 Sep;145(3): 312-316.

48. Kumar P, McKean MC. Evidence based paediatrics: review of BTS guidelines for the management of community acquired pneumonia in children. *J Infect* 2004 Feb; 48(2):134-318.

49. Pride NB, Permutt S, Riley RL, Bromberger-Barnea B. Determinants of maximal expiratory flow from the lungs. *J Appl Physiol* 1967 Nov; 23(5):646-662.

50. Sarnaik AP, Daphtary KM, Meert KL, Lieh-Lai MW, Heidemann SM. Pressure-controlled ventilation in children with severe status asthmaticus. *Pediatr Crit Care Med* 2004 Mar; 5(2):133-138.

Section 6

51. Saharan S, Lodha R, Kabra SK. Management of status asthmaticus in children. *Indian J Pediatr* 2010 Dec; 77(12):1417-1423.

52. Krieger BP. Hyperinflation and intrinsic positive end-expiratory pressure: less room to breathe. *Respiration* 2009; 77(3):344-350.

53. MacIntyre NR, Cheng KC, McConnell R. Applied PEEP during pressure support reduces the inspiratory threshold load of intrinsic PEEP. *Chest* 1997 Jan; 111(1):188-193.

54. Pelosi P, Gattinoni L. Respiratory mechanics in ARDS: a siren for physicians? *Intensive Care Med* 2000 June; 26(6):653-656.

55. Hess RD, Kacmarek, M Robert, (Ed.) Acute Lung Injury and Acute Respiratory Distress Syndrome. 2nd ed; *McGraw-Hill;* 2002.

56. Saharan S, Lodha R, Kabra SK. Management of acute lung injury/ARDS. *Indian J Pediatr* 2010 Nov; 77(11):1296-1302.

57. Pelosi P, Brazzi L, Gattinoni L. Prone position in acute respiratory distress syndrome. *Eur Respir J* 2002 Oct;20(4):1017-1028.

58. Curley MA, Thompson JE, Arnold JH. The effects of early and repeated prone positioning in pediatric patients with acute lung injury. *Chest* 2000 Jul; 118(1):156-163.

59. Adhikari NK, Burns KE, Friedrich JO, Granton JT, Cook DJ, Meade MO. Effect of nitric oxide on oxygenation and mortality in acute lung injury: systematic review and meta-analysis. *BMJ* 2007 Apr 14; 334(7597):779.

60. Prabhakaran P. Acute respiratory distress syndrome. *Indian Pediatr* 2010 Oct; 47(10): 861-868.

61. Duffett M, Choong K, Ng V, Randolph A, Cook DJ. Surfactant therapy for acute respiratory failure in children: a systematic review and meta-analysis. *Crit Care* 2007;11(3):66.

62. Brochard L, Rauss A, Benito S, Conti G, Mancebo J, Rekik N, *et al.* Comparison of three methods of gradual withdrawal from ventilatory support during weaning from mechanical ventilation. *Amer J Respir Crit Care Med* 1994 Oct;150(4):896-903.

63. Blackwood B, Alderdice F, Burns KE, Cardwell CR, Lavery G, O'Halloran P. Protocolized versus non-protocolized weaning for reducing the duration of mechanical ventilation in critically ill adult patients. *Cochrane Database Syst Rev.* 2010(5):CD006904.

64. Sinha SK, Donn SM. Weaning newborns from mechanical ventilation. *Semin Neonatol* 2002 Oct; 7(5):421-428.

65. Wittekamp BH, van Mook WN, Tjan DH, Zwaveling JH, Bergmans DC. Clinical review: post-extubation laryngeal edema and extubation failure in critically ill adult patients. *Crit Care* 2009;13(6):233.

66. Davies MW, Davis PG. Nebulized racemic epinephrine for extubation of newborn infants. *Cochrane Database Syst Rev* 2002(1):CD000506.

67. Nutman J, Brooks LJ, Deakins KM, Baldesare KK, Witte MK, Reed MD. Racemic versus l-epinephrine aerosol in the treatment of postextubation laryngeal edema: results from a prospective, randomized, double-blind study. *Crit Care Med* 1994 Oct; 22(10): 1591-1594.

68. Khemani RG, Randolph A, Markovitz B. Corticosteroids for the prevention and treatment of post-extubation stridor in neonates, children and adults. *Cochrane Database Syst Rev* 2009(3):CD001000.

69. Gardner DL, Shirland L. Evidence-based guideline for suctioning the intubated neonate and infant. *Neonatal Netw* 2009 Sep-Oct;28(5):281-302.

70. Muscedere J, Dodek P, Keenan S, Fowler R, Cook D, Heyland D. Comprehensive evidence-based clinical practice guidelines for ventilator-associated pneumonia: prevention. *J Crit Care* 2008 Mar;23(1):126-137.

71. Reines HD, Sade RM, Bradford BF, Marshall J. Chest physiotherapy fails to prevent postoperative atelectasis in children after cardiac surgery. *Ann Surg* 1982 Apr; 195(4):451-455.

72. Vandenplas Y, Diericx A, Blecker U, Lanciers S, Deneyer M. Esophageal pH monitoring data during chest physiotherapy. *J Pediatr Gastroenterol Nutr* 1991 Jul;13(1):23-26.

73. Raval D, Yeh TF, Mora A, Cuevas D, Pyati S, Pildes RS. Chest physiotherapy in preterm infants with RDS in the first 24 hours of life. *J Perinatol* 1987 Fall;7(4):301-304.

74. Krause MF, Hoehn T. Chest physiotherapy in mechanically ventilated children: a review. *Crit Care Med* 2000 May; 28(5):1648-51.

75. Fessler HE, Talmor DS. Should prone positioning be routinely used for lung protection during mechanical ventilation? *Respir Care* 2010 Jan; 55(1):88-99.

76. Girard TD, Bernard GR. Mechanical ventilation in ARDS: a state-of-the-art review. *Chest* 2007 Mar; 131(3):921-929.

77. Sweet DG, Halliday HL. The use of surfactant in 2009. *Arch Dis Child Educ Pract Ed* 2009 Jun; 94(3):78-83.

78. Gizzi C, Papoff P, Barbara CS, Cangiano G, Midulla F, Moretti C. Old and new uses of surfactant. *J Matern Fetal Neonatal Med* 2010 Oct;23 Suppl 3:41-44.

79. DiBlasi RM, Myers TR, Hess DR. Evidence-based clinical practice guideline: inhaled nitric oxide for neonates with acute hypoxic respiratory failure. *Respir Care* 2010 Dec; 55(12):1717-45.

80. Finer NN, Sun JW, Rich W, Knodel E, Barrington KJ. Randomized, prospective study of low-dose versus high-dose inhaled nitric oxide in the neonate with hypoxic

respiratory failure. *Pediatrics* 2001 Oct; 108(4): 949-955.

81. Finer NN, Barrington KJ. Nitric oxide for respiratory failure in infants born at or near term. *Cochrane Database Syst Rev* 2006(4): CD000399.

82. Dhand R. Special problems in aerosol delivery: artificial airways. *Respir Care* 2000 Jun;45(6):636-645.

83. Dhand R, Tobin MJ. Inhaled bronchodilator therapy in mechanically ventilated patients. *Amer J Respir Crit Care Med* 1997 Jul;156(1):3-10.

84. Keith RL, Pierson DJ. Complications of mechanical ventilation. A bedside approach. *Clin Chest Med* 1996 Sep; 17(3):439-451.

85. Baumann MH, Sahn SA. Medical management and therapy of bronchopleural fistulas in the mechanically ventilated patient. *Chest* 1990 Mar;97(3):721-728.

86. Haynes D, Baumann MH. Management of pneumothorax. *Semin Respir Crit Care Med* 2010 Dec; 31(6):769-780.

87. Eifinger F, Lenze M, Brisken K, Welzing L, Roth B, Koebke J. The anterior to midaxillary line between the 4th or 5th intercostal space (Buelau position) is safe for the use of thoracostomy tubes in preterm and term infants. *Paediatr Anaesth* 2009 Jun;19(6):612-617.

88. Bar-El Y, Ross A, Kablawi A, Egenburg S. Potentially dangerous negative intrapleural pressures generated by ordinary pleural drainage systems. *Chest* 2001 Feb; 119(2):511-514.

89. Davis PG, Morley CJ, Owen LS. Non-invasive respiratory support of preterm neonates with respiratory distress: continuous positive airway pressure and nasal intermittent positive pressure ventilation. *Semin Fetal Neonatal Med* 2009 Feb; 14(1):14-20.

90. Koyamaibole L, Kado J, Qovu JD, Colquhoun S, Duke T. An evaluation of bubble-CPAP in a neonatal unit in a developing country: effective respiratory support that can be applied by nurses. *J Trop Pediatr* 2006 Aug; 52(4):249-53.

91. Kahn DJ, Courtney SE, Steele AM, Habib RH. Unpredictability of delivered bubble nasal continuous positive airway pressure: role of bias flow magnitude and nares-prong air leaks. *Pediatr Res* 2007 Sep; 62 (3):343-347.

92. Gunlemez A, Isken T. Bubble CPAP must be used with care to avoid harm. *Arch Dis Child Fetal Neonatal Ed* 2008 Mar; 93(2):F170-F171.

93. Migliori C, Motta M, Angeli A, Chirico G. Nasal bilevel vs. continuous positive airway pressure in preterm infants. *Pediatr Pulmonol* 2005 Nov;40(5):426-430.

94. Owen LS, Morley CJ, Dawson JA, Davis PG. Effects of non-synchronised nasal intermittent positive pressure ventilation on spontaneous breathing in preterm infants. *Arch Dis Child Fetal Neonatal Ed* Feb 20, 2011.

95. Bhandari V, Gavino RG, Nedrelow JH, Pallela P, Salvador A, Ehrenkranz RA, et al. A randomized controlled trial of synchronized nasal intermittent positive pressure ventilation in RDS. *J Perinatol* 2007 Nov; 27(11):697-703.

96. Finer NN. Nasal cannula use in the preterm infant: oxygen or pressure? *Pediatrics* 2005 Nov;116(5): 1216-1217.

97. Clark RH, Gerstmann DR, Jobe AH, Moffitt ST, Slutsky AS, Yoder BA. Lung injury in neonates: causes, strategies for prevention, and long-term consequences. *J Pediatr* 2001 Oct;139(4):478-486.

98. Kraybill EN, Runyan DK, Bose CL, Khan JH. Risk factors for chronic lung disease in infants with birth weights of 751 to 1000 grams. *J Pediatr* 1989 Jul; 115(1):115-120.

Section 6

58

Emergency Procedures

Anu Thukral, Ashok K Deorari and Meharban Singh

Emergency procedures in children are often life-saving if performed in time and with due precautions. In general it is more time consuming to carry out a procedure in a child compared to an adult. Each unsuccessful attempt is traumatic not only for the child but also for the parents, doctors, nurses and assistants. The procedures are best learnt by observations and repetitive performance. The inherent risk of some procedures precludes their practice except upon a cadaver. Other procedures can be electively performed for the first time under optimal conditions and due supervision, on a living child who requires the procedure, keeping in mind that the operator may have to perform the same procedure in case of an emergency.

Most procedures are more difficult in infants because of their smaller size, and lack of cooperation. Patience is of vital importance and availability of an experienced assistant is an asset. A common problem in all pediatric procedures is the proper restraint of the infant. The restriction of an arm or leg movement is accomplished by swaddling the patient in a sheet. The usual "mummying" can be done by placing the infant on a sheet or blanket. The edge of the blanket is wrapped around the extended arm and trunk and tucked beneath the child. The opposite corner then immobilizes the other arm along the trunk and completely envelops the baby. The edges may be secured tightly using safety pins or leucoplast (Figure 58.1).

It is essential that consent is obtained prior to any procedure from the parent/ legal guardian of the child. It is best to have a flexible attitude as to whether the child's parents should be allowed during the procedure or not. Some children are anxious and need parental support. The nature of the procedure and operator's own confidence in coping with presence of parents should also be considered. It is advisable to be honest to the children if they are in a position to understand, and they should be told about the procedure. Talking to

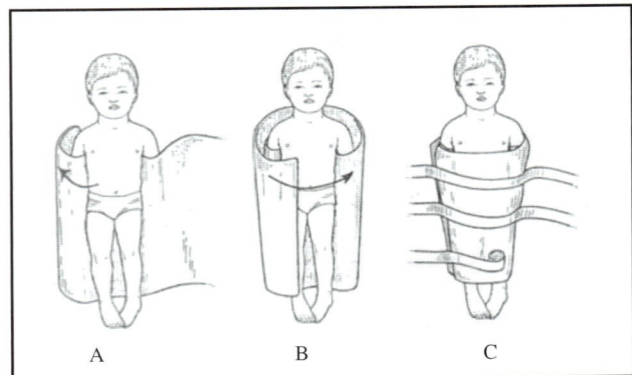

Figure 58.1 Mummy wrap of a child with a bed sheet

children during the procedure is often reassuring to them and helps to elicit better cooperation while the procedure is being conducted. It is always helpful to allay their fears about the procedure by affectionate and gentle handling.

For the painful and frightening procedures, it is better to sedate the child or give general anesthesia. Local infiltration of 1% lidocaine through skin, subcutaneous tissue, muscle and right upto the site to be punctured often reduces pain. Make sure that lidocaine is not injected into the blood vessel. Some of the commonly used sedatives at different ages in children are listed in Table 58.1.

Venipunctures

The procedure is required for obtaining venous blood samples for laboratory determinations and culture studies.

Technique

In older children a methodical inspection of upper extremities is performed with a particular attention to antecubital area. Median cubital vein is large, accessible and suitable for venipuncture but not for setting an intravenous line. If it is not seen or palpated, attention is next turned to branches of the median or basilic veins as they course over the volar surface of the forearm. If these are also

	Table 58.1 Commonly used sedatives in children		
Age	**Drug**	**Dosage (per dose)**	**Route**
Upto 1 year	Chlorpromazine hydrochloride	0.5 mg/kg	PO, IM
	Promethazine hydrochloride	0.5 mg/kg	PO, IM
	Chloral hydrate	5-20 mg/kg	PO
	Tricolofos sodium	10-20 mg/kg	PO
1-5 years	Chlorpromazine hydrochloride	0.5-4.0 mg/kg	PO, IM
	Chloral hydrate	5-20 mg/kg	PO
	Diazepam	0.2 mg/kg	IV, PO
	Pethidine	1-2 mg/kg	IM, IV
	Morphine	0.05-0.2 mg/kg	IV, IM
All ages	"Lytic cocktail" containing		
	Pethidine or meperidine,	2 mg/kg (maximum 50 mg)	IV, IM
	Chlorpromazine and	1 mg/kg (maximum 25 mg)	IV, IM
	Promethazine	1 mg/kg (maximum 25 mg)	IV, IM
	Ketamine hydrochloride	1-4 mg/kg IV, 5-15 mg/kg IM	IV, IM
	Morphine	0.05-0.2 mg/kg	IV, IM

Adapted from Drug Dosages in Children by Singh M and Deorari AK, *CBS Publishers & Distributors Pvt Ltd, New Delhi,* 9th edition, 2015, pp 144-151.

indistinct, dorsum of hand is searched for a vein. Alternative sites are saphenous vein on the medial aspect of the ankle at the medial malleolus and veins on the dorsum of feet. Flicking or slapping of the veins does not cause engorgement of the veins and may cause pain and hematoma formation.

Tourniquet is placed proximal to the site where venipuncture is to be performed so as to occlude venous drainage. Warming of limb, rubbing of alcohol, or clenching of fist may help to make the vein prominent. Site is prepared aseptically using spirit-iodine-spirit. Skin must be allowed to dry spontaneously before venipuncture.

A. *Peripheral venipuncture.* It is attempted after ascertaining that specific tubes and containers are available for blood collection. Use the non dominant hand to apply distal traction on the skin to stabilize the vein in the subcutaneous tissue. The needle and syringe are held at 10-15 degree to the skin and needle is briskly introduced beneath the dermis and advanced towards the vein. Flow of blood into the syringe indicates a successful attempt. Gentle steady suction is applied to collect requisite amount of blood. Thereafter, release the tourniquet and remove the needle. A small sterile gauze or cotton is placed at the puncture site and gentle pressure is applied for 2-3 minutes.

Complications. Cellulitis, hematoma formation, thrombosis and phlebitis.

B. *Femoral venipuncture.* In view of the inherent risks of femoral venipuncture (due to its deep location), it should be used as a last resort for collection of blood samples in neonates and infants. *It should never be used for administration of fluids and drugs.* The baby is restrained in frog's position. The femoral artery is located with thumb just below the midpoint of inguinal ligament. The femoral vein lies medial to the artery. Skin is pierced about 1-2 cm below the inguinal ligament directly over the femoral vein and needle is advanced at an angle of 30-45 degree with the skin while maintaining gentle negative suction. If no blood is obtained while needle is pushed forward, suction should be maintained as the needle is being withdrawn. After the procedure it is essential to apply firm pressure over the site of venipuncture for at least three to five minutes to safeguard against oozing and hematoma.

Complications. Septic arthritis, osteomyelitis, hematoma, internal bleeding and arterial spasm

Section 6

are recognized complications of femoral venipunctures.

C. **External Jugular Venipuncture.** Relatively short and obese neck of infants makes this procedure rather difficult. The external jugular vein courses in a line from the angle of the mandible to the middle of clavicle. The infant is restrained in a supine position and his head and neck are suspended beyond the edge of the table. The head is rotated to one side and supported by an assistant while shoulders are maintained firmly on the table. The infant or child is stimulated to cry which causes engorgement of the vessel. As soon as the vein is spotted, the skin is pierced immediately, over the vessel and needle advanced into the lumen while maintaining suction with the syringe. After the procedure, gentle but sufficient pressure should be applied over the puncture site and baby should be held in an upright position for two to three minutes.

Venous Catheterization

Venous catheterization follows venipuncture and when both phlebotomy and venous access for infusion is needed the procedure is combined. Operator must select a vein based either on visualization or palpation. It is worthless attempting the procdure in a blind manner. Thorough examination of patient's extremities is often rewarding. The purpose for establishing the intravenous line determines the choice of site. In hypovolemic shock, the largest and shortest line will provide the most rapid access for administration of fluids. Alternatively, a patient who requires an intravenous access solely for administration of parenteral antibiotics should have an appropriate line to serve those requirements. It should be remembered that a small volume of fluid can be infused through a large line, but a large volume cannot be given through a small line.

A. **Peripheral percutaneous venous catheterization**

Parenteral administration of fluids and medications, sampling and total parenteral nutrition can be administered through a peripheral vein. The fluids and electrolyte solutions can be infused for several days with less risk of leakage and dislodgement. It is feasible to administer drugs in larger volumes without repeated punctures. Total parenteral nutrition can be achieved through medicuts to meet nutritional requirements.

Technique. The commonly used sites are the antecubital vein or basilic veins located on the medial aspect of the volar surface of the forearm. For selection of other veins, refer to venipunctures *vide supra.*

For scalp vein puncture, shave and prepare an area on the infant's scalp with usual aseptic measures. A rubber band may be placed around the head as a tourniquet which will make the veins prominent. Enter the vein from above downwards along the flow of blood. After the vein is entered cut the rubber band tourniquet.

Catheter selection

(i) *Winged needle.* Butterfly scalp vein sets are available in 2 cm length and 16-25 gauges. They are particularly useful in infants and younger children.

(ii) *Catheter over needle.* Angiocath and medicuts are available in 2-5 cm length and 12-24 gauge needle sizes. They are stable with longer life expectancy as venous conduits. They are useful for administration of blood products and drugs when rapid and prolonged infusion of fluids is necessary.

(iii) *Catheter inside needle unit.* Intracaths are available in catheter lengths of 20-60 cm. The introducing needle size ranges from 14 to 21 gauge and catheter with the enclosed needle ranges from 16 to 22 gauge. These catheters can be used in all those situations when the catheter-over-needle units are used. They are particularly useful to establish central venous pressure (CVP) line because of the length of catheter.

Size selection/Gauge selection

It is important to remember that the flow in a conduit is directly proportional to the radius of the conduit raised to the fourth power and is inversely proportional to the length of the cartheter. Thus, a large bore catheter of short length will deliver far more fluid per unit time than a similar catheter of a greater length. A central line is, therefore, not an optimal line for delivering large amounts of fluids. The type of fluid to be infused must also be considered. Blood and blood products will flow with difficulty through catheters smaller than 20 gauge.

Procedure. Use restraint appropriately but do not apply a tight tourniquet. Vein is inspected and palpated. A soft compressible vein assures that the vein is not sclerosed or phlebitic. Before puncturing, the operator should ensure that all the necessary items and solutions to be infused are ready at hand. Prepare the site aseptically using spirit-iodine-spirit. If patient is unduly anxious or concerned, local anesthetic using 1% lignocaine is infiltrated. Local anesthesia is generally not necessary if catheter size is 20 gauge or smaller. The operator uses his nondominant hand to apply traction on the skin to firmly anchor the vein in the subcutaneous tissue.

(a) *Scalp vein.* Scalp vein set is attached to a syringe containing heparinised saline and flushed. The heparinised saline solution should be freshly prepared because stock solution may get contaminated by pathogenic microbes. Grasp the rubber finger grip (butterfly) of the needle and pierce the skin gently. The needle course is directed just under, and almost parallel to the skin. Coming over the vein, pierce it while applying gentle negative pressure on the needle by the syringe. The blood would appear in the tube immediately upon entry of the vein. Sometimes with 24-27 gauge needle and when the patient is in shock, the blood may not show in the tubing. Slowly flush the needle with saline and look for swelling proximal to the site of needle insertion and adjust the flow rate. Secure the needle and tubing to the site with adhesive tape as shown in Figure 58.2. Check flow rate regularly to prevent under/over infusion. Measured volume infusion sets (burette set) and infusion pumps are ideal in younger children.

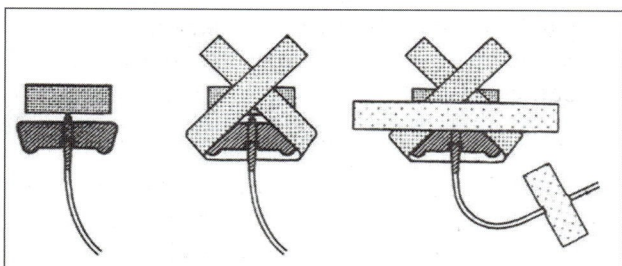

Figure 58.2 Technique to securely affix the butterfly needle

(b) *Catheter-needle.* If a large gauge catheter is to be used, the patient's skin may be pre-punctured or bored with an 18 gauge needle. This will facilitate passage of the plastic catheter through the dermis. The catheter is grasped between the thumb and index finger with its attached syringe resting against the palm of operator's hand. The vein may be approached from above, at a venous junction or from the side. The skin adjacent to the vein is briskly punctured with the needle-catheter

held approximately 10-15 degree to the skin or axis of the arm. Once beneath the dermis, the angle is narrowed so that the catheter is nearly flush with the axis of the vein. The catheter is advanced into the vein with the bevel facing up. When blood is seen in the needle hub, the catheter and needle are advanced along the course of the vein for additional 2-3 mm. If a syringe is attached to the catheter, it is aspirated to observe free return of blood. The plastic catheter is then advanced gently into the vein while the needle is held stationary. Slight pressure may be applied at the tip of the catheter to prevent backflow of blood while advancing the desired length of the catheter. The tourniquet is released, the needle is completely removed from the catheter and an intravenous solution is attached. Sterile dressing is placed at puncture site and the entry point of catheter. The catheter is secured by an adhesive tape. When scalp vein needle or catheter is removed, the site should be compressed for atleast two minutes and sterile dressing should then be applied.

Complications. Thrombosis and phlebitis followed by extravasations are the most common complications. Fluid overload may occur especially in neonates if measured volume burette or infusion pump is not used. Prolonged restraint is frequently necessary unless veins on the dorsum of the hand are used. This interferes with the activity of the child. Extravasations of fluid or blood must be identified early to prevent local complications. In neonates and compromised host, intravenous line may provide a source for nosocomial infections.

B. Subclavian vein catheterization

Indications. It is indicated for CVP monitoring, placement of Swan-Ganz line, percutaneous introduction of a pacemaker and rarely for intravenous infusion and hyper alimentation, hemodialysis and occasionally when it is impossible to establish peripheral venous access.

Position. The patient should be supine in a Trendelenburg position (10-20 degree elevation of feet) to distend the vein. The shoulders should be hyperextended by placing a rolled towel between the shoulder blades to elevate the vein more anteriorly. Head is rotated to the contra lateral side.

Anatomy. The subclavian vein lies immediately posterior to the medial segment of the clavicle. The vein follows a course running from the axilla, over the first rib and behind the clavicle at the junction of the medial and middle-thirds of the clavicle. It continues in the thorax to join the internal jugular vein and forms the innominate vein. The subclavian artery lies deep to it and is separated from it by the scalenus anterior muscle.

Procedure. Skin is prepared aseptically and allowed to dry. The angle formed by inter-section of the first rib and lower margin of clavicle is identified which is at the junction of medial and middle-thirds of clavicle. Subclavian vein is located at this point behind the clavicle and anterior to the first rib. Use a small caliber (18 to 20 gauge, 5 cm long) needle to localize the vein before proceeding with the 14 gauge needle. The needle should be directed 30 to 35 degree to the axis of the thorax towards a point 2 cm above the suprasternal notch. The smaller exploratory needle, attached to a 10 ml syringe, is advanced along this course to the inferior margin of the clavicle. When this is located, the needle should be directed downwards until it is just beneath the clavicle. Staying as close as possible to the inferior margin of the clavicle lessens the chances of pneumothorax. When the needle tip is beneath the clavicle, the angle formed by the needle shaft and the chest wall should be reduced so that the syringe and needle lie nearly parallel to the chest wall. The needle is then advanced towards the supraclavicular notch. Gentle negative pressure should be maintained so that the operator knows with the first gush of blood that the vein has been punctured.

Inserting the catheter. Once the vein has been located, a 14 gauge needle is introduced along the same route with an attached syringe. As soon as the vein is entered, the needle is advanced 2 to 3 mm more and held firmly by operator's nondominant hand. Catheter is introduced into the needle with due asepsis and needle is withdrawn over the catheter.

An alternative method uses the arrow or the cordis set. Complete prepackaged disposable sets are available, which include a small 18-gauge needle and a flexible wire. This needle is used to locate the subclavian vein as described *vide supra*. The flexible wire is introduced through the needle. The needle is then removed. The catheter is threaded over the guide wire and finally guide wire is removed. There are less chances of injury to the vital structures in the chest by this technique because a thinner needle is used. The catheter is sutured to the skin of the chest wall midway between clavicle and the nipple and dressed aseptically.

Complications. Puncture of pleura or lungs, pneumothorax, hemorrhage, hydrothorax, laceration of thoracic duct, subcutaneous emphysema and thrombosis of subclavian vein may occur.

Contraindications. The procedure should not be attempted if there is superior vena cava syndrome and a bleeding disorder.

C.   Internal jugular puncture

Indications. It is indicated for insertion of pacemakers, IVC occluding umbrellas, CVP/Swan-Ganz line placement and hyperalimentation.

Technique. Skin is prepared in the area posterior to the upper half of the sternocleidomastoid muscle. Head is held lower than the body, off the edge of the firm surface. The face is rotated 90 degrees to the opposite side. Extreme extension of the neck should be avoided as it tends to stretch and collapse the vein. A finger is placed in the suprasternal notch, slightly displacing the trachea away from the anticipated course of the needle. The needle, with the bevel facing upwards, enters the skin deeply under the posterior margin of sternocleidomastoid muscle at the junction of cephalic one-third and the middle-third.

The needle should traverse under the muscle but not through it. The negative pressure is applied to the syringe with non dominant hand and needle is slowly advanced along a course beneath the muscle and aimed towards the locator finger in the suprasternal notch. If blood is not obtained and the needle has reached the suprasternal notch as evidenced by locator finger, needle should be slowly withdrawn, maintaining negative pressure in the syringe. When the needle is completely withdrawn from the vein, gentle pressure must be applied over the middle of sternocleidomastoid muscle for atleast 5 minutes. The technique for introduction of a catheter is the same as that described under subclavian vein. Obtain a chest X-ray to confirm the position of the catheter tip and to rule out pneumothorax.

Complications. Hematoma, hydrothorax or hydromediastinum, air embolism thrombophlebitis and carotid puncture may occur. In addition, thoracic duct can be damaged while cannulating left internal juglar vein.

Intraosseous Infusion

Hypovolemic shock is a common emergency in children and is best managed by prompt administration of fluids, colloids and blood through an intravenous line. During shock, veins are often collapsed and difficult to puncture. Venesection is a time consuming procedure leading at times to fatal consequences. In these circumstances intraosseous infusion has been successfully employed in infants to save life.

Contraindications. Fracture of tibia/ long bone and cellulitis of insertion site

Procedure. After ensuring proper asepsis, 14 or 16 gauge Jamshidi bone marrow needle or hypodermic needle is inserted into the flat surface of tibial tuberosity. The trephine or standard bone marrow needles are easier to insert in bigger children. The alternative sites include tibial malleolus, iliac crest and femur. The needle is directed perpendicular to the skin and inserted into the bone till disappearance of resistance ("give") suggests that needle has entered the bone marrow. The properly placed needle would stand upright without support and would allow free infusion of fluids, colloids and blood. Medications can also be administered through this route (Figure 58.3). The bone marrow is abundantly supplied with sinusoids draining into large medullary venous channels that empty into the systemic venous system via nutrient and emissary veins. The circulation times of intraosseous and intravenous fluid injections are identical. The bone marrow can thus be considered as a large vein which does not collapse even in shock.

Complications. Subcutaneous leakage, osteomyelitis, cellulitis and pulmonary fat embolism are known hazards. In view of its serious hazards, the procedure should be used in a dire emergency. Medicut or venesection should be done as soon as the shock improves and veins are accessible.

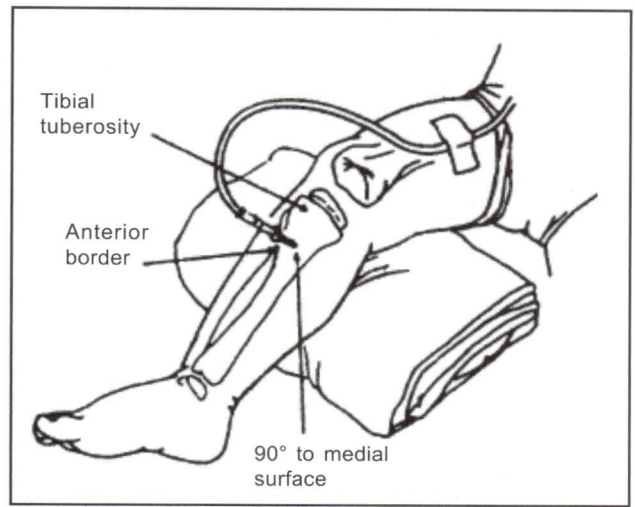

Figure 58.3 Procedure for setting up an intraosseous infusion

Venesection (cut down)

When the antecubital veins cannot be visualized and attempts to establish infusion line through a peripheral vein are unsuccessful, it is often safer to attempt venous cannulation by venesection rather than to proceed with the hazardous procedures of percutaneous placement of subclavian or internal jugular catheters.

Vein selection. The location of median basilic and median veins is already mentioned under venipuncture. Cephalic vein in the upper arm or deltopectoral groove, external jugular and saphenous vein anterior to the medial malleolus are alternative sites. Sapheno-femoral junction is located two finger breadths lateral and two finger breadths inferior to the pubic tubercle. It lies medial to the femoral artery. It is imperative that the catheter should be placed and secured in the proximal saphenous vein and not in the femoral vein. A catheter which is directly placed in the femoral vein will occlude total venous return of the leg.

Procedure. Proper restraint and sedation is necessary. Skin should be prepared aseptically. A small area is infiltrated with 1% lignocaine upto the vein. An incision is made perpendicular to and across the vein about 1.5 to 4.0 cm long. A hemostat is used and with repeated opening actions parallel to the vein, the subcutaneous tissues are teased and separated to expose the vein. The vein is picked up by a firm deep scooping run with a curved hemostat. Ligatures are tied around the distal portion of the vein. Ligatures are placed around the proximal portion of the vein to aid in traction. A stab wound is made through the skin approximately 2-3 cm distal to the site of initial incision. The catheter is introduced through this wound and the subcutaneous tissues prior to its introduction into the vein. This procedure reduces the chances of septic complications at the site of the incision. A small incision is made into the vein with iris scissors. A catheter with a rounded bevel is slipped into the vein and is tied with a ligature previously placed around the proximal portion of the vein. A skin suture tied distally around the catheter holds it in place. Incision wound is sutured, antibiotic powder is supplied and covered with a sterile gauze piece.

Complications They are similar to those pertaining to insertion of percutaneous line with additional risk of injury to neighbouring arteries in the groin.

Infusion rates. Ordinary IV drip sets deliver fluid at 62.5 ml/hr or 1500 ml/24 hr when infusion is given at 20 drops/min (20 drops/ml). Micro drip sets (measured volume burette sets) deliver fluids at 15 ml/hr when infusion is given at 20 drops/min (80 drops/ml). For infusion of very small volumes at a constant rate electronic infusion pumps must be used.

Central Venous Pressure (CVP) Monitoring

Central venous pressure is defined as the height at which a column of blood (or water) will stabilize above the supine patient's right atrium. The right atrium lies behind the sternum opposite 3rd and 4th ribs, at a depth of about one-fifth of the antero-posterior diameter of the chest.

Technique. Cannulate a major vein; femoral, subclavian, internal jugular or antecubital. The cannula should be at least 20 gauge or larger. The CVP cannula is connected by means of a three-way stopcock to an intravenous unit for infusion or an open plastic intravenous tube attached to a manometer. The manometer is taped to a centimeter ruler, and both are attached to an intravenous pole stand by means of rubber bands which allow free vertical movements of manometer. The zero mark on the ruler corresponds to the level of right atrium of the patient. The standard point of reference is designated as a point midway between the anterior and posterior chest walls and this level is marked clearly on the patient's thorax in the axilla with a marker. Alternatively the standard reference point is determined by "leveling" the sternal prominence at the second intercostal space (angle of Louis) with the 5 cm mark on the manometer scale (since the right atrium is assumed to be approximately 5 cm posterior to the sternal angle). The manometer can also be standardized at zero by placing it lower at a point against the lateral thoracic wall 5 cm below the sternal prominence. With the ruler and the attached manometer at the correct elevation (checked each time), the three way valve is turned to allow free flow of blood from the patient to the manometer. The meniscus level in the manometer is directly read as CVP (Figure 58.4).

Capillary Blood (Heel prick)

Indications. To obtain arterialized capillary blood for blood gas analysis, hematocrit, bilirubin, glucose and other biochemical estimations by micro methods.

Technique. Warm the heel with a cotton wool pledget soaked in sterile warm water at 40°C or hot towel. Prepare the site aseptically using spirit-iodine-spirit. Apply sterile liquid paraffin at the site of puncture so that a good sized drop of blood is formed. With the left hand, the foot should be

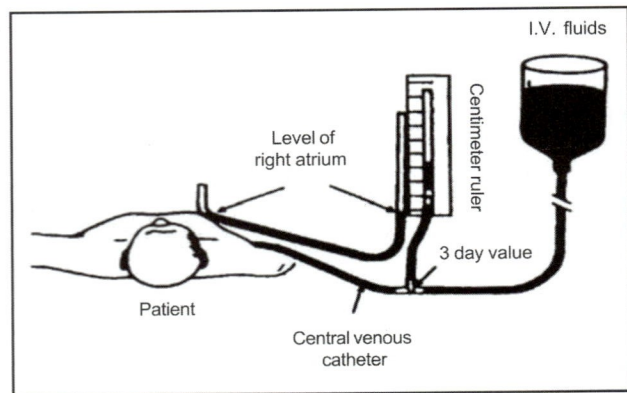

Figure 58.4 Technique to record central venous pressure. The zero mark of centimerter ruler should be placed opposite the level of right atrium

dorsiflexed and grasped alongwith the leg in such a way that engorged heel pulp stands out. Stab the heel laterally with a lancet to a depth of about 2 mm at sites indicated in Figure 58.5. Avoid inflicting puncture at the apex of heel, because painful scar may cause difficulty in walking later in life. Wipe the first drop (it contains tissue fluids which may contaminate the specimen) and subsequently collect the sample either in a heparinised capillary tube or a container. The alternate squeezing and releasing of calf facilitates milking out of blood. After collection of sample the site should be sealed aseptically with benozoin or an adhesive aseptically.

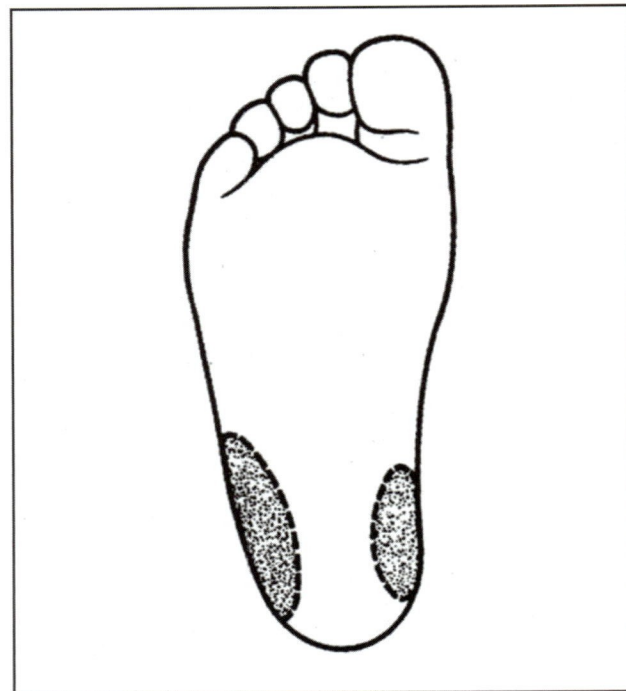

Figure 58.5 The shaded areas are the appropriate and safe sites for obtaining the sample of capillary blood from the heel

Vessel transillumination

Indications. To locate artery or vein for blood sampling or vessel cannulation.

Technique. In a dim lighted room put sterile tip probe of high intensity fibreoptic cold light source directly opposite to puncture site adjacent to vessel. Set light source at low intensity and increase as needed for visualization; the vessel is identified as dark linear structure with indistinct edges.

Radial Artery Puncture

Indications. Arterial puncture and cannulation is required for blood gas analysis and invasive blood pressure monitoring.

Prerequisite. Modified Allen's test is done to assess adequacy of collateral circulation through ulnar artery. Compress infants's hand with firm pressure (to blanch it) and simultaneously occlude the ipsilateral radial and ulnar arteries with index finger and thumb of other hand. After a few seconds, release the baby's hand and it should appear pale. Now release the pressure over the ulnar artery while maintaining firm pressure over the radial artery. Reperfusion of the entire palm should occur within few seconds if there is collateral circulation from ulnar artery. Radial artery cannulation should be done only if ulnar collateral circulation is satisfactory.

Technique. Prepare the site aseptically using spirit-iodine-spirit. Use a heparinized syringe attached to a disposable sterile 21-23 gauge needle. Keep the wrist extended and feel the radial artery just lateral to the tendon of flexor carpi radialis. Keep the left hand fingers on radial artery and with bevel facing upwards, needle should be inserted just superior to the proximal skin crease at an angle of 45 degree to the radial artery (Figure 58.6). The needle should be withdrawn while maintaining gentle suction till blood flows into the syringe. If the artery is missed, needle should be pushed again in either direction without withdrawing it from the skin. After collection of sample, site must be kept pressed for at least 5 minutes to avoid bleeding. Advance the cannula into the artery for 5-6 cm, attach three-way stopcock and infuse heparinised saline at 1.0 ml/hr through the infusion pump (Figure 58.7).

Temporal Artery Puncture

Technique. Prepare the site aseptically using spirit-iodine-spirit. Use a heparinised syringe attached to a disposable 21-23 gauge needle or a scalp vein set. The temporal artery is situated vertically in front of tragus of the ear and can be

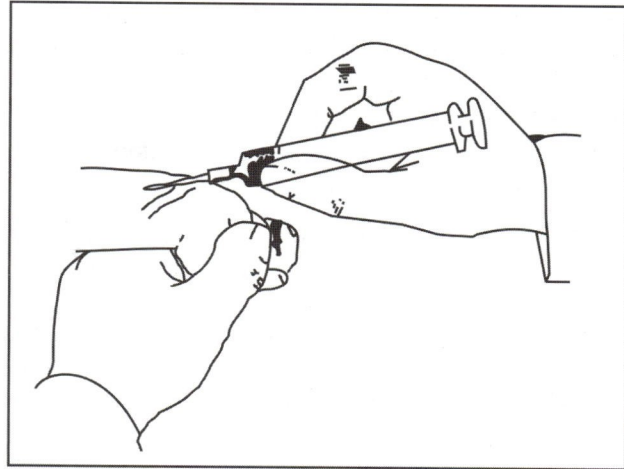

Figure 58.6 Direct puncturing of radial artery for collection of sample of arterial blood for gases

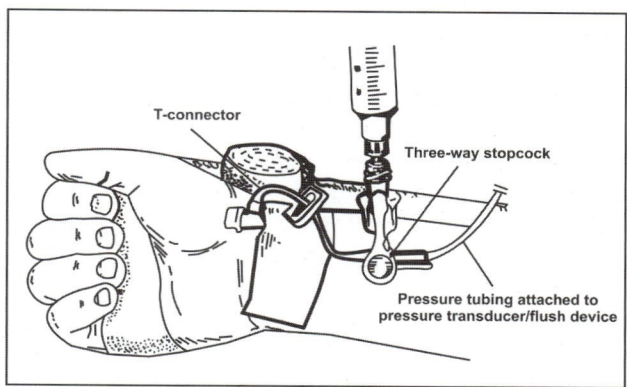

Figure 58.7 Radial artery indwelling catheter set up for continuous monitoring of arterial blood pressure and frequent blood sampling

located by palpation or by seeing the pulsations after removing the hair from the temporal region. The artery should be punctured against the flow of blood directing the needle from above downwards.

Umbilical Vessel Catheterization

Transparent polyvinyl infant feeding tubes with rounded end and a hold at the tip are used. The catheter size 4 or 5 Fr is suitable for artery and 7 or 8 Fr for the vein. The catheter is attached to a 10 ml syringe containing heparinized saline. A loose purse string ligature is placed around the base of the cord. The umbilical vein is usually located at about 12 o'clock position and often gapes. The two arteries stand out laterally as small whitish protrusions with obliterated lumens.

Umbilical Vein Catheterization

Indications. For exchange transfusion, rapid replacement of blood or fluids and rarely for setting up infusion when other sites fail. The infusion through umbilical veins should not be allowed to drip for more than 24 hours.

Technique. Restrain the infant by using a padded crucifix splint for fixing all the four limbs. Site is prepared aseptically using spirit-iodine-spirit. Drape the abdomen aseptically using sterile towels. The umbilical stump is held with a toothed forceps and opening of the vein is identified (Figure 58.8). Clot or debris is removed with forceps and its opening dilated with the closed point of small artery forceps. Select the appropriate sized catheter (5 Fr for <3.5 kg and 8 Fr for >3.5 kg). The catheter is marked with a thread for the appropriate distance to be inserted (20% of crown heel length). The catheter is gently pushed into the vein. If it sticks at a distance of 1-2 cm, gentle suction should be applied to suck out any additional clot followed by injection of heparinised saline. The umbilical stump is pulled downwards and the catheter is gently pushed forwards with occasional rotatory movements till a free flow of blood is obtained. If catheter is intended to be left *in-situ,* x-ray chest, postero-anterior and lateral views should be taken.

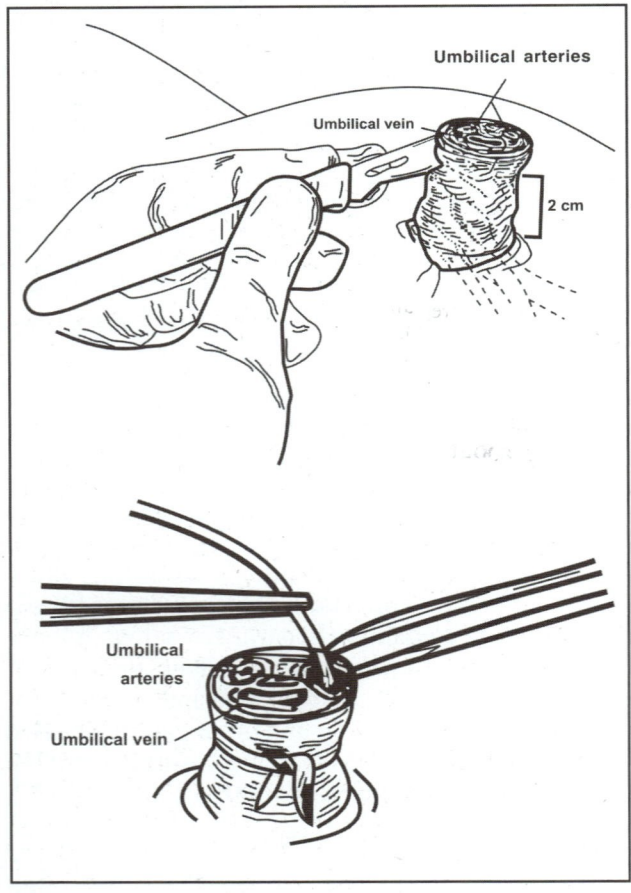

Figure 58.8 Identification of umbilical vessels and insertion of umbilical catheter

Ideally catheter tip should lie opposite D9-D10 vertebrae above the dome of right diaphragm. The desired length can be calculated by measuring the shoulder umbilical length (Figure 58.9). The venous catheter should never be left open to air for fear of air embolism. The free end of the catheter should be strapped to the abdominal wall away from the perineum to avoid contamination.

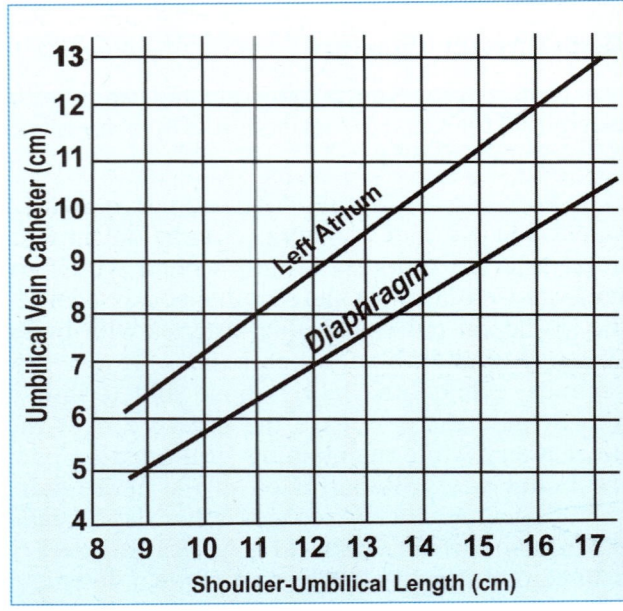

Figure 58.9 Desired umbilical venous catheter length using the shoulder umbilical length

Umbilical Artery Catheterization

Indications. For blood gas analysis in babies on assisted ventilation and invasive monitoring of blood pressure.

Technique. The umbilical stump is cut clean with a scalpel under asepsis. The stump should be grasped with a toothed forceps and opening of one of the umbilical arteries should be dilated with a metallic probe. Select the proper sized catheter (3.5 Fr for <1250 g and 5 Fr for >1250 g). Insert the catheter gently towards caudal direction. After inserting about 2 cm of catheter, the umbilical stump should be elevated superiorly and catheter pushed caudally till the desired length is cannulated. Refer to Table 58.2 and Figure 58.10 for the desired length of catheter to be inserted. The tip of the catheter may be positioned at a high or low site. In the former, the catheter tip lies at the lower thoracic aorta above the diaphragm between ductus arteriosus and origin of celiac axis (between T4-T11 vertebrae).

Section 6

Table 58.2 Optimal length of catheter to be passed for umbilical vessel catheterization		
Length of catheter (cm)	Venous catheter to reach IVC** (cm)	Arterial catheter to reach bifurcation of aorta*** (cm)
Crown heel length		
34	5.5	5.0
36	6.0	5.5
38	6.5	6.0
40	7.0	6.5
42	7.25	7.0
44	8.0	7.5
46	8.25	8.0
48	8.5	8.5
50	9.0	9.0
52	9.5	9.5
Shoulder umbilical length*		
10	5.5	5.5
11	6.0	6.0
12	6.75	6.75
13	7.5	7.5
14	8.25	8.5
15	8.75	9.25
16	9.5	10.0

*   Shoulder umbilical length is calculated from the lateral end of clavicle to a point vertically beneath it on the horizontal line drawn through umbilicus.

**   Resistance is usually met at the ductus venosus. The catheter should be passed 1-2 cm beyond the point of resistance.

***Resistance is often met at the junction of umbilical artery with internal iliac artery.

(Adapted from Dunn PM; *Arch Dis Child* 1966, 41: 69)

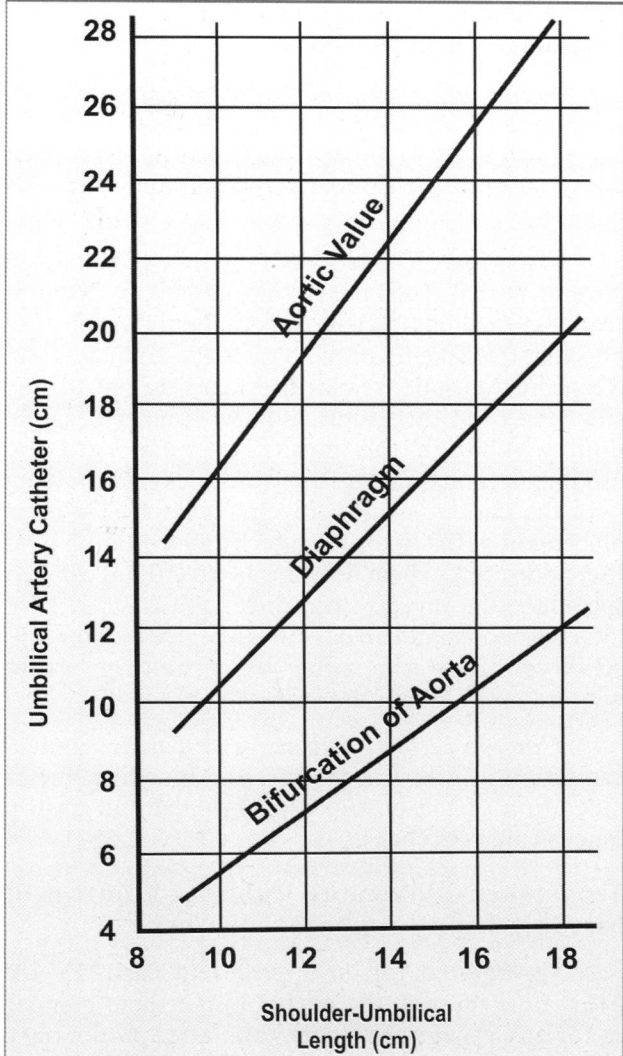

Figure 58.10 Desired umbilical arterial catheter length using the shoulder umbilical length

In the lower location of umbilical artery catheter, the tip is positioned in the abdominal aorta between inferior mesenteric artery and aortic bifurcation (opposite L4 vertebra). The lower location of catheter is associated with greater risk of blanching, cyanosis and gangrene of buttocks and legs. During and following the procedure, the feet should be examined for any evidence of discoloration and blanching. The purse string ligature at the base should be tightened and catheter stitched in place. The catheter is filled with heparinised saline and stoppered with a rubber cap. The umbilical area should be sprayed with an antibiotic powder and free end of the catheter should be strapped to the abdominal wall away from the perineum. For sampling, about 1 ml of blood and heparinised saline contained in the umbilical catheter is withdrawn, the sample should be collected in another heparinised syringe and the blood previously removed should be returned to the baby.

Complications. Sudden cyanosis or pallor of a part below the umbilicus especially the limbs, toes or buttock area may be related to embolism or spasm. If this complication develops, warm the opposite leg with warm towel. If the limb does not return to normal, the line should be removed and the attending physician should be notified. Other complications include thrombosis of the vessel, embolization, perforation of the vessel, air embolism, misplacement of catheter into the portal venous system, bleeding, infection, necrotizing enterocolitis and rarely extra hepatic portal hypertension in childhood.

Gastric Lavage

Indications. Poisoning (except kerosene, corrosives and petroleum products) and upper GI bleeding.

Technique. The length of the tube to be passed through nose is equivalent to the cumulative distance from external auditory meatus to the tip of the nose plus that from the tip of the nose to the xiphisternum. Restrain the patient with the head turned to one side. Pass the tube lubricated with normal saline gently through the mouth or nose into the esophagus, and then into the stomach synchronizing with the child's swallowing movements. Confirm placement of the tip of the tube by auscultating over the abdomen while injecting 10-20 ml of air. Introduce the lavage fluid under gravity and save total gastric aspirate in case of suspected poisonings. Always close the tube by pinching while withdrawing it from the stomach.

Complications. Reflex bradycardia, apnea, aspiration of gastric contents, and bleeding due to ulceration of the naso-oro-pharyngeal and gastric mucosa may occur.

Sengstaken-Blakemore Tube for Control of Bleeding from Esophageal Varices

Technique. Pass the appropriate sized (15, 18, 21Fr) tube through the nostril in the same manner as for any other nasogastric tube after preliminary sedation and restraining. In an uncooperative patient, a local anesthetic spray is used in the naso-pharynx. The tube should be lubricated with a water soluble lubricant. Pass the tube into stomach and inject 50-75 ml of air into the gastric balloon. Pull out the tube so that balloon sits snugly against gastroesophageal junction, and then tape it firmly on the face. Connect the esophageal balloon to a mercury manometer via the "Y" tube and inflate it to a pressure of 30 mm Hg. Maintain pressure for 24 hours with two five-minute periods of pressure release. The stomach should be lavaged with saline until clear aspirate is obtained. The control of hemorrhage may be checked periodically by aspirating stomach contents and pressure in the esophageal balloon may be released as soon as hemostasis is achieved. Keep nasogastric suction facility available round-the-clock. The saliva and secretions collecting above the esophageal balloon should be sucked periodically to prevent aspiration. If bleeding is not controlled by above maneuver, inflate the gastric balloon with up to 200 ml of air

to control gastric bleeding. Gavage feedings may substitute the intravenous fluids after 12-24 hours of control of hemorrhage.

Contraindications. The procedure is contraindicated if there is esophageal rupture or perforation, esophageal obstruction, obstructed nasopharynx and spinal cord injury.

Complications. Dislodgement of tube, major airway obstruction, pulmonary aspiration, esophago-gastric erosions, and esophageal rupture can occur.

Emergency Injection Sclerotherapy

Indications. To stop variceal bleeding by producing thrombosis of bleeding varix. Emergency sclerotherapy is often resorted to in case pitocin or balloon tamponade fail to stop bleeding due to esophageal varices.

Technique. Rigid fiberoptic endoscope can be used under general anesthesia. Flexible fiberoptic endoscope is preferred and can be used under sedation with diazepam and pentazocine. Buscopan (0.5 ml/kg) is given to relax GE junction to facilitate endoscopy.

After visualizing varices in the lower part of esophagus, sclerosant is injected. The scelerosant used include absolute alcohol, ethanolamine oleate, sodium morrhuate, sodium eteraclecyl and ethoxyskerol. The injection could be intravariceal, paravariceal or combined. Intravariceal injection is used when there is no bleb formation and after taking out the needle there is bleeding which can be stopped by pushing the endoscope in the stomach to compress the varix. This phenomenon occurs when injections are given for the first time and varices vary from Grade III to IV. When varices are sclerosed, paravariceal injection is given in the submucosa or mucosa but partially the injection may be intravariceal also. In one sitting 3 to 4 varices are injected with 5-10 ml of sclerosant. Injections are repeated after every 2-3 weeks till avariceal state is achieved. Injections can be given at weekly intervals also. Patients are followed every 2 months for repeat endoscopy to see the appearance of new varices in the esophagus, stomach and duodenum.

Complications. These include retrosternal discomfort, esophageal ulceration, perforation, and stricture formation, development of ectopic varices and rarely pulmonary thrombosis and extensive thrombosis extending to the splenoportal axis.

Spinal Puncture

Indications. The procedure is indicated to measure CSF pressure and to obtain a sample for cellular, chemical and bacteriological examination, to aid therapy by administration of spinal anesthetics and, occasionally, antibiotics or antitumor agents and for diagnostic purposes by injecting air (pneumo-encephalography), radio-opaque contrast material (myelography), or a radioactive substance (indium or radioactive iodinated serum albumin, RISA). In addition, it may be used to diagnose subarachnoid bleed or neoplastic invasion. It may also be used for cerebrospinal fluid removal (CSF) for relief of intracranial hypertension.

Contraindications. The procedure is risky in the presence of a raised intracranial pressure. In such a situation mannitol should be infused (unless contraindicated in a patient suspected to have intracranial bleeding) followed by guarded spinal puncture, keeping the head end low, and using a fine bore 22 or 23 gauge needle with a stylet and removing only a few drops of CSF for diagnostic purposes. *It is mandatory to examine the fundus in all patients before carrying out lumbar puncture.*

Technique. Ensure strict asepsis and proper restraint. Sudden movements of the patient when the needle is in the spinal canal may result in bleeding or tissue injury. Sitting position is preferred for premature babies because their CSF is under low pressure. In lateral position, assistant's left arm is around the child's legs and buttocks while the right hand is used to arch the back by holding below neck. Generally lumbar inter space at the level of the iliac crest (L3-L4) is chosen. However, lower space is used in infants due to a proportionately longer spinal cord. Spinal needle with stylet (sterile disposable needle 21 or 22 gauge for newborn and younger children) is introduced slowly in the midline with the bevel pointing upwards in order to avoid striking against the wall of the spinal canal with risk of rupturing blood vessels. A definite "give-in" sensation is perceived when dura is pierced.

Complications. Transtentorial herniation, back pain, bleeding, epidural, subdural or spinal hematoma, headache, iatrogenic infection, and spinal hematoma may occur.

Subdural Tap

Indications. To diagnose and drain subdural hematoma effusion and empyema.

Contraindications. Coagulopathy or bleeding disorder.

Technique. The procedure may be accomplished through an open fontanel, suture line or intact calvarium after making burr holes. Sedation and proper restraint are necessary. Shave head at least 5 cm posterior to the anterior fontanel and 5-10 cm lateral to the midline and forward upto the forehead. The lateral margins of the anterior fontanel are palpated along the coronal suture, and a site is chosen either as far lateral as possible or at the area of maximal transillumination. Under strict asepsis a gauge 20 subdural needle is carefully inserted perpendicular to the scalp through a depth of approximately 0.3-0.6 cm. A definite "pop" is felt upon entering the subdural space. The tap must be performed on both the sides. The tap is considered as negative when either no fluid or only a few drops of clear, colorless fluid with a protein content of normal CSF is obtained. A sterile benzoin gauze dressing should be tightly fixed with leukoplast, after the procedure.

Complications. Bleeding and infection may occur.

Ventricular Tap

Indications. To diagnose ventriculitis and intraventricular hemorrhage, to relieve acute rise of intracranial pressure in hydrocephalus and to visualize the ventricular system by contrast studies.

Technique. Initial steps are similar to a subdural tap. Needle is inserted from the lateral angle of anterior fontanel and is directed towards the nasion by pushing forwards and inwards piercing the dura and brain matter. Depending on the degree of ventricular dilatation and size of the baby, the ventricle is generally reached at a depth of about 2.5 cm. In children upto 3 years it may be possible to push in the needle through the sutures but in older children trephining is essential.

The CSF should be allowed to drip out spontanaously and no suction should be applied with a syringe. After removal of the needle, the baby should be made to sit up and CSF oozing stopped by local pressure. A sterile gauze dressing should be tightly fixed with sticking plaster or benzoin seal.

Complications. Trauma to the brain tissue and rarely superior saggital sinus may be entered.

Cisternal Puncture

Indications. Basal meningitis not diagnosed on a spinal or ventricular tap, when lumbar site is not available and for a contrast study.

Technique. Occipital region is shaved and prepared aseptically. Patient lies in the lateral position with a pillow under his head and chin is flexed so that the cervical spine is in line with thoracic spine. Skin is punctured immediately above the axial spine after lignocaine infiltration. It is advanced anteriorly and slightly upwards directed towards an imaginary line drawn from the external auditory canal to glabella till the needle touches the occipital bone. Approximate depth is noted and needle withdrawn upto but not out of the skin and reintroduced successively in a plane each time nearer to the auditory glabellar line till it touches the occiput or there is a sudden "give" and the CSF flows out on removal of stylet. The depth of the cistern varices from 1.5 cm in infants to 3-4 cm in adults.

Complications. Sudden death due to brain stem injury can occur. Procedure must be performed by an experienced neurosurgeon and with utmost care and caution.

Thoracocentesis

Indications. To remove air, fluid or blood from the pleural cavity and to instill medications.

Technique. The child should be sitting with head flexed, and arms folded in front of chest or over the head. The child may be made to lean over an attendant, table or pillow. The usual site of aspiration is the seventh or eighth intercostal space in the posterior axillary line below the angle of scapula. The site may be ascertained by percussion or from the chest film. Under strict asepsis, local anesthesia upto the level of pleura is given. Use a 16 or 17 gauge, short bevel needle about 7 to 8 cm long. A three-way stopcock should be attached to the needle which is connected to a 20 ml syringe and a piece of rubber tubing, which is clamped with a hemostat. The needle is inserted into the pleural cavity, piercing close to the upper border of the rib to avoid injury to the intercostal blood vessels which are located along the lower borders of ribs. After entering the pleural cavity, suction is applied with a syringe. If fluid is obtained the aspiration may be continued. After aspiration the needle is removed and a sterile dressing is applied to the site of the tap. A check X-ray chest must be taken after the procedure. For treatment of pneumothorax, a 16 gauge percutaneous catheter is introduced in a similar manner in the second intercostal space and connected to the closed under water seal attached to a slow suction machine. In older children a chest tube may be placed in the pleural cavity after surgical incision.

Complications. Pneumothorax, hemothorax, accidental lung puncture, air embolism and injury to intercostal vessels or nerves may occur.

Pericardiocentesis

Indications. Pericardial tamponade, symptomatic pericardial effusion, and pericardial biopsy

Contraindications. Skin infection at the site of needle insertion and severe bleeding disorder

Technique. Sedation and proper restraint are essential. Patient sits with a back rest. Under strict asepsis introduce the needle into the costo-xiphoid space on the left side close to the sternum and push the needle posteriorly and slightly upward into the pericardium. Needle should be advanced towards the shoulder with 15°-20° angle from the abdominal wall. Third, fourth or fifth intercostal spaces 1 to 2 cm left of the sternal border may also be used taking care to avoid injury to the internal mammary artery. If apex impulse is palpable puncture site should be just lateral to it within the lateral cardiac dullness; the needle is directed dorsally and medially.

The chest lead of an electrocardiogram may be attached to the needle. When the needle touches the myocardium, there will be an instant marked increase in the voltage and high QRS complexes indicating ventricular contact while P waves indicate atrial contact. If facilities are available for fluoroscopy or echocardiography, these can be employed for accurate insertion of the needle.

Intracardiac Injection

Indications. To give medications in a patient with cardiac arrest.

Technique. Pierce the chest just lateral to the left sternal border in the third to fifth intercostal space. A negative pressure is maintained on the syringe as the needle is pushed into the chest until blood is obtained. The medication is injected and needle quickly withdrawn. It is preferable to administer medications intravenously because intracardiac injections are hazardous and may lead to myocardial hematoma, necrosis and damage to coronary vessels. Epinephrine and lignocaine can also be administered intratracheally if patient is already intubated.

Defibrillation

Indications. Ventricular fibrillation, ventricular tachycardia with decompensation, supraventricular tachycardia with decompensation, atrial flutter, and atrial fibrillation.

Technique. Conscious patient should be restrained and sedated. Paddles are lubricated with a conducting jelly and DC shock 1-2 joules/kg body weight is given under continuous electrocardio-graphic monitoring. In ventricular fibrillation if there is no response the electrical current is doubled and two more applications are recommended before abandoning the procedure.

Abdominal Paracentesis

Indications. To relieve respiratory embarrass-ment caused by the presence of massive ascites and to ascertain the nature of ascites, or hemo-peritoneum for diagnostic purposes.

Technique. Empty the bladder before the procedure. Under asepsis and proper restraint make the child sit or lie in supine position and slightly rolled towards the side of procedure by placing a pillow on the opposite side. Introduce a 18-20 gauge needle at a point joining lateral one-third and medial two-thirds of a line drawn from the anterior superior iliac spine to umbilicus (Figure 58.11). The site selected may be infiltrated with 1% lignocaine upto the peritoneum.

While piercing the skin, subcutaneous tissue and muscle, keep changing the direction of the needle so that the holes produced are not in straight alignment. The zigzag track of needle would safeguard against leakage of ascitic fluid after the procedure. As soon as the peritoneum is entered, a hemostat should be clamped onto the needle at the level of skin surface to stabilize it.

Complications. Infection, perforation, hemorrhage, renal failure and hypotension may occur

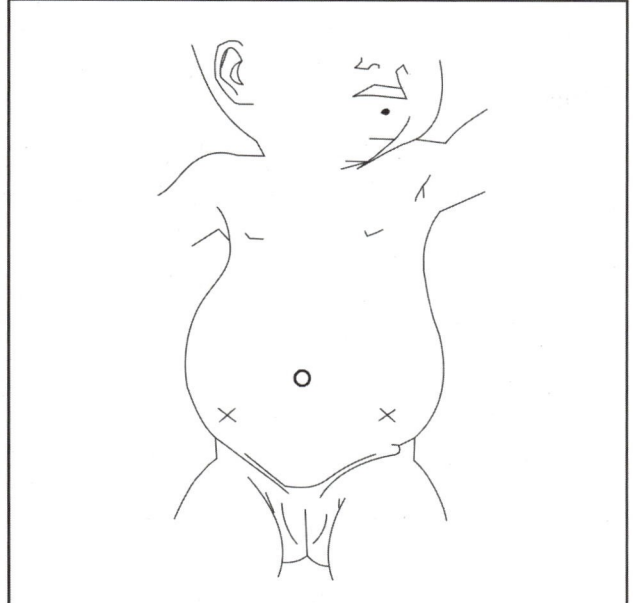

Figure 58.11 The site for paracentesis are marked with a cross

Liver Biopsy

Indications. Chronic viral hepatitis, suspected metabolic liver disease, deranged liver function tests for 3-6 months, unexplained jaundice, neonatal hepatitis/ cholestatic liver disease, suspected infiltrative or granulomatous disease, following a case of liver transplantation to evaluate and manage rejection.

Contraindications. Significant coagulopathy not corrected by FFP, cryoprecipitate and vitamin K, PT more than 3 sec. beyond control and INR >1.6, platelet count <50,000/mm^3, moderate to severe ascites, focal hepatic lesions (abscess, cyst, vascular lesion), In aforementioned situations, if biopsy is unavoidable it may be done contiously under ultrasound guidance. Empyema on the right side and infection of skin or subcutaneous tissues over hepatic area are absolute contraindications for biopsy.

Procedure

Patient should receive injection vitamin K 5 mg IM daily for children >1 year and 2 mg IM daily for children <1 year for 5 days before the procedure. All anticoagulants and aspirin should be stopped one week prior to the procedure. Hemoglobin should be atleast 10 gm/dl, and hematocrit should be >30. Obtain PT; PTT and platelet count in the morning on the day of liver biopsy. Do not proceed for biopsy if PT >2 sec of control, platelet count <50,000/mm^3, or the bleeding time is abnormal. Fasting for 4 hours in infants and 6 hours in children is required. Patient lies supine on a flat surface with right arm above the head. Biopsy site is selected and marked just anterior to right midaxillary line at the point of maximum dullness on percussion usually corresponding to 10th intercostal space in midaxillary line. A local anesthetic (2-5 ml of 1% lignocaine) is infiltrated subcutaneously along the upper margin of rib and through subcutaneous tissue upto the liver capsule. A small incision is made in the skin at biopsy site to facilitate entry of the biopsy needle. Skin should never be pierced in a drilling manner as it can lead to a very deep penetration and damage to surrounding vital organs as well as bleeding from laceration of liver. For neonates and small infants, a biopsy gun/needle (Trucut) of 18 G and for children a biopsy gun of 16 G (BARD/Boston scientific) should be used.

As soon as the resistance of liver tissue is felt, advance the gun not more than 0.5 cm. and then shoot holding the gun firmly. Withdraw the gun promptly and apply pressure dressing. Because Trucut needle requires more manipulation and

Section 6

remains in liver for a slightly longer time, it may be associated with an increased incidence of complications. It requires practice to coordinate the movements and complete the procedure within shortest time. After removing the trucut needle/biopsy gun, seal the puncture site with tincture or betadine gauze and pressure dressing.

Monitoring. Patient is positioned on right side approximately for 4 hours to compress the liver against abdominal wall, activity is limited for additional 8 to 12 hours post procedure. Vitals including heart rate, respiratory rate, blood pressure and capillary refill time are monitored every 15 minutes for 1 hour then every 30 min for 4 hours and then every 4 hr until discharge. Patient should be allowed oral feeds when he regains consciousness, earliest by 2 hours. Patient should ideally be discharged after 12 hours of the procedure and earliest by 6 hours.

Complications. Pain (pleuritic, peritoneal, diaphragmatic), hemorrhage (intraperitoneal, intrahepatic and/or subcapsular) hemobilia, bacteremia, sepsis and abscess formation, pneumothorax, subcutaneous emphysema, hemothorax and pleural effusion are recognized complications of the procedure.

Liver Abscess Tap

Indications. To diagnose and drain pyogenic or amebic liver abscess.

Technique. Proper sedation and restraint are necessary. Under strict asepsis, introduce a 16-18 gauge needle at the most prominent, fluctuant and tender point in the liver. Aspirate with negative pressure using 20 ml syringe. For an amebic liver abscess, which is commonly located in the right lobe posteriorly and superiorly, needle is introduced through 6th or 7th intercostal space in posterior or midaxillary line. Use of abdominal ultrasound helps in guiding the site and direction of the needle. After the tap apply sterile dressing at the site of puncture.

Suprapubic Bladder Puncture

Indications. To relieve acute retention and to collect uncontaminated urine specimen for examination and culture.

Technique. The procedure is feasible in infants below two years when distended urinary bladder is an abdominal organ. Restrain a sedated infant in a supine position. Confirm that the bladder is full by palpation and/or percussion. Prepare the site aseptically. Lignocaine 1% may be infiltrated locally.

The upper edge of the symphysis pubis is identified and 21-22 gauge needle attached to a syringe is inserted 1-2 cm above the symphysis. The needle is inserted vertically posteriorly towards the coccyx while constant gentle negative pressure is maintained in the syringe when the needle is advanced (Figure 58.12). Five to ten ml of urine is easily aspirated when bladder is entered. Sometimes the needle has to be rotated if it is occluded by the mucosa of the bladder.

Complications. Microscopic and even frank hematuria may occur following the procedure.

Uretheral Catheterization

Indications. Retention of urine, collection of urine sample for culture, to monitor urine output for accurate fluid balance and for radiological contrast studies.

Male. Strict asepsis must be observed. The penis is washed with soap and water or savlon and the meatus scrubbed with 1:2000 solution of chlorhexidine. Isolate the area with sterile drapes. Hands should be scrubbed and sterile gloves worn. Catheter is lubricated with 1% sterile lignocaine gel. Penis is held with the thumb and index finger of left hand with a sterile gauze and tip of catheter introduced into the urethra and advanced to the desired length. If the catheter fails to advance, it is withdrawn a little, twisted around and then reinserted. Having entered the bladder the catheter

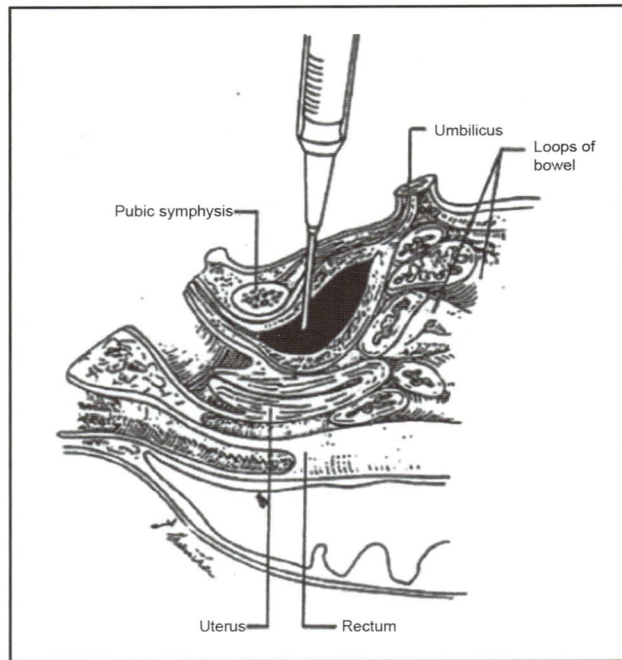

Figure 58.12 Needle is inserted vertically posteriorly just above the symphysis pubis for suprapubic bladder puncture

is connected to a sterile closed drainage system. After the procedure it is imperative to replace the prepuce over the glans penis otherwise paraphimosis may develop. A small protective dressing of ribbon gauze smeared with a greasy antiseptic preparation is applied to the external meatus.

Female. Labia majora are cleaned by swabbing from front backwards with 1:2000 chlorhexidine. The labia minora are separated with the thumb and index finger of left hand and cleaned with a swab. With a third swab, the region of the meatus is cleaned and swab left in place. Hands are washed again, sterile gloves worn and lubricated catheter is introduced, through the urethral orifice.

Skin Biopsy

The types of skin biopsy include shave biopsy, punch biopsy or excision/ incision biopsy.

Indications. For pedunculated lesions like seborrheic and actinic keratoses, intradermal nevi, or molluscum contagiosum etc. shave biopsy is required. For the diagnosis of systemic skin disorders like psoriasis, erythema multiforme, and connective tissue disorders punch biopsy is done.

Procedure. Skin needs to be effectively prepared to decrease the bacterial load. Lignocaine preferably without epinephrine should be infiltrated around the chosen site 3-5 minutes before biopsy.

Shave biopsy. After injection of anesthetic, the skin surrounding the lesion is pinched up with the thumb and middle finger to hold the lesion and aid hemostasis. The blade edge is kept parallel to the skin surface, the excision is then performed with one or more sweeping strokes. Just before the blade exits the skin, the lesion should be stablized with the index finger to avoid tearing the last bit of tissue. Hemostasis is achieved with 35% aluminum chloride solution.

Punch biopsy. Grasp a pinch of the skin between thumb and first two fingers. The punch is placed on the skin perpendicular to the surface. While applying gentle pressure, it is rotated back and forth and advanced to the hub. The edge is kept of the specimen is then gently grasped with a toothed forceps or "scooped" out by taking care not to crush the skin. Specimens for light microscopy should be fixed immediately in 10% aqueous formalin.

Peritoneal Dialysis

Indications

A. *Acute/chronic renal failure*

(i)   Blood urea > 100 mg/dL

(ii) Serum creatinine > 5-10 mg/dl

(iii) Hyperkalemia (> 6.5 mEq/L) not responding to pharmacological therapy

(iv) Fluid overload not responding to diuretics

(v)   Sensorial changes and deterioration of neurological status

(vi) Pulmonary edema

B. *Others*

(i)   Intoxications. Barbiturates and salicylates

(ii) Life-threatening electrolyte imbalance, hyper-natremia, hypercalcemia

Technique. Sedate the child and restrain him effectively preferably by immobilizing all the limbs to the four corners of bed. Bladder is emptied by catheterization and abdominal wall prepared aseptically. The catheter is usually placed in the midline few cm below the umbilicus. In an older child, the catheter is inserted lower down closer to the public symphysis. The site is anesthetized by injecting 1% lignocaine upto peritoneum. If there is no ascites distend the abdomen with 10 ml/kg dialysate using 17-20 gauge needle. Needle is withdrawn and a knife blade is used to enlarge the puncture wound in the skin. If ascites is present a very small incision is made in the skin and the trocar with catheter is introduced through it. The trocar with catheter is stabilized with the fingers of one hand on the skin while the other hand introduces the trocar through the abdominal wall with an alternating drilling motion. Penetration through the peritoneum is detected by a definite decrease in resistance and also by the appearance of fluid in the catheter when trocar is removed. The trocar is removed and catheter is retained in one of the gutters. All the fenestrations on the catheter must be within the peritoneal cavity. To achieve this, catheter length may have to be shortened at times. The catheter should be stabilized with the aid of a hemostat. There is no need to apply a purse string suture around the catheter. In case the leakage occurs from the peritoneal cavity, the fluid should be drained out of the body instead of extravasating in the abdominal wall.

Dialysate solution. The dialysate solution per 100 ml contains sodium chloride 0.5560 g, sodium

Section 6

acetate 0.4760 g, magnesium chloride 0.0152 g, calcium chloride 0.220 g, dextrose anhydrous 1.7 g and a preservative sodium metabisulfite 0.0150 g. It provides sodium 130 mEq/L, chloride 100 mEq/L, acetate 35 mEq/L. The neonates with ARF are often hypoxic and cannot metabolize lactate or acetate contained in the conventional dialysis solution. It is desirable to prepare a dialysis solution where lactate or acetate is replaced by bicarbonate. Since calcium may get precipitated in the solution containing bicarbonate it should not be incorporated in such a dialysate and administered separately intravenously.

Principles regarding administration of dialysate. Record weight prior to the procedure and every 12 hours. The patient may be placed on a weighing bed. Catheterize the bladder for measuring urine output. Warm the dialysate to body temperature and infuse it by gravity flow, placing the bottles 60-100 cm above the patient at a rate of 30-50 ml/kg/cycle. Volume should not exceed two liters per cycle. Each cycle should have a inflow time and outflow time of 5-10 minutes each. Let the dialysate equilibrate for 30-45 minutes in the abdominal cavity for effective exchange. Add 500 units heparin and 3 mEq potassium in one liter of dialysate. Potassium supplementations may be deferred for 5-6 hours in case of hyperkalemia. During dialysis the patient should receive the recommended parenteral fluids. Blood sugar, serum electrolytes, BUN, creatinine and calcium should be checked every 8 to 12 hours. In the presence of fluid overload use hypertonic dialysate by adding 50% glucose to usual 1.5% glucose containing dialysate solution to produce 4% to 7% glucose concentration. A solution containing 5% albumin enhances removal of salicylates while phenobarbitone elimination is increased with THAM and albumin. The usual total time taken for first dialysis is 48 hours. Daily culture of dialysate should be sent. At the end of procedure, microscopic examination, culture of dialysate and culture of catheter tip should be sent. Close the site of dialysis by sutures and keep it aseptic by use of bandages.

The most common problem encountered during the procedure is failure or slow drainage of dialysate from the abdomen. By repositioning of patient, flexion of knees and application of pressure over the abdomen, the fluid can usually be made to pool around the catheter and the catheter can be freed from obstructing omentum. Occasionally the catheter needs reprobing, flushing or replacement.

Complications. Leakage of fluid around catheter, respiratory embarrassment, poor outflow, hemorrhage, perforation, peritonitis, overhydration, dehydration, dyselectrolytemia, hypoproteinemia, pulmonary atelectasis, dysequilibrium syndrome and septicemia are recognised complications.

Contraindications. Fecal fistula, peritonitis, colostomy, abdominal surgery and severe chest infection are relative contraindications to the procedure.

Arthrocentesis

Indications. Septic arthritis, acute painful nontraumatized joint and effusion with suspicion of an occult fracture.

Technique. Under strict asepsis, prepare the skin over the site of aspiration. Drape with sterile towels. The skin and tissues upto the joint are infiltrated with 1% lignocaine using 25 gauge needle. A 18-gauge needle attached to 20 ml syringe is then introduced at a suitable site. When needle is introduced with a steady pressure through the subcutaneous tissue, a sudden change in resistance will be noticed when the needle point reaches the joint capsule. A perceptive "give" will be encountered once the joint is entered. The fluid should be aspirated with a gentle pressure and sent for examination. A dry sterile dressing should be placed over the aspiration site.

Contraindications. Cellulitis over a joint and bleeding diathesis are absolute contraindications.

Blood Transfusion

Indications. Severe blood loss, severe chronic anemia, severe burns, shock and to arrest the bleeding in a patient with deficiency of coagulation factors.

Technique. Select and prepare a proper site for percutaneous venipuncture with a needle not less than 20 gauge. Carefully check donor blood, bottle or bag should bear a compatibility label stating the patient's name, hospital, reference number, ward and blood group. Give detailed instructions to the nurse regarding the rate of flow. In acute emergencies it may be necessary to increase the rate of flow by using a positive pressure Martin pump or a simple blood pressure cuff around the plastic bag of blood.

Complications. Congestive heart failure; transfusion reactions (incompatibility, simple pyrexial reaction, allergic reaction, antibody production), infections like HBsAg and HCV hepatitis, malaria, cytomegalovirus, syphilis, AIDS, bacterial infections, thrombophlebitis, air embolism and disseminated intravascular coagulation are recognised complications.

Blood Substitutes

Plasma. It can be used without delay as a plasma expander. Dried plasma can be kept and reconstituted by adding sterile pyrogen free distilled water and shaking. Double strength plasma may be used in burns and shock. It also provides coagulation factors and proteins.

Dextrans. Polysaccharide polymers of varying molecular weight produce an osmotic pressure similar to plasma and is useful to tide over an emergency situation till blood or plasma is available. High molecular weight dextrans (70,000-1,10,000) are less effective in rapidly correcting hypovlemia but are longer acting since they are retained for a longer time in the circulation. Dextran 110 has the disadvantage of inducing marked rouleax formation of red blood cells which may lead to problems in grouping and cross matching. Low molecular weight dextrans (40,000) are faster in restoring plasma volume and being smaller molecules they are more readily excreted by the kidneys and their effect is short lived.

The prolonged administration of dextrans may be associated with occurrence of abnormal bleeding and this appears to be marked with high molecular weight dextrans. The total volume of dextran infused should not exceed 20-30 ml/kg/day.

Exchange Blood Transfusion

Indications. Rhesus isoimmunization, neonatal hyperbilirubinemia, partial exchange for anemia and polycythemia, disseminated intravascular coagulopathy, acute renal failure or hepatic failure, septicemia, hyperglycinemias and drug poisonings.

Technique. Restrain the neonate on a padded crucifix. Splint in such a manner that the legs and arms do not interfere. Fasten a stethoscope over the precordium with adhesive tape or attach the infant to a vital sign monitor. Body temperature should be maintained by using servo-controlled overhead heater. Oxygen and suction should be available. The stomach should be emptied before the procedure. Under strict asepsis, umbilical cord stump is cut off and vein is identified (it is largest in caliber, has the thinnest wall of the three vessels and is located at 12 o'clock position). Gently cannulate the umbilical vein upto a distance of 5-7 cm. Determine CVP by holding the free end of the catheter in a vertical position and measuring the column of blood above the skin surface. The procedure can be done by cannulating the radial artery (for removal of blood) and a peripheral vein

for infusing blood. In older children the procedure may be accomplished through the femoral vein or any other large central vein. Usually a two volume exchange is done. The catheter is attached to two three-way connectors so that leads are connected to the umbilical catheter, syringe, donor's blood and a sterile container for waste. Collect blood for hematocrit, bilirubin, sugar, electrolytes and culture before starting exchange transfusion. The blood should be warmed by immersing the bottle in a water bath at 37°C. Never use the boiling hot water bath for warming the blood. The blood is withdrawn with gentle suction and donor's blood is injected slowly in aliquots of 5 or 10 ml depending on the size of the baby. During the procedure, the bottle of donor's blood should be gently agitated from time to time to keep the cells and plasma mixed. The jammed syringes and blocked three-way connectors should be rinsed with heparinised saline (10 units of heparin/ml).

Accurate IN/OUT record and condition of the baby should be monitored closely. Whenever any untoward signs appear, such as restlessness, grunting, distressed respiration, heart rate above 180 or below 100 per minute and deterioration of the color of the baby, the procedure should be withheld till baby improves or abandoned altogether. After every 100 ml of blood exchanged, venous pressure should be checked. During exchange transfusion of a hydropic infant CVP should be monitored more frequently. When acid citrate dextrose (ACD) blood is being used for exchange transfusion, 1.0 ml of calcium gluconate should be injected slowly after every 50 ml of exchange. Routine use of sodium bicarbonate should be discouraged during exchange transfusion. After exchange transfusion samples for hematocrit, sugar, electrolytes, bilirubin and blood culture are taken. The catheter is removed and its tip is sent for culture. Apply compression bandage over the umbilical stump and keep a close watch on bleeding following the procedure. Routine prophylactic antibiotics are not indicated unless sepsis is suspected or multiple exchange blood transfusions are warranted.

Complications. The complications of the umbilical vein catheterization and in addition the known hazards of blood transfusion may be encountered. Congestive cardiac failure, shock, hypocalcemia, hyperkalemia, acidosis and cardiac arrest or arrhythmia may occur with the ACD blood. Hypoglycemia and bleeding may occur following exchange transfusion with heparinized blood. Hypothermia, anemia and oxygen toxicity may occur in neonates because adult hemoglobin (transfused blood) readily releases oxygen to the tissues by virtue of its poor affinity to bind oxygen. Splenic or portal vein thrombosis is a recognized complication later in childhood.

Plasmapheresis

Plasmapheresis implies selective removal of plasma of the patient with reinfusion of cellular constituents of blood back to the patient.

Indications. Antibody mediated diseases (ITP, Goodpasture's syndrome, autoimmune hemolytic anemia), immune-complex mediated diseases (Henoch-Schönlein purpura, immune complex mediated RPGN) and miscellaneous diseases, like Guillain-Barré syndrome, myasthenia gravis and hemolytic uremic syndrome, have been managed by plasmapheresis with variable results.

Technique. The procedure may be manual or automated. Manual procedure consists in collecting 5 ml/kg of patient's blood in a double bag, centrifugation is done to separate the plasma and cellular elements are reinfused back to the patient after suspending them in normal saline. Automated exchange is done with cell separators either as continuous flow (blood is withdrawn, centrifuged and cellular components returned in a continuous operation) or as discontinuous flow (each volume is drawn out, centrifuged and cellular constituents are returned back before next volume is withdrawn). Automated exchange is more efficient and simpler but is expensive. Small exchanges require replacement with crystalloids only (Ringer's lactate) but large exchanges require replacement with colloids (fresh plasma, 5% albumin).

Orotracheal Intubation

It is one of the most important and often a life saving procedure which every pediatrician must learn, practice and achieve perfection.

Pre-requisites. Foot-operated or electrical suction machine should be available. Proper laryngoscopes with appropriate sized disposable gamma-irradiated PVC endotracheal tubes of different sizes are mandatory. The conscious patient may need restraint and instillation of 1 ml of 1% lignocaine into the trachea with a 25-gauge needle inserted through tracheal rings to provide topical anesthesia. The approximate internal diameter of endotracheal tube is one-third of the tracheal outside diameter as assessed in the suprasternal notch. The size and length of endotracheal tubes needed at different ages are given in Chapter 3.

Technique. Before intubation, improve the oxygenation and condition of the child by administration of 100% oxygen through bag and mask for 3 to 4 minutes. The patient is kept supine upon a table or bed, with his head at the edge. The head is slightly extended (by placing a folded towel under the shoulders) with the mouth open and the jaw thrust forward. The technique depends on whether the blade of the laryngoscope is straight or curved. Straight blade (size 0 to 1) is preferred in an infant while curved blade (size 2-3) is used in an older child.

The laryngoscope is held in the left hand and placed in the right side of the mouth to displace the tongue to the left as the blade is swept to the left. The blade is advanced along the base of the tongue and the anterior wall of the pharynx until operator finds resistance at vallecula (with curved blade) or elevates the tip of epiglottis against anterior pharyngeal wall so as to visualize the larynx. The straight blade is designed to directly elevate the epiglottis and expose the larynx (Figure 58.13). A gentle pressure over the cricoid area (by the little and ring finger of hand holding laryngoscope or by an assistant) will occlude the esophagus and expose the glottic opening. With the right hand the endotracheal tube is introduced from the far right corner of the mouth towards the laryngeal opening and advanced into the trachea, 1 to 2 cm beyond the glottis. Laryngoscope is withdrawn and endotracheal tube is taped in place. To check position of tube, few puffs of air are blown into the tube with an Ambu bag and air entry in both the lungs is confirmed by auscultation. In case air entry is unequal, tube is withdrawn slightly. If laryngoscope is not available, an endotracheal tube may be inserted with the fingers of the hand, by locating the epiglottis and opening of the larynx and guiding the tube into place.

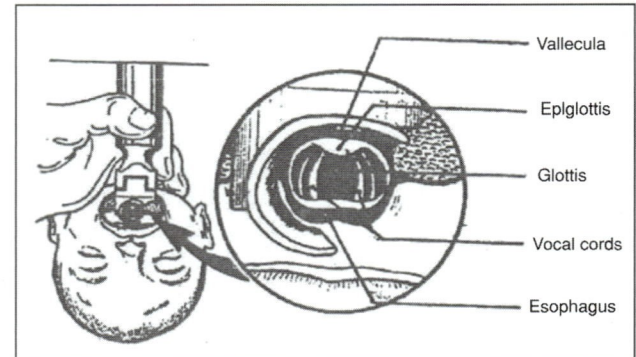

Figure 58.13 Anatomical land marks as seen during laryngoscopy. The blade of the laryngoscope should be lifted forward (not rotated) to expose the glottis

Nasotracheal Intubation

It is more difficult and cumbersome as compared to the orotracheal intubation but may be required when prolonged ventilation is anticipated. Polyvinyl endotracheal tube may be inserted through the nose and visualized in the pharynx, where it is grasped with a curved forceps and guided into the trachea, as in endotracheal intubation. Correct position of the head can often direct the tube into the trachea with little assistance.

Tracheostomy

Pending tracheostomy, the obstruction may be by-passed by inserting a wide gauge needle through the cricothyroid membrane between the Adams' apple and the cricoid cartilage below it. The needle is directed slightly downwards to avoid damage to the vocal cords (Figure 58.14). The needle may be replaced with a plastic IV cannula. This gives time to arrange for regular tracheostomy.

Indications. Laryngeal tissue swelling leading to obstruction, foreign body in the upper airways, injury to neck causing collapse of the larynx, paralysis of vocal cords, intercostal and diaphragmatic paralysis, respiratory center failure and major injury to the mandible and maxilla.

Technique. The patient lies flat with a pillow under his shoulders so as to extend head, as assistant holds the head firmly in the midline. If time allows and equipment is available, subcutaneous infiltration of the midline of the neck from the thyroid cartilage to the suprasternal notch is done. A midline vertical incision is made through the infiltrated skin and subcutaneous tissues, while the thumb and middle finger of the operator's other hand fix the trachea in the midline. The index finger palpates trachea through the incision (identified by the transverse ridges). With the help of knife and finger, dissection is carried out so as to separate muscles in the

midline. If the thyroid isthmus is prominent, it must be divided. The pretracheal fascia is then incised by taking care not to penetrate the wall between the trachea and esophagus, a vertical incision is made through the second, third and fourth tracheal rings. A tracheostomy tube of appropriate size is inserted into the trachea and tied into place around the neck. Trachea is cleared off secretions. Bleeding is controlled with pressure. Two or three sutures are placed above the tube. If prolonged tracheostomy is needed the tube is left in place for a week before changing it so that a tract will form, making replacement easy. The inner cannula is inspected and cleaned as often as needed. Moist gauze should be pinned over the tube opening to avoid formation of thick secretions and crusts. Before the tube is removed it should be blocked gradually for sufficient time to ensure that upper airway is adequate. This process may require several days as children often develop dependence on the tube.

After care of tracheostomy. A sterile, soft rubber catheter with one opening at the tip bevelled at a 45 degree angle is used for suction. Head is turned to the right to permit aspiration of the left bronchus and then to the left to permit suctioning of the right bronchus. Suction should be applied only while withdrawing the catheter. Crusting is avoided by maintaining good hydration of the patient and by using the moistened oxygen or air. Saline solution 0.5 ml, may occasionally be introduced directly into the tracheostomy tube and then immediately suctioned out. Tracheostomy site is cleaned with hydrogen peroxide diluted with equal amount of water using sterile cotton tipped swabs. Tracheostomy tube and dressings should be changed during every shift. It there is an inner cannula it should be removed and cleaned off debris every four hourly.

Care of the patient. Suctioning should be done initially every 10-15 minutes and later the interval is increased. Continuous humidification is necessary. During sleep a small pillow may be placed under the shoulders to prevent occlusion of the tracheostomy tube by flexion of the neck. Child should be carefully observed for evidences of cyanosis, respiratory distress and infection.

Bag and Mask Ventilation

It is very effective procedure for cardiopulmonary resuscitation of asphyxiated or apneic newborn babies and children. It is a life saving procedure and all the pediatricians should be skilled to provide effective bag and mask

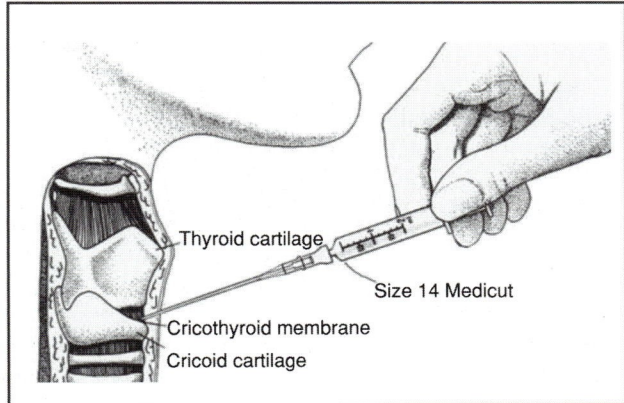

Figure 58.14 Landmarks for cricothyrotomy

ventilation. The anesthesia bags (flow inflating bags) are more effective to deliver higher concentrations (almost 100%) of oxygen but they are more difficult to use and require high flow rates of oxygen. Most pediatricians are conversant with self-inflating AMBU or Laerdal bags which are more convenient to use. It is possible to deliver 90 percent oxygen by attaching a corrugated tube or a bladder as a reservoir to the self-inflating bag.

Equipment. The pediatricians should be familiar with the type of bag and mask being used in their institution. The self-inflating bag as the name implies, inflates automatically without flow or oxygen or compressed air source. The salient components of self-inflating bag are shown in Figure 58.15. The capacity of bag for use in infants should not exceed 750 ml (250-750 ml) while larger (750-1500 ml) bags are used for older children. The air inlet is the largest opening, having one-way valve, and is located at the rear end. The oxygen reservoir (either corrugated tube or a closed rubber bladder) must be attached at the air inlet to deliver 100% oxygen to the infant. The oxygen inlet is located near the air inlet. It is a small nipple or projection to which oxygen tubing can be attached. The bag can, however, be used in an emergency without attaching oxygen but it will deliver only 21 percent of oxygen contained in the atmosphere. The air-oxygen mixture is forced out from the patient outlet to which an appropriate sized mask or endotracheal tube is attached. The one way valve assembly is positioned between the bag and patient outlet. It allows delivery of oxygen to the outlet when bag is squeezed but closes as soon as the bag is released so that exhaled air cannot reenter the bag. Due to

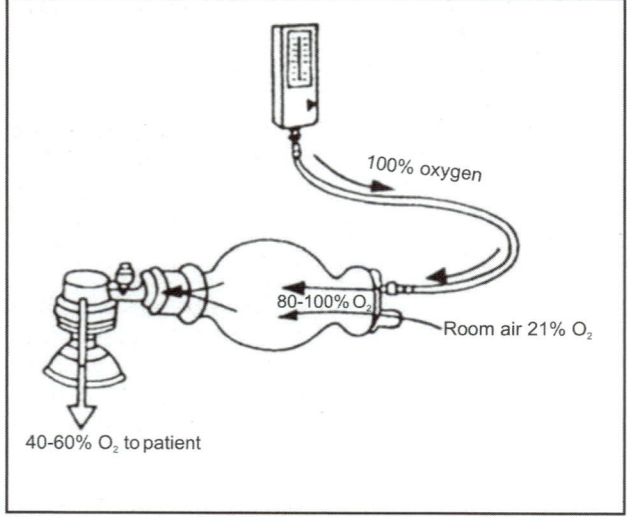

Figure 58.15 Self-inflating bag and mask assembly. See text for details

the presence of valve assembly, the self-inflating bag cannot be used for providing free-flow oxygen.

The self-inflating bags should have atleast one of the two safety mechanisms. The pop-off valve (pressure-release valve) can be set to actuate when inflation pressure exceeds 30-35 cm H_2O. In some self-inflating bags (especially Laerdal variety) there is a provision to attach a pressure gauge at a point located near the patient outlet. The gauge allows the person using the bag to control the pressure of the air or oxygen being delivered to the patient. The silicone-rubber bags and masks of Laerdal make are more sturdy and can withstand autoclaving and can be readily cleaned with antiseptic solutions. The self-inflating bag and masks available in the Indian market are unsatisfactory due to poor quality of rubber and inflatability of bag, lack of oxygen inlet and absence of any safety features including pop-off valve.

Different types, shapes and sizes (AMBU, OA, Rendell-Baker, Bennet, Laerdal, Ohio) of face masks are available. Soft circular masks with cushioned rim are preferable because they can form effective seal on the face, and are less likely to leak or cause damage to infant's eyes. The moulded triangular (anatomically shaped) masks are not preferred. The correct size of the mask for each infant should be chosen so that it snugly encloses the nose and mouth of the infant. The siliconized rubber masks can be more easily cleaned and sterilized as they can withstand boiling and autoclaving. The bag and mask assembly should be checked before hand while anticipating an asphyxiated baby. The bag should be squeezed while making an air tight seal of face mask with the palm of your hand to assess functioning of valve assembly, pop-off valve and leakage or tears in the bag. After attaching the pressure gauge one can practice and train oneself to deliver desired inspiratory pressure. One should be completely familiar with the types of bag and masks and other equipments being used in one's unit.

Indications. Bag and mask ventilation is indicated if an asphyxiated baby fails to establish satisfactory ventilation and cardiac status (heart rate < 100/ min) despite adequate suctioning and clearing of airways and tactile stimulation. Most asphyxiated neonates can be effectively resuscitated with a bag and mask ventilation alone. It is also indicated for cardiopulmonary resuscitation of critically sick neonates and children who are unable to maintain effective ventilation or develop prolonged apneic attacks. The infant is supported with bag and mask ventilations during brief periods while changing or suctioning the endotracheal tube in ventilated babies. Bag and mask ventilation is contraindicated in infants with diaphragmatic hernia because hernial contents will get overinflated by the procedure, resulting in further displacement of mediastinum and respiratory embarrassment.

Contraindications. The meconium stained babies should never be bagged unless effective tracheal suctioning has been achieved to suck out all traces of meconium from the air passages. When prolonged positive pressure ventilation is required, it is best to intubate the infant and attach him to a ventilator. Bag and mask ventilation should be avoided in infants with congenital diaphragmatic hernia.

Procedure. The infant should be positioned supine and neck slightly extended by placing a thin roll of towel under the shoulders. One should stand beyond the head end of the infant or to one side and should have unobstructed view of the chest and abdomen. After lifting the jaw, apply a proper sized mask to snuggly enclose the nose and mouth of the baby. The mask is held in place by the nondominant (left hand in a right handed person and *vice versa*) hand with the help of thumb and index finger while ring finger holds and lifts the chin of the baby. There should be no pressure either on the eyes or trachea. The face mask must establish an air tight seal with the face (Figure 58.16). Start compressing the bag with your finger tips (after connecting it to an oxygen source and attaching an oxygen reservoir) at a rate of 30-40/min depending upon the age of the child. The force of compression should be adjusted to the size of the child and compliance of lungs. The use of a manometer with

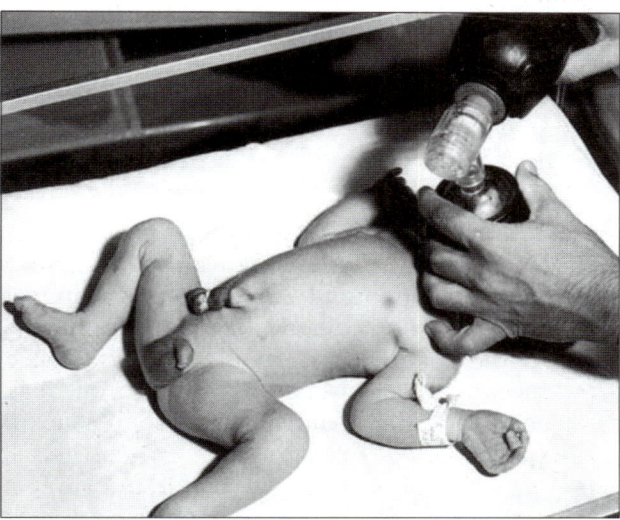

Figure 58.16 Bag and mask resuscitation. Most of the asphyxiated infants can be successfully resuscitated by this technique

a pop off valve helps to reduce the risk of pneumothorax due to overzealous bagging. There should be noticeable rise and fall of chest with each inflation. It should be associated with good air entry on both sides of the chest, improvement in color and heart rate. If the chest, does not expand adequately, reconfirm that face mask is forming an effective seal, airway is open and enough pressure is being applied on the bag which does not have any leakage or tears. Oropharyngeal airway may be inserted if a large tongue or glossoptosis and nasal obstruction (bilateral choanal atresia) are posing difficulties. When prolonged (>2 min) bag and mask ventilation is contemplated, it is preferable to insert an orogastric tube to aspirate the stomach contents in order to prevent abdominal distension.

During bag and mask ventilation of an asphyxiated baby at birth, check heart rate after every 15-20 seconds. To save time, heart rate is checked for 6 seconds only and multiplied by 10 to get heart rate/min. If despite adequate bag and mask ventilation with 100 percent oxygen (as evidenced by adequate bilateral expansion and deflation of chest with each bagging) the heart rate is not picking up and remains below 60/min, it is best to intubate the child (to provide bag and tube ventilation) and start external cardiac massage.

Pediatric basic life support (BLS) for cardiopulmonary arrest

Pediatric BLS uses the ABC approach. Sequential assessment followed by performance of actual motor skills is done in the areas of **A**irway, **B**reathing and **C**irculation, in that order. This is only the initial rescue management. If the child does not respond, advanced life support measures will have to be taken.

Airway

Opening of the airway should be accomplished immediately. Most often, the "head tilt-chin lift" maneuver is used. In cases with suspected neck injury, the above maneuver is avoided and replaced by a "Jaw-thrust" maneuver.

(i) *Head tilt–chin lift.* The neck is slightly extended and the head is tilted to place it into a neutral position by placing one hand onto the child's forehead. Index finger of the other hand (not thumb) is placed under the chin to lift the mandible up and outwards.

(ii) *Jaw thrust.* It is used for victims of neck injury and can be accomplished without extending the neck. Fingers of each hand are placed under the sides of lower jaw to lift it up and outwards. Remove any vomitus or foreign body, if visible. Do not close the mouth.

Breathing

After the airway is opened, determine if the child is breathing. If the child is breathing spontaneously, just maintain a proper airway. If no spontaneous breathing is detected, rescue breathing must be provided and airway kept patent concurrently. Place your mouth over the mouth and nose (in case of an infant) and over the mouth only in an older child. Create a seal. Pinch the nose in case of an older child. Give two breaths (1 to 1.5 seconds per breath). The correct volume for breath is assessed by adequacy of chest rise. If rescue breathing fails to produce chest expansion despite attempts at opening of the airway, suspect a foreign body airway obstruction.

Circulation

After the airway has been opened and two rescue breaths provided, determine the need for chest compressions. For this, check the pulse. If the pulse is not palpable or heart rate is < 60/min, begin chest compressions. The child should be on a firm surface. For a child of less than one year, the same method as used for neonates can be practised. For an older child aged 1 to 8 years, the compressions point is located two fingers above the subcostal notch. The heel of the hand placed along the long axis is used for compressions. Heel of the hand is placed over the lower half of sternum between the nipple line and xiphisternum taking care to avoid the xiphoid process. Chest is compressed to 1-1½ inches. The fingers of the compressing hand should not be touching the ribs. In a large child (more than 8 years), two hands are used for compression. One hand is placed over the other so that the heels of both hands are parallel to the fingers directed straight away from the rescuer. The compression rate is 80-100 times per minute and must always be accompanied by rescue breathing in a ratio of 5:1. After every fifth compression, a pause of 1 to 5 seconds is allowed for ventilation.

The new 2010 guidelines for cardiopulmonary resuscitation suggest that in older children and adults ABC should be replaced by CAB (Chest Compressions, Airway and Breathing). The rescuer should press the chest at least 1/3rd of anterior-posterior diameter or approximately $1\frac{1}{2}$ inches (4 cm) in infants and 2 inches (5 cm) in children at a rate of atleast 100 compressions per minute. If the rescuer is not trained in providing ventilations or is

unable to do to, he should continue with chest compressions alone until help arrives. However, in infants and young children ABC approach is preferred and is associated with better outcome.

Manual removal of Foreign Bodies

Foreign body should be suspected in cases of sudden respiratory distress associated with coughing, gagging, stridor, and cyanosis or wheezing. Don't try to remove the foreign bodies in upper airway by blind finger sweep; it may result in pushing back of the foreign body into the airway.

A. Back blows and chest thrusts.

Hold the infant face down on your forearm which in turn should rest on your thigh. Support the head of the child by firmly holding the jaw. Position the infant's head lower than the trunk. Deliver upto five blows with heel of your hand between the shoulder blades of the infant. Now turn the infant around to a supine position while firmly supporting the head and neck. Administer upto five quick chest thrusts in the similar manner and location used for chest compressions. The whole process can be repeated until the foreign body is expelled out.

B. Subdiaphragmatic abdominal thrusts (Heimlich's maneuver)

The maneuver increases the intrathoracic pressure and creates an artificial cough which forces the foreign body out of airway. Heimlich maneuver is not used in infants for the risk of liver injuries. It is carried out differently for conscious and unconscious children.

(i) *Conscious child.* Stand behind the child and encircle his torso by putting both arms directly under his axilla. Place the thumb side of one fist against the child's abdomen in midline slightly above navel and well below the xiphoid. With the other hand, grasp this fist and exert quick upward thrusts taking care not to touch the xiphoid process or lower rib margins. Each thrust should be forceful enough and intended to relieve the obstruction.

(ii) *Unconscious child.* Position the child in a supine position and kneel at the child's feet. Place the heel of one hand on the child's abdomen in the midline slightly above navel and well below rib cage. Place the second hand on top of the first and press into abdomen with a quick upward thrust.

Transillumination of chest

Indications. Detection of pneumothorax. A strong, presumptive diagnosis can be made without radiograph to avoid postponing treatment in an emergency.

Technique. A high intensity, fiberoptic probe is applied over skin of the chest wall in a darkened room and gradually moved over alternate sides of the chest. Normally, the ring of light surrounding the probe will extend about 1 cm. A larger or asymmetric ring of light suggests a pneumothorax. In a case of large pneumothorax the entire chest may light up. False negative transillumination may be seen in large infants with increased skin thickness, small collections of air, or situations where thymus gland is located against the chest wall. False positives are seen with subcutaneous edema, pneumomediastinum, lobar emphysema or extensive pulmonary interstitial emphysema.

REFERENCES

1. Allen P. Resuscitation: Airway management. In: Emergency Medicine; Harold L May (ed) *John Wiley and Sons,* 1984; p 897-916.

2. Avery GB (ed). In: Neonatology: Pathophysiology and Management of the Newborn. *Lippincott Company,* 1987.

3. Berg MD, Schexnayder SM, Chameides L, Terry M, Donoghue A, Hickey RW, et al. Pediatic basic life support:2010 American Heart Association Guidelines for Cardiopulmonary Resuscitation and Emergency Cardivascular Care. *Circulation* 2010; 122: S862-S875.

4. Brooks DC, Simpson GL. Circulatory support: Venous access. In: Emergency Medicine; Harold L May (ed). *John Wiley and Sons,* 1984; p 920-944.

5. Cote CJ, Jobes DR, Schwartz AJ, Ellison N. Two approaches to cannulation of a child's internal jugular vein. *Anesthesiology* 1979; 50: 371-373.

6. Deorari AK, Paul VK, Scotland J, *et al.* Practical Procedures for Newborn Nursery. *Noble Vision,* Ist edition 2001.

7. Fletcher MA, MacDonald MG. In: Atlas of Procedures in Neonatology, *JB Lippincott Compnay, Philadelphia,* 3ʳᵈ edition, 2002.

8. Harris MS, Little GA, Umbilical artery catheters. High, low, or no. *J Perinat Med* 1978; 6: 15-22.

9. Kellner GA, Smart JF, Percutaneous placement of catheters to monitor central venous pressure. *Anesthesiology* 1972; 36: 515-516.

10. Kohelet D, Goldberg A, Goldberg M. Depth of endotracheal tube placement in neonates. *J Pediatr* 1982; 101: 157-160.

11. Lissauer T (ed). In: Practical Procedures in Pediatric Emergencies. *MTP Press Limited* 1982; 273-295.

12. Shaw JCL. Arterial sampling from the radial artery in premature and fullterm infants. *Lancet* 1968; 2: 389-390.

13. Singh G. Intraosseous infusion in emergencies. *Indian Pediatr* 1987; 24: 686-688.

14. Singh M. Procedures. In: Care of the Newborn. *CBS Publishers & Distributors Pvt Ltd, New Delhi, 8ᵗʰ* edition, 2015, p 598-622.

15. Singh M. Nursing Procedures. In: Essential Pediatrics for Nurses. *CBS Publishers & Distributors Pvt Ltd, New Delhi,* third edition, 2014, p 434-461.

16. Symansky MR, Fox HA. Umbilical vessel catheterization: Indications, management and evaluation of the technique. *J Pediatr* 1972; 80: 820-826.

59

Compendium of Emergency Drugs

Meharban Singh

Administration of drugs is one of the most important responsibility of the nurse working in the pediatric intensive care unit. She should discharge this responsibility with utmost care, concern and caution. In order to avoid errors and accidents in administration of medicines to children, the following "5 rights" should be followed.

(i)   Right patient (check with mother or attendant)

(ii) Right medicine with valid expiry date (check twice)

(iii) Right dose and dilution (in case of intravenous medicines)

(iv) Right route of administration

(v)   Right timing of administration

In critically sick children admitted to PICU, drugs are administered through parenteral route. In life-threatening situations, intravenous route is preferred because absorption through intramuscular route is slow and erratic in children with hypotension, dehydration or shock. Intravenous medications should be administered with due aseptic precautions through an indwelling catheter to reduce the risk of leakage in the extravascular region. The drug should be appropriately diluted as per instructions by the manufacturer before administration. They can be injected as a slow bolus directly through the indwelling catheter or by puncturing the access port of the infusion set or through 3-way stopcock after wearing gloves and observing strict aseptic precautions. At times drugs are administered as a slow infusion over a period of 15-30 minutes through an infusion pump or microburrete set. The amount of diluent or flush fluid administered through intravenous medications should be recorded and subtracted from total daily fluid requirements as a safeguard against over infusion. When an injectable form of drug contains sodium, the amount of sodium being administered should be monitored. Some of the drugs can be added to the infusion bottle i.e. sodium bicarbonate, potassium chloride, calcium gluconate, inotropic agents etc. Drugs should not be added to the blood or blood products and TPN solution.

Drug/Emergency	Dose and route of administration	Remarks
ANAPHYLAXIS		
Epinephrine	0.01-0.03 ml/kg of 1:1000 sol IM, maximum dose 0.5 ml, may repeat every 15 min for 3 doses. It can be given IV or through endotracheal route in a dose of 0.1 ml/kg per dose in a child with shock or cardiac arrest. For larygeal edema due to anaphylaxis administer 0.1 ml/kg (max. 5 ml) of 1: 10,000 solution through a nebulizer	0.1-0.3 ml of 1:1000 sol can be infiltrated locally at the site of antigen entry.
Diphenhydramine hydrochloride	1.0-2.0 mg/kg IV slowly, may be repeated after 3 to 4 hr IM or PO for treatment of extrapyramidal side effects of phenothiazines and metoclopramide	Use with caution in patients with asthma, narrow angle glaucoma and urinary retention
Aminophylline	5 mg/kg IV loading dose diluted in 25 ml normal saline followed by 0.5-0.9 mg/kg/hr constant infusion for relief of bronchospasm	
Hydrocortisone sodium succinate	25-50 mg/kg IV (usually 100-3000 mg/dose) every 4-6 hr for 48-72 hours	The role is limited in the treatment of anaphylaxis
Dexamethasone	0.5 mg/kg IV (usually 4-12 mg/dose) q 6 hr	Useful for shock and cerebral edema

*For complete list of drugs with dosages, route of administration, proprietary formulations and their concentrations, please refer to *Drug Dosages in Children* by Singh M and Deorari AK, CBS Publishers & Distributors Pvt Ltd, New Delhi, 9th edition, 2015.

Drug/Emergency	Dose and route of administration	Remarks
ANTIDOTES, SPECIFIC		
Amyl nitrate	Pearls of vaporal to be inhaled every 2 min for 15-30 sec, followed by sodium nitrite 3% sol 0.2-0.4 ml/kg IV at a rate of 2.5-5.0 ml/min and sodium thiosulfate 25% sol 1-2 ml/kg IV over 10-20 min	For cyanide poisoning
Atropine	0.05 mg/kg IV or SC q 5-10 min till atropinisation occurs, maintain for 24 hr and taper in the next 24 hr	For organophosphate insecticide poisoning and propranolol overdose
B.A.L. (dimercaprol)	5 mg/kg IM stat; then 3 mg/kg IM q 4 hr for 2 days, 6 hr for 1 day, 12 hr for 7 days	For arsenic, gold, mercury and lead poisoning
Calcium disodium EDTA	50-75 mg/kg/day IM in 4 divided doses for 5 days	For arsenic, lead and copper poisoning
Chlorpromazine	1 mg/kg IM or IV	For amphetamine poisoning
d-Pencillamine	30-40 mg/kg/day (maximum 1g/day) PO in fruit juice in 3-4 div doses empty stomach for four weeks for lead poisoning and for one week for copper poisoning	
Deferoxamine	15 mg/kg/hr (maximum 80 mg/kg/d) IV in 100-200 ml of 5% dextrose in 6 hr, if wine colored urine persists, give 90 mg/kg over next 12 hr or till urine clears. Total dose should not exceed 6 g.	There is no role of oral deferoxamine for acute iron poisoning
Diphenhydramine hydrochloride	1-2 mg/kg IV q 30 min or IM q 3-4 hr upto maximum dose of 300 mg/day	For extrapyramidal reactions due to phenothiazines and metoclopramide
Ethanol	10 ml/kg 10% sol IV or 1.0/ml/kg of 95% sol in fruit juice PO for 4-5 days	For poisoning due to methanol and ethylene glycol
Flumazenil	Incremental doses of 0.02 mg/kg (maximum 0.2 mg/kg) or 0.1 mg, 0.2 mg, 0.3 mg, 0.5 mg at 1-min intervals IV until desired effect is achieved	Poisoning or toxicity due to benzodiazepines. Lack of response to a cumulative dose of 5 mg indicates that CNS depression is due to some other cause.
Methylene blue	0.2 ml/kg of 1% sol IV over 5-10 min. May be repeated after one hour upto maximum of 0.7 ml/kg	For toxic methemoglobinemia Urine becomes bluish-green in color
N-acetyl cysteine (NAC)	140 mg/kg 5% sol in water or fruit juice PO, then 70 mg/kg q 4 hr x 17 doses *Intravenous protocol*: 150 mg/kg loading dose in 5% dextrose slowly over 15 min, followed by maintenance dose of 50 mg/kg in 5% dextrose q 6-8 hr for 3 doses	For poisoning due to paracetamol
Naloxone hydrochloride	0.1 mg/kg IV or IM q 2-3 min upto 3 doses. After a satisfactory response repeat the dose every 5-10 min as long as opioid effect lasts. Maximum dose in children is 2 mg.	Poisoning due to opiates or its derivatives.
Oxygen	100% or hyperbaric oxygen till carboxyl hemoglobin level is <10%	Carbon monoxide suffocation.
Physostigmine	0.02 mg/kg/dose or 0.5 mg slow IV over 3 min or IM or SC. Repeat q 5 min till total of 2 mg	Poisoning or toxicity due to antichloinergic drugs
PAM or pralidoxine 2-pyridime aldozime methiodide	20-50 mg/kg IV or IM as 5% sol in normal saline, must be given within 48 hr of exposure. Repeat dose can be given after one hour followed by every 6-12 hr	For organophosphate insecticide poisoning
Prazosin	0.25 mg PO q 4-6 hr for 24 hr	Selective alpha-1-adrenergic blocking agent for scorpion bite
Protamine sulfate	Use 1 mg protamine sulfate as 1% sol IV slowly over 5 min to counteract 100 units of heparin. Give 2.5-5.0 mg/kg followed by 1.0-2.5 mg/kg IV q 4 hr. Protamine should be administered based on expected heparin amount because excess protamine also causes antiocoagulation	Antidote for heparin

Drug/Emergency	Dose and route of administration	Remarks
Pyridoxine	1.0 mg IV slowly over 30 min for each 1.0 mg of isoniazid upto a maximum of 500 mg if amount ingested is unknown.	
Vitamin K	5-10 mg IM or IV	Warfarin and dicumarol overdose

ARRHYTHMIAS

Supraventricular tachycardia	❑ Digitalize IV, refer to drugs for cardiopulmonary resuscitation	
	❑ Verapamil 0.1-0.3 mg/kg IV over 2 min, may repeat every 15 min upto maximum of 5 mg. Maintenance 1-2 mg/kg/every 8 hr. Oral dose: 4-8 mg/kg q 8 hr	Avoid in infants under one year and patients receiving beta blockers.
	❑ Propranolol 0.01-0.25 mg/kg slow IV every 10 min, for maintenance 0.5-1.0 mg/kg/day in 4 div doses PO	May cause hypoglycemia, bronchospasm, bradycardia
	❑ Adenosine 0.1 mg/kg IV push, increase bolus dose by 0.05 mg/kg q 2 min until a clinical response occurs or a maximum dose of 0.25 mg/kg or 12 mg is achieved	May cause bronchoconstriction in asthmatics
Auricular flutter/fibrillation	❑ Digitalize IV	
	❑ Quinidine sulfate test dose 2 mg/kg PO, 3-6 mg/kg/dose q 6 hr upto maximum of 5 doses per day	Avoid IV use
Ventricular tachycardia	❑ Lidocaine 1 mg/kg IV bolus, repeat q 5 min × 3 doses. 10-50 µg/kg/min constant infusion for maintenance	May cause seizures, coma and asystole
	❑ Bretylium tosylate 5-10 mg/kg IV over 10 min q 15 min upto maximum of 30 mg/kg	Do not give with digitalis.
	❑ Phenytoin 1.25 mg/kg IV q 5 min upto maximum of 15 mg/kg, maintenance dose 5-10 mg/kg/d q 12 hr IV or PO	Dilute only with normal saline, otherwise it crystallizes. IM absorption is very erratic
	❑ Procainamide 3-6 mg/kg/dose IV followed by constant infusion 0.02-0.08 mg/kg/min. Oral dose 50 mg/kg/d q 3-4 hr	It causes prolongation of PR, QRS, QT, Coomb's positive hemolytic anemia, and LE-like syndrome.
Complete heart block	❑ Atropine 0.01 mg/kg IV or SC, q 4-6 hr. Minimum dose 0.1 mg and maximum dose 1.0 mg	May be given through endotracheal tube
	❑ Isoproterenol 0.05-1.0 µg/kg/min as a constant infusion	

CARDIOPULMONARY RESUSCITATION (includes drugs for CCF)

Atropine	0.01 mg/kg/dose (minimum dose 0.1 mg) IV or SC	
Bretylium tosylate	Refer to drugs for arrhythmias	
Calcium gluconate (10%)	20-30 mg/kg/dose i.e. 0.25-0.5 ml/kg	Monitor heart rate, don't mix with sodium bicarbonate
Digitalis	*Total digitalizing dose*	
Premature neonate	10-20 µg/kg IV	
Full term neonate	30 µg/kg IV	
Infant	40-60 µg/kg PO or IV	
Child	40 µg/kg PO	
	Maintenance dose/day	
	4 µg/kg IV or PO q 24 hr	
	4-8 µg/kg IV or PO q 12 hr	
	10-20 µg/kg PO q 12 hr	
	5-10 µg/kg PO q 12 hr	
Dobutamine hydrochloride	5-20 µg/kg/min IV infusion, maximum 40 µg/kg/min	It also improve cardiac contractility. Do not mix with sodium bicarbonate. Titrate the dose to the desired effect.
Dopamine hydrochloride	5-20 µg/kg/min constant infusion, upto maximum of 50 µg/kg/min. Increase by increments of 5 µg/kg/min.	

$$\text{mg/100 ml of dobutamine/dopamine sol} = \frac{6 \times \text{weight in kg} \times \text{dose } (\mu g/kg/min)}{\text{Fluid infusion rate (ml/hr)}}$$

Drug/Emergency	Dose and route of administration	Remarks
Epinephrine	0.01 ml/kg/dose 1:1000 sol IM (0.01 mg/kg/dose). For IV use, dilute to 1: 10,000.	1: 1000 sol provides 1 mg/ml. Avoid intracardiac injection but can be instilled into the trachea in a dose of 0.5-1.0 ml/kg 1: 10,000 sol
Furosemide	1-2 mg/kg/dose IV or PO, upto 6 mg/kg/day q 12 hr	
Hydrocortisone sodium succinate	50 mg/kg IV every 6 hr	Used in patients with septic shock
Isoproterenol hydrochloride	Starting dose 0.1 µg/kg/min upto maximum of 1.0 mcg/kg/min	
Lidocaine	Refer to drugs for arrhythmias	
Naloxone hydrochloride	Refer to antidotes, specific	
Norepinephrine	Starting dose 0.1 µg/kg/min, maximum of 1.0 µg/kg/min	May cause renal ischemia
Sodium bicarbonate (7.5%)	1-2 mEq/kg/dose or 0.3 × kg × base deficit.	Establish ventilation before giving sodium bicarbonate. Do not add calcium gluconate, dopamine or epinephrine into sodium bicarbonate solution. Keep watch on serum sodium concentration.

CEREBRAL EDEMA (Raised ICP)

Phenobarbitone sodium	10-20 mg/kg IV stat, followed by maintenance dose of 5 mg/kg/d to maintain serum level between 20-40 mg/l	
Mannitol	5 ml/kg 20% sol IV stat in 30-60 min followed by 2 ml/kg q 8 hr	For diuresis the lowest dose (0.5 ml/kg) is given over 5 min.
Furosemide	Refer to drugs for cardiopulmonary resuscitation	
Dexamethasone	0.25 mg/kg (maximum 12 mg) IV q 6 hr	
Glycerol	0.5-1.0 g/kg PO q 6 hr	

CEREBRAL MALARIA

Quinine dihydrochloride	20 mg/kg of base is given in a concentration of 1mg/ml of normal saline or 5% dextrose. Infused over a period of 4 hours as a loading dose followed by 10 mg base/kg every 8 hourly as a slow infusion over 4 hours. Quinine dihydrochloride 12 mg of salt is equivalent to 10 mg of base. Shift to oral therapy as soon as possible. Give therapy for at least 7 days or upto 3 days after disappearance of asexual parasitemia	Watch for hypotension, cinchonism and hypoglycemia.
Artesunate	2.4 mg/kg IV bolus or IM stat, 12 hr, 24 hr and then once daily for total of 7 days. Available 60 mg vial is diluted with 0.6 ml of 7.5% sodium bicarbonate and made upto 5 ml with 5% dextrose. When patient is able to swallow oral medications are started along with doxycycline or tetracycline or clindamycin.	Avoid in G6PD dificiency and immunocompromised children
Artemether	3.2 mg/kg loading dose deep IM (Never IV) followed by 1.6 mg/kg once daily for 5 days. When patient is able to swallow, artemether is given orally along with doxycline or tetracycline or clindamycin	-do-

HYPERTENSIVE ENCEPHALOPATHY

Nifedipine	0.25-0.5 mg/kg per dose (maximum dose 10 mg) sublingual or oral q 6 hr	Flushing, headache, tachycardia
Hydralazine hydrochloride	0.1-0.2 mg/kg IM or IV, repeat after 4-6 hr. For maintenance 1.5-3.5 mg/kg/day in 4 div doses PO	Flushing, headache, tachycardia Avoid in porphyria, SLE and rheumatic valve disease

Section 6

Drug/Emergency	Dose and route of administration	Remarks
Reserpine	0.02 mg/kg/dose IM or PO q 12 hr, upto maximum of 0.07 mg/kg or 1.0 mg	Drowsiness, nasal congestion, GI bleeding
Diazoxide	1.0-3.0 mg/kg IV bolus, repeat q 5-15 min till blood pressure is controlled or maximum dose of 5 mg/kg is given	Hyperglycemia
Sodium nitroprusside	0.5-8.0 µg/kg/min IV constant infusion to titrate with blood pressure response. 50 mg is dissolved in one liter of 5% dextrose to provide a concentration of 50 µg/ml	Wrap bottle and infusion tubing in aluminium foil to prevent exposure of drug to light. Solution may appear brownish but if it is discolored blue, green, orange or red, it should be discarded
Amlodipine	0.05-0.1 mg/kg q 12-24 hr	Hendache, flushing and bradycardia
Nicardipine	0.5-4.0 µg/kg 1 min IV infusion upto maximum of 5 mg/hr	Flushing, headache, and tachycardia
Captopril	0.5-6.0 mg/kg/day in 2-3 div doses PO	Useful if plasma renin activity is high. Use with caution in patients with renal artery stenosis and volume depletion. The drug is not stable in solution and is available as tablets only.
Labetalol	0.25-1.0 mg/kg IV over 2 min, may repeat after 5 min or constant infusion 0.4-3.0 mg/kg/hr	Avoid in children with bronchial asthma, heart failure and hypoglycemia
Methyldopa	10-40 mg/kg/day in 3 div doses PO	Avoid in liver disease, pheochromocytoma, concomitant use of MAO inhibitors.
Furosemide	Refer to drugs for cardiopulmonary resuscitation	
Morphine sulfate	0.1-0.2 mg/kg IM. For continuous infusion 0.01-0.02 mg/kg/hr in neonates and 0.025-0.02 mg/kg/hr in older children	Useful in pulmonary edema

MUSCLE RELAXANTS

Drug/Emergency	Dose and route of administration	Remarks
Rocuronium	0.6-1.2 mg/kg IV or IM	Edrophonium, and neostigmine can reverse the effect of muscle relaxants
Succinylcholine	3 mg/kg IV in infants less than 1 year and 2 mg/kg IV in older children. Atropine should be used as a pretreatment in children below 5 years to prevent bradycardia	It is the drug of choice and has fast onset of action (< 1 min) and rapid recovery (5-10 min). Avoid using in children with family history of malignant hyperthermia and patients having hyperthermia, renal failure, burns and myopathy with elevated CPK.
Vecuronium	0.2-0.3 mg/kg IV every one hour as needed to maintain paralysis.	Onset of action is fast (60-90 sec) but recovery is delayed (90-120 min). Dose should be adjusted in children with hepatic dysfunction.

SEPSIS/MENINGITIS

Drug/Emergency	Dose and route of administration	Remarks
Aminoglycosides		Adjust the dose in renal dysfunction
Amikacin sulfate*	Preterm babies 0-7 days: 7.5 mg/kg/dose IV, IM q 12 hr Others: 10 mg/kg/dose IV, IM q 8-12 hr	
Gentamicin sulfate*	2.5 mg/kg/dose IV, IM q 8-12 hr	
Netilmicin	2.5 mg/kg/dose IV, IM q 8-12 hr	

Drug/Emergency	Dose and route of administration	Remarks
Streptomycin sulfate	20 mg/kg/dose 12 hr IM, upto maximum daily dose of 1000 mg.	Deafness may occur
Tobramycin	2.0 mg/kg/dose IV, IM q 8-12 hr	
Cephalosporins		Cross-sensitivity to penicillin
Cefaclor	5-10 mg/kg/dose q 6-8 hr oral	
Cefazoline sodium*	20 mg/kg/dose IV over 5-10 min infusion q 6 hr	
Cefepime	50-100 mg/kg/dose q 8-12 hr	Its antipseudomonal activity is similar to ceftazidime
Cefoperazone	25-100 mg/kg/dose IV q 8-12 hr	Does not cross the blood brain barrier
Cefotaxime sodium*	50 mg/kg/dose IV infusion over 15-30 min q 6-8 hr	
Ceftazidime*	50 mg/kg/dose IV, IM q 8 hr	
Ceftizoxime	50 mg/kg/dose IV, IM q 8 hr	Excellent for anerobes
Ceftriaxone sodium	50-70 mg/kg/dose IV or IM q 12-24 hr	
Cefuroxime axetil	25-50 mg/kg/dose IV, IM, PO q 6-8 hr	
Cephoxtin**	50 mg/kg/dose IV, IM.	Effective against *B. fragilis*
Moxalactum disodium	50 mg/kg/dose IV infusion over 15-30 min	
Lincosamides		
Clindamycin hydrochloride	0-7 days: 5 mg/kg/dose q 8 hr PO, IV >7 days: 5 mg/kg/dose q 6 hr PO, IV	Useful against MRSA, anerobic infections, *P. carinii* and toxoplasmosis
Lincomycin hydrochloride	5-10 mg/kg/dose q 12 hr IM, IV 7.5 mg/kg/dose q 6 hr PO	May cause pseudomembranous colitis
Macrolids		
Azithromycin	10 mg/kg single dose empty stomach oral on day 1 and 5 mg/kg during next 4-5 days. *Enteric fever*: 20 mg/kg/d for 7-14 days, *cholera*: 20 mg/kg single dose only	Gram-positive infections, typhoid fever, campylobacter enteritis, cat scratch disease, and cholera
Clarithromycin	15 mg/kg/d q 12 hr oral	Indicated in *H. pylori*, chlamydiae, mycoplasma, atypical mycobacteria, and *M. marinum* infection from sea water
Erythromycin	30-50 mg/kg/d q 6 hr PO. 5 mg/kg/dose IV infusion over 8 hr in normal saline or intermittent bolus over 30-60 min every 6-8 hr	Gram-positive infections and *Arcanobacterium haemolyticum*
Roxithromycin	5-8 mg/kg/d q 12 hr	Avoid concomitant use with ergotamine alkaloids
Penicillins		
Amoxycillin	25 mg/kg/dose q 6 hr PO	
Amoxycillin with potassium clavulanate	15-25 mg/kg/dose q 8 hr IV	Effective against beta-lactamase producing bugs
Ampicillin sodium trihydrate	Neonate: 25-50 mg/kg/dose IV Child: 25 mg/kg/dose, 50-100 mg/kg/dose IV for meningitis	
Carbenicillin**	100 mg/kg/dose IV (infused over 15 min), IM q 4-6 hr	Do not mix with gentamicin, may cause hypokalemia
Cloxacillin**	12.5-25 mg/kg/dose PO, IV q 4-6 hr	Crosses blood brain barrier
Methicillin**	25 mg/kg/dose, 50 mg/kg/dose for meningitis IV, IM	
Oxacillin sodium**	25 mg/kg/dose IV, IM	

* Every 12 hr for infants 0-7 days and every 8 hr for infants > 7 days

** Preterm upto 7 days, administer every 12 hr, term infant upto 7 days or preterm > 7 days every 8 hr and term infant after 7 days every 6 hr

Section 6

Drug/Emergency	Dose and route of administration	Remarks
Penicillin G, aqueous**	Neonates < 2 kg: 50,000 u/kg/day 12 hrly 1,00,000 u/kg/day 12 hrly for meningitis > 2 kg: 75,000 u/kg/day 8 hrly Older infants: 1,50,000 u/kg/day 8 hrly Children : 1,00,000- 2,50,000 u/kg/day every 6 hr 3,00,000 u/kg/day every 4 hrly for meningitis	Sodium and potassium content is 1.68 mEq per million units, rapid bolus injection may cause seizures.
Piperacillin with tazobactum	50-75 mg/kg/dose IV, IM q 6-8 hr	Active against Gram-negative and Gram-positive aerobic and anerobic bacteria
Ticarcillin disodium**	75 mg/kg/dose IV infusion over 15-30 min, IM q 6-8 hr	It is more active in-vitro against *Pseudomonas aeruginosa.*
Sulfas		
Trimethoprim-sulfamethoxazole	Neonate: 2 mg/kg TMP loading dose followed by 0.6 mg/kg q 12 hr PO, IV Child: 2.5-5.0 mg/kg of TMP q 12 hr PO, IV	Drug of choice for *Pneumocystis carinii*
Miscellaneous agents		
Amphotericin B	0.1 mg/kg IV test dose, 1.0 mg/kg/day IV infusion in 5% dextrose over 6 hr. Give till a total maximum dose of 30-35 mg/kg is reached *Lipsomal amphotericin B:* 1-3 mg/kg IV daily for 5 days followed by sixth dose on day 10	Protect against exposure to light, monitor serum potassium level during therapy and frequently change the IV site to prevent phlebitis
Aztreonam	30-50 mg/kg/dose IM, IV q 6-8 hr. Avoid below 1 week age.	Crosses blood brain barrier and is beta-lactamase stable
Chloramphenicol	25 mg/kg/dose IV, IM, PO (upto 2 weeks q 24 hr, 15-30 days q 12 hr; subsequently q 6-8 hr). Avoid below 1 week age.	Do not combine with gentamicin; monitor blood levels in neonates and maintain between 15-30 mcg/ml.
Ciprofloxacin	5-10 mg/kg/dose q 12 hr PO, IV	Caution in children
Colistin sulfate	5 mg/kg per dose q 6-8 hr PO	
Imipenem/cilastatin	20-30 mg/kg/dose IM or IV q 8 hr	Drug of choice for extended spectrum beta-lactamase producing microorganisms (ESBL). Use with caution in children with epilepsy
Meropenem	20 mg/kg/dose q 8-12 hr IV	Drug of choice for ESBL
Metronidazole	15 mg/kg loading dose PO, IV followed 24-48 hr later with 7.5 mg/kg/dose q 12 hr and after one week 15 mg/kg/dose q 12 hr	Useful for anerobic infections and antibiotic associated diarrhea
Ofloxacin	2.5-5 mg/kg/dose q 12 hr IV, PO	
Polymyxin B*	2.5-5.0 mg/kg/dose IV, IM	
Polymyxin E*	2.5 mg/kg/dose IV, IM	
Teicoplanin	10 mg/kg/dose q 12 hr for 3 doses, then 5-10 mg/kg q 24 hr IV bolus or infusion and IM	It has longer half life than vancomycin and can be given IM. Crosses blood brain barrier
Vancomycin hydrochloride*	10-15 mg/kg/dose IV over 60 min or longer infusion	Avoid bolus. Risk of ototoxicity, nephrotoxicity and "red man" syndrome
Tigecycline	1.5 mg/g stat followed by 1 mg/kg/d as IV infusion over 30-60 min for maintenance. Effective against MRSA, Gram-negative MDR, Acinetobacter ESBL, and Carbapenem resistant, *S. aureus*	Risk of hepatic toxicity

* Every 12 hr for infants 0-7 days and every 8 hr for infants > 7 days
** Preterm upto 7 days, administer every 12 hr, term infant upto 7 days or preterm > 7 days every 8 hr and term infant after 7 days every 6 hr

Drug/Emergency	Dose and route of administration	Remarks
STATUS ASTHMATICUS		
Epinephrine	Refer to drugs for anaphylaxis	
Terbutaline sulfate	5-10 µg/kg SC q 15 min x 3 doses, maintenance 0.1-0.15 mg/kg/day q 6-8 hr PO. Aerosol with 10% (10 mg/ml) respiratory solution, 0.03 ml/kg (2.5 mg <20 kg and 5.0 mg >20 kg) upto maximum of 1 ml diluted with 2 ml normal saline, pressurized aerosol 250-500 µg (1-2 puffs) 3-4 times/day	
Aminophylline	5-7 mg/kg IV diluted in 25-50 ml saline and given over 15-20 min as a loading dose, maintenance 0.65 mg/kg/hr constant infusion (maximum 0.85 mg/kg/hr in infants) or slow bolus q 6 hr. For maintenance 15-20 mg/kg/day q 8 hr, oral.	Avoid bolus and use lower dose if child is already receiving aminophylline. Maintain serum aminophylline level between 10-20 µg/ml. 1.0 mg/kg of aminophylline raises serum level by 2 µg/ml.
Salbutamol	0.1-0.4 mg/kg per dose q 8 hr PO *Aerosols:* Respiratory sol 0.5% (5 mg/ml) 0.01 –0.03 ml/kg upto maximum of 1 ml (2.5 mg diluted with 2 ml saline) 4 times/day, pressurized aerosol 100-200 µg (1-2 puffs) every 5 minutes upto 10-12 times or till relief followed by q 4-6 hr	Use low-pressure ultrasonic or wall mounted nebulizer. Monitor pulse rate and stop aerosol therapy if it exceeds 180/min.
Ipratropium bromide	2 puffs (20 ug/puff) every 5 min for a total of 10-20 puffs. 250 ug diluted in 3 ml normal saline is nebulized every 20 min for 3 doses	
Metaproterenol	5-10 mg in 2 ml saline as aerosol q 30 min x 4 doses. 2 mg/kg/day q 6-8 hr pO	
Orciprenaline	0.3-0.5 mg/kg/dose upto maximum of 1.0 mg/kg day PO, IM	
Bambuterol hydrochloride	Children 2-5 yr: 5 mg, 6-12 yr 10 mg single oral dose at night	Avoid below 2 yr
Budesonide	MDI 200-800 µg/d q 12 hr. For croup, 2 mg in 2.5 ml normal saline q 12 hr for 48 hr by nebulization	Useful for acute attack of bronchial asthma and maintenance therapy
Theophylline	15-25 mg/kg/d q 8 hr oral	Add-on therapy for severe attack
Hydrocortisone sodium succinate	10 mg/kg IV stat, followed by 5 mg/kg/day q 6 hr	The response is slow and maximal effect occurs after 2-3 days, taper therapy within 5-7 days
Dexamethasone phosphate (or betamethasone)	0.3 mg/kg IV stat, followed by 0.3 mg/kg/day q 6 hr	
Magnesium sulfate	30-70 mg/kg or 0.1 ml/kg of 50% solution in 30 ml N/5 saline IV infusion over 30 min. May be repeated every 6 hr for 3-4 doses	
Isoproterenol	0.1 mcg/kg/min constant IV infusion, increase dose at a rate of 0.1 mcg/kg/min every 15-20 min until there is clinical improvement or tachycardia (200 beats/min) or cardiac arrhythmia occurs.	
STATUS EPILEPTICUS		
Diazepam	0.2-0.5 mg/kg IV bolus over 1-2 min (maximum 10 mg) repeat at 15 min and 45 min if seizures persist. Rectal route: 0.3-0.5 mg/kg/dose	Watch for respiratory depression and hypotension
Lorazepam	0.05-0.1 mg/kg (upto max 4 mg) IV over 1-2 min, may repeat after 15 min	Risk of respiratory depression and hypotension is low, duration of effect is longer

* For complete list of drugs with dosages, route of administration, proprietary formulations and their concentrations, etc. please refer to Drug Dosages in Children by Singh M and Deorari AK, *CBS Publishers & Distributors Pvt Ltd, New Delhi*, 9th edition, 2015.

Drug/Emergency	Dose and route of administration	Remarks
Phenytoin sodium	20 mg/kg IV slowly at a rate of 1 mg/kg/min under cardiac monitoring, repeat 10 mg/kg after 1 hr and 4 hr if seizures persist. Dilute with normal saline and not dextrose.	Ensure serum concentration around 25 µg/ml. Watch for hypotension and arrhythmia
Fosphenytoin	15-20 mg phenytoin dose equivalents IV slowly at 3 mg/kg/min. Each 1.5 mg fosphenytoin = 1 mg phenytoin	It can be dissolved in 5% dextrose. There is less risk of hypotension and phlebitis.
Phenobarbitone sodium	20 mg/kg loading dose IV at 1 mg/kg/min, followed by maintenance of 5-10 mg/kg/day q 12-24 hr	Maintain serum concentration around 20-40 mg/l.
Midazolam	0.2 mg/kg IV bolus or IM followed by a continuous infusion of 1-2 mg/kg/hr. Intranasal 0.3 mg/kg, buccal route 0.3 mg/kg for domiciliary use	It is equally effective when given IM and through buccal route (0.2-0.5 mg/kg/dose)
Lidocaine	1-2 mg/kg IV bolus followed by a constant infusion at a rate of 3-5 mg/kg/hr	It does not cause any respiratory depression but experience is limited in children
Paraldehyde	150-200 mg/kg (0.1-0.2 ml/kg) loading dose IV over 15 min as 5% sol in normal saline, followed by 20 mg/kg /hr. May be given deep IM. Rectal dose is 0.3-0.5 ml/kg which can be repeated at 20 min intervals if seizures persist. For rectal administration it is diluted with equal volume of olive oil or coconut oil	Avoid use of plastic equipment for rectal use
Propofol	1-2 mg/kg bolus followed by 2-10 mg/kg/hr constant infusion for 12-24 hr	
Thiopental	5-10 mg/kg loading dose IV followed by 5 mg/kg/hr continuous infusion along with mechanical ventilation	
Valproate sodium	20 mg/kg loading dose followed by 5-10 mg/kg/dose q 8 hr. Dilute 1:1 in normal saline or 5% dextrose and give IV infusion slowly over 5 min (maximum 20 mg per minute). Rectal dose is 20 mg/kg	It is safe and effective. Give supplements of carnitine when using high doses

Appendices

1.1 Milligrams/Milliequivalents Conversions

$$\text{mEq/L (milliequivalents per liter)} = \frac{\text{mg per liter}}{\text{equivalent weight}}$$

$$\text{Equivalent weight} = \frac{\text{atomic weight}}{\text{valence of element}}$$

$$\text{mmoles/L (millimoles per liter)} = \frac{\text{mg per liter}}{\text{atomic weight}}$$

$$\text{mg/dl} = \frac{\text{mmol/L} \times \text{atomic weight}}{10}$$

Radical	mEq/L	mg/dl	mg/dl	mEq/L
Sodium	1	2.30	1	0.4348
Potassium	1	3.91	1	0.2558
Calcium	1	2.00	1	0.4988
Magnesium	1	1.21	1	0.8230
Chloride	1	3.55	1	0.2817
Ammonium	1	1.80	1	0.5556
Bicarbonate	1	6.10	1	0.1639
Lactate	1	8.90	1	0.1123
Phosphorus:				
Valence 1	1	3.10	1	0.3226
Valence 1.8	1	1.72	1	0.5814

Atomic Weights and Valencies

Radical	Atomic weight	Valence
Sodium	23	1
Potassium	39	1
Calcium	40	2
Magnesium	24	2
Phosphorus	31	1 and 1.8
Chloride	35.5	1

1.2 Conventional units/SI units[2, 5, 8]

The SI system (Systems International d' Units) has now been adopted in clinical biochemistry in the United Kingdom and many other countries and has replaced the empirical or conventional units (e.g. mg/dl, mEq/L). The SI unit uses mole or its fractions per liter (or cubic decimeter) to express concentration of biochemical substances.

$$\text{Number of moles (mol)} = \frac{\text{Weight in gram}}{\text{molecular weight}}$$

The decimal fractions of mole are millimoles (10^{-3}), micromoles (10^{-6}), nanomoles (10^{-9}) and picomoles (10^{-12}). The units of expression of concentration in SI units would be mmol/l, umol/l, nmol/l and pmol/l. When the molecular weight of a substance being measured is unknown or uncertain, the SI units will be in g or ml/l e.g. total serum protein of 7.0 g/dl would be expressed as 70 g/l.

Conversion of mEq/L to mmol/l

In the case of univalent ions such as Na and K, mEq/L is identical to mmol/L. For polyvalent ions the mEq/L unit is divided by the valency to obtain mmol/L value. For example, serum calcium of 5 mEq/L is expressed as 2.5 mmol/L.

Conversion of mg/dl to mmol/l

The method for conversion is to divide mg/dl value by the molecular weight (to convert mg to mmoles) and to multiply by 10 (to convert dl to liter). For example, the molecular weight of urea is 60 and of glucose 180. The blood urea and glucose concentrations of 30 mg/dl and 90 mg/dl respectively would be expressed as 5 mmol/l in SI units for both the constituents.

The SI unit of pressure is pascal (Pa) and kilopascal (kPa); one kilopascal is equivalent to 7.5 mm Hg. The unit of energy in SI system is joules (J) and kilojoules (kj); one kj is equivalent to 0.238 kcal.

1.3 Conversion Factors for SI Units for Selected Constituents[8]

Substance	Molecular weight	From SI units	To SI units
Bilirubin	584.7	u mol/l × 0.0585 = mg/dl	mg/dl × 17.1 = u mol/l
Calcium	40.08		
Plasma		mol/l × 4.008 = mg/dl	mg/dl × 0.250 = m mol/l
Urine		m mol/24 hr × 40.08 = mg/24 hr	mg/24 hr × 0.025 = m mol/l
Cholesterol	386.7	m mol/l × 38.6 = mg/dl	mg/dl × 0.0259 = m mol/l
Copper	63.54		
Plasma		u mol/l × 6.35 = ug/dl	ug/dl × 0.157 = u mol/l
Urine		u mol/24 hr × 63.5 = ug/24 hr	ug/24 hr × 0.0157 = u mol/24 hr
Creatinine	113.1		
Plasma		u mol/l × 0.0113 = mg/dl	mg/dl × 88.4 = u mol/l
Urine		m mol/24 hr × 0.113 = g/24 hr	g/24 hr × 8.84 = m mol/l
Glucose	180.2		
Plasma/blood		m mol/l × 18.02 = mg/dl	mg/dl × 0.0555 = m mol/l
Urine		m mol/l × 0.0180 = g/dl	g/dl × 55.5 = m mol/l
Iron and TIBC	55.85	u mol/l × 5.59 = ug/dl	ug/dl × 0.179 = u mol/l
Lead	207.2		
Blood		u mol/l × 20.7 = ug/dl	ug/dl × 0.0483 = u mol/l
Urine		u mol/24 hr × 207 = ug/24 hr	ug/24 hr × 0.0483 = u mol/24 hr
Magnesium	24.31		
Plasma		m mol/l × 2.43 = mg/dl	mg/dl × 0.411 = m mol/l
Urine		m mol/24 hr × 24.3 = mg/24 hr	mg/24 hr × 0.0411 = m mol/24 hr
Phosphate	30.97		
Serum		m mol/l × 3.10 = mg/dl	mg/dl × 0.323 = m mol/l hr
Urine		m mol/24 hr × 0.0310 = g/24 hr	g/24 hr × 32.3 = m mol/24 hr
Salicylate	138.1	m mol/l × 13.81 = mg/dl	mg/dl × 0.0724 = m mol/l
Thyroxine	776.9	n mol/l × 0.0777 = ug/dl	ug/dl × 12.87 = n mol/l
Triiodothyronine	651.01	n mol/l × 0.651 = ng/dl	ng/dl × 1.54 = n mol/l
Triglycerides	885.4	m mol/l × 88.5 = mg/dl	mg/dl × 0.113 = m mol/l
Uric acid	168.1	m mol/l × 16.81 = mg/dl	mg/dl × 0.595 = m mol/l
Urea	60.06	m mol/l × 6.01 = mg/dl	mg/dl × 0.166 = m mol/l

1.4 Weight and Measurement Conversion Tables[5]

Weight

Apothecary	Metric
1 grain	60 mg or 0.06 g
15 grains	1000 mg or 1.0 g
60 grains (1 dram)	4.0 g
8 drams (1 oz)	30.0 g
1 pound (16 oz)	480.0 g
2.2 pounds	1 kg

Liquid Measures

1 minim	0.06 ml
15 minims	1.0 ml
60 minims (1 fl dram)	3.7 ml
8 fl dram (1 fl oz)	30.0 ml
16 fl oz (1 pt)	500.0 ml
32 fl oz (1 qt)	1000.0 ml

Height and Weight Conversion Factors

To convert	Multiply by
Inches to centimeters	2.54
Inches to meters	0.0254
Feet to meters	0.3048
Pounds to kilograms	0.4535
Kilograms to pounds	2.2

Prefixes for Denoting Decimal Factors

Prefix	Symbol	Factor
Mega	M	10^6
Kilo	k	10^3
Hecto	h	10^2
Deka	da	10^1
Deci	d	10^{-1}
Centi	c	10^{-2}
Milli	m	10^{-3}
Micro	u	10^{-6}
Nano	n	10^{-9}
Pico	p	10^{-12}
Femto	f	10^{-15}

1.5 Thermometer Readings

The normal body temperature of 98.4°F corresponds to 36.9°C. To convert °F to °C subtract 32 and divide by 1.8. To convert °C to °F multiply by 1.8 and add 32.

Temperature Equivalents

Celsius	Fahrenheit	Celsius	Fahrenheit
35.0	95.0	38.6	101.4
35.4	95.7	39.0	102.2
35.8	96.4	39.4	102.9
36.0	96.8	39.8	103.6
36.4	97.5	40.2	104.3
36.8	98.2	40.6	105.1
37.0	98.6	41.0	105.8
37.4	99.3	41.4	106.5
37.8	100.0	41.8	107.2
38.2	100.7	42.0	107.6

Age	Mean systolic± 2 S.D.		Mean diastolic± S.D.	
	(kPa)	(mmHg)	(kPa)	(mmHg)
Newborn	10.6 ± 2.1	(80 ± 16)	6.1 ± 2.1	(46 ± 16)
6-12 months	11.8 ± 3.9	(89 ± 29)	8.0 ± 1.3	(60 ± 16)
1 year	12.8 ± 4.0	(96 ± 30)	8.8 ± 3.3	(66 ± 25)
2 years	13.2 ± 3.3	(99 ± 25)	8.5 ± 3.3	(64 ± 25)
3 years	13.3 ± 3.3	(100 ± 25)	8.9 ± 3.1	(67 ± 23)
4 years	13.2 ± 2.7	(99 ± 20)	8.6 ± 2.7	(65 ± 20)
5-6 years	12.5 ± 1.9	(94 ± 14)	7.3 ± 1.2	(55 ± 9)
6-7 years	13.3 ± 2.0	(100 ± 15)	7.5 ± 1.2	(56 ± 9)
7-8 years	13.6 ± 2.0	(102 ± 15)	7.5 ± 1.1	(56 ± 8)
8-9 years	14.0 ± 2.1	(105 ± 16)	7.6 ± 1.2	(57 ± 9)
9-10 years	14.2 ± 2.1	(107 ± 16)	7.6 ± 1.2	(57 ± 9)
10-11 years	14.8 ± 2.3	(111 ± 17)	7.7 ± 1.3	(58 ± 10)
11-12 years	15.0 ± 2.4	(113 ± 18)	7.8 ± 1.3	(59 ± 10)
12-13 years	15.3 ± 2.5	(115 ± 19)	7.8 ± 1.3	(59 ± 10)
13-14 years	15.7 ± 2.5	(118 ± 19)	8.0 ± 1.3	(60 ± 10)

APPENDIX 2 Normal Blood Pressure Values at Various Ages[7]

Blood pressure measurement should be made using a cuff covering two-thirds of the upper arm. (1 mmHg is approximately equal to 133 Pascals (pa) or one kilo Pascal = 7.5 mmHg)

APPENDIX 3 Nomogram for Calculating Body Surface Area

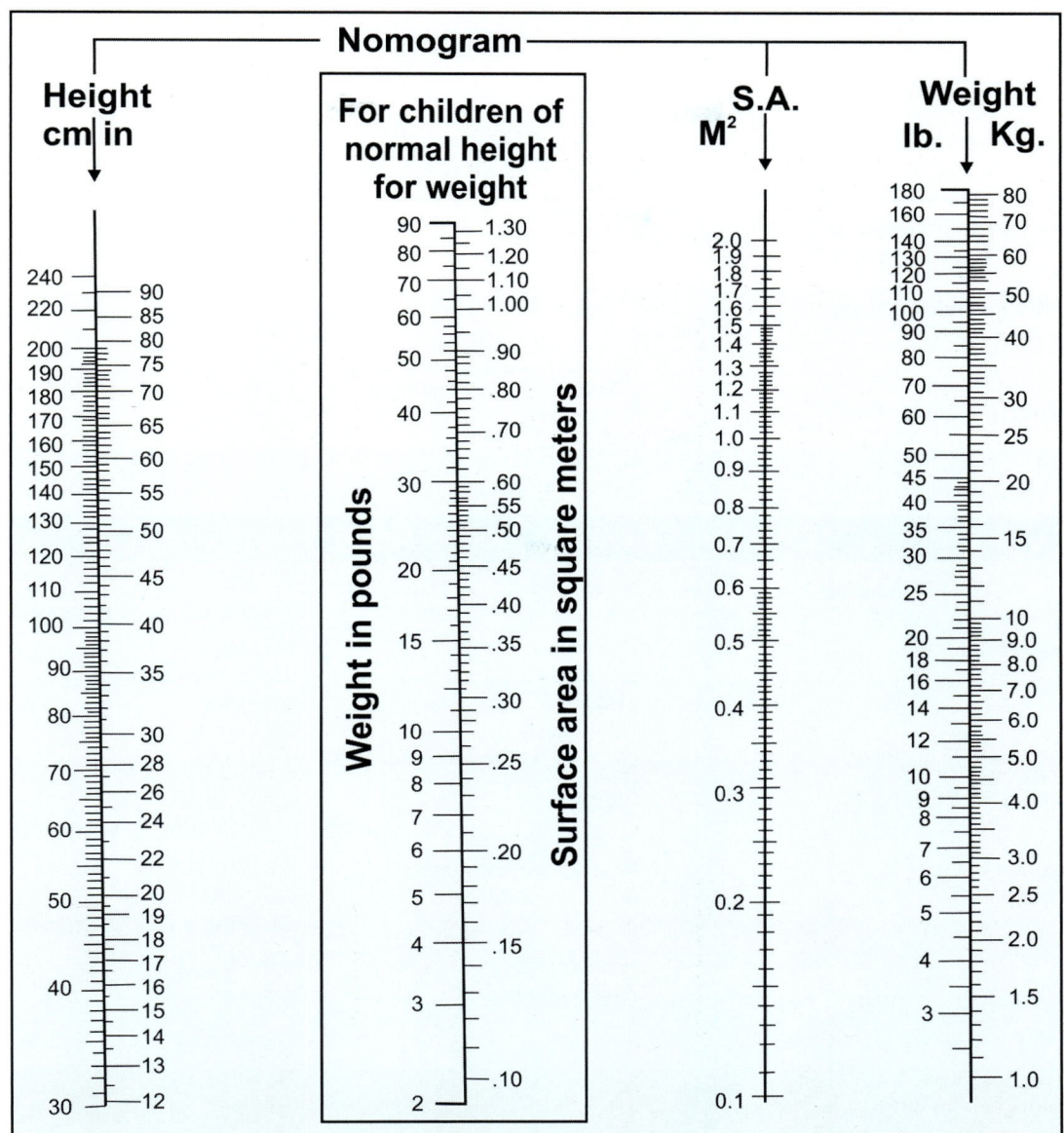

APPENDIX 4 Calculation of Approximate Surface Area from Weight in Children with Normal Physique	
Weight range (kg)	Approximate surface area (m²)
1-5	(0.05 × weight) + 0.05
6-10	(0.04 × weight) + 0.10
11-20	(0.03 × weight) + 0.20
21-40	(0.02 × weight) + 0.40

Lowe's formula: Surface area (m²) $= \sqrt[3]{\text{weight}^2 \text{ (kg)} \times 0.1}$

Costeff's formula: Surface area (m²) $= \dfrac{4w + 7}{w + 90}$ where w is weight in kg.

Mosteller's formula: Surface area (m²) $= \sqrt{\dfrac{\text{Height (cm)} \times \text{weight (kg)}}{3600}}$

APPENDIX 5 Reference Values of Urinalysis[2, 5]				
	Determination	Age	Normal range	
1.	Volume (ml/day)	Newborns Infants Children Adolescents	50-300 350-550 500-1000 700-1400	
2.	Specific gravity (random)	Infants Children	1.001-1.020 1.001-1.030 > 1.025 (after fluid restriction)	
3.	Osmolality (mOsm/l)	Prematures/newborns Infants & children	50-600 50-1400 >850 (after fluid restriction)	
4.	pH	Newborns & infants children	5.0-7.0 4.8-7.8	
5.	Sugar (qualitative)		Negative	
6.	Protein (qualitative) Quantitative (mg/dl)		Negative 10-100	
7.	Microscopic (per HPF) Leukocytes Erythrocytes Casts		0-4 rare rare	
8.	Addis count Leukocytes Erythrocytes Casts		< 10/mm³ < 5/mm³ Occasional hyaline	
9.	Colony count (colonies/ml)		Clean catch midstream	Catheterzation	Suprapubic bladder puncture
		Infants Children	< 1,000 < 10,000	Upto 100 Upto 100	0 0
10.	Sodium (mEq/kg/day)	Newborn Older	3.7 0.11-0.39	

APPENDIX 5 Reference Values of Urinalysis[2, 5] *(Contd.)*			
11.	Potassium (mEq/kg/day)	Newborn Older	2.3 2.0
12.	Creatinine (mg/kg/day)	Newborn/Infants Older	10-20 5-40
13.	Calcium (mg/kg/day)		4.0
14.	Phosphorus (mg/kg/day)		15.20

APPENDIX 6 Mean Urine Output at Different Ages			
Age	Normal urine output		Oliguria
	(ml/24 hr)	(ml/kg/hr)	(ml/kg/hr)
Newborn	250	2.5	<1.0
2 months	450	3.5	<1.25
1 year	500	2.0	<0.60
2 years	550	1.7	<0.50
4 years	650	1.7	<0.50
7 years	750	1.7	<0.45
11 years	1100	1.4	<0.40
14 years	1200	1.4	<0.40
Adult	1500	0.8	<0.30

Adapted from Black JA, Pediatric Emergencies. *Butterworths, London,* second edition 1987

APPENDIX 7 Normal Hematological Values[4]
(All values shown are means with the ranges in parentheses)

Age	Red blood cells per mm³	Hemoglobin (g%)	Hematocrit (%)	White blood cells per mm³	Neutrophils (%)	Lymphocytes (%)	Eosinophils (%)	Monocytes (%)	Reticulocytes (%)	Platelets per mm³	MVC (ft)	MCH (pg)	MCHC (%)
Birth	5.0-6.0 × 10⁶	17 (14-20)	55 (45-65)	18,000 (9,000-30,000)	60 (40-80)	32	2	7-14	5 (3-7)	1,00,000-3,00,000	94-118	32-40	34-36
1 week	Values fall within 3 months	17 (13-21)	54 (43-66)	12,000 (6-22,000)	90 (30-50)	46	3	7-14	2 (0-4)		88-108	32-40	34-36
2 weeks	--	16.5 (13-20)	50 (42-66)	12,000 (5-21,000)	40 (30-50)	48	3	6-12	1 (0-2)	150,000 to 450,000	86-106	32-40	34-36
3 months to 6 years	3.5-5.6 × 10⁶	12 (10.5-14)	38 (33-42)	10,000 (6-15,000)	42 (32-52)	51	2-3	4-8	1 (0-2)		76-88	24-30	30-36
Adult Females	3.9-5.6 × 10⁶	14 (12-16)	42 (37-47)	7500 (5-10,000)	60 (40-75)	30 (20-45)	1-6	2-10	0-2		76-96	27-32	30-35
Males	4.5-6.5 × 10⁶	16 (14-18)	46 (42-52)								76-96	27-32	30-35

In very low birth weight infants (BW <1500g) the mean Hb value falls from 18 g% at birth to 10 g% at six weeks (rising slowly thereafter) and mean corpuscular volume falls from 115 fl. to 95 fl. over the same period. Upto 34 to 36 weeks of fetal life 90 to 95 percent is fetal hemoglobin. Thereafter the proportion of fetal hemoglobin decreases at a rate of 3 to 4 percent/week, until 40 weeks when mean fetal hemoglobin is 75 percent and range 50 percent to 85 percent. To convert per mm³ to per liter, multiply by 10⁶.

APPENDIX 8 Simplified Coagulation Profile[4, 5]

Determination	Specimen	Age	Normal range
Activated clotting time	Hand held Water bath		1 min 50 sec to 2 min 30 sec 1 min 30 sec to 2 min 10 sec
Bleeding time (Ivy)		Premature/ Newborn Child	1-8 min 1-6 min
Clot retraction	Whole blood		40-94% at 2 hr
Clotting time (Lee-White) 2 tubes 3 tubes	Whole blood		 5-8 min 6-18 min
Fibrin degradation products (FDP)	Serum		<10 mcg/ml
Fibrinogen	Plasma	Cord Newborn Child	216 mg/dl 125-300 mg/dl 200-450 mg/dl
Fibrinolysin	Plasma		No lysis of clot in 2 hr
Partial thromboplastin time (PTT)*	Plasma	Premature Newborn Child	< 120 sec < 90 sec 20-40 sec
Prothrombin consumption	Serum		25 sec
Prothrombin time (PT)	Plasma	Newborn	< 17 sec 11-14 sec
Thrombin time	Plasma	Child	< 17 sec
Thromboplastin generation time (TGT)	Plasma	Premature Newborn Child	8-24 sec to 6 min 8-20 sec 8-16 sec

* Moderate deficiency of coagulation factors dependent upon vitamin K (II prothrombin; VII proconvertin; IX plasma thromboplastin component; X Stuart-Prower factor) occurs during the first day of life. Values return to near normal levels within one week. This deficiency may account for prolonged PTT, PT and TGT during this period.

APPENDIX 9 Reference Biochemical Values[5, 7, 8]			
Determination	**Specimen**	**Age/sex**	**Normal value**
1. Acetone (aceto acetic acid) (mg/dl)	Serum/ plasma	Qualitative Quantitative	Negative 0.3-3.0
2. Alanine aminotransferase (SGPT, 30°C) (u/l)	Serum	Newborn/Infant Thereafter; M F	5-28 6-12 4-17
3. Albumin (g/dl)	Serum	Newborn Child	2.5-3.5 4.0-5.0
4. Aldolase (Fructose 1-6 diphosphate, 37°C) (u/l)	Serum	Infant Child Adult	1.5-18.8 2.3-13.5 1.5-12.0
5. Ammonia (ug/dl)	Whole blood	Premature Newborn Child Thereafter	100-200 90-150 40-80 40-110
6. Amylase (37°C) (units/dl)	Serum		45-200 dye units
7. Antitrypsin, alpha-1 (mg/dl)	Serum	0-5 d1-9 yr	143-440 147-245
8. ASLO titer	Serum	Child	170-330 Todd units
9. Asparate aminotransferase (SGOT, 30°C) (u/l)	Serum	Newborn/Infant Thereafter; M F	5-40 7-21 6-18
10. Barbiturate (mg/dl)	Whole blood	Therapeutic 0.01-0.2 Coma level: Short acting > 1.0 Intermediate acting > 3, Long acting > 5	
11. Bilirubin, total (mg/dl) Direct (conjugated)	Serum	Cord 0-2 weeks Infant & Child	< 3 < 15 < 2 < 0.2
12. Calcium, total (mg/dl)	Serum	Cord Premature (1 wk) Newborn Infant Child Thereafter	8.2-11.1 6.1-11.0 5.9-10.7 9.0-11.0 8.8-10.8 8.5-10.4
13. Ceruloplasmin (mg/dl)	Serum	Newborn to 6 months 6 months-1 yr 1yr–12 yr Thereafter	1.0-3.0 15-50 30-65 25-43
14. Cholesterol (mg/dl)	Serum	1-3 yr 4-6 yr 7-14 yr	45-182 109-189 124-210
15. Copper (mcg/dl)	Serum	Newborn Infant & child Adolescent	20-70 30-150 90-240
16. Cortisol (RIA) (mcg/dl)	Plasma	8 A.M. 4 P.M.	5-20 2-15
17. Creatine kinase (iu/l)	Serum	Cord	10-300

(contd.)

APPENDIX 9 Reference Biochemical Values[5, 7, 8] *(Contd.)*

	Determination	Specimen	Age/sex		Normal value
18.	Creatinine (mg/dl)	Serum	Cord		0.6-1.2
			Infant		0.2-0.4
			Child		0.3-1.0
			Adolescent		0.5-1.0
			Adult:	M	0.6-1.2
				F	0.5-1.1
19.	Creatinine clearance (endogenous)	Serum and timed urine	Newborn		40-65 ml/min/1.73 m^2
			Child :	M	98-150
				F	95-125
20.	Fatty acids, free (mmol/l)	Serum			0.3-0.9 m mol/l
21.	Ferritin (ng/ml)	Serum	Newborn		25-200
			1 month		200-600
			2-5 months		50-200
			6 months – 16 yr		7-14
22.	Fetoproteins, alpha (mcg/ml)	Serum			1.0 < 2 times "multiple of the mean"
23.	Glucose, fasting (mg/dl)	Serum/ plasma	Cord		45-96
			Premature		40-60
			Neonate		40-80
			Child		60-100
			Thereafter		70-105
24.	Haptoglobin (mg/dl)	Serum/ plasma	Neonate		0-20
			Thereafter		40-180
25.	Hemoglobin (mg/dl)	Serum			0-3
26.	Hemoglobin, glycosylated (HbA1c)		1-5 yr		2.1-7.7%
			5-16 yr		3.0-6.2%
27.	Insulin, fasting (RIA) (m iu/l)	Serum	Newborn		< 8
			Adult		7-24
28.	Iron binding capacity (mcg/dl)	Serum	Newborn		60-175
			Infant		100-400
			Thereafter		250-400
29.	Iron, total (mcg/dl)	Serum	Newborn		100-250
			Infant		40-100
			Child		50-120
			Adult:	M	60-150
				F	50-130
30.	Lactate (m mol/l)	Whole blood	Venous		0.5-1.30
			Arterial		0.36-0.75
31.	Lactate dehydrogenase (LDH 30°C) (u/l)	Serum	Newborn		290-500
			Neonate		300-1500
			Infant		100-250
			Child		60-170
			Thereafter		40-90
32.	Lead (mcg/dl)	Whole blood	Children		< 10
			Toxic		> 100
33.	Lipase (olive oil, 37°C) (u/l)	Serum	Infant		9-105
			Thereafter		20-180
34.	Lipids, total (mg/dl)	Serum	Newborn–2 yrs		170-450
			2-14 yr		490-1000
			Thereafter		400-800

Appendices

(contd.)

APPENDIX 9 Reference Biochemical Values[5,7,8] (Contd.)

	Determination	Specimen	Age/sex		Normal value		

35.	Lipoproteins (mg/dl)	Plasma		Total	Alpha	Beta	Chylo
			Newborn	170-440	70-180	50-160	50-110
			Infant	240-800	80-280	120-450	50-250
			Thereafter	500-1100	150-330	225-540	100-270

	Determination	Specimen	Age/sex	Normal value
36.	Magnesium (mEq/L)	Serum	Newborn	1.4-2.2
			Thereafter	1.3-2.1
37.	Methemoglobin (g/dl)	Whole blood		0.0-0.3
38.	5' Nucleotidase (iu/l)	Serum		2.2-15.0
39.	Osmolality (m osm/kg)	Serum		289-308
40.	Osmolarity (m osm/l)	Serum		270-285
41.	Phosphatase, acid (iu/l)	Serum	Newborn–2wks	10.4 – 16.4
			2 wk–3 yrs	8.6 –12.6
			Thereafter: M	0.5 –11.0
			F	0.2-9.5
42.	Phosphatase, alkaline (iu/l)	Serum	Newborn	50-165
			Child	20-150
			Thereafter	20-70
43.	Phosphate, inorganic (mg/dl)	Serum	Cord	3.7-8.1
			Premature (1wk)	5.4-10.9
			Newborn	3.5-8.6
			Infant	4.5-6.7
			Child	4.5-5.5
			Thereafter	3.0-4.5
44.	Potassium (mEq/L)	Serum/ plasma	Premature (cord)	5.0-10.2
			Premature (24 hr)	3.0-6.0
			Newborn (cord)	5.6-12.0
			Newborn	3.7-5.0
			Infant	4.1-5.3
			Child	3.4-4.7
			Thereafter	3.5-5.3
45.	Protein bound iodine (PBI) (mcg/dl)	Serum		4.0-8.0
46.	Protein, total (g/dl)	Serum	Premature	4.3-7.6
			Newborn	4.6-7.6
			Child	6.2-8.0
			Thereafter	6.0-8.0
47.	Pyruvates (mEq/L)	Blood	Child	0.05-0.09
48.	Salicylates (mg/dl)	Serum		Negative: < 2.0
				Therapeutic: 10-20
				Toxic: >30
49.	Sodium (mEq/L)	Serum	Premature (cord)	116-140
			Premature (48 hr)	128-148
			Newborn (cord)	126-166
			Newborn	134-144
			Infant	139-146
			Child	138-145
			Thereafter	135-148
50.	Thyroxin (T4) (mcg/dl)	Serum	Cord blood	11.0-18.5
			Child	5.4-14.8
51.	Thyroid stimulating hormone (uU/ml)	Serum	Cord blood	2-12
			Newborn	3-18
			Thereafter	2-10

APPENDIX 9 Reference Biochemical Values[5, 7, 8] *(Contd.)*

	Determination	Specimen	Age/sex		Normal value
52.	Triiodo thyronine (T3) (ng/dl)	Serum	Cord blood		10-45
			Newborn		50-400
			Thereafter		100-250
53.	Triglycerides (mg/dl)	Serum	Newborn/Infant		5-40
			Adolescent		30-150
			Thereafter:	M	40-160
				F	35-135
54.	Urea nitrogen (mg/dl)	Serum/ plasma	Cord		21-40
			Premature (1 wk)		3-25
			Newborn		4-18
			Infant/child		5-18
			Thereafter		7-18
55.	Uric acid (mg/dl)	Serum/ plasma	Child		2.0-5.5
			Thereafter:	M	3.5-7.2
				F	2.6-6.0
56.	Zinc (mcg/dl)	Serum	Child		64-118

APPENDIX 10 Acid–Base Status (Arterial)[1, 9]

Parameter	Newborn	Infant	Child	Adult
pH	7.26-7.49	7.30-7.46	7.35-7.45	7.35-7.45
pCO_2 (mmHg)	30-40	27-40	30-45	32-48
HCO_3 (mEq/L)	17.2-23.6	19.0-23.9	16.3-23.9	18-23
paO_2 (mmHg)	55-95	85-110	85-110	85-110
O_2 saturation	40-90	95-98	95-98	95-98
Base excess	-10 to -2	-7 to -1	-4 to +2	-2 to +3

APPENDIX 11 Therapeutic and Toxic Range of Serum Drug Levels		
Drug	Therapeutic level	Toxic level
Acetaminophen	10-30 ug/ml	> 200 ug/ml
Amikacin	15-25 ug/ml	> 30 ug/ml
Carbamazepine	8-12 ug/ml	> 15 ug/ml
Chloramphenicol	10-25 ug/ml	> 30 ug/ml
Clonazepam	15-60 ng/ml	> 80 ng/ml
Diazepam	100-1000 ng/ml	> 5000 ng/ml
Digoxin	1.5-2.0 ng/ml	> 2.5 ng/ml
Ethosuximide	40-100 ug/ml	> 120 ug/ml
Gentamicin	4-8 ug/ml	> 10 ug/ml
Isoniazid	2-10 ug/ml	> 15 ug/ml
Kanamycin	15-25 ug/ml	> 30 ug/ml
Morphine	10-80 ng/ml	> 200 ng/ml
Phenobarbitone	15-40 ug/ml	> 40 ug/ml
Phenytoin	10-20 ug/ml	> 30 ug/ml
Salicylates	20-25 mg/dl	> 30 mg/dl
Theophylline	10-20 ug/ml	> 20 ug/ml
Valproic acid	50-100 ug/ml	> 100 ug/ml

APPENDIX 12 Cerebrospinal Fluid Constituents[1,2,10]					
Determination	Premature	Term infant		Infant	Child
		Day 1	Day 2		
Color	Clear or xanthochromic	Clear or xanthochromic	Clear or xanthochromic	Clear	Clear
Pressure (mm CSF)	50-80	50-80	50-80	40-150	70-200
Red blood cells (per mm³)	9 (0-1070)	23 (0-620)	3 (0-48)	0	0
Polymorphs (per mm³)	3 (0-70)	7 (0-26)	2 (0-5)	0	0
Lymphocytes (per mm³)	2 (0-20)	5 (0-16)	1 (0-4)	0-5	0-5
Protein (mg/dl)	63 (32-240)	73 (40-148)	47 (27-65)	15-40	15-40
Glucose* (mg/dl)	51 (32-78)	48 (35-64)	55 (48-62)	60-80	40-70
Chloride (mEq/L)	-	109-123	109-123	111-130	118-132
LDH (iu/l)	-	2.3-8.4	-	0-20	0-20
Lactate (mg/dl)	-	-	-	-	10-20
Ammonia (umol/l)	-	-	-	-	25-80

*Simultaneous blood sugar must be estimated, CSF sugar is approximately 60% of blood sugar.

APPENDIX 13 ECG Norms in Children

Appendix 13.1 PR intervals, with Rate and Age (and upper limits of normal)*

Rate	0-1 mo	1-6 mo	6 mo-1yr	1-3 yr	3-8 yr	8-12 yr	12-16 yr	Adult
< 60						0.16 (0.18)	0.16 (0.19)	0.17 (0.21)
60-80	0.10 (0.12)				0.15 (0.17)	0.15 (0.17)	0.15 (0.18)	0.16 (0.21)
80-100	0.10 (0.12)		(0.15)	0.13 (0.16)	0.14 (0.16)	0.15 (0.16)	0.15 (0.17)	0.15 (0.20)
100-120	0.10 (0.11)		0.11 (0.14)	0.12 (0.14)	0.14 (0.15)	0.15 (0.16)	0.15 (0.19)	
120-140	0.09 (0.11)	0.11 (0.14)	0.11 (0.14)	0.11 (0.14)	0.13 (0.15)	0.14 (0.15)		0.15 (0.18)
140-160	0.10 (0.11)	0.10 (0.13)	0.10 (0.13)	0.10 (0.12)	0.12 (0.14)			(0.17)
160-180		0.10 (0.12)	0.10 (0.12)					
>180	0.09	0.09 (0.11)						

*From Park MK, Guntheroth WG. How to Read Pediatric ECGs, *Chicago, Year Book Medical Publishers*, (ed. 2), 1987. (Used by permission).

Appendix 13.2 QRS Duration: Average (and upper limits) for Age*

	0-1mo	1-6 mo	6 mo-1 yr	1-3 yr	3-8 yr	8-12 yr	12-16 yr	Adult
Seconds	0.05 (0.07)	0.05 (0.07)	0.05 (0.07)	0.06 (0.07)	0.07 (0.08)	0.07 (0.09)	0.07 (0.10)	0.08 (0.10)

*Modified from Guntheroth WG. Pediatric Electrocardiography. *Philadelphia, WB Saunders Co*, 1965. (Used by permission).

Appendices

Appendix 13.3 R and S Voltages According to Lead and Age: Mean (and upper limits)*

Lead	0-1 mo	1-6 mo	6 mo-1yr	1-3 yr	3-8 yr	8-12 yr	12-16 yr	Young Adults
R voltage +								
I	4(8)	7(13)	8(16)	8(16)	7(15)	7(15)	6(13)	6(13)
II	6(14)	13(24)	13(27)	13(23)	13(22)	14(24)	14(24)	9(25)
III	8(16)	9(20)	9(20)	9(20)	9(20)	9(24)	9(24)	6(22)
aVR	3(7)	3(6)	3(6)	2(6)	2(5)	2(4)	2(4)	1(4)
aVL	2(7)	4(8)	5(10)	5(10)	3(10)	3(10)	3(12)	3(9)
aVF	7(14)	10(20)	10(16)	8(20)	10(19)	10(20)	11(21)	5(23)
V4R	6(12)	5(10)	4(8)	4(8)	3(8)	3(7)	3(7)	3(14)
V1	15(25)	11(20)	10(20)	9(18)	7(18)	6(16)	5(16)	3(14)
V2	21(30)	21(30)	19(28)	16(25)	13(28)	10(22)	9(19)	6(21)
V5	12(30)	17(30)	18(30)	19(36)	21(36)	22(36)	18(33)	12(33)
V6	6(21)	10(20)	13(20)	12(24)	14(24)	14(24)	14(22)	10(21)
S voltage +								
I	5(10)	4(9)	4(9)	3(8)	2(8)	2(8)	2(8)	1(6)
V4R	4(9)	4(12)	5(12)	5(12)	5(14)	6(20)	6(20)	
V1	10(20)	7(18)	8(16)	13(27)	14(30)	16(26)	15(24)	10(23)
V2	20(35)	16(30)	17(30)	21(34)	23(38)	23(38)	23(48)	14(36)
V5	9(30)	9(26)	8(20)	6(16)	5(14)	5(17)	5	
V6	4(12)	2(6)	2(4)	2(4)	1(4)	1(4)	1(5)	1 (13)

* From Park MK, Guntheroth WG. How to Read Pediatric ECGs, Chicago, Year Book Medical Publishers, (2nd ed.), 1987.

+ voltages are measured in millimeters, when IMV = 10 mm paper

Appendix 13.4 R/S Ratio According to Age. Mean, Lower and Upper Limits of Normal*

	Lead	0-1 mo	1-6 mo	6 mo-1yr	1-3yr	3-8yr	8-12yr	12-16yr	Adult
V1	LLN+	0.5	0.3	0.3	0.5	0.1	0.15	0.1	0.0
	Mean	1.5	1.5	1.2	0.8	0.65	0.5	0.3	0.3
	ULN++	19	S=0	6	2	2	1	1	1
V2	LLN	0.3	0.3	0.3	0.3	0.05	0.1	0.1	0.1
	Mean	1	1.2	1	0.8	0.5	0.5	0.5	0.2
	ULN	3	4	4	1.5	1.5	1.2	1.2	2.5
V6	LLN	0.1	1.5	2	3	2.5	2.5	2.5	2.5
	Mean	2	4	6	20	20	20	10	9
	ULN	S=0	S=0	S=0	S=0	S=0	S=0	S=0	S=0

*From Guntheroth WB, Pediatric Electrocardiography, *Philadelphia, WB Saunders Co.*, 1965.
+ Lower limits of normal
++ Upper limits of normal

APPENDIX 14 Calculation of Dose of Drugs in Children with Renal Failure

Estimated fraction of usual dose of drug required for a patient with a creatinine clearance of zero (dose fraction)

Drug	Dose Fraction	Drug	Dose Fraction
ANTIBIOTICS			
Amikacin	0.01	Lincomycin	0.4
Amoxyicillin	0.15	Methicillin	0.12
Ampicillin	0.1	Minocycline	0.9
Carbenicillin	0.1	Naficillin	0.4
Cephalexin	0.04	Oxacillin	0.25
Cephaloridine	0.08	Oxytetracycline	0.2
Cephalothin	0.02	Penicillin G	0.1
Cephazolin	0.06	Polymyxin B	0.12
Chloramphenicol	0.8	Rifampin	1.0
Clindamycin	0.8	Streptomycin	0.04
Cloxacillin	0.25	Sulfadiazine	0.45
Colistimethate	0.3	Sulfamethoxazole	0.85
Dicloxacillin	0.5	Tetracycline	0.12
Doxycycline	0.8	Tobramycin	0.02
Erythromycin	0.7	Tricarcillin	0.1
Gentamicin	0.02	Trimethoprim	0.45
Isonizid:		Vancomycin	0.03
Fast inactivators	0.8		
Slow inactivators	0.5		
Kanamycin	0.03		

(*contd.*)

Appendices

APPENDIX 14 Calculation of Dose of Drugs in Children with Renal Failure *(Contd.)*			
Estimated fraction of usual dose of drug required for a patient with a creatinine clearance of zero (dose fraction)			
Drug	**Dose Fraction**	**Drug**	**Dose Fraction**
CARDIAC GLYCOSIDES		MISCELLANEOUS DRUGS	
Digitoxin	0.7	Chlorpropamide	0.4
Digoxin	0.3	Lidocaine	0.9
		Sulfopyrazone	0.55

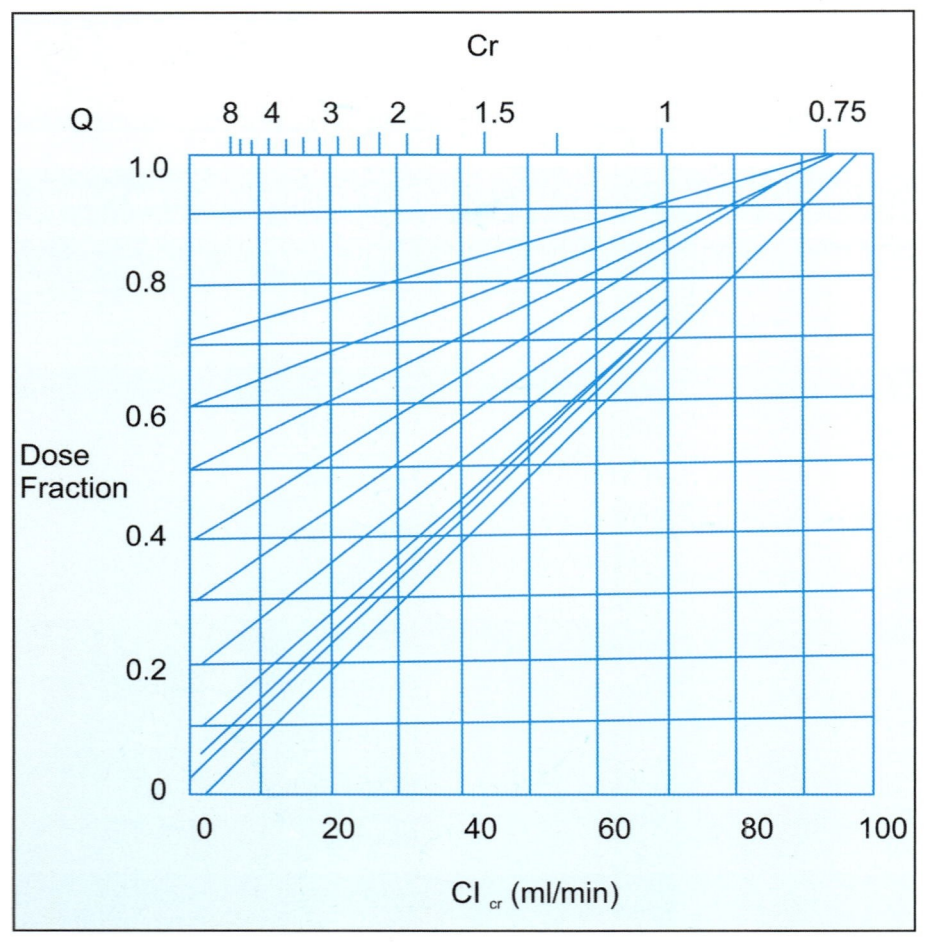

Nomogram in conjunction with Appendix 14 is used to calculate the dose of drugs which are exclusively excreted by kidneys in children with renal failure. The abscissa of nomogram gives creatinine clearance from 0-100 ml/min (bottom) and serum creatinine 0.75-8.0 mg/dl (top). The inordinate provides dose fraction to be used. For example, if a patient with a creatinine clearance of 50 ml/min requires penicillin G for an infection in which it is given in a dose of 1 million units/day to an individual with normal kidney function, then the approximate dose to this patient would be 5.5 million units. This dose is estimated by plotting the dose fraction for penicillin G (0.1 in appendix 15) on the left hand ordinate and connecting it to the vertical line corresponding to 50 ml/min creatinine clearance. When this point is extended horizontally to the left ordinate, it gives a dose fraction of 0.55. Hence penicillin G daily in this patient would be 0.55 × 10 million units i.e. 5.5 million units.

APPENDIX 15 Predicted Average Peak Expiratory Flow Rates on the Basis of Height in Normal Children*

Height (in)	Height (cm)	PEFR (L/min)		Height (in)	Height (cm)	PEFR (L/min)
43	109	147		56	142	320
44	112	160		57	144	334
45	114	173		58	147	347
46	117	187		59	149	360
48	122	214		60	152	373
49	124	227		61	154	387
50	127	240		63	159	413
51	129	254		64	162	427
52	132	267		65	164	440
53	134	280		66	167	454
54	137	293		67	170	467
55	139	307				

* At 100 cm height, average PEFR is about 100 L/min. For every 10 cm increase in height, add 50 L/min to get an approximate PEFR value. When PEFR is less than 80% of the predicted average or patient's known highest PEFR when well, it indicates that patient is unwell.

Adapted from Voter KZ, *Pediatric Review* 1996, 17(2): 53-63.

REFERENCES

1. Avery GB. Neonatology, Pathophysiology and Management of the Newborn. *JB Lippincott Co.,* 1987; pp 1344-1368.

2. Forfar JO, Arneil GC. Textbook of Pediatrics. *Churchill Livingstone, London* 3rd Ed., 1984; pp 1977-1991.

3. Nathan DG, Oski FA. Hematology of infancy and Childhood. *WB Saunders Company,* 1981; p 1568.

4. Nelson WE, Vaughan VC, McKay RJ, Behrman RE. Nelson Textbook of Pediatrics. *WB Saunders Company,* 11th Ed, 1981; pp 2075-2093.

5. Siggard Anderson O. Blood acid-base alignment nomogram. *Scand J Clin Lab Invest* 1963, Radiometer Reprint AS21.

6. Singh M. Care of the Newborn, 7th Ed, *Sagar Publications, New Delhi,* 2010, p 495-503.

7. Tietz NW. Fundamentals of Clinical Chemistry, 3rd, *WB Saunders* 1987; p 944-975.

8. Weisbrot IM, James LS, Prince CE, Holaday DA, Apgar V. Acid base homeostasis of the newborn infant during the first 24 hours of life. *J Pediatr* 1958; 52: 395-403.

9. Wolf H, Hoepffner L. The cerebrospinal fluid in newborn and premature infant. *World Neurol* 1961; 2: 871-874.

Index

Index

Other Outstanding Books of Professor Meharban Singh

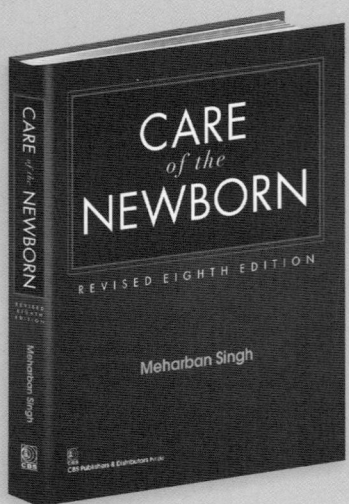

CARE of the NEWBORN

REVISED EIGHTH EDITION

Meharban Singh

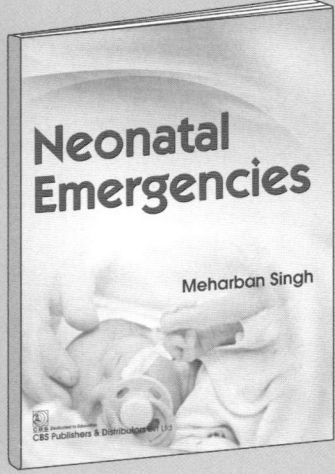

Neonatal Emergencies

Meharban Singh

CBS Publishers & Distributors Pvt Ltd

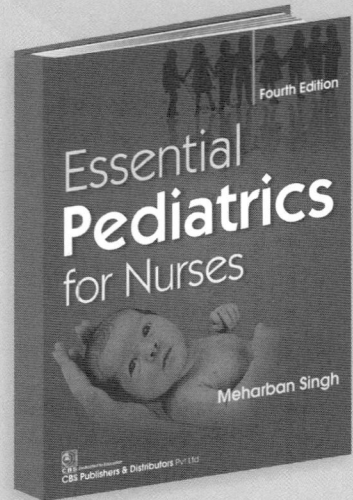

Fourth Edition

Essential Pediatrics for Nurses

Meharban Singh

CBS Publishers & Distributors Pvt Ltd

PEDIATRIC CLINICAL METHODS

Fifth Edition

Meharban Singh

CBS Publishers & Distributors Pvt Ltd

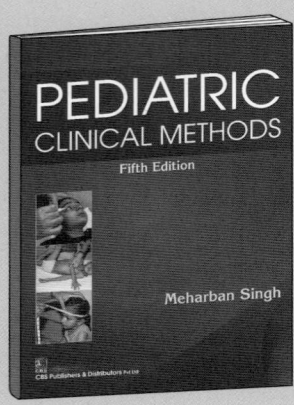

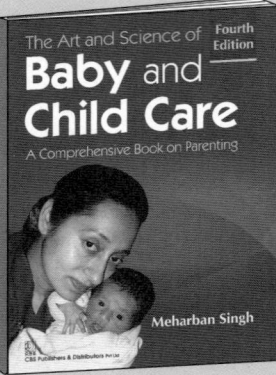

The Art and Science of Fourth Edition

Baby and Child Care

A Comprehensive Book on Parenting

Meharban Singh

CBS Publishers & Distributors Pvt Ltd

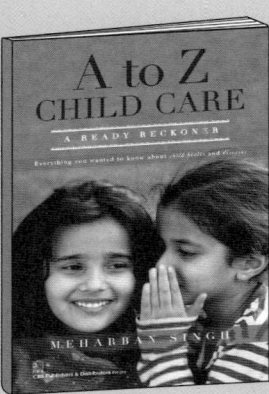

A to Z CHILD CARE

A READY RECKONER

Everything you wanted to know about child care and disease

MEHARBAN SINGH

CBS Publishers & Distributors Pvt Ltd

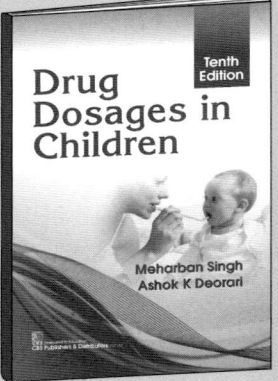

Tenth Edition

Drug Dosages in Children

Meharban Singh
Ashok K Deorari

CBS Publishers & Distributors

MEDICAL QUOTATIONS

Fourth Edition

by EMINENT PHYSICIANS and PHILOSOPHERS

MEHARBAN SINGH

CBS Publishers & Distributors Pvt Ltd

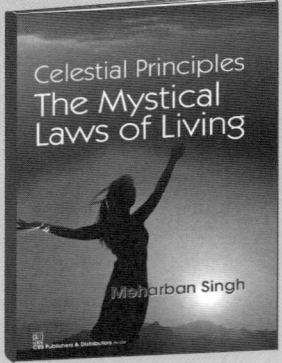

Celestial Principles The Mystical Laws of Living

Meharban Singh

CBS Publishers & Distributors Pvt Ltd

A Manual of Essential Pediatrics

Meharban Singh

Second Edition

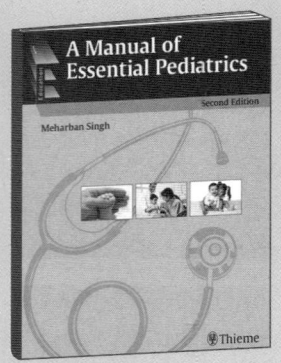

Thieme

बच्चों का स्वास्थ्य और उनकी देखभाल

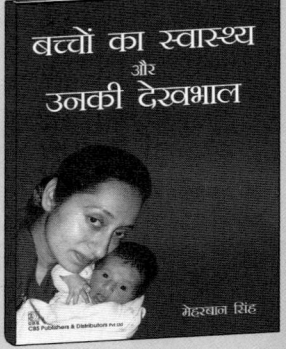

मेहरबान सिंह

CBS Publishers & Distributors Pvt Ltd

CBS Dedicated to Education

CBS Publishers & Distributors Pvt Ltd